Handbook of Health Physics and Radiological Health

THIRD EDITION

Handbook of Health Physics and Radiological Health

THIRD EDITION

EDITED BY

Bernard Shleien, Pharm.D., M.S.Hyg., CHP, FAPHA, FHPS

President, Scinta, Inc.
Silver Spring, Maryland

Lester A. Slaback, Jr., CHP

Gaithersburg, Maryland

Brian Kent Birky, Ph.D.

Health Physics Consultant affiliated with
Environmental Radiation Group
Applied Environmental Consulting, Inc.
Gainesville, Florida

Williams & Wilkins

A WAVERLY COMPANY

BALTIMORE • PHILADELPHIA • LONDON • PARIS • BANGKOK
BUENOS AIRES • HONG KONG • MUNICH • SYDNEY • TOKYO • WROCLAW

351 West Camden Street
Baltimore, Maryland 21201-2436

Accurate indications, adverse reactions, and dosage schedules for drugs are provided in this book, but it is possible that they may change. The reader is urged to review the package information data of the manufacturers of the medications mentioned.

Printed in the United States of America
(ISBN 0-683-18334-6)

98 99 00 01 02
1 2 3 4 5 6 7 8 9 10

This handbook is dedicated to all those who will be using it: health physicists, radiation protection workers; radiologist, medical radiation staffs, students, teachers; the host of allied personnel continually trying to better our common lot in a time of millenial hope and potential hazard

The Editors

FOREWORD

This book is an outgrowth of the *Radiological Health Handbook* that was originally developed in the early 1950s by staff members of the Short Course Training Program, Division of Radiological Health, U.S. Public Health Service. To state that it is an ''outgrowth,'' however, is an understatement. Dr. Bernard Shleien and his contributors have developed a Handbook that goes far beyond what the original authors could ever have envisioned. The current Handbook reflects not only improvements in the science of Health Physics and Radiological Health, but also a vastly superior method of organizing and presenting the data.

For these reasons, it is not surprising that *The Handbook of Health Physics and Radiological Health,* in its present configuration, is widely used throughout the world. Rather than representing a Handbook, as such, it now serves as a veritable encyclopedia on the subject. In fact, it probably represents the single most important book that professional health physicists need in their library, if they desire to have ready access to the latest information, concepts, and developments in the field. Making a major contribution to the success of the Handbook is the range of outstanding people in the field who have so willingly given of their time and efforts in support of Dr. Shleien in this effort.

Of all the people who might have undertaken such an effort, there are few, if any, who could have accomplished it in such a superb manner. Dr. Shleien, who received a doctorate in pharmacy at the University of Southern California, followed by post-doctoral training in radiological health at the Harvard School of Public Health, is an outstanding example of the multidisciplinary nature of the field of Health Physics and Radiological Health. Through the depth of his understanding of biology and chemistry, coupled with his knowledge of the physical sciences and engineering, he has been able to organize and present a wide range of information in a readily accessible and comprehensive manner. Professional health physics and radiological health personnel throughout the world owe him a deep debt of gratitude for his dedication and devotion. Through his efforts, he has ensured that people working in this field are provided with a sourcebook that is without parallel.

Dade W. Moeller, Ph.D.
Professor Emeritus
Harvard University

PREFACE

This handbook was conceived in order to fill the need of health physics practitioners, technicians, and students for an easy to use, practical handbook containing health physics and radiological health data. While briefer and more specific data sources are available on single subject areas, as are multi-volume compendia, there is no current up-to-date compilation of information useful on a daily basis by the health physicist.

A considerable effort has gone into ensuring the reliability of the information contained in this handbook. Users of this handbook are encouraged to inform Williams & Wilkins of omissions and errors.

We wish to acknowledge the pioneering efforts of Simon Kinsman who edited and compiled the first radiological handbook of this type and to James G. Terrill, Jr. and John C. Villforth who encouraged and directed him in those pursuits.

The chronology of publications of this book is as follows:

Publisher	*Color of Cover*	*Date*
U.S. Public Health Service	Blue	1960
U.S. Public Health Service	Gray	1970
Nuclear Lectern Associates	Pink	1984
Nuclear Lectern Associates	Pink	1986 Supplement
Scinta, Inc.	Black	1992

The 1970 U.S. Public Health Service publication was a reprinting of its 1960 edition. In 1984 an updating of material occurred which was added to in a thin supplement in 1986. A complete and thorough revision was published in 1992.

This volume has consequently and, in our opinion correctly so, been designated the Third Edition.

A WORD ABOUT UNITS AND REPRESENTATION OF RADIONUCLIDES

In the text and tables, data presentation is in International System of Units (SI) in many more cases than in the past. When SI units are employed, a footnote contains the conversion factor to conventional units.

International standards and guidelines are given in SI units, whereas United States regulations, standards and guidelines are given in conventional units or in conventional units with SI units following in parentheses. United States laws, rules and regulations which contain conventional units in the original Federal Regulatory Codes retain them in this book.

Radionuclide designations appear in more than one form in the text and tables. In text, the left superscript form, for example, 222Rn, is employed. This is not the case in tabular data presentations or in figures. In these cases various conventions for representing radionuclides may appear. This occurs because of the complexity of changing large computer files containing radionuclide data to hard copy and in order to save page space. The editors and publisher ask your indulgence for these variances from strict consistency.

ACKNOWLEDGMENTS

Acknowledgment must be made of the vital contributions provided by the contributors. Their cooperation, patience and expertise made this volume possible. The encouragement, support, and contributions of my wife Debra occurred every day and are special. My thanks to you all.

B. Shleien

Without the dedicated efforts of Dr. Shleien, as well as those of the many contributors, this publication would not, and could not exist. Also as an essential ingredient was the continued patience of my wife, Betty, for the time devoted to this project.

L. Slaback

I would like to acknowledge the efforts and technical submission of the following persons: S.M. Seltzer and J.H. Hubbell for interaction coefficients; T.E. Huston for lung dosimetry data and illustrations; K.F. Eckerman for dose conversion factors. I would also like to offer gratitude to my parents, Edgar and Belva Birky, for their love and support.

B. Birky

CONTRIBUTORS

Robert E. Alexander
Occupational Radiation Standards

Keith F. Eckerman
Radiation Dose Factors & Decay Products

David S. Kocher
Public and Environmental Standards and Guidelines

Jack S. Krohmer
Medical Radiation

William A. Miller
Radiation Risks

Timothy W. Osborne
Waste Disposal

Harold T. Peterson, Jr.
Environmental Monitoring and Atmospheric Dispersion

Robert Phillips
Medical Radiation Standards

Alan K. Roecklein
Occupational Radiation Standards

Genevieve S. Roessler
Glossaries

Ralph H. Thomas
Accelerator Health Physics

CONTENTS

CHAPTER 1

ESTIMATES OF RADIATION DOSES FROM VARIOUS SOURCES OF EXPOSURE

This chapter provides an overview of radiation doses to individuals and to the collective U.S. population from various sources of ionizing radiation. Summary tables present doses from occupational exposures and annual per capita doses from natural background, the healing arts, nuclear weapons, nuclear energy and consumer products. Although doses from non-ionizing radiation are not as yet readily available in a concise form, the major sources of non-ionizing radiation are listed.

TABLE OF CONTENTS

Table 1.1 Major Sources of Ionizing Radiation

Natural Background
- Cosmic radiation
- Terrestrial radiation

Healing Arts
- Medical
  - Medical diagnosis
  - Dental diagnosis
  - Therapy
- Radiopharmaceuticals
  - Medical diagnosis (*in vivo* and *in vitro*)
  - Therapy
  - Biological research

Atmospheric Weapons Tests

Industrial Activities
- Commercial power reactors
- Naval nuclear propulsion
- Fuel reprocessing
- Byproduct materials
- Mining and milling of radioactive ores
- Industrial radiography
- Gauges, static eliminators and industrial tracers
- Sterilizers

Research
- Particle accelerators
- X-ray diffraction units
- Electron microscopes
- Neutron generators
- Tracers

Consumer Products
- Building materials
- Tobacco

Miscellaneous
- Air travel
- Transport of radioactive materials

Table 1.2 Estimated Total Dose Equivalent for a Member of the Population in the United States and Canada[a] from Various Sources of Natural Background Radiation (Courtesy NCRP from Report 94, 1987)

	Dose Equivalent Rate ($mSv\ y^{-1}$)[b]			
Source	**Bronchial Epithelium**	**Other Soft Tissues**	**Bone Surfaces**	**Bone Marrow**
Cosmic	0.27	0.27	0.27	0.27
Cosmogenic	0.01	0.01	0.01	0.03
Terrestrial	0.28	0.28	0.28	0.28
Inhaled[c]	24	—	—	—
In the Body[d]	0.35	0.35	1.1	0.50
Rounded Totals	25	0.9	1.7	1.1

[a] The dose equivalent rates for Canada are about 20% lower for the Terrestrial and Inhaled components.

[b] 1 mSv = 100 mrem.

[c] Doses to other tissues from inhaled radionuclides included under ''In the Body.''

[d] Excluding the cosmogenic component shown separately.

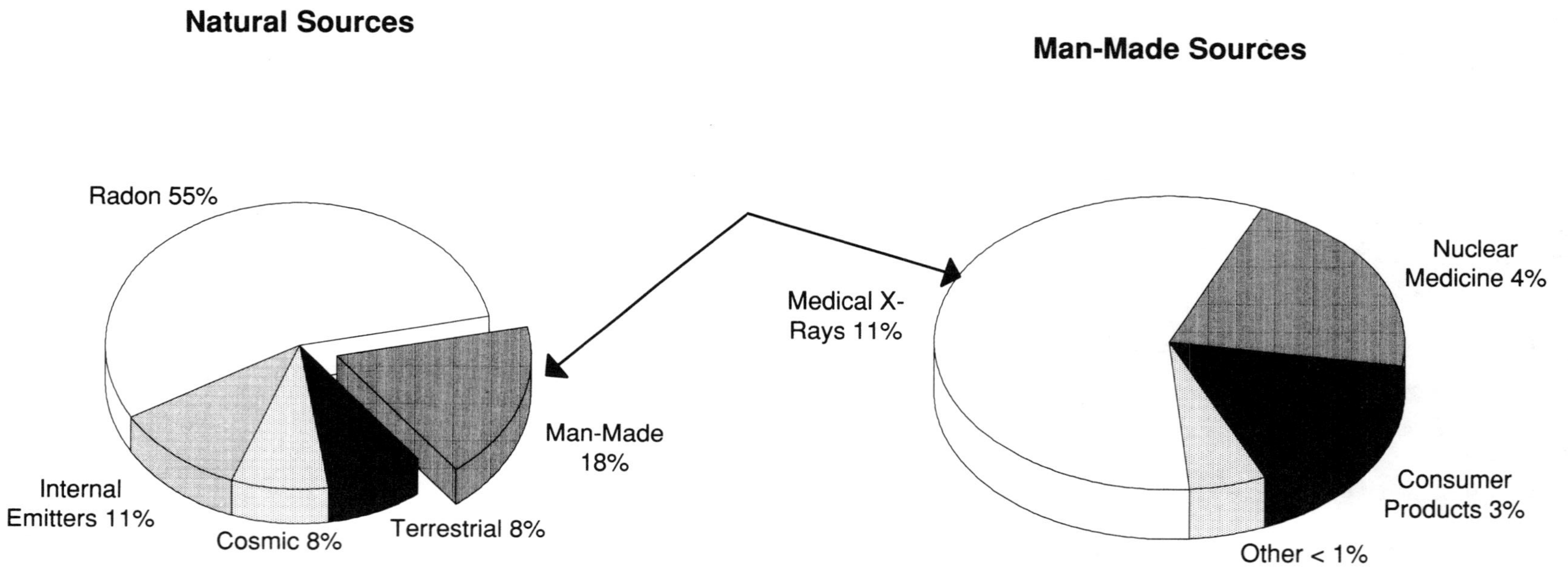

Other:	
Occupational	0.3%
Fallout	0.3%
Nuclear Power	0.1%
Miscellaneous	0.1%

Based on an average annual effective dose equivalent of 3.6 mSv (360 mrem) and a ground level radon concentration of about 40 Bqm^{-3} (1 pCi/l)

Figure 1.1 Radiation Exposure in the United States (Percentage of Total Effective Dose)

(After NCRP 93, 1987)

Table 1.2.1 Estimated Total Effective Dose Equivalent Rate for a Member of the Population in the United States and Canada[a] from Various Sources of Natural Background Radiation (After NCRP Report 94, 1987)

	Total Effective Dose Equivalent Rate ($mSvy^{-1}$)[b]					
Source	**Lung**	**Gonads**	**Bone Surfaces**	**Bone Marrow**	**Other Tissues[c]**	**Total**
w_T	0.12	0.25	0.03	0.12	0.48	1.0
Cosmic	0.03	0.07	0.008	0.03	0.13	0.27
Cosmogenic	0.001	0.002	—	0.004	0.003	0.01
Terrestrial	0.03	0.07	0.008	0.03	0.14	0.28
Inhaled[d]	2.0	—	—	—	—	2.0
In the body	0.04	0.09	0.03	0.06	0.17	0.40
Rounded totals	2.1	0.23	0.05	0.12	0.44	3.0

[a] The effective dose equivalent rates for Canada are about 20% lower for the Terrestrial and Inhaled components.
[b] 1 mSv = 100 mrem.
[c] This is an approximation derived by assuming that the rest of the organs had the same dose equivalent rate as the gonads, adding 0.17 $mSvy^{-1}$.
[d] Derived from calculations of ICRP Publication 32 (See NCRP Report 93, 1987).

Table 1.3 Dose Equivalent Rates to Lung Tissue from Inhaled Radionuclides (Courtesy NCRP from Report 94, 1987)

	Dose Equivalent Rate ($\mu Sv\ y^{-1}$)[a]		
Radionuclides	**Assumed Air Concentrations**	**Whole Lung**	**Bronchial Epithelium**
^{238}U–^{226}Ra	0.7 $\mu Bq/m^3$ (20 aCi/m^3)		0.1
^{222}Rn	40 Bq/m^3 (1 pCi/l)	200	
^{218}Po–^{214}Po	0.004 WL		24,000
^{210}Po	70 $\mu Bq/m^3$ (2 fCi/m^3)		8
^{232}Th–^{224}Ra	0.4 $\mu Bq/m^3$ (10 aCi/m^3)		0.2
^{220}Rn	0.2 Bq/m^3 (5 pCi/m^3)	0.1	
^{212}Pb–^{212}Po	0.07 Bq/m^3 (2 pCi/m^3)		400

[a] 1μSv = 100 μrem.

Table 1.4 Dose Equivalent Rates to Various Tissues from Natural Radionuclides Contained in the Body (Courtesy NCRP from Report 94, 1987)

	Dose Equivalent Rate (μSv y^{-1})[a,b,c]		
Radionuclides	Soft Tissue	Bone Surfaces	Bone Marrow
^{14}C	10	8	30
^{40}K	180	140	270
^{87}Rb	3	14	7
^{238}U–^{234}Th	4.6	3	0.4
^{230}Th	0.1	6	1
^{226}Ra	3	90	15
^{222}Rn	7	14	14
^{210}Pb–^{210}Po	140	700	140
^{232}Th	0.1	2	0.4
^{228}Ra–^{224}Ra	1.5	120	22
^{220}Rn	<0.1	—	—
Total	350	1,100	500

[a] 1 μSv = 100 μrem.
[b] In a few cases, individual organs may receive dose equivalent rates from individual radionuclides up to twice those shown for "Soft Tissues."
[c] These dose equivalent rates include the contribution from inhaled radionuclides.

Table 1.5 Mean Annual Bone Marrow Dose to Adults for All U.S. Radiographic Procedures: 1980 (Courtesy NCRP from Report 100, 1989)

	Active Marrow Dose (μGy)[a] per Examination			Mean Active Marrow Dose (μGy)[b]	
Examination	Shleien et al. (1978)	Rosenstein (1976)	Annual Exam Rate	Shleien et al. (1978)	Rosenstein (1976)
Skull	780	730	0.022	17	16
Head CT	220[b]	220[b]	0.015	33	33
Body CT	350[c]	350[c]	0.003	11	11
Chest	100	60	0.335	34	20
Abdomen (kidneys, ureters, bladder)	1,470	850	0.043	63	37
Biliary	1,680	1,260	0.019	32	24
Thoracic spine	2,470	1,210	0.010	25	12
Lumbar/lumbosacral spine	4,000	2,400	0.072	288	173
Full spine	640	350[d]	0.008	5	3
Upper gastrointestinal	5,350	3,640	0.042	225	153
Barium enema	8,750	5,690	0.027	236	154
Intravenous pyelogram	4,200	2,350	0.023	97	54
Pelvis, hip	830	390	0.026	22	10
Cervical spine & other head and neck	520	270	0.044	23	12
Dental	90	80	0.430	40	34
Total diagnostic radiology				1,151	746

[a] 1 Gy = 100 rad.
[b] Huda (1984).
[c] Huda (1984) and Ewen *et al* (1983).
[d] Kereiakes and Rosenstein (1980).

Table 1.6 Collective Effective Dose Equivalent from Diagnostic Medical X-Rays: United States 1980 (Courtesy NCRP from Report 100, 1989)

Examination Type	Examination H_E[a] (mSv)[b]	Examinations (in Thousands)	Collective H_E[a] (person-Sv)[c]
CT (head and body)	1.11	3,300	3,660
Chest	0.08	64,000	5,120
Skull	0.22	8,200	1,800
Cervical spine	0.20	5,100	1,020
Biliary	1.89	3,400	6,430
Lumbar spine	1.27	12,900	16,400
Upper gastrointestinal	2.44	7,600	18,500
Abdomen (kidneys, ureters, bladder)	0.56	7,900	4,420
Barium enema	4.06	4,900	19,900
Intravenous pyelogram	1.58	4,200	6,640
Pelvis	0.44[d]		
	0.64[d]	4,700	3,010
Hip	0.83		
Extremities	0.01	45,000	450
Other[e]	0.50	(8,400)	4,200
Rounded Total		92,000	

[a] H_E—Effective dose equivalent.
[b] 1 mSv = 100 mrem.
[c] 1 person-Sv = 100 person-rem.
[d] Double entry as per original report.
[e] Estimated from the average of all examinations.

Table 1.7 Factors Included in Calculation of Genetically Significant Dose (GSD) for 1980 by Sex and Examination Type[a] (Courtesy NCRP from Report 100, 1989)

Sex	Exam Type	Mean Gonadal Dose μGy (mrad)	Relative Frequency ($\times 10^{-3}$)	Relative Child Expectancy	GSD for Exam Type μGy (mrad)
Male	Head & neck	—[b]	40	0.57	—
	Chest	10 (1)	298	0.31	0.9 (0.09)
	Cervical spine	—	23	0.47	—
	Lumbar spine	2,180 (218)	59	0.15	19.3 (1.93)
	Hips/pelvis	6,000 (600)	18	0.38	41.0 (4.10)
	Upper extremities	—	106	0.65	—
	Lower extremities	150 (15)	119	0.70	12.5 (1.25)
	Abdomen (kidneys, ureters, bladder)	970 (97)	35	0.31	10.5 (1.05)
	Upper gastrointestinal & small bowel	10 (1)	28	0.22	0.1 (0.01)
	Barium enema	1,750 (175)	17	0.17	5.1 (0.51)
	Gall bladder	—	11	0.20	—
	Intravenous pyelogram	2,070 (207)	18	0.24	8.9 (0.89)
	Head CT	—	11	0.13	—
	Body CT	—	3	0.21	—
			Male Total		98 (9.8)
Female	Head & neck	—	32	0.41	—
	Chest	10 (1)	270	0.21	0.6 (0.06)
	Cervical spine	—	22	0.30	—
	Lumbar spine	7,210 (721)	56	0.21	84.8 (8.48)
	Hips/pelvis	2,100 (210)	25	0.21	11.0 (1.10)
	Upper extremities	—	72	0.15	—
	Lower extremities	—	103	0.41	—
	Abdomen (kidneys, ureters, bladder)	2,210 (221)	35	0.38	29.4 (2.94)
	Upper gastrointestinal & small bowel	1,710 (171)	39	0.26	17.3 (1.73)
	Barium enema	9,030 (903)	26	0.17	39.9 (3.99)
	Gall bladder	780 (78)	19	0.14	2.1 (0.21)
	Intravenous pyelogram	5,880 (588)	20	0.20	23.5 (2.35)
	Head CT	—	13	0.33	—
	Body CT	—	3	0.21	—
			Female Total		209 (20.9)

[a] There are a number of examination types which are usually included in the category of ''others'' which have not been included in this Table. Inclusion of these may increase the GSD by 10 to 20 percent.
[b] (—) indicates less than 0.01 μGy.

Table 1.8 Estimated Number and Collective Absorbed Thyroid Dose from Thyroid Scans and Uptakes in the U.S.[a] (Courtesy NCRP from Report 100, 1989)

Procedure	Number or Percent	
	1966	1981
Thyroid scans (total number)	150,000	519,400
$^{99m}TcO_4$	0	53%
^{123}I	0	37%
^{131}I	100%	10%
Thyroid uptakes with scan	150,000	413,000
Thyroid uptakes without scan	150,000	34,000
^{123}I	0	46%
^{131}I	100%	54%

Radionuclide	Collective Absorbed Dose(person-Gy)[b]	
	1966	1981
$^{99m}TcO_4$	—	3,600
^{123}I	—	5,700
^{131}I	181,400	129,800
Total collective thyroid absorbed dose	181,400	139,000

[a] Adapted from Rosenberg, et al. (1985).
[b] 1 person–Gy = 100 person-rad.

Table 1.9 Collective Absorbed Dose and Dose Equivalent to Organs (Other Than Thyroid) from Diagnostic Radionuclide Thyroid Scans and Uptakes in the U.S. in 1981[a,b]

(Courtesy NCRP from Report 100, 1989)

	Radiopharmaceutical			
	$^{99m}TcO_4$	^{123}I	^{131}I	Total
Ovary (person-Gy)[c]	216	7	9	232
Testes (person-Gy)[c]	65	2	4	71
Whole body (person-Gy)	252	14	96	362
Effective dose equivalent (person-Sv)	720	280	5,910	6,810

[a] Adapted from Rosenberg *et al* (1985).
[b] 1 person-Gy = 100 person-rad.
[c] Assumes that 60 percent of studies are performed on females and 40 percent on males.

Table 1.10 Relative Frequency of Nuclear Medicine Procedures (1991), Typical Activities Administered and Typical Dose (Courtesy NCRP from Report 124, 1996)

Procedure	Relative Frequency of Procedures[a] (percent)	Radiopharmaceutical	Activity Administered per Procedure (MBq)	Typical Dose to Patient (mGy)
Diagnostic				
Bone	20.6	^{99m}Tc medronate or oxidronate	740	1.3
Gastric emptying	4.6	^{99m}Tc sulfur colloid	40	0.2
Heart: Equilibrium radiocardiography	11.8	^{99m}Tc red cells	110	4.5
Heart: Myocardial perfusion	17.9	^{201}Tl thallous chloride	110	6.3
		^{99m}Tc sestamibi	1,110	5.0
		^{99m}Tc teboroxime	1,850	8.3
Hepatobiliary	2.9	^{99m}Tc disofenin	300	1.3
Kidney	9.6	^{131}I iodohippurate	15	0.4
		^{99m}Tc pentetate	370	0.6
		^{99m}Tc mertiatide	370	0.7
Lung perfusion	8.2	^{99m}Tc macro-aggregated albumin	110	0.5
Lung ventilation	7.3	^{133}Xe gas	370	0.14
		^{99m}Tc pentetate aerosol	740	1.6
Thyroid (25% uptake of iodine)	5.6	^{123}I Na iodide	15	0.4
		^{131}I Na iodide	4	0.7
		^{99m}Tc pertechnetate	185	0.7
Tumor/infection	3.8	^{67}Ga citrate	190	13.0
Other	5.7			
Therapeutic[b]				
Hyperthyroidism	1.8	^{131}I Na iodide	740	—[c]
Thyroid cancer	0.2	^{131}I Na iodide	3,700	—[c]

[a] Based on an unpublished survey (1991) of nuclear medicine facilities by Martin L. Nusynowitz, University of Texas Medical Branch at Galveston, Galveston, Texas.

[b] Treatment for hyperthyroidism and thyroid cancer estimated at 2 per 100 diagnostic procedures.

[c] Typical dose is meaningless in therapy. Dose to region of concern is the only consideration because that dose provides the benefit.

Table 1.10.1 Comparison of Collective Effective Dose Equivalent vs. Age-Weighted Collective Dose Equivalent for U.S. Nuclear Medicine Procedures in 1980 (Courtesy NCRP from Report 100, 1989)

Examination	H_E (mSv)	Exams ($\times 10^3$)	Collective Effective Dose Equivalent (person-Sv)[a]	Age-Weighted Collective Dose Equivalent (person-Sv)[a]
Brain	6.5	813	5,300	2,200
Hepatobiliary	3.7	180	700	300
Liver	2.4	1,424	3,400	1,300
Bone	4.4	1,811	8,000	2,900
Pulmonary	1.5	1,203	1,800	800
Thyroid	7.5	530	4,000	2,400
Renal	3.1	236	700	400
Tumor	12.2	121	1,500	600
Cardiovascular	7.1	961	6,800	2,600
Total			32,100	13,500
Per caput			140 μSv (14 mrem)	59 μSv (5.9 mrem)

[a] 1 Sv = 100 rem.

Table 1.11 Mean Dose Equivalent Commitments to the Year 2000 in the United States from Nuclear Testing through 1970[a] (Courtesy NCRP from Report 93, 1987)

Source	Dose Equivalent Commitment (μSv)[b]
External	
Whole Body	750
Internal	
^{90}Sr	
Marrow	450
Endosteal	650
^{137}Cs, Whole Body	150
$^{239,240}Pu$	
Lung	400
Bone	20
^{3}H, Whole Body	20
^{14}C, Whole Body	80[c]

[a] Most of this dose has already been received.
[b] 1 μSv = 0.1 mrem.
[c] This is the dose commitment to the year 2000. The total dose commitment, to be delivered over many generations, is 1.4 mSv (140 mrem).

Table 1.12 Global Components of Collective Dose Commitment to the World Population from Man-Made and Natural Sources of ^{14}C (Adapted from Till, 1983)

Date	Global Collective Dose Commitment (person-Sv)[a] Produced from ^{14}C Released by		
	Nuclear Power Industry	Nuclear Weapons Testing	Natural ^{14}C Produced Between 1975 and 2020
1975		3.4×10^5	
1990	1.8×10^4	5.3×10^5	2.8×10^4
2005	1.1×10^4	6.9×10^5	9.1×10^4
2025	4.3×10^4	9.2×10^5	2.2×10^5
2075	8.9×10^4	1.5×10^6	4.1×10^5
Infinite Time	1.9×10^6	3.2×10^7	8.8×10^6

[a] 1 person-Sv = 100 person-rem.

Table 1.13 Global Components of Collective Dose Commitment to the World Population from Man-Made and Natural Sources of ^{3}H (Adapted from Till, 1983)

Exposure Medium	Global Collective Dose Commitment (person-Sv)[a] Produced from ^{3}H Released by		
	Nuclear Power Industry and Consumer Products Between 1975 and 2020	Nuclear Weapons Testing	Natural ^{3}H Produced Between 1975 and 2020
Atmosphere	6.3×10^2	4.8×10^3	9.1×10^2
Deep Groundwater[b]	1.3×10^1	1.1×10^2	1.9×10^1
Freshwater Lakes and Streams[c]	1.6×10^4	5.2×10^3	9.9×10^2
Ocean Surface	3.9×10^1	1.1×10^1	2.1×10^1
Total	1.7×10^4	1.0×10^4	1.9×10^3

[a] 1 person-Sv = 100 person-rem.
[b] Contributes 20% of drinking water.
[c] Contributes 80% of drinking water.

Table 1.14 Summary of Average Annual Effective Dose Equivalents to the Maximally Exposed Individual Member of the Public Due to Airborne Radioactive Effluents from Fuel Cycle Facilities (Courtesy NCRP from Report 93, 1987)

Facility	Average Annual Effective Dose Equivalent (mSv)[a]	Basis of Estimate
Mining		
Open Pit	0.26	Model mine
Underground	0.61	Model mine
Milling	0.004–2.6	8 Typical mills
Conversion		
Wet	0.008	Plant, calculation
Dry	0.032	Plant, calculation
Enrichment	<0.001–0.004	All 3 plants
Fabrication	<0.001–0.007	All 7 plants
Nuclear Power Plants		
PWR	0.006	Model reactor
BWR	0.001	Model reactor
Low Level Waste Storage	<0.01	Maxey Flats, KY facility
Transportation	0.2	To support 1 model reactor

[a] 1 mSv = 100 mrem.

Table 1.15 Summary of Annual Collective Effective Dose Equivalents to Regional Populations Due to Radioactive Effluents in the Air and Water Pathways from Fuel Cycle Facilities (Courtesy NCRP from Report 93, 1987)

Facility	Average Collective Effective Dose Equivalent (person-Sv)[a]	Basis of Estimate
Mining		
Open Pit-Air	0.01	Model mine
Open Pit-Water	0.002	
Underground-Air	0.1	Model mine
Underground-Water	0.21	
Milling	0.62	Airborne effluent from model mill
Conversion		
Wet	0.004	Plant airborne effluent in 1980
Dry	0.029	Plant airborne effluent in 1980
Enrichment	0.00002–0.004	3 Plants, airborne effluent in 1981
Fabrication	0.0001–0.007	7 Plants, airborne effluent in 1980
Nuclear Power Plant		
Air	0.00003–0.13	47 Plants in 1980
Water	0–0.4	47 Plants in 1980
Low-Level Waste Storage	<0.04	Maxey Flats, KY facility (estimate)

[a] 1 person-Sv = 100 person-rem.

Table 1.16 Effective Dose Equivalents to Nearby Individuals and to Regional Populations from Air Emissions (Courtesy NCRP from Report 93, 1987)

Facility	Number of Persons Exposed	Organ or Tissue[a]	Annual Effective Dose Equivalent to Nearby Individuals (μSv)[b]	Annual Collective Effective Dose Equivalent (person-Sv)[c]
DOE Facilities				
Oak Ridge Reservation	4,200	Lung	500[d]	0.21
Savannah River Plant	24,000	Thyroid	50	0.04
				0.25
NRC Licensed Facilities and Non-DOE Federal Facilities				
Research and Test Reactors	340,000	Average all organs	10	3.4
Accelerator[e]	6,000	Average all organs	0.001	
Radiopharmaceutical Suppliers	30,000	Thyroid	3	0.003
AFRRI[f]	400	Average all organs	0.05	
U.S. Army Facilities (Two Reactors)	6,000	Spleen	0.3	—
U.S. Navy Facilities (Nine Shipyards)	4,000	Average all organs	0.2	—
Radiation Source Manufacturers	40,000	Average all organs	2	0.08
				3.5
Mineral Extraction Industry				
Aluminum Reduction Plants	3,400	Kidney	12	0.002
Copper Smelters	4,800	Lung	2	0.001
Zinc Smelters	125,000	Bone surface	0.2	0.007
Lead Smelters	14,000	Lung	50	0.08
				0.1
Rounded Total				4.0

[a] Organ with highest annual dose.
[b] 1 μSv = 0.1 mrem.
[c] 1 person-Sv = 100 person-rem.
[d] Recent surveys indicate much smaller values (ORNL, 1986).
[e] 6 MeV Van de Graaff.
[f] Armed Forces Radiobiology Research Institute.

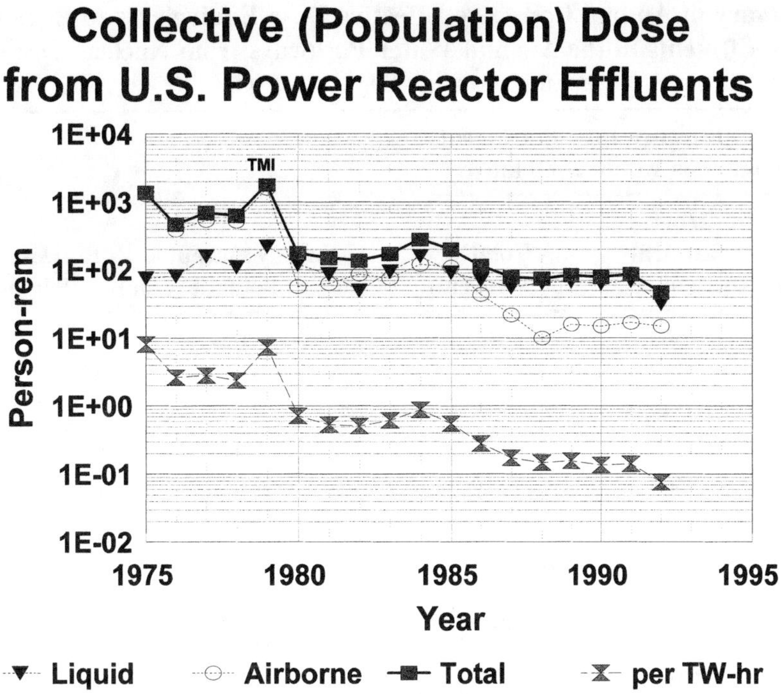

Figure 1.2 Annual Collective Effective Dose Equivalents to Regional Populations Due to Radioactive Effluents in the Air and Water Pathways from Nuclear Power Reactor Facilities (Data from NUREG/CR-2850. March 1996; see Table 1.17)

Table 1.17 Summary of Annual Collective Effective Dose Equivalents to Regional Populations Due to Radioactive Effluents in the Air and Water Pathways from Nuclear Power Reactors (Aberg and Baker, NUREG/CR-2850, March 1996)

	Collective Total Effective Dose Equivalent to the Population within 2–80 km				
Year	Liquid Effluent (person-rem)	Airborne Effluent (person-rem)	Total (person-rem)	Energy Output (Terawatt-hours[TW-hr])	Dose per Energy Unit (Person-rem per TW-hr)
1975	76	1300	1376	170	8.09
1976	82	390	472	180	2.62
1977	160	540	700	250	2.80
1978	110	530	640	270	2.37
1979	220	1600	1820	250	7.28
1980	120	57	177	250	0.71
1981	87	63	150	280	0.54
1982	50	87	137	270	0.51
1983	95	76	171	280	0.61
1984	160	120	280	320	0.88
1985	91	110	201	370	0.54
1986	71	44	115	410	0.28
1987	56	22	78	450	0.17
1988	65	10	75	510	0.15
1989	68	16	84	535	0.16
1990	63	15	78	570	0.14
1991	70	17	87	613	0.14
1992	32	15	47	616	0.08

Table 1.18 Radiation Exposure from Airborne Effluents from DOE Facilities in 1993 (From USDOE, 1995)

Facility (State)	Radionuclide Emission (curies)*				Calculated Annual Dose to Maximally-Exposed Individual (millirem/year)
	Tritium	Noble Gases	Transuranics	Other	
National Laboratories					
Argonne (IL)	3.5E + 01	2.2E + 01	2.6E − 05	3.2E + 02	6.0E − 05
Brookhaven (NY)	6.8E + 01	2.1E + 03	—	4.1E + 02	1.9E − 01
Hanford (WA)	1.3E + 01	—	4.1E − 03	8.2E − 03	6.3E − 03
Idaho NEL (ID)	1.1E + 02	2.6E + 03	6.8E − 06	3.2E + 01	1.1E − 02
Lawrence Berkeley (CA)	1.0E + 02	1.0E − 01	3.6E − 08	8.7E + 00	1.3E − 01
Lawrence Livermore (CA)	2.4E + 02	—	4.7E − 07	7.5E + 00	4.0E − 02
300 area	3.6E − 02	—	—	—	1.1E − 02
Los Alamos (NM)	1.7E + 03	1.8E + 02	4.1E − 05	2.3E + 04	5.6E + 00
Oak Ridge (TN)[1]	2.4E + 02	1.9E + 03	2.2E − 03	7.5E + 01	1.4E + 00
Sandia (NM)	7.0E − 05	4.5E + 00	1.6E − 11	1.0E + 00	1.6E − 03
Defense Programs Facilities					
Nevada Test Site (NV)	7.2E + 02	1.6E + 02	1.8E − 03	2.6E − 06	3.8E − 03
Pinellas (FL)	1.2E + 02	1.9E + 01	—	—	2.3E − 03
Pantex (TX)	3.1E − 01	—	—	—	5.7E − 05
Savannah River (SC)	1.9E + 05	3.2E − 02	2.5E − 03	2.5E − 02	1.8E − 01
Gaseous Diffusion Plants					
Paducah (KY)	—	—	4.9E − 06	4.5E − 03	2.3E − 03
Portsmouth (OH)	—	—	—	7.8E + 00	9.1E − 01
Naval Reactors Sites					
Bettis (PA)	—	—	9.6E − 09	1.1E − 05	1.3E − 03
KAPL-1 (NY)	—	7.3E − 01	2.57E − 07	1.3E − 05	2.1E − 03
KAPL-2 (NY)	—	1.4E + 00	—	—	1.7E − 02
KAPL-3 (CT)	—	3.3E − 02	—	—	1.2E − 03
Specialized Research Facilities					
Fermilab(Accelerator)(IL)	—	5.7E − 01	—	2.1E + 01	6.5E − 03
Princeton PPL(Fusion)(NJ)	3.0E + 01	1.8E + 00	—	1.2E + 00	2.7E − 02
Stanford Linear Accel. (CA)	—	1.7E − 01	—	1.9E + 00	9.3E − 03
Sites Undergoing Remediation					
Colonie (NY) CISS	0.0E + 00	0.0E + 00	0.0E + 00	4.6E − 06	—
Fernald (OH)	—	—	—	1.7E − 04	6.6E − 03
Rocky Flats (CO)	3.7E − 03	—	3.2E − 07	1.8E − 06	1.6E − 03
West Valley (NY)	3.2E − 02	—	6.7E − 07	4.1E − 05	2.0E − 04

* One curie equals 3.7×10^{10} becquerels.

[1] Includes the Oak Ridge National Laboratory, a defense programs facility (Y-12), and a former gaseous diffusion plant (K-25).

Table 1.19 Distribution of Occupational Doses for Selected Source Categories

(Thomas and Hagemeyer, 1996 for non-DOE; Smith et al., 1994 for DOE)

	Number of Workers with 1994 Doses (TEDE*) in Dose Range (rem or cSv)											Total Number Monitored	Number with Measurable Doses	Total Collective Dose (person-cSv)	Average TEDE (cSv)	Average TEDE Measurable (cSv)
	Not Meas.	Meas. −0.1	0.1–0.25	0.25–0.50	0.5–0.75	0.75–1.0	1.0–2.0	2.0–3.0	3.0–4.0	4.0–5.0	>5.0					
Nuclear Power Reactors																
Boiling Water (37)	30,322	15,898	8,036	6,754	3,719	2,191	2,306	198	6			69,430	39,108	12,092	0.17	0.31
Pressurized Water (72)	54,823	20,630	10,597	7,492	3,061	1,311	1,017	17				98,968	44,145	9,442	0.10	0.21
Total (109)	85,145	36,528	18,633	14,246	6,800	3,502	3,323	215	6			168,398	83,253	21,534	0.13	0.26
Industrial Radiography																
Single Location (29)	241	46	13	8	5	0	10	4	2	1		330	89	44	0.13	0.49
Multiple Location (111)	638	625	409	385	213	172	299	115	33	10	1	2,900	2,262	1,371	0.47	0.61
Total (139)	679	671	422	393	218	172	309	119	35	77	1	3,230	2,351	1,415	0.44	0.60
Isotope Manufacturing and Distribution																
Class ''A'' Broad (8)	1,256	402	104	78	51	39	100	74	29			2,133	877	544	0.26	0.62
Limited (36)	434	302	35	22	8	5	2					808	374	36	0.04	0.10
Total (44)	1,690	704	139	100	59	44	102	74	29			2,941	1,251	580	0.20	0.46
Low-Level Waste Disposal Sites																
NRC-licensed (2)	119	42	17	10	6	3	5					202	83	22	0.11	0.27
Independent Spent Fuel Storage Facility (1)	69	33	22	6	7	5	11	4	1			158	89	42	0.26	0.47
Fuel Fabrication Plants Total (8)	749	1423	373	326	197	117	306	92	13			3,596	2,847	1147	0.32	0.40
DOE Laboratory Contractor Employees and Visitors—1991	89700	28312	4084	1626	452	225	250	25	9	8	9	124,702	35,002	2944	0.024	0.084

* TEDE—Total Effective Dose Equivalent

Table 1.20 Summary of Average Annual Occupational Effective Dose Equivalents from High-LET Radiations (Courtesy NCRP from Report 101, 1989)

Occupational Category	Principal Radiations[a]	Number of Workers (Thousands) All	Exposed[b]	Year(s)	Average Annual Effective Dose Equivalent (mSv)[c] All	Exposed[b]	Annual Collective Effective Dose Equivalent (person-Sv)[d]
DOE	N	25		1979	2.6[e]		64[e]
Nuclear Power Plant							
Commercial	N		1.1[f]	1984		0.52[f]	0.6[f]
Commercial	N		0.083[g]	1984		0.32[g]	0.0[g]
Commercial	N		0.11[g]	1985		0.42[g]	0.1[g]
U.S. Navy	N	15	12	1984		0.24	2.9
Uranium Miner[h] (Total)	A		10	1977		10.0[i]	100
Production	A		5.9	1977		11.0[i]	65
Maintenance	A		1.8	1977		7.7[i]	14
Service	A		1.2	1977		7.0[i]	8.4
Salaried	A		1.4	1977		9.4[i]	13

[a] N for neutrons, A for alphas.
[b] Measurably exposed.
[c] 1 mSv = 100 mrem.
[d] 1 person-Sv = 100 person-rem, values less than 0.005 are recorded as zero.
[e] Approximated from the product of the dose mid-range and the number of people exposed. This probably overestimates both the collective and average doses.
[f] Data from 18 selected plants at 11 sites.
[g] Data from 5 plants.
[h] Data based on 62 underground mines.
[i] Conversion factor taken to be 2.4 Sv per Jhm^{-3} (0.85 rem) per WLM.

Table 1.21 Annual Collective Effective Dose Equivalents for U.S. Transportation of Radioactive Materials in the U.S. (1983)[a] (Courtesy NCRP from Report 93, 1987)

Transportation Mode	Number of Packages	Average TI[b] per Package	TIs Carried	Average Annual Collective Effective Dose Equivalent (person-Sv/TI)[c]	Annual Collective Effective Dose Equivalent (person-Sv)[c]
Air	604,000	0.34	202,000	0.000081	16
Highway	2,190,000	0.70	1,530,000	0.000089	140
Rail	6,900	0.74	5,100	0.000018	0.1
Other Unspecified	14,400	0.24	34,400	0.00002	0.7
Rounded Total					160

[a] Javits et al (1985) and U.S. Nuclear Regulatory Commission (1977).
[b] TI = Transport Index, defined in 1983 as the highest radiation dose rate (in mrem/h) at 1 m from any external surface of the package.
[c] 1 person-Sv = 100 person-rem.

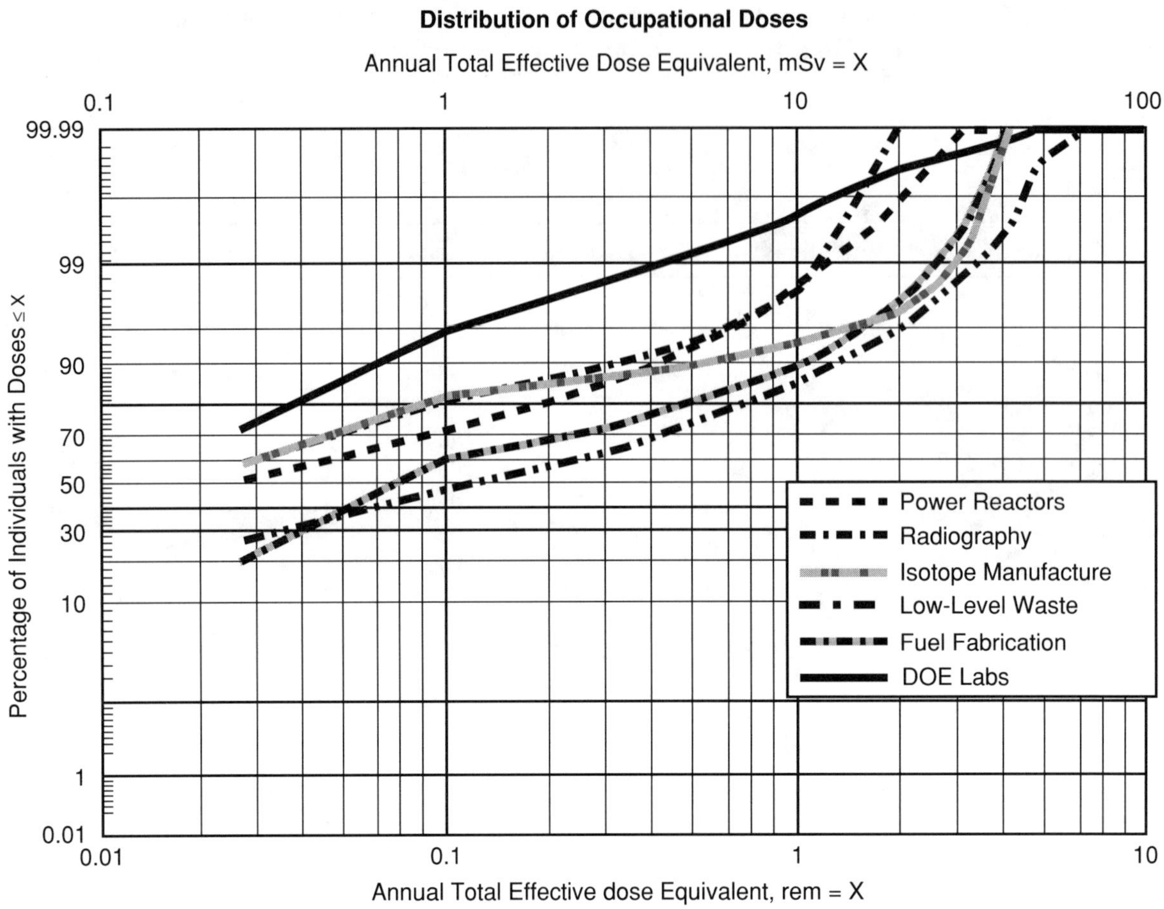

Figure 1.3 Cumulative Frequency Distribution of Annual Individual Dose Equivalents for Workers in Selected Occupational Categories (Based on all monitored workers)

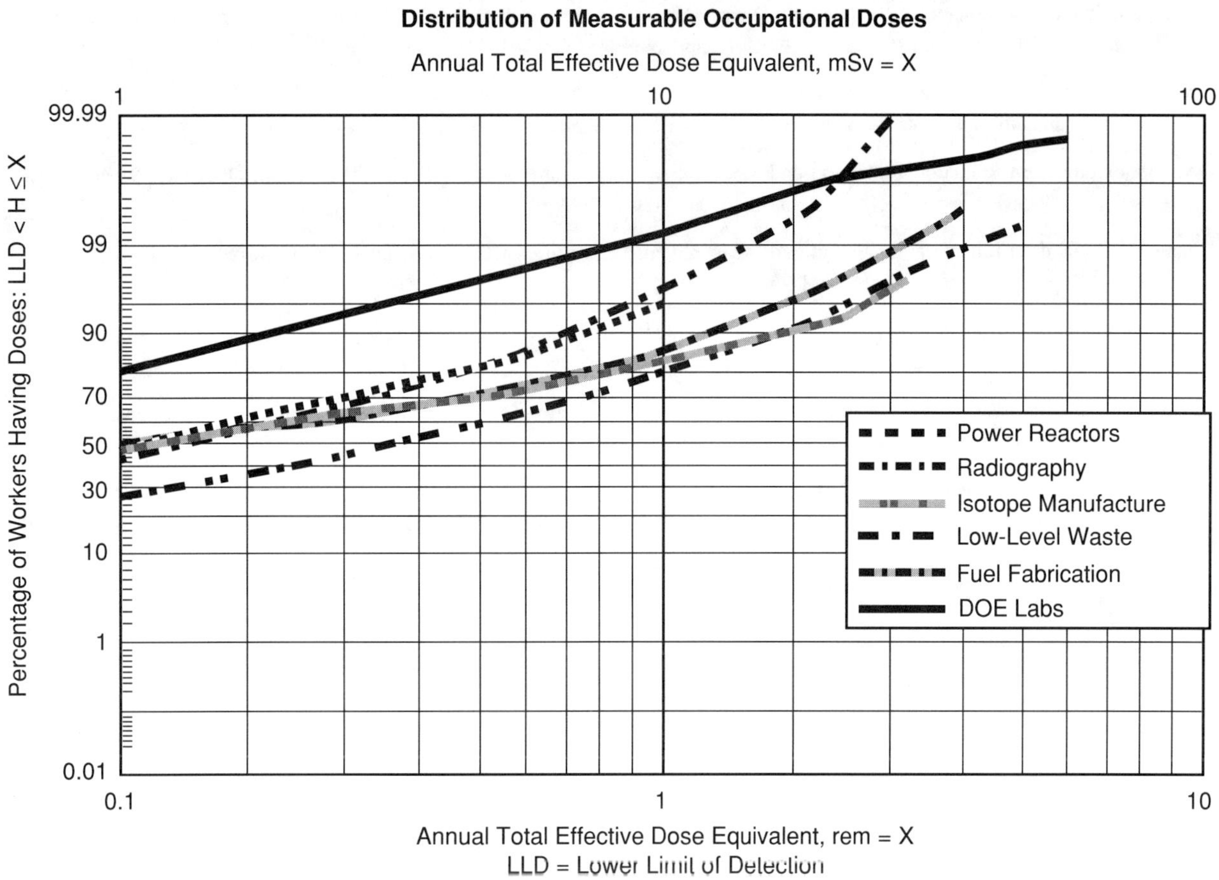

Figure 1.4 Cumulative Frequency Distribution of Annual Individual Dose Equivalents for Workers in Selected Occupational Categories (Based on workers with measurable doses)

References

Aaberg, R.L., Baker, D.A. (March 1996). *Dose Committments Due to Radioactive Releases from Nuclear Power Plant Sites in 1992.* Nuclear Regulatory Commission Report NUREG/CR-2850.

Ewen, V.K., Lackner, K., Fischer, P. ''Das Somatische Strahlenrisko bei Herzuntersuchungen mit der digitalenangiographic und der computertomographic.'' Fortschr Rontgenstr **139:**440, 1983.

Huda, W. ''Is energy imparted a good measure of the radiation risk associated with CT examinations?'' Phys. Med. Biol. **20:** 1137, 1984.

Javitz, H.S., Lyman, T.R., Maxwell, C., Myers, E.L., Thompson, C.R. (1985). *Transport of Radioactive Material in the United States: Results of a Survey to Determine the Magnitude and Characteristics of Domestic, Unclassified Shipments of Radioactive Materials,* Sandia National Laboratories Report SAND84-7174 (Springfield, Virginia: National Technical Information Services).

Kereiakes, J.G., Rosenstein, M. (1980). *Handbook of Radiation Doses in Nuclear Medicine and Diagnostic X-ray* (CRC Press, Boca Raton, Florida).

National Council on Radiation Protection and Measurements. Public Radiation Exposure from Nuclear Power Generation in the United States. NCRP Report No. 92; Bethesda, MD; December 30, 1987.

National Council on Radiation Protection and Measurements. Ionizing Radiation Exposure of the Population of the United States. NCRP Report No. 93; Bethesda, MD; September 1, 1987.

National Council on Radiation Protection and Measurements. Exposure of the Population in the United States and Canada from Natural Background Radiation. NCRP Report No. 94; Bethesda, MD; December 30, 1987.

National Council on Radiation Protection and Measurements. Radiation Exposure of the U.S. Population from Consumer Products and Miscellaneous Sources. NCRP Report No. 95; Bethesda, MD; December 30, 1987.

National Council on Radiation Protection and Measurements. Exposure of the U.S. Population from Diagnostic Medical Radiation. NCRP Report No. 100; Bethesda, MD; May 1, 1989.

National Council on Radiation Protection and Measurements. Exposure of the U.S. Population from Occupational Radiation. NCRP Report No. 101; Bethesda, MD; June 1, 1989.

National Council on Radiation Protection and Measurements. Risk Estimation for Radiation Protection. NCRP Report No. 115; Bethesda, MD; December 31, 1993.

National Council on Radiation Protection and Measurements. Radiation Protection in the Mineral Extraction Industry. NCRP Report No. 118; Bethesda, MD; November 30, 1993.

National Council on Radiation Protection and Measurements, Sources and Magnitude of Occupational and Public Exposures from Nuclear Medicine Procedures. NCRP Report No. 124; Bethesda, MD; March 11, 1996.

Nuclear Regulatory Commission. *Final Environmental Statement on Transportation of Radioactive Materials by Air and Other Modes.* NUREG-0170, Vol. 1; 1977.

Oak Ridge National Laboratory, Environmental Surveillance of the Oak Ridge Reservation and Surrounding Environs During 1985, Report ORNL-6271; Oak Ridge, TN; 1986.

Rosenberg, R., Mettler, F.A., Moseley, R.D., Parker, T.L., Williams, A.G., Christie, J.H., Kelsey, C.A. ''Collective absorbed dose to the U.S. population from radionuclide thyroid scanning and uptakes: Results of a 1981–1982 U.S. National Survey.'' *Radiology* **156:**183, 1985.

Rosenstein, M. *Organ Doses in Diagnostic Radiology*. Department of Health, Education and Welfare Publication FDA 76-8030. U.S. Government Printing Office, Washington, DC, 1976.

Shleien, B., Tucker, T.T., Johnson, D.W. ''The mean active bone marrow dose to the adult population of the United States from diagnostic radiology.'' *Health Phys* **34:**587, 1978.

Smith, M.H., Hui, T.E., Millet, W.H., Scholes, V.A. *Twenty-Third Annual Report: Radiation Exposures for DOE and DOE Contractor Employees—1990.* Department of Energy Report DOE/EH-0287P, 1994.

Thomas, M.L., Hagemeyer, D. *Occupational Radiation Exposure at Commercial Nuclear Power Reactors and Other Facilities—1994.* Nuclear Regulatory Commission Report NUREG-0713, January 1996.

Till, J.E., ''Chapter on models for special-case radionuclides,'' In *Radiological Assessment.* Nuclear Regulatory Commission. NUREG/CR-3332, ORNL-5968, 1983.

Till, J.E. *et al. Tritium—An Analysis of Key Environmental and Dosimetric Questions.* ORNL/TM-6990, Oak Ridge National Laboratory, Oak Ridge, Tenn, 1980.

U.S. Department of Energy. *Summary of Radionuclide Air Emissions from Department of Energy Facilities for CY 1993.* DOE/EH-0477, April 1995.

CHAPTER 2

COMMONLY USED UNITS, SIGNS, SYMBOLS, CONVERSION FACTORS AND CONSTANTS

Chapter 2 lists the metric system of measurements (SI), common chemical conventions, and the abbreviations, symbols and physical constants commonly employed in health physics and radiation protection. In addition to conversion factors for radiological units, the reader will also find, among others, conversion factors for physical parameters relating to area, volume, density, mass, and energy. New and old radiological units are listed. The chapter also presents the electromagnetic spectrum and the characteristics of its component radiations.

TABLE OF CONTENTS

Table 2.1 The International System of Units (SI) (After NIST Special Publication 330 1991)

Table 2.1.1 Introduction to SI Units

The 11th General Conference on Weights and Measurements (CGPM), 1960, by its Resolution 12, adopted the name *International System of Units*, with the international abbreviation SI, for this practical system of units of measurement, and laid down rules for the prefixes, the derived and supplementary units, and other matters, thus establishing a comprehensive specification for units of measurement.

SI units are divided into three classes: *base* units, *derived* units, and *supplementary* units. From the scientific point of view, division of SI units into these three classes is to a certain extent arbitrary, because it is not essential to the physics of the subject.

Nevertheless, the General Conference, considering the advantages of a single, practical, worldwide system of units for international relations, for teaching, and for scientific work, decided to base the International System on a choice of seven well-defined units which by convention are regarded as dimensionally independent: the meter, the kilogram, the second, the ampere, the kelvin, the mole, and the candela. These SI units are called *base units*.

The second class of SI units contains *derived units*, i.e., units that can be formed by combining base units according to the algebraic relations linking the corresponding quantities. The names and symbols of some units thus formed in terms of base units can be replaced by special names and symbols which can themselves be used to form expressions and symbols of other derived units.

The 11th CGPM (1960) admitted a third class of SI units, called *supplementary units* and containing the SI units of plane and solid angle.

The SI units of these three classes form a coherent set of units in the sense normally attributed to the word "coherent," i.e., a system of units mutually related by rules of multiplication and division without any numerical factor. Following the the Comité International des Poids et Measures (CIPM) Recommendation 1 (1969), the units of this coherent set of units are designated by the name *SI units*.

It is important to emphasize that each physical quantity has only one SI unit, even if the name of this unit can be expressed in different forms, but the inverse is not true: the same SI unit name can correspond to several different quantities.

Table 2.1.2 SI Base and Supplementary Units

Quantity	Name	Symbol
SI Base Units:		
length	meter	m
mass[a]	kilogram	kg
time	second	s
electric current	ampere	A
thermodynamic temperature	kelvin	K
amount of substance	mole	mol
luminous intensity	candela	cd
SI Supplementary Units:		
plane angle	radian	rad
solid angle	steradian	sr

[a] "Weight" in common parlance is often used to mean "mass."

Units for all other quantities are derived from these nine units. In table 2.1.3 are listed 19 SI derived units with special names which were derived from the base and supplementary units in a coherent manner, which means, in brief, that they are expressed as products and quotients of the nine base and supplementary units without numerical factors.

Table 2.1.3 SI Derived Units with Special Names

Quantity	SI Unit		
	Name	Symbol	Expression in Terms of Other Units
Frequency	hertz	Hz	s^{-1}
Force	newton	N	m/s^2
Pressure, stress	pascal	Pa	N/m^2
Energy, work, quantity of heat	joule	J	N m
Power, radiant flux	watt	W	J/s
Electric charge, quantity of electricity	coulomb	C	A s
Electric potential, potential difference, electromotive force	volt	V	W/A
Capacitance	farad	F	C/V
Electric resistance	ohm	Ω	V/A
Electric conductance	siemens	S	A/V
Magnetic flux	weber	Wb	V s
Magnetic flux density	tesla	T	Wb/m^2
Inductance	henry	H	Wb/A
Luminous flux	lumen	lm	cd sr
Illuminance	lux	lx	lm/m^2
Celsius temperature[a]	degree Celsius	°C	K
Activity (of a radionuclide)	becquerel	Bq	s^{-1}
Absorbed dose, specific energy imparted, kerma, absorbed dose index	gray	Gy	J/kg
Dose equivalent, dose equivalent index	sievert	Sv	J/kg

[a] In addition to the thermodynamic temperature (symbol T) expressed in kelvins (see Table 2.1.1), use is also made of Celsius temperature (symbol t) defined by the equation

$$t = T - T_o$$

where T_o = 273.15 K by definition. The unit "degree Celsius" is equal to the unit "kelvin," but "degree Celsius" is a special name in place of "kelvin" for expressing Celsius temperature. A temperature interval or a Celsius temperature difference can be expressed in degrees Celsius as well as in kelvins.

[b] The derived quantities to be expressed in the gray and the sievert have been revised in accordance with the recommendations of the International Commission on Radiation Units and Measurements (ICRU).

All other SI derived units, such as those in Tables 2.1.4 and 2.1.5, are similarly derived in a coherent manner from the supplementary, and special–name SI units.

Table 2.1.4 Examples of SI Derived Units Expressed in Terms of Base Units

Quantity	SI Unit	Unit Symbol
Area	square meter	m^2
Volume	cubic meter	m^3
Speed, velocity	meter per second	m/s
Acceleration	meter per second squared	m/s^2
Wave number	1 per meter	m^{-1}
Density, mass density	kilogram per cubic meter	kg/m^3
Specific volume	cubic meter per kilogram	m^3/kg
Current density	ampere per square meter	A/m^2
Magnetic field strength	ampere per meter	A/m
Concentration (of amount of substance)	mole per cubic meter	mol/m^3
Luminance	candela per square meter	cd/m^2

Table 2.1.5 Examples of SI Derived Units Expressed by Means of Special Names

Quantity	Name	Unit Symbol
Dynamic viscosity	pascal second	Pa s
Moment of force	newton meter	N m
Surface tension	newton per meter	N/m
Heat flux density, irradiance	watt per square meter	W/m^2
Heat capacity, entropy	joule per kelvin	J/K
Specific heat capacity, specific entropy	joule per kilogram kelvin	J/(kg K)
Specific energy	joule per kilogram	J/kg
Thermal conductivity	watt per meter kelvin	W/(m K)
Energy density	joule per cubic meter	J/m^3
Electric field strength	volt per meter	V/m
Electric charge density	coulomb per cubic meter	C/m^3
Electric flux density	coulomb per square meter	C/m^2
Permitivity	farad per meter	F/m
Permeability	henry per meter	H/m
Molar energy	joule per mole	J/mol
Molar entropy, molar heat capacity	joule per mole kelvin	J/(mol K)
Exposure (x and γ rays)	coulomb per kilogram	C/kg
Absorbed dose rate	gray per second	Gy/s

Certain units that are not part of the SI are used so widely that it is impractical to abandon them. The units that are accepted for continued use in the United States with the International System are listed in Table 2.1.6.

Table 2.1.6 Units in Use with the International System

Name	Symbol	Value in SI Unit
Minute (time)	min	1 min = 60 s
Hour	h	1 h = 60 min = 3,600 s
Day	d	1 d = 24 h = 86,400 s
Mean solar second	s	1.002738 sidereal s
Degree (angle)	°	$1° = (\pi/180)$ rad
Minute (angle)	′	$1' = (1/60)° = (\pi/10{,}800)$rad
Second (angle)	″	$1'' = (1/60)' = (\pi/648{,}000)$rad
Liter	l or L[a]	$1\ L = 1\ dm^3 = 10^{-3}\ m^3$
Metric ton	t	$1\ t = 10^3$ kg
Hectare (land area)[b]	ha	$1\ ha = 10^4\ m^2$
Electron volt[c]	eV	$1\ eV = 1.602 \times 10^{-19}$ J, approx.
Unified atomic mass unit[c]	u	$1\ u = 1.660\ 54 \times 10^{-27}$ kg, approx.

[a] Both L and l are international symbols for liter. Because "l" can easily be confused with the numeral "1" the symbol "L" is recommended for United States use.
[b] Unit in use temporarily with the International System
[c] Units used with the International System whose values in SI units are obtained experimentally.

Table 2.1.7 Examples of Conversion Factors from Non-SI Units to SI (From NBS Letter Circular LC1120, 1979)

Quantity	Name of Unit	Symbol for Unit	Definition in SI Units
Length	inch	in.	2.54×10^{-2} m
Length	nautical mile[a]	nmi	1852 m
Length	angstrom[a,b]	Å	10^{-10} m
Velocity	knot[a]	kn	(1852/3600) m/s
Cross Section	barn[a]	b	$10^{-28}\ m^2$
Acceleration	gal[a,b]	Gal	$10^{-2}\ m/s^2$
Mass	pound (avoirdupois)	lb	0.453 592 37 kg
Force	kilogram-force	kgf	9.806 65 N
Pressure	millimeter of mercury at 0°C	mm/Hg	133.322 Pa[c]
Pressure	atmosphere	atm	101 325 Pa
Pressure	torr	Torr	(101 325/760) Pa
Pressure	bar[a,b]	bar	10^5 Pa
Stress	pound-force per sq in	$lbf/in.^2$	6 894.757 Pa[c]
Energy	British thermal unit (Int. Table)	Btu	1055.056 J[c]
Energy	kilowatt hour	kWh	3.6×10^6 J
Energy	calorie (thermochemical)	cal	4.184 J
Activity (of a radionuclide)	curie[a]	Ci	3.7×10^{10} Bq
Exposure (x or γ rays)	roentgen[a]	R	$2.58 \times 10^{-4}\ C\ kg^{-1}$
Absorbed dose	rad[a]	rad	1×10^{-2} Gy
Dose equivalent	rem[a]	rem	1×10^{-2} Sv

[a] The CIPM has sanctioned the temporary use of these units.
[b] The use of these units is discouraged in the American National Standard for Metric Practice, Z210.1.
[c] Approximate, all other conversion factors are exact.

Table 2.2 The Electromagnetic Spectrum, Type of Radiation, Frequency, Wavelength and Photon Energy

Type of Radiation	Representative Frequency (Hz)	Equivalent Wavelength	Approximate Photon Energy
Electric waves	$<1 \times 10^5$	$>3 \times 10^5$ cm	$<4.1 \times 10^{-10}$ eV
Radio waves	1×10^5	3×10^5 cm	4.1×10^{-10} eV
	3×10^{10}	1.0 cm	1.24×10^{-4} eV
Infrared	3×10^{12}	0.01 cm	0.0124 eV
	3×10^{14}	10,000 Å	1.24 eV
Visible			
Red	4.3×10^{14}	7,000 Å	1.77 eV
Orange	4.64×10^{14}	6,470 Å	1.92 eV
Yellow	5.13×10^{14}	5,850 Å	2.12 eV
	5.22×10^{14}	5,750 Å	2.16 eV
Maximum visibility	5.4×10^{14}	5,560 Å	2.24 eV
Green	5.22×10^{14}	5,750 Å	2.16 eV
Blue	6.11×10^{14}	4,910 Å	2.53 eV
Violet	7.07×10^{14}	4,240 Å	2.93 eV
Ultraviolet	7.5×10^{14}	4,000 Å	3.1 eV
	3×10^{16}	100 Å	124 eV
X-ray[a]			
Low energy	3×10^{16}	100 Å	124 eV
Diagnostic and superficial therapy	3×10^{18}	1 Å	12.4 keV
Deep therapy	3×10^{19}	0.1 Å	0.124 MeV
	3×10^{20}	0.01 Å	1.24 MeV
Small betatron	3×10^{21}	0.001 Å	12.4 MeV
Large betatron	3×10^{22}	0.0001 Å	124 MeV
Proton synchrotron	3×10^{23}	0.00001 Å	1,240 MeV
Gamma rays	3×10^{18}	1 Å	12.4 keV
	3×10^{21}	0.001 Å	12.4 MeV
Cosmic photons	3×10^{21}	0.001 Å	10 MeV
	3×10^{22}	0.0001 Å	100 MeV

[a] Linear accelerators (linacs) are also sources of high energy X-rays, generally in the 4 to 10 MeV range, and electrons up to at least 45 MeV.

Table 2.3 Summary of New and Old Radiological Units (old units are in parens, obsolete units are in braces)

Quantity	Name	Symbol	Units
Activity	becquerel	Bq	$1\ s^{-1}$
	(curie)	Ci,{C}.	3.7×10^{10} Bq
	{rutherford}	{Rd}	$10^5\ min^{-1}$, 10^5 dpm
Absorbed Dose	gray	Gy	$J\ kg^{-1}$
	(rad)	rad	10^{-2} Gy
Dose Equivalent	sievert	Sv	$J\ kg^{-1}$
	(rem)	rem	10^{-2} Sv
Exposure	coulomb per kilogram		$C\ kg^{-1}$
	(roentgen)	R	$2.58 \times 10^{-4}\ C\ kg^{-1}$

Table 2.4 Fractions and Multiples Commonly Used with Radiological Units

Factor	Prefix	Symbol	Factor	Prefix	Symbol
10^{24}	yotta	Y	10^{-1}	deci	d
10^{21}	zetta	Z	10^{-2}	centi	c
10^{18}	exa	E	10^{-3}	milli	m
10^{15}	peta	P	10^{-6}	micro	μ
10^{12}	tera	T	10^{-9}	nano	n
10^{9}	giga	G	10^{-12}	pico	p
10^{6}	mega	M	10^{-15}	femto	f
10^{3}	kilo	k	10^{-18}	atto	a
10^{2}	hecto	h	10^{-21}	zepto	z
10^{1}	deka[a]	da	10^{-24}	yocto	y

[a] Outside the USA the spelling "deca" is extensively used.

Table 2.5 Greek Alphabet

A	α	Alpha	I	ι	Iota	P	ρ	Rho
B	β	Beta	K	κ	Kappa	Σ	σ, ς	Sigma
Γ	γ	Gamma	Λ	λ	Lambda	T	τ	Tau
Δ	δ	Delta	M	μ	Mu	Υ	υ	Upsilon
E	ϵ	Epsilon	N	ν	Nu	Φ	ϕ, φ	Phi
Z	ζ	Zeta	Ξ	ξ	Xi	X	χ	Chi
H	η	Eta	O	o	Omicron	Ψ	ψ	Psi
Θ	θ, ϑ	Theta	Π	π	Pi	Ω	ω	Omega

Table 2.6 Abbreviations

Absorbed dose of radiation	rad	Electrocardiogram	ECG
Alternating current	a–c	Electromagnetic unit	emu
Ampere	A	Electromotive force	emf
Angstrom	Å	Electrostatic unit	esu
Atmosphere	atm	Electron volt	eV
Atomic weight	at.wt	Erg(s)	erg(s)
Average	avg	Farad	F
Barn(s)	b	Feet, foot	ft
Becquerel	Bq	Figure	Fig.
Biological oxygen demand	BOD	Foot–pound	ft–lb
British thermal unit	Btu	Freezing point	fp
Boiling point	bp	Gastrointestinal	GI
Calorie	cal	Gallon	gal
Candela	cd	Gauss	G
Celsius temperature	°C	Giga (see footnote)	G
Centi (see footnote)	c	Gram	g
Centimeter	cm	Gram-molecule	mol
Centimeter-gram-second	cgs	Gravitational acceleration	g
Central nervous system	CNS	Gray	Gy
Circa	ca.	Hecto (see footnote)	h
Coulomb	C	Henry	H
Counts per minute	cpm	Hertz (cycle per second)	Hz
Counts per second	cps	Horsepower	hp
Cubic centimeter	cm^3	Hour	hr
Curie	Ci	Inch	in.
Day(s)	day(s)	Internal diameter	ID
Debye unit	D	Joule	J
Deci (see footnote)	d	Kelvin temperature	K
Decibel	dB	Kilo (see footnote)	k
Degree	°	Kilogram	kg
Degrees		Latitude	lat
Celsius and Centigrade	°C	Longitude	long.
Fahrenheit	°F	Liter	l or L
Kelvin	K	Logarithm	log
Deka (see footnote)	da	Logarithm (natural)	ln
Direct current	d–c	Lumen	lm
Disintegrations per minute	dpm	Lux	lx
Dyne	dyn		
Diameter—not abbreviated			

Table 2.6 Abbreviations (Continued)

Magnetomotive force	mmf	Radiofrequency	rf
Maximum	max	Relative humidity	rh
Maximum permissible dose	MPD	Relative biological effectiveness	RBE
Median lethal dose	LD_{50}	Revolutions per minute	rpm
Mega (see footnote)	M	Roentgen	R
Megohm	$M\Omega$	Roentgen-equivalent-man	rem
Melting point	mp	Root mean square	rms
Meter	m	Second(s)	s
Micrometer, micron	μm	Siemens	S
Micro (see footnote)	μ	Sievert	Sv
Mile	mile	Species	sp
Miles per hour	mph	Specific gravity	sp gr
Milli (see footnote)	m	Specific heat	sp ht
Minimum	min	Specific volume	sp vol
Minute(s)	min	Square foot	ft^2
Molar concentration	M	Standard deviation	S.D.
Mole	mol	Standard error	S.E.
Molecular weight	mol. wt	Standard temperature and pressure	STP
Month	month	Steradian	sr
Nano (see footnote)	n	Tesla	T
Newton	N	Temperature	temp
Normal concentration	N	Tera (see footnote)	T
Number	No.	Torr	torr
Ohm	Ω	Ultra-violet	UV
Ounce	oz	Versus	vs.
Outside diameter	OD	Volt	V
Parts per million	ppm	Volume	vol
Pascal	Pa	Volume by volume	v/v
Pico (see footnote)	p	Watt	W
Pound(s)	lb	Watt-hour	Wh
Pounds per square inch	psi	Weight	wt
Probability	P	Weber	Wb
Quality Factor	Q	Yard	yd
		Year	yr, y

NOTE: These symbols may be prefixed to any of the symbols denoting a unit of measure in the CGS system and this indicates a multiple or submultiple of the unit; e.g., kV-amp, μÅ, pCi, mmol and ns denote kilovolt-ampere, micro Angstrom, picocurie, millimole and nanosecond, respectively. Also, any unit of length may be written with exponent 2 or 3 to express the corresponding unit for measure of area of volume, e.g., m^2, ft^3 to designate square meter and cubic foot, respectively.

Table 2.7 Mathematical Signs and Symbols

$+$	plus, addition, positive	Δx	differential
$-$	minus, subtraction, negative	$\int_b^a f(x)\,dx$	definite integral of f(x)
$\pm$	plus or minus, positive or negative	$\int f(x)\,dx$	indefinite integral of f(x)
$\div$, /, —	division	$\sqrt{x}$	square root of x
$\times$, $\cdot$, ()	multiplication	$\sqrt[n]{x}$	nth root of x
(), []	collection (parentheses, brackets)	a^n	nth power of a
$=$	equal to	a^{-n}	reciprocal of nth power of a, $= 1/a^n$
$\neq$	not equal to	log, $\log_{10}$	common logarithm
$\equiv$	identical to	ln, $\log_e$	natural logarithm
$\approx$	equals approximately, congruent	e, ϵ	base of natural logs, 2.71828183 . . .
$>$	greater than	π	pi, 3.14159265 . . .
$\not>$	not greater than	$\angle$	angle
$\geq$, >=	greater than or equal to	$\perp$	perpendicular to
$<$	less than	$\parallel$	parallel to
$\not<$	not less than	n	any number
$\leq$, <=	less than or equal to	$\lvert n \rvert$	absolute value of n
$::$	proportional to	$\bar{n}$	average value of n
$:$	ratio	n°	n degrees
$\sim$	similar to	n'	n minutes (of a degree), n feet
$\propto$	varies, as proportional to	n''	n seconds (of a degree), n inches
$\rightarrow$	approaches	Σx_i	summation of x_i
∞	infinity	sin	sine (of an angle)
$\therefore$	therefore	cos	cosine (of an angle)
f(x)	function of x	tan	tangent (of an angle)
df(x)/dx	derivative	cot	cotangent (of an angle)

Table 2.8 The Chemical Elements (From HASL-300 1990)

Name	Symbol	Atomic Number	Atomic Weight	Name	Symbol	Atomic Number	Atomic Weight
Actinium	Ac	89	227.028	Bromine	Br	35	79.904
Aluminum	Al	13	26.9815	Cadmium	Cd	48	112.41
Americium	Am	95	(243.)[a]	Calcium	Ca	20	40.08
Antimony	Sb	51	121.75	Californium	Cf	98	(251.)
Argon	Ar	18	39.948	Carbon	C	6	12.011
Arsenic	As	33	74.9216	Cerium	Ce	58	140.12
Astatine	At	85	(210.)	Cesium	Cs	55	132.905
Barium	Ba	56	137.33	Chlorine	Cl	17	35.453
Berkelium	Bk	97	(247.)	Chromium	Cr	24	51.996
Beryllium	Be	4	9.01218	Cobalt	Co	27	58.9332
Bismuth	Bi	83	208.980	Copper	Cu	29	63.546
Boron	B	5	10.81	Curium	Cm	96	(247.)

Table 2.8 The Chemical Elements (Continued)

Name	Symbol	Atomic Number	Atomic Weight	Name	Symbol	Atomic Number	Atomic Weight
Dysprosium	Dy	66	162.50	Palladium	Pd	46	106.42
Einsteinium	Es	99	(252.)	Phosphorus	P	15	30.9738
Erbium	Er	68	167.26	Platinum	Pt	78	195.08
Europium	Eu	63	151.96	Plutonium	Pu	94	(244.)
Fermium	Fm	100	(257.)	Polonium	Po	84	(209.)
Fluorine	F	9	18.9984	Potassium	K	19	39.0938
Francium	Fr	87	(223.)	Praseodymium	Pr	59	140.908
Gadolinium	Gd	64	157.25	Promethium	Pm	61	(145.)
Gallium	Ga	31	69.72	Protactinium	Pa	91	231.036
Germanium	Ge	32	72.59	Radium	Ra	88	226.025
Gold	Au	79	196.967	Radon	Rn	86	(222.)
Hafnium	Hf	72	178.49	Rhenium	Re	75	186.207
Helium	He	2	4.00260	Rhodium	Rh	45	102.906
Holmium	Ho	67	164.930	Rubidium	Rb	37	85.4678
Hydrogen	H	1	1.00794	Ruthenium	Ru	44	101.07
Indium	In	49	114.82	Samarium	Sm	62	150.36
Iodine	I	53	126.905	Scandium	Sc	21	44.9559
Iridium	Ir	77	192.22	Selenium	Se	34	78.96
Iron	Fe	26	55.847	Silicon	Si	14	28.0855
Krypton	Kr	36	83.80	Silver	Ag	47	107.868
Lanthanum	La	57	138.906	Sodium	Na	11	22.9898
Lawrencium	Lr	103	(260.)	Strontium	Sr	38	87.62
Lead	Pb	82	207.2	Sulfur	S	16	32.06
Lithium	Li	3	6.941	Tantalum	Ta	73	180.948
Lutetium	Lu	71	174.967	Technetium	Tc	43	(98.)
Magnesium	Mg	12	24.305	Tellurium	Te	52	127.60
Manganese	Mn	25	54.9380	Terbium	Tb	65	158.925
Mendelevium	Md	101	(258.)	Thallium	Tl	81	204.383
Mercury	Hg	80	200.59	Thullium	Tm	69	168.934
Molybdenum	Mo	42	95.94	Thorium	Th	90	232.038
Neodymium	Nd	60	144.24	Tin	Sn	50	118.71
Neon	Ne	10	20.179	Titanium	Ti	22	47.88
Neptunium	Np	93	237.048	Tungsten	W	74	183.85
Nickel	Ni	28	58.69	Uranium	U	92	238.029
Niobium	Nb	41	92.9064	Vanadium	V	23	50.9415
Nitrogen	N	7	14.0067	Xenon	Xe	54	131.29
Nobelium	No	102	(259.)	Ytterbium	Yb	70	173.04
Osmium	Os	76	190.2	Yttrium	Y	39	88.9059
Oxygen	O	8	15.9994	Zinc	Zn	30	65.39
				Zirconium	Zr	40	91.224

[a] As indicated-original source table.

Table 2.9 List of Elements by Atomic Number

Atomic Number	Element	Symbol	Atomic Number	Element	Symbol
1	Hydrogen	H	42	Molybdenum	Mo
2	Helium	He	43	Technetium	Tc
3	Lithium	Li	44	Ruthenium	Ru
4	Beryllium	Be	45	Rhodium	Rh
5	Boron	B	46	Palladium	Pd
6	Carbon	C	47	Silver	Ag
7	Nitrogen	N	48	Cadmium	Cd
8	Oxygen	O	49	Indium	In
9	Fluorine	F	50	Tin	Sn
10	Neon	Ne	51	Antimony	Sb
11	Sodium	Na	52	Tellurium	Te
12	Magnesium	Mg	53	Iodine	I
13	Aluminum	Al	54	Xenon	Xe
14	Silicon	Si	55	Cesium	Cs
15	Phosphorus	P	56	Barium	Ba
16	Sulphur	S	57	Lanthanum	La
17	Chlorine	Cl	58	Cerium	Ce
18	Argon	Ar	59	Praseodymium	Pr
19	Potassium	K	60	Neodymium	Nd
20	Calcium	Ca	61	Promethium	Pm
21	Scandium	Sc	62	Samarium	Sm
22	Titanium	Ti	63	Europium	Eu
23	Vanadium	V	64	Gadolinium	Gd
24	Chromium	Cr	65	Terbium	Tb
25	Manganese	Mn	66	Dysprosium	Dy
26	Iron	Fe	67	Holmium	Ho
27	Cobalt	Co	68	Erbium	Er
28	Nickel	Ni	69	Thulium	Tm
29	Copper	Cu	70	Ytterbium	Yb
30	Zinc	Zn	71	Lutetium	Lu
31	Gallium	Ga	72	Hafnium	Hf
32	Germanium	Ge	73	Tantalum	Ta
33	Arsenic	As	74	Tungsten	W
34	Selenium	Se	75	Rhenium	Re
35	Bromine	Br	76	Osmium	Os
36	Krypton	Kr	77	Iridium	Ir
37	Rubidium	Rb	78	Platinum	Pt
38	Strontium	Sr	79	Gold	Au
39	Yttrium	Y	80	Mercury	Hg
40	Zirconium	Zr	81	Thallium	Tl
41	Niobium	Nb	82	Lead	Pb
			83	Bismuth	Bi
			84	Polonium	Po
			85	Astatine	At
			86	Radon	Rn
			87	Francium	Fr

Table 2.9 List of Elements by Atomic Number (Continued)

Atomic Number	Element	Symbol	Atomic Number	Element	Symbol
88	Radium	Ra	99	Einsteinium	Es
89	Actinium	Ac	100	Fermium	Fm
90	Thorium	Th	101	Mendelevium	Md
91	Protactinium	Pa	102	Nobelium	No
92	Uranium	U	103	Lawrencium	Lr
93	Neptunium	Np	104	Rutherfordium	Rf
94	Plutonium	Pu	105	Dubnium	Db
95	Americium	Am	106	Seaborgium	Sg
96	Curium	Cm	107	Bohrium	Bh
97	Berkelium	Bk	108	Hassium	Hs
98	Californium	Cf	109	Meitnerium	Mt

Table 2.10 The 1986 Recommended Values of the Fundamental Physical Constants (After Cohen and Taylor CODATA Bulletin 63 1986; Cohen and Taylor, 1989)

Quantity	Symbol	Value	Units	Relative Uncertainty ppm
Universal Constants				
Speed of light in vacuum	c	299 792 458	$m\ s^{-1}$	exact
Permeability of vacuum	μ_o	$4\pi \times 10^{-7}$	$N\ A^{-2}$	
		= 12.566 370 614...	$10^{-7}\ N\ A^{-2}$	exact
Permittivity of vacuum	$\in_o$	$1/\mu_o c^2$	$10^{-12}\ F\ m^{-1}$	exact
		= 8.854 187 817...		
Newtonian constant of gravitation	G	6.672 59(85)	$10^{-11}\ m^3 kg^{-1} s^{-2}$	128.
Planck constant	h	6.626 075 5(40)	10^{-34} J s	0.60
in electron volts, $h/[e]$		4.135 669 2(12)	10^{-15} eV s	0.30
$h/2\pi$	$\hbar$		1.054 572 66 (63) 10^{-34} J s	0.60
in electron volts, $\hbar/[e]$		6.582 122 0(20)	10^{-16} eV s	0.30
Planck mass $(\hbar c/G)^{1/2}$	m_p	2.176 71(14)	10^{-8} kg	64
Planck length, $\hbar/m_p c = (hG/c^3)^{1/2}$	l_p	1.616 05(10)	10^{-35} m	64
Planck time $l_p/c = (\hbar G/c^5)^{1/2}$	t_p	5.390 56(34)	10^{-44} s	64
Electromagnetic Constants				
Elementary charge	e	1.602 177 33(49)	10^{-19} C	0.30
	e/h	2.417 988 36(72)	$10^{14}\ A\ J^{-1}$	0.30
Magnetic flux quantum, $h/2e$	ϕ_o	2.067 834 61(61)	10^{-15} Wb	0.30
Josephson frequency—voltage quotient	$2e/h$	4.835 976 7(14)	$10^{14}\ Hz\ V^{-1}$	0.30
Quantized Hall conductance	e^2/h	3.874 046 14(17)	10^{-5} S	0.045
Quantized Hall resistance, $h/e^2 = \mu_o c/2a$	R_H	25 812.805 6(12)	Ω	0.045
Bohr magneton, $e\hbar/2m_e$	μ_B	9.274 015 4(31)	$10^{-24}\ J\ T^{-1}$	0.34
in electron volts, $\mu_B/[e]$		5.788 382 63(52)	$10^{-5}\ eV\ T^{-1}$	0.089
in hertz, μ_B/h		1.399 624 18(42)	$10^{10}\ Hz\ T^{-1}$	0.30
in wavenumbers, μ_B/hc		46.686 437(14)	$m^{-1}\ T^{-1}$	0.30
in kelvins, μ_B/K		0.671 709 9(57)	$K\ T^{-1}$	8.5
Nuclear magneton, $e\hbar/2sm_p$	μ_N	5.050 786 6(17)	$10^{-27}\ J\ T^{-1}$	0.34
in electron volts, $\mu_N/[e]$		3.152 451 66(28)	$10^{-8}\ eV\ T^{-1}$	0.089
in hertz, μ_N/h		7.622 591 4(23)	$MHz\ T^{-1}$	0.30
in wavenumbers, μ_N/hc		2.542 622 81(77)	$10^{-2}\ m^{-1}\ T^{-1}$	0.30
in kelvins, μ_N/K		3.658 246(31)	$10^{-4}\ K\ T^{-1}$	8.5
Atomic Constants				
Fine-structure constant, $\mu_o ce^2/2h$	α	7.297 353 08(33)	10^{-3}	0.045
inverse fine-structure constant	α^{-1}	137.035 989 5(61)		0.045
Rydberg constant, $m_e c\alpha^2/2h$	R_∞	10 973 731.534(13)	m^{-1}	0.0012
in hertz, $R_\infty c$		3.289 841 949 9(39)	10^{15} Hz	0.0012
in joules, $R_\infty hc$		2.179 874 1(13)	10^{-18} J	0.60
in eV, $R_\infty hc/[e]$		13.605 698 1(40)	eV	0.30
Bohr radius, $\alpha/4\pi R_\infty$	a_o	0.529 177 249(24)	10^{-10} m	0.045

Table 2.10 The 1986 Recommended Values of the Fundamental Physical Constants (Continued)

Quantity	Symbol	Value	Units	Relative Uncertainty ppm
Hartree energy, $e^2/4\pi\epsilon_o\alpha_o = 2R_\infty hc$	E_h	4.359 748 2(26)	10^{-18} J	0.60
in eV, $E_h/[e]$		27.211 396 1(81)	eV	0.30
Quantum of circulation	$h/2m_e$	3.636 948 07(33)	10^{-4} m^2 s^{-1}	0.089
	h/m_e	7.273 896 14(65)	10^{-4} m^2s^{-1}	0.089
Electron				
Mass	m_e	9.109 389 7(54)	10^{-31} kg	0.59
		5.485 799 03(13)	10^{-4} u	0.023
in electron volts, $m_ec^2/[e]$		0.510 999 06(15)	MeV	0.30
Electron-muon mass ratio	m_e/m_μ	4.836 332 18(71)	10^{-3}	0.15
Electron-proton mass ratio	m_e/m_p	5.446 170 13(11)	10^{-4}	0.020
Electron-deuteron mass ratio	m_e/m_d	2.724 437 07(6)	10^{-4}	0.020
Electron-α particle mass ratio	m_e/m_α	1.370 933 54(3)	10^{-4}	0.021
Specific charge	$-e/m_e$	1.758 819 62(53)	10^{11} C kg^{-1}	0.30
Molar mass	$M(e)$	5.485 799 03(13)	10^{-7} kg mol^{-1}	0.023
Compton wavelength, h/m_ec	λ_c	2.426 310 58(22)	10^{-12} m	0.089
$\lambda_c 2\pi = \alpha a_o = \alpha^2/4\pi R_{ii}$	λ_c	3.861 593 23(35)	10^{-13} m	0.089
Classical radius, $\alpha^2 a_o$	r_e	2.817 940 92(38)	10^{-15} m	0.13
Thomson cross section, $(8\pi/3)r_e^2$	σ_e	0.665 246 16(18)	10^{-28} m^2	0.27
Magnetic moment	μ_e	928.477 01(31)	10^{-26} J T^{-1}	0.34
in Bohr magnetons	μ_e/μ_B	1.001 159 652 193(10)		1×10^{-5}
in nuclear magnetons	μ_e/μ_N	1838.282 000(37)		0.020
Magnetic moment anomaly, $\mu_e\mu_B{}^{-1}$	a_e	1.159 652 193(10)	10^{-3}	0.0086
g-factor, $2(1 + a_e)$	g_e	2.002 319 304 386(20)		1×10^{-5}
Electron-muon magnetic moment ratio	μ_e/μ_μ	206.766 967(30)		0.15
Electron-proton magnetic moment ratio	μ_e/μ_p	658.210 688 1(66)		0.010
Muon				
Mass	m_μ	1.883 532 7(11)	10^{-28} kg	0.61
		0.113 428 913(17)	u	0.15
in electron volts, $m_\mu c^2/[e]$		105.658 389(34)	MeV	0.32
Muon-electron mass ratio	m_μ/m_e	206.768 262(30)		0.15
Molar mass	$M(\mu)$	1.134 289 13(17)	10^{-4} kg mol^{-1}	0.15
Magnetic moment	μ_μ	4.490 451 4(15)	10^{-26} J T^{-1}	0.33
in Bohr magnetons	μ_μ/μ_B	4.841 970 97(71)	10^{-3}	0.15
in nuclear magnetons	μ_μ/μ_N	8.890 598 1(13)		0.15
Magnetic moment anomaly, $[\mu_\mu/(e\hbar/2m_\mu)] - 1$	a_μ	1.165 923 0(84)	10^{-3}	7.2
g-factor, $2(1 + a_\mu)$	g_μ	2.002 331 846(17)		0.0084
Muon-proton magnetic moment ratio	μ_μ/μ_p	3.183 345 47(47)		0.15

(continued)

Table 2.10 The 1986 Recommended Values of the Fundamental Physical Constants (Continued)

Quantity	Symbol	Value	Units	Relative Uncertainty ppm
Proton				
Mass	m_p	1.672 623 1(10)	10^{-27} kg	0.59
		1.007 276 470(12)	μ	0.012
in electron volts, $m_pc^2/[e]$		938.272 31(28)	MeV	0.30
Proton-electron mass ratio	m_p/m_e	1836.152 701(37)		0.020
Proton-muon mass ratio	m_p/m_μ	8.880 244 4(13)		0.15
Specific charge	e/m_p	9.578 830 9(29)	10^7 C kg^{-1}	0.30
Molar mass	$M(p)$	1.007 276 470(12)	10^{-3} kg mol^{-1}	0.012
Compton wavelength, h/m_pc	$\lambda_{c,p}$	1.321 410 02(12)	10^{-15} m	0.089
$\lambda_{cp}/2\pi$	$\lambda_{\overline{cp}}$	2.103 089 37(19)	10^{-16} m	0.089
Magnetic moment	μ_p	1.410 607 61(47)	10^{-26} J T^{-1}	0.34
in Bohr magnetons	μ_p/μ_B	1.521 032 202(15)	10^{-3}	0.010
in nuclear magnetons	μ_p/μ_N	2.792 847 386(63)		0.023
Diamagnetic shielding correction for protons (H_2O, spherical sample, 25°C), $1 - \mu_p'/\mu_p$	σ_{H_2O}	25.689(15)	10^{-6}	—
Shielded proton moment (H_2O, spherical sample, 25°C)	μ_p'	1.410 571 38(47)	10^{-26} J T^{-1}	0.34
in Bohr magnetons	μ_p'/μ_B	1.520 993 129(17)	10^{-3}	0.011
in nuclear magnetons	μ_p'/μ_N	2.792 775 642(64)		0.023
Gyromagnetic ratio	γ_p	26 752.212 8(81)	10^4 s^{-1} T^{-1}	0.30
	$\gamma_p/2\pi$	42.577 469(13)	MHz T^{-1}	0.30
uncorrected (H_2O, spherical sample, 25°C)	γ_p'	26 751.525 5(81)	10^4 $^{-1}$ T^{-1}	0.30
	$\gamma_p/2\pi$	42.576 375(13)	MHz T^{-1}	0.30
Neutron				
Mass	m_n	1.674 928 6(10)	10^{-27} kg	0.59
		1.008 664 904(14)	μ	0.014
in electron volts, $m_nc^2/[e]$		939.565 63(28)	MeV	0.30
Neutron-electron mass ratio	m_n/m_e	1838.683 662(40)		0.022
Neutron-proton mass ratio	m_n/m_p	1.001 378 404(9)		0.009
Molar mass	$M(n)$	1.008 664 904(14)	10^{-3} kg mol^{-1}	0.014
Compton wavelength, h/m_nc	λ_{cm}	1.319 591 10(12)	10^{-15} m	0.089
$\lambda c_n/2\pi$	$\lambda_{\overline{c,n}}$	2.100 194 45(19)	10^{-16} m	0.089
Magnetic moment[a]	μ_n	0.966 237 07(40)	10^{-26} J T^{-1}	0.41
in Bohr magnetons	μ_n/μ_B	1.041 875 63(25)	10^{-3}	0.24
in nuclear magnetons	μ_n/μ_N	1.913 042 75(45)		0.24
Neutron-electron magnetic moment ratio	μ_n/μ_e	1.040 668 82(25)	10^{-3}	0.24
Neutron-proton magnetic moment ratio	μ_n/μ_p	0.684 979 34(16)		0.24

Table 2.10 The 1986 Recommended Values of the Fundamental Physical Constants (Continued)

Quantity	Symbol	Value	Units	Relative Uncertainty ppm
Deuteron				
Mass	m_d	3.343 586 0(20)	10^{-27} kg	0.59
		2.013 553 214(24)	u	0.012
in electron volts, $m_dc^2/[e]$		1875.613 39(57)	MeV	0.30
Deuteron-electron mass ratio	m_d/m_e	3670.483 014(75)		0.020
Deuteron-proton mass ratio	m_d/m_p	1.999 007 496(6)		0.003
Molar mass	$M(d)$	2.013 553 214(24)	10^{-3} kg mol^{-1}	0.012
Magnetic moment[a]	μ_d	0.433 073 75(15)	10^{-26} J T^{-1}	0.34
in Bohr magnetons	μ_d/μ_B	0.466 975 447 9(91)	10^{-3}	0.019
in nuclear magnetons	μ_d/μ_N	0.857 438 230(24)		0.028
Deuteron-electron magnetic moment ratio	μ_d/μ_e	0.466 434 546 0(91)	10^{-3}	0.019
Deuteron-proton magnetic moment ratio	μ_d/μ_p	0.307 012 203 5(51)		0.017
Physiochemical constants				
Avogadro constant	N_A, L	6.022 136 7(36)	10^{23} mol^{-1}	0.59
Atomic mass constant, $m(C^{12})/12$	m_u	1.660 540 2(10)	10^{-27} kg	0.59
in electron volts, $m_uc^2/[e]$		931.494 32(28)	MeV	0.30
Faraday constant	F	96 485.309(29)	C mol^{-1}	0.30
Molar Planck constant	N_Ah	3.990 313 23(36)	10^{-10} J s mol^{-1}	0.089
	N_Ahc	0.119 626 58(11)	J m mol^{-1}	0.089
Molar gas constant	R	8.314 510(70)	J mol^{-1} K^{-1}	8.4
Boltzmann constant, R/N_A	k	1.380 658(12)	10^{-23} J K^{-1}	8.5
in electron volts, $k/[e]$		8.617 385(73)	10^{-5} eV K^{-1}	8.4
in hertz, k/h		2.083 674(18)	10^{10} Hz K^{-1}	8.4
in wavenumbers, k/hc		69.503 87(59)	m^{-1} K^{-1}	8.4
Molar volume (ideal gas), RT/p (at 273.15 K, 101 325 Pa)	V_m	22 414.10(19)	cm^{3}mol^{-1}	8.4
Loschmidt constant, N_A/V_m	n_o	2.686 763(23)	10^{25} m^{-3}	8.5
Stefan-Boltzmann constant, $(\pi^2 / 60) k^4/h^3c^2$	σ	5.670 51(19)	10^{-8} W m^{-2} K^{-4}	34
First radiation constant, $2\pi hc^2$	c_1	3.741 774 9(22)	10^{-16} W m^2	0.60
Second radiation constant, hc/k	c_2	0.014 387 69(12)	m K	8.4
Wien displacement law constant, $\lambda_{max} T = c_2/4.965\ 114\ 23...$	b	2.897 756(24)	10^{-3} m K	8.4
Conversion factors and units				
Electron volt, $(e/C)J = [e]J$	eV	1.602 177 33(49)	10^{-19} J	0.30
Atomic mass unit (unified), $m_u = m(C^{12})/12$	u	1.660 540 2(10)	10^{-27} kg	0.59
Standard atmosphere	atm	101 325	Pa	exact
Standard acceleration of gravity	g_n	9.806 65	m s^{-2}	exact

(continued)

Table 2.10 The 1986 Recommended Values of the Fundamental Physical Constants (Continued)

Quantity	Symbol	Value	Units	Relative Uncertainty ppm
'As-maintained' electrical units				
BIPM-maintained ohm, Ω_{69-BI} *as of* 1 Jan 1985	Ω_{BI85}	$1 - 1.563(50) \times 10^{-6}$	Ω	
		= 0.999 998 437(50)	Ω	0.050
Drift rate of $\Omega_{69\text{-BI}}$	$d\Omega_{69\text{-}BI}/dt$	−0.0566(15)	$\mu\Omega$/yr	
BIPM maintained volt, *483 594 GHz(h/2e)*	V_{76}-*B1*	$1 - 7.59(30) \times 10^{-6}$	V	
		= 0.999 992 41(30)	V	0.30
BIPM maintained ampere, $A_{BIPM} = V_{76\text{-}BI}/\Omega_{69\text{-}BI}$	A_{BI85}	$1 - 6.03(30) \times 10^{-6}$	A	
		= 0.999 993 97(30)	A	0.30
X-ray standards				
Cu x-unit: $\lambda(CuK\alpha_1) \equiv 1537.400$ *xu*	$xu(CuK\alpha_1)$	1.002 077 89(70)	10^{-13} m	0.70
Mo x-unit: $\lambda(MoK\alpha_1) \equiv 707.831$ *xu*	$xu(MoK\alpha_1)$	1.002 099 38(45)	10^{-13} m	0.45
Å*: $\lambda(WK\alpha_1) \equiv 0.209\ 100$ Å*	Å*	1.000 014 81(92)	10^{-10} m	0.92
Lattice spacing of Si (in vacuum, 22.5°C)[b]	α	0.543 101 96(11)	nm	0.21
$d_{220} = \alpha/\sqrt{8}$	d_{220}	0.192 015 540(40)	nm	0.21
Molar volume of Si, $M(Si)/\rho(Si) = N_A\alpha^3/8$	$V_m(Si)$	12.058 817 9(89)	$cm^3\ mol^{-1}$	0.74

Digits in parentheses indicate the standard deviation uncertainty in the last digits of the given value.
Quantities in braces, such as [e], refer to the numerical value only.
[a] The scalar magnitude of the neutron moment is listed here. The neutron magnetic dipole is directed oppositely to that of the proton, and corresponds to the dipole associated with a spinning negative charge distribution. The vector sum $\mu_d = \mu_p + \mu_n$ is approximately satisfied.
[b] The lattice spacing of single-crystal Si can vary by parts in 10^7 depending on the preparation process. Measurements at the Physikalische-Technische Bundesanstalt in the Federal Republic of Germany indicate also the possibility of distortions from exact cubic symmetry of the order of 0.2 ppm.

Table 2.11 Elementary Particles: Long-Lived Particles (Stable or Decaying by Weak or Electromagnetic Transitions) (From Perkins 1982; adapted from Kelly et al., 1980)

Particle	Mass[a] (MeV)	Mean Life[a] (s)
γ	0	stable
Leptons		
ν_e	0(<50 eV)	stable
ν_p	0(<0.57)	
ν_τ	0(<250)	
$e^{\pm}$	0.511003($\pm$1)	stable
$\mu^{\pm}$	105.6595($\pm$2)	2.197($\pm$1) $\times 10^{-6}$
$\tau^{\pm}$	1784($\pm$4)	<2 $\times 10^{-12}$
Nonstrange mesons		
$\pi^{\pm}$	139.567($\pm$1)	2.603($\pm$2) $\times 10^{-8}$
π^{o}	134.963($\pm$4)	0.83($\pm$6) $\times 10^{-16}$
η	548.8($\pm$6)	(Width = 0.9 keV)
η'	958($\pm$1)	(Width = 0.3 MeV)
Strange mesons		
$K^{\pm}$	493.67($\pm$2)	1.237($\pm$3) $\times 10^{-8}$
K^{o}, $\overline{K}^{o}$	497.7($\pm$1)	50% K_S,50% K_L
K_S		0.892($\pm$2) $\times 10^{-10}$
K_L		5.18($\pm$4) $\times 10^{-8}$
Charmed mesons		
$D^{\pm}$	1868($\pm$1)	~2 $\times 10^{-13}$
D^{o}, $\overline{D}^{o}$	1863($\pm$1)	~4 $\times 10^{-13}$
Baryons		
p	938.280($\pm$3)	stable
n	939.573($\pm$3)	887 $\pm$ 14
Λ	1115.60($\pm$5)	2.63 ($\pm$2) $\times 10^{-10}$
Σ^{+}	1189.4($\pm$1)	0.800($\pm$4) $\times 10^{-10}$
Σ^{o}	1192.5($\pm$1)	6 $\times 10^{-20}$
Σ^{-}	1197.3($\pm$1)	1.48($\pm$1) $\times 10^{-10}$
Ξ^{o}	1314.7($\pm$7)	3.0($\pm$2) $\times 10^{-10}$
Ξ^{-}	1321.3($\pm$2)	1.64($\pm$2) $\times 10^{-10}$
Ω^{-}	1672.2($\pm$3)	0.82($\pm$3) $\times 10^{-10}$
Λ_c	2273.($\pm$6)	~7 $\times 10^{-13}$

[a] Errors given in a parentheses ($\pm$2) refer to the last decimal place.

Table 2.12 Conversion Factors

Multiply number of ⟶	by ⟶	to obtain number of
	Area	
barns	10^{-24} (absolute)	cm^2
circular mils	7.854×10^{-7}	$in.^2$
cm^2	10^{24} (absolute)	barns
cm^2	0.15499969	$in.^2$
cm^2	1.076×10^{-3}	ft^2
cm^2	10^{-4} (absolute)	m^2
ft^2	929.0341	cm^2
ft^2	144 (absolute)	$in.^2$
ft^2	0.09290341	m^2
$in.^2$	6.451626	cm^2
$in.^2$	6.944×10^{-3}	ft^2
$in.^2$	6.452×10^{-4}	m^2
m^2	1549.9969	$in.^2$
m^2	10.76387	ft^2
m^2	1.195985	yd^2
m^2	3.861×10^{-7}	sq mi
ha (hectare)	1.00×10^4	m^2
	Density	
cm^3/g	1.602×10^{-2}	ft^3/lb
ft^3/lb	62.43	cm^3/g
g/cm^3	62.43	lb/ft^3
lb/ft^3	1.602×10^{-2}	g/cm^3
$lb/in.^3$	27.68	g/cm^3
lb/gal	0.1198	g/cm^3
	Electrical	
amperes	1	Coulomb/s
amperes	2.998×10^9	esu/s
amperes	6.281×10^{18}	electrons/s
ampere-hours	3600	coulombs
to obtain number of ⟵	**by ⟵**	**Divide number of**

Table 2.12 Conversion Factors (Continued)

Multiply number of ⟶	by ⟶	to obtain number of
	Electrical	
ampere-hours	0.03731	faradays
coulombs	2.998×10^{9}	statcoulombs
coulombs	6.281×10^{18}	electronic charges
coulombs	1.036×10^{-5}	faradays
faradays/s	9.650×10^{4}	amperes
faradays	26.80	ampere-hours
faradays	9.650×10^{4}	coulombs
farads	10^{6}	microfarads
international amperes	0.999835 (absolute)	amperes
international volts	1.00033 (absolute)	volts
international ohms	1.000495 (absolute)	ohms
international volt faraday	9.654×10^{4}	joules
microfarads	10^{-6}	farads
microhms	10^{-12}	megohms
microhms	10^{-6}	ohms
watts	1	joules/s
	Energy	
Btu[a]	1.055056×10^{3}	joules (absolute)
Btu	0.25198	kg-cal
Btu	1.055056×10^{10}	ergs
Btu	2.930×10^{-4}	kW-hr
Btu/lb	0.556	g-cal/g
eV	1.6021×10^{-12}	ergs
eV	1.6021×10^{-19}	joules (absolute)
eV	10^{-3}	keV
eV	10^{-6}	MeV
ergs	10^{-7}	joules (absolute)
ergs	6.2418×10^{5}	MeV
ergs	6.2418×10^{11}	eV
to obtain number of ⟵	**by ⟵**	**Divide number of**

(continued)

[a] BTU are International unless otherwise specified.

Table 2.12 Conversion Factors (Continued)

Multiply number of ⟶	by ⟶	to obtain number of
	Energy	
ergs	1.0	dyne-cm
ergs	9.480×10^{-11}	Btu
ergs	7.375×10^{-8}	ft-lbf
ergs	2.390×10^{-8}	g-cal
ergs	1.020×10^{-3}	g-cm
gram-calories	3.968×10^{-3}	Btu
gram-calories	4.184×10^{7}	ergs
joule (≡W-s)	10^{7}	N m (Newton meter)
joules (absolute)	10^{7}	ergs
joules (absolute)	0.7376	ft-lbf
joules (absolute)	9.480×10^{-4}	Btu
g-cal/g	1.8	Btu/lb
kg-cal	3.968	Btu
kg-cal	3.087×10^{3}	ft-lbf
ft-lb	1.356	joules (abs)
ft-lb	3.239×10^{-4}	kg-cal
kW-hr	2.247×10^{19}	MeV
kW-hr	3.60×10^{13}	ergs
MeV	1.6021×10^{-6}	ergs
Energy to mass conversions under Miscellaneous		
	Fluid Flow Rates	
Gal (U.S.)/min	8.020834	ft^3/h
Gal (U.S.)/min	0.0630902	L/s
cm^3/s	2.118880×10^{-3}	ft^3/min
ft^3/h	7.865791	cm^3/s
ft^3/s	0.1246753	Gal (U.S.)/s
ft^3/s	101.9406	m^3/h
l/min	2.118880	ft^3/h
l/s	15.85032	Gal (U.S.)/min
to obtain number of ⟵	**by ⟵**	**Divide number of**

Table 2.12 Conversion Factors (Continued)

Multiply number of ⟶	by ⟶	to obtain number of
	Length	
angstroms (Å)	10^{-8}	cm
Å	10^{-10}	m
micrometers, micron (μm)	10^{-3}	mm
μm	10^{-4}	cm
μm	10^{-6}	m
μm	3.937×10^{-5}	in.
mm	10^{-1}	cm
cm	0.3937	in.
cm	3.2808×10^{-2}	ft
cm	10^{-2}	m
m	39.370	in.
m	3.2808	ft
m	1.0936	yd
m	10^{-3}	km
m	6.2137×10^{-4}	miles
km	0.62137	miles
mils	10^{-3}	in.
mils	2.540×10^{-3}	cm
in.	10^{3}	mils
in.	2.5400	cm
ft	30.480	cm
rods	5.500	yd
miles (U.S. Statute)	5280	ft
miles (U.S. Statute)	1760	yd
miles (U.S. Statute)	1.6094	km
n miles (nautical mile)	1.852	km
mile (international)	1.609344	km
rod (pole or patch)	16.5	ft
chain	66	ft
yd	.9144	m
fermi	1×10^{-15}	m
fathom	1.8288	m
A.U.	1.496×10^{11}	m
parsec	3.0867×10^{16}	m
to obtain number of ⟵	**by ⟵**	**Divide number of**

(continued)

Table 2.12 Conversion Factors (Continued)

Multiply number of ⟶	by ⟶	to obtain number of
	Mass	
mg	10^{-3}	g
mg	3.527×10^{-5}	oz avdp
mg	1.543×10^{-2}	grains
g	3.527×10^{-2}	oz avdp
g	10^{-3}	kg
g	2.205×10^{-3}	lb
kg	2.205	lb
kg	0.0685	slugs
kg	9.807×10^{5}	dynes
lb	4.448×10^{5}	dynes
lb	453.592	g
lb	0.45359237	kg
lb	16	oz avdp
lb	0.0311	slugs
u (unified—^{12}C scale)	$1.6605402 \times 10^{-27}$	kg
amu (physical—^{16}O scale)	1.65980×10^{-27}	kg
oz	28.35	g
oz	6.25×10^{-2}	lb
t (tonne = metric ton)	1.00×10^{3}	kg
Mass to energy conversions under miscellaneous		
	Miscellaneous	
temperature	°C = (°F − 32)/1.8 = (°F − 32) 5/9	
	°F = 1.8°C + 32 = (9/5) °C + 32	
	°K = °C + 273.16	
wavelength to energy conversion	keV = 12.40/Å	
	eV = 1.240×10^{-6}/m	
radians	57.296	degrees
eV	$1.60217733 \times 10^{-19}$	joule
eV	1.78258×10^{-33}	grams
eV	1.0735439×10^{-9}	u (amu)
erg	1.11265×10^{-21}	grams
proton masses	938.256	MeV
neutron masses	939.550	MeV
electron masses	511.006	keV
u (amu on ^{12}C scale)	931.478	MeV
to obtain number of ⟵	**by ⟵**	**Divide number of**

Table 2.12 Conversion Factors (Continued)

Multiply number of ⟶	by ⟶	to obtain number of
	Power	
Btu/hr	0.2162	ft-lbf/s
Btu/hr	0.0700	gm-cal/s
Btu/hr	3.929×10^{-4}	horsepower
Btu/hr (International)	0.2930711	watts
Btu/min	12.97	ft-lbf/s
Btu/min	0.02357	horsepower
Btu/min	0.01758	kilowatts
Btu/min	17.58	watts
cal/sec	4.187	watts
horsepower[b]	42.42	Btu/min
horsepower	33,000	ft-lbf/min
horsepower	550	ft-lbf/s
horsepower	10.69	kg-cal/min
horsepower	0.7457	kilowatts
horsepower	4.655×10^{15}	MeV/s
kg-cal/min	9.356×10^{-2}	horsepower
kilowatts	14.33	kg cal/min
kilowatts	1.341	horsepower
kilowatts	6.243×10^{15}	MeV/s
watts	10^{7}	ergs/s
watts	0.7376	ft-lbf/s
watts	3.414	Btu/hr
watts	0.05690	Btu/min
watts	0.01433	kg-cal/min
ergs s^{-1}	5.688×10^{-9}	Btu/min
ergs s^{-1}	4.425×10^{-6}	ft-lbf/min
ergs s^{-1}	1.433×10^{-9}	kg-cal/min
to obtain number of ⟵	**by ⟵**	**Divide number of**

(continued)

[b] All horsepower conversions based on 500 ft-lbf/s.

Table 2.12 Conversion Factors (Continued)

Multiply number of ⟶	by ⟶	to obtain number of
	Pressure	
atm	14.696	lb/in.^{2}
atm	760	mm Hg (0°C)
atm	76.0	cm Hg (0°C)
atm	1.01325	bars
atm	1.01325×10^5	Pa
atm	1.033227×10^3	g/cm^2
atm	29.92126	in. Hg (0°C)
cm Hg	0.4465	ft of H_2O
cm Hg	0.1934	lb/in.^{2}
cm Hg	1.316×10^{-2}	atm
cm Hg	0.4465	ft of H_2O
in. Hg	0.4912	lb/in.^{2}
mm Hg	133.322	Pa
g/cm^2	1.4223×10^{-2}	lb/in.^{2}
bars	10^6	dynes/cm^2
bars	10^5	Pa
bars	14.504	lb/in.^{2}
dynes/cm^2	1.4504×10^{-5}	lb/in.^{2}
dynes/cm^2	1.0197×10^{-3}	g/cm^2
lb/in.^{2}	27.673	in. of H_2O (4°C)
lb/in.^{2}	2.3066	ft. of H_2O (4°C)
lb/in.^{2}	6.805×10^{-2}	atm
lb/in.^{2}	2.036	in. Hg (0°C)
lb/in.^{2}	5.1715	cm Hg
lb/in.^{2}	51.715	mm Hg
ft of H_2O	2.230	cm Hg
Pa	1.0000	N/m^2
Torr	133.322	Pa
to obtain number of ⟵	**by ⟵**	**Divide number of**

Table 2.12 Conversion Factors (Continued)

Multiply number of ⟶	by ⟶	to obtain number of
	Radiological Units	
becquerel	2.703×10^{-11}	curies
becquerel	27.03	picocuries
curies	3.700×10^{10}	dis/sec (dps)
curies	2.220×10^{12}	dis/min (dpm)
curies	10^{3}	millicuries
curies	10^{6}	microcuries
curies	10^{12}	picocuries
curies	10^{-3}	kilocuries
curies	3.700×10^{10}	becquerel
nanocuries	37	becquerel
dis/min (dpm)	4.505×10^{-10}	millicuries
dis/min	4.505×10^{-7}	microcuries
dis/sec (dps)	2.703×10^{-8}	millicuries
dis/sec	2.703×10^{-5}	microcuries
gray	100	rad
kilocuries	10^{3}	curies
microcuries	3.700×10^{4}	dis/sec
microcuries	2.220×10^{6}	dis/min (dpm)
millicuries	3.700×10^{7}	dis/sec (dps)
millicuries	2.220×10^{9}	dis/min (dpm)
R	2.58×10^{-4}	C/kg of air (STP)
R	1	esu/cm^{3} of air (STP)
R	2.082×10^{9}	ion pairs/cm^{3} of air (STP)
R	1.610×10^{12}	ion pairs/g of air
R (33.7 eV/ion pr.)	7.02×10^{4}	MeV/cm^{3} of air (STP)
R (33.7 eV/ion pr.)	5.43×10^{7}	MeV/g of air
R (33.7 eV/ion pr.)	86.9	ergs/g of air
R (33.7 eV/ion pr.)	2.08×10^{-6}	g-cal/g of air
R (33.7 eV/ion pr.)	≈98	ergs/g of soft tissue
to obtain number of ⟵	**by ⟵**	**Divide number of**

(continued)

Table 2.12 Conversion Factors (Continued)

Multiply number of ⟶	by ⟶	to obtain number of
	Radiological Units	
rad	0.01	gray
rad	0.01	J/kg
rad	100	ergs/g
rad	8.071×10^4	MeV/cm^3 of air (STP)
rad	6.242×10^7	MeV/g
rad	10^{-5}	watt-sec/g
rad (33.7 eV/ion pr.)	2.39×10^9	ion prs/cm^3 of air (STP)
rem	0.01	sievert
μCi/cm^3 (μCi/ml)	2.22×10^{12}	dpm/m^3
μCi/cm^3	2.22×10^9	dpm/liter
dpm/m^3	0.4505	pCi/m^3
sievert	100	rem
	Time	
days	86,400	s
days	1440	min
years (365 days)	3.1536×10^7	s
years	5.256×10^5	min
years	8.760×10^3	h
work weeks	1.44×10^5	s
work weeks	40	h
work months	4.2	work weeks
work months	168	h
to obtain number of ⟵	**by ⟵**	**Divide number of**

Table 2.12 Conversion Factors (Continued)

Multiply number of ⟶	by ⟶	to obtain number of
	Velocity	
cm/sec	0.6000	m/min
cm/sec	0.0360	km/h
cm/sec	0.032808	ft/s
cm/sec	1.9685	ft/min
cm/sec	3.728×10^{-4}	mi/min
cm/sec	0.02237	mph
m/min	1.667	cm/s
m/min	5.468×10^{-2}	ft/s
m/min	3.728×10^{-2}	mph
ft/sec	18.29	m/min
ft/sec	0.6818	mph
ft/min	0.5080	cm/s
ft/min	1.667×10^{-2}	ft/s
ft/min	1.136×10^{-2}	mph
knot	1.852	km/h
knot	0.5144	m/s
mph	44.70	cm/s
mph	88	ft/min
mph	1.467	ft/s
mph	26.82	m/min
to obtain number of ⟵	**by ⟵**	**Divide number of**

(continued)

Table 2.12 Conversion Factors (Continued)

Multiply number of ⟶	by ⟶	to obtain number of
	Volume	
cm^3 (cc)	1.0000	ml
cm^3	6.10237×10^{-2}	$in.^3$
cm^3	10^{-6}	m^3
cm^3	1.000×10^{-3}	liters
cm^3	3.531467×10^{-5}	ft^3
m^3	35.31467	ft^3
m^3	2.642×10^2	gal
m^3	1.0000×10^3	liters
$in.^3$	16.387	cm^3
$in.^3$	5.787×10^{-4}	ft^3
$in.^3$	1.639×10^{-2}	liters
$in.^3$	4.329×10^{-3}	gal
ft^3	2.832×10^{-2}	m^3
ft^3	7.481	gal
ft^3	28.32	liters
ft^3	1728	$in.^3$
gal (U.S.)	231.0	$in.^3$
gal (U.S.)	0.13368	ft^3
gal (U.S.)	3785.3	cm^3
liters	33.8147	fluid oz
liters	1.05671	quarts
liters	0.26418	gal
gm moles (gas)	22.4	liters (STP)

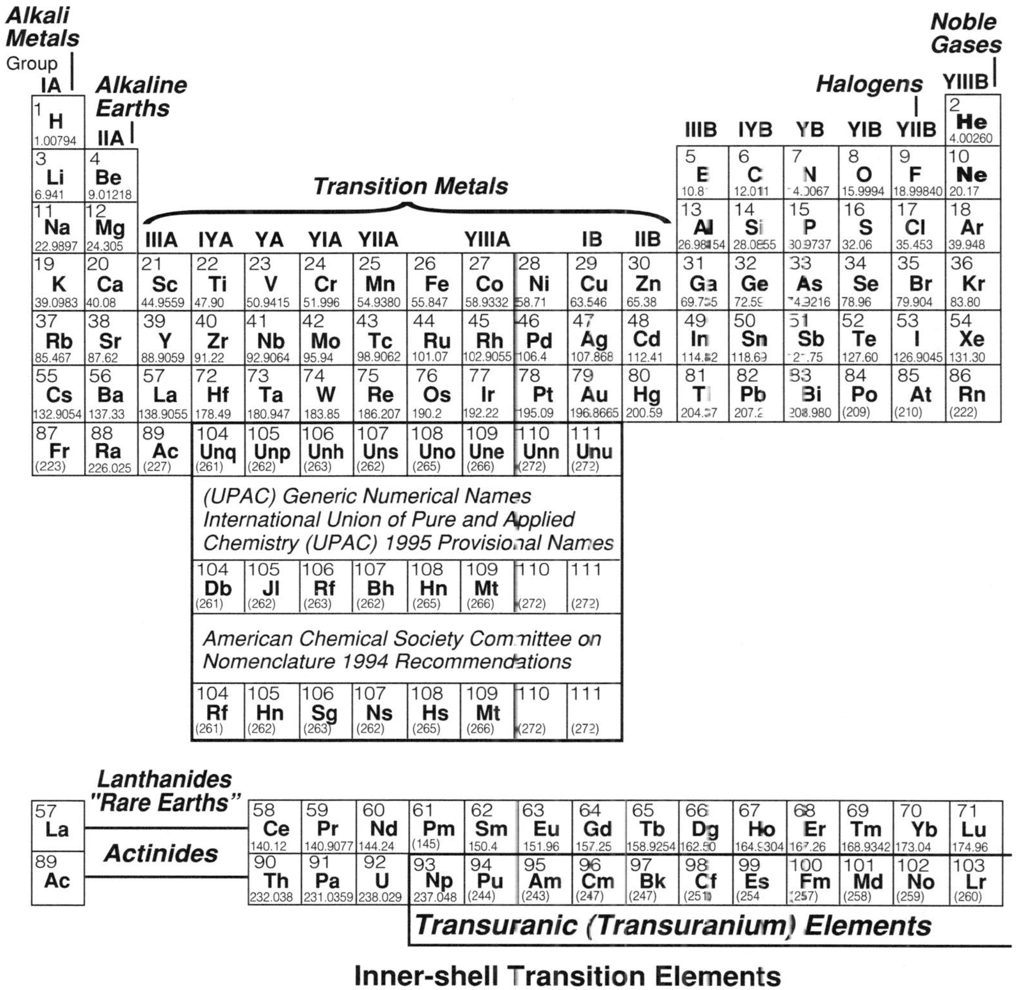

Elements by Chemical Symbol

Symbol	Element	Symbol	Element
Ac	Actinium	Mo	Molybdenum
Ag[1]	Silver	N	Nitrogen
Al	Aluminum	Na[2]	Sodium
Am	Americium	Nb	Niobium
AR	Argon	Nd	Neodymium
As	Arsenic	Ne	Neon
At	Astatine	Ni	Nickel
Au[3]	Gold	No	Nobelium
B	Boron	Np	Neptunium
Ba	Barium	O	Oxygen
Bi	Bismuth	Os	Osmium
Bk	Berkelium	P	Phosphorus
Br	Bromine	Pa	Protoactinium
C	Carbon	Pb[4]	Lead
Ca	Calcium	Pd	Palladium
Cd	Cadmium	Pm	Promethium
Ce	Cerium	Po	Polonium
Cf	Californium	Pr	Praseodymium
Cm	Curium	Pt	Platinum
Co	Cobalt	Pu	Plutonium
Cr	Chromium	Ra	Radium
Cs	Cesium	Rb	Rubidium
Cu[5]	Copper	Rd	Rutherfordium
Dy	Dysprosium	Re	Rhenium
Er	Erbium	Rh	Rhodium
Es	Einsteinium	Rn	Radon
Eu	Europium	Ru	Ruthenium
F	Fluorine	S	Sulfur
Fe[6]	Iron	Sb[7]	Antimony
Fm	Fermium	Sc	Scandium
Fr	Francium	Se	Selenium
Ga	Gallium	Si	Silicon
Gd	Gadolinium	Sm	Samarium
Ge	Germanium	Sn[8]	Tin
H	Hydrogen	Sr	Strontium
He	Helium	Ta	Tantalum
Hf	Hafnium	Tb	Terbium
Hg[9]	Mercury	Tc	Technectium
Ho	Holmium	Te	Tellurium
I	Iodine	Th	Thorium
In	Indium	Ti	Titanium
Ir	Iridium	Tl	Thallium
K[10]	Potassium	Tm	Thulium
K	Krypton	U	Uranium
Lr	Lanthanium	V	Vanadium
Li	Lithium	W[11]	Tungsten
Lr	Lawrencium	Xe	Xenon
Lu	Lutetium	Y	Yittrium
Md	Medelevium	Yb	Ytterbium
Mg	Magnesium	Zn	Zinc
Mn	Manganese	Zr	Zirconium

Symbols derived from Latin(L) or German(G)

1	L	*Argenium*	7	L	*Stibium*
2	L	*Natrium*	8	L	*Stannum*
3	L	*Aurium*	9	L	*Hydrargyrum*
4	L	*Plumbum*	10	L	*Kalium*
5	L	*Cuprum*	11	G	*Wolfram*
6	L	*Ferrum*			

Figure 2.1 The Periodic Table of the Elements

References

Cohen, E.R., Taylor, B.N. The 1986 adjustment of the fundamental physics constants, report of the CODATA Task Group on Fundamental Constants CODATA Bulletin No. 11; Pergamon Press; Elmsford, NY; 1986.

Cohen, E.R., Taylor, B.N. The 1986 adjustment of the fundamental constants, report of the CODATA Task Group on Fundamental Constants, CODATA Bulletin 63, Pergamon Press; Elmsford, NY; 1986.

Cohen, E.R., Taylor, B.N. ''The fundamental physical constants,'' *Physics Today*, BG8; August 1989.

HASL-300 27th Edition, Volume 1, *EML Procedures Manual*, Environmental Measurements Laboratory; New York; 1990.

Kelly, R.L. *et al.* ''Review of Particle Properties,'' Particle Data Group *Reviews of Modern Physics*; **51:**S1; April 1980.

National Institute of Standards and Technology. *The International System of Units (SI)*, Special Publication 330, 1991 Edition; Editor Barry N. Taylor; Gaithersburg, MD; 1991.

National Institute of Standards and Technology. *Guide for the Use of the International System of Units The Modernized Metric System*, Special Publication 811; 1995.

National Bureau of Standards ''Guidelines for the Use of the Modernized Metric System; the International System of Units,'' LC1120, p 13; *Dimensions/NBS*; December 1979.

Perkins, D.H. *Introduction to High Energy Physics*, 2nd Edition; Addison-Wesley Publishing Co.; Reading, MA; 1982.

CHAPTER 3

RULES OF THUMB AND USEFUL EQUATIONS

Useful ''rules of thumb'' for dose rates, exposure, and penetration from alpha and beta emitters, fallout, neutrons, and gamma and x-rays introduce some of the practical aspects of health physics in this chapter. The mathematical relationships important in determining radioactivity and radiation exposure are presented through a series of equations.

Also included in this chapter are commonly employed equations expressing logarithmic, and wave and quantum relationships, as well as those used in classical physics and electrostatics.

TABLE OF CONTENTS

Table 3.1 Rules-of-Thumb

Contents

Alpha Particles

It requires an alpha particle of at least 7.5 MeV to penetrate the protective layer of skin (0.07 mm thick).

Beta Particles and Electron Beams

(1) *It requires a beta particle of at least 70 keV to penetrate the protective layer of skin.*

(2) *Average Energy*

$\overline{E}\ (\beta^-) \approx 1/3\ E_{max}$ — The average of a beta energy distribution is approximately one-third its maximum energy.

$\overline{E}\ (\beta^+) \approx 0.44\ E_{max}$ — The average of a positron energy distribution is approximately 44% of its maximum energy.

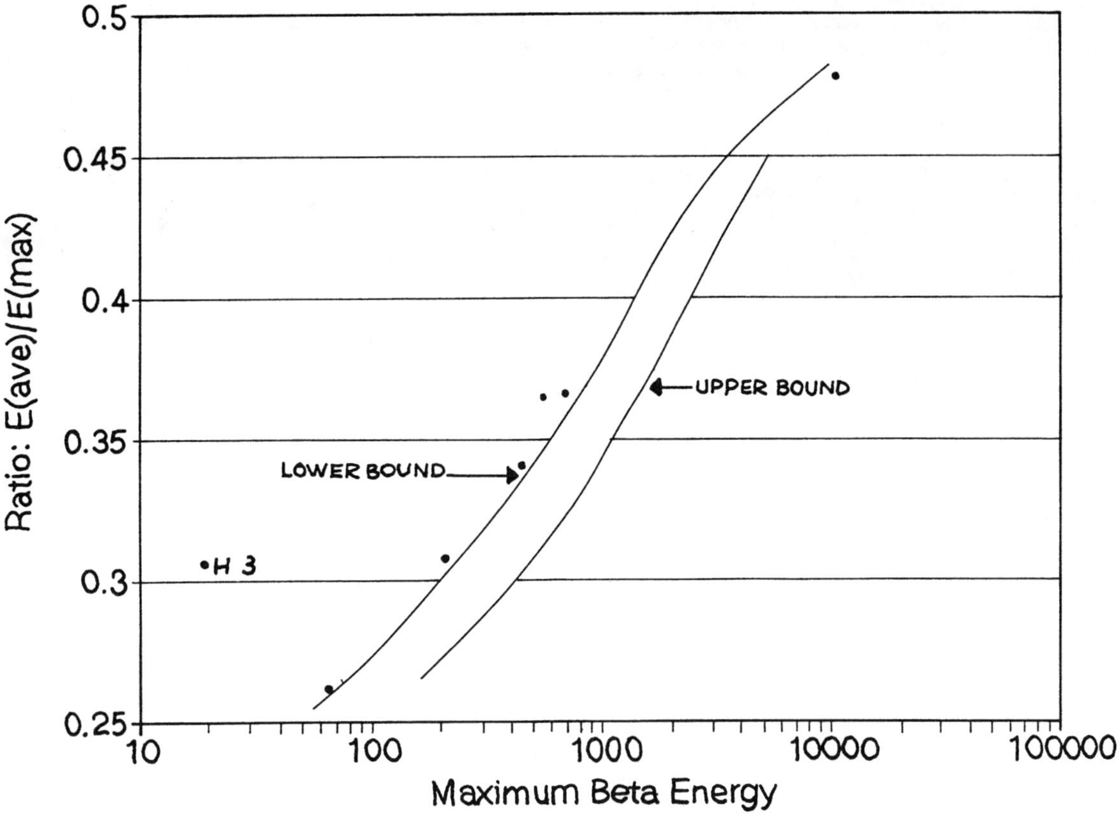

Figure 3.1.1 Illustration of Rule-of-Thumb (Personal Communication, Slaback, 1991)

(3) *Range in Air*

$Range_{air} \approx 12\ ft\ per\ MeV$

Example: E_{max} ^{32}P = 1.71 MeV
Maximum Range in Air ≈ 20 ft.

(4) *Range in Matter*

The range of beta particles in matter is approximately:

$$R(g/cm^2) \approx \frac{E_{max}}{2}$$

where R = range in g/cm^2 (range in cm times the density in g/cm^3
E_{max} = maximum energy in MeV (1–4 MeV energy range)

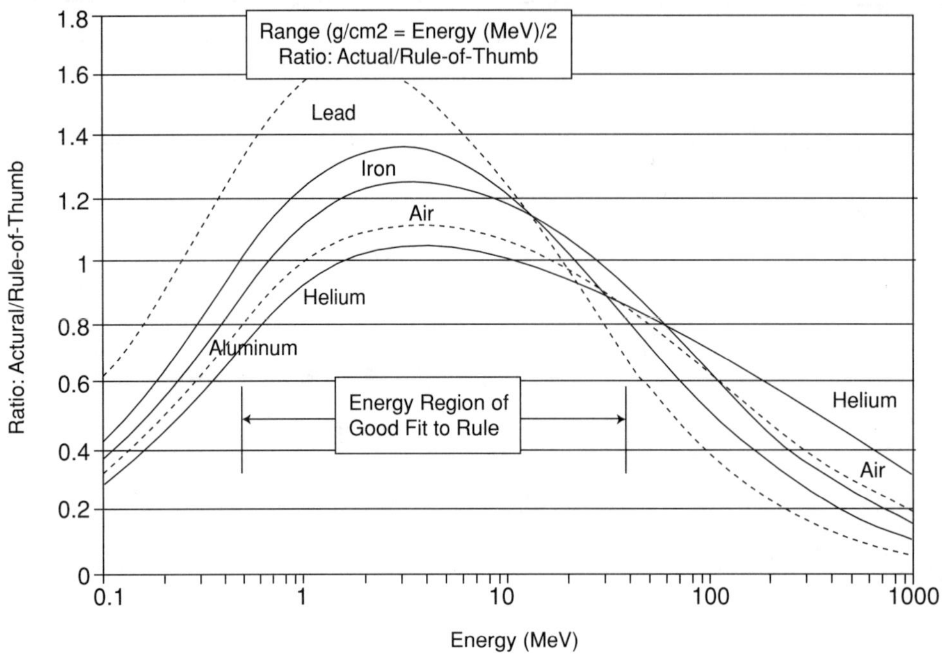

Figure 3.1.2 Illustration of Validity of Rule-of-Thumb (Personal Communication, Slaback, 1991)

(5) *Dose equivalent rate from an electron beam of flux density* ϕ *(electrons* $cm^{-2}\,s^{-1}$*)*:
(From IAEA Technical Report Series 188, 1979)

$H(rem/h) \approx 1.6 \times 10^{-4}\phi$ Approximate within $\pm$ 15% for E = 1 to 200 MeV

(6) *Dose Rate (in rad/hour) at One Centimeter from a Beta (* $\pm$ *) Point Source (neglecting self and air absorption)*

$Dose\ Rate_{1cm} \approx 300\ rad/h\ per\ mCi$ Example: Dose rate at 1 cm from 1 mCi of ^{32}P is approximately 300 rad/hour.

Dose rate at 1 cm from a point beta-ray source varies only slightly with beta energy.

(7) *Dose Rate (in rad/h) in a Solution*

$$Rate\ (in\ solution) \approx \frac{2.12\ \overline{E}C(rad/h)}{\rho}$$

where $\overline{E}$ = the average energy in MeV
C = the concentration in $\mu Ci/cm^3$
ρ = the density of the solution in g/cm^3.

The dose rate is about one-half this value at the surface of the solution.

Example: For ^{32}P with an average beta energy of 0.7 MeV, the dose rate from 1 $\mu Ci/cm^3$ in water is 1.48 rad/hour.

(8) *Surface Dose Rate Through the Skin*

For beta particle energies above 0.6 MeV, the dose rate through the nominal protective skin layer is 9 rad/h from a uniformly thin deposit of 1 $\mu Ci/cm^2$ of a beta emitting radionuclide. (See Chapter 13 for further beta dosimetric information.)

Bremsstrahlung

(1) *Average energy of "external" bremsstrahlung (NCRP, 1985)*

$$E_{ave} = 1.4 \times 10^{-7} Z E_{\beta}^{2} \text{ keV per } \beta$$

where Z = atomic number of the absorber
E_{β} = maximum energy of beta emitter, in keV

Example: For ^{32}P this average energy is 0.4 Z keV.

(2) *Average energy of "internal" bremsstrahlung (NCRP, 1985)*

$$E_{ave} \approx 1.5 \times 10^{-3} E_{\beta} \log(0.004\, E_{\beta} - 2.2)\ keV\ per\ \beta$$

Example: For ^{32}P this average energy is about 1.7 keV

(3) *Total bremsstrahlung dose rate (McLintock, 1994)*

$$\frac{6AE_{\beta}^{2}}{d^{2}} (Z + I)\, \mu_{en}\, \mu Svh^{-1}$$

where A = activity in MBq
E_{β} = maximum energy of the beta in MeV
Z = effective atomic number of the absorber
I accounts for the internal bremsstrahlung
μ_{en} = mass energy absorption coefficient
d = the distance from the source in cm.

Values of *Z* and *I* for Different External Absorbers

Absorber	*Z*	*I*[a]	*Z* + *I*
Perspex	5.9	5.4	11.3
Water	6.6	5.4	12
Pyrex	10	4	14
Steel	26	4.5	30.5
Brass	30	4	34
Lead	82	4	86

[a] Approximate values for energies from 0.16 keV (^{35}S) to 1.7 MeV (^{32}P).

Fallout (from Nuclear Weapons)

(1) *After exposure rates have begun to decrease, a rough idea of future rates can be gained by using the 7:10 rule. This rule is that for every seven-fold increase in time after detonation, there is a ten-fold decrease in exposure.*

Illustration:

Time (+H)	Decay	Radiation Intensity
1	—	1000 R/h
7	1/10	100 R/h
49	1/100	10 R/h
343	1/1000	1 R/h

Example: If a 50 R/hr radiation exposure rate exists at three hours after detonation, by the end of 21 hours, it will have decreased to 5 R/hr, and by the end of 147 hours, it will have decreased to 0.5 R/hr.

(2) *The exposure rate from fission products at any time (t) can be represented by:*

$$R(t) = It^{-1.2}$$

where I = the exposure rate at unit time
t = the time in same units

(Equation holds for t > 4 h and < 200 d)

Gamma and X-Rays

(1) *Exposure Rates from X- and Gamma Point Sources*

$$R_{ft} \approx 6\ CE\ (R/h\ at\ 1\ ft)$$

$$R_m \approx 0.53\ CE\ (R/h\ at\ 1\ m)$$

where C = curies
E = energy in MeV

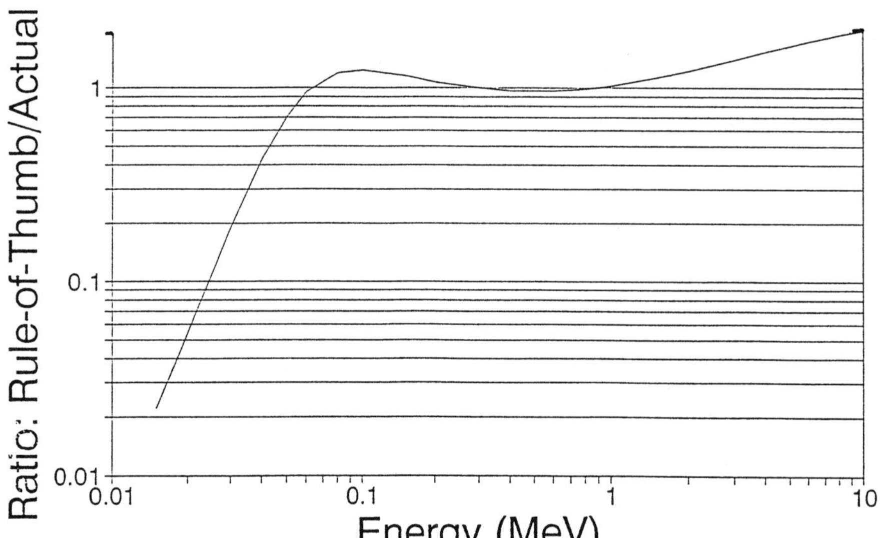

Figure 3.1.3 Illustration of Validity of 6CE Rule-of-Thumb (Personal Communication, Slaback, 1991)

The two above formulas are approximate only (within ±20%) and definitely cannot be used for x-ray and gamma energies outside the range 0.07 to 2 MeV.

(2) *Dose equivalent rate from a photon field of energy flux ψ (MeV $cm^{-2}\,s^{-1}$):*
(From IAEA Technical Report Series 88, 1979)

$H(rem/h) \approx 1.6 \times 10^{-6}\psi$ Valid to approx ± 15% for 0.1 to 2.5 MeV

(3) *Dose Rate to Tissue (rad/h) in an Infinite Medium Uniformly Contaminated by a Gamma Emitter*

$Dose\ Rate\ (rad/h) = 2.12\ EC/\rho$

where E = the average gamma energy per disintegration in MeV
C = the concentration in μCi/cm^3
ρ = the density of the medium in g/cm^3.

(4) *Exposure Rate from an X-Ray Machine*

Exposure rate (R/sec) at 2 feet from a diagnostic x-ray machine operated at 100 kVp and 100 milliampere seconds is approximately 2.3 R/sec.

Neutrons

(1) *Dose equivalent rate from a neutron field of flux density ϕ (neutrons $cm^{-2}\,s^{-1}$):*
(From IAEA Technical Report Series 188, 1979)

$H(rem/h) \approx 1.4 \times 10^{-4}\phi$ For an effective neutron energy of about 2 MeV

or

$$H(rem/h) \sim \frac{\phi}{7000}$$

(2) *For a point isotopic source of about 2 MeV*

$$H(rem/h) \approx \frac{Q}{30000\ \pi r^2}$$

where Q = number of neutrons emitted per second from a point source
r = distance in centimeters

(3) *Half Value Layer-Paraffin*

An approximate HVL for 1 MeV neutrons is 1.26 in. (3.2 cm) of paraffin; 2.72 in. (6.93 cm) for 5 MeV neutrons.

Radioactive Decay

(1) *The activity of any radionuclide is reduced to less than 1% after 7 half-lives, less than 0.1% after 10 half-lives.*

(2) *For radionuclides with half-lives greater than six days, the change in activity in 24 hours will be less than 10%.*

Table 3.2 Useful Equations

Contents

Air Sampling (Hickey, 1993)

$$C = \frac{\lambda^2 \mathrm{Nm}}{EFK\,(1 - e^{-\lambda T_s})\, e^{-\lambda T_d}\,(1 - e^{-\lambda T_g})}$$

$$MDC = \frac{\lambda^2\,(2.71 + 3.29\sqrt{R_b\, T_g\,(1 + T_g/T_b)}}{EFK\,(1 - e^{-\lambda T_s})\, e^{-\lambda T_d}\,(1 - e^{-\lambda T_g})}$$

where C = concentration (μCi cm^{-3} or Bq m^{-3})
MDC = minimum detectable concentration
N_n = $N_g - R_b\, T_g$ [net count rate]
N_g = gross count rate
R_b = background count rate
T_g = sample counting time (gross count)
T_s = sampling time
T_b = background count time
T_d = delay time between sampling and counting
λ = decay constant for radionuclide sampled
E = sampling efficiency
F = sampling flow rate (assumed to be constant, with units consistant with C and T)
K = detector factor (cpm per μCi, cps per Bq)

Beta Dose

(1) *The dose from beta radiation ($\beta^{\pm}$) is approximately:*
(From IAEA Technical Report Series 188, 1979)

$$H(rem/h) \approx rad/h \approx 300\ nCd^{-2}$$

where n = fraction of disintegrations where a beta is emitted
C = activity in curies
d = distance in feet

The equivalent metric rule is:

$$H(rem/h) \approx 30\ nCd^{-2}$$

where d = distance in meters

In SI units the rules become:

$$H(Sv/h) \approx Gy/h \approx 8 \times 10^{-12}\ nCd^{-2}$$
$$H(Sv/s) \approx Gy/s \approx 2 \times 10^{-15}\ nCd^{-2}$$

where C = activity in becquerels (Bq)
d = distance in meters
n = fraction of disintegrations that emit a beta ray

Beta Particle Counting

(1) *Self-Absorption*

$$\frac{R_0}{R} = \frac{1}{mx}(1 - e^{-mx})$$

where R_0 = measured counting rate
R = true counting rate
x = sample thickness (mg/cm^2)
m = absorption coefficient (cm^2/mg)[a]

Classical Physics

Unless otherwise noted, this section uses SI symbols and dimensions consistently as follows:

m = mass (kg)
v = velocity (m/s)
a = acceleration (m/s^2)
F = force (kg m/s^2 or newton)
r = radius of action (m)
s = distance (m)
t = time (s)

(1) *Linear Force*

$$F = ma = (kg)(m/s^2) = kg\ m/s^2 = newton\ (N)$$

(2) *Momentum*

$$p = mv = kg(m/s)$$

(3) *Conservation of Momentum* (any impact between Body A and Body B)

$$m_A V_{A_i} + m_B V_{B_i} = m_A V_{A_f} + m_B V_{B_f}$$

i = initial
f = final

(4) *Work*

$$W = Fs = mas = (kg)(m/s^2)(m) = kg\ m^2/s^2 = newton\text{-}m = joule\ (J)$$

[a] *Absorption coefficient.* Because of the continuous spectrum of particles emitted from a beta source, a fraction of the particles will be absorbed in the window of a mica-window counter and in the air between the counter and the source. As the first part of the absorption curve for a beta emitter is approximately linear on a semilogarithmic plot, this effect can be measured by counting the source with several thin absorbers and extrapolating through the thickness of the window and air to zero absorber. The slope of this line can be expressed as m in the equation $R/R_0 = e^{-mx}$ for use when the radionuclide is known. (R is the measured counting rate, R_0 is the extrapolated counting rate, and x is the combined effective thickness of the window and air.)

(5) *Energy*

$$E = (work) = Fs = (kg\ m/s^2)(m) = kg\ m^2/s^2 = joule$$

(6) *Kinetic Energy*

$$K.E. = 1/2\ mv^2 = (kg)(m/s)^2 = kg\ m^2/s^2 = joule$$

(7) *Conservation of Kinetic Energy* (elastic impact: Body A and Body B)

$$1/2\ m_A v_{A_i}^2 + 1/2\ m_B v_{B_i}^2 = 1/2\ m_A v_{A_f}^2 + 1/2\ m_B v_{B_f}^2$$

(8) *Power*

$$P = (work/time) = Fs/t = (kg\ m/s^2)(m)/s = J/s = watt\ (W)$$

Dead Time (Resolving time)

(1) *Resolving Time Correction (non-extendable)*

$$R = \frac{R_0}{1 - R_0\tau}$$

$$R_0 = \frac{R}{1 + R\tau}$$

where R = true counting rate (c/s)
R_0 = observed counting rate (c/s)
τ = resolving time, seconds

(2) *Resolving Time Correction (extendable)*

$$R_0 = Re^{-R\tau}$$

(3) *Resolving Time Determination (paired source)*

$$\tau = \frac{R_1 + R_2 - R_{1,2}}{2\ (R_1R_2)}$$

where τ = resolving time, seconds
R_1 = counting rate, source 1 (c/s)
R_2 = counting rate, source 2 (c/s)
$R_{1,2}$ = counting rate, combined sources 1 and 2 (c/s)

Note: Electronic methods offer more precise determination of the deadtime. (ICRU, 1994).

Electricity

The following units apply in this section:

Electric current in amperes (A) base SI unit
Work in joules (J)
Power in watts (W) or (J/s)

(1) *Electric Potential in volts (V)* $= W/A$ *or* JC^{-1}

(2) *Electric Charge or Quantity of Electricity in coulombs (C)* $= As$

(3) *Capacitance in farads (F)* $= CV^{-1}$

(4) *Electrical Resistance in ohms* (Ω) $= VA^{-1}$

Gamma Ray Exposure from Fixed Sources[b]

(1) *Exposure Rate* (from a point source)

(Equation assumes that the creation of one ion pair in air requires an average energy expenditure of 33.7 electron volts)

$$X = 194.3\ nC\bar{E}d^{-2}\left(\frac{\mu_{en}}{\rho}\right)$$

where X = exposure rate in R/hr
n = gamma quanta per disintegration
C = activity in curies
E = energy of gamma quanta in MeV
μ_{en}/ρ = mass energy absorption coefficient for gamma in air (STP) in cm^{-1}
d = distance in meters

(2) *Exposure Rate and Dose Rate, Approximate* (from any gamma point source)
(From IAEA Technical Report Series 88, 1979)

μ_{en}/ρ is taken as 0.00275 m^2/kg for energy range 0.07 to 2 MeV then:

$$H(rem/h) \approx R/h = 0.53\ nCEd^{-2}$$

where C = activity in curies
E = photon energy in MeV
n = gamma quanta per disintegration
d – distance in meters

This then gives:

$$R/h \approx 1/2\ nCEd^{-2}\ (d\ in\ meters)$$
$$R/h \approx 6\ nCEd^{-2}\ (d\ in\ feet)$$

In SI units these rules apply:

$$X\ (C\ kg^{-1}s^{-1}) \approx 1 \times 10^{-18}\ nBEd^{-2}$$
$$\dot{D}(Gy\ s^{-1}) \approx 35 \times 10^{-18}\ nBEd^{-2}$$
$$\dot{D}(Gy\ h^{-1}) \approx 1.26 \times 10^{-13}\ nBEd^{-2}$$

where d = distance in meters
B = activity in becquerels (Bq)
n = gamma quanta per disintegration
E = photon Energy in MeV
s = seconds
h = hours

(3) *Exposure Rate* (from point source of radium, 0.5 mm Pt)

$$mR/h \approx \frac{mg}{(yd)^2}$$

$$mR/h \approx \frac{8400\ mg}{cm^2}$$

where yd = distance to source (yd)
cm = distance to source (cm)
mg = number of mg of radium

[b] For Specific Gamma Ray *Dose Constants* Γ (mSv/h)/MBq at 1 meter see Chapter 6, Table 6.1.

(4) *Exposure Rate* (from any gamma point source)

$$mR/h = nI_{\gamma}/d^2$$

where n = number of millicuries
I_{γ} = mR/h at 1 meter per mCi
d = distance (meters)

(5) *Ratio of the finite to infinite semispherical-cloud photon dose rate* (Chabot, 1974)

$$f' = \mu_{en} R$$

where f′ = fraction of infinite cloud dose rate
μ_{en} = energy absorption coefficient
R = cloud radius

Between 0.2 MeV and 2 MeV this approximation is precise to ±10% up to 100 m.

Note that ICRP Report 30 uses the $(1 - e^{-\mu R})$ form, and applies a factor of 2 multiplier on the assumption that in a small room the geometry is no longer semispherical, i.e. it is a spherical geometry.

(6) *Exposure Rate* (from a line gamma emitter source)

$$\phi = \int_{Z_1}^{Z_2} \frac{S(dz)}{4\pi r^2}$$

$$\phi = \frac{S}{4\pi h}(\theta_2 - \theta_1)$$

where S = source activity in photons per second per unit line length (cm)
h = perpendicular distance from point of interest P, to the horizontal plane of source.
ϕ = flux at point of interest in photons per square centimeter per second
r = distance from source to point of interest, P
θ = angle in radians
$Z_2 - Z_1$ = line length of source in cm

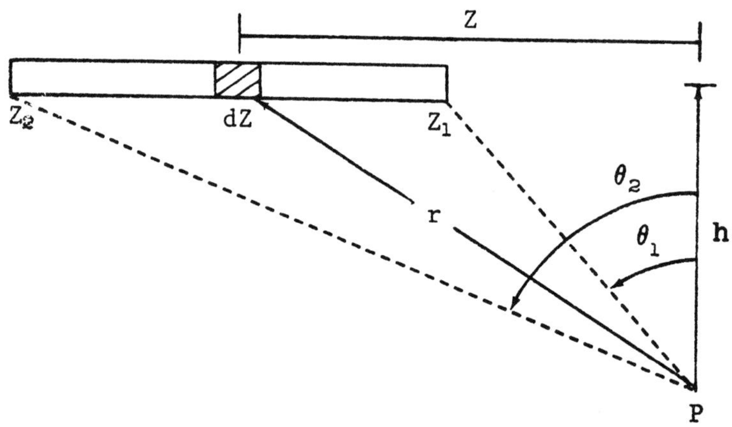

Figure 3.1.4 Exposure Rate (from a line gamma emitter source)

Geometry of a Counter

Point Source

$$G = 0.5\,(1 - \cos\alpha) = \sin^2 1/2\alpha$$

where $\alpha = \arc\tan\left(\frac{r}{d}\right)$

r = radius of counter window or phosphor

d = distance between counter and source (see "α" above)

G = geometry factor

Inverse Square Law (for point sources of gamma and x radiation)

The "inverse square law" states that radiation intensity from a point source varies inversely as the square of the distance from the source.

$$\frac{I_1}{I_2} = \frac{(R_2)^2}{(R_1)^2}$$

where I_1 = radiation intensity at distance R_1 from the source

I_2 = radiation intensity at distance R_2 from the source

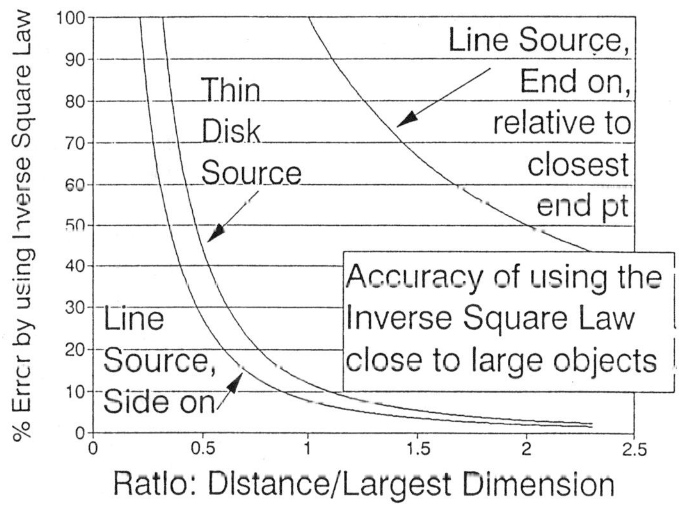

Figure 3.1.5 Accuracy of Using the Inverse Square Law Close to Large Objects (Personal Communication, Slaback, 1991)

Isotopic Dilution

Single Addition Method

$$w = w'\left(\frac{SpA'}{SpA} - 1\right)$$

where w = total weight of dilutent material (weight of stable material)

w′ = total weight of labeled material (weight of radioactive material)

SpA′ = specific activity of labeled material

SpA = specific activity of mixture

Logarithmic Relations

log N = The common logarithm of N, the exponent or power to which the base 10 must be raised to obtain a value N

ln N = The natural logarithm of N), the power to which the base 2.718 . . . (e) must be raised to obtain a value N

(1) $\log N = 0.4343 \ln N$

(2) $\ln N = 2.3026 \log N$

(3) $\log MN = \log M + \log N$

(4) $\log M/N = \log M - \log N$

(5) $\log N^a = a \log N$

(6) $\log \sqrt[a]{N} = (\log N)/a$

Neutron Activation Methods[c]

Thin Target

(A thin target is one which will not reduce the neutron flux by more than the error permitted for the experiment.)

$$A^{\phi} = k\sigma_{ac} fn(1 - e^{-\lambda t})\, e^{-\lambda\phi}$$

where A^{ϕ} = measured activity in net counts per second at time ϕ

ϕ = time increment between end of irradiation and the time at which the target is counted

k = efficiency of the counter for measuring the induced radioactivity

σ_{ac} = activation cross section for neutron capture by the target material, square centimeters per atom per neutron, averaged over the energy distribution of the neutron flux. In the case of 'thermal' neutrons, tabulated cross-sections are for neutrons with a velocity of 2200 ms^{-1}.

f = flux density of neutrons, neutrons per square centimeter per second

n = total number of target nuclei

λ = disintegration constant of radioactive material produced by the neutron reaction

t = time duration of exposure to neutron flux

e = base of natural logarithm (2.718 . . .)

[c] See Chapter 7, Table 7.21 for neutron activations of interest in health physics.

Radiation Absorption

(1) *Alpha Particle Range*

(a) For (E < 4 MeV)

$$R_a = 0.56E$$

where R_a = range in cm of air at 1 atm and 15°C
E = energy, MeV

NOTE: Good to +15%, −10% (Personal Communication Slaback, 1991)

(b) For (4 < E < 8 MeV)

$$R_a = 1.24E - 2.62$$

NOTE: Good to −10%, +4% (Personal Communication Slaback, 1991)

(2) *Beta Particle Range*

(a) For (0.01 ≤ E ≤ 2.5 MeV)

$$R = 0.412E^{1.265 - 0.0954 \ln E}$$

$$\ln E = 6.63 - 3.2376\,[10.2146 - \ln R]^{1/2}$$

where R = range in g/cm²
E = max. energy, MeV
(applicable to (a), (b), (c), and (d))

(b) For (E ≥ 2.5 MeV)

$$R - 0.530E - 0.106$$

(c) Sargent's Rule (E > 0.8 MeV)

$$R = 0.542E - 0.094$$

(d) Feather's rule (E > 0.6 MeV)

$$R = 0.542E - 0.133$$

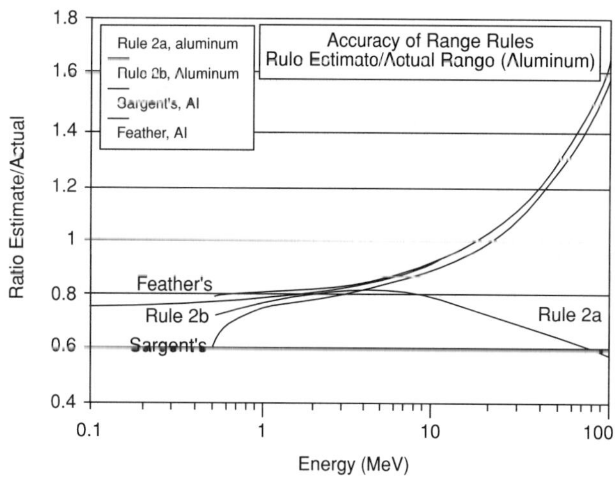

Figure 3.1.6 Accuracy of Range Rules Beta Particles—Aluminum (Personal Communication, Slaback, 1991)

(3) *Gamma Ray Attenuation*

The following symbols will be used in this section:

I_0 = original radiation exposure rate
I = attenuated radiation exposure rate
μ = linear attenuation coefficient (cm^{-1}) = $0.693/X^{1/2}$, or the mass attenuation coefficient $\times \rho$
μ/ρ = mass attenuation coefficient (cm^2/gm)
ρ = absorber density (gm/cm^3)
x = absorber thickness (cm)
$X^{1/2}$ = half-value layer of absorber (cm) (see ''μ'' above)
e = base of natural logarithms (2.718 . . .)
b = ''buildup'' factor

For monoenergetic or monochromatic narrow-beam radiation:

$$I = I_0 e^{-\mu x} \quad \text{or} \quad I = I_0 e^{-(\mu/\rho)(\rho)(x)}$$

For monoenergetic or monochromatic wide-beam radiation:

$$I = bI_0 e^{-\mu x}$$

(4) *Neutron Absorption* (for a collimated beam of monoenergetic neutrons)

$$I = I_0 e^{-\sigma N x}$$

where I_0 = initial neutron intensity
I = final neutron intensity
N = number of atoms per cm^3 in the absorber
σ = cross section (cm^2)
x = thickness of absorber (cm)
e = base of the natural logarithm (2.718 . . .)

Since this equation is only an approximation of neutron attenuation, average neutron energies can be used for determining the value of σ. The equation is not accurate enough to justify the use of neutron buildup factors.

(5) *Approximate Range—Energy Relation for Protons*
(From Segre, 1953)

$$R = \left(\frac{E}{9.3}\right)^{1.8}$$

where E = energy in MeV (few MeV to 200 MeV)
R = range in meters in air
$\pm 10\%$ for 2 − 200 MeV [$\pm 50\%$: 0.3 to 800 MeV]

Radioactive Decay (Physical and Biological)

The following symbols will be used in this section:

N_0 = number of nuclei at some original time
N = number of nuclei remaining after a time interval, t
I_0 = intensity of radiation at some original time
I = intensity of radiation after a time interval, t
A_0 = activity of sample at some original time
A = activity remaining after a time interval, t
λ = decay constant for the particular radioactive element
e = base of natural logarithms (2.718 . . .)
t = elapsed time

$T_{1/2}$ = half-life of a particular radioactive element
$n = t/T_{1/2}$ = number of half-lives

(1) $N = N_0 e^{-\lambda t}$ or $N = N_0 e^{-0.693t/T_{1/2}}$

(2) $A = A_0 e^{-\lambda t}$ or $A = A_0 e^{-0.693n}$

(3) $I = I_0 e^{-\lambda t}$ or $I = I_0(0.5)^n$

(4) *Decay Constant*

$$\lambda = 0.693/T_{1/2}$$

(5) *Biological Half-life*

$$T_b = \frac{0.693}{\lambda_b}$$

where λ_b = biological decay constant
T_b = biological half-life

(6) *Effective Half-life*

$$T_{eff} = \frac{(T_{1/2})(T_b)}{T_{1/2} + T_b}$$

where T_{eff} = effective half-life
$T_{1/2}$ = radioactive (physical) half-life
T_b = biological half-life

Specific Activity (Isotopic)

Specific Activity (dis/sec/gm)

$$\lambda N = 0.693N/T_{1/2}$$

where $T_{1/2}$ = half-life (seconds)
A = atomic weight (g/mole)
N = number of atoms per gram $= 6.02 \times 10^{23}/A$

Specific Activity (curies/gm)

$$\frac{\lambda N}{3.7 \times 10^{10}} = \frac{N \times 1.873 \times 10^{-11}}{T_{1/2}} = \frac{1.1275 \times 10^{13}}{AT_{1/2}\,(sec)} = \frac{3.575 \times 10^{5}}{AT_{1/2}\,(yrs)}$$

Statistics of Counting

(After Bleuler and Goldsmith, 1952)

C = number of counts, one observation
t = counting time, one observation
$\bar{C}$ = mean number of counts, series of observations
$\bar{t}$ = mean counting time, series of observations
n = number of observations
σ_c = theoretical standard deviation for a single observation
$\sigma_{\bar{c}}$ = theoretical standard deviation for an average number of counts in an interval
S_t = observed standard deviation of the time required to record a preset number of counts
S_c = observed mean standard deviation of the number of counts recorded in a preset time
R = average number of counts per unit time

(1) *Theoretical Standard Deviation*

$$\sigma_c = \sqrt{Rt} = \sqrt{C} \textit{ for single observation}$$

$$\sigma_{\bar{c}} = \sqrt{\frac{Rt}{n}} \cong \sqrt{\frac{C}{n}} \textit{ for average number of counts/interval}$$

(2) *Observed (Experimental) Standard Deviation*

(i) Series of observations, preset time

$$S_c = \left[\sum_{i=1}^{n} \frac{(C_i - \bar{C})^2}{(n - 1)} \right]^{1/2}$$

(ii) Series of observations, preset count

$$S_t = \left[\sum_{i=1}^{n} (t_i - \bar{t})^2/(n - 1) \right]^{1/2}$$

$$S_c = \left(\frac{\bar{C}}{\bar{t}} \right) S_t$$

(iii) Reliability factor

$$R.F. = \frac{S_c}{\sigma_{\bar{c}}}$$

(See Chapter 9 Figure 9.11 **Statistical Limits of Counter Reliability** for illustration of relationship between observed and theoretical standard deviation.)

Wave and Quantum Relations

Unless otherwise noted, symbols and dimensions in this section are used consistently as follows:

v = velocity of wave or particle (m/s)
h = Planck constant (6.6×10^{-34} J s)
υ = frequency of wave or quanta in hertz (s^{-1})
λ = wavelength (m)
λ_0 = wavelength of incident radiation in angstroms
λ_θ = wavelength of scattered radiation at angle θ in angstroms
E = energy in joules (J)
θ = angle between incident and scattered radiation
c = velocity of light (3×10^8 m s^{-1})
m = mass of particle (kg)
ϕ = work function (joules)

(1) *Wave Equation*

$$\textit{Wave velocity } (v \textit{ or } c) = \lambda \upsilon$$

(2) *Associated Wavelength of a Particle*

$$\text{Wavelength} = \lambda = \frac{h}{mv}$$

(3) *Photoelectric Equation*

$$E = \phi + \frac{1}{2}mv^2$$

(4) *Photon Energy*

$$E = hv$$

$$E = \frac{hc}{\lambda}$$

$$\text{Energy in electron volts} = \frac{1.2398 \times 10^4}{\text{Wavelength in angstroms}} = \frac{1.2398 \times 10^{-6}}{\lambda(m)}$$

(5) *Mass-Energy Relation*

$$E = mc^2$$

(6) *Momentum of Photon*

$$mv = \frac{h}{\lambda}$$

(7) *Compton Scattering of Gamma and X-Rays*

$$\lambda_\theta = \lambda_0 + 0.0242\ (1 - cos\theta)$$

(8) *Neutron Energy-Wavelength Relations*

$$E_T = kT = 8.61\ 10^{-5}\ T$$

$$\lambda_T = \frac{h}{\sqrt{2mE_T}}$$

$$\lambda_T\ (\mathring{A}) = \frac{0.286}{\sqrt{E_T}}$$

where k is the Boltzmann constant, E is in eV, T is in kelvin, Å $= 10^{-10}$ m.

References

Bleuler, E., Goldsmith, G. *Experimental Nucleonics.* Holt, Rinehart, and Winston, Inc.; New York; 1952.

Chabot, G., Skrable, K. *A Simple Formula for the Estimation of Surface Dose from Photons Emitted from a Finite Cloud. Health Physics* **27** (1) July, 1974.

Hickey, E.E., Stoetzel, G.A., Olsen, P.C., McGuire, S.A. *Air Sampling in the Workplace*, NUREG-1400, Nuclear Regulatory Commission, 1993.

ICRU. *Particle Counting in Radioactivity Measurements,* Report 52, International Commission on Radiation Units and Measurements, 1994.

McLintock, I.S., *Bremsstrahlung from Radionuclides (Practical Guidance for Radiation Protection).* HHSC Handbook No. 15, H and H Scientific Consultants Ltd., 1994.

NCRP. *Handbook of Radioactivity Measurements Procedures,* Report 58, National Council on Radiation Protection and Measurements, 1985.

Segre, E. *Experimental Nuclear Physics,* Vol. 1; John Wiley & Sons; 1953.

Swanson, W.P. *Radiological Safety Aspects of the Operation of Electron Linear Accelerators.* International Atomic Energy Agency (IAEA) Technical Series No. 188; Vienna; 1979.

CHAPTER 4

STANDARDS AND GUIDANCES FOR LIMITING IONIZING RADIATION EXPOSURE

This chapter is concerned with standards and guidances for limiting radiation exposures. It is divided into three sections, each of which has several parts. An outline of Chapter 4 follows:

Section 1: Ionizing Radiation—Standards and Guidances Applicable to the Public

Part A Radiation Protection Standards
Part B Environmental Radiation Standards
Part C Exempt Levels of Radioactivity
Part D Protective Action Guides for Accidents

Section 2: Ionizing Radiation—Standards Applicable to the Workplace

Section 3: Ionizing Radiation—Medical and Other Standards

This Chapter is intended to serve as a guide to the reader on the many radiation standards and guidances pertinent to health physicists. While up-to-date material available at the time of publication has been summarized here, the reader is directed to current published standards for the latest and most complete information.

Caution: This Chapter cites the latest available recommendations from the International Commission on Radiological Protection (ICRP) and the National Council on Radiation Protection and Measurements (NCRP). However, Federal agencies have not yet adopted some of these recommendations; therefore, use of the ICRP Publications 60 and 61, and recommendations of NCRP Report 116 may not be consistent with Federal regulations and should not be used for regulatory compliance purposes until they are officially adopted by the appropriate regulatory agency.

SECTION 1 IONIZING RADIATION—STANDARDS AND GUIDANCES APPLICABLE TO THE PUBLIC

This section presents information on current and proposed standards, recommendations, and guidances for limiting routine and accidental radiation exposures of the public. The information includes recommendations of the International Commission on Radiological Protection (ICRP) and the National Council on Radiation Protection and Measurements (NCRP), which are advisory bodies on radiation protection. It also includes standards and guidances developed by regulatory authorities in the U.S.: the Environmental Protection Agency (EPA), Nuclear Regulatory Commission (NRC), Department of Energy (DOE), and Food and Drug Administration (FDA).

In regard to routine radiation exposures of the public, it is important to distinguish between radiation protection standards and guidances (Part A) and environmental radiation standards and guidances (Part B). These standards, recommendations, or guidances specify limits on exposure that are regarded as necessary for protection of public health and should be met, except in the case of accidents or emergencies, regardless of cost. As used here, the terms ''radiation protection standard, recommendation, or guidances'' refer to standards, recommendations, or guidances that are generally applicable to all sources of exposure, exclusive of natural background radiation and deliberate medical practices.

On the other hand, the term ''environmental radiation standard or guidance'' refers to standards or guidances that specify limits on exposure for particular practices or sources. Most environmental radiation standards and guidances represent judgments regarding levels of public exposure from specified practices or sources that are reasonably achievable taking into account technical, economic, and social factors; that is, such standards usually are not based on the need for limitation of health risk per se. The one exception is the EPA standards for airborne emissions of radionuclides in 40 CFR Part 61, which are based on limits on lifetime risk for maximally exposed individuals and average individuals in large population groups. Standards for specific practices or sources involving man-made radionuclides are important because they provide a practical basis for ensuring that the radiation protection standards applicable to all sources of exposure will be met.

Information on current standards and recommendations on levels of radioactivity sufficiently low that they are or could be exempted from regulation is presented in Part C.

Protective action guides and recommendations applicable in radiation accidents are presented in Part D.

TABLE OF CONTENTS

Part A Radiation Protection Standards

(Following are summarized from the reference noted in bold print by David C. Kocher, Personal Communication, 1991. The material was revised and reviewed in 1997.)

Table 4.1 Radiation Standards and Guidances Applicable to the Public

The following tables present information on current recommendations on radiation protection standards for the public developed by the ICRP and NCRP and current radiation protection standards for the public established by the NRC and DOE.

Table 4.1.1 ICRP Recommendations on Radiation Protection of the Public (From ICRP Publication 60, 1991)

Limit on effective dose of 1 mSv (100 mrem) per year.

In special circumstances, higher dose could be allowed in single year, provided effective dose averaged over five years does not exceed 1 mSv (100 mrem) per year.

Limits on equivalent dose of 15 mSv (1.5 rem) per year to lens of the eye and 50 mSv (5 rem) per year to skin for prevention of deterministic effects.

Limits on effective dose and tissue weighting factors in definition of effective dose ensure that deterministic dose limit will be met for other organs and tissues (e.g., bone surfaces, thyroid).

Dose limits for limitation of stochastic effects are consistent with previous recommendations in ICRP Publications 26 (1977) and 45 (1985).

Other ICRP reports discuss recommendations on remedial actions for pre-existing exposure situations, including indoor radon and other natural sources, residual radioactivity, and accidents and emergencies; see ICRP Publications 63 (1993), 64 (1993), and 65 (1993).

Table 4.1.2 NCRP Recommendations on Radiation Protection of the Public[a]

NCRP Report No 116 (1993) For Public Exposures

Limit on annual effective dose of 1 mSv (100 mrem) for continuous exposure; and limit of 5 mSv (500 mrem) for infrequent exposure.

Limit on annual equivalent dose of 15 mSv (1.5 rem) to lens of the eye and 50 mSv (5 rem) to skin, hands, and feet.

Remedial action levels for natural sources: Average annual effective dose from external exposure, excluding medical practices but including naturally occurring sources, continuously exceeds 5 mSv (500 mrem); Average annual exposure to radon and its decay products exceeds 0.007 Jhm^{-3} [2 Working Level Months (WLM)].

Education and Training Exposures

Annual effective dose of less than 1 mSv (100 mrem). Annual equivalent dose limit to the skin, hands, and feet of 50 mSv (5 rem) and 15 mSv (1.5 rem) to the lens of the eye.

[a] Excluding medical and natural background radiation except as noted.

Table 4.1.3 NRC Radiation Protection Standards for the Public

10 CFR Part 20 (1994)

Dose limits:

- Limit on annual effective dose equivalent from external and internal exposure of 100 mrem (1 mSv), excluding dose from permissible releases of radionuclides into sanitary sewerage;
- Limit on effective dose equivalent from external exposure in any unrestricted area of 2 mrem (0.02 mSv) in any hour;
- Annual effective dose equivalents from external and internal exposure up to 500 mrem (5 mSv) may be permitted with prior NRC authorization.

Concentration limits:

- Annual average concentrations of radionuclides in gaseous and liquid effluents at boundary of unrestricted areas, as specified in Table 2 of Appendix B.
  - Concentration limits are based on annual effective dose equivalent from internal exposure for adults of 50 mrem (0.5 mSv), to ensure compliance with dose limit for all release pathways.

Table 4.1.4 DOE Radiation Protection Standards for the Public

DOE Order 5400.5 (1990)

Dose Limits:

- Limit on annual effective dose equivalent of 100 mrem (1 mSv);
- If avoidance of higher exposures is impractical, temporary limit on annual effective dose equivalent not to exceed 500 mrem (5 mSv) may be authorized;
- Limit on annual dose equivalent to any organ of 5 rem (50 mSv).

Concentration guides:

- For control of internal exposure, concentration guides for radionuclides in air and water in uncontrolled areas.
- For control of external exposure, concentration guides for noble gases and short-lived radionuclides in air in uncontrolled areas.
  - Concentration guides are based on limit on annual effective dose equivalent of 100 mrem (1 mSv).

SECTION 1 IONIZING RADIATION—STANDARDS AND GUIDANCES APPLICABLE TO THE PUBLIC

Part B Environmental Radiation Standards

(Environmental radiation standards were summarized by David C. Kocher, 1991, personal communication. The material was updated in 1997.)

The following tables present information on current standards and guidances established by the EPA, NRC, and DOE for limiting radiation exposures of the public from specific practices or sources.

Environmental radiation standards and guidances, which also may be referred to as source constraints, dose constraints, or authorized limits, may be grouped into the following categories:

- operations of uranium fuel-cycle facilities;
- radioactivity in drinking water;
- mill tailings and residual radioactivity;
- radioactive waste management and disposal;
- airborne radioactivity;
- indoor radon.

Table 4.1.5 NCRP Recommendation on Control of Individual Sources of Public Exposure to Man-Made Radionuclides

(From NCRP Report 116, 1993)

If member of the public could exceed 25% of limit on effective dose from exposure to single source, then site operator should ensure that effective dose to maximally exposed individuals from all sources does not exceed 1 mSv (100 mrem) per year on continuous basis.

Alternatively, no single source or set of sources under one control should result in effective dose exceeding 0.25 mSv (25 mrem) per year.

Recommendation assumes that individuals would not receive significant exposure from multiple sources and essentially provides limit on effective dose of 0.25 mSv (25 mrem) per year per source.

Table 4.1.6 NRC Design Objectives for Nuclear Power Reactors

10 CFR Part 50, Appendix I (1975)

Design objectives provide numerical guides for implementing requirement that releases of radioactivity from light-water-cooled nuclear power reactors shall be kept as low as reasonably achievable (ALARA).

Liquid effluents:

Limit on annual dose equivalent to whole body of 3 mrem (0.03 mSv);

Limit on annual dose equivalent to any organ of 10 mrem (0.1 mSv).

Gaseous effluents:

Limit on annual gamma absorbed dose in air of 10 mrad (0.1 mGy);

Limit on annual beta absorbed dose in air of 20 mrad (0.2 mGy);

Limit on annual dose equivalent to whole body of 5 mrem (0.05 mSv);

Limit on annual dose equivalent to skin of 15 mrem (0.15 mSv).

Releases of iodine and radionuclides in particulate form:

Limit on annual dose equivalent to any organ of 15 mrem (0.15 mSv).

If half of the annual design objectives are exceeded in a calendar quarter by operating reactors, then NRC requires reporting of releases and remedial action plans.

Table 4.1.7 EPA Standards for Operations of Uranium Fuel Cycle

40 CFR Part 190 (1977)

Standards apply to normal operations in milling of uranium ore, chemical conversion, fuel fabrication, electricity generation in nuclear power plants, and fuel reprocessing but do not apply to mining, waste disposal operations, transportation, and reuse of recovered special nuclear and byproduct materials.

Dose limits:

Limits on annual dose equivalent from all radionuclides except radon and its decay products of:

- 25 mrem (0.25 mSv) to whole body;
- 75 mrem (0.75 mSv) to thyroid;
- 25 mrem (0.25 mSv) to any other organ.

Release limits:

Limits on releases per GW (electrical)-year of electrical energy produced of:

- 50,000 Ci (2 PBq) for Kr-85;
- 5 mCi (0.2 GBq) for I-129;
- 0.5 mCi (0.02 GBq) for Pu-239 plus other alpha-emitting transuranic radionuclides with half-lives greater than 1 year.

Table 4.1.8 EPA Standards for Radioactivity in Community Drinking Water Systems

40 CFR Part 141 (1976)

Interim standards apply (1) to public or private water systems with at least 15 service connections or serving at least 25 persons and (2) at the tap rather than at the source.

Concentration limits:

Limit of 5 pCi/L (0.2 Bq/L) for Ra-226 plus Ra-228;

Limit of 15 pCi/L (0.6 Bq/L) for gross alpha-particle activity, including Ra-226 but excluding radon and uranium.

Dose limit:

Limit on annual dose equivalent to whole body or any organ of 4 mrem (0.04 mSv) from man made, beta/gamma-emitting radionuclides and NBS Handbook 69 shall be used to calculate the dose.

Proposed revisions of standards for radioactivity in drinking water issued in 1991 would apply to community and non-transient, non-community water systems and include:[a]

- separate concentration limits of 20 pCi/L (0.7 Bq/L) for Ra-226 and Ra-228;
- concentration limit of 20 μg/L for uranium, based primarily on prevention of chemical toxicity in the kidney;
- concentration limit of 300 pCi/L (11 Bq/L) for Rn-222.

[a] Note proposed, not final, rule as of January 1, 1997.

Table 4.1.9 DOE Standards for Radioactivity in Drinking Water

DOE Order 5400.5 (1990)

DOE drinking water supplies:

Limit on annual effective-dose equivalent from drinking water supplies operated by or for DOE of 4 mrem (0.04 mSv), excluding naturally occurring radionuclides.

Public or private drinking water supplies:

Liquid effluents from DOE activities will not cause public or private drinking water systems downstream of facility discharge to exceed concentration and dose limits in EPA drinking water standards (40 CFR Part 141).[a]

[a] The EPA drinking water standards are described in Table 4.1.9.

Table 4.1.10 EPA Standards for Uranium and Thorium Mill Tailings

40 CFR Part 192 (1995)

Standards apply to (1) control and cleanup of residual radioactive materials at inactive uranium processing sites or (2) management of uranium and thorium byproduct materials at active processing sites.

Releases of Rn-222:

Limit on annual average release rate to the atmosphere of 20 pCi/m^2s (0.7 Bq/m^2s); or

Limit on annual average concentration in air above background outside disposal site of 0.5 pCi/L (20 Bq/m^3).

Concentrations of Ra-226 in soil:

Limit of 5 pCi/g (0.2 Bq/g) averaged over the first 15 cm below the ground surface; and

Limit of 15 pCi/g (0.6 Bq/g) averaged over any 15-cm thick layers more than 15 cm below the ground surface.

Indoor radon decay-product concentration:

Limit of 0.03 Working Levels (WL) (6×10^{-7} J/m^3), including background, in any occupied or habitable building, with objective for remedial action of 0.02 WL (4×10^{-7} J/m^3).

Indoor gamma radiation level:

Limit of 20 μR per hour above background in any occupied or habitable building.

Groundwater protection requirements:

Limits on concentration in groundwater of 5 pCi/L (0.2 Bq/L) for radium-226 plus radium-228, 15 pCi/L (0.6 Bq/L) for gross alpha-particle activity; excluding radon and uranium, and 30 pCi/L (1.1 Bq/L) for U-234 plus U-238.

Thorium processing operations:

Limits on annual dose equivalent of 25 mrem (0.25 mSv) to whole body, 75 mrem (0.75 mSv) to thyroid, and 25 mrem (0.25 mSv) to any other organ.

Limits for uranium, Rn-222, and Ra-226 also apply to thorium, Rn-220, and Ra-228, respectively.

Standards for control of radon emissions shall be effective for up to 1,000 years, to extent reasonably achievable, and in any case for at least 200 years.

[a] The EPA drinking water standards are described in Table 4.1.9.

Table 4.1.11 DOE Standards for Residual Radioactivity

DOE Order 5400.5 (1990)

Requirements for control of residual radioactive material at DOE sites address (1) release of contaminated property for unrestricted use by the public, (2) interim storage of residual radioactive material, and (3) long-term management of uranium, thorium, and their decay products, but requirements do not apply to cleanup of inactive radioactive waste disposal sites.

Requirements involve hierarchy of:

- requirements for radiation protection of the public;
- generic or derived guidelines for acceptable levels of residual radioactivity that can be used if radiation protection requirements will be met;
- authorized limits on acceptable levels of residual radioactivity that are used if generic or derived guidelines would not ensure that radiation protection requirements will be met.

Requirements for radiation protection of the public:

Limit on annual effective dose equivalent from routine DOE operations and exposure to residual radioactive material of 100 mrem (1 mSv);

Higher annual doses from acute exposure are permitted, provided annual effective dose equivalent averaged over a lifetime is not expected to exceed 100 mrem (1 mSv);

Release of real property (i.e., land and structures) for unrestricted use by the public shall be governed by guidelines for residual radioactivity developed in Formerly Utilized Sites Remedial Action Program (FUSRAP) and remote Surplus Facilities Management Program (SFMP).[a]

Guidelines for residual radioactivity at FUSRAP and remote SFMP sites:

Limits on residual concentrations of radium and thorium in soil, airborne radon decay products in occupied or habitable structures on private property, and external gamma radiation inside buildings or habitable structures on a site as given in EPA mill tailings standards (40 CFR Part 192);[a]

Limits on residual concentrations of other radionuclides in soil shall be derived from dose limits in radiation protection requirements using prescribed site specific procedures and data.

Annual dose equivalent from residual radioactivity in soil and external gamma radiation, including exposure on open lands, shall comply with limits in radiation protection requirements.

Limits on residual radioactivity on surfaces of structures and equipment, based on NRC guidelines (1982) and NRC Regulatory Guide 1.86 (1974);[b]

Limits on residual concentrations of radionuclides in air and water such that applicable Federal and State standards will be met.

Guidelines for interim storage of residual radioactive material at FUSRAP and remote SFMP sites:[c]

Limits on Rn-222 concentrations in air above background of:

- 100 pCi/L (4 kBq/m^3) at any point within a site,
- 30 pCi/L (1 kBq/m^3) averaged over a year and over a site, and
- 3 pCi/L (0.1 kBq/m^3) averaged over a year at any location outside a site;

Limit on release rate of Rn-222 above background of 20 pCi/m^2s (0.7 Bq/m^2s);

Limits on radionuclide concentrations in groundwater or quantities of residual radioactive material as established in Federal or State standards;

Control and stabilization features designed to ensure, to extent reasonably achievable, effective life of 50 years with minimum life of at least 25 years.

Guidelines for long-term management of uranium, thorium, and their decay products:

Limits on Rn-222 release rate to the atmosphere and concentration in air outside boundary of contaminated areas as given in EPA mill tailings standards (40 CFR Part 192);[a]

Protection of groundwater in accordance with applicable Federal and State standards;

Design lifetime for control and stabilization features as given in EPA mill tailings standards (40 CFR Part 192);[a]

Control of access to site and prevention of misuse of onsite residual radioactive material by appropriate administrative controls and physical barriers designed to be effective, to extent reasonable, for at least 200 years.

[a] The EPA mill tailings standards are described in Table 4.1.10.

[b] Nuclear Regulatory Guide 1.86, Termination of Operating Licenses for Nuclear Reactors (1974).

[c] FUSRAP and remote SFMP sites are sites that were contaminated as a result of previous activities for Federal nuclear programs.

Table 4.1.12 Proposed EPA Guidance on Transuranium Elements in the Environment[a]

To update *proposed* guidance from 1977, EPA has developed draft interim recommendations on acceptable levels of transuranium elements above background. The 1987 draft recommendations include the following:

To extent practical, annual alpha absorbed dose from transuranium elements should be limited to 1 mrad (0.01 mGy) to pulmonary lung or 3 mrad (0.03 mGy) to bone, endosteal bone surfaces, or red bone marrow—Range I;

Doses above Range I but less than annual effective dose equivalent of 100 mrem (1 mSv) from all sources, excluding natural background and medical practices, are acceptable provided risks to population are justified, general surveillance and routine monitoring are implemented, and doses are maintained as low as reasonably achievable (ALARA)—Range II;

Doses above Range II but less than annual effective dose equivalent of 500 mrem (5 mSv) from all sources on intermittent basis require continuing monitoring and evaluation of individuals and limitations on access or use pending remedial actions—Range III;

Soil contamination level of 0.2 μCi/m^2 (7 kBq/m^2), to depth of 1 cm and for particle sizes less than 2 mm, and air concentration of 1 fCi/m^3 (0.04 mBq/m^3) for alpha-emitting transuranium elements provide screening levels for demonstrating compliance with Range I recommendations but do not define limits for implementing Range I recommendations.

Remedial actions should ensure compliance with applicable environmental standards (e.g., drinking water standards).

Recommendations do not provide general criteria for decontamination or decommissioning of sites or facilities, do not apply to the transient period during and immediately following accidents, and should not be used as limits for planned releases of transuranium elements.

[a] Note proposed, not final, rule as of January 1, 1997.

Table 4.1.13 EPA Standards for Management and Disposal of Spent Fuel, High-Level Waste, and Transuranic Waste

40 CFR Part 191 (1985, 1993)

Standards for management (except transportation) and storage:

For facilities regulated by NRC or Agreement States—

Limit on annual dose equivalent, including all operations covered by 40 CFR Part 190, of 25 mrem (0.25 mSv) to whole body, 75 mrem (0.75 mSv) to thyroid, or 25 mrem (0.25 mSv) to any other organ.

For facilities operated by DOE and not regulated by NRC or Agreement States—

Limit on annual dose equivalent of 25 mrem (0.25 mSv) to whole body or 75 mrem (0.75 mSv) to any other organ; or

Upon application for alternative standard, limit on annual dose equivalent from all sources, excluding natural background and medical practices, of 100 mrem (1 mSv) for continuous exposure or 500 mrem (5 mSv) for infrequent exposure.

Standards for disposal:

Containment requirements—

For 10,000 years after disposal, cumulative releases of radionuclides to accessible environment shall have a likelihood of (1) less than 1 chance in 10 of exceeding specified limits and (2) less than 1 chance in 1,000 of exceeding 10 times specified limits.

Assurance requirements—

To provide confidence that containment requirements will be met, qualitative requirements for maintaining active institutional controls, monitoring of disposal systems, use of permanent markers at disposal sites, use of engineered and natural barriers for waste isolation, avoidance of sites with valuable natural resources, and provision for retrieval of waste.

Individual protection requirements—

For 10,000 years after disposal, undisturbed performance of disposal system shall not cause effective dose equivalent to members of the public in accessible environment from all potential exposure pathways to exceed 15 mrem (0.15 mSv).

Groundwater protection requirements—

For 10,000 years after disposal, undisturbed performance of disposal system shall not cause levels of radioactivity in any underground source of drinking water in accessible environment to exceed limits specified in 40 CFR Part 141 as they exist when implementing agency determines compliance with requirements.

Table 4.1.14 NRC Standards for Near-Surface Land Disposal of Radioactive Waste

10 CFR Part 61 (1982)

Performance objectives:

Limit on annual dose equivalent beyond facility boundary of 25 mrem (0.25 mSv) to whole body, 75 mrem (0.75 mSv) to thyroid, or 25 mrem (0.25 mSv) to any other organ;

Qualitative requirement for protection of inadvertent intruders onto disposal site at any time after active institutional controls are removed (assumed to be 100 years after facility closure).

Technical requirements for waste classification:

Limits on radionuclide concentrations that are generally acceptable for near-surface land disposal—i.e., Class A and C limits for longer-lived radionuclides and Class A, B, and C limits for shorter-lived radionuclides.

Waste classification system is intended to provide protection of inadvertent intruders and is based on limit on annual dose equivalent of 0.5 rem (5 mSv) to whole body and bone or 1.5 rem (15 mSv) to any other organ for assumed scenarios for direct intrusion into disposal facilities.

Table 4.1.15 DOE Standards for Disposal of Low-Level Waste

DOE Order 5820.2A, Chapter III (1988)

Performance objectives:

Limit on annual effective dose equivalent beyond facility boundary of 25 mrem (0.25 mSv), with dose from airborne releases limited as specified in EPA's 40 CFR Part 62;[a]

Limit on annual effective dose equivalent for inadvertent intruders after loss of active institutional controls (at 100 years after facility closure) of 100 mrem (1 mSv) for continuous exposure or 500 mrem (5 mSv) for single, acute exposure;

Protection of groundwater resources consistent with Federal, State, and local requirements.

[a] The EPA standards for airborne emissions are discribed in Table 4.1.17.

Table 4.1.16 Suggested State Regulations for Control of Radiation—Licensing Requirements for Land Disposal of Radioactive Waste (From Conference of Radiation Control Program Directors, 1990)

Sec. M.19 Protection of the General Population from Releases of Radioactivity

Concentrations of radioactive material which may be released to the general environment in ground water, surface water, air, soil, plants, or animals shall not result in an annual dose exceeding an equivalent of 25 millirems (0.25 mSv) to the whole body, 75 millirems (0.75 mSv) to the thyroid, and 25 millirems (0.25 mSv) to any other organ of any member of the public. Reasonable effort should be made to maintain releases of radioactivity in effluents to the general environment as low as is reasonably achievable.

Table 4.1.17 EPA Standards for Airborne Emissions of Radionuclides

40 CFR Part 61 (1989–1996)

Limit on annual effective dose equivalent of 10 mrem (0.1 mSv) for:

- DOE facilities emitting any radionuclide other than radon, except for disposal facilities subject to 40 CFR Part 191 or 40 CFR Part 192 and excluding dose from Rn-222 and its decay products;
- non-DOE Federal facilities, except for disposal facilities subject to 40 CFR Part 191, inactive uranium mill tailings disposal sites subject to 40 CFR Part 192, or low-energy accelerators, but limit is 3 mrem (0.03 mSv) per year from iodine and dose from Rn-222 and its decay products is excluded from this statement.
- emissions of Rn-222 from underground uranium mines with production greater than specified values.

Limit on emission rate of Rn-222 of 20 pCi/m^2s (0.7 Bq/m^2s) from:

- DOE facilities for storage and disposal of material containing radium;
- phosphogypsum stacks;
- operating and inactive uranium mill tailings piles, except for inactive disposal sites licensed by NRC.

Limit on emissions of Po-210 from all calciners and nodulizing kilns at elemental phosphorus plants of 2 Ci (0.07 TBq) per year, or limit on total emissions from any plant of 4.5 Ci (0.17 TBq) per year when specified scrubbers are installed. Since standards were first issued in 1989, EPA has rescinded all standards that applied to NRC licensees, including standards for emissions of Rn-222 from inactive uranium mill tailings disposal sites (1994), standards for nuclear power reactors (1995), and standards for facilities other than nuclear power reactors (1996), based on finding that existing NRC regulations limit airborne emissions to an extent consistent with, or more restrictive than, EPA standards.

Table 4.1.18 Federal Guidance on Radon in Homes

Report EPA-86-004 (1986)

Guidance on radon concentration in homes above which mitigation of exposures is recommended:

- concentration of 4 pCi/L (0.15 kBq/m^3).

Guidance corresponds to concentration of radon decay products of about 0.02 WL (4×10^{-7} J/m^3).

Table 4.1.19 NRC Rulemaking on Decommissioning of Nuclear Facilities[a]

10 CFR Part 20 (1994)

In 1994, NRC issued *proposed* standards for decontamination and decommissioning of licensed nuclear facilities. NRC intends to base radiological criteria on limitation of dose (risk) to the public from unrestricted use of land, buildings, and equipment containing residual radioactive material.

(1) General provisions—
—application of radiological criteria for 1,000 years;
—reasonable expectation that residual radioactivity will not cause radioactivity in groundwater that is current or potential source of drinking water to exceed limits in EPA's 40 CFR Part 141.

(2) Sites will be considered acceptable for unrestricted use if—
—effective dose equivalent does not exceed 15 mrem (0.15 mSv) per year;
—residual radioactivity has been reduced to levels that are ALARA.

(3) If dose limit for unrestricted use is not technically achievable, license may be terminated under restricted conditions if—
—provisions for institutional controls would ensure that effective dose equivalent does not exceed 15 mrem (0.15 mSv) per year;
—effective dose equivalent would not exceed 100 mrem (1 mSv) per year for unrestricted use if institutional controls were no longer in effect.

(4) License normally will not be terminated if effective dose equivalent would exceed 100 mrem (1 mSv) per year for unrestricted use.

Proposed standards also include provisions for public participation in cleanup decisions.

[a] Proposed, not final, as of January 1, 1997.

SECTION 1 IONIZING RADIATION—STANDARDS AND GUIDANCES APPLICABLE TO THE PUBLIC

Part C Exempt Levels of Radioactivity

(Summarized by David C. Kocher, 1991)

The following tables present information on current standards and recommendations regarding levels of radiation or radioactivity which are sufficiently low that the sources or practices may be exempted from regulations for limiting exposures of the public to radioactive materials.

Table 4.1.20 NCRP Recommendations on Exemption

NCRP Report No. 116 (1993)—Negligible Individual Dose (NID)

Annual effective dose of 0.01 mSv (1 mrem) per source or practice.

Table 4.1.21 International Atomic Energy Agency Recommendations on Exemption Principles of Practice or Source within a Practice[a]

IAEA Safety Series No. 115 (1996)

A practice or a source within a practice may be exempted without further consideration, provided that, in all feasible situations (a) the effective dose expected to be incurred by any member of the public is of the order of 10 μSv (1 mrem) per year or less and (b) either the collective effective dose committed by one year of performance of the practice is no more than about 1 person-Sv or an assessment for the optimization of protection shows that exemption is the optimum option.

[a] A table presented in the reference gives exemption levels for specific radionuclides.

Table 4.1.22 Current Exemptions in NRC Standards

10 CFR Part 20, Radiation Protection Standards (1991)

Limits on concentrations or yearly releases of radionuclides for disposal into sanitary sewer systems, except limits do not apply to excreta from individuals undergoing medical treatment or therapy with radioactive material;

Limits on concentrations of H-3 and C-14 of 0.05 μCi/g (2 kBq/g) for land disposal of animal carcasses and materials used for liquid scintillation counting.

10 CFR Part 30, Domestic Licensing of Byproduct Material

Limits on exempt quantities and concentrations of byproduct material;

Exemptions for particular items containing specified amounts of byproduct material.

10 CFR Part 40, Domestic Licensing of Source Material

Limit on unimportant quantities of source material;

Exemptions for particular items containing specified amounts of source material.

10 CFR Part 71, Packaging and Transportation of Radioactive Material

Exemption from all requirements for any materials containing less than 2 nCi/g (0.07 kBq/g) of radioactivity;

Exemption from certain requirements for packages containing specified amounts of fissile material or americium and plutonium only.

SECTION 1 IONIZING RADIATION—STANDARDS AND GUIDANCE APPLICABLE TO THE PUBLIC

Part D Protective Action Guides for Accidents

The following tables present information on current guidances and recommendations regarding projected radiation doses to the public or measured levels of radioactivity in the environment from radiation accidents at which protective actions to avoid exposures are warranted. Available protective actions include sheltering, evacuation, stable iodine administration, control of foodstuffs and water, control of access to contaminated areas, decontamination of persons and areas, and permanent relocation of populations.

Protective actions usually are defined for the following three time phases following an accident:

- Early Phase—time period lasting from hours to days, when immediate decisions based on predictions of radiological conditions are required;
- Intermediate Phase—time period lasting from weeks to months after an accident has been brought under control, when environmental measurements can be used to assess the need for additional protective actions;
- Recovery Phase—time period lasting from months to years, when actions to reduce radioactivity to acceptable levels for permanent residence under normal conditions may be undertaken.

Part D discusses emergency action levels and appropriate actions and the Environmental Protection Agency and Food and Drug Administration's protective action guides for a gaseous plume, radioactivity in food, and use of potassium iodide as a thyroid blocking agent. Although the FDA protective action guidance on radioactivity in food has not been revised, it is likely that the levels allowed in food introduced into commerce following future accidents will be similar to those used by FDA following the Chernobyl accident or recommended by the Codex Alimentarius Commission. Hence, these are also included in the Chapter

Table 4.1.23 Basis for Emergency Action Levels for Nuclear Power Facilities (From Nuclear Regulatory Commission NUREG-0654, FEMA-REP-1, 1980)

Classes

Four classes of Emergency Action Levels have been established. The classes are:

Notification of Unusual Event
Alert
Site Area Emergency
General Emergency

The rationale for the notification and alert classes is to provide early and prompt notification of minor events which could lead to more serious consequences given operator error or equipment failure or which might be indicative of more serious conditions which are not yet fully realized. A gradation is provided to assure more extension preparations for more serious indicators. The site area emergency class reflects conditions where some significant releases are likely or are occurring but where a core melt situation is not indicated based on current information. In this situation full mobilization of emergency personnel in the near site environs is indicated as well as dispatch of monitoring teams and associated communications. The general emergency class involves actual or imminent substantial core degradation or melting with the potential loss of containment. The immediate action for this class is sheltering (staying inside) rather than evacuation until an assessment can be made that (1) an evacuation is indicated and (2) evacuation, if indicated, can be completed prior to significant release and transport of radioactive material to the affected areas.

Prompt Notification

Prompt notification of offsite authorities is intended to indicate within about 15 minutes for the unusual event class and sooner (consistent with the need for other emergency actions) for other classes. The time is measured from the time at which operators recognize that events have occurred which make declaration of an emergency class appropriate.

NOTIFICATION OF UNUSUAL EVENT

Class Description	*Licensee Actions*	*State and/or Local Offsite Authority Actions*
Unusual events are in process or have occurred which indicate a potential degradation of the level of safety of the plant. No releases of radioactive material requiring offsite response or monitoring are expected unless further degradation of safety systems occurs. *Purpose* Purpose of offsite notification is to (1) assure that the first step in any response later found to be necessary has been carried out, (2) bring the operating staff to a state of readiness, and (3) provide systematic handling of unusual events information and decision making.	1. Promptly inform State and/or local offsite authorities of nature of unusual condition as soon as discovered 2. Augment on-shift resources as needed 3. Assess and respond 4. Escalate to a more severe class, if appropriate **or** 5. Close out with verbal summary to offsite authorities; followed by written summary within 24 hours	1. Provide fire or security assistance if requested 2. Escalate to a more severe class, if appropriate 3. Stand by until verbal closeout

Table 4.1.23 Basis for Emergency Action Levels for Nuclear Power Facilities (Continued)

Class Description	*Licensee Actions*	*State and/or Local Offsite Authority Actions*
ALERT		
Events are in process or have occurred which involve an actual or potential substantial degradation of the level of safety of the plant. Any releases expected to be limited to small fractions of the EPA Protective Action Guideline exposure levels. *Purpose* Purpose of offsite alert is to (1) assure that emergency personnel are readily available to respond if situation becomes more serious or to perform confirmatory radiation monitoring, if required, and (2) provide offsite authorities current status information.	1. Promptly inform State and/or local authorities of alert status and reason for alert as soon as discovered. 2. Augment resources and activate on-site Technical Support Center and on-site operational support center. Bring Emergency Operations Facility (EOF) and other key emergency personnel to standby status 3. Assess and respond 4. Dispatch on-site monitoring teams and associated communications 5. Provide periodic plant status updates to offsite authorities (at least every 15 minutes) 6. Provide periodic meteorological assessments to offsite authorities and, if any releases are occurring, dose estimates for actual releases 7. Escalate to a more severe class, if appropriate 8. Close out or recommend reduction in emergency class by verbal summary to offsite authorities followed by written summary within 8 hours of closeout or class reduction	1. Provide fire or security assistance if requested 2. Augment resources and bring primary response centers and Emergency Broadcast System (EBS) to standby status 3. Alert to standby status key emergency personnel including monitoring teams and associated communications 4. Provide confirmatory offsite radiation monitoring and ingestion pathway dose projections if actual releases substantially exceed technical specification limits 5. Escalate to a more severe class, if appropriate 6. Maintain alert status until verbal closeout or reduction of emergency class

(continued)

Table 4.1.23 Basis for Emergency Action Levels for Nuclear Power Facilities (Continued)

Class Description	*Licensee Actions*	*State and/or Local Offsite Authority Actions*
SITE AREA EMERGENCY Events are in process or have occurred which involve actual or likely major failures of plant functions needed for protection of the public. Any releases not expected to exceed EPA Protective Action Guideline exposure levels except near site boundary. *Purpose* Purpose of the site area emergency declaration is to (1) assure that response centers are manned, (2) assure that monitoring teams are dispatched, (3) assure that personnel required for evacuation of near-site areas are at duty stations if situation becomes more serious, (4) provide consultation with offsite authorities, and (5) provide updates for the public through offsite authorities.	1. Promptly inform State and/or local offsite authorities of site area emergency status and reason for emergency as soon as discovered 2. Augment resources by activating on-site Technical Support Center, on-site operational support center and near-site Emergency Operations Facility (EOF) 3. Assess and respond 4. Dispatch on-site and offsite monitoring teams and associated communications 5. Dedicate an individual for plant status updates to offsite authorities and periodic briefings (perhaps joint with offsite authorities) 6. Make senior technical and management staff onsite available for consultation with NRC and State on a periodic basis 7. Provide meteorological and dose estimates to offsite authorities for actual releases via a dedicated individual or automated data transmission. 8. Provide release and dose projections based on available plant condition information and foreseeable contingencies 9. Escalate to *general emergency* class, if appropriate **or** 10. Close out or recommend reduction in emergency class by briefing of offsite authorities at EOF and by phone followed by written summary within 8 hours of closeout or class reduction	1. Provide any assistance requested 2. If sheltering near the site is desirable, activate public notification system within at least two miles of the plant 3. Provide public within about 10 miles periodic updates on emergency status 4. Augment resources by activating primary response centers 5. Dispatch key emergency personnel including monitoring teams and associated communications 6. Alert to standby status other emergency personnel (e.g., those needed for evacuation) and dispatch personnel to near-site duty stations 7. Provide offsite monitoring results to licensee, DOE, and others and jointly assess them 8. Continuously assess information from licensee and offsite monitoring with regard to changes to protective actions already initiated for public and mobilizing evacuation resources 9. Recommend placing milk animals within 2 miles on stored feed and assess need to extend distance 10. Provide press briefings, perhaps with licensee 11. Escalate to *general emergency* class, if appropriate 12. Maintain site area emergency status until closeout or reduction of emergency class

Table 4.1.23 Basis for Emergency Action Levels for Nuclear Power Facilities (Continued)

Class Description	*Licensee Actions*	*State and/or Local Offsite Authority Actions*
GENERAL EMERGENCY Events are in process or have occurred which involve actual or imminent substantial core degradation or melting with potential for loss of containment integrity. Releases can be reasonably expected to exceed EPA Protective Action Guideline exposure levels offsite for more than the immediate site area. *Purpose* Purpose of the general emergency declaration is to (1) initiate predetermined protective actions for the public, (2) provide continuous assessment of information from licensee and offsite organization measurements, (3) initiate additional measures as indicated by actual or potential releases, (4) provide consultation with offsite authorities and (5) provide updates for the public through offsite authorities	1. Promptly inform State and local offsite authorities of general emergency status and reason for emergency as soon as discovered (Parallel notification of State/local) 2. Augment resources by activating on-site Technical Support Center, on-site operational support center and near site Emergency Operations Facility (EOF) 3. Assess and respond 4. Dispatch on-site and offsite monitoring teams and associated communications 5. Dedicate an individual for plant status updates to offsite authorities and periodic press briefings (perhaps joint with offsite authorities) 6. Make senior technical and management staff onsite available for consultation with NRC and State on a periodic basis 7. Provide meteorological and dose estimates to offsite authorities for actual releases via a dedicated individual or automated data 8. Provide release and dose projections based on available plant condition information and foreseeable contingencies 9. Close out or recommend reduction of emergency class by briefing of offsite authorities at EOF and by phone followed by written summary within 8 hours of closeout or class reduction.	1. Provide any assistance requested 2. Activate immediate public notification of emergency status and provide public periodic updates 3. Recommend sheltering for 2 mile radius and 5 miles downwind and assess need to extend distances. Consider advisability of evacuation (projected time available vs. estimated evacuation times) 4. Augment resources by activating primary response centers 5. Dispatch key emergency personnel including monitoring teams and associated communications 6. Dispatch key emergency personnel to duty stations within 5 mile radius and alert all others to standby status 7. Provide offsite monitoring results to licensee, DOE and others and jointly assess them 8. Continuously assess information from licensee and offsite monitoring with regard to changes to protective actions already initiated for public and mobilizing evacuation resources 9. Recommend placing milk animals within 10 miles on stored feed and assess need to extend distance 10. Provide press briefings, perhaps with licensee 11. Maintain general emergency status until closeout or reduction of emergency class

Table 4.1.24 Generic Action Levels for Foodstuffs[a] (International Atomic Energy Agency from Safety Series No. 115, Vienna, Austria, 1996)

Radionuclides	Foods Destined for General Consumption (kBq/kg)	Milk, Infant Foods and Drinking Water (kBq/kg)
Cs-134, Cs-137, Ru-103, Ru-106, Sr-89	1	1
I-131		0.1
Sr-90	0.1	
Am-241, Pu-238, Pu-239	0.01	0.001

[a] The Table is based on, and consistent with, the Codex Alimentarius Commission's guideline levels for radionuclides in food moving in international trade following accidental contamination (Joint FAO/WHO Food Standards Programme, Codex Alimentarius Commission, Codex Alimentarius, Volume 1 (1991) Section 6.1, 'Levels for Radionuclides'), but it is limited to the nuclides usually considered relevant to emergency exposure situations.

Table 4.1.25 Radionuclides in Imported Foods: Levels of Concern Adopted Following the Chernobyl Accident (Food and Drug Administration 1986 and U.S. Department of Agriculture, 1986)

	Levels of Concern (pCi/kg)		
	Infant Food	Other Foods	Meat & Poultry
	Food and Drug Administration (FDA)		U.S. Department of Agriculture (USDA)
^{131}I	1,500	8,000	1,500
$^{134}Cs + ^{137}Cs$	10,000	10,000	75,000 (10,000)[a]

[a] The USDA level of 75,000 pCi/kg was reduced to 10,000 pCi/kg to agree with the FDA level in October 1986.

Table 4.1.26 Protective Action Guides for Radioactivity in Food (Food and Drug Administration *Federal Register* Vol. 47, 47073, 1982)

Preventive Protective Action Guides:

The *Preventive PAG* is applicable to incidents where protective actions causing minimal impact are justified. These protective actions, such as placing cows on stored feed, prevent or reduce concentrations of radioactivity in food.

Dose commitments at which protective actions having minimal impact should be taken:

- 1.5 rem (15 mSv) to thyroid;
- 0.5 rem (5 mSv) to whole body, bone marrow, or any other organ.

Emergency Protective Action Guides:

The *Emergency PAG* is applicable to incidents where protective actions of high impact are justified because of the greater projected health hazards.

Dose commitment at which food containing radioactivity should be isolated and responsible officials determine if condemnation or another disposition is appropriate:

- 15 rem (150 mSv) to thyroid;
- 5 rem (50 mSv) to whole body, bone marrow, or any other organ.

The FDA guidance includes derived Response Levels equivalent to the Preventive and Emergency Protective Action Guides for ^{131}I, ^{134}Cs, ^{137}Cs, ^{89}Sr, and ^{90}Sr. Response Levels for the grass-cow-milk pathway are given for:

- initial activity per unit area deposited on the ground;
- activity per unit mass in forage (fresh weight);
- peak activity concentration in milk;
- total activity intake in foodstuffs.

Table 4.1.27 Potassium Iodide as a Thyroid-Blocking Agent in a Radiation Emergency: Final Recommendations on Use (Food and Drug Administration *Federal Register* Vol. 47, 25158, June 28, 1982)

Based on its consideration of comments received and its analysis of available information, FDA concludes in the final recommendations that risks from the short-term use of relatively low doses of potassium iodide for thyroid blocking in a radiation emergency are outweighed by the risks of radioiodine-induced thyroid nodules or cancer at a projected dose to the thyroid gland of 25 rem. FDA recommends that potassium iodide in doses of 130 milligrams (mg) per day for adults and children above 1 year and 65 mg per day for children below 1 year of age be considered for thyroid blocking in radiation emergencies in those persons who are likely to receive a projected radiation dose of 25 rem or greater to the thyroid gland from radioiodines released into the environment. To have the greatest effect in decreasing the accumulation of radioiodine in the thyroid gland, these doses of potassium iodide should be administered immediately before or after exposure.

Table 4.1.28 EPA Protective Action Guides (From EPA 400-R-92-001, 1992)

Early Phase:

Evacuation or sheltering for effective dose equivalents from external and internal exposure of 1–5 rem (10–50 mSv), with protective actions normally initiated at 1 rem (10 mSv), and committed dose equivalents to the thyroid and skin may be 5 and 50 times larger, respectively;

Administration of stable iodine for committed dose equivalent to the thyroid from radioiodine of 25 rem (250 mSv);

For workers performing emergency services, limits on effective dose equivalent from external and internal exposure of—

- 5 rem (50 mSv) for all activities;
- 10 rem (100 mSv) while protecting valuable property, provided lower dose is not practical;
- 25 rem (250 mSv) during lifesaving or protection of large populations, provided lower dose is not practical;
- >25 rem (250 mSv) during lifesaving or protection of large populations only on a voluntary basis to persons fully aware of risks involved.

Intermediate Phase:

Relocation of general population for effective dose equivalent from external and internal exposure in the first year above 2 rem (20 mSv), and beta dose to skin may be up to 50 times higher;

Application of simple dose reduction techniques for effective dose equivalent in the first year below 2 rem (20 mSv) to reduce doses as low as practicable;

Protective Action Guides for radioactivity in food as given in 1982 FDA recommendations (see Table 4.1.25).

Protective Action Guides for radioactivity in drinking water are under development.

Longer-Term Objectives:

Effective dose equivalent in any single year after the first should not exceed 0.5 rem (5 mSv);

Cumulative effective dose equivalent over 50 years, including first and second years, should not exceed 5 rem (50 mSv).

For reactor accidents, Protective Action Guide of 2 rem (20 mSv) in first year is expected to provide assurance that longer-term objectives will be met, but additional Protective Action Guides for long-term recovery phase have not been developed.

Table 4.1.29 Recommended Protective Actions to Reduce Whole Body and Thyroid Dose from Exposure to a Gaseous Plume (From EPA 520/1-75-001-A, 1990)

Projected Dose (Rem) to the Population		Recommended Action[a]	Comments
Whole body Thyroid	<1 <5	No planned protective actions.[b] State may issue an advisory to seek shelter and await further instructions. Monitor environmental radiation levels.	Previously recommended protective actions may be reconsidered or terminated.
Whole body Thyroid	1 to <5 5 to <25	Seek shelter as a minimum. Consider evacuation. Evacuate unless constraints make it impractical. Monitor environmental radiation levels. Control access.	If constraints exist, special consideration should be given for evacuation of children and pregnant women.
Whole body Thyroid	5 and above 25 and above	Conduct mandatory evacuation. Monitor environmental radiation levels and adjust area for mandatory evacuation based on these levels. Control access	Seeking shelter would be an alternative if evacuation were not immediately possible.
Projected Dose (Rem) to Emergency Team Workers			
Whole body Thyroid	25 125[c]	Control exposure of emergency team members to these levels except for lifesaving missions. (Appropriate controls for emergency workers, include time limitations, respirators, and stable iodine.)	Although respirators and stable iodine should be used where effective to control dose to emergency team workers, thyroid dose may not be a limiting factor for lifesaving missions.
Whole body	75	Control exposure of emergency team members performing lifesaving missions to this level. (Control of time of exposure will be most effective.)	

[a] These actions are recommended for planning purposes. Protective action decisions at the time of the incident must take existing conditions into consideration.

[b] At the time of the incident, officials may implement low-impact protective actions in keeping with the principle of maintaining radiation exposures as low as reasonably achievable.

[c] No specific upper limit is given for thyroid exposure since in the extreme case complete thyroid loss might be an acceptable penalty for a life saved. However, this would not be necessary if respirators and/or thyroid protection for rescue personnel are available as the result of adequate planning.

Table 4.1.30 ICRP Recommendations for Protection Following Radiation Accidents (From ICRP Publication 63, 1993)

ICRP Publication 63 (1993)

Current recommendations on intervention levels for early and intermediate phases in ICRP Publication 63 (1993) include:

- dose levels above which intervention is almost always justified;
- ranges below justified intervention levels within which optimized intervention levels are expected to be found.

(1) Recommendations for early phase countermeasures
Justified intervention levels of:

- 50 mSv (5 rem) effective dose for sheltering;
- 500 mSv (50 rem) equivalent dose to thyroid for administration of stable iodine;
- 500 mSv (50 rem) effective dose or 5,000 mSv (500 rem) equivalent dose to skin for evacuation during first week.

Range of optimized values should be not more than factor of 10 lower than justified value for each type of intervention.

(2) Recommendations for intermediate phase countermeasures
For relocation:

- Justified intervention level of 1000 mSv (100 rem) effective dose;
- range of optimized values for 5–15 mSv (0.5–1.5 rem) effective dose per month for prolonged exposure.

For restriction of single foodstuff:

- justified intervention level of 10 mSv (1 rem) effective dose in a year;
- range of optimized values of radionuclide concentrations in foodstuff of 1,000–10,000 Bq/kg for beta/gamma-emitters and 10–100 Bq/kg for alpha emitters (1 Bq = 27 pCi).

ICRP also discusses available countermeasures for long-term recovery phase and optimization of dose level for withdrawal of countermeasures based on cost-benefit analysis, but specific recommendations on dose levels are not given.

Table 4.1.31 NCRP Guidance for Life-Saving Activities (NCRP 116, 1993)

- Only actions involving life-saving justify acute exposures that are significantly in excess of the annual effective dose limit.
- Exposures not involving life-saving should be controlled at occupational dose limits. Where this is not possible, a limit of 0.5 Sv effective dose and 5 Sv skin effective dose are recommended.

SECTION 2 IONIZING RADIATION—IN THE WORKPLACE

Standards and guidance for limiting ionizing radiation exposure to radiation workers include the Nuclear Regulatory Commission's revised 10 CFR Part 20 (1991) and Federal Radiation Protection Guidance, *Federal Register* 52:1987. Both are basic to occupational radiation protection in the United States. Similar guidance is also provided in NCRP 116.

A synopsis of each appears in the following tables. As is always the case for rules having legal status, the full regulation must be consulted along with license conditions and/or technical specifications to assure compliance.

''**Caution:** This Chapter cites the latest available recommendations from the International Commission on Radiological Protection (ICRP) and the National Council on Radiation Protection and Measurements (NCRP). However, Federal agencies have not yet adopted some of these recommendations; therefore, use of the ICRP Publications 60 and 61, and recommendations of NCRP Report 116 may not be consistent with Federal regulations and should not be used for regulatory compliance purposes until they are officially adopted by the appropriate regulatory agency.'' National Council on Radiation Protection and Measurements report (NCRP Report No. 106) is concerned with limits for exposure to ''hot particles'' on the skin and is also presented in this section.

Although its publication date was prior to the ICRP and NRC requirements, the NCRP's occupational guidance in its Report 91 is reflective of more recent developments than 10CFR20 and reflects parallel but differing recommendations to those of the ICRP. NCRP has discussed these recommendations further in NCRP Report 116.

TABLE OF CONTENTS

Table 4.2.1 Radiation Limits for Workers; Federal Radiation Protection Guidance (After *Federal Register* Vol. 52, No. 17; January 27, 1987) [52 FR 2822]

RECOMMENDATIONS

The following recommendations are made for the guidance of Federal agencies in their conduct of programs for the protection of workers from ionizing radiation.

1. There should not be any occupational exposure of workers to ionizing radiation without the expectation of an overall benefit from the activity causing the exposure. Such activities may be allowed provided exposure of workers is limited in accordance with these recommendations.
2. No exposure is acceptable without regard to the reason for permitting it, and it should be general practice to maintain doses from radiation to levels below the limiting values specified in these recommendations. Therefore, it is fundamental to radiation protection that a sustained effort be made to ensure that collective doses, as well as annual, committed, and cumulative lifetime individual doses, are maintained as low as reasonably achievable (ALARA), economic and social factors being taken into account.
3. In addition to the above recommendations, radiation doses received as a result of occupational exposure should not exceed the *limiting values for assessed dose to individual workers* specified below. These are given separately for protection against different types of effects on health and apply to the sum of doses from external and internal sources of radiation. For cancer and genetic effects, the limiting value is specified in terms of a derived quantity called the effective dose equivalent. For other health effects, the limiting values are specified in terms of the dose equivalent[a] to specific organs or tissues.

   Cancer and Genetic Effects. The effective dose equivalent, H_E, received in any year by an adult worker should not exceed 5 rem (0.05 sievert).[b] The effective dose equivalent is defined as:

   $$H_E = \sum_T W_T H_T,$$

   where W_T is a weighting factor and H_T is the annual dose equivalent averaged over organ or tissue T. Values of W_T, and their corresponding organs and tissues are the same as those in table 13.1.3.

   For the case of uniform irradiation of the whole body, where H_T may be assumed the same for each organ or tissue, the effective dose equivalent is equal to the dose equivalent to the whole body.

   Other Health Effects. In addition to the limitation on effective dose equivalent, the dose equivalent, H_T, received in any year by an adult worker should not exceed 15 rem (0.15 sievert) to the lens of the eye, and 50 rem (0.5 sievert) to any other organ, tissue (including the skin), or extremity[c] of the body.

   Additional limiting values which apply to the control of dose from internal exposure to radionuclides in the workplace are specified in Recommendation 4. Continued exposure of a worker at or near the limiting values for dose received in any year over substantial portions of a working lifetime should be avoided. This should normally be accomplished through application of appropriate radiation protection practices established under Recommendation 2.

---

[a] "Dose equivalent" is the product of the absorbed dose, a quality factor which varies with the energy and type of radiation, and other modifying factors, as defined by the International Commission on Radiation Units and Measurements.

[b] The unit of dose equivalent in the system of special quantities for ionizing radiation currently in use in the United States is the "rem." In the recently adopted international system (SI) the unit of dose equivalent is the "sievert." One sievert = 100 rem.

[c] "Extremity" means the forearms and hands, or the lower legs and feet.

NOTE: DOE Order 5480.11 titled "Radiation Protection for Occupational Workers" contains departmental guidance on radiation protection of occupational workers. A proposed rule, 10 CFR 835 (FR 64334 Vol. 56 No. 236 December 9, 1991), initiates the codification process.

Table 4.2.1 Radiation Limits for Workers; Federal Radiation Protection Guidance (Continued)

4. As the primary means for controlling internal exposure to radionuclides, agencies should require that radioactive materials be contained, to the extent reasonably achievable, so as to minimize intake. In controlling internal exposure consideration should also be given to concomitant external exposure.

   The control of necessary exposure of adult workers to radioactive materials in the workplace should be designed, operated, and monitored with sufficient frequency to ensure that, as a result of intake of radionuclides in a year, the following *limiting values for control of the workplace* are satisfied: (a) the anticipated magnitude of the committed effective dose equivalent from such intake plus any annual effective dose equivalent from external exposure will not exceed 5 rem (0.05 sievert), and (b) the anticipated magnitude of the committed dose equivalent to any organ or tissue from such intake plus any annual dose equivalent from external exposure will not exceed 50 rem (0.5 sievert). The committed effective dose equivalent from internal sources of radiation, $H_{E,50}$, is defined as:

$$H_{E,50} = \sum_{T} W_T H_{T,50},$$

   where W_T is defined as in Recommendation 3 and the committed dose equivalent, $H_{T,50}$, is the sum of all dose equivalents to organ or tissue T that may accumulate over an individual's anticipated remaining lifetime (taken as 50 years) from radionuclides that are retained in the body. These conditions on committed doses should provide the primary basis for the control of internal exposure to radioactive materials.[d]

   In circumstances where assessment of actual intake for an individual worker shows the above conditions for control of intake have not been met, agencies should require that appropriate corrective action be taken to assure control has been reestablished and that future exposure of the worker is appropriately managed. Provision should be made to assess annual dose equivalents due to radionuclides retained in the body from such intake for as long as they are significant for ensuring conformance with the limiting values specified in Recommendation 3.

5. Occupational dose equivalents to individuals under the age of eighteen should be limited to one-tenth of the values specified in Recommendations 3 and 4 for adult workers.

6. Exposure of an unborn child should be less than that of adult workers. Workers should be informed of current knowledge of risks to the unborn[e] from radiation and of the responsibility of both employers and workers to minimize exposure of the unborn. The dose equivalent to an unborn as a result of occupational exposure of a woman who has declared that she is pregnant should be maintained as low as reasonably achievable, and in any case should not exceed 0.5 rem (0.005 sievert) during the entire gestation period. Efforts should be made to avoid substantial variation above the uniform monthly exposure rate that would satisfy this limiting value. The limiting value for the unborn does not create a basis for discrimination, and should be achieved in conformance with the provisions of Title VII of the Civil Rights Act of 1964, as amended, regarding discrimination in employment practices, including hiring, discharge, compensation, and terms, conditions, or privileges of employment.

7. Individuals occupationally exposed to radiation and managers of activities involving radiation should be instructed on the basic risks to health from ionizing radiation and on basic radiation protection principles. This should, as a minimum, include instruction on the somatic (including *in utero*) and genetic effects of ionizing radiation, the recommendations set forth in Federal radiation protection guidance for occupational exposure and applicable regulations and operating procedures which implement this guidance, the general levels of risk and appropriate radiation protection practices for their work situations, and the responsibilities of individual workers to avoid and minimize exposure. The degree and type of instruction that is appropriate will depend on the potential radiation exposures involved.

(continued)

[d] When these conditions on intake of radioactive materials have been satisfied, it is not necessary to assess contributions from such intakes to annual doses in future years, and, as an operational procedure, such doses may be assigned to the year of intake for the purpose of assessing compliance with Recommendation 3.

[e] The term ''unborn'' is defined to encompass the period commencing with conception and ending with birth.

Table 4.2.1 Radiation Limits for Workers; Federal Radiation Protection Guidance (Continued)

8. Appropriate monitoring of workers and the work place should be performed and records kept to ensure conformance with these recommendations. The types and accuracy of monitoring methods and procedures utilized should be periodically reviewed to assure that appropriate techniques are being competently applied.

   Maintenance of a cumulative record of lifetime occupational doses for each worker is encouraged. For doses due to intake of radioactive materials, the committed effective dose equivalent and the quantity of each radionuclide in the body should be assessed and recorded, to the extent practicable. A summary of annual, cumulative, and committed effective dose equivalents should be provided each worker on no less than an annual basis; more detailed information concerning his or her exposure should be made available upon the worker's request.
9. Radiation exposure control measures should be designed, selected, utilized, and maintained to ensure that anticipated and actual doses meet the objectives of this guidance. Establishment of administrative control levels[f] below the limiting values for control may be useful and appropriate for achieving this objective. Reference levels[g] may also be useful to determine the need to take such actions as recording, investigation, and intervention. Since such administrative control and reference levels will often involve ALARA considerations, they may be developed for specific categories of workers or work situations. Agencies should encourage the establishment of measures by which management can assess the effectiveness of ALARA efforts, including, where appropriate, local goals for limiting individual and collective occupational doses. Supervision should be provided on a part-time, full-time, or task-by-task basis as necessary to maintain effective control over the exposure of workers.
10. The numerical values recommended herein should not be deliberately exceeded except during emergencies, or under unusual circumstances for which the Federal agency having jurisdiction has carefully considered the reasons for doing so in light of these recommendations. If Federal agencies authorize dose equivalents greater than these values for unusual circumstances, they should make any generic procedures specifying conditions under which such exposures may occur publicly available or make specific instances in which such authorization has been given a matter of public record.

The following notes are provided to clarify application of the above recommendations:

1. Occupational exposure of workers does not include that due to normal background radiation and exposure as a patient of practitioners of the healing arts.
2. The existing Federal guidance (34 FR 576 and 36 FR 12921) for limiting exposure of underground miners to radon decay products applies independently of, and is not changed by, these recommendations.
3. The values specified by the International Commission on Radiological Protection (ICRP) for quality factors and dosimetric conventions for the various types of radiation, the models for reference persons, and the results of their dosimetric methods and metabolic models may be used for determining conformance to these recommendations.
4. ''Annual Limits on Intake'' (ALIs)[h] and/or ''Derived Air Concentrations'' (DACs) may be used to limit radiation exposure from intake of or immersion in radionuclides. The ALI or DAC for a single radionuclide is the maximum intake in a year or average air concentration for a working year, respectively, for a reference person that, in the absence of any external dose, satisfies the conditions on committed effective dose equivalent and committed dose equivalent of Recommendation 4. ALIs and DACs may be derived for different chemical or physical forms of radioactive materials.
5. The numerical values provided by these recommendations do not apply to workers responsible for the management of or response to emergencies.

[f] Administrative control levels are requirements determined by a competent authority or the management of an institution or facility. They are not primary limits, and may therefore be exceeded, upon approval of competent authority or management, as situations dictate.

[g] Reference levels are not limits, and may be expressed in terms of any useful parameter. They are used to determine a course of action, such as recording, investigation, or intervention, when the value of a parameter exceeds, or is projected to exceed, the reference level.

[h] ICRP recommendation in ICRP 61 employs the same concept for ALIs. NCRP Publication 116 introduces ''Annual Reference Levels of Intake'' (ARLI) at the same effective dose level as recommended by the ICRP.

Table 4.2.2 Radiation Limits for Workers—Synopsis of Major Changes in the Revised 10 CFR Part 20 (Contributed by Robert E. Alexander, 1991; Updated by Alan K. Roecklein, 1996)

A major revision of 10 CFR Part 20, Standards for Radiation Protection, was published in the Federal Register on May 21, 1991 [Vol. 56, No. 98, 23360–23474]. Below is a synopsis of the important changes. NRC licensees were required to implement the new rule by January 1, 1994.

To assure compliance, the full regulation must be implemented along with license conditions and/or technical specifications. Official NRC guidance regarding acceptable methods of compliance may be found in the preamble also published with the rule and in a number of Regulatory Guides issued by the NRC in connection with publication of the rule. Copies of the Regulatory Guides mentioned in this section can be obtained by writing Office of Administration, Distribution and Services Section, U.S. Nuclear Regulatory Commission Washington D.C. 20555-0011 or by fax at (301) 415–2260. § 20.1006 states clearly that no interpretation of the meaning of the Part 20 regulations is binding upon the Commission other than written interpretations by the NRC General Counsel.

Several clarifying amendments have been made to 10 CFR Part 20, since its publication. Some of the more important changes are as follows:

- A declared pregnant woman must now inform the licensee, rather than her employer, because the licensee is responsible for controlling the dose to the embryo/fetus of the declarant.
- The definition of High Radiation Area and Very High Radiation Area are revised to make it clear that the relevant radiation levels are from sources external to the body.
- The term *eye dose equivalent* is deleted and the term *lens dose equivalent* is added to the regulations to eliminate confusion with ''effective dose equivalent'' (EDE).
- §20.1206(a) is revised so that PSEs are authorized in exceptional situations when alternatives that might avoid any additional dose estimated to result from the PSE are unavailable or impractical.
- In §20.1208, dose to the embryo/fetus, language in changed to ''dose equivalent'' to the embryo/fetus to clarify what dose is limited.
- Section 1502 (a)(2) is revised to separate minors and declared pregnant women to recognize that the term of pregnancy is 9 months rather than 1 year. The criteria for monitoring are also changed to ''likely to receive a dose equivalent in excess of 0.1 rem (1mSv).'' Thus the criterion for badging is set so that it is unlikely to exceed the public dose limit of 100 mRem rather than the more restrictive and difficult to measure 50 mRem.
- §20.2101, regarding records is revised to permit licensees to record quantities in SI units in parentheses following each of the special units specification paragraphs (a) of this section.

SUBPART A GENERAL PROVISIONS

§ 20.1001 Purpose

In paragraph (b) of this section the following statement appears: ''However, nothing in this part shall be construed as limiting action that may be necessary to protect health and safety.''

§ 20.1008 Implementation

This section explains the effect of the new rule on license conditions and technical specifications. This information may be summarized as follows. A technical specification or license condition must be replaced because of the rule only if both of two conditions are met: (1) the technical specification or license condition was not an exemption from the old rule, and (2) the new rule is more restrictive than the technical specification or license condition.

SUBPART B RADIATION PROTECTION PROGRAMS

§ 20.1101 Radiation Protection Programs

Licensees are required to develop, document and implement a radiation protection program ''commensurate with the scope and extent of licensed activities and sufficient to ensure compliance with'' the new Part 20. Documentation is covered in § 20.2102, where it is stated that ''the provisions of the program'' are to be included. Since implementation is required by the rule, the program commitments are inspectable and enforceable. However, the programs do not have to be submitted to the NRC for review and approval. These commitments are, in effect, licensee-specific regulations written and approved by the licensees themselves. This approach to regulation provides for a high degree of subjectivity as needed, for example, in the implementation of the occupational ALARA concept.

The content and implementation of a program have to be reviewed at least annually. § 20.2102 states that ''Audits and other reviews of program content and implementation'' must be recorded. For licensees subject to 10 CFR Part 50, the word *audit* indicates that reviews performed pursuant to § 20.1101 may be subject to the audit requirements of Appendix B, XVIII. The question of who can perform these reviews and audits is not specifically answered in the rule; this answer is expected to be forthcoming in a regulatory guide.

The new ALARA rule is also imposed by § 20.1101, which contains [for the first time in Part 20] a prescriptive directive that licensees are to use procedures and engineering controls to achieve occupational doses and doses to members of the public that are ALARA. Since implementation of the ALARA concept is highly subjective, the ALARA rule uses indefinite, performance terminology that can be made more specific by individual licensees as they develop this section of their programs. *Sound radiation protection principles* must be used *to the extent practicable.*

The new Part 20 is based primarily on ICRP Publications 26 and 30. In ICRP Publication 26 occupational dose limits are coupled with *optimization,* a term synonymous with ALARA. However, optimization is defined as a technique to identify, for a dose-reduction measure, the point above which the dose allowed is not ALARA because the dose is too high and below which the dose is not ALARA because the cost is too high. Optimization raises a question as to whether, in the name of ALARA, dose reduction efforts should be continued beyond the point where costs become too high. The Commission's position on this question regarding public protection is given in the preamble as quoted below:

> The Commission agrees that there would be advantages to establishing such a ''floor,'' below which efforts to further reduce doses would not be necessary.

This statement indicates that, for implementation of the occupational ALARA concept, the Commission also would not necessarily object to written ALARA programs which include a reasonable ''floor'' for worker protection.

Practicable means possible or feasible, able to be done, capable of being used. *Practical* is synonymous with judicious [the use of discrete judgement] and sensible [the use of sound reason and common sense]. The word *practical* is much more consistent with the term *reasonably achievable,* with the ALARA definition in § 20.1003, with statements made in the preamble about ALARA, and with the term *optimization* as defined by the ICRP. Many NRC personnel are known to favor judicious and sensible dose-reduction decisions.

SUBPART C OCCUPATIONAL DOSE LIMITS

§ 20.1201 Occupational Dose Limits for Adults

These limits are applicable to anyone other than members of the public. The limits for minors and declared pregnant women are lower than those established for other workers. Subsequent to publishing the new Part 20 changes were made to the definition of occupational and public dose so that both are independent of where an individual is and are determined by whether or not the dose is received in the course of employment in which the individuals assigned duties involve exposure to radiation or to radioactive material. 10 CFR Part 19, § 19.12, now requires training in radiation protection commensurate with the hazards present for anyone who in the course of employment is likely to receive in a year an occupational dose in excess of 100 mRem (1mSv). Paragraph 20.1201(a) establishes an annual dose limit of 5 rems for the total effective dose equivalent (TEDE). The TEDE is the sum of the deep dose equivalent (DDE), measured at a depth of 1 cm, and the committed effective dose equivalent (CEDE) to a person. If only one organ is significantly irradiated, the CEDE is the familiar committed dose equivalent (CDE) multiplied by the specified weighting, or radiation sensitivity, factor w_T for the organ (see Table 13.1.3). The CEDE for a person, according to ICRP Publication 26, is the sum of such CEDEs for 11 organs. No organ or tissue is allowed to receive more than 50 rems, DDE plus CDE, in a year. Since it is possible with certain radionuclides to exceed this limit even when the TEDE is less than 5 rems, 50 rems in a year serves as a regulatory cap. It is intended to prevent non-stochastic effects. Neutron quality factors remain essentially unchanged.

The annual limit for the lens is 15 rems DE at a depth of 0.3 cm. For the skin, the annual limit is 50 rems shallow dose equivalent (SDE); the dose to the extremities is, of course, controlled by the skin dose limit, measured at 0.007 cm. § 20.1201 (c) states that the DDE and SDE ''must be for the part of the body receiving the highest exposure.'' The extremities now include the joints and more distal tissues.

The definitions in § 20.1003 have removed ''or less'' from the specified depths.

§ 20.1202 Compliance with Requirements for Summation of External and Internal Doses

In § 20.1502, licensees are required to provide individual monitoring for a worker likely to receive more than 10% of the annual limits on external dose; and, for a worker likely to receive in a year more than 10% of the radionuclide intake limit, monitoring of the intake and assessment of the CEDE is required. If monitoring for both external and internal dose is required, the doses must be summed to demonstrate compliance with the TEDE limit. Once the DDE and CEDE are determined, summation is a simple exercise in arithmetic. It is the new requirement to determine, record and report the CEDE that requires preparation.

Regulatory Guide 8.34 ''Monitoring Criteria and Methods to Calculate Occupational Radiation Doses.'' was published in July 1992 and provides additional guidance on this subject.

§ 20.1204 Determination of Internal Exposure

Suitable and timely measurements of radionuclide concentrations in air, of radionuclide depositions in the body, or combinations of these are required to determine compliance with the TEDE limit. In several places in Part 20 it is made clear that 1 Annual Limit on Intake (ALI) is equal to 2000 DAC-hours, and that each of these is in turn equal to 5 rem CEDE. DAC is the acronym for Derived Air Concentration, the term replacing Maximum Permissible Concentration. Once the intake is decided upon, calculation of the CEDE is also a matter of simple arithmetic.

A stochastic ALI is defined as the microcurie intake in a year that will deliver to the reference man a CEDE of 5 rem. A non-stochastic ALI is the intake in a year that will deliver a CDE of 50 rem to the most highly exposed organ. The Part 20 ALI for a radionuclide is the smaller of the stochastic or non-stochastic ALIs. Appendix B provides the stochastic ALI for each nuclide and the non-stochastic ALI as well when and only when it is the smaller value. Calculation of a missing non-stochastic ALIs is simple; it is the ratio of the 50-rem limit to the largest dose conversion factor h, in rem/microcurie inhaled, listed for any organ for the nuclide. The values of h used by the ICRP in the calculation of the ALIs may be found in ''Limiting Values of Radionuclide Intake and Air Concentration and Dose Conversion Factors for Inhalation, Submersion, and Ingestion,'' EPA-520/1-88-020, Federal Guidance Report No. 11, September, 1988. Acceptable methods of converting bioassay results to intake may be found in ''Interpretation of Bioassay Measurements,'' NUREG/CR-4884, July, 1987

Although for a given nuclide the non-stochastic ALI may be the smallest, licensees are not required to use this ALI in the calculation of the CEDE. Pursuant to § 20.1204(h)(2) the larger stochastic ALI may be used in such cases, resulting in a smaller (and correct) CEDE. The only condition is that it must be demonstrated that no organ or tissue received, from all radionuclides combined, a CDE larger than 50 rem.

Regulatory Guide 8.34 ''Monitoring Criteria and Methods to Calculate Occupational Radiation Doses.'' was published in July 1992 and provides additional guidance on this subject.

§ 20.1206 Planned Special Exposures

A licensee may permit a worker in one year to receive, in addition to the limits specified in Paragraph 20.1201(a), planned special exposures [PSEs] not to exceed these limits provided that the lifetime doses from PSEs do not exceed five times these limits. The intent is to provide operational flexibility as might be essential, for example, for plant safety purposes. PSE doses are recorded separately and have no effect on routine exposure accounting. PSEs are approved [in advance and in writing] by the licensee rather than the NRC; a contractor employee's PSE must be approved by the actual employer also. Stringent conditions are imposed.

PSEs may be approved only under exceptional conditions and must comply with at least one of two tests: alternatives must be unavailable or impractical. If a licensee should authorize a PSE, and as a result a worker received more than 5 rem TEDE from routine doses and the PSE combined, it would mean an overexposure unless the NRC agreed, after the fact, that all of the viable alternatives were either unavailable or impractical.

Work involving PSEs may be assigned; the regulation does not require volunteers. PSEs are considered to be safe because the risk is proportional to the lifetime dose rather than to the dose during any one year. Affected workers must be informed of the purpose of the planned operation and of their radiation risk. They must also be instructed in measures to maintain their doses ALARA. In an unusual departure from common federal agency non-encroachment practices, the NRC requires licensees to include associated industrial hygiene and safety hazards in the information given to the affected workers.

Certain workers are not allowed to receive the entire PSE doses. Excess doses, i.e., the amount of dose in excess of regulatory limits that has been received as a result of overexposures, accidents or emergencies must be subtracted. For example, the excess TEDE received during the current year must be subtracted from the 5-rem PSE limit, and the excess TEDE received at any time must be subtracted from the 25-rem lifetime PSE limit. A worker for whom a complete exposure record was unobtainable is not eligible for PSEs [§ 20.2104(e)(2)]. See also § 20.2104(b) regarding the determination of prior dose.

The licensee must provide a dose report to the affected worker(s) within 30 days from the date of the exposure. § 20.2204 requires a written report to the NRC within 30 days of the PSE. This report must include all of the extensive information required by § 20.2105 to be recorded:

1. The exceptional circumstances, i.e., the alternatives analysis;
2. Copies of the signed authorizations;
3. What actions were necessary;
4. Why they were necessary;
5. How doses were maintained ALARA;
6. What individual and collective doses were expected and those actually received.

Regulatory Guide 8.35, ''Planned Special Exposures'' was published in June 1992 and provides additional guidance on the use of PSEs.

§ 20.1207 Occupational Dose Limits for Minors

The dose limits for minors are 10% of those established for adults.

§ 20.1208 Dose to an Embryo/Fetus

The human organism from conception to birth is defined in § 20.1003 as an embryo/fetus. Although the term *dose* is used in Paragraph 20.1208 in connection with the limit for the embryo/fetus, it is clear from the context that the word is not used as defined in § 20.1003, i.e., as a generic term including the absorbed dose, DE, EDE, CDE, CEDE, or TEDE. The unit *rem* is used, but a clear distinction of the quantity is provided only in the case of radiation originating outside the body of the mother, viz., the DDE. For radiation originating from radionuclides inside the mother's body or within the embryo/fetus itself, use of the absorbed dose would preclude appropriate addition of the different types of radiation. Since weighting factors have not been determined for the organs of the embryo/fetus, the effective dose is not in any manner intended. Since the term *committed* as used with *dose* is defined in § 20.1003 as specifying a 50-year integrated dose, and since a child's status as a fetus ends at birth, the committed dose is not intended. Regulatory Guide 8.36, ''Radiation Dose to the Embryo/Fetus,'' was published in July 1992 and confirms these considerations.

This limit is 0.5 rem. It includes three sources. First, sources external to the mother's body; the dose to be assigned for the embryo/fetus is the DDE to the mother. Second, sources internal to the mother but external to the embryo/fetus, such as gamma emitters deposited in organs near the uterus and in the placenta. Third, radionuclides transferred from the blood of the mother to the blood of the embryo/fetus and subsequently deposited in the organs of the embryo/fetus. The regulatory guide provides acceptable DE determination assumptions, methods and the necessary parameters to perform the required calculations.

A cushion is provided in an attempt to preserve the employability of the mother. The embryo/fetus is allowed to receive an additional 50 mrem even though the limit has already been exceeded at the time the pregnancy is declared. If at this time the dose is just below 0.5 rem, the cushion is also allowed. Allowing the cushion was considered to be safe because microcephaly, the biological effect to be prevented, is believed to have a threshold much higher than the limit. This effect has not been observed at absorbed doses of less than about 20 rad. The preamble states that the threshold is believed to lie between 20 and 40 rad.

Section 20.1208(b) requires licensees to make efforts to, in effect, avoid doses to declared pregnant women in excess of about 55 mrem in a month. The primary problem addressed here is avoidance of a large dose to the embryo/fetus during the time microcephaly is most likely to be caused by radiation, i.e., the eighth to the fifteenth week. The rule can be successful after the declaration of pregnancy but not before recognition of the pregnancy by the mother. Protection of the embryo/fetus between the eighth week and pregnancy recognition is not regulated in a special manner by Part 20 but may be provided through cooperation between the prospective mother and her employer.

SUBPART D RADIATION DOSE LIMITS FOR MEMBERS OF THE PUBLIC

For the first time a dose limit is established in Part 20 for members of the public. [The 0.5-rem value in the old Part 20 was a licensing criterion.] § 20.1301 establishes the limit as 0.1 rem TEDE in a year. The familiar limit of 2 mrem in an hour in any unrestricted area is retained. The quantity is not given, but external sources are specified. Since the DDE quantity is not used, the SDE is by inference the appropriate quantity, meaning that beta radiation must be included. No distance from the radiation source is specified. Thus if the source is located off site, NRC inspectors are authorized to select arbitrarily the distance at which compliance is to be determined. The former limit of 0.1-rem in 7 consecutive days has been eliminated since this dose is now the annual limit.

The newly defined *controlled area* lies between the restricted and unrestricted area, including administrative offices, grounds, etc. Personnel in controlled areas are limited to 0.1 rem TEDE in a year unless they are performing duties assigned by the licensee.

Two methods of compliance with the 0.1-rem TEDE limit are given as licensee options in § 20.1302(b). Licensees may demonstrate that the individual member of the public receiving the highest, actual TEDE received less than 0.1 rem during the year. Alternatively, a licensee may demonstrate: (1) that the concentration of liquid and gaseous effluents, averaged over 1 year, did not exceed Appendix B values (these values are based on a TEDE of 50 mrem); and (2) that 2-mrem SDE in an hour could not have been received by an individual continuously present in an unrestricted area; and (3) that the SDE in a year to such an individual could not have exceeded 50 mrem. Two additional methods of compliance are given in the preamble to the rule: (1) compliance with the EPA regulation 40 CFR Part 190, and (2) compliance with the design criteria given in 10 CFR Part 50, Appendix I.

It should be noted that almost all exposure limits in Part 20 are specified as doses rather than as dose rates. NRC inspectors are not authorized to impose periods of time shorter than those specified in the rule unless shorter periods appear in license conditions, orders, or other Commission directives.

SUBPART F SURVEYS AND MONITORING

§ 20.1501 General

Licensees are required to perform surveys as reasonable under the circumstances to evaluate existing radiation levels, concentration and quantities of radioactive materials that can be measured. They must also survey for *potential* radiological hazards that could be present and must in some manner be anticipated during the survey process. Pursuant to 20.2103(a), survey recording requirements apply to potential hazard surveys; in § 20.1003 the definition of *surveys* now includes potential hazards. No follow-up action is specified in Part 20, but inspectors will undoubtedly look into this aspect of protection. Elimination of the hazard is preferred but, if that is not reasonable, action can be taken to reduce the probability of trouble and to ensure that those affected know what to do just in case. By excluding potential hazards that have an exceedingly low probability of occurrence or would have exceedingly low consequences, this new rule can have a favorable and well accepted impact on a radiation protection program.

The instrument calibration rule given in § 20.1501(b) is quite liberal; it does not require, for example, that the strength of the calibration source be known. Licensees, of course, are not prohibited from developing their own ''rules'' in their written programs. On a positive note, calibration is not required for instruments that are used only as detectors [i.e., not used to quantitatively measure dose or disintegration rates].

Regulatory Guide 8.34 ''Monitoring Criteria and Methods to Calculate Occupational Radiation Doses'' was published in July 1992 and provides additional guidance on this subject.

SUBPART G CONTROL OF EXPOSURE FROM EXTERNAL SOURCES IN RESTRICTED AREAS

§ 20.1601 Control of Access to High Radiation Areas

The term ''entrance and access point'' has been redefined to include portals (undefined) of sufficient size to permit human entry irrespective of the intended use of the portal. The term is used in § 20.1601(a) where it is stated that one or more of three specific features must be provided at each entrance or access point for a high radiation area. Although these features are not new, application at portals is. Many licenses contain elaborations based on the old rule. In accordance with § 20.1008(d), if a license condition provided an exemption from the old rule, the exemption remains in effect. Otherwise, if the expanded definition will make the new rule more restrictive than the license condition, the license condition will be superseded (§ 20.1008 (b) and compliance under the new definition may be enforced. The three specific features mentioned above are: (1) an automatic dose-rate reduction device upon entry, (2) visible or audible alarm signals, or (3) locked entryways. [As used in this paragraph immediately above, the term license condition includes technical specifications.]

Continuous electronic surveillance capable of preventing unauthorized entry has been added as an acceptable alternate to the three features.

§ 20.1602 Control of Access to Very High Radiation Areas

Each licensee is required, at entrance and access points to very high radiation areas, to institute measures additional (unspecified) to those provided for high radiation areas.

§ 20.1602 Control of Access to Very High Radiation Areas—Irradiators

In paragraph (a), subparagraph (2)(ii) now requires that the ''other authorized individual'' who must be alerted by entry alarms has to be physically present.

Regulatory Guide 8.38, ''Control of Access to High and Very High Radiation Areas in Nuclear Power Plants'' was published in June 1993 and provides additional guidance on this issue.

SUBPART H RESPIRATORY PROTECTION AND CONTROLS TO RESTRICT INTERNAL EXPOSURE IN RESTRICTED AREAS

Subpart H is currently under revision by the NRC as well as Regulatory Guide 8.15 and NUREG 0041. The changes under consideration incorporate recent ANSI recommendations and would simplify the rule structure.

§ 20.1701 Use of Process or Other or Other Engineering Controls

This rule requires licensees to use controls such as containment and/or ventilation to limit concentrations of radioactive material in the air in restricted areas. The prominent position of the rule in the Subpart indicates the Commission's position that keeping radionuclides out of the workplace air is intended to be the first line of defense.

§ 20.1702 Use of Other Controls

This section divides the workplace into two types of areas: those in which the concentration is sufficiently low that posting as an Airborne Radioactivity Area is not required, and areas where such posting is required. [Posting is required if a worker without a respirator could receive an exposure exceeding 12 DAC-hours (0.6% ALI) while present during a week.] Under specific conditions, a licensee may be able to demonstrate that it is not *practicable,* using such controls, to maintain concentrations sufficiently low that posting is not required. When this happens licensees may employ alternative measures [access control, exposure time limitations, respirators, or other controls] to limit intakes. The position assigned to respirators in these sections suggests a Commission position that they are virtually to be the last resort. The monitoring effort [air sampling, bioassays] where posting is required must exceed the effort where posting is not required.

This section contains a directive that the total effective dose equivalent [TEDE] must be ALARA when the alternative methods are relied upon. Under certain conditions a respirator can slow a worker's progress and increase the time needed to complete a task. If the concentration is low and the external radiation dose rate is high, the TEDE can be increased by the respirator, potentially to the disadvantage of the worker's health. Compliance with this rule would prevent an unnecessarily high TEDE as caused by overly zealous protection against internal dose.

§ 20.1703 Use of Individual Respiratory Protective Equipment

Paragraph (a) is written in a manner to eliminate a practice by a few licensees who divide plant areas into those where the Commission's respirator rules apply (because protection factors are employed) and those where the rules do not. Any licensee who uses respiratory protective equipment to limit intakes pursuant to § 20.1702 is now subject to all of the provisions of § 20.1703.

Subparagraph (a)(3)(i) establishes stringent performance requirements for air sampling: it must be sufficient to identify the hazard, permit proper equipment selection, and evaluate actual intakes. The rule does not use the word *representative* and deliberately stops short of requiring the use of lapel air samplers. However, the word *actual* is exacting, inspectable, and enforceable. [The subparagraph uses the word *potential* in reference to hazard identification; air samples, of course, provide information about existing hazards only, and licensees will undoubtedly be expected to perform air sampling to identify these hazards.]

Subparagraph (a)(3)(ii) requires bioassays, as appropriate, in the conduct of the respiratory protection program. A very clear interpretation appears on page 23377 of the Federal Register Notice preamble. A bioassay is required, to verify the performance of the respirator, if the intake would have exceeded 10% of the ALI before credit was taken for a protection factor.

Subparagraph (a)(3)(v) now requires a determination by a physician that a worker is physically able to use respiratory protective equipment *before* initial fit testing.

Paragraph (b) is changed in only one important respect. A sentence has been added which permits a licensee to use a respirator with a protection factor too low to comply with the ''peak concentration'' rule [which has been retained] if that is necessary to maintain the TEDE ALARA.

§ 20.1704(b)(2) warns that the Commission may impose further restrictions to limit the extent to which respiratory protective equipment is employed rather than process or other engineering controls.

SUBPART I STORAGE AND CONTROL OF LICENSED MATERIAL

For *any* amount of licensed radioactive material in controlled or unrestricted areas, §§ 20.1801 and 20.1802 require licensees to secure stored materials from unauthorized removal or access and to maintain constant surveillance over materials not in storage.

SUBPART J PRECAUTIONARY PROCEDURES

§ 20.1901 Caution Signs

Black is now allowed for the radiation symbol. Where high temperatures exist, no color is required. Etching and stamping is permitted. Although the wording on required signs is prescribed, licensees are permitted to add wording as considered necessary to warn against potential hazards.

§ 20.1902 Posting Requirements

An improvement has been made regarding the requirements for posting radiation and high radiation areas. The old Part 20 required posting if a major portion of the body could in an hour receive the specified dose criterion. Inspectors have tended to insist on posting based on contact dose rate measurements. The new Part 20 definitions specify a distance of 30 cm for the measurements—>5 mrem DE in an hour for radiation areas and >100 mrem DE in an hour for high radiation areas. Since the DE quantity includes the DDE and SDE, beta radiation is included in the posting criteria. The criterion of >100 mrem in 5 consecutive days has been dropped. A change was made in the required wording for radiation areas; use of the word ''caution'' is specified, prohibiting continued use of the word ''danger''. For high radiation area signs, licensees may choose between the words ''caution'' and ''danger.'' But it is the preference of the NRC staff that ''caution'' be reserved for the lower dose rate areas, with ''danger'' reserved for higher dose rates; dose rates in high radiation areas can be as high as 500 rads per hour at 1 meter. Very high radiation areas are now defined (>500 rads in an hour at 1 meter), and the prescribed wording for the sign is ''grave danger.''

Posting as an airborne radioactivity area is required where the DAC is exceeded and where a worker with no respirator could receive while present 0.6% of an ALI or 12 DAC-hours in a week. Other than changes in the concentration values, there is essentially no change from the previous requirement.

Under the old rule posting as a radioactive material(s) area was required where 10 times Appendix C values or more were used or stored; in the cases of natural uranium or thorium the requirement was 100 times Appendix C values or more. The new rule uses ''10 times Appendix C values'' for all nuclides including natural uranium and thorium. For both natural uranium and natural thorium, in the old and new Appendix C, the value is 100 μCi. Thus posting is now required for smaller quantities of these materials—by an order of magnitude. Licenses should check other radionuclide changes as well.

§ 20.1903 Exemptions to Posting Requirements

One posting exemption has been eliminated. In § 20.204(d) the old rule exempted from posting and access control requirements areas that were high radiation areas only because of materials packaged and labeled for shipment in accordance with DOT regulations. This rule now appears in § 20.1601(e), and the exemption is for access control only.

With regard to patients in hospitals, words added to the new rule limit that exemption from posting to patients who ''have been treated with sealed or unsealed radioactive material in quantities less than 30 millicuries, or the measured dose rate at 1 meter from the patient is less than 0.005 rem (0.05 mSv) per hour . . .'' and to conditions under which the ALARA provisions of the licensee's radiation protection program have been met.

§ 20.1904 Labeling Containers

Where the labeling of containers is required (no change), the new § 20.1904(a) includes an additional example of the type of information that must be provided, viz., the radionuclide(s) present. In the preamble, page 23380, it is stated that ''mixed fission products'' and ''fission and activation products'' may be regarded for these labeling purposes as radionuclides.

§ 20.1905 Exemptions to Labeling Requirements

Exempt concentration values are now specified in a new Table 3 of Appendix B. Examples have been added in paragraph (e) to clarify types of containers exempt from labeling where a readily available written record is used to warn workers rather than labels. A new paragraph (f) exempts from labeling installed manufacturing or process equipment.

§ 20.1906 Procedures for Receiving and Opening Packages

The package reception and notification requirements of paragraph (a) of this section now apply only to Type A quantities as defined in § 71.4 and Appendix A of Part 71. The package monitoring requirement is extended to include those labeled as containing radioactive material. When a package requiring monitoring is delivered after normal working hours, monitoring is now required not later than 3 hours from the beginning of the next working day; the 18-hour rule is eliminated for such cases, but the limiting ''as soon as practicable'' rule remains.

SUBPART K WASTE DISPOSAL

The most important change in this Subpart for many licensees is the elimination in § 20.2003(a) of the authorization to discharge (with one exception) *any* amount of readily dispersible insoluble radioactive material into sanitary sewer systems. With this absolute prohibition, some licensees are subject to the seemingly impossible task of demonstrating compliance for diminutive insoluble particles of low curie content. The exception is insoluble material in readily dispersible biological material.

SUBPART L RECORDS

§ 20.2101 General Provisions

Paragraph (a) requires licensees to continue using the special units, curie, rad and rem, and to clearly indicate the units of all quantities on records required by Part 20. Paragraph (b) requires a clear distinction among the quantities entered on records required by Part 20, for example, when the word ''dose'' or the unit ''rem'' are used. The use of other units concurrently with the special units is now encouraged. The roentgen is not mentioned at all in Part 20 or the preamble. It can be used concurrently with the rem, if the licensee determines the relationship between the two.

Clear indication of quantity units and clear distinction among quantities can in many cases be achieved: (1) by including the quantity intended whenever the rem unit is used, (2) by using the word ''dose'' as defined in § 20.1003, i.e., as a collective noun including all the dose quantities, and (3) by using the appropriate quantity acronym rather than the word ''dose'' when the quantity is not clear in the text.

§ 20.2102 Records of Radiation Protection Programs

This section refers to the requirement in § 20.1101(a) to prepare a written radiation protection program. Regarding the content, the program description is to include ''the provisions of the program.'' Regarding the annual program review, the word audit is also used here, possibly bringing to bear any NRC directives on required auditing.

§ 20.2103 Records of Surveys

While this section is not changed, the definition of ''surveys'' in § 20.1003 has been changed to include associated calculations and potential hazard surveys. § 20.1501, cited in this section, also includes potential radiological hazard surveys.

§ 20.2104 Determination of Prior Occupational Dose

Subsequent to publication of the new Part 20, a change was made to §20,2104 (a). The words ''. . . may enter the licensee's restricted or controlled area and . . .'' are deleted so that determination of prior occupational dose is required only if an individual is likely to receive an occupational dose requiring monitoring pursuant to §20.1502. Subparagraph (a)(2) requires licensees to ''attempt'' to obtain the lifetime cumulative dose of a worker for whom monitoring is required. Subparagraph (c)(2) limits this attempt to contacting the most recent employer. Recording of the dose information on NRC Form 4 is required by paragraph (d) and space is also provided on NRC Form 5. However, no use is made of these lifetime data in the new Part 20 regulatory control program where the focus is on the current year. Lifetime dose records as accepted must be signed by the individual and countersigned by an appropriate official of the most recent employer. The countersignature is not required for accepting current-year records.

Paragraph (c) permits licensees to accept prior-dose records from the ''most recent employer'', possibly leaving the impression that accepting records from the facility at which a worker was most recently exposed would not be acceptable. This interpretation was not intended. Accepting records from the facility at which a worker was most recently exposed is not mentioned and is not prohibited.

§ 20.2106 Records of Individual Monitoring Results

Licensees are required to maintain annual records of doses received by all individuals for whom dose or intake determination was required, e.g., those likely to receive in excess of 10% of the applicable limits. Records of doses received during planned special exposures, accidents and emergency conditions are also required. These records must include:

1. The DDE, eye DE, SDE to the skin, SDE to the extremities;
2. The intake or body burden;
3. The CEDE;
4. Information specific for the individual that was used to calculate the CEDE;
5. The TEDE (if both external and internal monitoring was required);
6. The sum of the DDE and the CDE to the organ receiving the highest total.

The CEDE and CDE are assigned to the year of intake; the intakes are not considered again in subsequent NRC Form 5.

Paragraph (c) incorporates NRC Form 5 instructions into Part 20 (but not NRC Form 4). Paragraph (e) requires the NRC Form 5 for an embryo/fetus to be maintained with that of the declared pregnant woman. The declaration of pregnancy must also be kept on file, separately if desired.

Revision 1 to regulatory Guide 8.7, ''Instructions for Recording and Reporting Occupational Radiation Exposure Data,'' was published June 1992 and provides detailed guidance for complying with these requirements.

§ 20.2107 Records of Dose to Individual Members of the Public

Licensees are now required to maintain records sufficient to demonstrate compliance with the new 0.1-rem (TEDE) annual limit for members of the public.

§ 20.2110 Form of Records

The following new requirements have been added:

> ''The record may also be stored in electronic media with the capability for producing legible, accurate and complete records during the required retention period. Records such as letters, drawings, specifications, must include all pertinent information such as stamps, initials, and signatures. The licensee shall maintain adequate safeguards against tampering with and loss of records.''

SUBPART M REPORTS

§ 20.2201 Reports of Theft or Loss of Licensed Material

Immediate notification of the NRC Operations Center (301-951-0550) is now required if the aggregate quantity lost or stolen is equal to or greater than 1,000 times the quantity specified in Appendix C. A 30-day follow-up report is required if the quantity still missing exceeds 10 times the Appendix C value.

§ 20.2202 Notification of Incidents

Immediate notification criteria are now: a TEDE of 25 rem, an eye DE of 75 rem, or an SDE (sic) of 250 rad. Twenty-four hour notification criteria are now: a TEDE of 5 rem, an eye DE of 15 rem, and an SDE of 50 rem.

If a release of radioactive material *inside* or outside of a restricted area occurs, immediate notification of the NRC Operations Center by telephone is required if an individual present for twenty-four hours could have received an intake of 5 ALIs (about 417 × DAC averaged over twenty-four hours). Twenty-four notification is required if this intake could have been 1 ALI (about 83.4 × DAC). These notifications are not required if the release occurs in a location ''where personnel are not normally stationed during routine operations.''

§ 20.2203 Reports of Exposures, Radiation Levels, and Concentrations of Radioactive Material Exceeding the Limits

Paragraph (a) now provides (in most cases) more time for submitting reportable event notifications. The 30-day time period now begins at the time the licensee learns of the event rather than at the time the event occurs. The following new limits are now included in the list of reportable events: the TEDE limit for adults, minors, embryo/fetus of a declared pregnant woman, and an individual member of the public.

In an important departure from the old rule, a licensee who submits a report pursuant to this section must include the schedule for taking corrective action to achieve conformance with regulations and/or license conditions violated [§ 20.2203(b)(1)(iv)].

Section 20.2205, ''Reports to Individuals of Exceeding Dose Limits,'' has been added. When a licensee is required to report to the Commission any exposure of an identified occupationally exposed individual or an identified member of the public, the licensee must also provide a copy of the report to the individual.

§ 20.2206 Reports of Individual Monitoring

The annual statistical summary and termination dose reports to the NRC have been eliminated. However, for each individual for whom monitoring was required, an annual report to the NRC containing the information recorded on NRC Form 5 is required for certain licensees. Licensees are given an additional month to submit this report, i.e., until April 30th. The revised § 19.13(b) requires an annual report to each worker for whom dose recording was required. This report must contain the information required to be recorded by § 20.2106. The use of electronic media for submitting reports to the NRC is authorized.

Table 4.2.3 ICRP Dose Quantities for Protection Against External Radiations Guidance on the 1990 Recommendations of ICRP (With Permission Clark M.J. NRPB Bulletin No. 141, April 1993)

The Board's guidance on dose quantities used in radiological protection[a] supports the Statement and associated recommendations. This comprehensive document replaces earlier guidance[b] given on this topic. It is important to note that, until the Health and Safety Executive gives formal direction on the new quantities, it is necessary to retain the use of the current dosimetric quantities for monitoring in the workplace. Current legislation in the UK concerning radiological protection is in accordance with the Basic Safety Standards[c] of the European Communities which are based on the previous ICRP recommendations of Publication 26. Implementation of the new ICRP recommendations into legislation will take some time.

Basic Dosimetric Quantities for Radiological Protection

The fundamental dosimetric quantity in radiological protection is the absorbed dose, D, the energy absorbed per unit mass. This quantity has units of joules per kilogram (J kg^{-1}) which are given the special name of gray (Gy). Absorbed dose has traditionally been defined at a point in tissue but, in Publication 60, ICRP defined a quantity D_T as the average absorbed dose over a tissue or organ for the purpose of risk estimation. The use of an average dose as an indicator of the probability of subsequent deleterious health effects of radiation is justified from the biological evidence for the occurrence of stochastic health effects.

Biological studies have shown that the probability of stochastic health effects of radiation depends not only on the absorbed dose but also on the type and energy of the radiation causing the dose. This can be accommodated by weighting the absorbed dose by a factor related to the type of radiation and its energy. Prior to Publication 60 ICRP recommended that the weighting factor be applied to the absorbed dose at a point, and it was called the quality factor, Q. The weighted absorbed dose was referred to as the dose equivalent. In Publication 60 a new quantity of equivalent dose was defined, with absorbed dose averaged over a tissue or organ and modified by a radiation weighting factor, W_R, due to radiation of type R incident on the body or emitted by radionuclides in the body. The symbol H_T is used for equivalent dose and is given by

$$H_T = \sum_R W_R D_{T,R}$$

where $D_{T,R}$ is the absorbed dose averaged over a tissue or organ T, due to radiation of type R. ICRP recommended the use of radiation weighting factors, W_Rs, based on a review of the biological information, a variety of exposure circumstances and calculations of operational dose equivalent quantities.

The value of the radiation weighting factor for a specified type and energy of radiation has been selected by ICRP to reflect the relative biological effectiveness (RBE) of the radiation in producing stochastic health effects at low doses. Observed RBE values for stochastic effects of ionising radiation cover a range and, following an extensive review in Publication 60, ICRP specified values for W_R, based on the type and energy of the radiation incident on the body or of the radiation emitted by radionuclides in the body. The Board has recommended the adoption of the values for W_R given in Table 4.2.3.1.

[a] NPRB. "Dose quantities for protection against external radiations." *Doc NRPB*, **4:** 3; 1993.

[b] NPRB. "New quantities recommended by ICRU for practical use in radiological protection and their implementation in the United Kingdom." Chilton; *NRPB-GS5,* 1986.

[c] CEC. Basic Safety Standards. *Off J Euro Commun* **L246; 23:** 1 72 (1980).

[d] ICRU. "Determination of dose equivalents resulting from external radiation sources." Bethesda, Maryland, ICRU Report 39 (1985).

[e] ICRU. Measurement of dose equivalents resulting from external photon and electron radiation. Bethesda, Maryland, ICRU Report 47 (1992).

[f] ICRP. Statement from the 1985 Paris Meeting. ICRP Publication 45. *Ann ICRP,* **15:** No. 3, i–ii; 1985.

Table 4.2.3.1 ICRP Values for w_R[a]

Type and Energy Range	Radiation Weighting Factor, w_R
Photons, all energies	1
Electrons and muons, all energies	1
Protons, other than recoil protons of energy > 2 MeV	5
Alpha particles, fission fragments, heavy nuclei	20
Neutrons of energy E (MeV)[a]	$5 + 17 \exp[-(\ln 2E)^2/6]$

[a] Here the Board has placed emphasis on the smooth fit function for w_R values for neutrons, instead of the step function values given in Table A.2 of ICRP Publication 60. The Board considers that the difficulties in applying step function values in practice mean that the numerical smooth fit equation is more suitable.

ICRP has recommended a new relationship between the quality factor, $Q(L)$, and unrestricted linear energy transfer, L, to reflect the higher RBE values for intermediate energy neutrons. A simple relationship has been chosen to allow for the lack of precise information on radiation effects in man (for example, there are no human RBE data for neutrons), and in appreciation of practical aspects of radiation protection. Different quality factors for different photon energies have not been recommended but the reduced effectiveness of heavy ions of L greater than 100 keV μm^{-1} has been recognised. The Q-L relationship recommended by ICRP is given in Table 4.2.3.2.

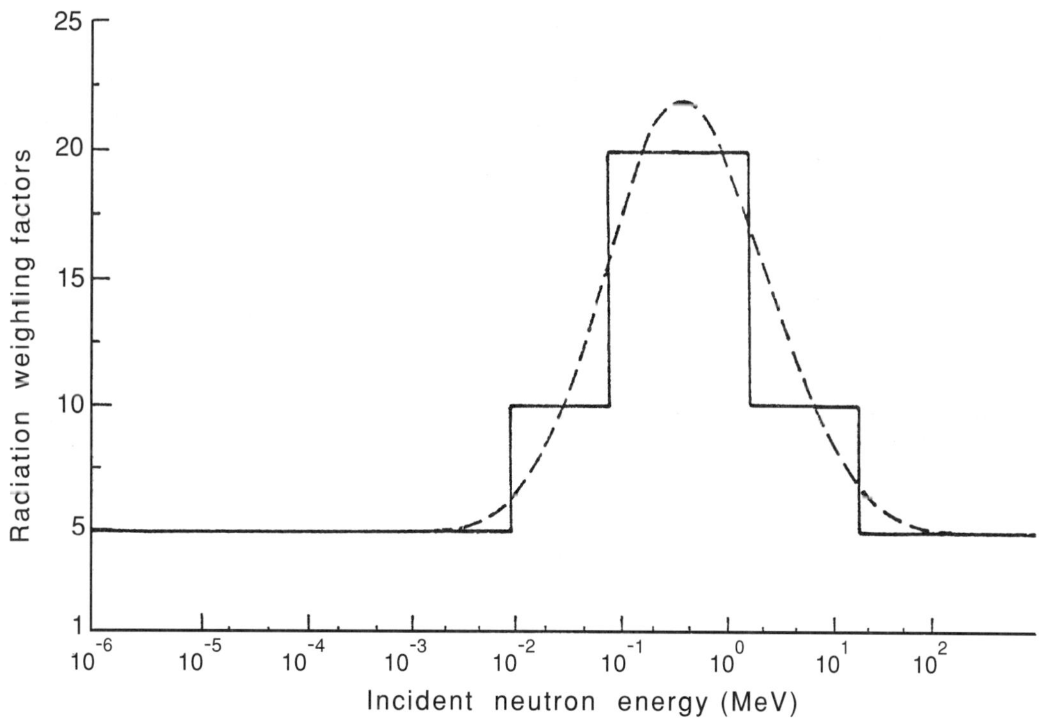

Figure 4.2.1 Radiation Weighting Factors for Neutrons

The smooth curve is to be treated as an approximation.

Table 4.2.3.2 Comparison of Old and New ICRP Quantities and Quality Factor (Q) Values[a]

(With permission from J. Radiol. Prot., 1993)

	Old ICRP		New ICRP	
Limiting quantities	Effective Dose Equivalent Dose Equivalent in specific organs		Effective Dose Equivalent Dose in specific organs	
Value of Q	Collision stopping power, L_∞ (keV μm^{-1})	Q	Unrestricted linear energy transfer, L (keV μm^{-1})	$Q(L)$
	3.5 (and less)	1	<10	1
	7	2	10–100	$0.32L-2.2$
	23	5	>100	$300/\sqrt{L}$
	53	10		
	175 (and above)	20		

[a] This table is not in review article above.

It is important to note that the Q-L relationship is used almost exclusively for the purposes of external radiation monitoring by means of the operational quantities, defined by ICRU (the International Commission on Radiation Units and Measurement), and is not used for calculating effective doses.

Effective Dose

The incidence of stochastic health effects of radiation has been shown to depend on the organ or tissue irradiated. Some organs are more susceptible to radiation damage than others, and have a greater risk of producing cancer or other deleterious effects. ICRP has therefore developed another quantity to reflect the differing risks, which is derived from equivalent dose. Each organ or tissue is weighted according to its observed susceptibility to stochastic health effects using a tissue weighting factor, W_T. This factor represents the relative contribution of the organ or tissue to the total detriment from stochastic effects, compared to that from uniform irradiation of the whole body. The weighted equivalent dose is called the effective dose, E, and has units of J kg^{-1} with the special name of sievert (Sv). It is given by the expression

$$E = \sum_T W_T H_T$$

where H_T is the equivalent dose in tissue or organ T and W_T is the appropriate weighting factor for tissue T. Given the definition of equivalent dose,

$$E = \sum_T W_T \sum_R W_R D_{T,R}$$

and it is also assumed by ICRP that W_T values are independent of radiation type and W_R values are independent of tissue, therefore

$$E = \sum_R = W_R \sum_T W_T D_{T,R}$$

where $D_{T,R}$ is the mean absorbed dose in tissue or an organ T delivered by radiation R. In both expressions, the radiation R is that incident on the body or emitted by a source within the body.

The tissue weighting factors recommended by ICRP in Publication 60 are given in Table 4.2.3.3

Table 4.2.3.3 IRCP Tissue Weighting Factors, w_T[a,b]

Tissue or Organ	Tissue Weighting Factor, w_T
Gonads	0.20
Bone marrow (red)	0.12
Colon	0.12
Lung	0.12
Stomach	0.12
Bladder	0.05
Breast	0.05
Liver	0.05
Oesophagus	0.05
Thyroid	0.05
Skin	0.01
Bone surface	0.01
Remainder[c]	0.05

[a] Tissue weighting factor used in 10 CFR-Part 20 differ, See Table 13.1.3.
[b] Adapted by NCRP, 1993 and 1993a.
[c] Muscle, ST wall, SI wall, LLI wall, kidneys, pancreas, spleen, thymus, uterus, adrenals and bladder wall.

Operational Quantities

The quantities equivalent dose and effective dose are defined by ICRP in order to determine the scale of the risk of health effects associated with exposure to radiation. The quantities are impossible to measure in practice and so, for the purposes of monitoring external radiations, it is common practice to use operational dose equivalent quantities defined by its sister Commission, ICRU. Operational dose equivalent quantities incorporate the definition of absorbed dose at a point either in the ICRU sphere or in the body of a person wearing a personal dosemeter[d]. The *Q-L* relationship is then used to weight the absorbed dose at a point in tissue, rather than using W_R values recommended by ICRP applied to a mean absorbed dose to an organ or tissue. It is a general principle that operational quantities should not underestimate effective doses and should avoid any excessive overestimation.

The dose equivalent quantities recommended by ICRU for area monitoring are defined in a tissue equivalent phantom which has become known as the ICRU sphere[d]. This phantom is a 30 cm diameter tissue equivalent sphere with a density of 1 g cm^{-3} and a mass composition of 76.2% oxygen, 11.1% carbon, 10.1% hydrogen and 2.6% nitrogen. Two quantities for area monitoring were specified by ICRU—the ambient dose equivalent, $H^*(d)$, and the directional dose equivalent, $H'(d)$. Both quantities can be used for strongly and weakly penetrating radiations. The operational dose equivalent quantities for use in personal dosimetry are the individual dose equivalent penetrating, $H_p(s)$, and individual dose equivalent superficial, $H_s(d)$, based on definitions given by ICRU in 1985[d]. In recent publications, ICRU has made changes to the definitions[e] and the new quantity is the personal dose equivalent, $H_p(d)$. This quantity can be used for measurements of superficial and deep organs, depending on the chosen value of the depth in tissue, d. The subscript in H_p now stands for 'personal' rather than 'penetrating'.

Relationships Between Quantities

The relationships between the limit quantities used for radiological protection and operational quantities are discussed in detail in the Board's document[a] for photons, neutrons and electrons. For photon radiations, the implications of the new ICRP quantities of equivalent dose, H_T, and effective dose, E, are small. The differences between effective dose, E, and the quantity recommended previously in 1977 in ICRP Publication 26, H_E, for uniform irradiation of the body are less than 10% for most monoenergic photon energies and irradiation geometries. The operational quantities, defined by ICRU for area and personal monitoring in the workplace, will provide reasonable estimates of E for photon radiations, without underestimation or excessive overestimation. In contrast, for neutron radiations there are more significant implications, because calculations show that E can be between two and four times larger than H_E as defined in Publication 26 for monoenergetic neutrons of up to 2 MeV in various irradiation geometries (although in 1985 ICRP did propose an increase in the value of the quality factor for neutrons[f], but this recommendation was not adopted in the UK or in other EC countries). The increase in E relative to H_E will have significant implications for those calculating doses from neutron radiations but, in practice, operational quantities will still provide an overestimate of E for most neutron energies and irradiation geometries, and for observed neutron spectra in the workplace. The overestimate is less significant for E than it was for H_E as defined in Publication 26 for most neutron energies, because the operational quantities have not increased proportionately as a result of the new ICRP recommendations.

Impact on Instrument and Dosemeter Designs

The impact of ICRP Publication 60 on instrument and dosemeter designs is slight from the point of view of the required variation of response with radiation energy and angle of incidence. This is the case for both photon and neutron radiations. However, ICRP as well as defining new dose limiting quantities has also reduced the corresponding dose limit for effective dose from 50 mSv per year to 20 mSv per year averaged over defined periods of 5 years. Thus, more attention will need to be paid in future to low doses, i.e. the dose threshold of dosemeters will need to be as low as 0.1 mSv with uncertainties in measurements limited to about a factor of two at this level. This is certainly achievable for photon dosemeters but will be more difficult for neutron dosemeters in view of the increased weighting factors.

For hand-held instruments used to monitor the workplace, compliance with the average limit of 20 mSv per year implies a requirement to be able to monitor dose rates of less than 10 μSv h^{-1} routinely. As far as photons are concerned there are no insurmountable problems in achieving the sensitivity. However, this is not the case for neutrons and basic design changes will be necessary to produce instruments capable of routinely measuring neutron dose rates in the range 1–10 μSv h^{-1}.

Recommendations

The Board recommends that the dose quantities of equivalent dose, H_T, and effective dose, E, defined by ICRP in Publication 60 be adopted as the primary limit quantities in radiological protection. As it is not possible to measure these quantities directly, operational dose equivalent quantities, first defined by ICRU in 1985, should be used for the practical measurement of external radiations in the workplace. Instruments and personal dosemeters should be designed to measure the operational dose equivalent quantities and appropriate type test and calibration procedures should be adopted. Measurements of operational dose equivalent quantities will normally provide an overestimate of primary limit quantities and, in some situations, the overestimate may be excessive. If, as a result, assessed exposures are close to limits, measurements of energy spectra and irradiation geometry can be used to obtain a more accurate measure of the limit quantity effective dose. For measurements of external radiation in the environment from natural or artificial sources, operational dose equivalent quantities will overestimate effective doses to a significant extent, mainly because of the irradiation geometry. In these circumstances measurements of a primary field quantity (e.g., air kerma or absorbed dose to air) should be carried out and conversion coefficients applied to obtain effective doses.

Table 4.2.4 Quantities Used in Radiological Protection: 1993 Update (With Permission Dodd, D.H. and Robinson, C.A. NRPB Bulletin No 141, 1993)

The Board's response to the publication of the 1990 Recommendations of ICRP[a] has been published[b] together with practical guidance on its application[c]. This paper summarises the quantities and units used by the Board, for ease of reference.

Radiological protection practice involves a number of dose and risk-related quantities. The intention of this article is to define some of those most frequently encountered and to explain, where appropriate, how definitions and terminology have changed with the new ICRP recommendations that have been endorsed by the Board. The different measures of dose are described and their application to different radiological protection situations is discussed.

The quantities used in assessments of dose and risk may be divided into two categories: individual dosimetric quantities and collective quantities. The individual quantities are used in assessments of doses from one or more sources to an individual and in comparisons with dose limits, constraints and investigation levels. Collective quantities are derived from primary dosimetric quantities. Collective quantities are generally used in source-related assessments, where the aim is to determine the impact of a particular source on the population, rather than on individuals. Each type of quantity is discussed in turn.

Before going on to discuss radiological protection quantities in more detail, it is useful to consider briefly the types of health effect which may result from radiation exposure. ICRP distinguishes between two types of effect: deterministic and stochastic.

If a sufficient number of irradiated cells are killed or prevented from reproducing and functioning normally, then there will be an observable effect, reflecting a loss of tissue function. The probability of causing such an effect will be zero at small doses, but above some level of dose (the threshold) will increase steeply to unity (100%). This type of effect is now termed **deterministic** (previously known as non-stochastic).

The other type of effect is termed **stochastic**. These effects may occur when the irradiated cell is modified rather than killed. In an exposed individual these modified cells may result in the manifestation of malignant conditions (cancers). If the damage occurs in a germ cell hereditary effects may arise in the progeny of the exposed person. These effects are of many different kinds and severity. A general assumption is made that over a limited range of dose there is a simple proportional relationship between dose and probability of effect which implies that stochastic effects can never be eliminated, their occurrence can only be minimised. At levels of dose and dose rate normally encountered from controlled sources deterministic effects are very unlikely to occur. As a result protection measures are generally aimed at reducing the probability of stochastic effects, and the definition of radiological protection quantities reflects this priority.

In order to quantify the health effects of radiation, ICRP has used the terms harm and detriment. **Harm** is used to denote clinically observable, deleterious effects that are expressed in individuals (*somatic effects*) or their descendants (*hereditary effects*). **Detriment** is a complex concept combining the probability, severity and time of expression of harm.

Individual Dosimetric Quantities

Absorbed Dose

A fundamental assumption in describing in a quantitative way the interaction of radiation with matter is that the relevant measure is the energy deposited per unit mass. This is termed the **absorbed dose** and its units are the joule per kilogram, which are given the name gray (Gy). The absorbed dose is given by

$$D = \frac{d\bar{\varepsilon}}{dm}$$

---

[a] ICRP. 1990 Recommendations of the International Commission on Radiological Protection. ICRP Publication 60. Ann. ICRP, 4, No. 1:1–5; 1991.

[b] NRPB Board Statement. 1990 Recommendations of the International Commission on Radiological Protection. Doc. NPRB, 4, No. 1:1–5; 1993.

[c] NRPB. 1990 Recommendations of the International Commission on Radiological Protection. Recommendations for the practical application of the Board's Statement. Doc NRPB, 4, No. 1:7–22; 1993.

where $d\bar{\varepsilon}$ is the mean energy imparted by ionising radiation to matter in a volume element and dm is the mass of matter in that volume element. Absorbed dose is defined in terms that allow it to be specified at a point but ICRP uses it to mean the average dose over a tissue or organ. The use of the average dose as an indicator of the probability of subsequent stochastic effects depends on the linearity of the relationship between the probability of inducing an effect and the dose (the dose-response relationship)—a reasonable approximation over a limited range of dose. The dose-response relationship is not linear for deterministic effects, so the average absorbed dose is not directly relevant to deterministic effects unless the dose is fairly uniformly distributed over the tissue or organ.

Absorbed dose is a physical quantity which does not fully reflect the possible biological effects of ionising radiation. These effects depend not only on the energy deposited per unit mass of tissue, but also on the type and energy of radiation and the tissue affected. In order to take account of these factors ICRP has established radiation and tissue weighting factors and two additional dose quantities. The term **equivalent dose** has been applied to the tissue- or organ-averaged absorbed dose modified by radiation weighting factors, W_R values. The term **effective dose** refers to the equivalent dose further modified by tissue weighting factors, W_T values. These quantities are analogous to the terms dose equivalent and effective dose equivalent included in previous ICRP publications[a]. It should be emphasised that equivalent dose in a tissue or organ is a measure of the probability of stochastic effects to that tissue or organ, whereas effective dose is the sum of the contributions each organ or tissue makes to the total detriment due to effects resulting from irradiation of the whole body.

The values of both W_R and W_T are dependent on current knowledge of radiobiology and may change from time to time. ICRP has stated that these quantities may be assumed to refer to the values currently recommended, if additional information to the contrary is not provided. ICRP also stated in Publication 60 that the earlier values of dose equivalent and effective dose equivalent need not be corrected for the new weighting factors, and that these values may be added to equivalent and effective doses without adjustments.

ICRP historically made provision for the possibility of additional weighting factors by the inclusion of a dimensional factor N, in the definition of effective dose equivalent. In practice N has been assigned a value of unity and ICRP has decided to omit N from the definition of effective dose in its new recommendations.

Equivalent Dose

Previously, ICRP used the quantity dose equivalent *at a point, H*, but has now adopted the term equivalent dose, H_T, to represent the product of the absorbed dose averaged over a tissue or organ and the radiation weighting factor of W_R. The equivalent dose in tissue T is given by

$$H_T = \sum_R W_R D_{T,R}$$

where W_R is the radiation weighting factor and $D_{T,R}$ is the average absorbed dose in the tissue or organ T due to radiation R incident on the body or emitted by radionuclides in the body. The units of equivalent dose are the joule per kilogram and have the name sievert (Sv).

ICRP has selected the value of the radiation weighting factor for a specified type and energy of radiation to be representative of values of the relative biological effectiveness of the radiation in inducing stochastic effects at low doses. The **relative biological effectiveness** (RBE) of one radiation compared with another is the inverse ratio of the absorbed doses producing the same degree of a defined biological endpoint.

The values of W_R are broadly compatible with those used for the quality factor Q, which are related to the quantity **linear energy transfer** (LET), which is a measure of the density of ionisation along the track of an ionising particle. ICRP originally intended that the relationship was to provide a rough indication of the variation of values of Q with changes in radiation, but it was often interpreted to imply spurious precision which it is hoped will not be inferred from the new radiation weighting factors. The W_R values are based on a review of biological information in a variety of exposure circumstances, and calculations of operational dose equivalent quantities.

Effective Dose

The relationship between the probability of occurrence of stochastic effects and equivalent dose is found to depend on the organ or tissue irradiated. It is therefore appropriate to define a further quantity, derived from equivalent dose, to indicate the combination of different doses to several different tissues in a way that is likely to correlate well with the total of the stochastic effects. In order to take account of some of these, ICRP has included four components in assessing the relative contributions of organs to the total detriment: the probability of attributable fatal cancer, the weighted probability of attributable non-fatal cancer, the weighted probability of severe hereditary effects, and the relative length of life lost. The relative contributions of the organs to the total detriment form the basis of the ICRP tissue weighting factors, W_Ts. These factors represent the relative contribution of each organ or tissue to the total health detriment resulting from uniform irradiation of the whole body. ICRP now uses the term effective dose, E, to refer to the sum of the weighted equivalent doses. The units of effective dose are the joule per kilogram, which are given the name sievert (Sv). The effective dose, E, is given by

$$E = \sum_T W_T \sum_R W_R D_{T,R}$$

where $D_{T,R}$ is the mean absorbed dose in the tissue or organ T due to radiation R and W_T and W_R are the tissue weighting factors and radiation weighting factors, respectively, as defined earlier.

Committed Equivalent Dose and Committed Effective Dose

For irradiation following intakes of radionuclides, the absorbed dose will be delivered over time as the radionuclide decays. The time distribution of the absorbed dose rate depends on the radionuclide, its form, the mode of intake, and the tissue within which it is incorporated. ICRP has defined the **committed equivalent dose,** $H_T(\tau)$, to be the time integral of the equivalent dose rate in organ T; τ is the integration time in years following the intake and unless otherwise specified is taken to be 50 years for adults, and from intake to age 70 years for children.

$$H_T(\tau) = \int_{t_0}^{t_0+\tau} H_T(\tau)\mathrm{d}t$$

The **committed effective dose,** $E(\tau)$, is the sum of the committed equivalent doses to the individual organs, multiplied by the appropriate weighting factors:

$$E(\tau) = \sum_T W_T H_T(\tau)$$

Operational Quantities

The quantities equivalent and effective dose are not directly measurable. As a result, operational quantities are required for measurement purposes. ICRP makes reference to four operational quantities of the International Commission on Radiation Units and Measurement (ICRU) which has defined operational quantities for area and individual monitoring[d]. For area monitoring, ICRU has defined two quantities: **ambient dose equivalent** $H^*(d)$, and **directional dose equivalent,** $H'(d)$. Both refer to the dose equivalent at a depth d within a 30 cm diameter of tissue equivalent material, known as the ICRU sphere. For individual monitoring, two additional quantities were defined. The **individual dose equivalent penetrating** is appropriate for organs and tissues situated deep within the body, and the **individual dose equivalent superficial** is appropriate for organs and tissues which are nearer to the surface and likely to be irradiated by both weakly and strongly penetrating radiation. Instead of the two quantities defined for individual monitoring, a simplified concept called **personal dose equivalent,** $H_p(d)$, has recently been defined by ICRU[e], appropriate for both strongly and weakly penetrating radiation, depending on the value of depth d.

Collective and Source Related Quantities

Collective equivalent dose and collective effective dose

ICRP has stated that the collective quantities can be thought of as representing the total consequences of the exposure of a population or group, but that their use in this way should be limited to situations in which the consequences are truly proportional to both the dosimetric quantity and the number of people exposed, and in which an appropriate probability coefficient is available. As such, these quantities are not appropriate in situations in which deterministic effects are possible or where the probability of individual stochastic effects approaches unity.

Collective equivalent dose is defined to express the total radiation exposure of a specific tissue or organ in a group of individuals. The collective equivalent dose in tissue T is given by

$$S_T = \int_0^\infty H_T \frac{\mathrm{d}N}{\mathrm{d}H_T} \mathrm{d}H_T$$

[d] ICRU. Determination of dose equivalents resulting from external radiation sources. Bethesda, MD, ICRU Report 39; 1985.

[e] ICRU. Determination of dose equivalents from external radiation sources. Part 2. Bethesda, MD, ICRU, Report 43; 1988.

where $(dN/H_T)dH_T$ is the number of individuals receiving an equivalent dose between H_T and $H_T + dH_T$ or

$$S_T = \sum_i \overline{H_{T,i}} N_i$$

where N_i is the number of individuals in population subgroup i, receiving mean organ equivalent dose, $\overline{H_{T,i}}$.

Collective effective dose is a measure of the radiation exposure of a population. The quantity has been defined as

$$S = \int_0^\infty E \frac{dn}{dE} dE \quad \text{or} \quad \sum_i \overline{E_i} N_i$$

where E_i is the mean effective dose to subgroup i.

Neither the definition of collective equivalent dose nor that of collective effective dose explicitly specifies the time over which the dose is delivered. Therefore, the time period and population over which the collective equivalent dose is summed or integrated should be specified. If the integration is not over infinite time, the quantity is described as being truncated at a defined time. The word commitment is no longer needed to refer to the collective dose integrated to infinity.

Dose Commitment

The dose commitment is a calculational tool, $H_{C,T}$ or E_C. It can be assessed for a critical group as well as the whole world population. It is defined as the infinite time integral of the ***per caput dose rate,*** H_T or E, due to a specified event, which is a unit of practice. In the case of an indefinite practice at a constant rate, the maximum annual *per caput* dose rate, H_T or E, in the future for the specified population will be equal to the dose commitment from one year of practice, irrespective of changes in the population size. If the practice is continued over a finite time τ, the maximum future *per caput* annual dose will be equal to the corresponding truncated dose commitment.

$$H_{C,T}(\tau) = \int_0^\tau H_T(\tau)dt \quad \text{or} \quad E_C(\tau) = \int_0^\tau E(t)dt$$

Table 4.2.5 ICRP Secondary and Derived Limits for the Control of Internal Dose

(Courtesy ICRP after Publication 30, 1978)

Reference Man

The standards for control of internal dose for workers are derived for an adult person of stated anatomical and physiological features which are defined in the report of the ICRP Task Group on Reference Man (ICRP Publication 23) (see tables 12.6 through 12.15).

Committed Dose Equivalent (H_{50})

The committed dose equivalent (H_{50}) in a particular organ or tissue is the total dose equivalent to which that organ or tissue would be committed during the 50 years after intake of a radionuclide.

Annual Limit on Intake (ALI)[a,b]

The annual limit on intake (ALI) of a radionuclide is a secondary limit designed to meet the basic limits for occupational exposure. ALI is the greatest value of the annual intake I which satisfies both of the following inequalities

$$I \sum_T W_T(H_{50,T} \text{ per unit intake}) \leq 0.05 \text{ Sv}$$

$$I(H_{50,T} \text{ per unit intake}) \leq 0.5 \text{ Sv}$$

where I (in Bq) is the annual intake of the specified radionuclide either by ingestion on inhalation; W_T is the weighting factor for tissue (T) (see table 4.2.1.3); and $H_{50,T}$ per unit intake (in Sv Bq^{-1}) is the committed dose equivalent in tissue (T) from the intake of unit activity of the radionuclide by the specified route.

Application of Annual Limits on Intake

(a) Values of ALI are estimated for exposure, both by ingestion and inhalation, to the specified radionuclide. Any daughter radionuclides produced in the body after intake of the specified radionuclide are taken into account. When the intake consists of a mixture of radionuclides, and/or exposure occurs both by ingestion and inhalation, the values of ALI do not directly apply. In all such cases it is recommended that intakes in any one year should be controlled so that the dose limits (table 4.2.3) are not exceeded. For occupational exposures[a], the 1990 ICRP recommendations (table 4.2.3) limit the effective dose to 0.1 Sv in a five year period (average annual value of 0.02 Sv) with a limit of 0.05 Sv in any single year and includes annual limits on the equivalent dose to skin and hands of 0.5 Sv and to the lens of the eye of 0.15 Sv. The latter are important in relation to external radiation of the body. In the case of internal exposure, the annual limit on intake is based on a committed effective dose of 0.02 Sv. Thus, the annual limit of intake (ALI) for any radionuclide is obtained by dividing the annual average effective dose limit (0.02 Sv) by the committed effective dose $E(50)$, resulting from the intake of 1 Bq of that radionuclide.

For exposure to a mixture of radionuclides the following inequality must be satisfied:

$$\sum_j \left(\frac{I_j}{ALI_j}\right)_{ING} + \sum_j \left(\frac{I_j}{ALI_j}\right)_{INH} + \sum_{j'} \frac{U_{j'}}{2000\ DAC(Submersion)_{j'}} \leq 1$$

where $(I_j)_{ING}$ is the intake of radionuclide j by ingestion in any one year;
$(I_j)_{INH}$ is the intake of a radionuclide j by inhalation in any one year;
$(ALI_j)_{ING}$ is the Annual Limit on Intake for radionuclide j by ingestion;
$(ALI_j)_{INH}$ is the Annual Limit on Intake for radionuclide j by inhalation;
$U_{j'}$ is $\int C_{j'}(t)\,dt$, where t has units of hours, $C_{j'}(t)$ is the concentration of radionuclide j' in which the man is submerged at time t and the time integral is over 1 year of practice (see Chapters 3 and 8);
$DAC(Submersion)_{j'}$ is the Derived Air Concentration (Submersion) for any relevant radionuclide j', and 2000 is the number of hours in a working year.

(b) Values of ALI and of H_{50} per unit intake are intended for use in the control of occupational exposure and are based on the parameters of a Reference Man. However, when there is reason to believe that a particular individual has taken in more than the ALI, and it is thought necessary to estimate the resulting committed dose equivalent, it is recommended that his age and known biological parameters should be taken into account as far as is practicable.

Derived Air Concentration (DAC)[a]

The limit for inhalation of a radionuclide is the appropriate ALI. The concentration of a radionuclide in air during any year is limited as follows

$$\int C(t)\,B(t)\,\mathrm{d}t \le \text{ALI Bq}$$

where at any time t,

C(t) (in Bq m^{-3}) is the concentration of the radionuclide in air;

B(t) (in m^3 per unit time) is the volume of air breathed by the worker per unit time, and the limits on integration are over a working year.

The value of *B(t)* depends on the type of work being performed and for heavy work it could be more than twice the reference value for ''light activity'' given in ICRP Publication 23 (see Table 12.6).

For convenience, the Commission recommends values of derived air concentration (DAC). The DAC for any radionuclide is defined as that concentration in air (Bq m^{-3}) which, if breathed by Reference Man for a working year of 2000 h (50 weeks at 40 h per week) under conditions of ''light activity'', would result in the ALI by inhalation.

$$\begin{aligned}\text{DAC} &= \text{ALI}/(2000 \times 60 \times 0.02)\\ &= \text{ALI}/2.4 \times 10^3\ \text{Bq m}^{-3}\end{aligned}$$

where 0.02 m^3 is the volume of air breathed at work by Reference Man per minute under conditions of ''light activity''.

In the unlikely event of a person being exposed continuously to a DAC, and breathing air at a rate which is on average greater than 0.02 m^3 per min, the activity inhaled in a working year would be more than the ALI. In this respect, it is emphasized that the ALI is the overriding limit and the derived limit DAC should always be used circumspectly.

Derived Air Concentration for Submersion, DAC (Submersion)

For operations involving exposure to radioactive noble gases and elemental tritium, values are given for the derived air concentration for submersion of a Reference Man in a cloud of the gas, DAC(Submersion).

DAC(Submersion) for Elemental Tritium

Exposure to elemental tritium in air during any year is limited by consideration of stochastic effects in the lung as follows

$$W_{Lung}\dot{H}_{Lung}\int C(t)\,\mathrm{d}t \le 0.05\ \text{Sv}$$

where: W_{Lung} is the weighting factor for lung (see table 4.2.1.3); $\dot{H}_{Lung}$ (in Sv m^3 Bq^{-1} h^{-1}) is the dose-equivalent rate to lung from exposure to unit concentration of tritium in air (i.e., 1 Bq m^{-3}); and *C(t)* (in Bq m^{-3}) is the concentration of elemental tritium in air at any time t and the limits on integration are over a working year.

For convenience, the Commission recommends a value of DAC for elemental tritium which is 1/2000th of the greatest value of $\int C(t)\,\mathrm{d}t$ that satisfies relationship. A worker may be exposed to concentrations of elemental tritium in air greater than the DAC provided that the conditions in relationship above are satisfied.

DAC(Submersion) for a Radioactive Noble Gas

Exposure to a radioactive noble gas, other than radon and thoron which are the subject of a separate report, during any year is limited by consideration of external exposure of the body as follows

$$\sum_T W_T\dot{H}_T\int C(t)\,\mathrm{d}t \le 0.05\ \text{Sv}$$

and $\dot{H}_T \int C(t)\,\mathrm{d}t \le 0.5$ Sv

and $\dot{H}_{Lens} \int C(t)\,\mathrm{d}t \le 0.3$ Sv (changed to 0.15 Sv by ICRP 61, 1981, see table 4.2.3)

where $C(t)$ (in Bq m^{-3}) is the concentration of the radioactive noble gas in air at any time t and the limits on integration are over a working year;
W_T is the weighting factor for tissue (T) and has the values shown in table 4.2.1.3.
$\dot{H}_T$ (in Sv m^3 Bq^{-1} h^{-1}) is the dose-equivalent rate in any tissue (T), and
$\dot{H}_{Lens}$ is the corresponding value for the lens of the eye, resulting from submersion of Reference Man in unit concentration of the noble gas in air (i.e., 1 Bq m^{-3}).

For convenience the Commission recommends a value of DAC for a radioactive noble gas which is 1/2000th of the greatest value of $\int C(t)\,dt$ that satisfies relationship above. (2000 is the number of hours in a working year.) A worker may be exposed to concentrations of a noble gas in air greater than the DAC provided that the conditions in relationship are satisfied.

[a] International Commission on Radiological Protection and Measurements Publication 61 1990.
[b] NCRP Publication 116 introduces ''Annual Reference Levels of Intake'' (ARLI) at the same effective dose level as recommended by the ICRP.

Table 4.2.6 ICRP Conceptual Framework (After Clarke with permission of author, 1991)

The ICRP's recommendations are based on prevention of deterministic effects by keeping doses below their threshold level, and by assuring that reasonable actions are taken to limit the occurrence of stochastic effects to acceptable levels. The ICRP's conceptual framework promotes the assessment of the effectiveness of radiation protection by relating it to individual doses from a single source (source-related); or to individual doses from all relevant sources (individual-related).

Source-related assessments permit evaluation of whether a radiation activity's advantages outweigh its disadvantages. Individual-related assessments are made to discern if the total dose from all sources is too high.

Activities which *add* radiation exposures are called *practices*. Those which *subtract* radiation exposure are called *intervention*.

The following principles recommended by the ICRP are relevant to *practices*.

- A practice involving exposure should produce sufficient benefit to offset the radiation detriment it causes—*justification*.
- For any source, doses or the likelihood of being exposed should be as low as reasonably achievable (ALARA) and constrained by doses to individuals and risks to individuals from potential exposures—*optimization*.
- Individual exposure from all sources susceptible to control are subject to dose limits and some control of risk from potential exposures—*dose and risk limits*.

The ICRP introduced the concept of a *constraint* to dose or risk. A *constraint* is an individual-related criterion applied to a single source to ensure that the dose limits are not exceeded. A dose *constraint* is a boundary on the optimization of a specific source. It is a fraction of the dose limit and may be seen as a regulatory requirement, not a design target or operational investigation level.

In accidents or emergencies *intervention* is achieved through countermeasures. Countermeasures have disadvantages, so they need to be justified—their benefits must outweigh their risks. Social disruption and anxiety produced by the countermeasure need to be considered.

The general principles for intervention recommended by the ICRP are:

- Any intervention must do more good than harm so the reduction in radiation detriment must exceed the harm and social cost of the intervention.
- The scale and duration of the intervention should be such that the net benefit of the reduction in dose, less the cost of intervention, should be as large as reasonably achievable.

The ICRP believes that *effective dose* is an adequate surrogate for detriment to an individual and *collective effective dose* for a population.

Table 4.2.7 ICRP Dose Limits (Courtesy ICRP after Publication 60 1991)

ICRP dose limits are applicable to occupational and public exposures. The dose limit is set such that continued exposure at a dose just above the limit would be unacceptable on any reasonable basis. Continued exposure just below the limit is tolerated but not encouraged, so that acceptable doses are somewhat below the limit.

The limits for workers apply to all occupational situations including mishaps and misjudgments in plant operations and planned and unplanned maintenance and decommissioning of nuclear plants.

1. Deterministic Effects
   Annual limits for workers are 150 mSv for the lens and 500 mSv for the skin and extremities (unchanged from previous limits). (Deterministic limits for members of the public are given in table 4.1.1.)
2. Stochastic Effects
   Figure 4.2.2 shows the annual risk of death from radiation-induced cancer at various dose rates received between the ages of 18 to 65 years. Because a multiplicative risk model is employed, the trends follow the probability of death for the general population.

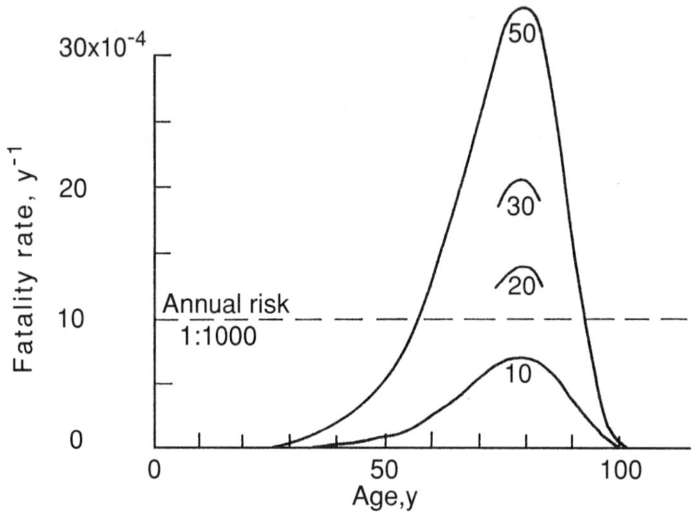

Figure 4.2.2 Annual Risk of Death from Radiation-Induced Cancer for 10, 20, 30 and 50 mSv y^{-1} Received from Age 18 to 65 Years

The annual risk of death found in conventional industries is 1×10^{-3} per year. This figure would be exceeded at an age in the mid-50 years age group for someone receiving 50 mSv y^{-1} and in the mid-60 age group for someone receiving 20 mSv y^{-1}.

In addition to cancer fatalities, non-fatal cancers (about 20% of the number of fatalities) and hereditary defects (also about 20% of the fatality rate) were added to obtain a total detriment.

The ICRP chosen effective dose limit of 1 Sv over a working life is the upper limit of tolerability, i.e., just short of being an unacceptable level. The rate of delivery of radiation is not to exceed an effective dose of 50 mSv in any single year or 100 mSv in any five (5) year period (20 mSv y^{-1} averaged over 5 years). An additional admonition is that continued exposure at the limit would be acceptable only after a careful cost-benefit analysis indicates the risk to be justified.

Values for the annual limit on intake (ALI) for radionuclides for a *committed effective dose* of 20 mSv are published in the recommendation. The ALI are based on stochastic effects only, a separate limit for the ALI based on deterministic effects not being required.

Occupational exposure for women who are not pregnant is the same as that for men. However, if a woman is, or may be, pregnant, additional controls have to be considered to protect the unborn child. The ICRP policy is to provide a standard of protection for any conceptus broadly comparable with that provided for members of the public. This will be achieved if the woman is working the normal system of protection before the pregnancy is declared. Once pregnancy has been declared, the conceptus should be protected by applying a supplementary dose limit to the surface of the woman's abdomen of 2 mSv for the remainder of the pregnancy and by restricting intakes of radionuclides to one-twentieth of an ALI.

The ICRP limits for members of the public are discussed in section 4.1 of this handbook.

Table 4.2.8 Practical Implementation of ICRP Recommendations (After Clarke with permission of author, 1991)

A. Classification of Workplaces

A *controlled area* is one under normal working conditions including minor mishaps, where workers are required to follow established radiation protection procedures. A *supervised area* is one in which working practices are reviewed, but no special work procedures are normally required. The distinction between these areas should be defined by management after considering the potential for variability of external exposures and intake of radionuclides. A *controlled area* would be one in which routine environmental workplace monitoring is not sufficient to predict individual worker doses with confidence. If environmental monitoring does not adequately reflect individual exposures, the work area should be considered a *controlled area* and individual monitoring is required for external and internal doses. If environmental monitoring is sufficient, but doses may exceed limits for the public, the area should be considered a *supervised area.* Persons working within these areas are regarded as occupationally exposed.

B. Exemption from Regulatory Control

For sources that can be controlled, the ICRP recommends exemption if individual doses are unlikely to exceed 10 μSv y^{-1} and the collective dose is not more than 1 person Sv per year of practice.

C. Skin Doses

The recommended annual limit is 500 mSv averaged over 1 cm^2 regardless of the area exposed. The nominal depth is 7 mg cm^{-2}. This *effective dose* provides sufficient protection against stochastic deterministic effects. In practice, monitoring is done at representative locations and over large areas. This limit applied to the skin of the face provides protection to the lens of the eye against beta particles, and can also be applied to the hands and feet.

Table 4.2.9 Summary of NCRP Occupational Recommendations[a,b] (Courtesy NCRP from Report 116, 1993)

A number of modifications of the Council's earlier recommendations on limits for exposure to ionizing radiation (NCRP, 1987) have been made. These modifications and a summary of the current recommendations are presented here.

For occupational exposures:

1. The NCRP recommends that the cumulative effective dose not exceed the age of the individual in years $\times$ 10 mSv.
2. The NCRP continues the use of the annual limit of 50 mSv but only as a limit on the annual rate of effective dose.[c]
3. For the exposure of pregnant women under occupational conditions, it is recommended that there be a limitation on the rate of equivalent dose to the embryo-fetus of no more than 0.5 mSv in a month. With this recommendation, there is no need for a limit on the total equivalent dose received by the embryo-fetus.
4. The NCRP continues to recommend explicitly that all dose limits apply to the sum of external and internal exposures; the external exposures being assessed through the effective dose and the internal exposures assessed on the basis of the committed effective dose.
5. New facilities and the introduction of new practices should be designed to limit annual effective doses to workers to a fraction of the 10 mSv y^{-1} implied by the lifetime dose limit.
6. In this Report the NCRP introduces Annual Reference Levels of Intake (ARLI) at the same effective dose level as recommended by the ICRP for Annual Limits on Intake (ALI) of 20 mSv for workers.

Another important change is the introduction of the radiation weighting factors (W_R) which range from 1 for all photon energies up to 20 for 1 MeV neutrons and alpha particles. Also, in the interest of providing a uniform approach to radiation protection, the new definitions and concepts given in ICRP Publication 60 (ICRP, 1991) have been adopted wherever practical.

[a] The NCRP recommendations for public exposures are found in Table 4.1.2.

[b] The NCRP established a boundary below which the dose can be dismissed from considerations. See Table 4.1.18.

[c] Based on stochastic effects.

For deterministic effects, the following annual equivalent dose limits are recommended:

150 mSv for the crystalline lens of the eye, and 500 mSv for localized areas of the skin, the hands and feet. These limits apply whether an individual tissue or organ is exposed selectively or together with other tissues or organs. Such discrete limits are required for the hands, for example, since limitation based on stochastic risks alone (effective dose) would permit several sievert per year, which could eventually result in deterministic effects.

Table 4.2.10 Recommendations on Radiation Exposure Limits for the Special Case of a Hot Particle on the Skin (Courtesy NCRP from Report No. 106 1989)

It is *recommended* that:

1. *A limit for exposure to hot particles be based on ensuring that acute deep ulceration of the skin be prevented and that this be accomplished by a limit based on the time integral of the beta particles emitted due to the activity of the particle in contact with the skin,*
2. *Exposure to the skin from a ''point'' particle or a particle of unknown size but less than 1 mm in diameter be limited to 10^{10} beta particles emitted from the radionuclides contained in the particle. For the case where 1 beta particle is emitted per disintegration, this limit may be expressed as 10 GBq s or 75 μCi h. For a particle for which the self absorption can be measured or calculated, the limit can be increased by the ratio of the beta particles emitted by the radionuclides divided by the beta particles emitted from the surface of the particle. Alternatively, the limit can be expressed as 10^{10} beta particles emitted from the surface of the particle,*
3. *Exposure in excess of the limit should require periodic medical evaluation of the exposed site for a period of approximately four weeks in order to determine what effect, if any occurs.* If an ulcer occurs, the decision on allowing the exposed individual to work should be based on the same criteria one would apply to any open wound. The affected individual should be aware that the risk of skin cancer from such events is extremely small.

The basis for this recommendation is data obtained primarily from beta particle emissions from irradiated fuel particles. The probability for serious tissue damage from particles containing ^{60}Co is no greater than that for particles containing irradiated fuel and is likely to be much less due to the shorter range of the ^{60}Co beta particle.

The recommendations in this report are intended for application to hot particles in contact with the skin. When a given hot particle is not in contact, it produces lower doses in the skin; also the radiation field changes less rapidly with distance, both laterally and with depth. Under these circumstances, a given hot particle is expected to produce less harm.

When hot particles are found on a person, they are not always in contact with the skin. They may, for example, be on clothing or in the hair. Regardless of where they are found, due to their considerable mobility, their past positions and movements are not known and cannot be determined. In general, therefore, to be conservative, it is recommended that a hot particle be assumed to have been in contact with the skin throughout the possible irradiation period. In cases where it can be determined that the hot particle was never in contact with the skin (for example, if it were between two layers of clothing) dose limits for exposure of large areas of the skin should be applied. The circumstance in which skin is irradiated by hot particles not directly on the skin requires further study.

There are wide variations in the data on which recommendations for limits of exposure of the skin to hot particles must be based. Additional research is occurring presently and should be continued on both the biological effects of hot particles and the dosimetry of hot particles. Results from this ongoing work may well eventually provide sufficient new information to further support these recommendations or to require their review at a later time.

Table 4.2.11 Derivation of an Exposure Limit for a Hot Particle on the Skin

(Courtesy NCRP from Report No. 106, 1989)

A recommended limit should be for point sources to allow for the potential of encountering hot particles of very small size and essentially no self absorption. A recommendation for point sources is a conservative one because self absorption in larger particles, such as those actually used in the experiments, would always result in a lower beta particle emission rate from the surface of the particle. Figure 4.2.7.1 gives the calculated point source dose rates for $^{235}UC_2$ spheres of various diameters at a depth of 100 μm (Ulberg and Kochendorfer, 1966). A point source would have to emit about one third the number of beta particles to produce the same dose at 100 μm depth as the 100 μm particles used by Forbes and Mikhail. Hence, the acute deep ulceration threshold estimated for point sources of irradiated nuclear fuel particles on human skin is estimated to be:

$$3 \times 10^{10} \times \frac{1}{3} = 10^{10} \textit{ beta particles}$$

If each disintegration is assumed to emit one beta particle, this limit can be expressed as 10 GBq s, or in traditional units as 75 μCi h.

It is not unusual in setting radiation protection limits to provide a specific safety factor or element of conservatism. This approach is warranted when the endpoint to be avoided or minimized is a serious health consequence. In the present case, however, the selected endpoint to be prevented, acute deep ulceration of minute areas of the skin, is not a serious health consequence. The cost both in additional whole body radiation exposure due to frequent surveillance of workers and in money that would be required to comply with a limit employing a safety factor is not justified in this case. Therefore, an explicit safety factor has not been incorporated into these recommendations.

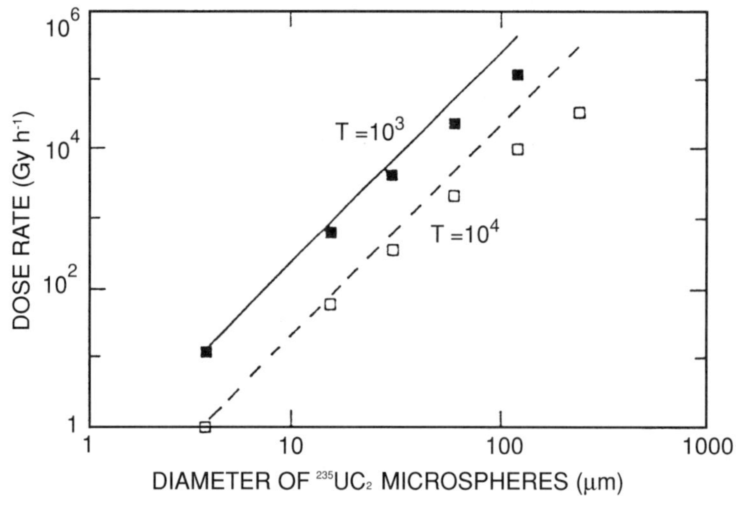

Figure 4.2.11.1 Dose Rate From ^{235}U Microspheres The points are the dose rates calculated by Ulberg and Kochendorfer (1966) at 100 μm distance from activated $^{235}UC_2$ microspheres of different diameters for time (T) equal to 10^3 and 10^4 seconds after removal from the reactor. The lines represent the dose rates that would have been produced by point sources (no self absorption) with the same activities.

SECTION 3 IONIZING RADIATION—MEDICAL AND OTHER (Contributed by Robert A. Phillips, personal communication, 1996)

The Food and Drug Administration is responsible for promulgation of Federal regulations applicable to radiation emitting devices. Their regulations, published in the *Code of Federal Regulations 21 Subchapter J-Radiological Health*, are abstracted here. While these abstracts are intended to give the reader insight into the particular regulation, they are not intended as a guide to ensure compliance. The original regulation needs to be consulted for this purpose. Short extracts are presented relevant to television receivers, cathode ray tubes, diagnostic x-ray systems, standby storage capacitors, mammography units, fluoroscopic equipment, computed tomographs, and cabinet x-ray systems.

Recommendations for the safe and efficacious use of medical radiation is contained in the National Commission on Radiation Protection and Measurements (NCRP) Report No. 102. This report is concerned with minimizing the radiation dose to patients, radiation workers and members of the public from medical radiation. It is summarized here.

TABLE OF CONTENTS

Government Regulation of Radiation Sources—Medical and Other

Government regulation of radiation sources occurs at several levels and is distributed among several agencies. The federal government regulates electronic products that emit radiation under the Food, Drug and Cosmetic Act (FD&C Act), formally the Radiation Control for Health and Safety Act of 1968 (RCHSA). Medical devices, including those that emit radiation, are also regulated under the Medical Device Amendments to the FD&C Act of 1976. Mammography devices are also regulated under the Mammographic Quality Standards Act of 1992. Naturally occurring radioactive materials are not regulated at the federal level and the users of radiation emitting products are regulated by the individual states. These This regulation is guided by the ''Suggested State Regulations'' published by the Council of State Radiation Program Directors. Guidance is also supplied by voluntary standards organizations such as the National Council on Radiation Protection and Measurements.

Radiation Emitting Devices—The Radiation Control for Health and Safety Act of 1968

The FDA through its Center for Devices and Radiological Health promulgates regulations covering radiation emitting devices. These are regulations are found in the Code of Federal Regulations 21 (21 CFR) Subchapter J-Radiological Health. The exact citation is 21 CFR 1000 to 1050. The division of Subpart J and a brief summary or selected excerpts of each major section follow. The regulations apply to the manufacture and distribution of these devices.

21 CFR Section	Title
1000	General Provisions
1010	Performance Standards for Electronic Products: General
1020	Performance Standards for Ionizing Radiation Emitting Products
1020.10	Television receivers
1020.20	Cold-cathode gas discharge tubes
1020.30	Diagnostic x-ray systems and their major components
1020.31	Radiographic equipment
1020.32	Fluoroscopic equipment
1020.33	Computed tomography (CT) equipment
1020.40	Cabinet x-ray systems
1030	Performance Standards for Microwave and Radio frequency Emitting Products
1040	Performance Standards for Light-Emitting Products
1040.10	Laser products
1040.11	Specific purpose laser products
1040.20	Sunlamp products and ultraviolet lamps intended for use in sunlamp products
1040.30	High-intensity mercury vapor discharge lamps
1050	Performance Standards for Sonic, Infrasonic, and Ultrasonic Radiation-Emitting Products

Section 21 CFR 1000—General

This section opens the entire Subchapter J. It provides general provisions, statements of policy and interpretation, radiation protection recommendations (gonadal shielding, diagnostic radiology quality assurance, and administratively required dental x-ray examinations). The general provisions section provides definitions that are used throughout the subchapter. The statement of policy and interpretation provides examples of products subject to the RCHSA. This section is worth reviewing if you are involved with a device that may be covered. The recommendations provide the agency's position on the prudent use of radiation in several areas. These do not have the force of law, i.e., are not requirements, but recommendation. Part 1002 describes records and reports that are required by the regulations. Part 1003 describes obligations to report defects or failures to comply. Part 1004 covers manufacturer's obligation to repurchase, repair, or replace defective electronic products. Part 1005 covers importation of electronic products.

Part 1010 Performance Standards for Electronic Products: General

¶ 1010.2 Certification (a)—Every manufacturer of an electronic product for which an applicable standard is in effect under this sub-chapter shall furnish to the dealer or distributer, at the time of delivery of such product, the certification that such product conforms to all applicable standards under this sub-chapter.

¶ 1020.10 Television Receivers

(c) *Requirements*—(1) *Exposure rate limit.* (1) Radiation exposure rates produced by the television receiver shall not exceed 0.5 milliroentgens per hour at a distance of five (5) centimeters from any point on the external surface of the receiver, as measured in accordance with this section.

¶ 1020.20 Cold-Cathode Gas Discharge Tubes

(c) *Requirements*—(1) *Exposure rate limit.* (1) Radiation exposure rates produced by cold-cathode gas discharge tubes shall not exceed 10 mR/hr at a distance of thirty (30) centimeters from any point on the external surface of the tube, as measured in accordance with this section.

¶ 1020.30 Diagnostic x-ray systems and their major components

(k) Leakage radiation from the diagnostic source assembly. The leakage radiation from the diagnostic source assembly measured at a distance of 1 meter in any direction from the source shall not exceed 2.58 $\times$ 10^{-5} columbs per kilogram (C/kg) (100 milliroentgens (mR)) in 1 hour when the tube is operated at the leakage technique factors. If the maximum rated peak tube potential of the tube housing assembly is greater than the maximum rated peak tube potential for the diagnostic source assembly, positive means shall be provided to limit the maximum x-ray tube potential to that of the diagnostic source assembly. Compliance shall be determined by measurements averaged over an area of 100 square centimeters with no linear dimension greater that 20 centimeters.

(l) Radiation from components other than the diagnostic source assembly. The radiation emitted by a component other than the diagnostic source assembly shall not exceed 5.16 $\times$ 10^{-7} C/kg (2 mR) in 1 hour at 5 centimeters from any accessible surface of the component when it is operated in an assembled x-ray system under any conditions for which it is designed. Compliance shall be determined by measurements over an area of 100 square centimeters with no linear dimension greater than 20 centimeters.
(m) Beam quality—(1) *Half-value layer.* The half-value layer (HVL) of the useful beam for a given x-ray tube potential shall not be less than the appropriate value shown in Table 4.3.1 under ''Specified dental systems,'' for any dental system designed for use with intraoral image receptors and manufactured after December 1, 1980; and under ''Other x-ray systems,'' for all other x-ray systems subject to this section. If it is necessary to determine such HVL at an x-ray tube potential which is not listed in Table I, linear interpolation or extrapolation may be made. Positive means shall be provided to insure that at least the minimum filtration needed to achieve the above beam quality requirements in the useful beam during exposure.

Table 4.3.1 Diagnostic X-Ray Systems and Their Major Components—Beam Quality and Half-Value Layer

X-Ray Tube Voltage (kilovolt peak)		Minimum HVL (millimeters of aluminum)	
Designed Operating Range	**Measured Operating Potential**	**Specified Dental Systems**	**Other X-ray Systems**
Below 51	30	1.5	0.3
	40	1.5	0.4
	50	1.5	0.5
51 to 70	51	1.5	1.2
	60	1.5	1.3
	70	1.5	1.5
Above 70	71	2.1	2.1
	80	2.3	2.3
	90	2.5	2.5
	100	2.7	2.7
	110	3.0	3.0
	120	3.2	3.2
	130	3.5	3.5
	140	3.8	3.8
	150	4.1	4.1

(n) Aluminum equivalent of material between patient and image receptor. Except when used in a CT system, the aluminum equivalent of each of the items listed in Table 4.3.2, which are used between the patient and the image receptor, may not exceed the indicated limits. Compliance shall be determined by x-ray measurements made at a potential of 100 kilovolts peak and with an x-ray beam that has an HVL of 2.7 millimeters of aluminum. This requirement applies to the front panel(s) of cassette holders and film changers provided by the manufacturer for patient support or for prevention of foreign object intrusion. It does not apply to screens and their associated mechanical support panels or grids.

Table 4.3.2 Diagnostic X-Ray Systems and Their Major Components—Aluminum Equivalent of Material Between Patient and Image Receptor

Item	Aluminum Equivalent (millimeters)
Front panel(s) of cassette holder (total of all)	1.0
Front panel(s) of film changer (total of all)	1.0
Cradle	2.0
Tabletop, stationary, without articulated joint(s)	1.0
Tabletop, movable, without articulated joint(s) (including stationary subtop)	1.5
Tabletop, with radiolucent panel having one articulated joint	1.5
Tabletop, with radiolucent panel having two or more articulated joints	2.0
Tabletop, cantilevered	2.0
Tabletop, radiation therapy simulator	5.0

¶ 1020.31 Radiographic Equipment

(l) Radiation from capacitor energy storage equipment. Radiation emitted from the x-ray tube shall not exceed:

1. 8.6×10^{-9} C/kg (0.03 mR) in 1 minute at 5 centimeters from any accessible surface of the diagnostic source assembly, with the beam-limiting device fully open, the system fully charged, and the exposure switch, timer, or any discharge mechanism not activated. Compliance shall be determined by measurements over an area of 100 square centimeters with no linear dimension greater than 20 centimeters: and

2. 2.58×10^{-5} C/kg (100 mR) in 1 hour at 100 centimeters from the x-ray source, with the beam-limiting device fully open, when the system is discharged through the x-ray tube either manually or automatically by use of a discharge switch or deactivation of the input power. Compliance shall be determined by measurements of the maximum exposure per discharge multiplied by the total number of discharges in 1 hour (duty cycle). The measurement shall be averaged over an area of 100 square centimeters with no linear dimension greater than 20 centimeters.

(m) Transmission limit for image receptor supporting devices used for mammography. For x-ray systems manufactured after September 5, 1978, which are designed only for mammography, the transmission of the primary beam through any image receptor support provided with the system shall be limited such that the exposure 5 centimeters from any accessible surface beyond the plane of the image receptor supporting the device does not exceed 2.58×10^{-8} C/kg (0.1 mR) for each activation of the tube. Exposure shall be measured with the system operated at the minimum SID for which it is designed. Compliance shall be determined at the maximum rated peak tube potential for the system and at the maximum rated product of the tube current and exposure time (mAs) for the peak tube potential. Compliance shall be determined by measurements over an area of 100 square centimeters with no linear dimension greater than 20 centimeters.

¶ 1020.32 Fluoroscopic Equipment

(a) Primary protective barrier—(1) *Limitation of useful beam.* The fluoroscopic imaging assembly shall be provided with a primary protective barrier which intercepts the entire cross section of the useful beam at any SID. The x-ray tube used for fluoroscopy shall not produce x-rays unless the barrier is in position to intercept the entire useful beam. The exposure rate due to transmission through the barrier with the attenuation block in the useful beam combined with radiation from the image intensifier if provided, shall not exceed 3.34×10^{-3} percent of the entrance exposure rate, at a distance of 10 centimeters from any accessible surface of the fluoroscopic imaging assembly beyond the plane of the image receptor. Radiation therapy simulation systems shall be exempt from this requirement provided the systems are intended only for remote control operation and the manufacturer sets forth instructions for assemblers with respect to control location as part of the information required in ¶ 1020.30(g). Additionally, the manufacturer shall provide to users, pursuant to ¶ 1020.30(h)(1)(I), precautions concerning the importance of remote control operation.

(d) Entrance exposure rates. For equipment manufactured before May 19, 1995, the following requirements apply:

1. *Equipment with automatic exposure rate control (AERC).* Fluoroscopic equipment that is provided with AERC shall not be operable at any combination of tube potential and current that will result in an exposure rate in excess of 2.58×10^{-3} coulomb per kilogram (C/kg) per minute (10 roentgens per minute (10 R/min) at the point where the useful beam enters the patient, except:

(i) During recording of fluoroscopic images, or

(ii) When an optional high-level control is provided. When so provided, the equipment shall not be operable at any combination of tube potential and current that will result in an exposure of 1.29×10^{-3} C/kg per minute (5 R/min) at the point where the useful beam enters the patient, unless, the high-level control is activated. Special means of activation of high-level controls shall be required. The high-level control shall be operable only when continuous manual activation is provided by the operator. A continuous signal audible to the fluoroscopist shall indicate that the high-level control is being employed

2. *Equipment without AERC (manual mode).* Fluoroscopic equipment that is not provided with AERC shall not be operable at any combination of tube potential and current that will result in an exposure rate in excess of 1.29×10^{-3} C/kg per minute (5 R/min) at the point where the center of the useful beam enters the patient, except:
   (i) During recording of fluoroscopic images, or
   (ii) When an optional high-level control is activated. Special means of activation of high-level controls shall be required. The high-level control shall be operable only when continuous manual activation is provided by the operator. A continuous signal audible to the fluoroscopist shall indicate that the high-level control is being employed.

3. *Equipment with both an AERC mode and a manual mode.* Fluoroscopic equipment that is provided with both an AERC and a manual control shall not be operable at any combination of tube potential and current that will result in an exposure rate in excess of 2.58×10^{-3} coulomb per kilogram (C/kg) per minute (10 roentgens per minute (10 R/min)) at the point where the useful beam enters the patient, except:
   (i) During recording of fluoroscopic images, or
   (ii) When the mode or modes have an optional high-level control, in which case that mode or modes shall not be operable at any combination of tube potential and current that will result in an exposure of 1.29×10^{-3} C/kg per minute (5 R/min) at the point where the useful beam enters the patient, unless, the high-level control is activated. Special means of activation of high-level controls shall be required. The high-level control shall be operable only when continuous manual activation is provided by the operator. A continuous signal audible to the fluoroscopist shall indicate that the high-level control is being employed.

(e) Entrance rate exposure limits. For equipment manufactured on or after May 19, 1995, the following requirements apply:

1 Fluoroscopic equipment operable at any combination of tube potential and current that results in an exposure rate greater that 1.29×10^{-3} C/kg per minute (5 R/min) at the point where the center of the useful beam enters the patient shall be equipped with AERC. Provisions for manual selection of technique factors may be provided.

2 Fluoroscopic equipment shall not be operable at any combination of tube potential and current that results in an exposure rate in excess of 2.58×10^{-3} C/kg per minute (10 R/min) at the point where the center of the useful beam enters the patient except:
   (i) During the recording of images from an image-intensifier tube using photographic film or a video camera when the x-ray source is operating in pulsed mode.
   (ii) When an optional high-level control is activated. When the high-level control is activated, the equipment shall not be operable at any combination of tube potential and current that results in an exposure rate in excess of 5.16×10^{-3} C/kg per minute (20 R/min) at the point where the center of the useful beam enters the patient. Special means of activation of high-level controls shall be required. The high-level control shall be operable only when continuous manual activation

is provided by the operator. A continuous signal audible to the fluoroscopist shall indicate that the high-level control is being employed.

¶ 1020.33 Computed Tomography Equipment

This section is primarily a reporting requirement. The manufacturer must make certain measurements on the device and provide them in the device labeling.

(h) Beam-on and shutter status indicators. (1) Means shall be provided on the control and on or near the housing of the scanning mechanism to provide visual indication when and only when the x rays are produced and, if applicable, whether the shutter is open or closed. If the x-ray production period is less than one half second, the indication of x-ray production shall be activated for one-half second. Indicators at or near the housing of the scanning mechanism shall be discernable from any point external to the patient opening where insertion of any part of the human body into the primary beam is possible.

(2) For systems that allow high-voltage to be applied to the x-ray tube continuously and that control emission of x-rays with a shutter, the radiation emitted may not exceed 100 milliroentgens (2.58×10^{-5} coulomb/kilogram) in 1 hour at any point 5 centimeters outside the external surface of the housing of the scanning mechanism when the shutter is closed. Compliance shall be determined by measurements averaged over 100 square centimeters with no linear dimension greater than 20 centimeters.

¶ 1020.40 Cabinet X-ray Systems

(c) *Requirements—(1) Emission limits*

(i) Radiation emitted from the cabinet x-ray system shall not exceed an exposure of 0.5 milliroentgen in one hour at a point 5 centimeters outside the external surface.

(ii) Compliance with the exposure limit in paragraph (c)(1)(i) of this section shall be determined by measurements averaged over a cross-sectional area of ten square centimeters with no linear dimension greater that 5 centimeters, with the cabinet x-ray system operated at those combinations of tube potential, current, beam orientation, and conditions of scatter radiation which produce the maximum x-ray exposure at the external surface, and with the door(s) and access panel(s) fully closed as well as fixed at any other position(s) which will allow the generation of x radiation.

Part 1030 Performance Standards for Microwave and Radio Frequency Emitting Products

¶ 1030.10 Microwave Ovens

(c) *Requirements* (1) *Power density limit.* The equivalent plane-wave power limit density existing in the proximity of the external oven shall not exceed 1 milliwatt per square centimeter at any point 5 centimeters or more from the external surface of the oven, measured prior to acquisition by a purchaser, and thereafter, 5 milliwatts per square centimeter at any such point.

Part 1040 Performance Standards for Light-Emitting Products

¶ 1040.10 Laser products

(d) *Accessible emission limits.* Accessible emission limits for laser radiation in each class are specified in Tables 4.3.3, 4.3.3.1, 4.3.3.2, 4.3.3.3., and 4.3.3.4 of this paragraph. The factors are given in Table IV of this paragraph, with selected numerical values in Table V of this paragraph. Accessible emission limits for collateral radiation are specified in Table VI of this paragraph.

Notes applicable to Tables I, II-A, II, III-A, and III-B:

1. The factors k_1 and k_2 are wavelength-dependent correction factors determined from Table IV.
2. The variable t in the expressions of emission limits is the magnitude of the sampling interval in units of seconds.

Table 4.3.3 Class I Accessible Emission Limits for Laser Radiation

Wavelength (nanometers)	Emission duration (seconds)	Class I—Accessible Emission Limits (value)	(unit)	(quantity)**
≥180 but ≤400	≤3.0 × 10^4	$2.4 \times 10^{-5} k_1 k_2$*	Joules (J)*	radiant energy
	>3.0 × 10^4	$8.0 \times 10^{-10} k_1 k_2$*	Watts (W)*	radiant power
>400 but ≤1400	>1.0 × 10^{-9} to 2.0 × 10^{-5}	$2.0 \times 10^{-7} k_1 k_2$	J	radiant energy
	>2.0 × 10^{-5} to 1.0 × 10^1	$7.0 \times 10^{-4} k_1 k_2 t^{3/4}$	J	radiant energy
	>1.0 × 10^1 to 1.0 × 10^4	$3.9 \times 10^{-3} k_1 k_2$	J	radiant energy
	>1.0 × 10^4	$3.9 \times 10^{-7} k_1 k_2$	W	radiant power
	and also (See paragraph (d)(4) of this section)			
	>1.0 × 10^{-9} to 1.0 × 10^1	$10 k_1 k_2 t^{1/3}$	$Jcm^{-2}sr^{-1}$	integrated radiance
	>1.0 × 10^1 to 1.0 × 10^4	$20 k_1 k_2$	$Jcm^{-2}sr^{-1}$	integrated radiance
	>1.0 × 10^4	$2.0 \times 10^{-3} k_1 k_2$	$Wcm^{-2}sr^{-1}$	radiance
>1400 but ≤2500	>1.0 × 10^{-9} to 1.0 × 10^{-7}	$7.0 \times 10^{-5} k_1 k_2$	J	radiant energy
	>1.0 × 10^{-7} to 1.0 × 10^1	$4.4 \times 10^{-3} k_1 k_2 t^{1/4}$	J	radiant energy
	>1.0 × 10^1	$7.9 \times 10^{-4} k_1 k_2$	W	radiant power
>2500 but ≤1.0 × 10^6	>1.0 × 10^{-9} to 1.0 × 10^{-7}	$1.0 \times 10^{-2} k_1 k_2$	Jcm^{-2}	radiant exposure
	>1.0 × 10^{-7} to 1.0 × 10^1	$5.6 \times 10^{-1} k_1 k_2 t^{1/4}$	Jcm^{-2}	radiant exposure
	>1.0 × 10^1	$1.0 \times 10^{-1} k_1 k_2 t$	Jcm^{-2}	radiant exposure

* Class I accessible emission limits for wavelengths equal to or greater than 180 nm but less than or equal to 400 nm shall not exceed the Class I accessible limits for the wavelengths greater than 1400 nm but less than or equal to 1.0 × 10^6 nm with k_1 and k_2 of 1.0 for comparable sampling intervals.

** Measurement parameters and test conditions shall be in accordance with paragraphs (d)(1), (2), (3), and (4), and (e) of this section.

Table 4.3.3.1 Class IIa Accessible Emission Limits for Laser Radiation

Class IIa Accessible Limits are Identical to Class I Accessible Emission Limits Except Within the Following Range of Wavelengths and Emission Durations

Wavelength (nanometers)	Emission Duration (seconds)	Class IIa—Accessible Limits (value)	(unit)	(quantity)*
>400 but ≤710	>1.0 × 10^3	3.9×10^{-6}	W	radiant power

* Measurement parameters and test conditions shall be in accordance with paragraphs (d)(1), (2), (3), and (4), and (e) of this section.

Table 4.3.3.2 Class II Accessible Emission Limits for Laser Radiation

Class II Accessible Limits are Identical to Class I Accessible Emission Limits Except Within the Following Range of Wavelengths and Emission Durations

Wavelength (nanometers)	Emission Duration (seconds)	Class II—Accessible Limits		
		(value)	(unit)	(quantity)*
>400 but ≤710	$>2.5 \times 10^{-1}$	1.0×10^{-3}	W	radiant power

* Measurement parameters and test conditions shall be in accordance with paragraphs (d)(1), (2), (3), and (4), and (e) of this section.

Table 4.3.3.3 Class IIIa Accessible Emission Limits for Laser Radiation

Class IIIa Accessible Limits are Identical to Class I Accessible Emission Limits Except Within the Following Range of Wavelengths and Emission Durations

Wavelength (nanometers)	Emission Duration (seconds)	Class IIIa—Accessible Limits		
		(value)	(unit)	(quantity)*
>400 but ≤710	$>3.8 \times 10^{-4}$	5.0×10^{-3}	W	radiant power

* Measurement parameters and test conditions shall be in accordance with paragraphs (d)(1), (2), (3), and (4), and (e) of this section.

Table 4.3.3.4 Class IIIb Accessible Emission Limits for Laser Radiation

Wavelength (nanometers)	Emission Duration (seconds)	Class IIIb—Accessible Limits		
		(value)	(unit)	(quantity)*
≥180 but ≤400	$\leq 2.5 \times 10^{-1}$	$3.8 \times 10^{-4}k_1k_2$	J	radiant energy
	$>2.5 \times 10^{-1}$	$1.5 \times 10^{-3}k_1k_2$	W	radiant energy
>400 but ≤1400	$>1.0 \times 10^{-9}$ to 2.5×10^{-1}	$10k_1k_2t^{1/3}$	Jcm^{-2}	radiant exposure
		to a maximum value of 10	Jcm^{-2}	radiant exposure
	$>2.5 \times 10_{-1}$	$5.0 \times 10_{-1}$	W	radiant power
>1400 but ≤1.0×10^6	$>1.0 \times 10^{-9}$ to 1.0×10^1	10	Jcm^{-2}	radiant exposure
	$>1.0 \times 10^1$	5.0×10^{-1}	W	radiant power

* Measurement parameters and test conditions shall be in accordance with paragraphs (d)(1), (2), (3), and (4), and (e) of this section.

Table 4.3.4 Values of Wavelength Dependent Correction Factors k_1 and k_2

Wavelength (nanometers)	k_1	k_2		
180 to 302.4	1.0	1.0		
>302.4 to 315	$10\left[\frac{\lambda - 302.4}{5}\right]$	1.0		
>315 to 400	330.0	1.0		
>400 to 700	1.0	1.0		
>700 to 800	$10\left[\frac{\lambda - 700}{515}\right]$	if: $t \leq \frac{10100}{\lambda - 699}$ then: $k_2 = 1.0$	if: $\frac{10100}{\lambda - 699} < t \leq 10^4$ then: $k_2 = \frac{t(\lambda - 699)}{10100}$	if: $t > 10^4$ then: $k_2 = \frac{\lambda - 699}{1.01}$
>800 to 1060	$10\left[\frac{\lambda - 700}{515}\right]$			
>1060 to 1400	5.0	if: $t \leq 100$ then: $k_2 = 1.0$	if: $100 < t \leq 10^4$ then: $k_2 = \frac{t}{100}$	if: $t > 10^4$ then: $k_2 = 100$
>1400 to 1535	1.0	1.0		
>1535 to 1545	$t \leq 10^{-7}$ $k_1 = 100.0$ $t > 10^{-7}$ $k_1 = 1.0$	1.0		
> 1545 to 1.0×10^6	1.0	1.0		

Note: The variables in the expressions are the magnitudes of the sampling interval(t), in units of seconds, and the wavelength (γ), in units of nanometers.

Table 4.3.5 Selected Numerical Solutions for k_1 and k_2

Wavelength (nanometers)	k_1	k_2				
		$t \leq 100$	$t = 300$	$t = 1000$	$t = 3000$	$t \geq 10,000$
180	1.0					
300	1.0					
302	1.0					
303	1.32					
304	2.09					
305	3.31					
306	5.25					
307	8.32					
308	13.2					
309	20.9					
310	33.1			1.0		
311	52.5					
312	83.2					
313	132.0					
314	209.0					
315	330.0					
400	330.0					
401	1.0					
500	1.0					
600	1.0					
700	1.0					
710	1.05	1	1	1.1	3.3	11.0
720	1.09	1	1	2.1	6.3	21.0
730	1.14	1	1	3.1	9.3	31.0
740	1.20	1	1.2	4.1	12.0	41.0
750	1.25	1	1.5	5.0	15.0	50.0
760	1.31	1	1.8	6.0	18.0	60.0
770	1.37	1	2.1	7.0	21.0	70.0
780	1.43	1	2.4	8.0	24.0	80.0
790	1.50	1	2.7	9.0	27.0	90.0
800	1.56	1	3.0	10.0	30.0	100.0
850	1.95	1	3.0	10.0	30.0	100.0
900	2.44	1	3.0	10.0	30.0	100.0
950	3.05	1	3.0	10.0	30.0	100.0
1000	3.82	1	3.0	10.0	30.0	100.0
1050	4.78	1	3.0	10.0	30.0	100.0
1060	5.00	1	3.0	10.0	30.0	100.0
1100	5.00	1	3.0	10.0	30.0	100.0
1400	5.00	1	3.0	10.0	30.0	100.0
1500	1.0					
1540	100.0*					
1600	1.0			1.0		
1.0×10^6	1.0					

* The factor $k_1 = 100.0$ when $t \leq 10^{-7}$ and $k_1 = 1.0$ when $t > 10^{-7}$

Note: The variable (t) is the magnitude of the sampling interval in units of seconds.

Table 4.3.6 Accessible Emission Limits for Collateral Radiation From Laser Products

1. *Accessible emission limits* for collateral radiation having wavelengths greater than 180 nanometers but less than or equal to 1.0×10^6 nanometers are identical to the accessible emission limits of Class I laser radiation, as determined from Tables I and IV in this paragraph.
   i. In the wavelength range of less than or equal to 400 nanometers, for all emission durations;
   ii. In the wavelength range of greater than 400 nanometers, for all emission durations less than or equal to 1×10^3 seconds and, when applicable under paragraph (f)(8) of this section, for all emission durations.
2. *Accessible emission limit* for collateral radiation within the x-ray range of wavelengths is 0.5 milliroentgen in an hour, averaged over a cross-section parallel to the external surface of the product, having an area of 10 square centimeters with no dimension greater than 5 centimeters.

The reader is referred to 21 CFR 1040.10 for the additional limit tables.

Part 1050 Performance Standards for Sonic, Infrasonic, and Ultrasonic Radiation-Emitting Products

These Paragraphs and sections provide for informational material, performance, and certain design features (interlocks) applicable to sunlamps. There are no emission limits. Note: The ultrasound standard (21 CFR 1050.10) covers therapy products only.

The Medical Device Amendments of 1976 to the Food, Drug and Cosmetic Act

This law, passed in 1976 and amended in 1990 and 1992, is intended to assure that medical devices sold in the United States are safe and effective for their intended use when used in accordance with their labeling. It applies to manufacturers of medical devices and regulates device labeling. There are no direct regulations pertaining to radiation output or safety.

Definition

Section 201(h) of the Federal Food, Drug, and Cosmetic Act defines the term ''device'' as ''an instrument, apparatus, implement, machine, contrivance, implant, in vitro reagent, or other similar or related article, including any component, part, or accessory, which is—

- recognized in the official National Formulary, or in the United States Pharmacopeia, or in any supplement to them,
- intended for use in the diagnosis of disease or other conditions, or in the cure, mitigation, treatment, or prevention of disease, in man or other animals, or intended to affect the structure or any function of the body of man or other animals, and

which does not achieve any of its primary purposes through chemical action within or on the body of man or other animals and which is not dependent upon being metabolized for achievement of any of its principle intended purposes.''

The Medical Device Amendments of 1076 expanded the definition of 'device' to include:

- devices intended for use in the diagnosis of conditions other than disease, such as pregnancy, and
- in vitro diagnostic products, including those previously regulated as drugs.

Device Classifications

The Act called for the classification into three classes, all devices that were on the market at the time of the passage of the Act (May 28, 1976). The classes were based of a risk model.

Class I, ''General Controls'' includes devices for which controls other than special controls or premarket approval are sufficient to assure safety and effectiveness. General controls include regulations that prohibit adulteration or misbranding; require domestic device manufacturers, initial importer, and distributors to register their establishments and list their devices; grant authority to ban certain devices; provide for notification of risks and of repair, replacement, or refund; restrict the sale, distribution, or use of certain devices; and govern Good Manufacturing Practices, records and reports, and inspection.

Class II, ''Special Controls'' include general controls but where general controls alone are insufficient to provide reasonable assurance of safety and effectiveness and for which sufficient information exists to establish special controls to provide this assurance. Until a special control is established, only general controls apply. Examples of special controls are mandatory performance standards, voluntary performance standards, and post-marketing studies.

Class III, 'Premarket Approval'': include general controls but where insufficient information exists to assure that general controls and special controls provide reasonable assurance of safety and effectiveness. Generally, class III devices are those represented to be life sustaining or supporting, those implanted in the body, or those presenting potential for unreasonable risk of illness or injury. New class III devices must have approved Premarket Approval Applications (PMAs) prior to distribution. Until PMAs are called for by regulation, preamendment class III devices (those on the market prior to May 28, 1976) are called for by regulation, preamendment class III devices are subject only to general controls.

Routes to Marketing Clearance

New devices are automatically classified into class III unless they can be shown to be ''substantially equivalent'' to a device marketed prior to May 28, 1976. In this case they assume the classification of their predicate. If a new device can not be shown to be substantially equivalent, it needs an approved PMA to be distributed.

Section 510(k) of the FD&C Act requires those device manufacturers who must register to notify FDA of their intent to market a device. This process is known as premarket notification. It allows FDA to determine whether the device is equivalent to a device already placed into one of the three classification categories. The device under review cannot be commercially marketed until the manufacturer (or the importer) receives a specific letter from FDA that finds the device substantially equivalent. The process determines that the new device is equivalent to the predicate device, hence the safety and effectiveness is assured by the device class. FDA must make a decision (i.e., request more information, or find the device class III) within 90 days.

Class III device are subject to premarket approval requirements of section 515 of the FD&C Act. This process is similar to a new drug approval. In a premarket approval application the manufacturer must demonstrate with data that the device is safe and effective for its indicated use when used according to its labeling. Most PMAs are reviewed by FDA and an outside advisory group of medical experts prior to a decision. FDA should reach a decision within 180 days.

Section 520(g) of the FD&C Act allows FDA to exempt devices intended solely for investigational use from certain requirements of the FD&C Act in order to allow for the shipment and use on human subjects. Regulations governing the investigational device exemption process are found in 21 CFR 812.

Mammography Quality Standards Act (MQSA) of 1992

This act was passed to improve the quality of mammography preformed in the United States. Interim regulations (21 CFR 900) were promulgated on December 21, 1993. These addressed the areas of accreditation (Subpart A) and Quality Standards and Certification (Subpart B). The regulations apply to the performance of the equipment and the mammographic facility, quality assurance, personnel qualifications, inspection, and records.

¶ 900.12 Quality Standards

(c) *Dose.* The average glandular dose delivered during a single cranio-caudal view of an accepted phantom simulating a 4.5 centimeter thick, compressed breast consisting of 50 percent glandular and 50 percent adipose tissue, shall not exceed 3.0 milliGray (0.3 rad) per exposure for screen-film mammography procedures and 4.0 milliGray (0.4 rad) per exposure for xeromammography procedures. The dose shall be determined at least annually under technique factors and conditions that are used to produce the phantom images submitted for accreditation.

NATIONAL COUNCIL ON RADIATION PROTECTION AND MEASUREMENTS

NCRP Report 102—Medical Radiation Protection Recommendations
(Summarized by Jack S. Krohmer)

General Considerations

Medical radiation protection is concerned with minimizing the radiation dose equivalent to patients, radiation workers and members of the public. Obviously the lowest doses to these three groups would exist if no radiation was used in medical procedures, however, if this alternative was chosen, the diagnosis and treatment of disease would be seriously compromised. Thus, since the use of radiation and radiation sources in medical procedures is mandated, methods for the protection of all involved persons have been developed. Very broadly, these include the employment of trained and experienced workers who use good safety practices and equipment with well engineered safety features, in properly shielded facilities.

Radiation protection of the *patient* requires many medical and technical decisions. Medical decisions include a determination of:

a. the *need* for the examination or treatment

b. possible *contraindications*, e.g., pregnancy

c. selection of the *most appropriate procedure*

These decisions must be made by the physician, using his professional judgment, and *in consultation with the patient.*

Technical decisions include the choice of *appropriate equipment and technique.* (NOTE:) The equipment must be in proper working condition and maintained under quality assurance program.

Radiation protection of *radiation workers* and nearby members of the *public* are generally achieved by:

a. *increasing the distance* of the individual from the source of radiation.

b. *reducing the time* the individual is near the source.

c. *using protective barriers* between the individual and the source.

GENERAL GUIDELINES IN THE CLINICAL USES OF RADIATION

In *diagnostic* radiation procedures the dose to the patient should be kept to a minimum consistent with clinical objectives, but bearing in mind that too low a dose may compromise the examination. In *therapeutic* radiation procedures the dose to the selected site of treatment should be as prescribed while keeping the dose to all other locations in the patient to a minimum. In order to achieve these goals the following recommendations are presented for the guidance of the medical users:

a. The useful radiation beam *shall* be limited to the smallest area practicable and consistent with the objectives of the examination or treatment.

b. The kilovoltage and source-skin distance and filtration employed in *diagnostic* examinations and *therapeutic* procedures *should* be as large as practical and consistent with objectives of the study.

c. Protection of the embryo or fetus of pregnant women should be given special consideration during diagnostic or therapeutic procedures. In practice, the timeliness and importance of *medical needs* should be the primary considerations in determining the time of the exam and technique details when irradiating these patients.

d. Sensitive body organs (e.g., lens of eye, gonads) should be shielded whenever they are likely to be in the useful beam of radiation providing that this shielding does not compromise diagnostic information or proper treatment.

e. Fluoroscopy should be reserved for the study of dynamics, spatial relationships, guidance in spot-film recording and simulation in radiation therapy.

f. All image recording devices and media should be as sensitive as is consistent with the requirements of the examination.

g. Care should be taken to align the radiation beam with the patient and image receptor in diagnostic studies.

h. No person should routinely hold patients during diagnostic examinations. When a patient must be held in position for these studies, a mechanical supporting or restraining device should be used. If such use of mechanical means is not possible and human support or restraint must be used, the individual holding the patient should be chosen so that cumulative doses will be held within applicable limits.

i. Only persons whose presence is necessary shall be in the diagnostic or low energy (below 150 kV) therapy x-ray rooms during exposure. All such persons shall be protected (e.g., provided with leaded aprons, leaded gloves and/or portable shields).

j. Persons, other than the patient, shall not be in high energy (over 150 kV) therapy rooms during exposure.

k. Proper useful beam filtration should be used for all diagnostic and therapeutic procedures.

l. The operator shall stand behind the provided barrier and shall observe the patient during all diagnostic and therapeutic procedures.

m. The maximum source-skin-distance (SSD) consistent with medical requirements of the procedure should be used for both diagnostic and therapeutic procedures. For diagnostic procedures, other than dental procedures, distances less than 12 inches shall not be used.

n. Radiation source systems, imaging systems, film and film processors should be subjected to appropriate quality assurance programs.

SPECIAL CHARGE TO MEDICAL RADIATION USERS

All individuals who use medical radiation sources for diagnosis or treatment of disease should understand the manner in which the radiation source operates and should know the dose rate and the approximate dose administered to the patient for each procedure.

RADIATION PROTECTION SURVEYS

Medical radiation sources and installations shall be subjected to a radiation protection survey prior to initial use, after any changes in equipment or procedures, and periodically thereafter. A proper radiation protection survey should include:

a. *Investigation.* Collection and examination of information regarding radiation source(s), their intended uses, safeguards present or planned and written procedures.

b. *Inspection.* Verification of the presence of sources, their condition, their uses, operability and integrity of safeguards, and adherence of personnel to written procedures.

c. *Measurement.* Measurement of radiation fields and surface and/or airborne contamination depending on the type of installation. (NOTE: When radiation fields are measured, primary barrier evaluations are made with no phantom in the useful beam and secondary barrier evaluations are made with a phantom in the useful beam and the largest beam possible.)

d. *Evaluation and Recommendation.* Measurement results are converted by means of operational factors into a form which can be directly compared with dose equivalent limits or leakage limits. Results of this comparison and the inspection findings are used to evaluate the safety status of the installation. Recommendations are made regarding remedial action and resurvey after corrective action has been taken.

e. *Records and Reports.* All findings and results are recorded and reported to responsible individuals.

PROTECTION METHODS

When a *qualified expert* finds that there is a reasonable probability that a person in or near a diagnostic or therapeutic installation may receive more than 10% of the applicable dose limit, then one or more of the following actions should be taken:

a. Measure dose rate and apply appropriate workload, use factor and occupancy factors to calculate the potential cumulative dose equivalent to occupants of the area.

b. Use personnel monitoring equipment to evaluate dose equivalent received by occupants of the area.

c. Add shielding (e.g., leaded aprons, leaded gloves and portable shields) to reduce radiation levels to acceptable values.

d. Impose restrictions on the use of equipment and/or degrees of occupancy of surrounding areas to reduce radiation levels to acceptable values.

SAFETY FEATURE TEST FREQUENCIES

All personnel interlocks, ''ON-OFF'' beam control mechanisms, safety and warning devices on radiation therapy or diagnostic installations shall be tested and serviced weekly. Patient protection interlocks shall be checked daily. Results of tests should be recorded.

RADIATION WARNING SIGNS

Proper radiation warning signs shall be posted at appropriate locations around radiation therapy or diagnostic installations. When such signs are deemed to be a source of apprehension to patients and their relatives, the signs may be omitted, providing personnel occupying the area are informed of the radiation levels present and providing entry to the area is strictly enforced.

VERIFICATION OF ADHERENCE TO RESTRICTIONS

If the design and/or approved use of a therapy or diagnostic installation depends upon restrictions in the Use Factor and Occupancy Factor attributed to the primary barriers, it shall be determined that the restrictions are actually observed.

ADMINISTRATIVE RESPONSIBILITIES

Each medical radiation installation shall have an administrative director who shall be responsible for the radiation safety of patients, workers and the public. This director will assure that radiation sources under his jurisdiction are used only by persons competent to use them. The director will also see that appropriate instruction of personnel in safe operating procedures are provided and that rules for radiation safety are available.

DEMONSTRATION EXPOSURES

Deliberate exposure of an individual to the useful beam for training or demonstration purposes shall not be permitted unless there is also a valid medical reason for that exposure.

QUALIFIED EXPERTS

Qualified experts for radiation protection, calibration of equipment and quality assurance in the medical radiation field are as follows:

a. For radiation protection, a person having the knowledge and training to measure ionizing radiation, to evaluate safety techniques and to advise regarding radiation protection needs. (For example, persons certified in an appropriate field by the American Board of Radiology, the American Board of Health Physics, the American Board of Medical Physics, the American Board of Science in Nuclear Medicine or persons determined to have equivalent qualifications.)

b. For radiation therapy calibrations, a person having, in addition to the above qualifications, training and experience in the clinical application of radiation physics to radiation therapy. (For example, persons certified in Radiological Physics, X-Ray and Radium Physics or Therapeutic Radiological Physics by the American Board of Radiology (or in Radiation Oncology Physics by the American Board of Medical Physics) or persons determined to have equivalent qualifications).

c. For diagnostic x-ray performance evaluations, a person having, in addition to the qualifications of part (a) above, training and experience in the physics of diagnostic radiology. (For example, persons certified in Radiological Physics, or X-Ray and Radium Physics or Diagnostic Radiological Physics by the American Board of Radiology (or persons certified in Imaging Physics by the American Board of Medical Physics) or persons determined to have equivalent qualifications).

Not in NCRP 102 but recognized as having expertise.

PERSONNEL MONITORING

Personnel monitoring devices and procedures in the medical radiation field are essentially the same as for any field in which radiation sources are used. The one unique situation which occurs in medical radiation protection has to do with the placement of the radiation monitors when protective aprons are worn, for example, in medical fluoroscopic procedures. In these situations the following paragraph should be used:

> Practice on the positioning of the dosimeter varies from facility to facility, with some placing a single dosimeter under protective aprons, when they are worn, and others placing the single dosimeter outside of protective aprons. In other instances, two dosimeters are used, one under and one outside of protective aprons. If only one dosimeter is worn under the apron, it will approximate the dose to most internal organs but it will underestimate the dose to the head and neck (including the thyroid gland). If only one dosimeter is worn and it is worn outside the apron, it will approximate the dose to the head and neck but it will overestimate the dose to the organs covered by the apron. In either case, if only one dosimeter is worn, the Radiation Safety Officer (RSO) should calculate the *effective dose equivalent* using what is known of the ratio of the exposure received under the apron to that received outside the apron. In facilities where two dosimeters are worn, one under and one outside the apron, the *effective dose equivalent* can be more readily calculated. If two dosimeters are worn, *the RSO must adopt a method for combining the two readings to yield a single estimate of the effective dose equivalent*. When no apron is worn, the dosimeter should be worn on the trunk of the body at waist level or above where it will be representative of the most highly exposed part of the surface of the trunk.

SUGGESTED STATE REGULATIONS FOR CONTROL OF RADIATION: VOLUME 1 IONIZING RADIATION

(From Conference of Radiation Control Program Directors 1990)

The Suggested State Regulations for Control of Radiation (SSRCR) were initially published in 1962 by the Council of State Governments with the advice and assistance of the Atomic Energy Commission and the Public Health Service. The 8th edition of the SSRCR was prepared by the Conference of Radiation Control Program Directors, Inc., Nuclear Regulatory Commission, Environmental Protection Agency and the Food and Drug Administration. Additional technical assistance was provided by individuals from State radiation control programs, Department of Energy, Department of Transportation and Federal Emergency Management Agency.

The SSRCR require the licensing of all radioactive material and the registration of all other sources of ionizing radiation. Applicable federal statutes require that certain state regulations be compatible with, identical to, or as effective as, federal regulations. Some of the provisions in this edition were developed or revised to reflect compatibility with current NRC regulations for use by Agreement States that assume regulatory responsibility over source, byproduct, and certain special nuclear material under Section 274b of the Atomic Energy Act of 1954 as amended. Further certain provisions have been prepared to not conflict with electronic product performance standards issued by the Food and Drug Administration under Section 358 of the Public Health Service Act.

Section 274 of the Atomic Energy Act was enacted by Congress on September 23, 1959 to recognize the interests of the States in the safe use of atomic energy, to clarify the respective responsibilities of State and Federal Governments, and to provide a mechanism for States to enter into formal agreements

---

effective dose equivalent: The sum over specified tissues of the products of the dose equivalent in a tissue (T) and the weighting factor for that tissue.

with the Atomic Energy Commission (AEC), and later, its successor, the Nuclear Regulatory Commission (NRC), under which the States assume regulatory authority over byproduct, source, and small quantities of special nuclear materials, collectively referred to as agreement materials. The mechanism by which the NRC discontinues and the States assume regulatory authority over agreement materials is an agreement between the Governor of a State and the Commission. Before entering into an Agreement, the Governor is required to certify that the State has a regulatory program that is adequate to protect the public health and safety and compatible with NRC programs. In addition, the Commission must perform an independent evaluation and make a finding that the State's program is adequate from the health and safety standpoint and compatible with Commission's regulatory program.

It should be stressed that these are suggested state regulations and the regulations of the applicable state should be consulted in any specific situation. An index of the SSRCR parts and excerpted provisions of interest are provided in the following tables.

Parts of the SSRCR

Part A	General Provisions
Part B	Registration of Radiation Machine Facilities and Services (Draft revision 1994)
Part C	Licensing of Radioactive Material
Part D	Standards for Protection Against Radiation
Part E	Radiation Safety Requirements for Industrial Radiographic Operations
Part F	X-Rays in the Healing Arts (Draft revision 1995)
Part G	Use of Radionuclides in the Healing Arts
Part H	Radiation Safety Requirements for Analytical X-Ray Equipment
Part I	Radiation Safety Requirements for Particle Accelerators
Part J	Notices, Instructions, and Reports to Workers; Inspections
Part M	Licensing Requirements for Land Disposal of Radioactive Waste
Part T	Transportation of Radioactive Material
Part U	Licensing Requirements for Source Material Milling Facilities
Part W	Radiation Safety Requirements for Wireline Service Operations and Subsurface Tracer Studies

Part E Radiation Safety Requirements for Industrial Radiographic Operations

Sec. E.101 Limits on Levels of Radiation for Radiographic Exposure Devices and Storage Containers

Radiographic exposure devices measuring less than 4 inches (10 cm) from the sealed source storage position to any exterior surface of the device shall have no radiation level in excess of 50 milliroentgens (1.29×10^{-5} C/kg) per hour at 6 inches (15 cm) from any exterior surface of the device. Radiographic exposure devices measuring a minimum of 4 inches (10 cm) from the sealed source storage position to any exterior surface of the device, and all storage containers for sealed sources or outer containers for radiographic exposure devices, shall have no radiation level in excess of 200 milliroentgens (5.16×10^{-5} C/kg) per hour at any exterior surface, and 10 milliroentgens (2.58×10^{-6} C/kg) per hour at 39.4 inches (1 m) from any exterior surface. The radiation levels specified are with the sealed source in the shielded position.

Part F X-Rays in the Healing Arts

(Revised Part F Use of Diagnostic X-Rays In The Healing Arts from 1995 Draft follow)

Sec. F.8 Therapeutic X-Ray Systems of Less than One MeV

(a) *Equipment Requirements*

(1) *Leakage Radiation.* When the tube is operated at its leakage technique factors, the leakage radiation shall not exceed the value specified at the distance specified for the classification of that x-ray system.

(i) *Contact Therapy Systems.* Leakage radiation shall not exceed 100 milliroentgens (25.8 μC/kg) per hour at 5 centimeters from the surface of the tube housing assembly.

(ii) *0–150 kVp Systems.* Systems which were manufactured or installed prior to [the effective date of F.8] shall have a leakage radiation which does not exceed 1 roentgen (0.258 mC/kg) in 1 hour at 1 meter from the source.

(iii) *0–150 kVp Systems.* Systems which are manufactured on or after [the effective date of F.8] shall have a leakage radiation which does not exceed 100 milliroentgens (25.8 μC/kg) in 1 hour at 1 meter from the source.

(iv) *151 to 999 kVp Systems.* The leakage radiation shall not exceed 1 roentgen (0.258 mC/kg) in 1 hour at 1 meter from the source except systems that operate in excess of 500 kVp may have a leakage radiation at 1 meter from the source not to exceed 0.1 percent of the useful beam 1 meter from the source.

Sec. F.9 X-Ray and Electron Therapy Systems with Energies of One MeV and Above.

(b) *Requirements for Equipment*

(1) *Leakage Radiation to the Patient Area.*

(i) New equipment shall meet the following requirements.

(*a*) For operating conditions producing maximum leakage radiation, the absorbed dose in rads (grays) due to leakage radiation, including x-rays, electrons, and neutrons, at any point in a circular plane of 2 meters radius centered on and perpendicular to the central axis of the beam at the isocenter or normal treatment distance and outside the maximum useful beam size shall not exceed 0.1 percent of the maximum absorbed dose in rads (grays) of the unattenuated useful beam measured at the point of intersection of the central axis of the beam and the plane surface. Measurements excluding those for neutrons shall be averaged over an area up to but not exceeding 100 square centimeters at the positions specified. Measurements of the portion of the leakage radiation dose contributed by neutrons shall be averaged over an area up to but not exceeding 200 square centimeters.

(2) *Leakage Radiation Outside the Patient Area for New Equipment.*

(i) The absorbed dose in rads (grays) due to leakage radiation except in the area specified in F.9(b)(1)(i)(*a*) when measured at any point 1 meter from the path of the charged particle, before the charged particle strikes the target or window, shall not exceed 0.1 percent for x-ray leakage nor 0.05 percent for neutron leakage of the maximum absorbed dose in rads (grays) of the unattenuated useful beam measured at the point of intersection of the central axis of the beam and the circular plane specified in F.9(b)(1)(i)(*a*).

(ii) The registrant shall determine or obtain from the manufacturer, the actual leakage radiation existing at the positions specified in F.9(b)(2)(i) for specified operating conditions. Radiation measurements excluding neutrons shall be averaged over an area up to but not exceeding 100 square centimeters. Neutron measurements shall be averaged over an area up to but not exceeding 200 square centimeters.

Part F Use of Diagnostic X-Rays In The Healing Arts from Draft revision 1995

Section F.3 General and Administrative Requirements

(a) Radiation Safety Requirements

(ii) Individuals who will be operating x-ray systems shall be adequately instructed in the safe operating procedures for diagnostic purposes

Section F.4 General Requirements for All Diagnostic X-ray Systems

(c) *Leakage Radiation from the Diagnostic Source Assembly.* The leakage radiation from the diagnostic source assembly measured at a distance of 1 meter in any direction from the source shall not exceed 25.8 μC/kg (100 milliroentgens) in 1 hour when the x-ray tube is operated at its leakage technique factors. Compliance shall be determined by measurements averaged over an area of 100 square centimeters with no linear measurement greater than 20 centimeters.

(d) *Radiation from Components Other Than the Diagnostic Source Assembly.* The radiation emitted by a component other than the diagnostic source assembly shall not exceed 0.5 μC/kg (2 milliroentgens) in 1 hour at 5 centimeters from any accessible surface of the component when it is operated in an assembled x-ray system under any conditions for which it was designed. Compliance shall be determined by measurements averaged over an area of 100 square centimeters with no linear measurement greater than 20 centimeters.

Section F.5 Fluoroscopic X-Ray Systems

Exposure rate limits

(i) Entrance Exposure Rate Allowed Limits.

(1) Fluoroscopic equipment which is provided with automatic *exposure* rate control shall not be operable at any combination of tube potential and current which will result in an *exposure* rate in excess of 2.6 mC/kg (10 roentgens) per minute at the point where the center of the useful beam enters the patient, except:

(a) During recording of fluoroscopic images, or

(b) When an optional high-level control is provided. When so provided, the equipment shall not be operable at an *exposure* rate of 1.3 mC/kg (5 roentgens) per minute at the point where the useful beam combination of tube potential and current which will result in an enters the patient unless the high-level control is activated. Special means of activation of high level controls shall be required. The high-level control shall be operable only when continuous manual activation is provided by the operator. A continuous signal audible to the fluoroscopist shall indicate that the high-level control is being employed.

(2) Fluoroscopic equipment which is not provided with automatic *exposure* rate control shall not be operable at any combination of tube potential and current which will result in an *exposure* rate in excess of 1.3 mC/kg (5 roentgens) per minute at the point where the center of the useful beam enters the patient, except:

(a) During recording of fluoroscopic images, or

(b) When an optional high-level control is provided. When so provided, the equipment shall not be operable at an *exposure* rate of 1.3 mC/kg (5 roentgens) per minute at the point where the useful beam combination of tube potential and current which will result in an enters the patient unless the high-level control is activated. Special means of activation of high level controls shall be required. The high-level control shall be operable only when continuous manual activation is provided by the operator. A continuous signal audible to the fluoroscopist shall indicate that the high-level control is being employed.

Part G Use of Radionuclides in the Healing Arts

Sec. G.26 Release of Patients Containing Radiopharmaceuticals or Permanent Implants.

(a) A licensee shall not authorize release from confinement for medical care any patient administered a radiopharmaceutical until either:
  (1) The dose rate from the patient is less than 5 millirems (50 μSv) per hour at a distance of 1 meter; or
  (2) The activity in the patient is less than 30 millicuries (1.11 GBq).

(b) A licensee shall not authorize release from confinement for medical care any patient administered a permanent implant until the dose rate from the patient is less than 5 millirems (50 μSv) per hour at a distance of 1 meter.

Specific Requirement for the Use of Radiopharmaceuticals for Therapy
Sec. G.38 Safety Precautions

(7) Survey the patient's room and private sanitary facility for removable contamination with a radiation detection survey instrument before assigning another patient to the room. The room must not be reassigned until removable contamination is less than 200 disintegrations per minute (3.33 Bq) per 100 square centimeters.

Specific Requirements for the Use of a Sealed Source in Teletherapy
Sec. G.59 Radiation Surveys for Teletherapy Facilities.

(a) Before medical use, after each installation of a teletherapy source, and after making any change for which an amendment is required by G.50, the licensee shall perform radiation surveys with an operable radiation measurement survey instrument calibrated in accordance with G.17 (calibration and check of survey instruments) to verify that:
  (1) The maximum and average radiation levels at 1 meter from the teletherapy source with the source in the ''off'' position and the collimator set for a normal treatment field do not exceed 10 millirems (100 μSv) per hour, respectively; and
  (2) With the teletherapy source in the ''on'' position with the largest clinically available treatment field and with a scattering phantom in the primary beam of radiation, that
    (I) Radiation levels in restricted areas are not likely to cause personnel exposures in excess of the limits specified in D.101 of these regulations (i.e., occupational limits); and
    (ii) Radiation levels in unrestricted areas do not exceed the limits specified in D.105 (a) of these regulations (i.e., public limits).

Part H Radiation Safety Requirements for Analytical X-Ray Equipment

Sec. H.3 Equipment Requirements

(f) *Radiation Source Housing.* Each radiation source housing shall be subject to the following requirements:
  (1) Each x-ray tube housing shall be equipped with an interlock that shuts off the tube if it is removed from the radiation source housing or if the housing is disassembled.
  (2) Each radioactive source housing or port cover or each x-ray tube housing shall be so constructed that, with all shutters closed, the radiation measured at a distance of 5 centimeters from its surface is not capable of producing a dose in excess of 2.5 millirems (0.025 mSv) in one hour. For systems utilizing x-ray tubes, this limit shall be met at any specified tube rating.

(g) *Generator Cabinet.* Each x-ray generator shall be supplied with a protective cabinet which limits leakage radiation measured at a distance of 5 centimeters from its surface such that it is not capable of producing a dose in excess of 0.25 millirem (2.5 μSv) in one hour.

References

Alexander, R.E. *Synopsis of Major Changes in the Revised 10CFR Part 20.* The Alexander Corporation; Fairfax, VA; 1991.

Alexander, R.E. Personal communication; 1991.

British Committee on Radiological Units and Measurements. (BCRU). *J Radiol Pro* **13:**71–73, 1993.

Clark, R.H. ''Response by NRPB to the 1990 recommendations of the ICRP,'' National Radiation Protection Board; *Radiological Protection Bulletin* **141:** April 1993.

Dodd, D.H., Robinson C.A. ''Quantities used in radiological protection: 1993 update; National Radiation Protection Board,'' Radiological Protection Bulletin **14:** April 1993.

Clarke, R.H. Supplement to the *Radiological Protection Bulletin*, No. 119, National Radiological Protection Board; Oxon, UK; 1991.

Code of Federal Regulations 21, Parts 800 to 1200; Revised as of April 1, 1996.

Codex Alimentarius Commission ''Contaminants: Guideline levels for radionuclides in food following accidental nuclear contamination for use in international trade,'' CAC/Vol XVII Ed 1, Supplement 1, Joint FAO/WHO Food Standards Programme, Food and Agriculture Organization, World Health Organization; Rome; 1989.

Department of Agriculture. ''Radionuclide screening values for monitoring imported meat products,'' Food Safety and Inspection Service; Washington, DC; 1986.

Department of Energy. ''Management of low-level waste,'' in *Radioactive Waste Management*, Order 5820.2A, 1988.

Department of Energy, ''Radiation protection of the public and the environment,'' Order 5400.5; 1990.

Dodd, D.H., Robinson, C.A. NRPB Bulletin No. 141; 1993.

Environmental Protection Agency. ''Federal radiation protection guidance for occupational exposure,'' *Fed. Register* **52:**2822; 1987.

Environmental Protection Agency. ''Part 141—National interim primary drinking water regulations,'' in Title 40 of *Code of Federal Regulations*, published annually by U.S. Government Printing Office, Washington, DC; see also *Fed Register* **41:**28402; 1976.

Environmental Protection Agency. ''Part 190—Environmental radiation protection standards for nuclear power operations,'' in Title 40 of *Code of Federal Regulations*, published annually by U.S. Government Printing Office, Washington, DC; see also *Fed Register* **42:**2858 1977.

Environmental Protection Agency. ''Proposed guidance on dose limits for persons exposed to transuranium elements in the general environment,'' EPA 520/4-77-016 1977.

Environmental Protection Agency. ''Part 192—Health and environmental protection standards for uranium and thorium mill tailings,'' in Title 40 of *Code of Federal Regulations*, published annually by U.S. Government Printing Office, Washington, DC; see also *Fed Register* **48:**602 1983 and *Fed. Registr.* **48:**45946; 1983.

Environmental Protection Agency. ''Part 191—Environmental radiation protection standards for management and disposal of spent nuclear fuel, high-level and transuranic waste,'' in Title 40 of *Code of Federal Regulations*, published annually by U.S. Government Printing Office, Washington, DC; see also *Fed Register* 50, 38066; 1985.

Environmental Protection Agency and Department of Health and Human Services. *A Citizen's Guide to Radon*, OPA-86-004; 1986.

Environmental Protection Agency. ''Interim recommendations on doses to persons exposed to transuranium elements in the general environment,'' draft report; Washington, DC; 1987.

Environmental Protection Agency, ''Part 61—National emission standards for hazardous air pollutants,'' in Title 40 of *Code of Federal Regulations*, published annually by U.S. Government Printing Office, Washington, DC; see also *Fed Register* 54, 51695; 1989.

Environmental Protection Agency 40CFR "Part 61, National emissions standards for hazardous air pollutants, polonium—210 emissions from elemental phosphorus plants: Final Rule," *Fed Register* **56:**244, 65934; 1991.

Environmental Protection Agency, "Manual of Protective Action Guides and Protective Actions for Nuclear Incidents," EPA 400-R-92-001 1992.

Environmental Protection Agency 40CFR, "Part 61, National emissions standards for hazardous air pollutants; national emission standards for radon emission from phosphogypsum stacks: Final Rule," *Fed Register* **57:**107, 23305; 1992.

Environmental Protection Agency 40CFR, "Part 191, Environmental radiation protection standards for the management and disposal of spent nuclear fuel, high-level and transuranic radioactive wastes: Final rule" *Fed Register* **58:**242, 66398; 1993.

Environmental Protection Agency 40CFR. "Part 61, National emissions standards for hazardous air pollutants: Final rule," *Fed Register* **59:**135, 36281; 1994. International Atomic Energy Agency, Safety Series No. 115,

Everything You Always Wanted to Know About Medical Device Requirements and Weren't Afraid to Ask, 4th ed, HHS Publication FDA 92-4173; 1992.

Food and Drug Administration. *Code of Federal Regulations 21, Subchapter J-Radiological Health*; April 1, 1990.

Food and Drug Administration, "Accidental radioactive contamination of human food and animal feeds; recommendations for state and local agencies," *Fed Register* **47:**47073; 1982.

Food and Drug Administration, "Radionuclides in imported foods—levels of concern," Compliance Policy Guide 7119.14, *Import Foods*, Rockville, MD; 1986.

Food and Drug Administration, "Potassium iodide as a thyroid blocking agent in a radiation emergency: Final recommendations on use," *Fed. Register* **47:**28158; 1982.

Forbes, P.D., Mikhail, S.Z. "Acute lesions in skin produced by radioactive microspheres," oral presentation at the annual meeting of the Radiation Research Society, 1970, abstract in *Radiat Res* **39:**493.

International Atomic Energy Agency. "International basic safety standards for protection against ionizing radiation and for the safety of radiation sources," IAEA Safety Series 115, IAEA, Vienna; 1996.

International Commission on Radiological Protection, "Recommendations of the International Commission on Radiological Protection," ICRP Publication 26, *Ann ICRP* **1:**3, Pergamon Press; Oxford; 1977.

International Commission on Radiological Protection. "Limits for intakes of radionuclides by workers," ICRP Publication 30 Part 1, *Ann ICRP* **2:**3/4; Pergamon Press; Oxford; 1978.

International Commission on Radiological Protection. "Protection of the public in the event of major radiation accidents: Principles for planning," ICRP Publication 40, *Ann ICRP* **14:**2, Pergamon Press; Oxford; 1984.

International Commission on Radiological Protection. "Statement from the 1985 Paris Meeting of the International Commission on Radiological Protection," in ICRP Publication 45, *Ann ICRP* **15:**3, Pergamon Press; Oxford; 1985.

International Commission on Radiological Protection. "1990 Recommendations of the International Commission on Radiological Protection," ICRP Publication 60, *Ann ICRP* **21:**1–3; Pergamon Press; Oxford; 1991.

International Commission on Radiological Protection. "Annual Limits on Intake of Radionuclides by Workers Based on the 1990 Recommendations," ICRP Publication 61; Pergamon Press; Oxford; 1990.

International Commission on Radiology Protection. *Principles for Intervention for Protection of the Public in a Radiological Emergency*. Pergamon Press; Oxford; ICRP Publication 63; *Ann ICRP* **20:**4; 1993.

International Commission on Radiological Protection. *Protection for Potential Exposure: A Conceptual Framework*. Pergamon Press; Oxford; ICRP Publication 64; *Ann ICRP* **23:**1; 1993.

International Commission on Radiological Protection. *Protection Against Radon—222 at Home and at Work*. Pergamon Press; Oxford; ICRP Publication 64; *Ann ICRP* **23:**2; 1993.

ICRU. ''Determination of dose equivalents resulting from external radiation sources.'' Bethesda, MD, ICRU Report 39; 1985.

ICRU. Determination of dose equivalents from external radiation sources. Part 2. Bethesda, MD, ICRU, Report 43; 1988.

Kocher, D.C. Personal communication; 1991.

National Council on Radiation Protection and Measurements. ''Evaluation of risk estimates for radiation protection purposes, NCRP Report No. 115, NCRP, Bethesda, MD; 1993a.

National Council on Radiation Protection and Measurements. ''Limitation of exposure to ionizing radiation,'' NCRP Report No. 116, NCRP, Bethesda, MD; 1993.

National Council on Radiation Protection and Measurements. ''Recommendations on limits for exposure to ionizing radiation,'' NCRP Report No. 91, NCRP, Bethesda, MD; 1987.

National Council on Radiation Protection and Measurements. ''Medical x-ray, electron beam and gamma-ray protection for energies up to 50 MeV (equipment design, performance and use),'' NCRP Report No. 102, NCRP, Bethesda, MD; 1989.

National Council on Radiation Protection and Measurements. ''Limit for exposure to 'hot particles' on the skin,'' NCRP Report No. 106; NCRP; Bethesda, MD; 1989.

National Council on Radiation Protection and Measurements. ''Limitations of exposure to ionizing radiators,'' NCRP Report No. 116, NCRP; Bethesda, MD; 1993.

NRPB. Board Statement. ''1990 Recommendations of the International Commission on Radiological Protection.'' *Doc NRPB* **4:**1–5; 1993.

NRPB. ''1990 Recommendations of the International Commission on Radiological Protection. Recommendations for the practical application of the board's statement.'' *Doc NRPB*, **4:**7–22; 1993.

Nuclear Regulatory Commission. ''Termination of operating licenses for nuclear reactors,'' *Regulatory Guide* **1.86**; 1974.

Nuclear Regulatory Commission. ''Appendix I—Numerical guides for design objectives and limiting conditions for operation to meet the criterion 'as low as is reasonably achievable' for radioactive material in light-water-cooled nuclear power reactor effluents,'' in ''Part 50—Domestic licensing of production and utilization facilities,'' in Title 10 of *Code of Federal Regulations*, published annually by U.S. Government Printing Office, Washington, DC; see also *Fed Register* **40:**19442; 1975.

Nuclear Regulatory Commission. ''Criteria for preparation and evaluation of radiological emergency response plans and preparedness in support of nuclear power plants,'' NUREG-0654, FEMA-REP-1, Rev. 1, Appendix 1; November 1980.

Nuclear Regulatory Commission. ''Guidelines for decontamination of facilities and equipment prior to release for unrestricted use or termination of licenses for byproduct, source or special nuclear material,'' 1982.

Nuclear Regulatory Commission. ''Part 61—Licensing requirements for land disposal of radioactive waste,'' in Title 10 of *Code of Federal Regulations*, published annually by U.S. Government Printing Office, Washington, DC; see also *Fed Registdr* **47:**57446; 1982.

Nuclear Regulatory Commission. ''Below regulatory concern,'' policy statement, *Fed Register* 55, 27522 1990.

Nuclear Regulatory Commission. ''Part 30—Rules of general applicability to domestic licensing of byproduct material,'' in Title 10 of *Code of Federal Regulations*, published annually by U.S. Government Printing Office, Washington, DC.

Nuclear Regulatory Commission. ''Part 40—Domestic licensing of source material,'' in Title 10 of *Code of Federal Regulations*, published annually by U.S. Government Printing Office, Washington, DC.

Nuclear Regulatory Commission. ''Part 71—Packaging and transportation of radioactive material,'' in Title 10 of *Code of Federal Regulations*, published annually by U.S. Government Printing Office, Washington, DC.

Nuclear Regulatory Commission. ''10 CFR Part 20—Standards for protection against radiation,'' Final Rule, *Fed Register* **56:** 23360; 1991.

Phillips, R.A. Personal communication; 1966.

Radiological Criteria for Decommissioning. 10 CFR Part 20, *Fed Register* **V59:**161; 1994.

Roecklein, A.K. Personal Communication 1996.

Suggested State Regulations for Control of Radiation. *Volume 1; Ionizing Radiation; Conference of Radiation Control Program Directors, Inc*; 8th Edition; June 1990.

Suggested State Regulations for Control of Radiation. *Part B, Registration of Radiation Machine Facilities and Services; Draft Revision*; 1994.

Suggested State Regulations for Control of Radiation. *Part F, Use of Diagnostic Xrays in the Healing Arts; Draft Revision*; 1995

Suggested State Regulations for Control of Radiation. *Part G, Use of Radionuclides in the Healing Arts*, Draft Revision; 1995.

Suggested State Regulations for Control of Radiation. *Part H, Radiation Safety Requirements for Analytical Xray Equipment*, Draft Revision; 1995.

Suggested State Regulations for Control of Radiation. *Part M, Licensing Requirements for Land Disposal of Radioactive Waste*, Draft Revision; 1995.

Ulbert, J.C., Kochendorfer, D.B. *Model for Estimating Beta Dose to Tissue from Particle Debris in Aerospace Nuclear Applications*, USNDRL-TR-1107; United States Technical Information Service; Springfield, VA; 1966.

Vennert, J. "The 1990 recommendations of the International Commission on Radiological Protection," Note. *J Radiol Prot* **11:**199–203; 1991.

CHAPTER 5

INTERACTION OF RADIATION WITH MATTER

Attenuation coefficients and density are physical characteristics of matter essential for radiation shielding and dose calculations. For flexibility, both mass and mass energy-absorption coefficients are listed in this chapter for a continuum of photon energy interactions with pertinent elements found in shielding materials and tissue. Specific mass attenuation coefficients are provided for materials such as concrete, lucite, polyethylene, Bakelite, Pyrex glass and lead as well as tissues such as bone and muscle. Coefficients are provided above and below edges for better interpolation. Mass attenuation coefficients of compounds and mixtures use simple additivity for elements according to their proportions by weight, but mass energy-absorption coefficients are adjusted for matrix effects. The attenuation coefficients for the three mechanisms by which radiation interacts with matter (photoelectric, Compton and pair production) are provided in graphical form for lead and water. For practical values on the transmission of radiation from various sources through many materials see Chapter 6.

TABLE OF CONTENTS

Table 5.1 Mass Attenuation and Energy-Absorption Coefficients (cm^2/g)[a] (From Hubbell and Seltzer, 1995)

Photon Energy (MeV)	Hydrogen μ/ρ (cm^2/g)	Z = 1 μ_{en}/ρ (cm^2/g)	Photon Energy (MeV)	Lithium μ/ρ (cm^2/g)	Z = 3 μ_{en}/ρ (cm^2/g)
1.00000E − 03	7.217E + 00	6.820E + 00	1.00000E − 03	2.339E + 02	2.335E + 02
1.50000E − 03	2.148E + 00	1.752E + 00	1.50000E − 03	6.668E + 01	6.629E + 01
2.00000E − 03	1.059E + 00	6.643E − 01	2.00000E − 03	2.707E + 01	2.672E + 01
3.00000E − 03	5.612E − 01	1.693E − 01	3.00000E − 03	7.549E + 00	7.249E + 00
4.00000E − 03	4.546E − 01	6.549E − 02	4.00000E − 03	3.114E + 00	2.840E + 00
5.00000E − 03	4.193E − 01	3.278E − 02	5.00000E − 03	1.619E + 00	1.364E + 00
6.00000E − 03	4.042E − 01	1.996E − 02	6.00000E − 03	9.875E − 01	7.477E − 01
8.00000E − 03	3.914E − 01	1.160E − 02	8.00000E − 03	5.054E − 01	2.888E − 01
1.00000E − 02	3.854E − 01	9.849E − 03	1.00000E − 02	3.395E − 01	1.387E − 01
1.50000E − 02	3.764E − 01	1.102E − 02	1.50000E − 02	2.176E − 01	3.910E − 02
2.00000E − 02	3.695E − 01	1.355E − 02	2.00000E − 02	1.856E − 01	1.885E − 02
3.00000E − 02	3.570E − 01	1.863E − 02	3.00000E − 02	1.644E − 01	1.138E − 02
4.00000E − 02	3.458E − 01	2.315E − 02	4.00000E − 02	1.551E − 01	1.131E − 02
5.00000E − 02	3.355E − 01	2.709E − 02	5.00000E − 02	1.488E − 01	1.237E − 02
6.00000E − 02	3.260E − 01	3.053E − 02	6.00000E − 02	1.438E − 01	1.361E − 02
8.00000E − 02	3.091E − 01	3.620E − 02	8.00000E − 02	1.356E − 01	1.588E − 02
1.00000E − 01	2.944E − 01	4.063E − 02	1.00000E − 01	1.289E − 01	1.776E − 02
1.50000E − 01	2.651E − 01	4.813E − 02	1.50000E − 01	1.158E − 01	2.098E − 02
2.00000E − 01	2.429E − 01	5.254E − 02	2.00000E − 01	1.060E − 01	2.290E − 02
3.00000E − 01	2.112E − 01	5.695E − 02	3.00000E − 01	9.210E − 02	2.481E − 02
4.00000E − 01	1.893E − 01	5.860E − 02	4.00000E − 01	8.249E − 02	2.552E − 02
5.00000E − 01	1.729E − 01	5.900E − 02	5.00000E − 01	7.532E − 02	2.569E − 02
6.00000E − 01	1.599E − 01	5.875E − 02	6.00000E − 01	6.968E − 02	2.559E − 02
8.00000E − 01	1.405E − 01	5.739E − 02	8.00000E − 01	6.121E − 02	2.499E − 02
1.00000E + 00	1.263E − 01	5.556E − 02	1.00000E + 00	5.503E − 02	2.419E − 02
1.25000E + 00	1.129E − 01	5.311E − 02	1.25000E + 00	4.921E − 02	2.312E − 02
1.50000E + 00	1.027E − 01	5.075E − 02	1.50000E + 00	4.476E − 02	2.210E − 02
2.00000E + 00	8.769E − 02	4.650E − 02	2.00000E + 00	3.830E − 02	2.028E − 02
3.00000E + 00	6.921E − 02	3.992E − 02	3.00000E + 00	3.043E − 02	1.753E − 02
4.00000E + 00	5.806E − 02	3.523E − 02	4.00000E + 00	2.572E − 02	1.561E − 02
5.00000E + 00	5.049E − 02	3.174E − 02	5.00000E + 00	2.257E − 02	1.422E − 02
6.00000E + 00	4.498E − 02	2.905E − 02	6.00000E + 00	2.030E − 02	1.316E − 02
8.00000E + 00	3.746E − 02	2.515E − 02	8.00000E + 00	1.725E − 02	1.167E − 02
1.00000E + 01	3.254E − 02	2.247E − 02	1.00000E + 01	1.529E − 02	1.066E − 02
1.50000E + 01	2.539E − 02	1.837E − 02	1.50000E + 01	1.252E − 02	9.182E − 03
2.00000E + 01	2.153E − 02	1.606E − 02	2.00000E + 01	1.109E − 02	8.385E − 03

[a] μ/ρ includes the photoelectric, coherent (Rayleigh) and incoherent (Compton) scattering, and the electron-position production cross-sections. The latter includes both production in the field of the nucleus as well as that of the atomic electrons. Photonuclear cross-sections, nuclear-resonance scattering, and Delbrück scattering are not included.

Table 5.1 Mass Attenuation and Energy-Absorption Coefficients (Continued)

Photon Energy (MeV)	Beryllium	Z = 4	Photon Energy (MeV)	Boron	Z = 5
	μ_{en}/ρ (cm²/g)	μ_{en}/ρ (cm²/g)		μ/ρ (cm²/g)	μ_{en}/ρ (cm²/g)
1.00000E − 03	6.041E + 02	6.035E + 02	1.00000E − 03	1.229E + 03	1.228E + 03
1.50000E − 03	1.797E + 02	1.791E + 02	1.50000E − 03	3.766E + 02	3.759E + 02
2.00000E − 03	7.469E + 01	7.422E + 01	2.00000E − 03	1.597E + 02	1.591E + 02
3.00000E − 03	2.127E + 01	2.090E + 01	3.00000E − 03	4.667E + 01	4.617E + 01
4.00000E − 03	8.685E + 00	8.367E + 00	4.00000E − 03	1.927E + 01	1.886E + 01
5.00000E − 03	4.369E + 00	4.081E + 00	5.00000E − 03	9.683E + 00	9.332E + 00
6.00000E − 03	2.527E + 00	2.260E + 00	6.00000E − 03	5.538E + 00	5.223E + 00
8.00000E − 03	1.124E + 00	8.839E − 01	8.00000E − 03	2.346E + 00	2.072E + 00
1.00000E − 02	6.466E − 01	4.255E − 01	1.00000E − 02	1.255E + 00	1.006E + 00
1.50000E − 02	3.070E − 01	1.143E − 01	1.50000E − 02	4.827E − 01	2.698E − 01
2.00000E − 02	2.251E − 01	4.780E − 02	2.00000E − 02	3.014E − 01	1.084E − 01
3.00000E − 02	1.792E − 01	1.898E − 02	3.00000E − 02	2.063E − 01	3.506E − 02
4.00000E − 02	1.640E − 01	1.438E − 02	4.00000E − 02	1.793E − 01	2.084E − 02
5.00000E − 02	1.554E − 01	1.401E − 02	5.00000E − 02	1.665E − 01	1.737E − 02
6.00000E − 02	1.493E − 01	1.468E − 02	6.00000E − 02	1.583E − 01	1.680E − 02
8.00000E − 02	1.401E − 01	1.658E − 02	8.00000E − 02	1.472E − 01	1.785E − 02
1.00000E − 01	1.328E − 01	1.836E − 02	1.00000E − 01	1.391E − 01	1.940E − 02
1.50000E − 01	1.190E − 01	2.157E − 02	1.50000E − 01	1.243E − 01	2.255E − 02
2.00000E − 01	1.089E − 01	2.353E − 02	2.00000E − 01	1.136E − 01	2.453E − 02
3.00000E − 01	9.463E − 02	2.548E − 02	3.00000E − 01	9.862E − 02	2.654E − 02
4.00000E − 01	8.471E − 02	2.620E − 02	4.00000E − 01	8.834E − 02	2.731E − 02
5.00000E − 01	7.739E − 02	2.639E − 02	5.00000E − 01	8.065E − 02	2.749E − 02
6.00000E − 01	7.155E − 02	2.627E − 02	6.00000E − 01	7.460E − 02	2.737E − 02
8.00000E − 01	6.286E − 02	2.565E − 02	8.00000E − 01	6.549E − 02	2.671E − 02
1.00000E + 00	5.652E − 02	2.483E − 02	1.00000E + 00	5.890E − 02	2.586E − 02
1.25000E + 00	5.054E − 02	2.373E − 02	1.25000E + 00	5.266E − 02	2.472E − 02
1.50000E + 00	4.597E − 02	2.268E − 02	1.50000E + 00	4.791E − 02	2.362E − 02
2.00000E + 00	3.938E − 02	2.083E − 02	2.00000E + 00	4.108E − 02	2.171E − 02
3.00000E + 00	3.138E − 02	1.806E − 02	3.00000E + 00	3.284E − 02	1.889E − 02
4.00000E + 00	2.664E − 02	1.617E − 02	4.00000E + 00	2.798E − 02	1.698E − 02
5.00000E + 00	2.347E − 02	1.479E − 02	5.00000E + 00	2.476E − 02	1.562E − 02
6.00000E + 00	2.121E − 02	1.377E − 02	6.00000E + 00	2.248E − 02	1.461E − 02
8.00000E + 00	1.819E − 02	1.233E − 02	8.00000E + 00	1.945E − 02	1.322E − 02
1.00000E + 01	1.627E − 02	1.138E − 02	1.00000E + 01	1.755E − 02	1.232E − 02
1.50000E + 01	1.361E − 02	1.001E − 02	1.50000E + 01	1.495E − 02	1.104E − 02
2.00000E + 01	1.227E − 02	9.294E − 03	2.00000E + 01	1.368E − 02	1.039E − 02

[a] μ/ρ includes the photoelectric, coherent (Rayleigh) and incoherent (Compton) scattering, and the electron-position production cross-sections. The latter includes both production in the field of the nucleus as well as that of the atomic electrons. Photonuclear cross-sections, nuclear-resonance scattering, and Delbrück scattering are not included.

(continued)

Table 5.1 Mass Attenuation and Energy-Absorption Coefficients (Continued)

Photon Energy (MeV)	Carbon (graphite) μ/ρ (cm²/g)	Z = 6 μ_{en}/ρ (cm²/g)	Photon Energy (MeV)	Nitrogen μ/ρ (cm²/g)	Z = 7 μ_{en}/ρ (cm²/g)
1.00000E − 03	2.211E + 03	2.209E + 03	1.00000E − 03	3.311E + 03	3.306E + 03
1.50000E − 03	7.002E + 02	6.990E + 02	1.50000E − 03	1.083E + 03	1.080E + 03
2.00000E − 03	3.026E + 02	3.016E + 02	2.00000E − 03	4.769E + 02	4.755E + 02
3.00000E − 03	9.033E + 01	8.963E + 01	3.00000E − 03	1.456E + 02	1.447E + 02
4.00000E − 03	3.778E + 01	3.723E + 01	4.00000E − 03	6.166E + 01	6.094E + 01
5.00000E − 03	1.912E + 01	1.866E + 01	5.00000E − 03	3.144E + 01	3.086E + 01
6.00000E − 03	1.095E + 01	1.054E + 01	6.00000E − 03	1.809E + 01	1.759E + 01
8.00000E − 03	4.576E + 00	4.242E + 00	8.00000E − 03	7.562E + 00	7.170E + 00
1.00000E − 02	2.373E + 00	2.078E + 00	1.00000E − 02	3.879E + 00	3.545E + 00
1.50000E − 02	8.071E − 01	5.627E − 01	1.50000E − 02	1.236E + 00	9.715E − 01
2.00000E − 02	4.420E − 01	2.238E − 01	2.00000E − 02	6.178E − 01	3.867E − 01
3.00000E − 02	2.562E − 01	6.614E − 02	3.00000E − 02	3.066E − 01	1.099E − 01
4.00000E − 02	2.076E − 01	3.343E − 02	4.00000E − 02	2.288E − 01	5.051E − 02
5.00000E − 02	1.871E − 01	2.397E − 02	5.00000E − 02	1.980E − 01	3.217E − 02
6.00000E − 02	1.753E − 01	2.098E − 02	6.00000E − 02	1.817E − 01	2.548E − 02
8.00000E − 02	1.610E − 01	2.037E − 02	8.00000E − 02	1.639E − 01	2.211E − 02
1.00000E − 01	1.514E − 01	2.147E − 02	1.00000E − 01	1.529E − 01	2.231E − 02
1.50000E − 01	1.347E − 01	2.449E − 02	1.50000E − 01	1.353E − 01	2.472E − 02
2.00000E − 01	1.229E − 01	2.655E − 02	2.00000E − 01	1.233E − 01	2.665E − 02
3.00000E − 01	1.066E − 01	2.870E − 02	3.00000E − 01	1.068E − 01	2.873E − 02
4.00000E − 01	9.546E − 02	2.950E − 02	4.00000E − 01	9.557E − 02	2.952E − 02
5.00000E − 01	8.715E − 02	2.969E − 02	5.00000E − 01	8.719E − 02	2.969E − 02
6.00000E − 01	8.058E − 02	2.956E − 02	6.00000E − 01	8.063E − 02	2.956E − 02
8.00000E − 01	7.076E − 02	2.885E − 02	8.00000E − 01	7.081E − 02	2.886E − 02
1.00000E + 00	6.361E − 02	2.792E − 02	1.00000E + 00	6.364E − 02	2.792E − 02
1.25000E + 00	5.690E − 02	2.669E − 02	1.25000E + 00	5.693E − 02	2.669E − 02
1.50000E + 00	5.179E − 02	2.551E − 02	1.50000E + 00	5.180E − 02	2.550E − 02
2.00000E + 00	4.442E − 02	2.345E − 02	2.00000E + 00	4.450E − 02	2.347E − 02
3.00000E + 00	3.562E − 02	2.048E − 02	3.00000E + 00	3.579E − 02	2.057E − 02
4.00000E + 00	3.047E − 02	1.849E − 02	4.00000E + 00	3.073E − 02	1.867E − 02
5.00000E + 00	2.708E − 02	1.710E − 02	5.00000E + 00	2.742E − 02	1.734E − 02
6.00000E + 00	2.469E − 02	1.607E − 02	6.00000E + 00	2.511E − 02	1.639E − 02
8.00000E + 00	2.154E − 02	1.468E − 02	8.00000E + 00	2.209E − 02	1.512E − 02
1.00000E + 01	1.959E − 02	1.380E − 02	1.00000E + 01	2.024E − 02	1.434E − 02
1.50000E + 01	1.698E − 02	1.258E − 02	1.50000E + 01	1.782E − 02	1.332E − 02
2.00000E + 01	1.575E − 02	1.198E − 02	2.00000E + 01	1.673E − 02	1.285E − 02

[a] μ/ρ includes the photoelectric, coherent (Rayleigh) and incoherent (Compton) scattering, and the electron-position production cross-sections. The latter includes both production in the field of the nucleus as well as that of the atomic electrons. Photonuclear cross-sections, nuclear-resonance scattering, and Delbrück scattering are not included.

Table 5.1 Mass Attenuation and Energy-Absorption Coefficients (Continued)

Photon Energy (MeV)	Oxygen μ/ρ (cm²/g)	Z = 8 μ_{en}/ρ (cm²/g)	Photon Energy (MeV)	Fluorine μ/ρ (cm²/g)	Z = 9 μ_{en}/ρ (cm²/g)
1.00000E − 03	4.590E + 03	4.576E + 03	1.00000E − 03	5.649E + 03	5.615E + 03
1.50000E − 03	1.549E + 03	1.545E + 03	1.50000E − 03	1.979E + 03	1.969E + 03
2.00000E − 03	6.949E + 02	6.926E + 02	2.00000E − 03	9.047E + 02	9.005E + 02
3.00000E − 03	2.171E + 02	2.158E + 02	3.00000E − 03	2.888E + 02	2.870E + 02
4.00000E − 03	9.315E + 01	9.221E + 01	4.00000E − 03	1.256E + 02	1.244E + 02
5.00000E − 03	4.790E + 01	4.715E + 01	5.00000E − 03	6.514E + 01	6.424E + 01
6.00000E − 03	2.770E + 01	2.708E + 01	6.00000E − 03	3.789E + 01	3.716E + 01
8.00000E − 03	1.163E + 01	1.116E + 01	8.00000E − 03	1.602E + 01	1.548E + 01
1.00000E − 02	5.952E + 00	5.565E + 00	1.00000E − 02	8.205E + 00	7.776E + 00
1.50000E − 02	1.836E + 00	1.545E + 00	1.50000E − 02	2.492E + 00	2.186E + 00
2.00000E − 02	8.651E − 01	6.179E − 01	2.00000E − 02	1.133E + 00	8.796E − 01
3.00000E − 02	3.779E − 01	1.729E − 01	3.00000E − 02	4.487E − 01	2.451E − 01
4.00000E − 02	2.585E − 01	7.530E − 02	4.00000E − 02	2.828E − 01	1.036E − 01
5.00000E − 02	2.132E − 01	4.414E − 02	5.00000E − 02	2.214E − 01	5.747E − 02
6.00000E − 02	1.907E − 01	3.207E − 02	6.00000E − 02	1.920E − 01	3.903E − 02
8.00000E − 02	1.678E − 01	2.468E − 02	8.00000E − 02	1.639E − 01	2.676E − 02
1.00000E − 01	1.551E − 01	2.355E − 02	1.00000E − 01	1.496E − 01	2.394E − 02
1.50000E − 01	1.361E − 01	2.506E − 02	1.50000E − 01	1.298E − 01	2.417E − 02
2.00000E − 01	1.237E − 01	2.679E − 02	2.00000E − 01	1.176E − 01	2.554E − 02
3.00000E − 01	1.070E − 01	2.877E − 02	3.00000E − 01	1.015E − 01	2.729E − 02
4.00000E − 01	9.566E − 02	2.953E − 02	4.00000E − 01	9.073E − 02	2.800E − 02
5.00000E − 01	8.729E − 02	2.971E − 02	5.00000E − 01	8.274E − 02	2.815E − 02
6.00000E − 01	8.070E − 02	2.957E − 02	6.00000E − 01	7.649E − 02	2.801E − 02
8.00000E − 01	7.087E − 02	2.887E − 02	8.00000E − 01	6.717E − 02	2.734E − 02
1.00000E + 00	6.372E − 02	2.794E − 02	1.00000E + 00	6.037E − 02	2.645E − 02
1.25000E + 00	5.697E − 02	2.669E − 02	1.25000E + 00	5.399E − 02	2.527E − 02
1.50000E + 00	5.185E − 02	2.551E − 02	1.50000E + 00	4.915E − 02	2.416E − 02
2.00000E + 00	4.459E − 02	2.350E − 02	2.00000E + 00	4.228E − 02	2.226E − 02
3.00000E + 00	3.597E − 02	2.066E − 02	3.00000E + 00	3.422E − 02	1.964E − 02
4.00000E + 00	3.100E − 02	1.882E − 02	4.00000E + 00	2.960E − 02	1.797E − 02
5.00000E + 00	2.777E − 02	1.757E − 02	5.00000E + 00	2.663E − 02	1.685E − 02
6.00000E + 00	2.552E − 02	1.668E − 02	6.00000E + 00	2.457E − 02	1.607E − 02
8.00000E + 00	2.263E − 02	1.553E − 02	8.00000E + 00	2.195E − 02	1.508E − 02
1.00000E + 01	2.089E − 02	1.483E − 02	1.00000E + 01	2.039E − 02	1.451E − 02
1.50000E + 01	1.866E − 02	1.396E − 02	1.50000E + 01	1.846E − 02	1.382E − 02
2.00000E + 01	1.770E − 02	1.360E − 02	2.00000E + 01	1.769E − 02	1.357E − 02

[a] μ/ρ includes the photoelectric, coherent (Rayleigh) and incoherent (Compton) scattering, and the electron-position production cross-sections. The latter includes both production in the field of the nucleus as well as that of the atomic electrons. Photonuclear cross-sections, nuclear-resonance scattering, and Delbrück scattering are not included.

(continued)

Table 5.1 Mass Attenuation and Energy-Absorption Coefficients (Continued)

	Photon Energy (MeV)	Sodium Z = 11 μ/ρ (cm²/g)	Sodium Z = 11 μ_{en}/ρ (cm²/g)		Photon Energy (MeV)	Magnesium Z = 12 μ/ρ (cm²/g)	Magnesium Z = 12 μ_{en}/ρ (cm²/g)
	1.00000E − 03	6.542E + 02	6.522E + 02		1.00000E − 03	9.225E + 02	9.203E + 02
	1.03542E − 03	5.960E + 02	5.941E + 02		1.14237E − 03	6.474E + 02	6.452E + 02
	1.07210E − 03	5.429E + 02	5.410E + 02		1.30500E − 03	4.530E + 02	4.509E + 02
K	1.07210E − 03	6.435E + 03	6.320E + 03	K	1.30500E − 03	5.444E + 03	5.310E + 03
	1.50000E − 03	3.194E + 03	3.151E + 03		1.50000E − 03	4.004E + 03	3.918E + 03
	2.00000E − 03	1.521E + 03	1.504E + 03		2.00000E − 03	1.932E + 03	1.899E + 03
	3.00000E − 03	5.070E + 02	5.023E + 02		3.00000E − 03	6.585E + 02	6.499E + 02
	4.00000E − 03	2.261E + 02	2.238E + 02		4.00000E − 03	2.974E + 02	2.937E + 02
	5.00000E − 03	1.194E + 02	1.178E + 02		5.00000E − 03	1.583E + 02	1.561E + 02
	6.00000E − 03	7.030E + 01	6.915E + 01		6.00000E − 03	9.381E + 01	9.227E + 01
	8.00000E − 03	3.018E + 01	2.941E + 01		8.00000E − 03	4.061E + 01	3.965E + 01
	1.00000E − 02	1.557E + 01	1.499E + 01		1.00000E − 02	2.105E + 01	2.036E + 01
	1.50000E − 02	4.694E + 00	4.313E + 00		1.50000E − 02	6.358E + 00	5.925E + 00
	2.00000E − 02	2.057E + 00	1.759E + 00		2.00000E − 02	2.763E + 00	2.432E + 00
	3.00000E − 02	7.197E − 01	4.928E − 01		3.00000E − 02	9.306E − 01	6.855E − 01
	4.00000E − 02	3.969E − 01	2.031E − 01		4.00000E − 02	4.881E − 01	2.815E − 01
	5.00000E − 02	2.804E − 01	1.063E − 01		5.00000E − 02	3.292E − 01	1.451E − 01
	6.00000E − 02	2.268E − 01	6.625E − 02		6.00000E − 02	2.570E − 01	8.820E − 02
	8.00000E − 02	1.796E − 01	3.761E − 02		8.00000E − 02	1.951E − 01	4.671E − 02
	1.00000E − 01	1.585E − 01	2.931E − 02		1.00000E − 01	1.686E − 01	3.410E − 02
	1.50000E − 01	1.335E − 01	2.579E − 02		1.50000E − 01	1.394E − 01	2.766E − 02
	2.00000E − 01	1.199E − 01	2.635E − 02		2.00000E − 01	1.245E − 01	2.761E − 02
	3.00000E − 01	1.029E − 01	2.771E − 02		3.00000E − 01	1.065E − 01	2.871E − 02
	4.00000E − 01	9.185E − 02	2.833E − 02		4.00000E − 01	9.492E − 02	2.928E − 02
	5.00000E − 01	8.372E − 02	2.845E − 02		5.00000E − 01	8.647E − 02	2.938E − 02
	6.00000E − 01	7.736E − 02	2.830E − 02		6.00000E − 01	7.988E − 02	2.921E − 02
	8.00000E − 01	6.788E − 02	2.760E − 02		8.00000E − 01	7.008E − 02	2.848E − 02
	1.00000E + 00	6.100E − 02	2.669E − 02		1.00000E + 00	6.296E − 02	2.753E − 02
	1.25000E + 00	5.454E − 02	2.549E − 02		1.25000E + 00	5.629E − 02	2.629E − 02
	1.50000E + 00	4.968E − 02	2.437E − 02		1.50000E + 00	5.129E − 02	2.514E − 02
	2.00000E + 00	4.282E − 02	2.249E − 02		2.00000E + 00	4.426E − 02	2.322E − 02
	3.00000E + 00	3.487E − 02	1.997E − 02		3.00000E + 00	3.613E − 02	2.067E − 02
	4.00000E + 00	3.037E − 02	1.842E − 02		4.00000E + 00	3.159E − 02	1.915E − 02
	5.00000E + 00	2.753E − 02	1.743E − 02		5.00000E + 00	2.873E − 02	1.819E − 02
	6.00000E + 00	2.559E − 02	1.675E − 02		6.00000E + 00	2.681E − 02	1.756E − 02
	8.00000E + 00	2.319E − 02	1.595E − 02		8.00000E + 00	2.445E − 02	1.683E − 02
	1.00000E + 01	2.181E − 02	1.552E − 02		1.00000E + 01	2.313E − 02	1.646E − 02
	1.50000E + 01	2.023E − 02	1.508E − 02		1.50000E + 01	2.168E − 02	1.614E − 02
	2.00000E + 01	1.970E − 02	1.496E − 02		2.00000E + 01	2.127E − 02	1.609E − 02

[a] μ/ρ includes the photoelectric, coherent (Rayleigh) and incoherent (Compton) scattering, and the electron-position production cross-sections. The latter includes both production in the field of the nucleus as well as that of the atomic electrons. Photonuclear cross-sections, nuclear-resonance scattering, and Delbrück scattering are not included.

Table 5.1 Mass Attenuation and Energy-Absorption Coefficients (Continued)

	Photon Energy (MeV)	Aluminum μ/ρ (cm^2/g)	Z = 13 μ_{en}/ρ (cm^2/g)		Photon Energy (MeV)	Silicon μ/ρ (cm^2/g)	Z = 14 μ_{en}/ρ (cm^2/g)
	1.00000E − 03	1.185E + 03	1.183E + 03		1.00000E − 03	1.570E + 03	1.567E + 03
	1.50000E − 03	4.022E + 02	4.001E + 02		1.50000E − 03	5.355E + 02	5.331E + 02
	1.55960E − 03	3.621E + 02	3.600E + 02		1.83890E − 03	3.092E + 02	3.070E + 02
K	1.55960E − 03	3.957E + 03	3.829E + 03	K	1.83890E − 03	3.192E + 03	3.059E + 03
	2.00000E − 03	2.263E + 03	2.204E + 03		2.00000E − 03	2.777E + 03	2.669E + 03
	3.00000E − 03	7.880E + 02	7.732E + 02		3.00000E − 03	9.784E + 02	9.516E + 02
	4.00000E − 03	3.605E + 02	3.545E + 02		4.00000E − 03	4.529E + 02	4.427E + 02
	5.00000E − 03	1.934E + 02	1.902E + 02		5.00000E − 03	2.450E + 02	2.400E + 02
	6.00000E − 03	1.153E + 02	1.133E + 02		6.00000E − 03	1.470E + 02	1.439E + 02
	8.00000E − 03	5.033E + 01	4.918E + 01		8.00000E − 03	6.468E + 01	6.313E + 01
	1.00000E − 02	2.623E + 01	2.543E + 01		1.00000E − 02	3.389E + 01	3.289E + 01
	1.50000E − 02	7.955E + 00	7.487E + 00		1.50000E − 02	1.034E + 01	9.794E + 00
	2.00000E − 02	3.441E + 00	3.094E + 00		2.00000E − 02	4.464E + 00	4.076E + 00
	3.00000E − 02	1.128E + 00	8.778E − 01		3.00000E − 02	1.436E + 00	1.164E + 00
	4.00000E − 02	5.685E − 01	3.601E − 01		4.00000E − 02	7.012E − 01	4.782E − 01
	5.00000E − 02	3.681E − 01	1.840E − 01		5.00000E − 02	4.385E − 01	2.430E − 01
	6.00000E − 02	2.778E − 01	1.099E − 01		6.00000E − 02	3.207E − 01	1.434E − 01
	8.00000E − 02	2.018E − 01	5.511E − 02		8.00000E − 02	2.228E − 01	6.896E − 02
	1.00000E − 01	1.704E − 01	3.794E − 02		1.00000E − 01	1.835E − 01	4.513E − 02
	1.50000E − 01	1.378E − 01	2.827E − 02		1.50000E − 01	1.448E − 01	3.086E − 02
	2.00000E − 01	1.223E − 01	2.745E − 02		2.00000E − 01	1.275E − 01	2.905E − 02
	3.00000E − 01	1.042E − 01	2.816E − 02		3.00000E − 01	1.082E − 01	2.932E − 02
	4.00000E − 01	9.276E − 02	2.862E − 02		4.00000E − 01	9.614E − 02	2.968E − 02
	5.00000E − 01	8.445E − 02	2.868E − 02		5.00000E − 01	8.748E − 02	2.971E − 02
	6.00000E − 01	7.802E − 02	2.851E − 02		6.00000E − 01	8.077E − 02	2.951E − 02
	8.00000E − 01	6.841E − 02	2.778E − 02		8.00000E − 01	7.082E − 02	2.875E − 02
	1.00000E + 00	6.146E − 02	2.686E − 02		1.00000E + 00	6.361E − 02	2.778E − 02
	1.25000E + 00	5.496E − 02	2.565E − 02		1.25000E + 00	5.688E − 02	2.652E − 02
	1.50000E + 00	5.006E − 02	2.451E − 02		1.50000E + 00	5.183E − 02	2.535E − 02
	2.00000E + 00	4.324E − 02	2.266E − 02		2.00000E + 00	4.480E − 02	2.345E − 02
	3.00000E + 00	3.541E − 02	2.024E − 02		3.00000E + 00	3.678E − 02	2.101E − 02
	4.00000E + 00	3.106E − 02	1.882E − 02		4.00000E + 00	3.240E − 02	1.963E − 02
	5.00000E + 00	2.836E − 02	1.795E − 02		5.00000E + 00	2.967E − 02	1.878E − 02
	6.00000E + 00	2.655E − 02	1.739E − 02		6.00000E + 00	2.788E − 02	1.827E − 02
	8.00000E + 00	2.437E − 02	1.678E − 02		8.00000E + 00	2.574E − 02	1.773E − 02
	1.00000E + 01	2.318E − 02	1.650E − 02		1.00000E + 01	2.462E − 02	1.753E − 02
	1.50000E + 01	2.195E − 02	1.631E − 02		1.50000E + 01	2.352E − 02	1.746E − 02
	2.00000E + 01	2.168E − 02	1.633E − 02		2.00000E + 01	2.338E − 02	1.757E − 02

[a] μ/ρ includes the photoelectric, coherent (Rayleigh) and incoherent (Compton) scattering, and the electron-position production cross-sections. The latter includes both production in the field of the nucleus as well as that of the atomic electrons. Photonuclear cross-sections, nuclear-resonance scattering, and Delbrück scattering are not included.

(continued)

Table 5.1 Mass Attenuation and Energy-Absorption Coefficients (Continued)

	Photon Energy (MeV)	Phosphorus μ/ρ (cm²/g)	Z = 15 μ_{en}/ρ (cm²/g)		Photon Energy (MeV)	Sulfur μ/ρ (cm²/g)	Z = 16 μ_{en}/ρ (cm²/g)
	1.00000E − 03	1.913E + 03	1.910E + 03		1.00000E − 03	2.429E + 03	2.426E + 03
	1.50000E − 03	6.547E + 02	6.522E + 02		1.50000E − 03	8.342E + 02	8.314E + 02
	2.00000E − 03	3.018E + 02	2.996E + 02		2.00000E − 03	3.853E + 02	3.828E + 02
	2.14550E − 03	2.494E + 02	2.473E + 02		2.47200E − 03	2.168E + 02	2.145E + 02
K	2.14550E − 03	2.473E + 03	2.343E + 03	K	2.47200E − 03	2.070E + 03	1.935E + 03
	3.00000E − 03	1.118E + 03	1.074E + 03		3.00000E − 03	1.339E + 03	1.265E + 03
	4.00000E − 03	5.242E + 02	5.079E + 02		4.00000E − 03	6.338E + 02	6.066E + 02
	5.00000E − 03	2.860E + 02	2.782E + 02		5.00000E − 03	3.487E + 02	3.360E + 02
	6.00000E − 03	1.726E + 02	1.682E + 02		6.00000E − 03	2.116E + 02	2.046E + 02
	8.00000E − 03	7.660E + 01	7.457E + 01		8.00000E − 03	9.465E + 01	9.171E + 01
	1.00000E − 02	4.035E + 01	3.912E + 01		1.00000E − 02	5.012E + 01	4.847E + 01
	1.50000E − 02	1.239E + 01	1.179E + 01		1.50000E − 02	1.550E + 01	1.477E + 01
	2.00000E − 02	5.352E + 00	4.939E + 00		2.00000E − 02	6.708E + 00	6.235E + 00
	3.00000E − 02	1.700E + 00	1.422E + 00		3.00000E − 02	2.113E + 00	1.809E + 00
	4.00000E − 02	8.096E − 01	5.850E − 01		4.00000E − 02	9.872E − 01	7.466E − 01
	5.00000E − 02	4.916E − 01	2.965E − 01		5.00000E − 02	5.849E − 01	3.779E − 01
	6.00000E − 02	3.494E − 01	1.735E − 01		6.00000E − 02	4.053E − 01	2.199E − 01
	8.00000E − 02	2.324E − 01	8.083E − 02		8.00000E − 02	2.585E − 01	1.000E − 01
	1.00000E − 01	1.865E − 01	5.068E − 02		1.00000E − 01	2.020E − 01	6.052E − 02
	1.50000E − 01	1.432E − 01	3.188E − 02		1.50000E − 01	1.506E − 01	3.516E − 02
	2.00000E − 01	1.250E − 01	2.899E − 02		2.00000E − 01	1.302E − 01	3.080E − 02
	3.00000E − 01	1.055E − 01	2.870E − 02		3.00000E − 01	1.091E − 01	2.983E − 02
	4.00000E − 01	9.359E − 02	2.892E − 02		4.00000E − 01	9.665E − 02	2.991E − 02
	5.00000E − 01	8.511E − 02	2.891E − 02		5.00000E − 01	8.781E − 02	2.984E − 02
	6.00000E − 01	7.854E − 02	2.869E − 02		6.00000E − 01	8.102E − 02	2.959E − 02
	8.00000E − 01	6.884E − 02	2.793E − 02		8.00000E − 01	7.098E − 02	2.878E − 02
	1.00000E + 00	6.182E − 02	2.698E − 02		1.00000E + 00	6.373E − 02	2.780E − 02
	1.25000E + 00	5.526E − 02	2.575E − 02		1.25000E + 00	5.697E − 02	2.652E − 02
	1.50000E + 00	5.039E − 02	2.462E − 02		1.50000E + 00	5.193E − 02	2.535E − 02
	2.00000E + 00	4.358E − 02	2.279E − 02		2.00000E + 00	4.498E − 02	2.349E − 02
	3.00000E + 00	3.590E − 02	2.049E − 02		3.00000E + 00	3.715E − 02	2.118E − 02
	4.00000E + 00	3.172E − 02	1.921E − 02		4.00000E + 00	3.293E − 02	1.993E − 02
	5.00000E + 00	2.915E − 02	1.846E − 02		5.00000E + 00	3.036E − 02	1.923E − 02
	6.00000E + 00	2.747E − 02	1.801E − 02		6.00000E + 00	2.872E − 02	1.884E − 02
	8.00000E + 00	2.552E − 02	1.760E − 02		8.00000E + 00	2.682E − 02	1.850E − 02
	1.00000E + 01	2.452E − 02	1.747E − 02		1.00000E + 01	2.589E − 02	1.845E − 02
	1.50000E + 01	2.364E − 02	1.754E − 02		1.50000E + 01	2.517E − 02	1.864E − 02
	2.00000E + 01	2.363E − 02	1.771E − 02		2.00000E + 01	2.529E − 02	1.889E − 02

[a] μ/ρ includes the photoelectric, coherent (Rayleigh) and incoherent (Compton) scattering, and the electron-position production cross-sections. The latter includes both production in the field of the nucleus as well as that of the atomic electrons. Photonuclear cross-sections, nuclear-resonance scattering, and Delbrück scattering are not included.

Table 5.1 Mass Attenuation and Energy-Absorption Coefficients (Continued)

	Photon Energy (MeV)	Chlorine μ/ρ (cm²/g)	Z = 17 μ_{en}/ρ (cm²/g)		Photon Energy (MeV)	Argon μ/ρ (cm²/g)	Z = 18 μ_{en}/ρ (cm²/g)
	1.00000E − 03	2.832E + 03	2.829E + 03		1.00000E − 03	3.184E + 03	3.180E + 03
	1.50000E − 03	9.771E + 02	9.742E + 02		1.50000E − 03	1.105E + 03	1.102E + 03
	2.00000E − 03	4.520E + 02	4.494E + 02		2.00000E − 03	5.120E + 02	5.093E + 02
	2.82240E − 03	1.774E + 02	1.752E + 02		3.00000E − 03	1.703E + 02	1.682E + 02
K	2.82240E − 03	1.637E + 03	1.506E + 03		3.20290E − 03	1.424E + 02	1.403E + 02
	3.00000E − 03	1.473E + 03	1.361E + 03	K	3.20290E − 03	1.275E + 03	1.153E + 03
	4.00000E − 03	7.037E + 02	6.626E + 02		4.00000E − 03	7.572E + 02	6.979E + 02
	5.00000E − 03	3.901E + 02	3.711E + 02		5.00000E − 03	4.225E + 02	3.953E + 02
	6.00000E − 03	2.384E + 02	2.282E + 02		6.00000E − 03	2.593E + 02	2.449E + 02
	8.00000E − 03	1.075E + 02	1.034E + 02		8.00000E − 03	1.180E + 02	1.125E + 02
	1.00000E − 02	5.725E + 01	5.510E + 01		1.00000E − 02	6.316E + 01	6.038E + 01
	1.50000E − 02	1.784E + 01	1.700E + 01		1.50000E − 02	1.983E + 01	1.886E + 01
	2.00000E − 02	7.739E + 00	7.227E + 00		2.00000E − 02	8.629E + 00	8.074E + 00
	3.00000E − 02	2.425E + 00	2.114E + 00		3.00000E − 02	2.697E + 00	2.382E + 00
	4.00000E − 02	1.117E + 00	8.756E − 01		4.00000E − 02	1.228E + 00	9.907E − 01
	5.00000E − 02	6.483E − 01	4.433E − 01		5.00000E − 02	7.012E − 01	5.020E − 01
	6.00000E − 02	4.395E − 01	2.570E − 01		6.00000E − 02	4.664E − 01	2.904E − 01
	8.00000E − 02	2.696E − 01	1.148E − 01		8.00000E − 02	2.760E − 01	1.280E − 01
	1.00000E − 01	2.050E − 01	6.745E − 02		1.00000E − 01	2.043E − 01	7.344E − 02
	1.50000E − 01	1.480E − 01	3.639E − 02		1.50000E − 01	1.427E − 01	3.703E − 02
	2.00000E − 01	1.266E − 01	3.067E − 02		2.00000E − 01	1.205E − 01	2.998E − 02
	3.00000E − 01	1.054E − 01	2.898E − 02		3.00000E − 01	9.953E − 02	2.757E − 02
	4.00000E − 01	9.311E − 02	2.887E − 02		4.00000E − 01	8.776E − 02	2.727E − 02
	5.00000E − 01	8.453E − 02	2.874E − 02		5.00000E − 01	7.958E − 02	2.708E − 02
	6.00000E − 01	7.795E − 02	2.847E − 02		6.00000E − 01	7.335E − 02	2.679E − 02
	8.00000E − 01	6.826E − 02	2.767E − 02		8.00000E − 01	6.419E − 02	2.601E − 02
	1.00000E + 00	6.128E − 02	2.671E − 02		1.00000E + 00	5.762E − 02	2.510E − 02
	1.25000E + 00	5.478E − 02	2.549E − 02		1.25000E + 00	5.150E − 02	2.394E − 02
	1.50000E + 00	4.994E − 02	2.436E − 02		1.50000E + 00	4.695E − 02	2.288E − 02
	2.00000E + 00	4.328E − 02	2.258E − 02		2.00000E + 00	4.074E − 02	2.123E − 02
	3.00000E + 00	3.585E − 02	2.043E − 02		3.00000E + 00	3.384E − 02	1.927E − 02
	4.00000E + 00	3.188E − 02	1.931E − 02		4.00000E + 00	3.019E − 02	1.827E − 02
	5.00000E + 00	2.950E − 02	1.871E − 02		5.00000E + 00	2.802E − 02	1.777E − 02
	6.00000E + 00	2.798E − 02	1.839E − 02		6.00000E + 00	2.667E − 02	1.753E − 02
	8.00000E + 00	2.628E − 02	1.819E − 02		8.00000E + 00	2.517E − 02	1.742E − 02
	1.00000E + 01	2.549E − 02	1.824E − 02		1.00000E + 01	2.451E − 02	1.754E − 02
	1.50000E + 01	2.496E − 02	1.861E − 02		1.50000E + 01	2.418E − 02	1.800E − 02
	2.00000E + 01	2.520E − 02	1.899E − 02		2.00000E + 01	2.453E − 02	1.842E − 02

[a] μ/ρ includes the photoelectric, coherent (Rayleigh) and incoherent (Compton) scattering, and the electron-position production cross-sections. The latter includes both production in the field of the nucleus as well as that of the atomic electrons. Photonuclear cross-sections, nuclear-resonance scattering, and Delbrück scattering are not included.

(continued)

Table 5.1 Mass Attenuation and Energy-Absorption Coefficients (Continued)

	Photon Energy (MeV)	Potassium μ/ρ (cm^2/g)	Z = 19 μ_{en}/ρ (cm^2/g)		Photon Energy (MeV)	Calcium μ/ρ (cm^2/g)	Z = 20 μ_{en}/ρ (cm^2/g)
	1.00000E − 03	4.058E + 03	4.053E + 03		1.00000E − 03	4.867E + 03	4.861E + 03
	1.50000E − 03	1.418E + 03	1.415E + 03		1.50000E − 03	1.714E + 03	1.710E + 03
	2.00000E − 03	6.592E + 02	6.563E + 02		2.00000E − 03	7.999E + 02	7.966E + 02
	3.00000E − 03	2.198E + 02	2.174E + 02		3.00000E − 03	2.676E + 02	2.650E + 02
	3.60740E − 03	1.327E + 02	1.306E + 02		4.00000E − 03	1.218E + 02	1.197E + 02
K	3.60740E − 03	1.201E + 03	1.065E + 03		4.03810E − 03	1.187E + 02	1.166E + 02
	4.00000E − 03	9.256E + 02	8.304E + 02	K	4.03810E − 03	1.023E + 03	8.887E + 02
	5.00000E − 03	5.189E + 02	4.752E + 02		5.00000E − 03	6.026E + 02	5.373E + 02
	6.00000E − 03	3.205E + 02	2.974E + 02		6.00000E − 03	3.731E + 02	3.387E + 02
	8.00000E − 03	1.469E + 02	1.383E + 02		8.00000E − 03	1.726E + 02	1.600E + 02
	1.00000E − 02	7.907E + 01	7.490E + 01		1.00000E − 02	9.341E + 01	8.744E + 01
	1.50000E − 02	2.503E + 01	2.370E + 01		1.50000E − 02	2.979E + 01	2.804E + 01
	2.00000E − 02	1.093E + 01	1.023E + 01		2.00000E − 02	1.306E + 01	1.220E + 01
	3.00000E − 02	3.413E + 00	3.045E + 00		3.00000E − 02	4.080E + 00	3.665E + 00
	4.00000E − 02	1.541E + 00	1.272E + 00		4.00000E − 02	1.830E + 00	1.538E + 00
	5.00000E − 02	8.679E − 01	6.454E − 01		5.00000E − 02	1.019E + 00	7.822E − 01
	6.00000E − 02	5.678E − 01	3.730E − 01		6.00000E − 02	6.578E − 01	4.520E − 01
	8.00000E − 02	3.251E − 01	1.628E − 01		8.00000E − 02	3.656E − 01	1.958E − 01
	1.00000E − 01	2.345E − 01	9.161E − 02		1.00000E − 01	2.571E − 01	1.085E − 01
	1.50000E − 01	1.582E − 01	4.346E − 02		1.50000E − 01	1.674E − 01	4.876E − 02
	2.00000E − 01	1.319E − 01	3.378E − 02		2.00000E − 01	1.376E − 01	3.639E − 02
	3.00000E − 01	1.080E − 01	3.015E − 02		3.00000E − 01	1.116E − 01	3.146E − 02
	4.00000E − 01	9.495E − 02	2.959E − 02		4.00000E − 01	9.783E − 02	3.060E − 02
	5.00000E − 01	8.600E − 02	2.929E − 02		5.00000E − 01	8.851E − 02	3.019E − 02
	6.00000E − 01	7.922E − 02	2.895E − 02		6.00000E − 01	8.148E − 02	2.979E − 02
	8.00000E − 01	6.929E − 02	2.807E − 02		8.00000E − 01	7.122E − 02	2.884E − 02
	1.00000E + 00	6.216E − 02	2.707E − 02		1.00000E + 00	6.388E − 02	2.780E − 02
	1.25000E + 00	5.556E − 02	2.581E − 02		1.25000E + 00	5.709E − 02	2.650E − 02
	1.50000E + 00	5.068E − 02	2.467E − 02		1.50000E + 00	5.207E − 02	2.532E − 02
	2.00000E + 00	4.399E − 02	2.290E − 02		2.00000E + 00	4.524E − 02	2.352E − 02
	3.00000E + 00	3.666E − 02	2.084E − 02		3.00000E + 00	3.780E − 02	2.147E − 02
	4.00000E + 00	3.282E − 02	1.985E − 02		4.00000E + 00	3.395E − 02	2.052E − 02
	5.00000E + 00	3.054E − 02	1.935E − 02		5.00000E + 00	3.170E − 02	2.007E − 02
	6.00000E + 00	2.915E − 02	1.914E − 02		6.00000E + 00	3.035E − 02	1.992E − 02
	8.00000E + 00	2.766E − 02	1.910E − 02		8.00000E + 00	2.892E − 02	1.997E − 02
	1.00000E + 01	2.704E − 02	1.928E − 02		1.00000E + 01	2.839E − 02	2.022E − 02
	1.50000E + 01	2.687E − 02	1.983E − 02		1.50000E + 01	2.838E − 02	2.088E − 02
	2.00000E + 01	2.737E − 02	2.029E − 02		2.00000E + 01	2.903E − 02	2.140E − 02

[a] μ/ρ includes the photoelectric, coherent (Rayleigh) and incoherent (Compton) scattering, and the electron-position production cross-sections. The latter includes both production in the field of the nucleus as well as that of the atomic electrons. Photonuclear cross-sections, nuclear-resonance scattering, and Delbrück scattering are not included.

Table 5.1 Mass Attenuation and Energy-Absorption Coefficients (Continued)

	Photon Energy (MeV)	Titanium μ/ρ (cm^2/g)	Z = 22 μ_{en}/ρ (cm^2/g)		Photon Energy (MeV)	Iron μ/ρ (cm^2/g)	Z = 26 μ_{en}/ρ (cm^2/g)
	1.00000E − 03	5.869E + 03	5.860E + 03		1.00000E − 03	9.085E + 03	9.052E + 03
	1.50000E − 03	2.096E + 03	2.091E + 03		1.50000E − 03	3.399E + 03	3.388E + 03
	2.00000E − 03	9.860E + 02	9.824E + 02		2.00000E − 03	1.626E + 03	1.620E + 03
	3.00000E − 03	3.323E + 02	3.295E + 02		3.00000E − 03	5.576E + 02	5.535E + 02
	4.00000E − 03	1.517E + 02	1.494E + 02		4.00000E − 03	2.567E + 02	2.536E + 02
	4.96640E − 03	8.380E + 01	8.188E + 01		5.00000E − 03	1.398E + 02	1.372E + 02
K	4.96640E − 03	6.878E + 02	5.684E + 02		6.00000E − 03	8.484E + 01	8.265E + 01
	5.00000E − 03	6.838E + 02	5.657E + 02		7.11200E − 03	5.319E + 01	5.133E + 01
	6.00000E − 03	4.323E + 02	3.691E + 02	K	7.11200E − 03	4.076E + 02	2.978E + 02
	8.00000E − 03	2.023E + 02	1.793E + 02		8.00000E − 03	3.056E + 02	2.316E + 02
	1.00000E − 02	1.107E + 02	1.001E + 02		1.00000E − 02	1.706E + 02	1.369E + 02
	1.50000E − 02	3.587E + 01	3.311E + 01		1.50000E − 02	5.708E + 01	4.896E + 01
	2.00000E − 02	1.585E + 01	1.465E + 01		2.00000E − 02	2.568E + 01	2.260E + 01
	3.00000E − 02	4.972E + 00	4.488E + 00		3.00000E − 02	8.176E + 00	7.251E + 00
	4.00000E − 02	2.214E + 00	1.904E + 00		4.00000E − 02	3.629E + 00	3.155E + 00
	5.00000E − 02	1.213E + 00	9.737E − 01		5.00000E − 02	1.958E + 00	1.638E + 00
	6.00000E − 02	7.661E − 01	5.634E − 01		6.00000E − 02	1.205E + 00	9.555E − 01
	8.00000E − 02	4.052E − 01	2.422E − 01		8.00000E − 02	5.952E − 01	4.104E − 01
	1.00000E − 01	2.721E − 01	1.312E − 01		1.00000E − 01	3.717E − 01	2.177E − 01
	1.50000E − 01	1.649E − 01	5.393E − 02		1.50000E − 01	1.964E − 01	7.961E − 02
	2.00000E − 01	1.314E − 01	3.726E − 02		2.00000E − 01	1.460E − 01	4.825E − 02
	3.00000E − 01	1.043E − 01	3.007E − 02		3.00000E − 01	1.099E − 01	3.361E − 02
	4.00000E − 01	9.081E − 02	2.861E − 02		4.00000E − 01	9.400E − 02	3.039E − 02
	5.00000E − 01	8.191E − 02	2.804E − 02		5.00000E − 01	8.414E − 02	2.914E − 02
	6.00000E − 01	7.529E − 02	2.756E − 02		6.00000E − 01	7.704E − 02	2.836E − 02
	8.00000E − 01	6.572E − 02	2.661E − 02		8.00000E − 01	6.699E − 02	2.714E − 02
	1.00000E + 00	5.891E − 02	2.561E − 02		1.00000E + 00	5.995E − 02	2.603E − 02
	1.25000E + 00	5.263E − 02	2.439E − 02		1.25000E + 00	5.350E − 02	2.472E − 02
	1.50000E + 00	4.801E − 02	2.330E − 02		1.50000E + 00	4.883E − 02	2.360E − 02
	2.00000E + 00	4.180E − 02	2.166E − 02		2.00000E + 00	4.265E − 02	2.199E − 02
	3.00000E + 00	3.512E − 02	1.989E − 02		3.00000E + 00	3.621E − 02	2.042E − 02
	4.00000E + 00	3.173E − 02	1.913E − 02		4.00000E + 00	3.312E − 02	1.990E − 02
	5.00000E + 00	2.982E − 02	1.884E − 02		5.00000E + 00	3.146E − 02	1.983E − 02
	6.00000E + 00	2.868E − 02	1.879E − 02		6.00000E + 00	3.057E − 02	1.997E − 02
	8.00000E + 00	2.759E − 02	1.899E − 02		8.00000E + 00	2.991E − 02	2.050E − 02
	1.00000E + 01	2.727E − 02	1.933E − 02		1.00000E + 01	2.994E − 02	2.108E − 02
	1.50000E + 01	2.762E − 02	2.013E − 02		1.50000E + 01	3.092E − 02	2.221E − 02
	2.00000E + 01	2.844E − 02	2.067E − 02		2.00000E + 01	3.224E − 02	2.292E − 02

[a] μ/ρ includes the photoelectric, coherent (Rayleigh) and incoherent (Compton) scattering, and the electron-position production cross-sections. The latter includes both production in the field of the nucleus as well as that of the atomic electrons. Photonuclear cross-sections, nuclear-resonance scattering, and Delbrück scattering are not included.

(continued)

Table 5.1 Mass Attenuation and Energy-Absorption Coefficients (Continued)

	Photon Energy (MeV)	Copper μ/ρ (cm^2/g)	Z = 29 μ_{en}/ρ (cm^2/g)		Photon Energy (MeV)	Gallium μ/ρ (cm^2/g)	Z = 31 μ_{en}/ρ (cm^2/g)
	1.00000E − 03	1.057E + 04	1.049E + 04		1.00000E − 03	1.697E + 03	1.692E + 03
	1.04695E − 03	9.307E + 03	9.241E + 03		1.05613E − 03	1.492E + 03	1.487E + 03
	1.09610E − 03	8.242E + 03	8.186E + 03		1.11540E − 03	1.312E + 03	1.307E + 03
L1	1.09610E − 03	9.347E + 03	9.282E + 03	L3	1.11540E − 03	3.990E + 03	3.955E + 03
	1.50000E − 03	4.418E + 03	4.393E + 03		1.12877E − 03	4.887E + 03	4.842E + 03
	2.00000E − 03	2.154E + 03	2.142E + 03		1.14230E − 03	5.664E + 03	5.611E + 03
	3.00000E − 03	7.488E + 02	7.430E + 02	L2	1.14230E − 03	7.405E + 03	7.332E + 03
	4.00000E − 03	3.473E + 02	3.432E + 02		1.21752E − 03	7.138E + 03	7.070E + 03
	5.00000E − 03	1.899E + 02	1.866E + 02		1.29770E − 03	6.358E + 03	6.299E + 03
	6.00000E − 03	1.156E + 02	1.128E + 02	L1	1.29770E − 03	7.206E + 03	7.139E + 03
	8.00000E − 03	5.255E + 01	5.054E + 01		1.50000E − 03	5.087E + 03	5.044E + 03
	8.97890E − 03	3.829E + 01	3.652E + 01		2.00000E − 03	2.515E + 03	2.496E + 03
K	8.97890E − 03	2.784E + 02	1.824E + 02		3.00000E − 03	8.857E + 02	8.782E + 02
	1.00000E − 02	2.159E + 02	1.484E + 02		4.00000E − 03	4.130E + 02	4.082E + 02
	1.50000E − 02	7.405E + 01	5.788E + 01		5.00000E − 03	2.266E + 02	2.229E + 02
	2.00000E − 02	3.379E + 01	2.788E + 01		6.00000E − 03	1.382E + 02	1.352E + 02
	3.00000E − 02	1.092E + 01	9.349E + 00		8.00000E − 03	6.302E + 01	6.082E + 01
	4.00000E − 02	4.862E + 00	4.163E + 00		1.00000E − 02	3.421E + 01	3.250E + 01
	5.00000E − 02	2.613E + 00	2.192E + 00		1.03671E − 02	3.099E + 01	2.936E + 01
	6.00000E − 02	1.593E + 00	1.290E + 00	K	1.03671E − 02	2.214E + 02	1.344E + 02
	8.00000E − 02	7.630E − 01	5.581E − 01		1.50000E − 02	8.537E + 01	6.135E + 01
	1.00000E − 01	4.584E − 01	2.949E − 01		2.00000E − 02	3.928E + 01	3.059E + 01
	1.50000E − 01	2.217E − 01	1.027E − 01		3.00000E − 02	1.281E + 01	1.061E + 01
	2.00000E − 01	1.559E − 01	5.781E − 02		4.00000E − 02	5.726E + 00	4.810E + 00
	3.00000E − 01	1.119E − 01	3.617E − 02		5.00000E − 02	3.076E + 00	2.560E + 00
	4.00000E − 01	9.413E − 02	3.121E − 02		6.00000E − 02	1.868E + 00	1.518E + 00
	5.00000E − 01	8.362E − 02	2.933E − 02		8.00000E − 02	8.823E − 01	6.613E − 01
	6.00000E − 01	7.625E − 02	2.826E − 02		1.00000E − 01	5.197E − 01	3.497E − 01
	8.00000E − 01	6.605E − 02	2.681E − 02		1.50000E − 01	2.387E − 01	1.193E − 01
	1.00000E + 00	5.901E − 02	2.562E − 02		2.00000E − 01	1.619E − 01	6.463E − 02
	1.25000E + 00	5.261E − 02	2.428E − 02		3.00000E − 01	1.123E − 01	3.782E − 02
	1.50000E + 00	4.803E − 02	2.316E − 02		4.00000E − 01	9.325E − 02	3.156E − 02
	2.00000E + 00	4.205E − 02	2.160E − 02		5.00000E − 01	8.236E − 02	2.920E − 02
	3.00000E + 00	3.599E − 02	2.023E − 02		6.00000E − 01	7.487E − 02	2.793E − 02
	4.00000E + 00	3.318E − 02	1.989E − 02		8.00000E − 01	6.466E − 02	2.631E − 02
	5.00000E + 00	3.177E − 02	1.998E − 02		1.00000E + 00	5.767E − 02	2.506E − 02
	6.00000E + 00	3.108E − 02	2.027E − 02		1.25000E + 00	5.139E − 02	2.371E − 02
	8.00000E + 00	3.074E − 02	2.100E − 02		1.50000E + 00	4.692E − 02	2.260E − 02
	1.00000E + 01	3.103E − 02	2.174E − 02		2.00000E + 00	4.113E − 02	2.110E − 02
	1.50000E + 01	3.247E − 02	2.309E − 02		3.00000E + 00	3.538E − 02	1.986E − 02
	2.00000E + 01	3.408E − 02	2.387E − 02		4.00000E + 00	3.280E − 02	1.966E − 02
					5.00000E + 00	3.156E − 02	1.985E − 02
					6.00000E + 00	3.099E − 02	2.021E − 02
					8.00000E + 00	3.086E − 02	2.108E − 02
					1.00000E + 01	3.130E − 02	2.191E − 02
					1.50000E + 01	3.300E − 02	2.339E − 02
					2.00000E + 01	3.479E − 02	2.425E − 02

[a] μ/ρ includes the photoelectric, coherent (Rayleigh) and incoherent (Compton) scattering, and the electron-position production cross-sections. The latter includes both production in the field of the nucleus as well as that of the atomic electrons. Photonuclear cross-sections, nuclear-resonance scattering, and Delbrück scattering are not included.

Table 5.1 Mass Attenuation and Energy-Absorption Coefficients (Continued)

	Photon Energy (MeV)	Germanium Z = 32 μ/ρ (cm^2/g)	μ_{en}/ρ (cm^2/g)		Photon Energy (MeV)	Arsenic Z = 33 μ/ρ (cm^2/g)	μ_{en}/ρ (cm^2/g)
	1.00000E − 03	1.893E + 03	1.887E + 03		1.00000E − 03	2.121E + 03	2.116E + 03
	1.10304E − 03	1.502E + 03	1.496E + 03		1.15026E − 03	1.523E + 03	1.517E + 03
	1.21670E − 03	1.190E + 03	1.185E + 03		1.32310E − 03	1.092E + 03	1.087E + 03
L3	1.21670E − 03	4.389E + 03	4.343E + 03	L3	1.32310E − 03	4.513E + 03	4.459E + 03
	1.23215E − 03	4.734E + 03	4.684E + 03		1.34073E − 03	4.469E + 03	4.416E + 03
	1.24780E − 03	4.974E + 03	4.922E + 03		1.35860E − 03	4.452E + 03	4.398E + 03
L2	1.24780E − 03	6.698E + 03	6.622E + 03	L2	1.35860E − 03	6.093E + 03	6.015E + 03
	1.32844E − 03	6.348E + 03	6.279E + 03		1.50000E − 03	5.227E + 03	5.164E + 03
	1.41430E − 03	5.554E + 03	5.495E + 03		1.52650E − 03	4.997E + 03	4.938E + 03
L1	1.41430E − 03	6.287E + 03	6.221E + 03	L1	1.52650E − 03	5.653E + 03	5.585E + 03
	1.50000E − 03	5.475E + 03	5.420E + 03		2.00000E − 03	2.931E + 03	2.902E + 03
	2.00000E − 03	2.711E + 03	2.688E + 03		3.00000E − 03	1.049E + 03	1.039E + 03
	3.00000E − 03	9.613E + 02	9.527E + 02		4.00000E − 03	4.920E + 02	4.862E + 02
	4.00000E − 03	4.497E + 02	4.445E + 02		5.00000E − 03	2.709E + 02	2.667E + 02
	5.00000E − 03	2.472E + 02	2.433E + 02		6.00000E − 03	1.656E + 02	1.622E + 02
	6.00000E − 03	1.509E + 02	1.477E + 02		8.00000E − 03	7.573E + 01	7.330E + 01
	8.00000E − 03	6.890E + 01	6.660E + 01		1.00000E − 02	4.115E + 01	3.928E + 01
	1.00000E − 02	3.742E + 01	3.564E + 01		1.18667E − 02	2.577E + 01	2.425E + 01
	1.11031E − 02	2.811E + 01	2.653E + 01	K	1.18667E − 02	1.792E + 02	1.008E + 02
K	1.11031E − 02	1.981E + 02	1.157E + 02		1.50000E − 02	9.856E + 01	6.371E + 01
	1.50000E − 02	9.152E + 01	6.256E + 01		2.00000E − 02	4.564E + 01	3.310E + 01
	2.00000E − 02	4.222E + 01	3.178E + 01		3.00000E − 02	1.506E + 01	1.198E + 01
	3.00000E − 02	1.385E + 01	1.126E + 01		4.00000E − 02	6.760E + 00	5.537E + 00
	4.00000E − 02	6.207E + 00	5.152E + 00		5.00000E − 02	3.635E + 00	2.983E + 00
	5.00000E − 02	3.335E + 00	2.759E + 00		6.00000E − 02	2.203E + 00	1.783E + 00
	6.00000E − 02	2.023E + 00	1.642E + 00		8.00000E − 02	1.030E + 00	7.837E − 01
	8.00000E − 02	9.501E − 01	7.184E − 01		1.00000E − 01	5.971E − 01	4.155E − 01
	1.00000E − 01	5.550E − 01	3.803E − 01		1.50000E − 01	2.622E − 01	1.399E − 01
	1.50000E − 01	2.491E − 01	1.288E − 01		2.00000E − 01	1.719E − 01	7.350E − 02
	2.00000E − 01	1.661E − 01	6.865E − 02		3.00000E − 01	1.150E − 01	4.043E − 02
	3.00000E − 01	1.131E − 01	3.891E − 02		4.00000E − 01	9.414E − 02	3.261E − 02
	4.00000E − 01	9.327E − 02	3.193E − 02		5.00000E − 01	8.259E − 02	2.966E − 02
	5.00000E − 01	8.212E − 02	2.930E − 02		6.00000E − 01	7.483E − 02	2.813E − 02
	6.00000E − 01	7.452E − 02	2.790E − 02		8.00000E − 01	6.440E − 02	2.628E − 02
	8.00000E − 01	6.426E − 02	2.618E − 02		1.00000E + 00	5.735E − 02	2.494E − 02
	1.00000E + 00	5.727E − 02	2.489E − 02		1.25000E + 00	5.106E − 02	2.355E − 02
	1.25000E + 00	5.101E − 02	2.353E − 02		1.50000E + 00	4.661E − 02	2.243E − 02
	1.50000E + 00	4.657E − 02	2.242E − 02		2.00000E + 00	4.093E − 02	2.096E − 02
	2.00000E + 00	4.086E − 02	2.094E − 02		3.00000E + 00	3.539E − 02	1.984E − 02
	3.00000E + 00	3.524E − 02	1.977E − 02		4.00000E + 00	3.296E − 02	1.974E − 02
	4.00000E + 00	3.275E − 02	1.962E − 02		5.00000E + 00	3.187E − 02	2.005E − 02
	5.00000E + 00	3.158E − 02	1.987E − 02		6.00000E + 00	3.141E − 02	2.049E − 02
	6.00000E + 00	3.107E − 02	2.027E − 02		8.00000E + 00	3.146E − 02	2.148E − 02
	8.00000E + 00	3.103E − 02	2.120E − 02		1.00000E + 01	3.207E − 02	2.241E − 02
	1.00000E + 01	3.156E − 02	2.208E − 02		1.50000E + 01	3.405E − 02	2.404E − 02
	1.50000E + 01	3.340E − 02	2.364E − 02		2.00000E + 01	3.603E − 02	2.495E − 02
	2.00000E + 01	3.528E − 02	2.452E − 02				

[a] μ/ρ includes the photoelectric, coherent (Rayleigh) and incoherent (Compton) scattering, and the electron-position production cross-sections. The latter includes both production in the field of the nucleus as well as that of the atomic electrons. Photonuclear cross-sections, nuclear-resonance scattering, and Delbrück scattering are not included.

(continued)

Table 5.1 Mass Attenuation and Energy-Absorption Coefficients (Continued)

	Photon Energy (MeV)	Bromine μ/ρ (cm²/g)	Z = 35 μ_{en}/ρ (cm²/g)		Photon Energy (MeV)	Molybdenum μ/ρ (cm²/g)	Z = 42 μ_{en}/ρ (cm²/g)
	1.00000E − 03	2.624E + 03	2.618E + 03		1.00000E − 03	4.942E + 03	4.935E + 03
	1.50000E − 03	1.002E + 03	9.964E + 02		1.50000E − 03	1.925E + 03	1.918E + 03
	1.54990E − 03	9.255E + 02	9.200E + 02		2.00000E − 03	9.593E + 02	9.531E + 02
L3	1.54990E − 03	4.289E + 03	4.223E + 03		2.52020E − 03	5.415E + 02	5.358E + 02
	1.57278E − 03	3.838E + 03	3.780E + 03	L3	2.52020E − 03	1.979E + 03	1.924E + 03
	1.59600E − 03	3.587E + 03	3.534E + 03		2.57212E − 03	1.854E + 03	1.802E + 03
L2	1.59600E − 03	5.097E + 03	5.014E + 03		2.62510E − 03	1.750E + 03	1.703E + 03
	1.68644E − 03	4.595E + 03	4.523E + 03	L2	2.62510E − 03	2.433E + 03	2.360E + 03
	1.78200E − 03	3.969E + 03	3.910E + 03		2.74267E − 03	2.183E + 03	2.119E + 03
L 1	1.78200E − 03	4.495E + 03	4.427E + 03		2.86550E − 03	1.961E + 03	1.906E + 03
	2.00000E − 03	3.407E + 03	3.360E + 03	L1	2.86550E − 03	2.243E + 03	2.179E + 03
	3.00000E − 03	1.231E + 03	1.216E + 03		3.00000E − 03	2.011E + 03	1.956E + 03
	4.00000E − 03	5.815E + 02	5.740E + 02		4.00000E − 03	9.703E + 02	9.475E + 02
	5.00000E − 03	3.213E + 02	3.163E + 02		5.00000E − 03	5.450E + 02	5.328E + 02
	6.00000E − 03	1.968E + 02	1.930E + 02		6.00000E − 03	3.373E + 02	3.295E + 02
	8.00000E − 03	9.026E + 01	8.756E + 01		8.00000E − 03	1.565E + 02	1.522E + 02
	1.00000E − 02	4.912E + 01	4.706E + 01		1.00000E − 02	8.576E + 01	8.275E + 01
	1.34737E − 02	2.176E + 01	2.033E + 01		1.50000E − 02	2.854E + 01	2.684E + 01
K	1.34737E − 02	1.471E + 02	7.668E + 01		1.99995E − 02	1.308E + 01	1.193E + 01
	1.50000E − 02	1.119E + 02	6.336E + 01	K	1.99995E − 02	7.950E + 01	3.293E + 01
	2.00000E − 02	5.266E + 01	3.502E + 01		2.00000E − 02	7.950E + 01	3.293E + 01
	3.00000E − 02	1.753E + 01	1.328E + 01		3.00000E − 02	2.810E + 01	1.664E + 01
	4.00000E − 02	7.900E + 00	6.267E + 00		4.00000E − 02	1.294E + 01	8.757E + 00
	5.00000E − 02	4.264E + 00	3.431E + 00		5.00000E − 02	7.037E + 00	5.074E + 00
	6.00000E − 02	2.582E + 00	2.068E + 00		6.00000E − 02	4.274E + 00	3.178E + 00
	8.00000E − 02	1.198E + 00	9.185E − 01		8.00000E − 02	1.962E + 00	1.477E + 00
	1.00000E − 01	6.861E − 01	4.890E − 01		1.00000E − 01	1.096E + 00	8.042E − 01
	1.50000E − 01	2.899E − 01	1.634E − 01		1.50000E − 01	4.208E − 01	2.693E − 01
	2.00000E − 01	1.838E − 01	8.378E − 02		2.00000E − 01	2.423E − 01	1.316E − 01
	3.00000E − 01	1.186E − 01	4.360E − 02		3.00000E − 01	1.379E − 01	5.919E − 02
	4.00000E − 01	9.563E − 02	3.398E − 02		4.00000E − 01	1.047E − 01	4.117E − 02
	5.00000E − 01	8.328E − 02	3.036E − 02		5.00000E − 01	8.848E − 02	3.437E − 02
	6.00000E − 01	7.515E − 02	2.851E − 02		6.00000E − 01	7.851E − 02	3.104E − 02
	8.00000E − 01	6.443E − 02	2.640E − 02		8.00000E − 01	6.619E − 02	2.764E − 02
	1.00000E + 00	5.728E − 02	2.496E − 02		1.00000E + 00	5.837E − 02	2.567E − 02
	1.25000E + 00	5.094E − 02	2.350E − 02		1.25000E + 00	5.167E − 02	2.390E − 02
	1.50000E + 00	4.650E − 02	2.237E − 02		1.50000E + 00	4.713E − 02	2.263E − 02
	2.00000E + 00	4.089E − 02	2.092E − 02		2.00000E + 00	4.163E − 02	2.118E − 02
	3.00000E + 00	3.552E − 02	1.991E − 02		3.00000E + 00	3.675E − 02	2.046E − 02
	4.00000E + 00	3.327E − 02	1.995E − 02		4.00000E + 00	3.496E − 02	2.084E − 02
	5.00000E + 00	3.229E − 02	2.036E − 02		5.00000E + 00	3.439E − 02	2.153E − 02
	6.00000E + 00	3.194E − 02	2.090E − 02		6.00000E + 00	3.440E − 02	2.231E − 02
	8.00000E + 00	3.218E − 02	2.207E − 02		8.00000E + 00	3.523E − 02	2.382E − 02
	1.00000E + 01	3.293E − 02	2.314E − 02		1.00000E + 01	3.650E − 02	2.513E − 02
	1.50000E + 01	3.521E − 02	2.507E − 02		1.50000E + 01	3.978E − 02	2.731E − 02
	2.00000E + 01	3.738E − 02	2.618E − 02		2.00000E + 01	4.264E − 02	2.840E − 02

[a] μ/ρ includes the photoelectric, coherent (Rayleigh) and incoherent (Compton) scattering, and the electron-position production cross-sections. The latter includes both production in the field of the nucleus as well as that of the atomic electrons. Photonuclear cross-sections, nuclear-resonance scattering, and Delbrück scattering are not included.

Table 5.1 Mass Attenuation and Energy-Absorption Coefficients (Continued)

	Photon Energy (MeV)	Silver μ/ρ (cm²/g)	Z = 47 μ_{en}/ρ (cm²/g)		Photon Energy (MeV)	Cadmium μ/ρ (cm²/g)	Z = 48 μ_{en}/ρ (cm²/g)
	1.00000E − 03	7.039E + 03	7.029E + 03		1.00000E − 03	7.350E + 03	7.340E + 03
	1.50000E − 03	2.790E + 03	2.782E + 03		1.50000E − 03	2.931E + 03	2.922E + 03
	2.00000E − 03	1.401E + 03	1.393E + 03		2.00000E − 03	1.473E + 03	1.466E + 03
	3.00000E − 03	5.136E + 02	5.073E + 02		3.00000E − 03	5.414E + 02	5.350E + 02
	3.35110E − 03	3.887E + 02	3.827E + 02		3.53750E − 03	3.575E + 02	3.517E + 02
L3	3.35110E − 03	1.274E + 03	1.223E + 03	L3	3.53750E − 03	1.152E + 03	1.103E + 03
	3.43632E − 03	1.200E + 03	1.151E + 03		3.63101E − 03	1.083E + 03	1.036E + 03
	3.52370E − 03	1.126E + 03	1.082E + 03		3.72700E − 03	1.013E + 03	9.715E + 02
L2	3.52370E − 03	1.547E + 03	1.479E + 03	L2	3.72700E − 03	1.389E + 03	1.324E + 03
	3.66203E − 03	1.409E + 03	1.348E + 03		4.00000E − 03	1.170E + 03	1.118E + 03
	3.80580E − 03	1.282E + 03	1.229E + 03		4.01800E − 03	1.157E + 03	1.106E + 03
L1	3.80580E − 03	1.468E + 03	1.406E + 03	L1	4.01800E − 03	1.324E + 03	1.264E + 03
	4.00000E − 03	1.305E + 03	1.252E + 03		5.00000E − 03	7.685E + 02	7.383E + 02
	5.00000E − 03	7.385E + 02	7.122E + 02		6.00000E − 03	4.793E + 02	4.619E + 02
	6.00000E − 03	4.610E + 02	4.457E + 02		8.00000E − 03	2.254E + 02	2.174E + 02
	8.00000E − 03	2.164E + 02	2.092E + 02		1.00000E − 02	1.244E + 02	1.197E + 02
	1.00000E − 02	1.193E + 02	1.149E + 02		1.50000E − 02	4.178E + 01	3.952E + 01
	1.50000E − 02	3.998E + 01	3.780E + 01		2.00000E − 02	1.920E + 01	1.776E + 01
	2.00000E − 02	1.836E + 01	1.695E + 01		2.67112E − 02	8.809E + 00	7.863E + 00
	2.55140E − 02	9.527E + 00	8.534E + 00	K	2.67112E − 02	5.065E + 01	1.821E + 01
K	2.55140E − 02	5.539E + 01	2.031E + 01		3.00000E − 02	3.765E + 01	1.594E + 01
	3.00000E − 02	3.668E + 01	1.660E + 01		4.00000E − 02	1.778E + 01	9.812E + 00
	4.00000E − 02	1.720E + 01	9.869E + 00		5.00000E − 02	9.779E + 00	6.115E + 00
	5.00000E − 02	9.444E + 00	6.066E + 00		6.00000E − 02	5.975E + 00	4.001E + 00
	6.00000E − 02	5.766E + 00	3.938E + 00		8.00000E − 02	2.751E + 00	1.957E + 00
	8.00000E − 02	2.651E + 00	1.907E + 00		1.00000E − 01	1.524E + 00	1.096E + 00
	1.00000E − 01	1.470E + 00	1.062E + 00		1.50000E − 01	5.593E − 01	3.753E − 01
	1.50000E − 01	5.426E − 01	3.622E − 01		2.00000E − 01	3.038E − 01	1.813E − 01
	2.00000E − 01	2.972E − 01	1.751E − 01		3.00000E − 01	1.571E − 01	7.580E − 02
	3.00000E − 01	1.560E − 01	7.392E − 02		4.00000E − 01	1.129E − 01	4.868E − 02
	4.00000E − 01	1.131E − 01	4.803E − 02		5.00000E − 01	9.250E − 02	3.838E − 02
	5.00000E − 01	9.321E − 02	3.822E − 02		6.00000E − 01	8.064E − 02	3.339E − 02
	6.00000E − 01	8.153E − 02	3.347E − 02		8.00000E − 01	6.670E − 02	2.854E − 02
	8.00000E − 01	6.766E − 02	2.881E − 02		1.00000E + 00	5.826E − 02	2.597E − 02
	1.00000E + 00	5.921E − 02	2.632E − 02		1.25000E + 00	5.129E − 02	2.387E − 02
	1.25000E + 00	5.217E − 02	2.425E − 02		1.50000E + 00	4.673E − 02	2.247E − 02
	1.50000E + 00	4.754E − 02	2.284E − 02		2.00000E + 00	4.139E − 02	2.099E − 02
	2.00000E + 00	4.209E − 02	2.135E − 02		3.00000E + 00	3.698E − 02	2.051E − 02
	3.00000E + 00	3.754E − 02	2.082E − 02		4.00000E + 00	3.559E − 02	2.114E − 02
	4.00000E + 00	3.606E − 02	2.142E − 02		5.00000E + 00	3.536E − 02	2.206E − 02
	5.00000E + 00	3.577E − 02	2.232E − 02		6.00000E + 00	3.563E − 02	2.300E − 02
	6.00000E + 00	3.601E − 02	2.324E − 02		8.00000E + 00	3.691E − 02	2.477E − 02
	8.00000E + 00	3.723E − 02	2.499E − 02		1.00000E + 01	3.853E − 02	2.625E − 02
	1.00000E + 01	3.882E − 02	2.647E − 02		1.50000E + 01	4.253E − 02	2.869E − 02
	1.50000E + 01	4.276E − 02	2.889E − 02		2.00000E + 01	4.587E − 02	2.985E − 02
	2.00000E + 01	4.609E − 02	3.005E − 02				

[a] μ/ρ includes the photoelectric, coherent (Rayleigh) and incoherent (Compton) scattering, and the electron-position production cross-sections. The latter includes both production in the field of the nucleus as well as that of the atomic electrons. Photonuclear cross-sections, nuclear-resonance scattering, and Delbrück scattering are not included.

(continued)

Table 5.1 Mass Attenuation and Energy-Absorption Coefficients (Continued)

	Photon Energy (MeV)	Tin	Z = 50		Photon Energy (MeV)	Tellurium	Z = 52
		μ/ρ (cm²/g)	μ_{en}/ρ (cm²/g)			μ/ρ (cm²/g)	μ_{en}/ρ (cm²/g)
	1.00000E − 03	8.157E + 03	8.144E + 03		1.00000E − 03	8.434E + 03	8.419E + 03
	1.50000E − 03	3.296E + 03	3.287E + 03		1.00300E − 03	8.380E + 03	8.365E + 03
	2.00000E − 03	1.665E + 03	1.657E + 03		1.00600E − 03	8.326E + 03	8.311E + 03
	3.00000E − 03	6.143E + 02	6.077E + 02	M1	1.00600E − 03	8.684E + 03	8.668E + 03
	3.92880E − 03	3.114E + 02	3.058E + 02		1.50000E − 03	3.608E + 03	3.598E + 03
L3	3.92880E − 03	9.285E + 02	8.845E + 02		2.00000E − 03	1.832E + 03	1.824E + 03
	4.00000E − 03	9.393E + 02	8.945E + 02		3.00000E − 03	6.792E + 02	6.726E + 02
	4.15610E − 03	8.469E + 02	8.074E + 02		4.00000E − 03	3.297E + 02	3.240E + 02
L2	4.15610E − 03	1.145E + 03	1.084E + 03		4.34140E − 03	2.678E + 02	2.625E + 02
	4.30764E − 03	1.060E + 03	1.002E + 03	L3	4.34140E − 03	7.882E + 02	7.460E + 02
	4.46470E − 03	9.712E + 02	9.221E + 02		4.47465E − 03	7.504E + 02	7.078E + 02
L1	4.46470E − 03	1.117E + 03	1.059E + 03		4.61200E − 03	6.995E + 02	6.629E + 02
	5.00000E − 03	8.471E + 02	8.064E + 02	L2	4.61200E − 03	9.445E + 02	8.880E + 02
	6.00000E − 03	5.294E + 02	5.065E + 02		4.77280E − 03	8.782E + 02	8.237E + 02
	8.00000E − 03	2.500E + 02	2.400E + 02		4.93920E − 03	8.062E + 02	7.600E + 02
	1.00000E − 02	1.384E + 02	1.327E + 02	L1	4.93920E − 03	9.292E + 02	8.744E + 02
	1.50000E − 02	4.664E + 01	4.413E + 01		5.00000E − 03	9.014E + 02	8.487E + 02
	2.00000E − 02	2.146E + 01	1.990E + 01		6.00000E − 03	5.721E + 02	5.423E + 02
	2.92001E − 02	7.760E + 00	6.876E + 00		8.00000E − 03	2.702E + 02	2.578E + 02
K	2.92001E − 02	4.360E + 01	1.514E + 01		1.00000E − 02	1.501E + 02	1.433E + 02
	3.00000E − 02	4.121E + 01	1.490E + 01		1.50000E − 02	5.078E + 01	4.802E + 01
	4.00000E − 02	1.942E + 01	9.835E + 00		2.00000E − 02	2.341E + 01	2.175E + 01
	5.00000E − 02	1.070E + 01	6.314E + 00		3.00000E − 02	7.878E + 00	6.997E + 00
	6.00000E − 02	6.564E + 00	4.211E + 00		3.18138E − 02	6.738E + 00	5.929E + 00
	8.00000E − 02	3.029E + 00	2.101E + 00	K	3.18138E − 02	3.719E + 01	1.251E + 01
	1.00000E − 01	1.676E + 00	1.189E + 00		4.00000E − 02	2.064E + 01	9.480E + 00
	1.50000E − 01	6.091E − 01	4.119E − 01		5.00000E − 02	1.145E + 01	6.330E + 00
	2.00000E − 01	3.260E − 01	1.990E − 01		6.00000E − 02	7.041E + 00	4.306E + 00
	3.00000E − 01	1.639E − 01	8.179E − 02		8.00000E − 02	3.255E + 00	2.195E + 00
	4.00000E − 01	1.156E − 01	5.138E − 02		1.00000E − 01	1.801E + 00	1.256E + 00
	5.00000E − 01	9.374E − 02	3.980E − 02		1.50000E − 01	6.492E − 01	4.409E − 01
	6.00000E − 01	8.113E − 02	3.417E − 02		2.00000E − 01	3.429E − 01	2.132E − 01
	8.00000E − 01	6.662E − 02	2.878E − 02		3.00000E − 01	1.679E − 01	8.646E − 02
	1.00000E + 00	5.800E − 02	2.601E − 02		4.00000E − 01	1.163E − 01	5.326E − 02
	1.25000E + 00	5.095E − 02	2.379E − 02		5.00000E − 01	9.328E − 02	4.055E − 02
	1.50000E + 00	4.638E − 02	2.233E − 02		6.00000E − 01	8.022E − 02	3.440E − 02
	2.00000E + 00	4.112E − 02	2.085E − 02		8.00000E − 01	6.538E − 02	2.854E − 02
	3.00000E + 00	3.686E − 02	2.044E − 02		1.00000E + 00	5.669E − 02	2.559E − 02
	4.00000E + 00	3.561E − 02	2.115E − 02		1.25000E + 00	4.967E − 02	2.327E − 02
	5.00000E + 00	3.548E − 02	2.213E − 02		1.50000E + 00	4.518E − 02	2.179E − 02
	6.00000E + 00	3.583E − 02	2.312E − 02		2.00000E + 00	4.009E − 02	2.033E − 02
	8.00000E + 00	3.724E − 02	2.496E − 02		3.00000E + 00	3.606E − 02	1.998E − 02
	1.00000E + 01	3.895E − 02	2.649E − 02		4.00000E + 00	3.494E − 02	2.075E − 02
	1.50000E + 01	4.315E − 02	2.901E − 02		5.00000E + 00	3.492E − 02	2.177E − 02
	2.00000E + 01	4.662E − 02	3.018E − 02		6.00000E + 00	3.534E − 02	2.279E − 02
					8.00000E + 00	3.683E − 02	2.466E − 02
					1.00000E + 00	3.860E − 02	2.620E − 02
					1.50000E + 01	4.290E − 02	2.873E − 02
					2.00000E + 01	4.642E − 02	2.989E − 02

[a] μ/ρ includes the photoelectric, coherent (Rayleigh) and incoherent (Compton) scattering, and the electron-position production cross-sections. The latter includes both production in the field of the nucleus as well as that of the atomic electrons. Photonuclear cross-sections, nuclear-resonance scattering, and Delbrück scattering are not included.

Table 5.1 Mass Attenuation and Energy-Absorption Coefficients (Continued)

	Photon Energy (MeV)	Iodine μ/ρ (cm²/g)	Z = 53 μ_{en}/ρ (cm²/g)		Photon Energy (MeV)	Cesium μ/ρ (cm²/g)	Z = 55 μ_{en}/ρ (cm²/g)
	1.00000E − 03	9.096E + 03	9.078E + 03		1.00000E − 03	9.365E + 03	9.343E + 03
	1.03542E − 03	8.465E + 03	8.448E + 03		1.03199E − 03	8.775E + 03	8.754E + 03
	1.07210E − 03	7.863E + 03	7.847E + 03		1.06500E − 03	8.214E + 03	8.194E + 03
M1	1.07210E − 03	8.198E + 03	8.181E + 03	M2	1.06500E − 03	8.685E + 03	8.663E + 03
	1.50000E − 03	3.919E + 03	3.908E + 03		1.13851E − 03	7.576E + 03	7.557E + 03
	2.00000E − 03	1.997E + 03	1.988E + 03		1.21710E − 03	6.584E + 03	6.567E + 03
	3.00000E − 03	7.420E + 02	7.351E + 02	M1	1.21710E − 03	6.888E + 03	6.870E + 03
	4.00000E − 03	3.607E + 02	3.548E + 02		1.50000E − 03	4.335E + 03	4.322E + 03
	4.55710E − 03	2.592E + 02	2.537E + 02		2.00000E − 03	2.226E + 03	2.216E + 03
L3	4.55710E − 03	7.550E + 02	7.121E + 02		3.00000E − 03	8.319E + 02	8.246E + 02
	4.70229E − 03	7.123E + 02	6.724E + 02		4.00000E − 03	4.055E + 02	3.994E + 02
	4.85210E − 03	6.636E + 02	6.270E + 02		5.00000E − 03	2.303E + 02	2.251E + 02
L2	4.85210E − 03	8.943E + 02	8.375E + 02		5.01190E − 03	2.290E + 02	2.237E + 02
	5.00000E − 03	8.430E + 02	7.903E + 02	L3	5.01190E − 03	6.674E + 02	6.248E + 02
	5.18810E − 03	7.665E + 02	7.198E + 02		5.18274E − 03	6.184E + 02	5.763E + 02
L1	5.18810E − 03	8.837E + 02	8.283E + 02		5.35940E − 03	5.645E + 02	5.299E + 02
	6.00000E − 03	6.173E + 02	5.822E + 02	L2	5.35940E − 03	7.692E + 02	7.142E + 02
	8.00000E − 03	2.922E + 02	2.777E + 02		5.53401E − 03	7.146E + 02	6.610E + 02
	1.00000E − 02	1.626E + 02	1.548E + 02		5.71430E − 03	6.556E + 02	6.108E + 02
	1.50000E − 02	5.512E + 01	5.208E + 01	L1	5.71430E − 03	7.547E + 02	7.015E + 02
	2.00000E − 02	2.543E + 01	2.363E + 01		6.00000E − 03	6.711E + 02	6.253E + 02
	3.00000E − 02	8.561E + 00	7.622E + 00		8.00000E − 03	3.214E + 02	3.029E + 02
	3.31694E − 02	6.553E + 00	5.744E + 00		1.00000E − 02	1.793E + 02	1.697E + 02
K	3.31694E − 02	3.582E + 01	1.188E + 01		1.50000E − 02	6.104E + 01	5.753E + 01
	4.00000E − 02	2.210E + 01	9.616E + 00		2.00000E − 02	2.822E + 01	2.623E + 01
	5.00000E − 02	1.232E + 01	6.573E + 00		3.00000E − 02	9.507E + 00	8.502E + 00
	6.00000E − 02	7.579E + 00	4.518E + 00		3.59846E − 02	5.863E + 00	5.102E + 00
	8.00000E − 02	3.510E + 00	2.331E + 00	K	3.59846E − 02	3.143E + 01	1.017E + 01
	1.00000E − 01	1.942E + 00	1.342E + 00		4.00000E − 02	2.381E + 01	9.185E + 00
	1.50000E − 01	6.978E − 01	4.742E − 01		5.00000E − 02	1.340E + 01	6.618E + 00
	2.00000E − 01	3.663E − 01	2.295E − 01		6.00000E − 02	8.248E + 00	4.653E + 00
	3.00000E − 01	1.771E − 01	9.257E − 02		8.00000E − 02	3.836E + 00	2.464E + 00
	4.00000E − 01	1.217E − 01	5.650E − 02		1.00000E − 01	2.124E + 00	1.438E + 00
	5.00000E − 01	9.701E − 02	4.267E − 02		1.50000E − 01	7.589E − 01	5.154E − 01
	6.00000E − 01	8.313E − 02	3.598E − 02		2.00000E − 01	3.941E − 01	2.502E − 01
	8.00000E − 01	6.749E − 02	2.962E − 02		3.00000E − 01	1.863E − 01	1.000E − 01
	1.00000E + 00	5.841E − 02	2.646E − 02		4.00000E − 01	1.257E − 01	6.003E − 02
	1.25000E + 00	5.111E − 02	2.399E − 02		5.00000E − 01	9.912E − 02	4.463E − 02
	1.50000E + 00	4.647E − 02	2.243E − 02		6.00000E − 01	8.431E − 02	3.717E − 02
	2.00000E + 00	4.124E − 02	2.092E − 02		8.00000E − 01	6.789E − 02	3.014E − 02
	3.00000E + 00	3.716E − 02	2.059E − 02		1.00000E + 00	5.854E − 02	2.671E − 02
	4.00000E + 00	3.607E − 02	2.142E − 02		1.25000E + 00	5.108E − 02	2.408E − 02
	5.00000E + 00	3.608E − 02	2.250E − 02		1.50000E + 00	4.641E − 02	2.246E − 02
	6.00000E + 00	3.655E − 02	2.357E − 02		2.00000E + 00	4.121E − 02	2.091E − 02
	8.00000E + 00	3.815E − 02	2.553E − 02		3.00000E + 00	3.725E − 02	2.064E − 02
	1.00000E + 01	4.002E − 02	2.714E − 02		4.00000E + 00	3.625E − 02	2.153E − 02
	1.50000E + 01	4.455E − 02	2.980E − 02		5.00000E + 00	3.635E − 02	2.268E − 02
	2.00000E + 01	4.823E − 02	3.101E − 02		6.00000E + 00	3.689E − 02	2.380E − 02
					8.00000E + 00	3.860E − 02	2.583E − 02
					1.00000E + 01	4.057E − 02	2.750E − 02
					1.50000E + 01	4.529E − 02	3.026E − 02
					2.00000E + 01	4.910E − 02	3.152E − 02

[a] μ/ρ includes the photoelectric, coherent (Rayleigh) and incoherent (Compton) scattering, and the electron-position production cross-sections. The latter includes both production in the field of the nucleus as well as that of the atomic electrons. Photonuclear cross-sections, nuclear-resonance scattering, and Delbrück scattering are not included.

(continued)

Table 5.1 Mass Attenuation and Energy-Absorption Coefficients (Continued)

	Photon Energy (MeV)	Barium Z = 56 μ/ρ (cm²/g)	μ_{en}/ρ (cm²/g)		Photon Energy (MeV)	Cerium Z = 58 μ/ρ (cm²/g)	μ_{en}/ρ (cm²/g)
	1.00000E − 03	8.543E + 03	8.521E + 03		1.00000E − 03	9.711E + 03	9.679E + 03
	1.03063E − 03	7.990E + 03	7.969E + 03		1.08876E − 03	7.991E + 03	7.964E + 03
	1.06220E − 03	7.465E + 03	7.445E + 03		1.18540E − 03	6.563E + 03	6.541E + 03
M3	1.06220E − 03	8.547E + 03	8.524E + 03	M3	1.18540E − 03	7.545E + 03	7.519E + 03
	1.09882E − 03	7.957E + 03	7.935E + 03		1.22832E − 03	6.984E + 03	6.960E + 03
	1.13670E − 03	7.404E + 03	7.384E + 03		1.27280E − 03	6.465E + 03	6.442E + 03
M2	1.13670E − 03	7.837E + 03	7.815E + 03	M2	1.27280E − 03	6.853E + 03	6.829E + 03
	1.21224E − 03	6.861E + 03	6.841E + 03		1.35222E − 03	6.031E + 03	6.010E + 03
	1.29280E − 03	5.985E + 03	5.968E + 03		1.43660E − 03	5.293E + 03	5.273E + 03
M1	1.29280E − 03	6.255E + 03	6.237E + 03	M1	1.43660E − 03	5.532E + 03	5.512E + 03
	1.50000E − 03	4.499E + 03	4.485E + 03		1.50000E − 03	5.033E + 03	5.015E + 03
	2.00000E − 03	2.319E + 03	2.308E + 03		2.00000E − 03	2.607E + 03	2.595E + 03
	3.00000E − 03	8.696E + 02	8.622E + 02		3.00000E − 03	9.857E + 02	9.776E + 02
	4.00000E − 03	4.246E + 02	4.184E + 02		4.00000E − 03	4.811E + 02	4.745E + 02
	5.00000E − 03	2.414E + 02	2.361E + 02		5.00000E − 03	2.740E + 02	2.684E + 02
	5.24700E − 03	2.135E + 02	2.084E + 02		5.72340E − 03	1.943E + 02	1.892E + 02
L3	5.24700E − 03	6.098E + 02	5.689E + 02	L3	5.72340E − 03	5.454E + 02	5.046E + 02
	5.43204E − 03	5.634E + 02	5.263E + 02		6.00000E − 03	4.908E + 02	4.550E + 02
	5.62360E − 03	5.169E + 02	4.835E + 02		6.16420E − 03	4.554E + 02	4.228E + 02
L2	5.62360E − 03	7.016E + 02	6.486E + 02	L2	6.16420E − 03	6.188E + 02	5.665E + 02
	5.80333E − 03	6.507E + 02	6.025E + 02		6.35359E − 03	5.756E + 02	5.278E + 02
	5.98880E − 03	6.013E + 02	5.577E + 02		6.54880E − 03	5.332E + 02	4.899E + 02
L1	5.98880E − 03	6.930E + 02	6.412E + 02	L1	6.54880E − 03	6.149E + 02	5.633E + 02
	6.00000E − 03	6.898E + 02	6.383E + 02		8.00000E − 03	3.732E + 02	3.458E + 02
	8.00000E − 03	3.334E + 02	3.127E + 02		1.00000E − 02	2.082E + 02	1.945E + 02
	1.00000E − 02	1.860E + 02	1.754E + 02		1.50000E − 02	7.143E + 01	6.690E + 01
	1.50000E − 02	6.347E + 01	5.972E + 01		2.00000E − 02	3.312E + 01	3.073E + 01
	2.00000E − 02	2.938E + 01	2.730E + 01		3.00000E − 02	1.119E + 01	1.005E + 01
	3.00000E − 02	9.904E + 00	8.875E + 00		4.00000E − 02	5.215E + 00	4.496E + 00
	3.74406E − 02	5.498E + 00	4.768E + 00		4.04430E − 02	5.066E + 00	4.359E + 00

[a] μ/ρ includes the photoelectric, coherent (Rayleigh) and incoherent (Compton) scattering, and the electron-position production cross-sections. The latter includes both production in the field of the nucleus as well as that of the atomic electrons. Photonuclear cross-sections, nuclear-resonance scattering, and Delbrück scattering are not included.

Table 5.1 Mass Attenuation and Energy-Absorption Coefficients (Continued)

	Photon Energy (MeV)	Barium μ/ρ (cm²/g)	Z = 56 μ_{en}/ρ (cm²/g)		Photon Energy (MeV)	Cerium μ/ρ (cm²/g)	Z = 58 μ_{en}/ρ (cm²/g)
K	3.74406E − 02	2.919E + 01	9.346E + 00	K	4.04430E − 02	2.635E + 01	8.272E + 00
	4.00000E − 02	2.457E + 01	8.842E + 00		5.00000E − 02	1.520E + 01	6.569E + 00
	5.00000E − 02	1.379E + 01	6.534E + 00		6.00000E − 02	9.447E + 00	4.847E + 00
	6.00000E − 02	8.511E + 00	4.660E + 00		8.00000E − 02	4.409E + 00	2.677E + 00
	8.00000E − 02	3.963E + 00	2.501E + 00		1.00000E − 01	2.445E + 00	1.597E + 00
	1.00000E − 01	2.196E + 00	1.470E + 00		1.50000E − 01	8.687E − 01	5.862E − 01
	1.50000E − 01	7.828E − 01	5.309E − 01		2.00000E − 01	4.452E − 01	2.865E − 01
	2.00000E − 01	4.046E − 01	2.583E − 01		3.00000E − 01	2.039E − 01	1.134E − 01
	3.00000E − 01	1.891E − 01	1.028E − 01		4.00000E − 01	1.342E − 01	6.664E − 02
	4.00000E − 01	1.265E − 01	6.125E − 02		5.00000E − 01	1.041E − 01	4.851E − 02
	5.00000E − 01	9.923E − 02	4.521E − 02		6.00000E − 01	8.757E − 02	3.970E − 02
	6.00000E − 01	8.410E − 02	3.743E − 02		8.00000E − 01	6.962E − 02	3.145E − 02
	8.00000E − 01	6.744E − 02	3.011E − 02		1.00000E + 00	5.961E − 02	2.750E − 02
	1.00000E + 00	5.803E − 02	2.657E − 02		1.25000E + 00	5.181E − 02	2.456E − 02
	1.25000E + 00	5.058E − 02	2.388E − 02		1.50000E + 00	4.701E − 02	2.281E − 02
	1.50000E + 00	4.592E − 02	2.224E − 02		2.00000E + 00	4.177E − 02	2.118E − 02
	2.00000E + 00	4.078E − 02	2.069E − 02		3.00000E + 00	3.792E − 02	2.096E − 02
	3.00000E + 00	3.692E − 02	2.044E − 02		4.00000E + 00	3.705E − 02	2.194E − 02
	4.00000E + 00	3.598E − 02	2.135E − 02		5.00000E + 00	3.727E − 02	2.316E − 02
	5.00000E + 00	3.612E − 02	2.250E − 02		6.00000E + 00	3.792E − 02	2.434E − 02
	6.00000E + 00	3.669E − 02	2.363E − 02		8.00000E + 00	3.981E − 02	2.645E − 02
	8.00000E + 00	3.844E − 02	2.566E − 02		1.00000E + 01	4.194E − 02	2.816E − 02
	1.00000E + 01	4.042E − 02	2.731E − 02		1.50000E + 01	4.699E − 02	3.094E − 02
	1.50000E + 01	4.518E − 02	3.003E − 02		2.00000E + 01	5.103E − 02	3.216E − 02
	2.00000E + 01	4.902E − 02	3.126E − 02				

[a] μ/ρ includes the photoelectric, coherent (Rayleigh) and incoherent (Compton) scattering, and the electron-position production cross-sections. The latter includes both production in the field of the nucleus as well as that of the atomic electrons. Photonuclear cross-sections, nuclear-resonance scattering, and Delbrück scattering are not included.

(continued)

Table 5.1 Mass Attenuation and Energy-Absorption Coefficients (Continued)

	Photon Energy (MeV)	Gadolinium μ/ρ (cm²/g)	Z = 64 μ_{en}/ρ (cm²/g)		Photon Energy (MeV)	Tungsten μ/ρ (cm²/g)	Z = 74 μ_{en}/ρ (cm²/g)
	1.00000E − 03	2.291E + 03	2.281E + 03		1.00000E − 03	3.683E + 03	3.671E + 03
	1.08867E − 03	1.960E + 03	1.949E + 03		1.50000E − 03	1.643E + 03	1.632E + 03
	1.18520E − 03	1.668E + 03	1.658E + 03		1.80920E − 03	1.108E + 03	1.097E + 03
M5	1.18520E − 03	1.931E + 03	1.919E + 03	M5	1.80920E − 03	1.327E + 03	1.311E + 03
	1.20109E − 03	2.527E + 03	2.510E + 03		1.84014E − 03	1.911E + 03	1.883E + 03
	1.21720E − 03	3.961E + 03	3.934E + 03		1.87160E − 03	2.901E + 03	2.853E + 03
M4	1.21720E − 03	4.764E + 03	4.731E + 03	M4	1.87160E − 03	3.170E + 03	3.116E + 03
	1.50000E − 03	5.041E + 03	5.008E + 03		2.00000E − 03	3.922E + 03	3.853E + 03
	1.54400E − 03	4.701E + 03	4.670E + 03		2.28100E − 03	2.828E + 03	2.781E + 03
M3	1.54400E − 03	5.432E + 03	5.395E + 03	M3	2.28100E − 03	3.279E + 03	3.226E + 03
	1.61454E − 03	4.900E + 03	4.867E + 03		2.42350E − 03	2.833E + 03	2.786E + 03
	1.68830E − 03	4.421E + 03	4.391E + 03		2.57490E − 03	2.445E + 03	2.407E + 03
M2	1.68830E − 03	4.694E + 03	4.662E + 03	M2	2.57490E − 03	2.599E + 03	2.558E + 03
	1.78195E − 03	4.164E + 03	4.136E + 03		2.69447E − 03	2.339E + 03	2.301E + 03
	1.88080E − 03	3.691E + 03	3.666E + 03		2.81960E − 03	2.104E + 03	2.071E + 03
M1	1.88080E − 03	3.854E + 03	3.829E + 03	M1	2.81960E − 03	2.194E + 03	2.160E + 03
	2.00000E − 03	3.360E + 03	3.337E + 03		3.00000E − 03	1.902E + 03	1.873E + 03
	3.00000E − 03	1.292E + 03	1.280E + 03		4.00000E − 03	9.564E + 02	9.405E + 02
	4.00000E − 03	6.380E + 02	6.296E + 02		5.00000E − 03	5.534E + 02	5.423E + 02
	5.00000E − 03	3.653E + 02	3.584E + 02		6.00000E − 03	3.514E + 02	3.428E + 02
	6.00000E − 03	2.305E + 02	2.246E + 02		8.00000E − 03	1.705E + 02	1.643E + 02
	7.24280E − 03	1.429E + 02	1.379E + 02		1.00000E − 02	9.691E + 01	9.204E + 01
L3	7.24280E − 03	3.844E + 02	3.452E + 02		1.02068E − 02	9.201E + 01	8.724E + 01
	7.57876E − 03	3.427E + 02	3.088E + 02	L3	1.02068E − 02	2.334E + 02	1.966E + 02
	7.93030E − 03	3.049E + 02	2.755E + 02		1.08548E − 02	1.983E + 02	1.684E + 02
L2	7.93030E − 03	4.149E + 02	3.665E + 02		1.15440E − 02	1.689E + 02	1.444E + 02
	8.00000E − 03	4.068E + 02	3.595E + 02	L2	1.15440E − 02	2.312E + 02	1.889E + 02
	8.37560E − 03	3.631E + 02	3.223E + 02		1.18186E − 02	2.268E + 02	1.797E + 02

[a] μ/ρ includes the photoelectric, coherent (Rayleigh) and incoherent (Compton) scattering, and the electron-position production cross-sections. The latter includes both production in the field of the nucleus as well as that of the atomic electrons. Photonuclear cross-sections, nuclear-resonance scattering, and Delbrück scattering are not included.

Table 5.1 Mass Attenuation and Energy-Absorption Coefficients (Continued)

	Photon Energy (MeV)	Gadolinium μ/ρ (cm^2/g)	Z = 64 μ_{en}/ρ (cm^2/g)		Photon Energy (MeV)	Tungsten μ/ρ (cm^2/g)	Z = 74 μ_{en}/ρ (cm^2/g)
L1	8.37560E − 03	4.190E + 02	3.702E + 02		1.20998E − 02	2.065E + 02	1.699E + 02
	1.00000E − 02	2.693E + 02	2.416E + 02	L1	1.20998E − 02	2.382E + 02	1.948E + 02
	1.50000E − 02	9.335E + 01	8.538E + 01		1.50000E − 02	1.389E + 02	1.172E + 02
	2.00000E − 02	4.363E + 01	3.994E + 01		2.00000E − 02	6.573E + 01	5.697E + 01
	3.00000E − 02	1.484E + 01	1.333E + 01		3.00000E − 02	2.273E + 01	1.991E + 01
	4.00000E − 02	6.920E + 00	6.033E + 00		4.00000E − 02	1.067E + 01	9.240E + 00
	5.00000E − 02	3.859E + 00	3.242E + 00		5.00000E − 02	5.949E + 00	5.050E + 00
	5.02391E − 02	3.812E + 00	3.199E + 00		6.00000E − 02	3.713E + 00	3.070E + 00
K	5.02391E − 02	1.864E + 01	5.585E + 00		6.95250E − 02	2.552E + 00	2.049E + 00
	6.00000E − 02	1.175E + 01	4.722E + 00	K	6.95250E − 02	1.123E + 01	3.212E + 00
	8.00000E − 02	5.573E + 00	2.937E + 00		8.00000E − 02	7.810E + 00	2.879E + 00
	1.00000E − 01	3.109E + 00	1.849E + 00		1.00000E − 01	4.438E + 00	2.100E + 00
	1.50000E − 01	1.100E + 00	7.197E − 01		1.50000E − 01	1.581E + 00	9.378E − 01
	2.00000E − 01	5.534E − 01	3.584E − 01		2.00000E − 01	7.844E − 01	4.913E − 01
	3.00000E − 01	2.410E − 01	1.409E − 01		3.00000E − 01	3.238E − 01	1.973E − 01
	4.00000E − 01	1.517E − 01	8.039E − 02		4.00000E − 01	1.925E − 01	1.100E − 01
	5.00000E − 01	1.139E − 01	5.650E − 02		5.00000E − 01	1.378E − 01	7.440E − 02
	6.00000E − 01	9.371E − 02	4.483E − 02		6.00000E − 01	1.093E − 01	5.673E − 02
	8.00000E − 01	7.252E − 02	3.399E − 02		8.00000E − 01	8.066E − 02	4.028E − 02
	1.00000E + 00	6.120E − 02	2.893E − 02		1.00000E + 00	6.618E − 02	3.276E − 02
	1.25000E + 00	5.262E − 02	2.530E − 02		1.25000E + 00	5.577E − 02	2.761E − 02
	1.50000E + 00	4.759E − 02	2.325E − 02		1.50000E + 00	5.000E − 02	2.484E − 02
	2.00000E + 00	4.228E − 02	2.144E − 02		2.00000E + 00	4.433E − 02	2.256E − 02
	3.00000E + 00	3.865E − 02	2.129E − 02		3.00000E + 00	4.075E − 02	2.236E − 02
	4.00000E + 00	3.802E − 02	2.241E − 02		4.00000E + 00	4.038E − 02	2.363E − 02
	5.00000E + 00	3.844E − 02	2.374E − 02		5.00000E + 00	4.103E − 02	2.510E − 02
	6.00000E + 00	3.928E − 02	2.502E − 02		6.00000E + 00	4.210E − 02	2.649E − 02
	8.00000E + 00	4.147E − 02	2.725E − 02		8.00000E + 00	4.472E − 02	2.886E − 02
	1.00000E + 01	4.384E − 02	2.902E − 02		1.00000E + 01	4.747E − 02	3.072E − 02
	1.50000E + 01	4.943E − 02	3.188E − 02		1.50000E + 01	5.384E − 02	3.360E − 02
	2.00000E + 01	5.385E − 02	3.306E − 02		2.00000E + 01	5.893E − 02	3.475E − 02

[a] μ/ρ includes the photoelectric, coherent (Rayleigh) and incoherent (Compton) scattering, and the electron-position production cross-sections. The latter includes both production in the field of the nucleus as well as that of the atomic electrons. Photonuclear cross-sections, nuclear-resonance scattering, and Delbrück scattering are not included.

(continued)

Table 5.1 Mass Attenuation and Energy-Absorption Coefficients (Continued)

	Photon Energy (MeV)	Mercury μ/ρ (cm^2/g)	Z = 80 μ_{en}/ρ (cm^2/g)		Photon Energy (MeV)	Lead μ/ρ (cm^2/g)	Z = 82 μ_{en}/ρ (cm^2/g)
	1.00000E − 03	4.830E + 03	4.817E + 03		1.00000E − 03	5.210E + 03	5.197E + 03
	1.50000E − 03	2.174E + 03	2.161E + 03		1.50000E − 03	2.356E + 03	2.344E + 03
	2.00000E − 03	1.184E + 03	1.172E + 03		2.00000E − 03	1.285E + 03	1.274E + 03
	2.29490E − 03	8.773E + 02	8.660E + 02		2.48400E − 03	8.006E + 02	7.895E + 02
M5	2.29490E − 03	9.925E + 02	9.778E + 02	M5	2.48400E − 03	1.397E + 03	1.366E + 03
	2.33947E − 03	1.407E + 03	1.378E + 03		2.53429E − 03	1.726E + 03	1.682E + 03
	2.38490E − 03	2.151E + 03	2.101E + 03		2.58560E − 03	1.944E + 03	1.895E + 03
M4	2.38490E − 03	2.316E + 03	2.261E + 03	M4	2.58560E − 03	2.458E + 03	2.390E + 03
	2.60577E − 03	2.257E + 03	2.202E + 03		3.00000E − 03	1.965E + 03	1.913E + 03
	2.84710E − 03	2.080E + 03	2.030E + 03		3.06640E − 03	1.857E + 03	1.808E + 03
M3	2.84710E − 03	2.400E + 03	2.343E + 03	M3	3.06640E − 03	2.146E + 03	2.090E + 03
	3.00000E − 03	2.117E + 03	2.069E + 03		3.30130E − 03	1.796E + 03	1.748E + 03
	3.27850E − 03	1.704E + 03	1.666E + 03		3.55420E − 03	1.496E + 03	1.459E + 03
M2	3.27850E − 03	1.808E + 03	1.767E + 03	M2	3.55420E − 03	1.585E + 03	1.546E + 03
	3.41712E − 03	1.638E + 03	1.600E + 03		3.69948E − 03	1.442E + 03	1.405E + 03
	3.56160E − 03	1.486E + 03	1.454E + 03		3.85070E − 03	1.311E + 03	1.279E + 03
M1	3.56160E − 03	1.549E + 03	1.515E + 03	M1	3.85070E − 03	1.368E + 03	1.335E + 03
	4.00000E − 03	1.179E + 03	1.153E + 03		4.00000E − 03	1.251E + 03	1.221E + 03
	5.00000E − 03	6.869E + 02	6.710E + 02		5.00000E − 03	7.304E + 02	7.124E + 02
	6.00000E − 03	4.387E + 02	4.272E + 02		6.00000E − 03	4.672E + 02	4.546E + 02
	8.00000E − 03	2.140E + 02	2.065E + 02		8.00000E − 03	2.287E + 02	2.207E + 02
	1.00000E − 02	1.221E + 02	1.164E + 02		1.00000E − 02	1.306E + 02	1.247E + 02
	1.22839E − 02	7.266E + 01	6.821E + 01		1.30352E − 02	6.701E + 01	6.270E + 01
L3	1.22839E − 02	1.780E + 02	1.437E + 02	L3	1.30352E − 02	1.621E + 02	1.291E + 02
	1.32113E − 02	1.464E + 02	1.197E + 02		1.50000E − 02	1.116E + 02	9.100E + 01
	1.42087E − 02	1.209E + 02	9.988E + 01		1.52000E − 02	1.078E + 02	8.807E + 01
L2	1.42087E − 02	1.663E + 02	1.289E + 02	L2	1.52000E − 02	1.485E + 02	1.131E + 02
	1.45206E − 02	1.674E + 02	1.233E + 02		1.55269E − 02	1.416E + 02	1.083E + 02
	1.48393E − 02	1.501E + 02	1.173E + 02		1.58608E − 02	1.344E + 02	1.032E + 02

[a] μ/ρ includes the photoelectric, coherent (Rayleigh) and incoherent (Compton) scattering, and the electron-position production cross-sections. The latter includes both production in the field of the nucleus as well as that of the atomic electrons. Photonuclear cross-sections, nuclear-resonance scattering, and Delbrück scattering are not included.

Table 5.1 Mass Attenuation and Energy-Absorption Coefficients (Continued)

	Photon Energy (MeV)	Mercury μ_{en}/ρ (cm²/g)	Z = 80 μ_{en}/ρ (cm²/g)		Photon Energy (MeV)	Lead μ/ρ (cm²/g)	Z = 82 μ_{en}/ρ (cm²/g)
L1	1.48393E − 02	1.728E + 02	1.340E + 02	L1	1.58608E − 02	1.548E + 02	1.180E + 02
	1.50000E − 02	1.681E + 02	1.307E + 02		2.00000E − 02	8.636E + 01	6.899E + 01
	2.00000E − 02	8.123E + 01	6.647E + 01		3.00000E − 02	3.032E + 01	2.536E + 01
	3.00000E − 02	2.841E + 01	2.410E + 01		4.00000E − 02	1.436E + 01	1.211E + 01
	4.00000E − 02	1.342E + 01	1.141E + 01		5.00000E − 02	8.041E + 00	6.740E + 00
	5.00000E − 02	7.504E + 00	6.321E + 00		6.00000E − 02	5.021E + 00	4.149E + 00
	6.00000E − 02	4.683E + 00	3.878E + 00		8.00000E − 02	2.419E + 00	1.916E + 00
	8.00000E − 02	2.259E + 00	1.782E + 00		8.80045E − 02	1.910E + 00	1.482E + 00
	8.31023E − 02	2.055E + 00	1.607E + 00	K	8.80045E − 02	7.683E + 00	2.160E + 00
K	8.31023E − 02	8.464E + 00	2.384E + 00		1.00000E − 01	5.549E + 00	1.976E + 00
	1.00000E − 01	5.279E + 00	2.043E + 00		1.50000E − 01	2.014E + 00	1.056E + 00
	1.50000E − 01	1.909E + 00	1.036E + 00		2.00000E − 01	9.985E − 01	5.870E − 01
	2.00000E − 01	9.456E − 01	5.661E − 01		3.00000E − 01	4.031E − 01	2.455E − 01
	3.00000E − 01	3.834E − 01	2.342E − 01		4.00000E − 01	2.323E − 01	1.370E − 01
	4.00000E − 01	2.224E − 01	1.304E − 01		5.00000E − 01	1.614E − 01	9.128E − 02
	5.00000E − 01	1.555E − 01	8.711E − 02		6.00000E − 01	1.248E − 01	6.819E − 02
	6.00000E − 01	1.210E − 01	6.536E − 02		8.00000E − 01	8.870E − 02	4.644E − 02
	8.00000E − 01	8.679E − 02	4.493E − 02		1.00000E + 00	7.102E − 02	3.654E − 02
	1.00000E + 00	6.993E − 02	3.563E − 02		1.25000E + 00	5.876E − 02	2.988E − 02
	1.25000E + 00	5.814E − 02	2.936E − 02		1.50000E + 00	5.222E − 02	2.640E − 02
	1.50000E + 00	5.179E − 02	2.605E − 02		2.00000E + 00	4.606E − 02	2.360E − 02
	2.00000E + 00	4.575E − 02	2.339E − 02		3.00000E + 00	4.234E − 02	2.322E − 02
	3.00000E + 00	4.207E − 02	2.307E − 02		4.00000E + 00	4.197E − 02	2.449E − 02
	4.00000E + 00	4.172E − 02	2.436E − 02		5.00000E + 00	4.272E − 02	2.600E − 02
	5.00000E + 00	4.246E − 02	2.586E − 02		6.00000E + 00	4.391E − 02	2.744E − 02
	6.00000E + 00	4.362E − 02	2.730E − 02		8.00000E + 00	4.675E − 02	2.989E − 02
	8.00000E + 00	4.643E − 02	2.975E − 02		1.00000E + 01	4.972E − 02	3.181E − 02
	1.00000E + 01	4.937E − 02	3.165E − 02		1.50000E + 01	5.658E − 02	3.478E − 02
	1.50000E + 01	5.613E − 02	3.460E − 02		2.00000E + 01	6.206E − 02	3.595E − 02
	2.00000E + 01	6.154E − 02	3.576E − 02				

[a] μ/ρ includes the photoelectric, coherent (Rayleigh) and incoherent (Compton) scattering, and the electron-position production cross-sections. The latter includes both production in the field of the nucleus as well as that of the atomic electrons. Photonuclear cross-sections, nuclear-resonance scattering, and Delbrück scattering are not included.

(continued)

Table 5.1 Mass Attenuation and Energy-Absorption Coefficients (Continued)

	A-150 Tissue-Equivalent Plastic				Adipose Tissue (ICRU-44)		
	Photon Energy (MeV)	μ/ρ (cm^2/g)	μ_{en}/ρ (cm^2/g)		Photon Energy (MeV)	μ/ρ (cm^2/g)	μ_{en}/ρ (cm^2/g)
	1.00000E − 03	2.259E + 03	2.256E + 03		1.00000E − 03	2.628E + 03	2.623E + 03
	1.50000E − 03	7.282E + 02	7.267E + 02		1.03542E − 03	2.392E + 03	2.387E + 03
	2.00000E − 03	3.183E + 02	3.172E + 02		1.07210E − 03	2.176E + 03	2.171E + 03
	3.00000E − 03	9.652E + 01	9.576E + 01	11K	1.07210E − 03	2.182E + 03	2.177E + 03
	4.00000E − 03	4.081E + 01	4.021E + 01		1.50000E − 03	8.622E + 02	8.601E + 02
	4.03810E − 03	3.966E + 01	3.907E + 01		2.00000E − 03	3.800E + 02	3.787E + 02
20K	4.03810E − 03	5.629E + 01	5.326E + 01		2.47200E − 03	2.053E + 02	2.043E + 02
	5.00000E − 03	3.069E + 01	2.901E + 01	16K	2.47200E − 03	2.072E + 02	2.060E + 02
	6.00000E − 03	1.813E + 01	1.708E + 01		2.64140E − 03	1.707E + 02	1.696E + 02
	8.00000E − 03	7.914E + 00	7.337E + 00		2.82240E − 03	1.405E + 02	1.396E + 02
	1.00000E − 02	4.186E + 00	3.771E + 00	17K	2.82240E − 03	1.420E + 02	1.409E + 02
	1.50000E − 02	1.394E + 00	1.106E + 00		3.00000E − 03	1.188E + 02	1.178E + 02
	2.00000E − 02	7.068E − 01	4.605E − 01		4.00000E − 03	5.054E + 01	4.983E + 01
	3.00000E − 02	3.481E − 01	1.378E − 01		5.00000E − 03	2.587E + 01	2.531E + 01
	4.00000E − 02	2.562E − 01	6.411E − 02		6.00000E − 03	1.494E + 01	1.446E + 01
	5.00000E − 02	2.198E − 01	4.018E − 02		8.00000E − 03	6.300E + 00	5.917E + 00
	6.00000E − 02	2.008E − 01	3.095E − 02		1.00000E − 02	3.268E + 00	2.935E + 00
	8.00000E − 02	1.803E − 01	2.561E − 02		1.50000E − 02	1.083E + 00	8.103E − 01
	1.00000E − 01	1.680E − 01	2.520E − 02		2.00000E − 02	5.677E − 01	3.251E − 01
	1.50000E − 01	1.485E − 01	2.736E − 02		3.00000E − 02	3.063E − 01	9.495E − 02
	2.00000E − 01	1.353E − 01	2.937E − 02		4.00000E − 02	2.396E − 01	4.575E − 02
	3.00000E − 01	1.173E − 01	3.159E − 02		5.00000E − 02	2.123E − 01	3.085E − 02
	4.00000E − 01	1.049E − 01	3.245E − 02		6.00000E − 02	1.974E − 01	2.567E − 02
	5.00000E − 01	9.579E − 02	3.265E − 02		8.00000E − 02	1.800E − 01	2.358E − 02
	6.00000E − 01	8.857E − 02	3.249E − 02		1.00000E − 01	1.688E − 01	2.433E − 02
	8.00000E − 01	7.777E − 02	3.172E − 02		1.50000E − 01	1.500E − 01	2.737E − 02
	1.00000E + 00	6.992E − 02	3.070E − 02		2.00000E − 01	1.368E − 01	2.959E − 02
	1.25000E + 00	6.253E − 02	2.934E − 02		3.00000E − 01	1.187E − 01	3.194E − 02
	1.50000E + 00	5.691E − 02	2.805E − 02		4.00000E − 01	1.062E − 01	3.283E − 02
	2.00000E + 00	4.880E − 02	2.578E − 02		5.00000E − 01	9.696E − 02	3.304E − 02
	3.00000E + 00	3.907E − 02	2.247E − 02		6.00000E − 01	8.965E − 02	3.289E − 02
	4.00000E + 00	3.335E − 02	2.025E − 02		8.00000E − 01	7.873E − 02	3.211E − 02
	5.00000E + 00	2.958E − 02	1.867E − 02		1.00000E + 00	7.078E − 02	3.108E − 02
	6.00000E + 00	2.690E − 02	1.751E − 02		1.25000E + 00	6.330E − 02	2.970E − 02
	8.00000E + 00	2.338E − 02	1.592E − 02		1.50000E + 00	5.760E − 02	2.839E − 02
	1.00000E + 01	2.117E − 02	1.489E − 02		2.00000E + 00	4.940E − 02	2.610E − 02
	1.50000E + 01	1.819E − 02	1.346E − 02		3.00000E + 00	3.955E − 02	2.275E − 02
	2.00000E + 01	1.675E − 02	1.275E − 02		4.00000E + 00	3.377E − 02	2.050E − 02
					5.00000E + 00	2.995E − 02	1.891E − 02
					6.00000E + 00	2.725E − 02	1.773E − 02
					8.00000E + 00	2.368E − 02	1.612E − 02
					1.00000E + 01	2.145E − 02	1.509E − 02
					1.50000E + 01	1.843E − 02	1.365E − 02
					2.00000E + 01	1.698E − 02	1.293E − 02

[a] μ/ρ includes the photoelectric, coherent (Rayleigh) and incoherent (Compton) scattering, and the electron-position production cross-sections. The latter includes both production in the field of the nucleus as well as that of the atomic electrons. Photonuclear cross-sections, nuclear-resonance scattering, and Delbrück scattering are not included.

Table 5.1 Mass Attenuation and Energy-Absorption Coefficients (Continued)

Air, Dry (Near Sea Level)

	Photon Energy (MeV)	μ/ρ (cm^2/g)	μ_{en}/ρ (cm^2/g)
	1.00000E − 03	3.606E + 03	3.599E + 03
	1.50000E − 03	1.191E + 03	1.188E + 03
	2.00000E − 03	5.279E + 02	5.262E + 02
	3.00000E − 03	1.625E + 02	1.614E + 02
	3.20290E − 03	1.340E + 02	1.330E + 02
18K	3.20290E − 03	1.485E + 02	1.460E + 02
	4.00000E − 03	7.788E + 01	7.636E + 01
	5.00000E − 03	4.027E + 01	3.931E + 01
	6.00000E − 03	2.341E + 01	2.270E + 01
	8.00000E − 03	9.921E + 00	9.446E + 00
	1.00000E − 02	5.120E + 00	4.742E + 00
	1.50000E − 02	1.614E + 00	1.334E + 00
	2.00000E − 02	7.779E − 01	5.389E − 01
	3.00000E − 02	3.538E − 01	1.537E − 01
	4.00000E − 02	2.485E − 01	6.833E − 02
	5.00000E − 02	2.080E − 01	4.098E − 02
	6.00000E − 02	1.875E − 01	3.041E − 02
	8.00000E − 02	1.662E − 01	2.407E − 02
	1.00000E − 01	1.541E − 01	2.325E − 02
	1.50000E − 01	1.356E − 01	2.496E − 02
	2.00000E − 01	1.233E − 01	2.672E − 02
	3.00000E − 01	1.067E − 01	2.872E − 02
	4.00000E − 01	9.549E − 02	2.949E − 02
	5.00000E − 01	8.712E − 02	2.966E − 02
	6.00000E − 01	8.055E − 02	2.953E − 02
	8.00000E − 01	7.074E − 02	2.882E − 02
	1.00000E + 00	6.358E − 02	2.789E − 02
	1.25000E + 00	5.687E − 02	2.666E − 02
	1.50000E + 00	5.175E − 02	2.547E − 02
	2.00000E + 00	4.447E − 02	2.345E − 02
	3.00000E + 00	3.581E − 02	2.057E − 02
	4.00000E + 00	3.079E − 02	1.870E − 02
	5.00000E + 00	2.751E − 02	1.740E − 02
	6.00000E + 00	2.522E − 02	1.647E − 02
	8.00000E + 00	2.225E − 02	1.525E − 02
	1.00000E + 01	2.045E − 02	1.450E − 02
	1.50000E + 01	1.810E − 02	1.353E − 02
	2.00000E + 01	1.705E − 02	1.311E − 02

Bakelite

Photon Energy (MeV)	μ/ρ (cm^2/g)	μ_{en}/ρ (cm2/g)
1.00000E − 03	2.484E + 03	2.480E + 03
1.50000E − 03	8.027E + 02	8.010E + 02
2.00000E − 03	3.512E + 02	3.500E + 02
3.00000E − 03	1.065E + 02	1.057E + 02
4.00000E − 03	4.494E + 01	4.433E + 01
5.00000E − 03	2.288E + 01	2.237E + 01
6.00000E − 03	1.315E + 01	1.272E + 01
8.00000E − 03	5.521E + 00	5.162E + 00
1.00000E − 02	2.860E + 00	2.545E + 00
1.50000E − 02	9.552E − 01	6.961E − 01
2.00000E − 02	5.089E − 01	2.779E − 01
3.00000E − 02	2.824E − 01	8.135E − 02
4.00000E − 02	2.241E − 01	3.988E − 02
5.00000E − 02	2.000E − 01	2.754E − 02
6.00000E − 02	1.866E − 01	2.340E − 02
8.00000E − 02	1.707E − 01	2.200E − 02
1.00000E − 01	1.602E − 01	2.292E − 02
1.50000E − 01	1.424E − 01	2.594E − 02
2.00000E − 01	1.300E − 01	2.809E − 02
3.00000E − 01	1.127E − 01	3.033E − 02
4.00000E − 01	1.009E − 01	3.118E − 02
5.00000E − 01	9.210E − 02	3.138E − 02
6.00000E − 01	8.516E − 02	3.124E − 02
8.00000E − 01	7.478E − 02	3.049E − 02
1.00000E + 00	6.723E − 02	2.951E − 02
1.25000E + 00	6.013E − 02	2.821E − 02
1.50000E + 00	5.472E − 02	2.696E − 02
2.00000E + 00	4.694E − 02	2.479E − 02
3.00000E + 00	3.761E − 02	2.163E − 02
4.00000E + 00	3.215E − 02	1.951E − 02
5.00000E + 00	2.854E − 02	1.802E − 02
6.00000E + 00	2.599E − 02	1.692E − 02
8.00000E + 00	2.264E − 02	1.543E − 02
1.00000E + 01	2.055E − 02	1.447E − 02
1.50000E + 01	1.775E − 02	1.315E − 02
2.00000E + 01	1.641E − 02	1.249E − 02

[a] μ/ρ includes the photoelectric, coherent (Rayleigh) and incoherent (Compton) scattering, and the electron-position production cross-sections. The latter includes both production in the field of the nucleus as well as that of the atomic electrons. Photonuclear cross-sections, nuclear-resonance scattering, and Delbrück scattering are not included.

(continued)

Table 5.1 Mass Attenuation and Energy-Absorption Coefficients (Continued)

Bone, Cortical (ICRU-44)

	Photon Energy (MeV)	μ/ρ (cm^2/g)	μ_{en}/ρ (cm^2/g)
	1.00000E − 03	3.781E + 03	3.772E + 03
	1.03542E − 03	3.452E + 03	3.444E + 03
	1.07210E − 03	3.150E + 03	3.143E + 03
11K	1.07210E − 03	3.156E + 03	3.149E + 03
	1.18283E − 03	2.434E + 03	2.429E + 03
	1.30500E − 03	1.873E + 03	1.869E + 03
12K	1.30500E − 03	1.883E + 03	1.878E + 03
	1.50000E − 03	1.295E + 03	1.291E + 03
	2.00000E − 03	5.869E + 02	5.846E + 02
	2.14550E − 03	4.824E + 02	4.803E + 02
15K	2.14550E − 03	7.114E + 02	6.961E + 02
	2.30297E − 03	5.916E + 02	5.789E + 02
	2.47200E − 03	4.907E + 02	4.805E + 02
16K	2.47200E − 03	4.962E + 02	4.857E + 02
	3.00000E − 03	2.958E + 02	2.897E + 02
	4.00000E − 03	1.331E + 02	1.303E + 02
	4.03810E − 03	1.296E + 02	1.269E + 02
20K	4.03810E − 03	3.332E + 02	3.006E + 02
	5.00000E − 03	1.917E + 02	1.757E + 02
	6.00000E − 03	1.171E + 02	1.085E + 02
	8.00000E − 03	5.323E + 01	4.987E + 01
	1.00000E − 02	2.851E + 01	2.680E + 01
	1.50000E − 02	9.032E + 00	8.388E + 00
	2.00000E − 02	4.001E + 00	3.601E + 00
	3.00000E − 02	1.331E + 00	1.070E + 00
	4.00000E − 02	6.655E − 01	4.507E − 01
	5.00000E − 02	4.242E − 01	2.336E − 01
	6.00000E − 02	3.148E − 01	1.400E − 01
	8.00000E − 02	2.229E − 01	6.896E − 02
	1.00000E − 01	1.855E − 01	4.585E − 02
	1.50000E − 01	1.480E − 01	3.183E − 02
	2.00000E − 01	1.309E − 01	3.003E − 02
	3.00000E − 01	1.113E − 01	3.032E − 02
	4.00000E − 01	9.908E − 02	3.069E − 02
	5.00000E − 01	9.022E − 02	3.073E − 02
	6.00000E − 01	8.332E − 02	3.052E − 02
	8.00000E − 01	7.308E − 02	2.973E − 02
	1.00000E + 00	6.566E − 02	2.875E − 02
	1.25000E + 00	5.871E − 02	2.745E − 02
	1.50000E + 00	5.346E − 02	2.623E − 02
	2.00000E + 00	4.607E − 02	2.421E − 02
	3.00000E + 00	3.745E − 02	2.145E − 02
	4.00000E + 00	3.257E − 02	1.975E − 02
	5.00000E + 00	2.946E − 02	1.864E − 02
	6.00000E + 00	2.734E − 02	1.788E − 02
	8.00000E + 00	2.467E − 02	1.695E − 02
	1.00000E + 01	2.314E − 02	1.644E − 02
	1.50000E + 01	2.132E − 02	1.587E − 02
	2.00000E + 01	2.068E − 02	1.568E − 02

Breast Tissue (ICRU-44)

	Photon Energy (MeV)	μ/ρ (cm^2/g)	μ_{en}/ρ (cm^2/g)
	1.00000E − 03	3.263E + 03	3.255E + 03
	1.03542E − 03	2.975E + 03	2.967E + 03
	1.07210E − 03	2.710E + 03	2.703E + 03
11K	1.07210E − 03	2.716E + 03	2.709E + 03
	1.50000E − 03	1.088E + 03	1.085E + 03
	2.00000E − 03	4.842E + 02	4.825E + 02
	2.14550E − 03	3.961E + 02	3.946E + 02
15K	2.14550E − 03	3.983E + 02	3.967E + 02
	2.30297E − 03	3.250E + 02	3.235E + 02
	2.47200E − 03	2.649E + 02	2.636E + 02
16K	2.47200E − 03	2.686E + 02	2.670E + 02
	2.64140E − 03	2.221E + 02	2.204E + 02
	2.82240E − 03	1.831E + 02	1.818E + 02
17K	2.82240E − 03	1.845E + 02	1.831E + 02
	3.00000E − 03	1.546E + 02	1.533E + 02
	4.00000E − 03	6.625E + 01	6.540E + 01
	5.00000E − 03	3.407E + 01	3.341E + 01
	6.00000E − 03	1.972E + 01	1.918E + 01
	8.00000E − 03	8.320E + 00	7.899E + 00
	1.00000E − 02	4.295E + 00	3.937E + 00
	1.50000E − 02	1.378E + 00	1.094E + 00
	2.00000E − 02	6.889E − 01	4.394E − 01
	3.00000E − 02	3.403E − 01	1.260E − 01
	4.00000E − 02	2.530E − 01	5.792E − 02
	5.00000E − 02	2.186E − 01	3.666E − 02
	6.00000E − 02	2.006E − 01	2.881E − 02
	8.00000E − 02	1.808E − 01	2.470E − 02
	1.00000E − 01	1.688E − 01	2.478E − 02
	1.50000E − 01	1.493E − 01	2.734E − 02
	2.00000E − 01	1.361E − 01	2.945E − 02
	3.00000E − 01	1.179E − 01	3.173E − 02
	4.00000E − 01	1.055E − 01	3.260E − 02
	5.00000E − 01	9.631E − 02	3.281E − 02
	6.00000E − 01	8.904E − 02	3.266E − 02
	8.00000E − 01	7.820E − 02	3.188E − 02
	1.00000E + 00	7.031E − 02	3.086E − 02
	1.25000E + 00	6.287E − 02	2.949E − 02
	1.50000E + 00	5.721E − 02	2.818E − 02
	2.00000E + 00	4.910E − 02	2.592E − 02
	3.00000E + 00	3.937E − 02	2.264E − 02
	4.00000E + 00	3.369E − 02	2.045E − 02
	5.00000E + 00	2.995E − 02	1.891E − 02
	6.00000E + 00	2.731E − 02	1.779E − 02
	8.00000E + 00	2.384E − 02	1.626E − 02
	1.00000E + 01	2.169E − 02	1.529E − 02
	1.50000E + 01	1.882E − 02	1.395E − 02
	2.00000E + 01	1.746E − 02	1.330E − 02

[a] μ/ρ includes the photoelectric, coherent (Rayleigh) and incoherent (Compton) scattering, and the electron-position production cross-sections. The latter includes both production in the field of the nucleus as well as that of the atomic electrons. Photonuclear cross-sections, nuclear-resonance scattering, and Delbrück scattering are not included.

Table 5.1 Mass Attenuation and Energy-Absorption Coefficients (Continued)

	Calcium Fluoride				Calcium Sulfate		
	Photon Energy (MeV)	μ/ρ (cm^2/g)	μ_{en}/ρ (cm^2/g)		Photon Energy (MeV)	μ/ρ (cm^2/g)	μ_{en}/ρ (cm^2/g)
	1.00000E − 03	5.248E + 03	5.228E + 03		1.00000E − 03	4.163E + 03	4.153E + 03
	1.50000e − 03	1.843E + 03	1.836E + 03		1.50000E − 03	1.429E + 03	1.425E + 03
	2.00000E − 03	8.509E + 02	8.472E + 02		2.00000E − 03	6.529E + 02	6.503E + 02
	3.00000E − 03	2.779E + 02	2.757E + 02		2.47200E − 03	3.627E + 02	3.606E + 02
	4.00000E − 03	1.237E + 02	1.220E + 02	16K	2.47200E − 03	7.993E + 02	7.659E + 02
	4.03810E − 03	1.204E + 02	1.187E + 02		3.00000E − 03	4.961E + 02	4.774E + 02
20K	4.03810E − 03	5.848E + 02	5.151E + 02		4.00000E − 03	2.289E + 02	2.215E + 02
	5.00000E − 03	3.410E + 02	3.070E + 02		4.03810E − 03	2.231E + 02	2.159E + 02
	6.00000E − 03	2.100E + 02	1.919E + 02	20K	4.03810E − 03	4.895E + 02	4.431E + 02
	8.00000E − 03	9.642E + 01	8.965E + 01		5.00000E − 03	2.820E + 02	2.595E + 02
	1.00000E − 02	5.194E + 01	4.867E + 01		6.00000E − 03	1.727E + 02	1.606E + 02
	1.50000E − 02	1.651E + 01	1.546E + 01		8.00000E − 03	7.858E + 01	7.394E + 01
	2.00000E − 02	7.255E + 00	6.692E + 00		1.00000E − 02	4.210E + 01	3.977E + 01
	3.00000E − 02	2.313E + 00	2.002E + 00		1.50000E − 02	1.329E + 01	1.247E + 01
	4.00000E − 02	1.077E + 00	8.405E − 01		2.00000E − 02	5.831E + 00	5.352E + 00
	5.00000E − 02	6.311E − 01	4.298E − 01		3.00000E − 02	1.876E + 00	1.587E + 00
	6.00000E − 02	4.311E − 01	2.512E − 01		4.00000E − 02	8.928E − 01	6.645E − 01
	8.00000E − 02	2.674E − 01	1.137E − 01		5.00000E − 02	5.381E − 01	3.403E − 01
	1.00000E − 01	2.048E − 01	6.741E − 02		6.00000E − 02	3.788E − 01	2.001E − 01
	1.50000E − 01	1.491E − 01	3.681E − 02		8.00000E − 02	2.474E − 01	9.290E − 02
	2.00000E − 01	1.278E − 01	3.112E − 02		1.00000E − 01	1.962E − 01	5.732E − 02
	3.00000E − 01	1.067E − 01	2.944E − 02		1.50000E − 01	1.487E − 01	3.443E − 02
	4.00000E − 01	9.437E − 02	2.933E − 02		2.00000E − 01	1.293E − 01	3.057E − 02
	5.00000E − 01	8.570E − 02	2.920E − 02		3.00000E − 01	1.088E − 01	2.981E − 02
	6.00000E − 01	7.905E − 02	2.892E − 02		4.00000E − 01	9.653E − 02	2.994E − 02
	8.00000E − 01	6.924E − 02	2.811E − 02		5.00000E − 01	8.777E − 02	2.989E − 02
	1.00000E + 00	6.217E − 02	2.715E − 02		6.00000E − 01	8.100E − 02	2.964E − 02
	1.25000E + 00	5.558E − 02	2.591E − 02		8.00000E − 01	7.100E − 02	2.884E − 02
	1.50000E + 00	5.065E − 02	2.476E − 02		1.00000E + 00	6.377E − 02	2.787E − 02
	2.00000E + 00	4.380E − 02	2.290E − 02		1.25000E + 00	5.701E − 02	2.660E − 02
	3.00000E + 00	3.606E − 02	2.058E − 02		1.50000E + 00	5.193E − 02	2.542E − 02
	4.00000E + 00	3.184E − 02	1.927E − 02		2.00000E + 00	4.488E − 02	2.350E − 02
	5.00000E + 00	2.923E − 02	1.850E − 02		3.00000E + 00	3.679E − 02	2.102E − 02
	6.00000E + 00	2.753E − 02	1.804E − 02		4.00000E + 00	3.232E − 02	1.958E − 02
	8.00000E + 00	2.553E − 02	1.758E − 02		5.00000E + 00	2.954E − 02	1.869E − 02
	1.00000E + 01	2.450E − 02	1.743E − 02		6.00000E + 00	2.770E − 02	1.814E − 02
	1.50000E + 01	2.356E − 02	1.745E − 02		8.00000E + 00	2.547E − 02	1.753E − 02
	2.00000E + 01	2.351E − 02	1.759E − 02		1.00000E + 01	2.428E − 02	1.727E − 02
					1.50000E + 01	2.305E − 02	1.711E − 02
					2.00000E + 01	2.282E − 02	1.716E − 02

[a] μ/ρ includes the photoelectric, coherent (Rayleigh) and incoherent (Compton) scattering, and the electron-position production cross-sections. The latter includes both production in the field of the nucleus as well as that of the atomic electrons. Photonuclear cross-sections, nuclear-resonance scattering, and Delbrück scattering are not included.

(continued)

Table 5.1 Mass Attenuation and Energy-Absorption Coefficients (Continued)

	Concrete, Ordinary				Eye Lens (ICRU-44)		
	Photon Energy (MeV)	μ/ρ (cm^2/g)	μ_{en}/ρ (cm^2/g)		Photon Energy (MeV)	μ/ρ (cm^2/g)	μ_{en}/ρ (cm^2/g)
	1.00000E − 03	3.466E + 03	3.456E + 03		1.00000E − 03	3.599E + 03	3.588E + 03
	1.03542E − 03	3.164E + 03	3.156E + 03		1.03542E − 03	3.282E + 03	3.273E + 03
	1.07210E − 03	2.889E + 03	2.880E + 03		1.07210E − 03	2.992E + 03	2.984E + 03
11K	1.07210E − 03	2.978E + 03	2.968E + 03	11K	1.07210E − 03	2.998E + 03	2.989E + 03
	1.18283E − 03	2.302E + 03	2.295E + 03		1.50000E − 03	1.206E + 03	1.203E + 03
	1.30500E − 03	1.775E + 03	1.769E + 03		2.00000E − 03	5.386E + 02	5.368E + 02
12K	1.30500E − 03	1.781E + 03	1.775E + 03		2.14550E − 03	4.410E + 02	4.393E + 02
	1.50000E − 03	1.227E + 03	1.223E + 03	15K	2.14550E − 03	4.432E + 02	4.414E + 02
	1.55960E − 03	1.104E + 03	1.100E + 03		2.30297E − 03	3.619E + 02	3.603E + 02
13K	1.55960E − 03	1.176E + 03	1.169E + 03		2.47200E − 03	2.952E + 02	2.938E + 02
	1.69350E − 03	9.419E + 02	9.365E + 02	16K	2.47200E − 03	3.007E + 02	2.989E + 02
	1.83890E − 03	7.525E + 02	7.482E + 02		2.64140E − 03	2.485E + 02	2.469E + 02
14K	1.83890E − 03	1.631E + 03	1.587E + 03		2.82240E − 03	2.053E + 02	2.038E + 02
	2.00000E − 03	1.368E + 03	1.333E + 03	17K	2.82240E − 03	2.067E + 02	2.051E + 02
	3.00000E − 03	4.646E + 02	4.552E + 02		3.00000E − 03	1.733E + 02	1.719E + 02
	3.60740E − 03	2.804E + 02	2.751E + 02		4.00000E − 03	7.446E + 01	7.353E + 01
19K	3.60740E − 03	2.911E + 02	2.844E + 02		5.00000E − 03	3.834E + 01	3.764E + 01
	4.00000E − 03	2.188E + 02	2.139E + 02		6.00000E − 03	2.221E + 01	2.163E + 01
	4.03810E − 03	2.131E + 02	2.084E + 02		8.00000E − 03	9.372E + 00	8.931E + 00
20K	4.03810E − 03	2.520E + 02	2.415E + 02		1.00000E − 02	4.829E + 00	4.458E + 00
	5.00000E − 03	1.401E + 02	1.348E + 02		1.50000E − 02	1.531E + 00	1.242E + 00
	6.00000E − 03	8.401E + 01	8.094E + 01		2.00000E − 02	7.510E − 01	4.988E − 01
	7.11200E − 03	5.187E + 01	4.995E + 01		3.00000E − 02	3.570E − 01	1.421E − 01

[a] μ/ρ includes the photoelectric, coherent (Rayleigh) and incoherent (Compton) scattering, and the electron-position production cross-sections. The latter includes both production in the field of the nucleus as well as that of the atomic electrons. Photonuclear cross-sections, nuclear-resonance scattering, and Delbrück scattering are not included.

Table 5.1 Mass Attenuation and Energy-Absorption Coefficients (Continued)

	Concrete, Ordinary			Eye Lens (ICRU-44)		
	Photon Energy (MeV)	μ/ρ (cm²/g)	μ_{en}/ρ (cm²/g)	Photon Energy (MeV)	μ/ρ (cm²/g)	μ_{en}/ρ (cm²/g)
26K	7.11200E − 03	5.415E + 01	5.153E + 01	4.00000E − 02	2.590E − 01	6.418E − 02
	8.00000E − 03	3.878E + 01	3.689E + 01	5.00000E − 02	2.209E − 01	3.961E − 02
	1.00000E − 02	2.045E + 01	1.937E + 01	6.00000E − 02	2.013E − 01	3.035E − 02
	1.50000E − 02	6.351E + 00	5.855E + 00	8.00000E − 02	1.803E − 01	2.518E − 02
	2.00000E − 02	2.806E + 00	2.462E + 00	1.00000E − 01	1.679E − 01	2.490E − 02
	3.00000E − 02	9.601E − 01	7.157E − 01	1.50000E − 01	1.482E − 01	2.719E − 02
	4.00000E − 02	5.058E − 01	2.995E − 01	2.00000E − 01	1.350E − 01	2.922E − 02
	5.00000E − 02	3.412E − 01	1.563E − 01	3.00000E − 01	1.169E − 01	3.146E − 02
	6.00000E − 02	2.660E − 01	9.554E − 02	4.00000E − 01	1.046E − 01	3.231E − 02
	8.00000E − 02	2.014E − 01	5.050E − 02	5.00000E − 01	9.547E − 02	3.252E − 02
	1.00000E − 01	1.738E − 01	3.649E − 02	6.00000E − 01	8.827E − 02	3.237E − 02
	1.50000E − 01	1.436E − 01	2.897E − 02	8.00000E − 01	7.752E − 02	3.160E − 02
	2.00000E − 01	1.282E − 01	2.868E − 02	1.00000E + 00	6.969E − 02	3.058E − 02
	3.00000E − 01	1.097E − 01	2.969E − 02	1.25000E + 00	6.232E − 02	2.922E − 02
	4.00000E − 01	9.783E − 02	3.024E − 02	1.50000E + 00	5.671E − 02	2.793E − 02
	5.00000E − 01	8.915E − 02	3.033E − 02	2.00000E + 00	4.869E − 02	2.570E − 02
	6.00000E − 01	8.236E − 02	3.015E − 02	3.00000E + 00	3.908E − 02	2.247E − 02
	8.00000E − 01	7.227E − 02	2.940E − 02	4.00000E + 00	3.349E − 02	2.033E − 02
	1.00000E + 00	6.495E − 02	2.843E − 02	5.00000E + 00	2.981E − 02	1.883E − 02
	1.25000E + 00	5.807E − 02	2.716E − 02	6.00000E + 00	2.722E − 02	1.774E − 02
	1.50000E + 00	5.288E − 02	2.595E − 02	8.00000E + 00	2.383E − 02	1.626E − 02
	2.00000E + 00	4.557E − 02	2.395E − 02	1.00000E + 01	2.174E − 02	1.534E − 02
	3.00000E + 00	3.701E − 02	2.120E − 02	1.50000E + 01	1.896E − 02	1.407E − 02
	4.00000E + 00	3.217E − 02	1.951E − 02	2.00000E + 01	1.767E − 02	1.346E − 02
	5.00000E + 00	2.908E − 02	1.840E − 02			
	6.00000E + 00	2.697E − 02	1.763E − 02			
	8.00000E + 00	2.432E − 02	1.669E − 02			
	1.00000E + 01	2.278E − 02	1.617E − 02			
	1.50000E + 01	2.096E − 02	1.559E − 02			
	2.00000E + 01	2.030E − 02	1.539E − 02			

[a] μ/ρ includes the photoelectric, coherent (Rayleigh) and incoherent (Compton) scattering, and the electron-position production cross-sections. The latter includes both production in the field of the nucleus as well as that of the atomic electrons. Photonuclear cross-sections, nuclear-resonance scattering, and Delbrück scattering are not included.

(continued)

Table 5.1 Mass Attenuation and Energy-Absorption Coefficients (Continued)

Glass, Borosilicate ("Pyrex")

	Photon Energy (MeV)	μ/ρ (cm^2/g)	μ_{en}/ρ (cm^2/g)
	1.00000E − 03	3.164E + 03	3.155E + 03
	1.03542E − 03	2.887E + 03	2.879E + 03
	1.07210E − 03	2.634E + 03	2.627E + 03
11K	1.07210E − 03	2.800E + 03	2.790E + 03
	1.50000E − 03	1.152E + 03	1.148E + 03
	1.55960E − 03	1.037E + 03	1.033E + 03
13K	1.55960E − 03	1.079E + 03	1.073E + 03
	1.69350E − 03	8.629E + 02	8.583E + 02
	1.83890E − 03	6.883E + 02	6.845E + 02
14K	1.83890E − 03	1.776E + 03	1.723E + 03
	2.00000E − 03	1.500E + 03	1.457E + 03
	3.00000E − 03	5.123E + 02	5.011E + 02
	3.60740E − 03	3.098E + 02	3.036E + 02
19K	3.60740E − 03	3.133E + 02	3.067E + 02
	4.00000E − 03	2.355E + 02	2.307E + 02
	5.00000E − 03	1.260E + 02	1.235E + 02
	6.00000E − 03	7.500E + 01	7.337E + 01
	8.00000E − 03	3.269E + 01	3.178E + 01
	1.00000E − 02	1.705E + 01	1.642E + 01
	1.50000E − 02	5.217E + 00	4.828E + 00
	2.00000E − 02	2.297E + 00	1.995E + 00
	3.00000E − 02	7.987E − 01	5.684E − 01
	4.00000E − 02	4.341E − 01	2.361E − 01
	5.00000E − 02	3.022E − 01	1.235E − 01
	6.00000E − 02	2.417E − 01	7.648E − 02
	8.00000E − 02	1.890E − 01	4.230E − 02
	1.00000E − 01	1.657E − 01	3.209E − 02
	1.50000E − 01	1.389E − 01	2.727E − 02
	2.00000E − 01	1.246E − 01	2.757E − 02
	3.00000E − 01	1.069E − 01	2.885E − 02
	4.00000E − 01	9.540E − 02	2.946E − 02
	5.00000E − 01	8.696E − 02	2.957E − 02
	6.00000E − 01	8.035E − 02	2.941E − 02
	8.00000E − 01	7.052E − 02	2.868E − 02
	1.00000E + 00	6.337E − 02	2.774E − 02
	1.25000E + 00	5.667E − 02	2.650E − 02
	1.50000E + 00	5.160E − 02	2.533E − 02
	2.00000E + 00	4.447E − 02	2.337E − 02
	3.00000E + 00	3.611E − 02	2.069E − 02
	4.00000E + 00	3.140E − 02	1.904E − 02
	5.00000E + 00	2.838E − 02	1.795E − 02
	6.00000E + 00	2.632E − 02	1.721E − 02
	8.00000E + 00	2.373E − 02	1.629E − 02
	1.00000E + 01	2.223E − 02	1.579E − 02
	1.50000E + 01	2.045E − 02	1.522E − 02
	2.00000E + 01	1.982E − 02	1.503E − 02

Lithium Fluoride

Photon Energy (MeV)	μ/ρ (cm^2/g)	μ_{en}/ρ (cm^2/g)
1.00000E − 03	4.200E + 03	4.175E + 03
1.50000E − 03	1.467E + 03	1.460E + 03
2.00000E − 03	6.698E + 02	6.667E + 02
3.00000E − 03	2.135E + 02	2.121E + 02
4.00000E − 03	9.282E + 01	9.188E + 01
5.00000E − 03	4.815E + 01	4.742E + 01
6.00000E − 03	2.802E + 01	2.742E + 01
8.00000E − 03	1.187E + 01	1.142E + 01
1.00000E − 02	6.101E + 00	5.733E + 00
1.50000E − 02	1.884E + 00	1.612E + 00
2.00000E − 02	8.792E − 01	6.494E − 01
3.00000E − 02	3.727E − 01	1.826E − 01
4.00000E − 02	2.486E − 01	7.890E − 02
5.00000E − 02	2.020E − 01	4.541E − 02
6.00000E − 02	1.791E − 01	3.223E − 02
8.00000E − 02	1.563E − 01	2.385E − 02
1.00000E − 01	1.441E − 01	2.229E − 02
1.50000E − 01	1.260E − 01	2.332E − 02
2.00000E − 01	1.145E − 01	2.484E − 02
3.00000E − 01	9.899E − 02	2.663E − 02
4.00000E − 01	8.853E − 02	2.734E − 02
5.00000E − 01	8.076E − 02	2.749E − 02
6.00000E − 01	7.467E − 02	2.736E − 02
8.00000E − 01	6.557E − 02	2.671E − 02
1.00000E + 00	5.894E − 02	2.585E − 02
1.25000E + 00	5.271E − 02	2.470E − 02
1.50000E + 00	4.798E − 02	2.361E − 02
2.00000E + 00	4.122E − 02	2.173E − 02
3.00000E + 00	3.321E − 02	1.907E − 02
4.00000E + 00	2.857E − 02	1.733E − 02
5.00000E + 00	2.554E − 02	1.614E − 02
6.00000E + 00	2.343E − 02	1.528E − 02
8.00000E + 00	2.069E − 02	1.414E − 02
1.00000E + 01	1.903E − 02	1.345E − 02
1.50000E + 01	1.687E − 02	1.253E − 02
2.00000E + 01	1.592E − 02	1.211E − 02

[a] μ/ρ includes the photoelectric, coherent (Rayleigh) and incoherent (Compton) scattering, and the electron-position production cross-sections. The latter includes both production in the field of the nucleus as well as that of the atomic electrons. Photonuclear cross-sections, nuclear-resonance scattering, and Delbrück scattering are not included.

Table 5.1 Mass Attenuation and Energy-Absorption Coefficients (Continued)

	Lung Tissue (ICRU 44)				Muscle, Skeletal (ICRU-44)		
	Photon Energy (MeV)	μ/ρ (cm^2/g)	μ_{en}/ρ (cm^2/g)		Photon Energy (MeV)	μ/ρ (cm^2/g)	μ_{en}/ρ (cm^2/g)
	1.00000E − 03	3.803E + 03	3.791E + 03		1.00000E − 03	3.719E + 03	3.709E + 03
	1.03542E − 03	3.469E + 03	3.459E + 03		1.03542E − 03	3.393E + 03	3.383E + 03
	1.07210E − 03	3.164E + 03	3.155E + 03		1.07210E − 03	3.094E + 03	3.085E + 03
11K	1.07210E − 03	3.176E + 03	3.167E + 03	11K	1.07210E − 03	3.100E + 03	3.091E + 03
	1.50000E − 03	1.283E + 03	1.280E + 03		1.50000E − 03	1.251E + 03	1.247E + 03
	2.00000E − 03	5.746E + 02	5.727E + 02		2.00000E − 03	5.594E + 02	5.574E + 02
	2.14550E − 03	4.707E + 02	4.690E + 02		2.14550E − 03	4.581E + 02	4.564E + 02
15K	2.14550E − 03	4.752E + 02	4.732E + 02	15K	2.14550E − 03	4.626E + 02	4.606E + 02
	2.30297E − 03	3.883E + 02	3.865E + 02		2.30297E − 03	3.776E + 02	3.762E + 02
	2.47200E − 03	3.170E + 02	3.154E + 02		2.47200E − 03	3.085E + 02	3.069E + 02
16K	2.47200E − 03	3.226E + 02	3.206E + 02	16K	2.47200E − 03	3.140E + 02	3.121E + 02
	2.64140E − 03	2.668E + 02	2.650E + 02		2.64140E − 03	2.597E + 02	2.579E + 02
	2.82240E − 03	2.204E + 02	2.189E + 02		2.82240E − 03	2.145E + 02	2.130E + 02
17K	2.82240E − 03	2.248E + 02	2.229E + 02	17K	2.82240E − 03	2.160E + 02	2.143E + 02
	3.00000E − 03	1.888E + 02	1.870E + 02		3.00000E − 03	1.812E + 02	1.796E + 02
	3.60740E − 03	1.103E + 02	1.091E + 02		3.60740E − 03	1.057E + 02	1.046E + 02
19K	3.60740E − 03	1.125E + 02	1.110E + 02	19K	3.60740E − 03	1.100E + 02	1.083E + 02
	4.00000E − 03	8.306E + 01	8.181E + 01		4.00000E − 03	8.127E + 01	7.992E + 01
	5.00000E − 03	4.296E + 01	4.210E + 01		5.00000E − 03	4.206E + 01	4.116E + 01
	6.00000E − 03	2.497E + 01	2.431E + 01		6.00000E − 03	2.446E + 01	2.377E + 01
	8.00000E − 03	1.058E + 01	1.010E + 01		8.00000E − 03	1.037E + 01	9.888E + 00
	1.00000E − 02	5.459E + 00	5.067E + 00		1.00000E − 02	5.356E + 00	4.964E + 00
	1.50000E − 02	1.721E + 00	1.423E + 00		1.50000E − 02	1.693E + 00	1.396E + 00
	2.00000E − 02	8.316E − 01	5.740E − 01		2.00000E − 02	8.205E − 01	5.638E − 01
	3.00000E − 02	3.815E − 01	1.635E − 01		3.00000E − 02	3.783E − 01	1.610E − 01
	4.00000E − 02	2.699E − 01	7.286E − 02		4.00000E − 02	2.685E − 01	7.192E − 02
	5.00000E − 02	2.270E − 01	4.393E − 02		5.00000E − 02	2.262E − 01	4.349E − 02
	6.00000E − 02	2.053E − 01	3.282E − 02		6.00000E − 02	2.048E − 01	3.258E − 02
	8.00000E − 02	1.826E − 01	2.625E − 02		8.00000E − 02	1.823E − 01	2.615E − 02
	1.00000E − 01	1.695E − 01	2.550E − 02		1.00000E − 01	1.693E − 01	2.544E − 02
	1.50000E − 01	1.493E − 01	2.748E − 02		1.50000E − 01	1.492E − 01	2.745E − 02
	2.00000E − 01	1.359E − 01	2.945E − 02		2.00000E − 01	1.358E − 01	2.942E − 02
	3.00000E − 01	1.177E − 01	3.167E − 02		3.00000E − 01	1.176E − 01	3.164E − 02
	4.00000E − 01	1.053E − 01	3.252E − 02		4.00000E − 01	1.052E − 01	3.249E − 02
	5.00000E − 01	9.607E − 02	3.272E − 02		5.00000E − 01	9.598E − 02	3.269E − 02
	6.00000E − 01	8.882E − 02	3.257E − 02		6.00000E − 01	8.874E − 02	3.254E − 02
	8.00000E − 01	7.800E − 02	3.179E − 02		8.00000E − 01	7.793E − 02	3.177E − 02
	1.00000E + 00	7.013E − 02	3.077E − 02		1.00000E + 00	7.007E − 02	3.074E − 02
	1.25000E + 00	6.271E − 02	2.940E − 02		1.25000E + 00	6.265E − 02	2.938E − 02
	1.50000E + 00	5.706E − 02	2.810E − 02		1.50000E + 00	5.701E − 02	2.808E − 02
	2.00000E + 00	4.900E − 02	2.586E − 02		2.00000E + 00	4.896E − 02	2.584E − 02
	3.00000E + 00	3.935E − 02	2.262E − 02		3.00000E + 00	3.931E − 02	2.259E − 02
	4.00000E + 00	3.374E − 02	2.048E − 02		4.00000E + 00	3.369E − 02	2.045E − 02
	5.00000E + 00	3.005E − 02	1.898E − 02		5.00000E + 00	3.000E − 02	1.895E − 02
	6.00000E + 00	2.746E − 02	1.789E − 02		6.00000E + 00	2.741E − 02	1.786E − 02
	8.00000E + 00	2.407E − 02	1.643E − 02		8.00000E + 00	2.401E − 02	1.639E − 02
	1.00000E + 01	2.198E − 02	1.551E − 02		1.00000E + 01	2.192E − 02	1.547E − 02
	1.50000E + 01	1.922E − 02	1.427E − 02		1.50000E + 01	1.915E − 02	1.421E − 02
	2.00000E + 01	1.794E − 02	1.367E − 02		2.00000E + 01	1.786E − 02	1.361E − 02

[a] μ/ρ includes the photoelectric, coherent (Rayleigh) and incoherent (Compton) scattering, and the electron-position production cross-sections. The latter includes both production in the field of the nucleus as well as that of the atomic electrons. Photonuclear cross-sections, nuclear-resonance scattering, and Delbrück scattering are not included.

(continued)

Table 5.1 Mass Attenuation and Energy-Absorption Coefficients (Continued)

Ovary ICRU-44)

	Photon Energy (MeV)	μ/ρ (cm^2/g)	μ_{en}/ρ (cm^2/g)
	1.00000E − 03	3.835E + 03	3.823E + 03
	1.03542E − 03	3.499E + 03	3.489E + 03
	1.07210E − 03	3.191E + 03	3.182E + 03
11K	1.07210E − 03	3.203E + 03	3.194E + 03
	1.50000E − 03	1.295E + 03	1.291E + 03
	2.00000E − 03	5.800E + 02	5.780E + 02
	2.14550E − 03	4.752E + 02	4.734E + 02
15K	2.14550E − 03	4.796E + 02	4.776E + 02
	2.30297E − 03	3.920E + 02	3.902E + 02
	2.47200E − 03	3.200E + 02	3.184E + 02
16K	2.47200E − 03	3.237E + 02	3.218E + 02
	2.64140E − 03	2.677E + 02	2.660E + 02
	2.82240E − 03	2.211E + 02	2.196E + 02
17K	2.82240E − 03	2.240E + 02	2.223E + 02
	3.00000E − 03	1.880E + 02	1.864E + 02
	3.60740E − 03	1.098E + 02	1.086E + 02
19K	3.60740E − 03	1.119E + 02	1.105E + 02
	4.00000E − 03	8.261E + 01	8.142E + 01
	5.00000E − 03	4.269E + 01	4.185E + 01
	6.00000E − 03	2.479E + 01	2.414E + 01
	8.00000E − 03	1.049E + 01	1.002E + 01
	1.00000E − 02	5.410E + 00	5.019E + 00
	1.50000E − 02	1.705E + 00	1.407E + 00
	2.00000E − 02	8.247E − 01	5.669E − 01
	3.00000E − 02	3.796E − 01	1.614E − 01
	4.00000E − 02	2.693E − 01	7.196E − 02
	5.00000E − 02	2.269E − 01	4.349E − 02
	6.00000E − 02	2.054E − 01	3.258E − 02
	8.00000E − 02	1.828E − 01	2.617E − 02
	1.00000E − 01	1.698E − 01	2.548E − 02
	1.50000E − 01	1.496E − 01	2.751E − 02
	2.00000E − 01	1.361E − 01	2.950E − 02
	3.00000E − 01	1.179E − 01	3.172E − 02
	4.00000E − 01	1.055E − 01	3.258E − 02
	5.00000E − 01	9.624E − 02	3.278E − 02
	6.00000E − 01	8.898E − 02	3.263E − 02
	8.00000E − 01	7.814E − 02	3.185E − 02
	1.00000E + 00	7.026E − 02	3.083E − 02
	1.25000E + 00	6.282E − 02	2.946E − 02
	1.50000E + 00	5.717E − 02	2.815E − 02
	2.00000E + 00	4.909E − 02	2.591E − 02
	3.00000E + 00	3.942E − 02	2.266E − 02
	4.00000E + 00	3.380E − 02	2.052E − 02
	5.00000E + 00	3.010E − 02	1.902E − 02
	6.00000E + 00	2.750E − 02	1.792E − 02
	8.00000E + 00	2.411E − 02	1.646E − 02
	1.00000E + 01	2.202E − 02	1.554E − 02
	1.50000E + 01	1.924E − 02	1.429E − 02
	2.00000E + 01	1.797E − 02	1.369E − 02

Polyethylene

Photon Energy (MeV)	μ/ρ (cm^2/g)	μ_{en}/ρ (cm^2/g)
1.00000E − 03	1.894E + 03	1.892E + 03
1.50000E − 03	5.999E + 02	5.988E + 02
2.00000E − 03	2.593E + 02	2.584E + 02
3.00000E − 03	7.743E + 01	7.678E + 01
4.00000E − 03	3.242E + 01	3.189E + 01
5.00000E − 03	1.643E + 01	1.598E + 01
6.00000E − 03	9.432E + 00	9.032E + 00
8.00000E − 03	3.975E + 00	3.635E + 00
1.00000E − 02	2.088E + 00	1.781E + 00
1.50000E − 02	7.452E − 01	4.834E − 01
2.00000E − 02	4.315E − 01	1.936E − 01
3.00000E − 02	2.706E − 01	5.932E − 02
4.00000E − 02	2.275E − 01	3.196E − 02
5.00000E − 02	2.084E − 01	2.442E − 02
6.00000E − 02	1.970E − 01	2.236E − 02
8.00000E − 02	1.823E − 01	2.265E − 02
1.00000E − 01	1.719E − 01	2.423E − 02
1.50000E − 01	1.534E − 01	2.789E − 02
2.00000E − 01	1.402E − 01	3.029E − 02
3.00000E − 01	1.217E − 01	3.276E − 02
4.00000E − 01	1.089E − 01	3.368E − 02
5.00000E − 01	9.947E − 02	3.390E − 02
6.00000E − 01	9.198E − 02	3.375E − 02
8.00000E − 01	8.078E − 02	3.295E − 02
1.00000E + 00	7.262E − 02	3.190E − 02
1.25000E + 00	6.495E − 02	3.049E − 02
1.50000E + 00	5.910E − 02	2.914E − 02
2.00000E + 00	5.064E − 02	2.677E − 02
3.00000E + 00	4.045E − 02	2.328E − 02
4.00000E + 00	3.444E − 02	2.091E − 02
5.00000E + 00	3.045E − 02	1.921E − 02
6.00000E + 00	2.760E − 02	1.794E − 02
8.00000E + 00	2.383E − 02	1.620E − 02
1.00000E + 01	2.145E − 02	1.506E − 02
1.50000E + 01	1.819E − 02	1.344E − 02
2.00000E + 01	1.658E − 02	1.260E − 02

[a] μ/ρ includes the photoelectric, coherent (Rayleigh) and incoherent (Compton) scattering, and the electron-position production cross-sections. The latter includes both production in the field of the nucleus as well as that of the atomic electrons. Photonuclear cross-sections, nuclear-resonance scattering, and Delbrück scattering are not included.

Table 5.1 Mass Attenuation and Energy-Absorption Coefficients (Continued)

Polymethyl Methacrylate, "Lucite"			Polystyrene		
Photon Energy (MeV)	**μ/ρ (cm²/g)**	**μ_{en}/ρ (cm²/g)**	**Photon Energy (MeV)**	**μ/ρ (cm²/g)**	**μ_{en}/ρ (cm²/g)**
1.00000E − 03	2.794E + 03	2.788E + 03	1.00000E − 03	2.040E + 03	2.038E + 03
1.50000E − 03	9.153E + 02	9.131E + 02	1.50000E − 03	6.462E + 02	6.450E + 02
2.00000E − 03	4.037E + 02	4.024E + 02	2.00000E − 03	2.792E + 02	2.783E + 02
3.00000E − 03	1.236E + 02	1.228E + 02	3.00000E − 03	8.338E + 01	8.271E + 01
4.00000E − 03	5.247E + 01	5.181E + 01	4.00000E − 03	3.489E + 01	3.435E + 01
5.00000E − 03	2.681E + 01	2.627E + 01	5.00000E − 03	1.767E + 01	1.721E + 01
6.00000E − 03	1.545E + 01	1.498E + 01	6.00000E − 03	1.013E + 01	9.730E + 00
8.00000E − 03	6.494E + 00	6.114E + 00	8.00000E − 03	4.252E + 00	3.915E + 00
1.00000E − 02	3.357E + 00	3.026E + 00	1.00000E − 02	2.219E + 00	1.918E + 00
1.50000E − 02	1.101E + 00	8.324E − 01	1.50000E − 02	7.738E − 01	5.200E − 01
2.00000E − 02	5.714E − 01	3.328E − 01	2.00000E − 02	4.363E − 01	2.075E − 01
3.00000E − 02	3.032E − 01	9.645E − 02	3.00000E − 02	2.640E − 01	6.246E − 02
4.00000E − 02	2.350E − 01	4.599E − 02	4.00000E − 02	2.183E − 01	3.264E − 02
5.00000E − 02	2.074E − 01	3.067E − 02	5.00000E − 02	1.986E − 01	2.421E − 02
6.00000E − 02	1.924E − 01	2.530E − 02	6.00000E − 02	1.870E − 01	2.172E − 02
8.00000E − 02	1.751E − 01	2.302E − 02	8.00000E − 02	1.725E − 01	2.160E − 02
1.00000E − 01	1.641E − 01	2.368E − 02	1.00000E − 01	1.624E − 01	2.296E − 02
1.50000E − 01	1.456E − 01	2.657E − 02	1.50000E − 01	1.448E − 01	2.632E − 02
2.00000E − 01	1.328E − 01	2.872E − 02	2.00000E − 01	1.322E − 01	2.857E − 02
3.00000E − 01	1.152E − 01	3.099E − 02	3.00000E − 01	1.147E − 01	3.088E − 02
4.00000E − 01	1.031E − 01	3.185E − 02	4.00000E − 01	1.027E − 01	3.175E − 02
5.00000E − 01	9.410E − 02	3.206E − 02	5.00000E − 01	9.379E − 02	3.196E − 02
6.00000E − 01	8.701E − 02	3.191E − 02	6.00000E − 01	8.672E − 02	3.182E − 02
8.00000E − 01	7.641E − 02	3.116E − 02	8.00000E − 01	7.615E − 02	3.106E − 02
1.00000E + 00	6.870E − 02	3.015E − 02	1.00000E + 00	6.847E − 02	3.006E − 02
1.25000E + 00	6.143E − 02	2.882E − 02	1.25000E + 00	6.123E − 02	2.874E − 02
1.50000E + 00	5.591E − 02	2.755E − 02	1.50000E + 00	5.573E − 02	2.747E − 02
2.00000E + 00	4.796E − 02	2.533E − 02	2.00000E + 00	4.777E − 02	2.524E − 02
3.00000E + 00	3.844E − 02	2.210E − 02	3.00000E + 00	3.822E − 02	2.199E − 02
4.00000E + 00	3.286E − 02	1.995E − 02	4.00000E + 00	3.261E − 02	1.979E − 02
5.00000E + 00	2.919E − 02	1.843E − 02	5.00000E + 00	2.889E − 02	1.824E − 02
6.00000E + 00	2.659E − 02	1.731E − 02	6.00000E + 00	2.626E − 02	1.708E − 02
8.00000E + 00	2.317E − 02	1.579E − 02	8.00000E + 00	2.278E − 02	1.550E − 02
1.00000E + 01	2.105E − 02	1.482E − 02	1.00000E + 01	2.060E − 02	1.448E − 02
1.50000E + 01	1.820E − 02	1.348E − 02	1.50000E + 01	1.763E − 02	1.305E − 02
2.00000E + 01	1.684E − 02	1.282E − 02	2.00000E + 01	1.620E − 02	1.232E − 02

[a] μ/ρ includes the photoelectric, coherent (Rayleigh) and incoherent (Compton) scattering, and the electron-position production cross-sections. The latter includes both production in the field of the nucleus as well as that of the atomic electrons. Photonuclear cross-sections, nuclear-resonance scattering, and Delbrück scattering are not included.

(continued)

Table 5.1 Mass Attenuation and Energy-Absorption Coefficients (Continued)

	Testis (ICRU-44)				Tissue, Soft (ICRU 44)		
	Photon Energy (MeV)	μ/ρ (cm^2/g)	μ_{en}/ρ (cm^2/g)		Photon Energy (MeV)	μ/ρ (cm^2/g)	μ_{en}/ρ (cm^2/g)
	1.00000E − 03	3.824E + 03	3.812E + 03		1.00000E − 03	3.712E + 03	3.701E + 03
	1.03542E − 03	3.489E + 03	3.479E + 03		1.03542E − 03	3.386E + 03	3.376E + 03
	1.07210E − 03	3.182E + 03	3.173E + 03		1.07210E − 03	3.087E + 03	3.079E + 03
11K	1.07210E − 03	3.194E + 03	3.184E + 03	11K	1.07210E − 03	3.099E + 03	3.090E + 03
	1.50000E − 03	1.291E + 03	1.288E + 03		1.50000E − 03	1.251E + 03	1.247E + 03
	2.00000E − 03	5.783E + 02	5.763E + 02		2.00000E − 03	5.596E + 02	5.577E + 02
	2.14550E − 03	4.737E + 02	4.719E + 02		2.14550E − 03	4.583E + 02	4.566E + 02
15K	2.14550E − 03	4.759E + 02	4.740E + 02	15K	2.14550E − 03	4.650E + 02	4.629E + 02
	2.30297E − 03	3.889E + 02	3.872E + 02		2.30297E − 03	3.800E + 02	3.782E + 02
	2.47200E − 03	3.174E + 02	3.159E + 02		2.47200E − 03	3.102E + 02	3.086E + 02
16K	2.47200E − 03	3.211E + 02	3.193E + 02	16K	2.47200E − 03	3.158E + 02	3.137E + 02
	2.64140E − 03	2.654E + 02	2.638E + 02		2.64140E − 03	2.612E + 02	2.594E + 02
	2.82240E − 03	2.193E + 02	2.178E + 02		2.82240E − 03	2.158E + 02	2.142E + 02
17K	2.82240E − 03	2.222E + 02	2.205E + 02	17K	2.82240E − 03	2.188E + 02	2.169E + 02
	3.00000E − 03	1.864E + 02	1.849E + 02		3.00000E − 03	1.836E + 02	1.819E + 02
	3.60740E − 03	1.088E + 02	1.077E + 02		3.60740E − 03	1.073E + 02	1.061E + 02
19K	3.60740E − 03	1.109E + 02	1.095E + 02	19K	3.60740E − 03	1.105E + 02	1.089E + 02
	4.00000E − 03	8.188E + 01	8.071E + 01		4.00000E − 03	8.161E + 01	8.030E + 01
	5.00000E − 03	4.229E + 01	4.147E + 01		5.00000E − 03	4.224E + 01	4.135E + 01
	6.00000E − 03	2.456E + 01	2.391E + 01		6.00000E − 03	2.456E + 01	2.389E + 01
	8.00000E − 03	1.039E + 01	9.916E + 00		8.00000E − 03	1.042E + 01	9.935E + 00
	1.00000E − 02	5.357E + 00	4.967E + 00		1.00000E − 02	5.379E + 00	4.987E + 00
	1.50000E − 02	1.689E + 00	1.392E + 00		1.50000E − 02	1.699E + 00	1.402E + 00
	2.00000E − 02	8.182E − 01	5.606E − 01		2.00000E − 02	8.230E − 01	5.663E − 01
	3.00000E − 02	3.778E − 01	1.596E − 01		3.00000E − 02	3.790E − 01	1.616E − 01
	4.00000E − 02	2.687E − 01	7.125E − 02		4.00000E − 02	2.688E − 01	7.216E − 02
	5.00000E − 02	2.266E − 01	4.315E − 02		5.00000E − 02	2.264E − 01	4.360E − 02
	6.00000E − 02	2.053E − 01	3.240E − 02		6.00000E − 02	2.048E − 01	3.264E − 02
	8.00000E − 02	1.828E − 01	2.611E − 02		8.00000E − 02	1.823E − 01	2.617E − 02
	1.00000E − 01	1.699E − 01	2.547E − 02		1.00000E − 01	1.693E − 01	2.545E − 02
	1.50000E − 01	1.497E − 01	2.753E − 02		1.50000E − 01	1.492E − 01	2.745E − 02
	2.00000E − 01	1.363E − 01	2.952E − 02		2.00000E − 01	1.358E − 01	2.942E − 02
	3.00000E − 01	1.180E − 01	3.175E − 02		3.00000E − 01	1.175E − 01	3.164E − 02
	4.00000E − 01	1.055E − 01	3.261E − 02		4.00000E − 01	1.052E − 01	3.249E − 02
	5.00000E − 01	9.633E − 02	3.281E − 02		5.00000E − 01	9.598E − 02	3.269E − 02
	6.00000E − 01	8.906E − 02	3.266E − 02		6.00000E − 01	8.873E − 02	3.254E − 02
	8.00000E − 01	7.822E − 02	3.188E − 02		8.00000E − 01	7.793E − 02	3.176E − 02
	1.00000E + 00	7.032E − 02	3.086E − 02		1.00000E + 00	7.006E − 02	3.074E − 02
	1.25000E + 00	6.288E − 02	2.949E − 02		1.25000E + 00	6.265E − 02	2.938E − 02
	1.50000E + 00	5.722E − 02	2.818E − 02		1.50000E + 00	5.701E − 02	2.807E − 02
	2.00000E + 00	4.914E − 02	2.593E − 02		2.00000E + 00	4.895E − 02	2.583E − 02
	3.00000E + 00	3.945E − 02	2.268E − 02		3.00000E + 00	3.931E − 02	2.259E − 02
	4.00000E + 00	3.382E − 02	2.053E − 02		4.00000E + 00	3.369E − 02	2.045E − 02
	5.00000E + 00	3.012E − 02	1.903E − 02		5.00000E + 00	3.000E − 02	1.895E − 02
	6.00000E + 00	2.752E − 02	1.793E − 02		6.00000E + 00	2.741E − 02	1.786E − 02
	8.00000E + 00	2.411E − 02	1.646E − 02		8.00000E + 00	2.401E − 02	1.639E − 02
	1.00000E + 01	2.202E − 02	1.554E − 02		1.00000E + 01	2.193E − 02	1.547E − 02
	1.50000E + 01	1.924E − 02	1.428E − 02		1.50000E + 01	1.915E − 02	1.422E − 02
	2.00000E + 01	1.796E − 02	1.368E − 02		2.00000E + 01	1.787E − 02	1.362E − 02

[a] μ/ρ includes the photoelectric, coherent (Rayleigh) and incoherent (Compton) scattering, and the electron-position production cross-sections. The latter includes both production in the field of the nucleus as well as that of the atomic electrons. Photonuclear cross-sections, nuclear-resonance scattering, and Delbrück scattering are not included.

Table 5.1 Mass Attenuation and Energy-Absorption Coefficients (Continued)

Tissue, Soft (ICRU Four-Component)			Water, Liquid		
Photon Energy (MeV)	μ/ρ (cm^2/g)	μ_{en}/ρ (cm^2/g)	Photon Energy (MeV)	μ/ρ (cm^2/g)	μ_{en}/ρ (cm^2/g)
1.00000E − 03	3.829E + 03	3.818E + 03	1.00000E − 03	4.078E + 03	4.065E + 03
1.50000E − 03	1.286E + 03	1.283E + 03	1.50000E − 03	1.376E + 03	1.372E + 03
2.00000E − 03	5.755E + 02	5.736E + 02	2.00000E − 03	6.173E + 02	6.152E + 02
3.00000E − 03	1.792E + 02	1.781E + 02	3.00000E − 03	1.929E + 02	1.917E + 02
4.00000E − 03	7.681E + 01	7.598E + 01	4.00000E − 03	8.278E + 01	8.191E + 01
5.00000E − 03	3.947E + 01	3.880E + 01	5.00000E − 03	4.258E + 01	4.188E + 01
6.00000E − 03	2.283E + 01	2.226E + 01	6.00000E − 03	2.464E + 01	2.405E + 01
8.00000E − 03	9.604E + 00	9.163E + 00	8.00000E − 03	1.037E + 01	9.915E + 00
1.00000E − 02	4.937E + 00	4.564E + 00	1.00000E − 02	5.329E + 00	4.944E + 00
1.50000E − 02	1.558E + 00	1.266E + 00	1.50000E − 02	1.673E + 00	1.374E + 00
2.00000E − 02	7.616E − 01	5.070E − 01	2.00000E − 02	8.096E − 01	5.503E − 01
3.00000E − 02	3.604E − 01	1.438E − 01	3.00000E − 02	3.756E − 01	1.557E − 01
4.00000E − 02	2.609E − 01	6.474E − 02	4.00000E − 02	2.683E − 01	6.947E − 02
5.00000E − 02	2.223E − 01	3.987E − 02	5.00000E − 02	2.269E − 01	4.223E − 02
6.00000E − 02	2.025E − 01	3.051E − 02	6.00000E − 02	2.059E − 01	3.190E − 02
8.00000E − 02	1.813E − 01	2.530E − 02	8.00000E − 02	1.837E − 01	2.597E − 02
1.00000E − 01	1.688E − 01	2.501E − 02	1.00000E − 01	1.707E − 01	2.546E − 02
1.50000E − 01	1.490E − 01	2.732E − 02	1.50000E − 01	1.505E − 01	2.764E − 02
2.00000E − 01	1.356E − 01	2.936E − 02	2.00000E − 01	1.370E − 01	2.967E − 02
3.00000E − 01	1.175E − 01	3.161E − 02	3.00000E − 01	1.186E − 01	3.192E − 02
4.00000E − 01	1.051E − 01	3.247E − 02	4.00000E − 01	1.061E − 01	3.279E − 02
5.00000E − 01	9.593E − 02	3.267E − 02	5.00000E − 01	9.687E − 02	3.299E − 02
6.00000E − 01	8.870E − 02	3.252E − 02	6.00000E − 01	8.956E − 02	3.284E − 02
8.00000E − 01	7.789E − 02	3.175E − 02	8.00000E − 01	7.865E − 02	3.206E − 02
1.00000E + 00	7.003E − 02	3.073E − 02	1.00000E + 00	7.072E − 02	3.103E − 02
1.25000E + 00	6.262E − 02	2.937E − 02	1.25000E + 00	6.323E − 02	2.965E − 02
1.50000E + 00	5.699E − 02	2.806E − 02	1.50000E + 00	5.754E − 02	2.833E − 02
2.00000E + 00	4.893E − 02	2.582E − 02	2.00000E + 00	4.942E − 02	2.608E − 02
3.00000E + 00	3.929E − 02	2.258E − 02	3.00000E + 00	3.969E − 02	2.281E − 02
4.00000E + 00	3.367E − 02	2.044E − 02	4.00000E + 00	3.403E − 02	2.066E − 02
5.00000E + 00	2.998E − 02	1.894E − 02	5.00000E + 00	3.031E − 02	1.915E − 02
6.00000E + 00	2.739E − 02	1.785E − 02	6.00000E + 00	2.770E − 02	1.806E − 02
8.00000E + 00	2.400E − 02	1.638E − 02	8.00000E + 00	2.429E − 02	1.658E − 02
1.00000E + 01	2.191E − 02	1.546E − 02	1.00000E + 01	2.219E − 02	1.566E − 02
1.50000E + 01	1.913E − 02	1.420E − 02	1.50000E + 01	1.941E − 02	1.441E − 02
2.00000E + 01	1.785E − 02	1.360E − 02	2.00000E + 01	1.813E − 02	1.382E − 02

[a] μ/ρ includes the photoelectric, coherent (Rayleigh) and incoherent (Compton) scattering, and the electron-position production cross-sections. The latter includes both production in the field of the nucleus as well as that of the atomic electrons. Photonuclear cross-sections, nuclear-resonance scattering, and Delbrück scattering are not included.

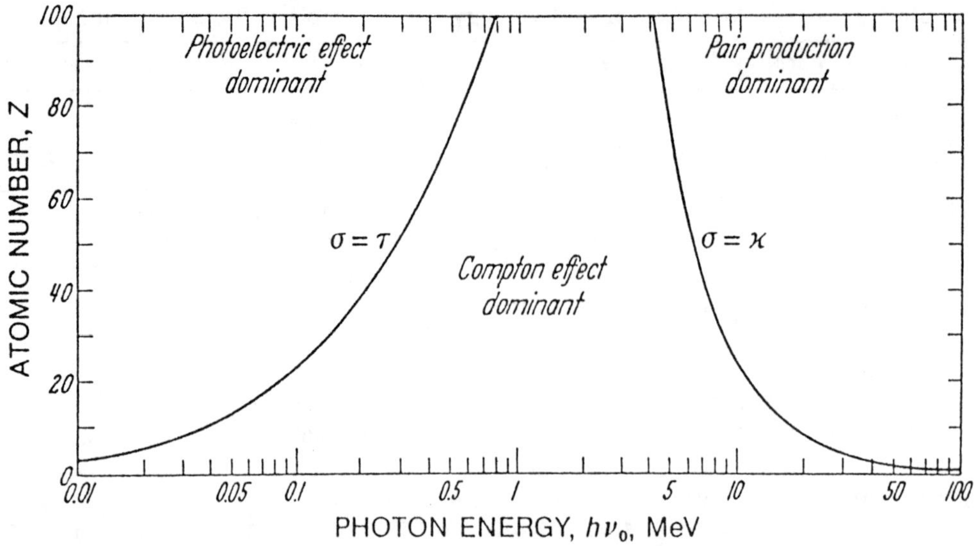

Figure 5.1 Photon Energy, $h\nu_\alpha$ (MeV). Locus of equal atomic cross section for Compton and photoelectric interactions ($\sigma = \tau$), and for Compton and pair-production interactions ($\sigma = \kappa$). The incident photon energy is $h\nu_0$, and Z is the atomic number of the atoms in the absorber. Compton collisions have larger cross sections than any other mode of interaction in the entire domain of medium-energy photons marked ''Compton effect dominant''. (Courtesy NCRP from Report 108, 1991)

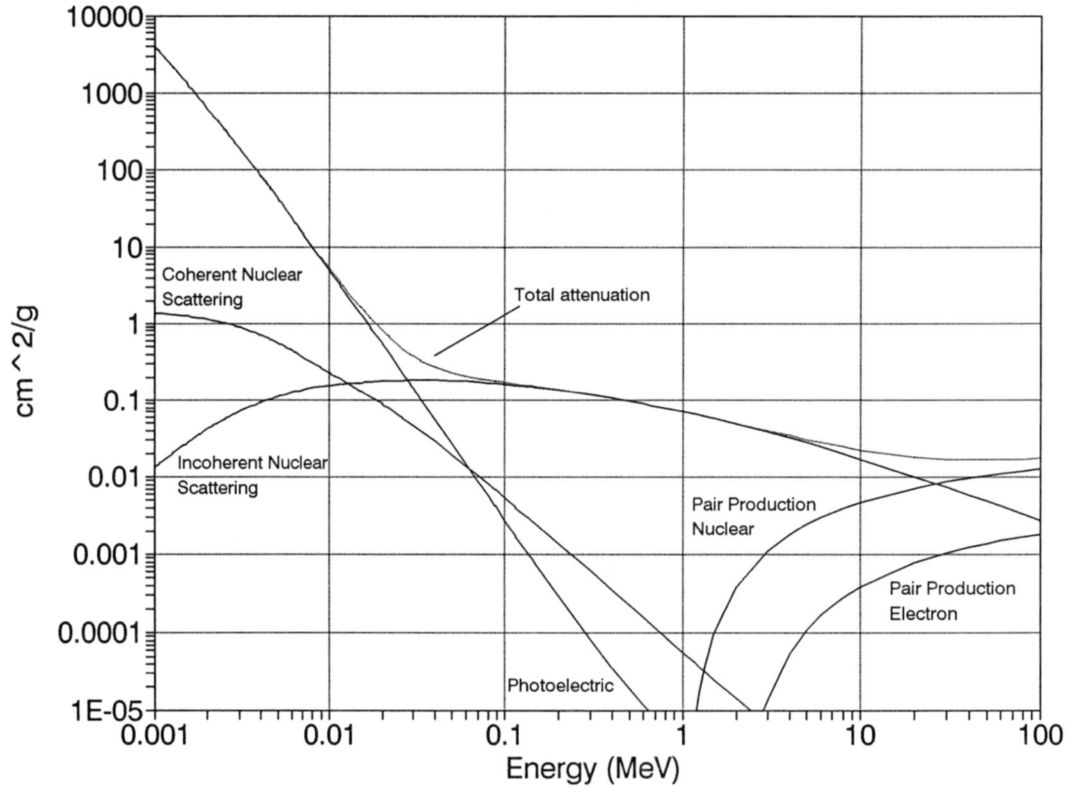

Figure 5.2 Mass Attenuation Coefficients for Photons in Water (Based on data from Berger and Hubbell, 1987)

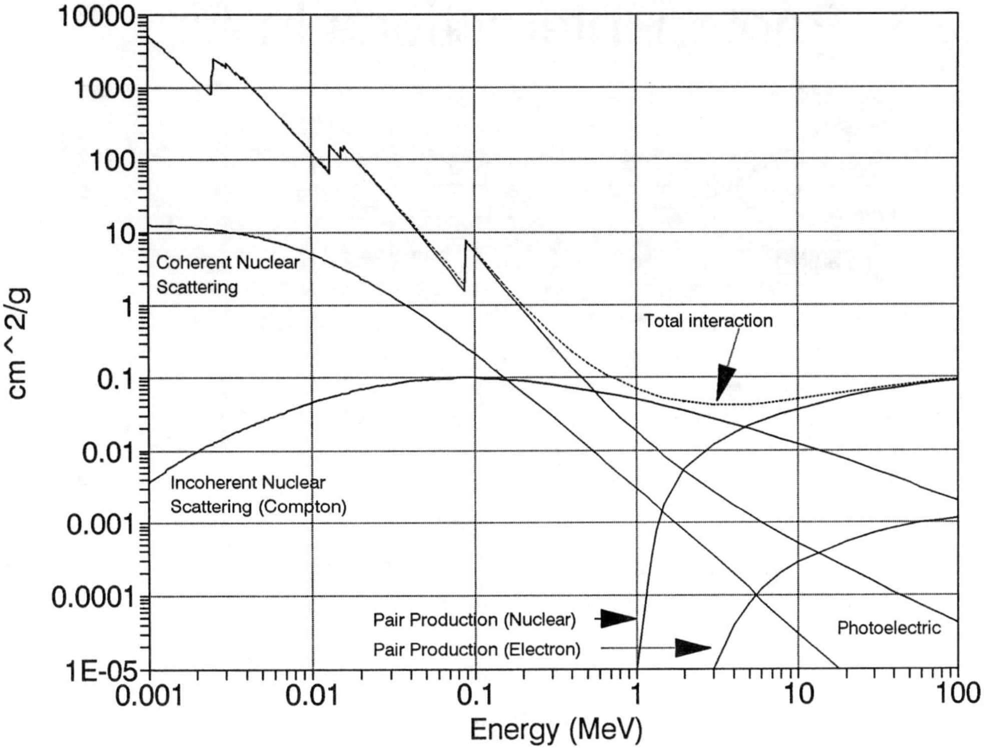

Figure 5.3 Mass Attenuation Coefficients for Photons in Lead (Based on data from Berger and Hubbell, 1987)

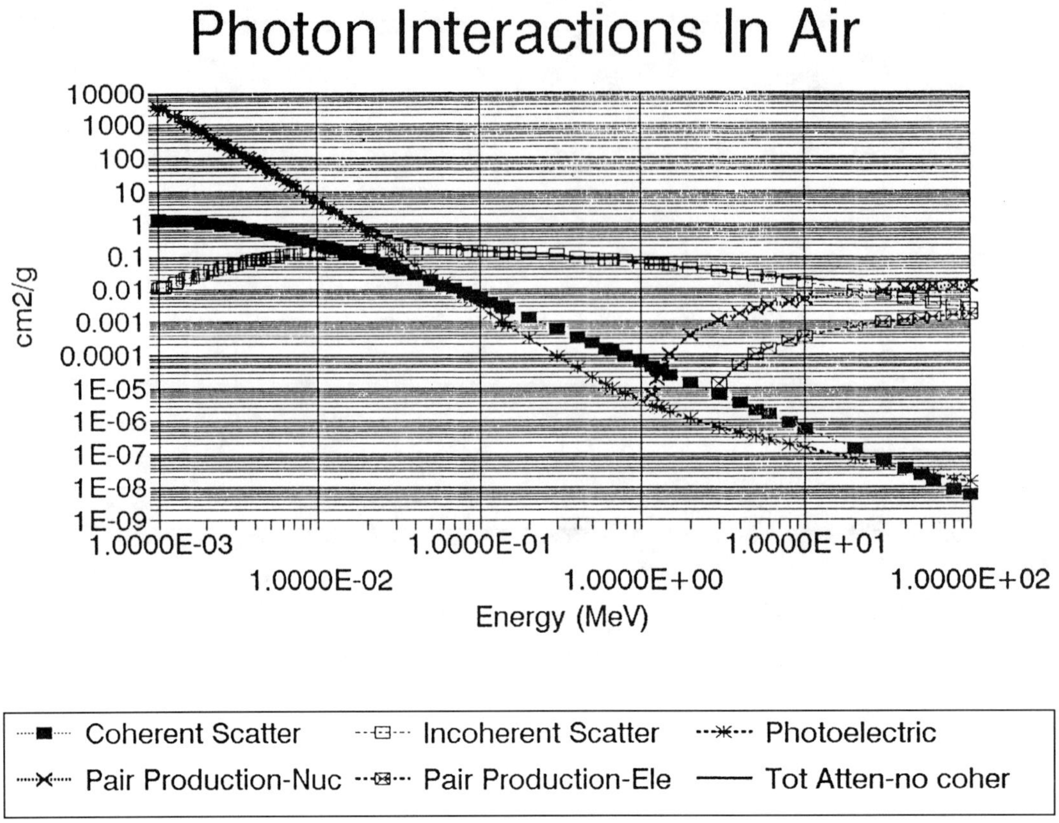

Figure 5.4 Mass Attenuation Coefficients for Photons in Air (Based on data from Burger and Hubbell, 1987)

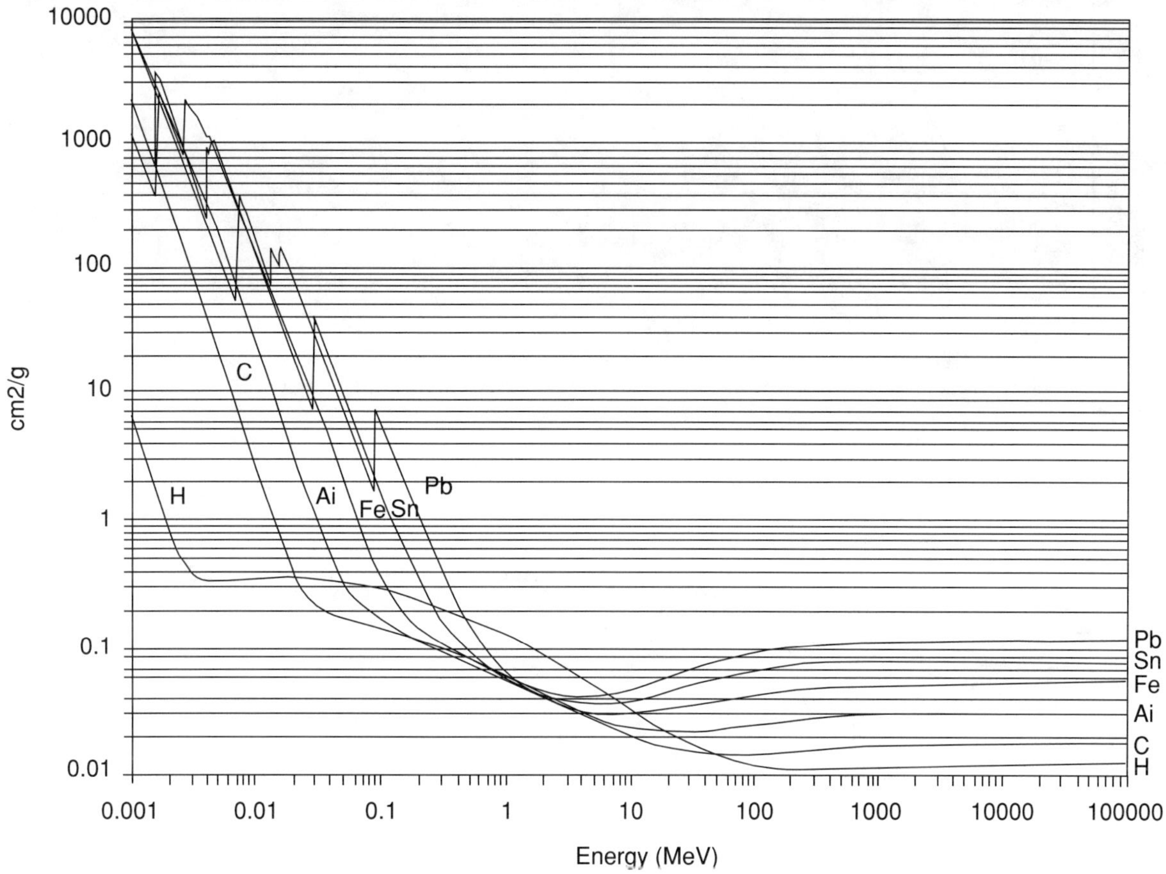

Figure 5.5 Mass Attenuation Coefficient (Without Coherent Scattering) for Selected Elements (Slaback personal communication, 1991, after Berger and Hubbell, 1987)

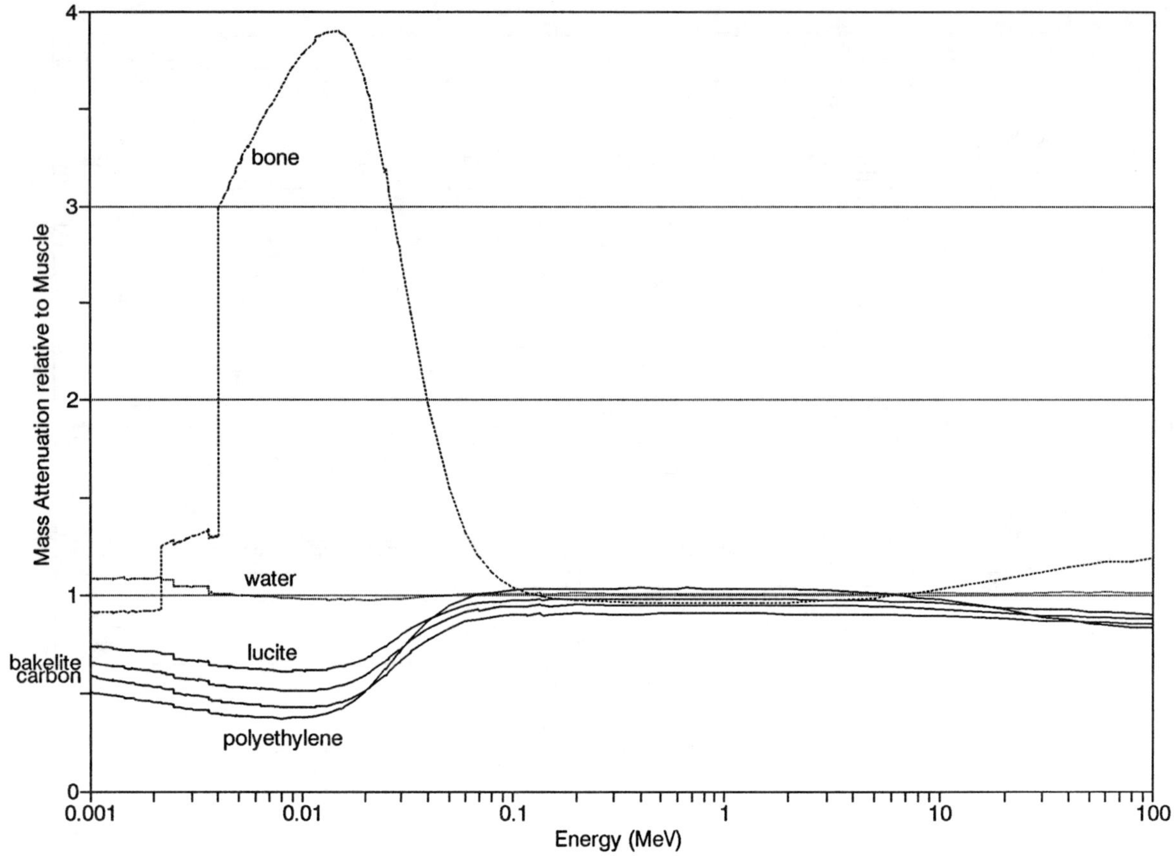

Figure 5.6 Photon Mass Attenuation Coefficient (Without Coherent Scattering) Relative to Muscle

(Slaback personal communication based on data from Berger and Hubbell, 1987)

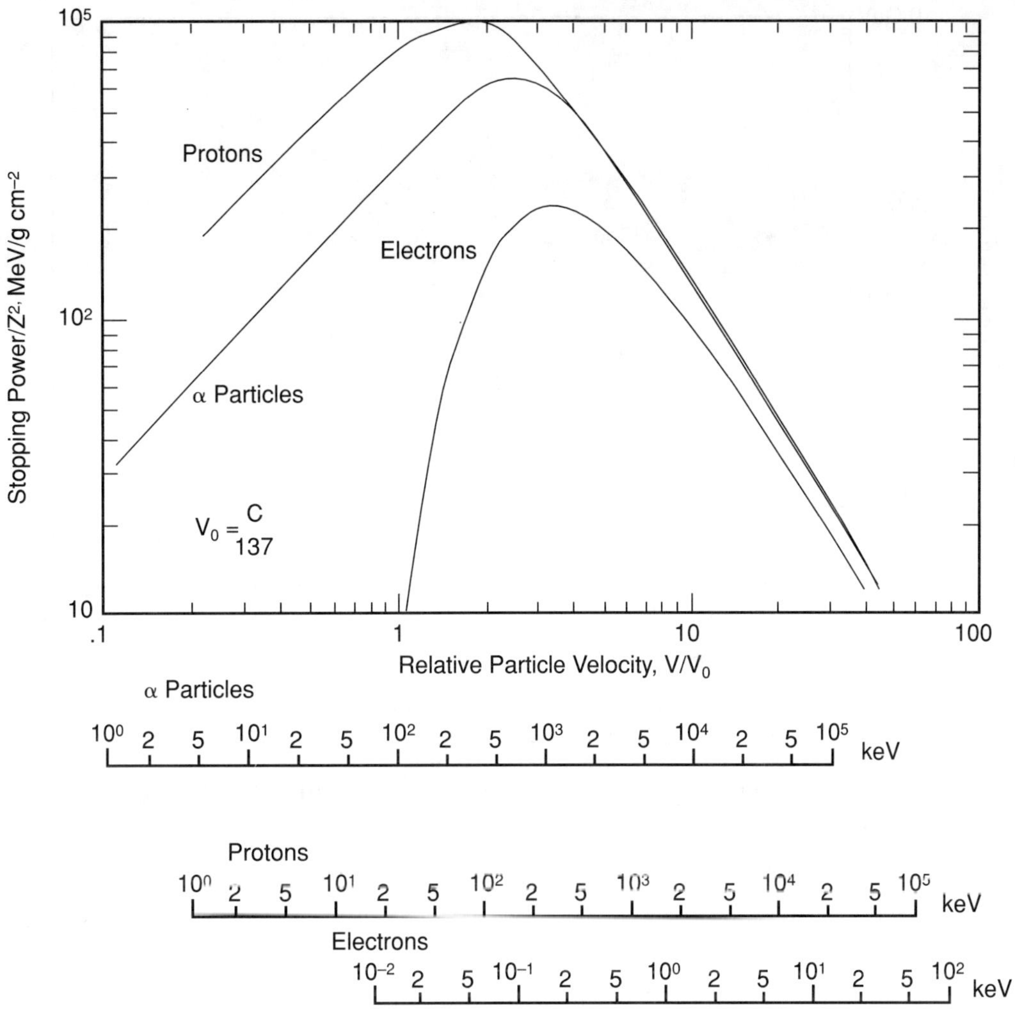

Figure 5.7 Mass Collision Stopping Power of Electrons, Protons and Alpha Particles. Divided by z^2 for electrons, protons, and alpha particles in water vapor as functions of particle velocity expressed as the ratio of the particle velocity, v, to the Bohr velocity, $v_o = c/137$. Particle-energy scales are shown below the figure. (Courtesy NCRP from Report 108, 1991) (After Berger, 1978)

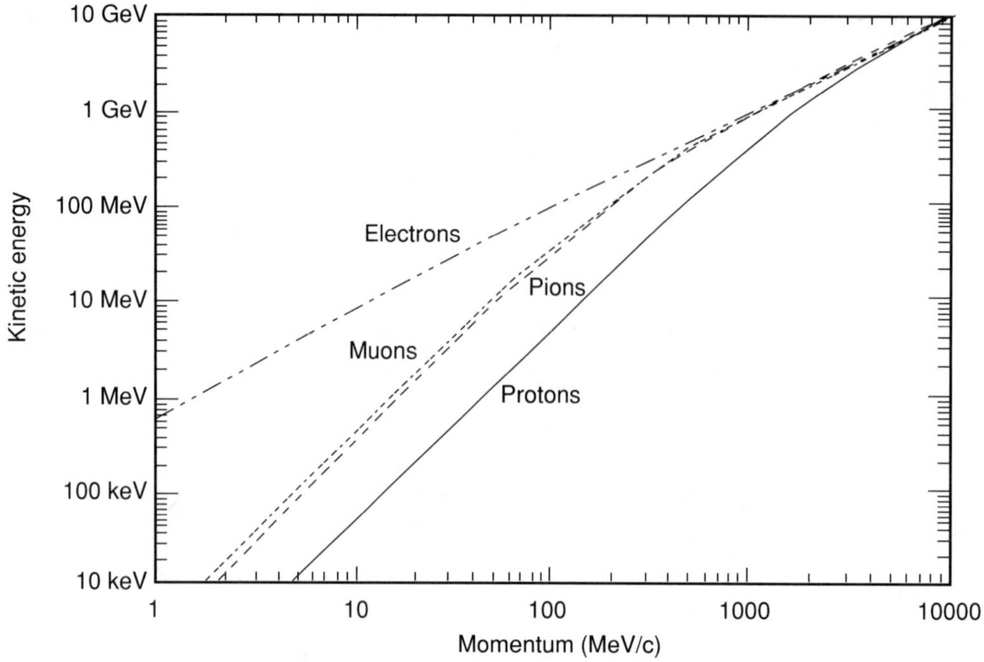

Relation between energy and momentum for
different types of high-energy particles.

Figure 5.8 Relation Between Energy and Momentum for Different Types of High-Energy Particles

(Private communication Sullivan, Cern., 1992)

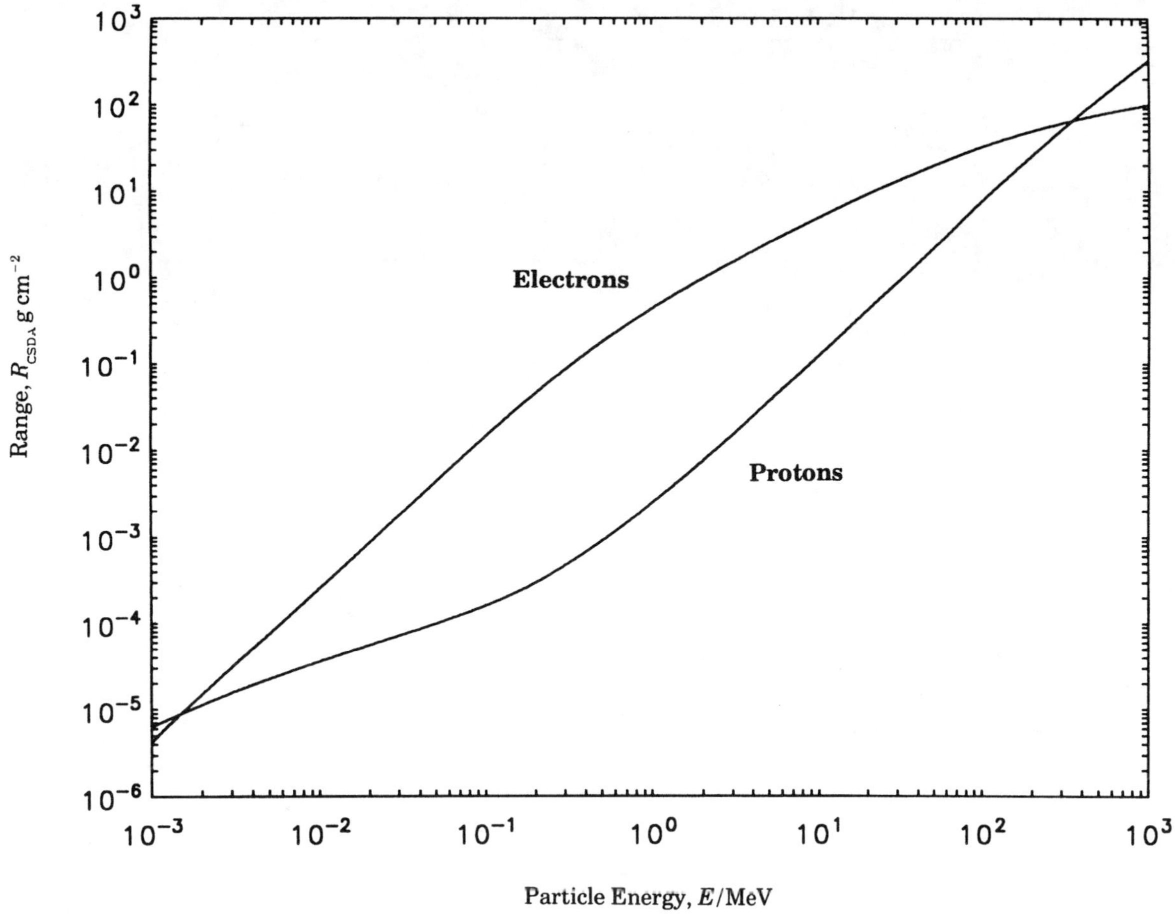

Figure 5.8.1 Plots of Range (R_{csda}) Versus Energy for Electrons and Protons Absorbed in Water
(From ICRU Report 46 based on data from Seltzer, 1989.)

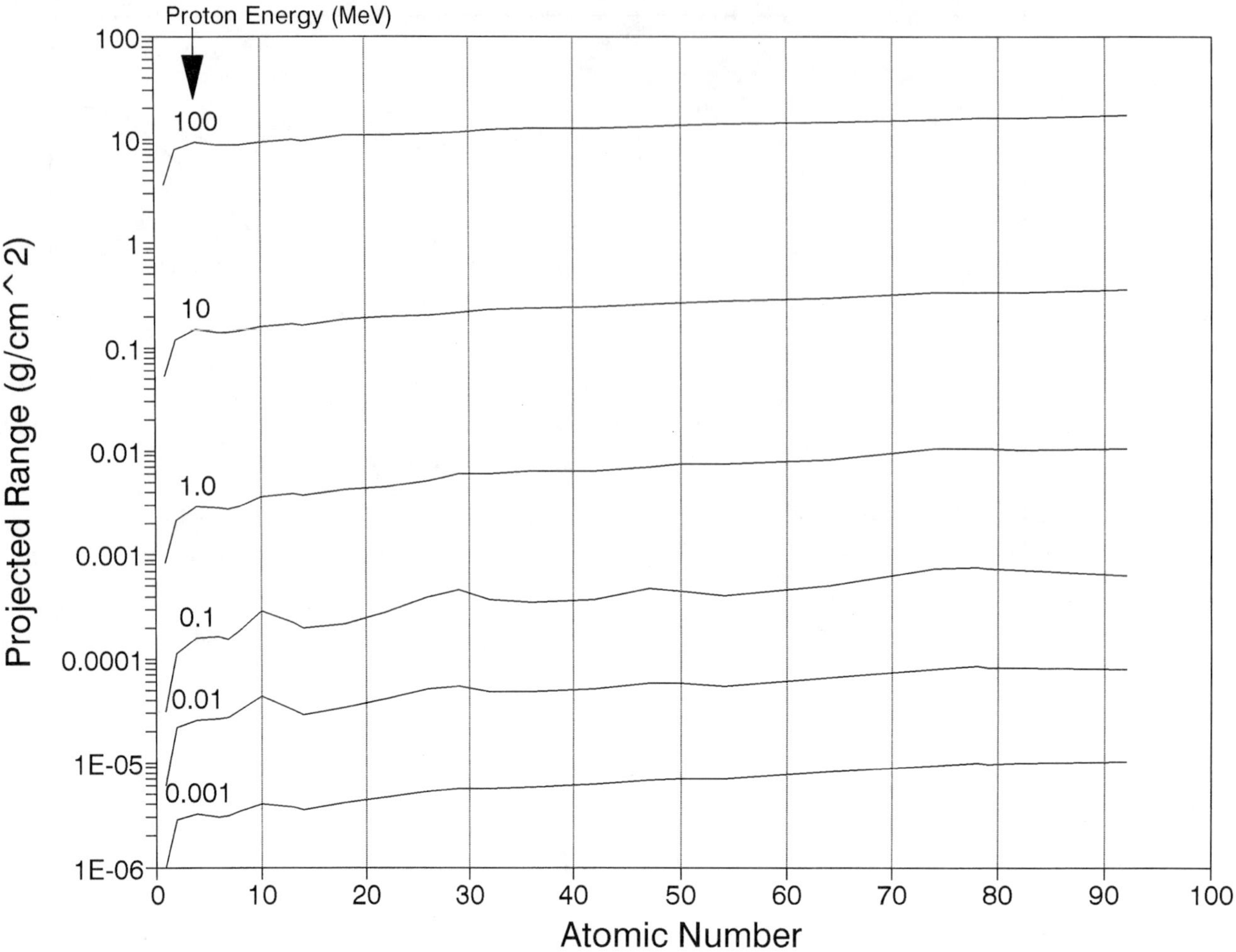

Figure 5.8.2 Proton Range for Selected Energies (Berger, 1992)

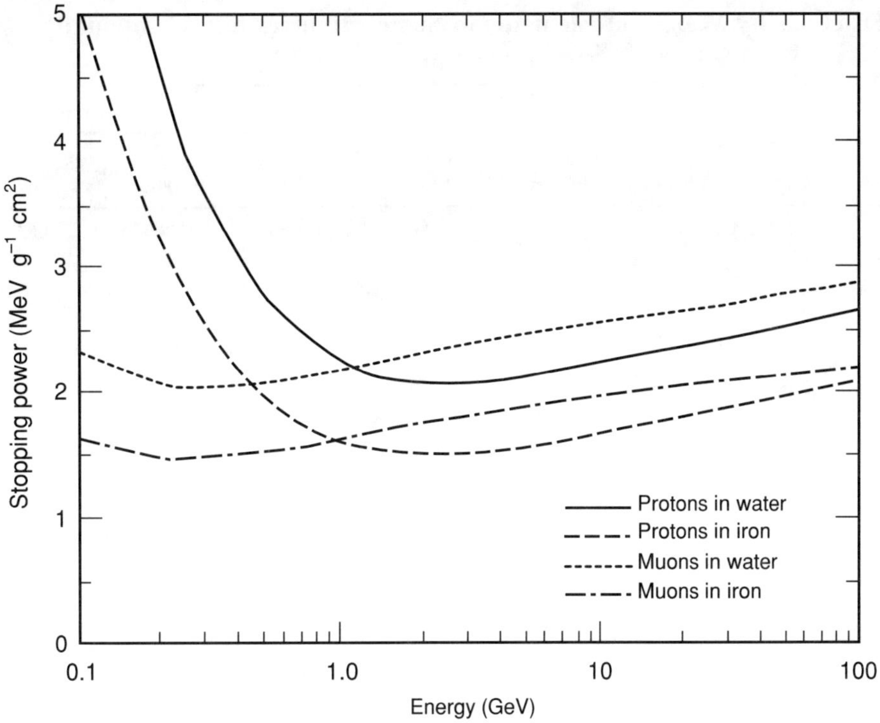

The stopping power of protons and muons in water and iron as a function of particle energy.

Figure 5.9 The Stopping Power of Protons and Muons in Water (Solid Curves) and Iron (Dashed Curves) as a Function of Particle Energy (Private communication Sullivan, Cern., 1992)

Table 5.2 Fractions by Weight of Elements in Some Mixtures and Compounds (Hubbel and Seltzer, 1995)

						Concrete[b]			
Element Z	**Symbol**	**Water**	**Silicon Dioxide[a]**	**Sodium Iodide[a]**	**Air (dry) Sea Level**	**Ordinary**	**Barytes**	**Magnetite**	**Ferro-phosphorus**
1	H	0.1119				0.0056	0.0069	0.0062	0.0050
3	Li								
5	B								
6	C				0.000124				0.0005
7	N				0.755268				
8	O	0.8881	0.5326		0.231781	0.4981	0.3381	0.3345	0.0846
9	F								
11	Na			0.1534		0.0171			
12	Mg					0.0026	0.0011	0.0066	0.0010
13	Al					0.0457	0.0039	0.0273	0.0040
14	Si		0.4674			0.3151	0.0100	0.0347	0.0280
15	P							0.0002	0.2066
16	S					0.0013	0.1039	0.0010	
17	Cl								
18	Ar				0.012827				
19	K					0.0192			
20	Ca					0.0829	0.0477	0.0677	0.0421
22	Ti							0.0270	
23	V							0.0017	
24	Cr							0.0008	0.0005
25	Mn							0.0007	0.0250
26	Fe					0.0124	0.0457	0.4916	0.6028
28	Ni								
53	I			0.8466					
56	Ba						0.4426		

[a] (From Hubbel, NBS 29 1969)

[b] (From Foderaro, 1978)

Table 5.2 Fractions by Weight of Elements in Some Mixtures and Compounds (Continued)

Element Z	Symbol	Bone (ICRU-44) Cortical	Muscle (ICRU-44) Skeletal	Polystyrene	Lucite[a]	Polyethylene	Bakelite	Pyrex Glass	A-150 TEP	Adipose Tissue (ICRU-44)
1	H	0.034	0.102	0.077421	0.0805	0.143716	0.057444		0.1013	0.114
3	Li									
5	B							0.0401		
6	C	0.155	0.143	0.922579	0.5999	0.856284	0.774589		0.7755	0.598
7	N	0.042	0.034						0.0351	0.007
8	O	0.435	0.71		0.3196		0.167968	0.5396	0.0523	0.278
9	F								0.0174	
11	Na	0.001	0.001					0.0282		0.001
12	Mg	0.002								
13	Al							0.0116		
14	Si							0.3772		
15	P	0.103	0.002							
16	S	0.003	0.003							0.001
17	Cl		0.001							0.001
18	Ar									
19	K		0.004					0.0033		
20	Ca	0.225							0.0184	
22	Ti									
23	V									
24	Cr									
25	Mn									
26	Fe									
28	Ni									
53	I									
56	Ba									

[a] (From Hubbel, NBS 29 1969)
[b] (From Foderaro, 1978)

(continued)

Table 5.2 Fractions by Weight of Elements in Some Mixtures and Compounds (Continued)

Element Z	Symbol	Breast Tissue (ICRU-44)	Calcium Fluoride	Calcium Sulfate	Eye Lens (ICRU-44)	Lithium Fluoride	Lung Tissue (ICRU-44)	Ovary (ICRU-44)	Testis (ICRU-44)	Soft Tissue (ICRU-44)
1	H	0.106			0.096		0.103	0.105	0.106	0.102
3	Li					0.267585				
5	B									
6	C	0.332			0.195		0.105	0.093	0.099	0.143
7	N	0.03			0.057		0.031	0.024	0.02	0.034
8	O	0.527		0.470081	0.646		0.749	0.768	0.766	0.708
9	F		0.486672			0.732415				
11	Na	0.001			0.001		0.002	0.002	0.002	0.002
12	Mg									
13	Al									
14	Si									
15	P	0.001			0.001		0.002	0.002	0.001	0.003
16	S	0.002		0.235534	0.003		0.003	0.002	0.002	0.003
17	Cl	0.001			0.001		0.003	0.002	0.002	0.002
18	Ar									
19	K						0.002	0.002	0.002	0.003
20	Ca		0.513328	0.294385						
22	Ti									
23	V									
24	Cr									
25	Mn									
26	Fe									
28	Ni									
53	I									
56	Ba									

[a] (From Hubbel, NBS 29 1969)
[b] (From Foderaro, 1978)

Table 5.3 Classification of Photon Interactions (After Hubbell NSRDS-NBS 29, 1969)

		Scattering	
Type of interaction ⇒⇒ **Interaction with ⇓⇓⇓**	**Absorption**	**Elastic (Coherent)**	**Inelastic (Incoherent)**
I Atomic Electrons	**Photoelectric Effect** $\tau_{pe}\begin{cases}\sim Z^4 \text{ (low energy)}\\ \sim Z^5 \text{ (high energy)}\end{cases}$	*Rayleigh Scattering* $\sigma_R \sim Z^2$ (low energy limit)	**Compton Scattering** $\sigma \sim Z$
II Nucleons	*Photonuclear Reactions* (γ,n), (γ,p), (γ,f), etc. $\sigma_{pn} \sim Z$ $(h\nu \gtrsim 10$ MeV)	Elastic Nuclear Scattering	Nuclear Resonance Scattering
III Electric field of surrounding charged particles	**Pair Production** a. **Field of Nucleus** $\kappa_n \sim Z^2$ ($h\nu \geq 1.02$ MeV) b. *Field of Electron* $\kappa_e \sim Z$ ($h\nu \geq 2.04$ MeV)	Delbrück Scattering	
IV Mesons	Photomeson Production $h\nu \gtrsim 140$ MeV		

[a] Bolded entries indicate major effects contributing to photon attenuation in matter. Italicized items indicate additional effects which contribute more than 1 percent over particular energy ranges.

Table 5.4 Density of Common Materials (After Handbook of Chemistry and Physics, 1991; Trout et al. 1961; IAEA Tech, Rept. Series 188, 1979; Hubbel, NBS 29, 1969; Foderaro, 1978; and Hubbel and Seltzer, 1995)

Material	Density Range (g cm^{-3})	Normal Density (g cm^{-3})
A-150 Tissue Equiv. Plastic	—	1.127
Adipose tissue (ICRU-44)	—	0.95
Air	—	0.0012929
Air (dry, sea level)	—	0.001205
Aluminum	—	2.7
Asbestos	2.0–2.8	—
Asphalt	1.1–1.5	—
Blood, whole (ICRU-44)	—	1.06
Bone, cortical (ICRU-44)	—	1.92
Bakelite (typical)	1.2–1.7	—
Breast tissue (ICRU-44)	—	1.02
Brick (soft)	1.4–1.9	1.65
Brick (hard)	1.8–2.3	2.05
Calcium fluoride	—	3.18
Calcium sulfate	—	2.96
Cement	2.7–3.0	—
Cesium iodide	—	4.51
Clay	1.8–2.6	—
Concretes:		
Ordinary (silicacious)	2.2–2.4	2.35
Barite (barytes)	3.0–3.8	—
Ferrophosphorus	—	4.68
Ilmenite	2.9–3.9	—
Iron (shot, punchings, etc.)	4.0–6.0	—
Limonite (Goethite)	2.6–3.7	—
Magnetite	2.9–4.0	—
Copper		8.96
Earth	1.5–1.9	1.7
Ebonite	—	1.15
Eye lens (ICRU-44)	—	1.07
Gelatin	—	1.27
Glass (common)	2.4–2.8	—
Glass (flint)	2.9–5.9	—
Granite	2.60–2.76	2.65
Graphite	2.30–2.72	—
Gypsum	2.31–2.33	—
Lead	—	11.35
Limestone	1.87–2.76	2.46

Table 5.4 Density of Common Materials (Continued)

Material	Density Range ($g\ cm^{-3}$)	Normal Density ($g\ cm^{-3}$)
Linoleum	—	1.18
Lithium fluoride	—	2.635
Lucite	—	1.19
Lung tissue (ICRU-44)	—	1.05
Marble	2.47–2.86	2.7
Muscle, skeletal (ICRU-44)	—	1.05
Ovary (ICRU-44)	—	1.05
Paraffin	0.87–0.91	—
Plaster, sand	—	1.54
Polyethylene	—	0.92
Polystyrene	1.05–1.07	—
Pressed wood: Pulp board	—	0.19
Pyrex glass	—	2.23
Sandstone	—	1.90
Slate	2.6–3.3	—
Steel	—	7.8
Testis (ICRU-44)	—	1.04
Tile	1.6–2.5	—
Tissue, soft (ICRU-44)	—	1.06
Water	—	1
Water (heavy)	—	1.105
Wood:		
Oak	0.60–0.90	—
White Pine	0.35–0.50	—
Yellow Pine	0.37–0.60	—

Table 5.5 Radiation Parameters of Selected Composite Materials (Courtesy IAEA from Technical Report Series 188, 1979)

Material		Density[a]	Radiation[b] Length		Minimum Collision[c] Stopping Power		Critical[d] Energy	Attenuation Coeff[e] at Compton Minimum		Geometrical[f] Cross Section	Nuclear[f] Collision Length	
		($g\ cm^{-3}$)	($g\ cm^{-2}$)	(cm)	($MeV\ cm^2\ g^{-1}$)	(MeV)	(MeV)	Coeff ($cm^3\ g^{-2}$)	Energy (MeV)	(barns)	($g\ cm^{-2}$)	(cm)
Deuterium ($^2H_2$)		0.165 L	126.1	764	1.874	1.95	403	0.00555	300	0.074	45.1	273
Water (H_2O)		1.000 L	36.08	36.1	1.852	1.55	92	0.0166	55	0.51	59.2	59
Air[h]		(1.205 G)	36.61	30380	1.653	1.20	102	0.0160	45	—	61.2	50800
CO_2		(1.79 G)	36.20	20220	1.658	1.25	100	0.0161	43	1.19	61.3	34200
Polyethylene $(CH_2)_n$		0.92–0.95	44.78	47.9	1.906	1.65	119	0.0140	70	—	56.1	60
Plexiglass (Lucite) $(C_5H_8O_2)_n$		1.16–1.20	40.55	34.4	1.774	1.55	100	0.0151	55	—	58.3	49
Polystyrene $(C_8H_8O_2)_n$		1.03–1.07	41.10	39.1	1.783	1.60	109	0.0142	60	—	58.5	56
Mylar $(C_5H_4O_2)_n$		1.39	39.95	28.7	1.73	1.6	110	0.0151	60	—	59.1	43
Nylon $(C_6N_{11}NO)_n$		1.09–1.14	41.92	37.6	1.83	1.6	115	0.0146	60	—	57.6	52
Bakelite $(C_7H_5O)_n$		1.3–1.4	41.77	30.9	1.74	1.6	110	0.0147	55	—	58.5	43
Cellulose $(C_6H_{10}O_5)_n$	(amorph	1.3–1.6)	38.75	26.7	1.77	1.6	110	0.0155	55	—	59.2	41
	(wood	0.5–0.9)		55.4								85
Film emulsion[h]		3.815	11.33	2.97	1.296	1.20	22.3	—	—	—	83.5	22
Muscle[h]		1.00	36.66	36.7	1.829	1.55	112	0.0164	50	—	59.2	59
Bone[h]		1.7–2.0	30.49	16.5	1.709	1.50	81.9	0.0189	37	—	61.6	33
SiO_2		2.32	27.05	11.7	1.583	1.25	66	0.0202	27	1.53	65.3	28
$CaCO_3$	(marble	2.5–2.9)	24.03	8.9	—	—	—	0.0219	25	2.51	66.2	25
$BaSO_4$	(barite	4.5)	11.64	2.59	—	—	—	0.0322	7.3	4.72	82.1	18
Concrete[h]		2.35	25.71	10.9	1.58	1.25	—	0.0209	25	—	65.8	28
Pyrex glass[h]		2.23	28.17	12.6	1.58	1.25	—	0.0195	30	—	64.7	29
LiF		2.64	39.25	14.9	1.473	1.55	81	0.0149	43	0.70	61.1	23
NaI		3.67	9.49	2.59	1.179	1.15	17.4	0.0348	5.3	2.71	91.9	25

[a] The densities of most solids listed may be quite variable. Where critical, the density of the material used should be measured. L: The density is given for the liquid state (at boiling point for deuterium, and 20°C for water). G: Gas at STP (in units of g liter^{-1}).
[b] Radiation lengths (in g cm^{-2}). The *median* density indicated is used to obtain the equivalent in cm.
[c] Minimum collision stopping power for *electrons* (values for heavy particles are generally 10–15% greater), and kinetic energy at which it occurs. The values of stopping power with four significant figures are from Berger and Seltzer (1964, 1966).
[d] Critical energy from Berger and Seltzer (1964). Critical energy, defined as kinetic energy at which mean values of electron collision and radiative energy losses are equal. Data are interpolated from Table II of Berger and Seltzer (1964). The critical energy (in MeV) may also be approximated by the convenient formula $E_c = 800/(Z + 1.2)$.
[e] Values of attenuation coefficient are interpolated from Storm and Israel (1970) or Hubbell (1969). The Compton minimum is defined as the photon energy at which the attenuation coefficient is minimum. Values given for the minimum attenuation coefficient are based on Storm and Israel (1970) for $Z > 3$. For $Z \leq 3$, the compilation by Hubbell (1969) is used. As the minima are generally broad, the energies shown should be considered uncertain by about ±10% for $1 \leq Z \leq 10$, by ±5% for $10 < Z \leq 20$, and ±2% for higher Z.
[f] Nuclear total cross-sections, based on the parameterization of Carlson et al. (1973) with nuclear radius (in centimeters) $R = 1.23 \times 10^{-13} A^{1/3}$ and nuclear absorption length $X_{on} = 3.05 \times 10^{13}$ cm, corresponding to 21 GeV/c. The corresponding collision lengths are obtained from $L_{coll} = A/(N_A\alpha)$. The nuclear *absorption* lengths (not shown) correspond to inelastic processes only and are larger, for example, by factors of about 1.5, 1.7 and 1.9 for Al, Fe and Pb, respectively. The data given here are reasonably representative of real n-nucleus (and p-nucleus) cross-sections (to within ±10%) as low as 150 MeV kinetic energy, and are considerably more accurate than this at higher energies. The geometrical cross-sections indicated are for molecules. The *median* density indicated is used to obtain the equivalent in cm.
[h] *First column: Material*
Composition assumed (by weight), normalized to unit density:
Air: (N:O:Ar) = (0.755:0.232:0.013)
Film emulsion: (H:C:N:O:S:Br:Ag:I) = (0.0141:0.0723:0.0193:0.0661:0.0019:0.3491:0.4741:0. 0031)
Muscle: (H:C:N:O:Na:Mg:P:S:K:Ca) = (0.102:0.123:0.0350:0.7289:0.0008:0.0002:0.002:0.005:0.003:0.0001)
Bone: (H:C:N:O:Mg:P:S:Ca) = (0.064:0.278:0.027:0.41:0.002:0.07:0.002:0.147)
Concrete: (H:O:Na:Mg:Al:Si:S:K:Ca:Fe) = (0.0056:0.4983:0.0171:0.0024:0.0456:0.3158:0. 0012:0.0192:0.0826:0.0122)
Pyrex glass: (B:O:Na:Al:Si:K) = (0.0401:0.5396:0.0282:0.0116:0.3772:0.0033)

Table 5.6 Attenuation of Beta Ray Dose, Relative to air, for Low Z Media[a] (From Atomic Energy of Canada Ltd. Cross et al., 1982)

Medium	Relative Stopping Power	$\bar{Z}$	Relative Attenuation (η_{air})	Medium	Relative Stopping Power	$\bar{Z}$	Relative Attenuation (η_{air})
Be	0.927	4.0	0.83	Methane	1.352	4.0	1.22
Ethane	1.288	4.33	1.18	Anthracene	1.088	5.47	1.03
Polyethylene	1.205	4.75	1.12	Methyl Methacrylate	1.114	5.85	1.06
Polystyrene	1.118	5.29	1.04	Mylar	1.066	6.24	1.03
Carbon	1.007	6.00	0.96	ICRP Muscle	1.136	6.65	1.11
Water	1.150	6.60	1.12				
Air	1.00	7.36	1.00	ICRP Adipose Tissue	1.169	5.35	1.10
"Bone"	1.063	8.74	1.09				
Al	0.890	13.0	1.00	CO_2	1.002	7.45	0.99
Ar	0.808	18.0	1.00	Teflon (CF_2)	1.032	8.25	1.05
				LiF	0.965	7.50	0.968
				Calcium	0.884	20.0	1.13

[a] Values of relative attenuation in the left half of table were calculated from Spencer 1959.

References

Atomic Energy of Canada Limited. *Tables of Beta-Ray Dose Distributions in Water, Air and Other Media.* Cross, W.G.; Ing, H.; Freedman, N.O., Mainville, J., eds. AECL-7617; Chalk River Nuclear Laboratories; Chalk River, Ontario; 1982.

Berger, M.J., Hubbell, J.H. *XCOM: Photon Cross Sections on a Personal Computer.* NBSIR 87–3597; National Bureau of Standards; 1987.

Berger, M.J., Seltzer, S.M. *Tables of Energy Losses and Ranges of Electrons and Positrons.* Rep. NASA SP-3012, National Aeronautics and Space Administration; Washington, DC; 1964.

Berger, M.J., Seltzer, S.M. *Additional Stopping Power and Range Tables for Protons. Mesons, and Electrons*, Rep NASA SP-3036, National Aeronautics and Space Administration; Washington, DC; 1966.

Berman, R.L. *Atlas of Photoneutron Cross Sections Obtained with Monoenergetic Photons Atomic Data and Nuclear Tables*, **15:**319; 1975.

Carlson, P.J., Diddens, A.N., Monnig, F., and Schopper, H. ''Total np and nN cross sections.'' In Hellwege, K.-H., ed. *Numerical Data and Functional Relationships in Science and Technology.* (Landolt-Bornstein), Group I; *Nuclear and Particle Physics*, Vol. 7, *Elastic and Charge Exchange Scattering of Elementary Particles*, 14–21; Springer-Verlag; Berlin; 1973.

Chemical Rubber Co. *Handbook of Chemistry and Physics*, 71st ed., 1990–1991; Chemical Rubber Co.; Boca Raton, FL; 1991.

Cross *et al.* 1982.

Evans, R.D. *The Atomic Nucleus.* McGraw-Hill, New York; 1955.

Foderaro, A. *The Photon Shielding Manual, Second Edition.* Pennsylvania State University; State College, PA; 1978.

Hubbell, J.H., and Seltzer, S.M. *Tables of X-Ray Mass Attenuation Coefficients and Mass Energy-Absorption Coefficients 1 keV to 20 MeV for Elements Z=1 to 92 and 48 Additional Substances of Dosimetric Interest.* NISTIR 5632, National Institute of Standards and Technology, Gaithersburg, MD; 1995.

Hubbell, J.H. *Photon Cross Sections, Attenuation Coefficients, and Energy Absorption Coefficients from 10 keV to 100 GeV.* NSRDS-NBS 29, National Bureau of Standards; 1969.

International Atomic Energy Agency. *Radiological Safety Aspects of the Operation of Electron Linear Accelerators.* IAEA Technical Reports Series No. 188, Vienna; 1979.

International Commission on Radiation Units and Measurements (ICRU). *Photon, Electron, Proton and Neutron Interaction Data for Body Tissues*, Bethesda, MD; 1992.

Jaeger, R.G., Blizard, E.P., Chilton, A.B., *et al.*, eds. *Engineering Compendium on Radiation Shielding*, Vol. 1, *Shielding Fundamentals and Methods.* Springer-Verlag; Berlin; 1968.

National Bureau of Standards. *Physical Aspects of Irradiation.* Handbook 85; 1964.

National Council on Radiation Protection and Measurements (NCRP). *Conceptual Basis for Calculations of Absorbed Dose Distributions*, Report No. 108; Bethesda, MD; 1991.

Seltzer, S.M. Private communication to the ICRU; 1989.

Spencer, L.V. *Energy Dissipation by Fast Electrons*, National Bureau of Standards; Monograph **1,** 1959.

Storm, E., Israel, H.I. ''Photon cross sections from 0.001 to 100 MeV for elements 1 through 100,'' Los Alamos Scientific Laboratory Rep. LA-3753, UC-34, Physics, TID4500 (1967); *Nucl Data Tables* **A7:**565; 1970.

Sullivan, Cern. Private communication to Thomas R.H.; 1992.

Trout, E. Dale, *et al.* ''Conventional building materials as protective barriers,'' *Radiology*, **76:**2:237–244; 1961.

CHAPTER 6

EXPOSURE AND SHIELDING FROM EXTERNAL RADIATION

This chapter opens with specific gamma-ray constants and the mean attenuation coefficients for selected radionuclides important in radiation assessment and protection. The bulk of the material in this chapter deals with shielding information and practical values for the transmission of radiation through different materials from common radiation sources and x-ray machines. Parameters are given for shielding calculations (half-value layers for gamma and x-ray radiations at varying energies for various materials and buildup factors), as well as ranges of electrons, alpha particles and protons in various materials.

Attenuation through lead, concrete and other materials is illustrated in tables and graphs for x-ray energies in the diagnostic and therapeutic range. Shielding requirements for primary and secondary barriers for three phase x-ray generators and for mammography units are presented. Similar tables are given for ^{60}Co and ^{137}Cs. Also included are percentage backscatter of x-rays from patients and calculated exposure rates from patients containing selected radionuclides at various distances.

The chapter concludes with information on shielding for accelerator facilities, that is: broad beam transmission through lead, concrete and steel, and TVLs for bremsstrahlung. Additional information concerning new shielding materials and aggregates is provided.

TABLE OF CONTENTS

Table 6.1 General Shielding Principles (From Slaback, personal communication, 1996)

Source geometry:
When sources are small or limited in area, do local shielding before doing large area shielding (i.e., shield the source).

Gamma shielding:
For large gamma shields where space and floor loading is not a restriction—use concrete, as much as is needed. When the volume of the shield must be reduced, consider iron (steel), lead, tungsten (in that order of expense). For very specific source spectra, the higher atomic number shielding materials might have an extra consideration.

Fast/non-thermal neutron spectra:
Hydrogenous material is required in order to thermalize the neutrons so they can be captured. The choice is determined by the cost and required physical properties (rigidity, combustibility, ease of adding shielding additives—shot, boron, etc.). If space is critical then hydrogen density is the primary factor, with high density polyethylene being the prime choice. If the neutrons are being 'removed' by scattering (e.g., shutters), a combination of hydrogenous and a high Z material would be used.

Thermal neutrons:
The choice of thermal neutron capture material basically depends on the number of neutrons being stopped, i.e., on the resultant gamma field. Where the flux is high, use ^{6}Li compounds. For lesser fluxes, or where the neutron captures are inside gamma shielding, use boron. Cadmium (2450 barns) is used in special situations, e.g., reducing low neutron fluxes for background control, for 'shaping' thermal neutron fields in a sharply defined manner where its characteristic as a metal is critical. Where the highest attenuation in the minimum space is required use the material with the highest cross-section—gadolinium (49000 barns) or enriched ^{157}Gd (255000 barns).

Mixed gamma—neutron fields:
The specific mixture of gamma and neutron shielding materials depends upon the relative intensities of the radiation types. In general, concrete as a bulk shield will do the job, except in very specialized situations, e.g., high-energy accelerator shielding. For any shield that must truly be optimized to minimize bulk for a desired reduction factor there is no general answer. To simply do a better job than concrete while keeping costs reasonable, the shield simply needs a higher hydrogen density (add more water, paraffin, etc), a higher mass density (add iron, lead), and better thermal neutron absorbing material (B, Li). Paraffin-shot and layered polyethylene-steel both achieve this end.

Special issues:
Neutrons impinging on steel surfaces produce significant high-energy prompt gamma sources that are difficult to shield. Covering such surfaces with borated-aluminum, Boroflex® or Li compounds reduces this problem. For shielding purposes cold neutrons are the same as thermal neutrons.

Table 6.1 General Shielding Principles (Continued)

Material	Primary shield use	Advantages	Disadvantages
Iron	Gamma	Cheap, available in many forms and thicknesses, reasonable density (7.8), good structural characteristics, easy to form.	Activates in neutron fields, not as good as lead in terms of attenuation per unit thickness (because of lead's higher density) or even per unit weight (because of lead's higher attenuation coefficient). Leaks intermediate energy neutrons.
Lead	Gamma	Cheap, easy to form, moderately high density (11.5), nonactivating if reactor grade is selected (low in impurities).	Toxic metal, severe, restrictions on disposal as radioactive waste. Some impurities neutron activate.
Tungsten	Gamma	Highest available density (19.3) in a commonly available metal, good activation characteristics.	Very expensive, difficult to form.
Water	Neutron*, gamma	Cheap, transparent, good hydrogen density for neutron shielding, density of 1 requires lots of thickness for gammas.	Can flow (i.e., leak out of container) and evaporate. Needs 12 times the thickness of lead to have the same attenuation.
Paraffin	Neutron*. gamma	Cheap, easily formed, good hydrogen density; can have various additives easily mixed in by the user, no neutron activation issues.	Combustible, final form not rigid (i.e., can flow or deform). Same as water in regard to gamma shielding. Neutron capture by H produces a hard-to-shield 2-MeV gamma.
Polyethylene	Neutron*, gamma	Easily shaped, machined; good hydrogen density; can be manufactured with selected additives, does not activate.	Not cheap, only semirigid (large sections need support), a fuel in a fire.

* Hydrogen serves to reduce the neutron energy to thermal energies, after which the neutron is captured. The element in which it is captured (e.g., H, B, Li) determines the characteristics of the radiation produced by that capture process.

(continued)

Table 6.1 General Shielding Principles (Continued)

Material	Primary shield use	Advantages	Disadvantages
Concrete	Gamma, neutron*	Cheap, good structural characteristics, density = 2.4 [but can be increased to 4+ with the addition of magnetite (iron ore)], best choice when space is not a concern, acceptable hydrogen density for neutrons, stable at elevated temperatures.	Activates. Care must be taken to avoid voids. Large shields must be reinforced to avoid cracks. Large shields can have voids.
H – 0.33 b	Neutron*	Available in many materials, good for reducing energy of neutrons.	Low thermal capture cross-section, produces high-energy gamma.
Boron nat B – 765 b ^{10}B – 3838 b	Thermal neutrons	High cross-section, easily added to many materials. The gamma produced (0.48 Me) is easier to shield than the H capture gamma (2 MeV). Does not result in a radioactive product.	Difficult to add to materials in a high concentration, enriched ''B (which is the high cross-section isotope of boron) is expensive.
BAl BORAL®	Thermal neutrons	BORAL® is BC4 sandwiched between aluminum, ^{10}BAl is a boron-aluminum alloy. Both can be made in many shapes.	BAl has a limited B concentration compared to BORAL®. Both are expensive. BORAL® is very difficult to cut and shape.
Lithium (^{6}Li) nat Li – 71 b ^{6}Li – 941 b	Thermal neutrons	The neutron absorption process does not produce any gammas. Can be mixed with other materials. Lithium enriched in ^{6}Li is available.	Not as high a cross-section as boron. Each absorbed neutron produced a tritium atom (but this should be a minor issue). The high absorption cross-section isotope (^{6}Li) is expensive.
Cadmium 2450 barns	Thermal neutrons	A metal, easily formed with sharp edges for beam definition, very high cross-sect (a thin piece stops all thermal neutrons).	Metal is toxic. Long-lived radioactive nuclide is produced. Neutron capt. produces high-energy gammas that are difficult to shield.

* Hydrogen serves to reduce the neutron energy to thermal energies, after which the neutron is captured. The element in which it is captured (e.g., H, B, Li) determines the characteristics of the radiation produced by that capture process.

Table 6.2 Specific Gamma-Ray Dose Constants for Selected Nuclides Important to Radiological Assessment and Protection (After Unger and Trubey ORNL/RSIC-45, 1981)

The unshielded gamma ray dose-equivalent rate at 1 meter from a point source, i.e., the specific gamma ray dose constant, is a useful quantity in radiation protection applications. An extensive compilation of the nuclear data required to compute this constant is available (Kocher, 1981) for approximately 500 nuclides important to dosimetry and radiological assessment applications, and it has been used to compute a table of the specific gamma ray dose constants. In addition, the mean attenuation coefficient was computed.

The data were computed on a different basis from earlier tabulations (Nachtigall, 1969). The dose equivalent rate is given in SI units as mSv h^{-1} for a unit source of 1 MBq. To convert to the previous common normalization, one may note that 1 mCi is equal to 37 MBq and 1 Sv is equal to 100 rem. That is, to convert data in units of (mSv h^{-1}) per MBq to (mrem h^{-1}) per μCi, multiply by 3.7.

A second difference is that the conversion of gamma ray flux density was taken to be:

$$\ln D(E) = A + B (\ln E) + C (\ln E)^2 + F (\ln E)^3 \qquad (\text{rem h}^{-1})(\text{cm}^2 - \text{s}) \qquad (1)$$

where the energy is in units of MeV, and the constants are given in Table 6.2.1 taken from ANSI 1977.

The specific gamma ray dose constant, Γ, was summed over n according to:

$$\Gamma = (\tfrac{1}{4}\pi R^2)\Sigma S_i D(E_i) \qquad (\text{rem h}^{-1} \text{ per Bq}) \qquad (2)$$

where R = 100 cm,
n = number of gamma rays emitted by the nuclide,
S_i = emission probability of each gamma ray,
E_i = energy of the gamma ray (MeV),
$D(E_i)$ = dose rate per unit flux density from Eq. 1.

Only gamma rays of energies greater than 0.01 MeV were included.

The mean attenuation coefficient[a] was determined by first computing the thickness of lead required for 95% attenuation, i.e.,

$$0.05\Gamma = \Sigma \Gamma_i \exp(-\mu(E_i)t) \qquad (3)$$

where $\Gamma_i = S_i D(E_i)/(4\pi R^2)$
μE_i = linear attenuation coefficient (Hubbell 1969) for lead,
t = thickness required (cm).

The value of t was determined by an iterative procedure, i.e., Newton's method. The value of the mean attenuation coefficient was determined by solving the following equation for μ:

$$0.05 = \exp(-\mu t).$$

The results, presented in Table 6.2.2 were computed using computer-readable data (Kocher, 1981) available as DLC-80/DRALIST from the Radiation Shielding Information Center. The computations were performed using a computer program, SPEC-GAM, programmed by the first author for the ORNL Engineering Physics Information Centers (EPIC) Data General Eclipse S/130 computer in FORTRAN.

[a] An alternative description of μ as employed in Table 6.2.2 might be the effective attenuation coefficient for lead at 95% attenuation.

Table 6.2.1 Gamma-Ray Flux-to-Dose Rate Conversion Factors Polynomial Coefficients in Analytic Form

$$\ln D(E) = A + Bx + Cx^2 + Fx^3$$

$D(E) = (\text{rem h}^{-1})(\text{cm}^2\ \text{s})$, E = Photon Energy in MeV and x = ln E (After Unger and Trubey ORNL/RSIC-45, 1981)

Photon Energy (Mev)	A	B	C	F
0.01 to 0.03	−20.477	−1.7454		
0.03 to 0.5	−13.626	−0.57117	−1.0954	−0.24897
0.5 to 5.0	−13.133	0.72008	−0.033603	
5.0 to 15.0	−12.791	0.28309	0.10873	

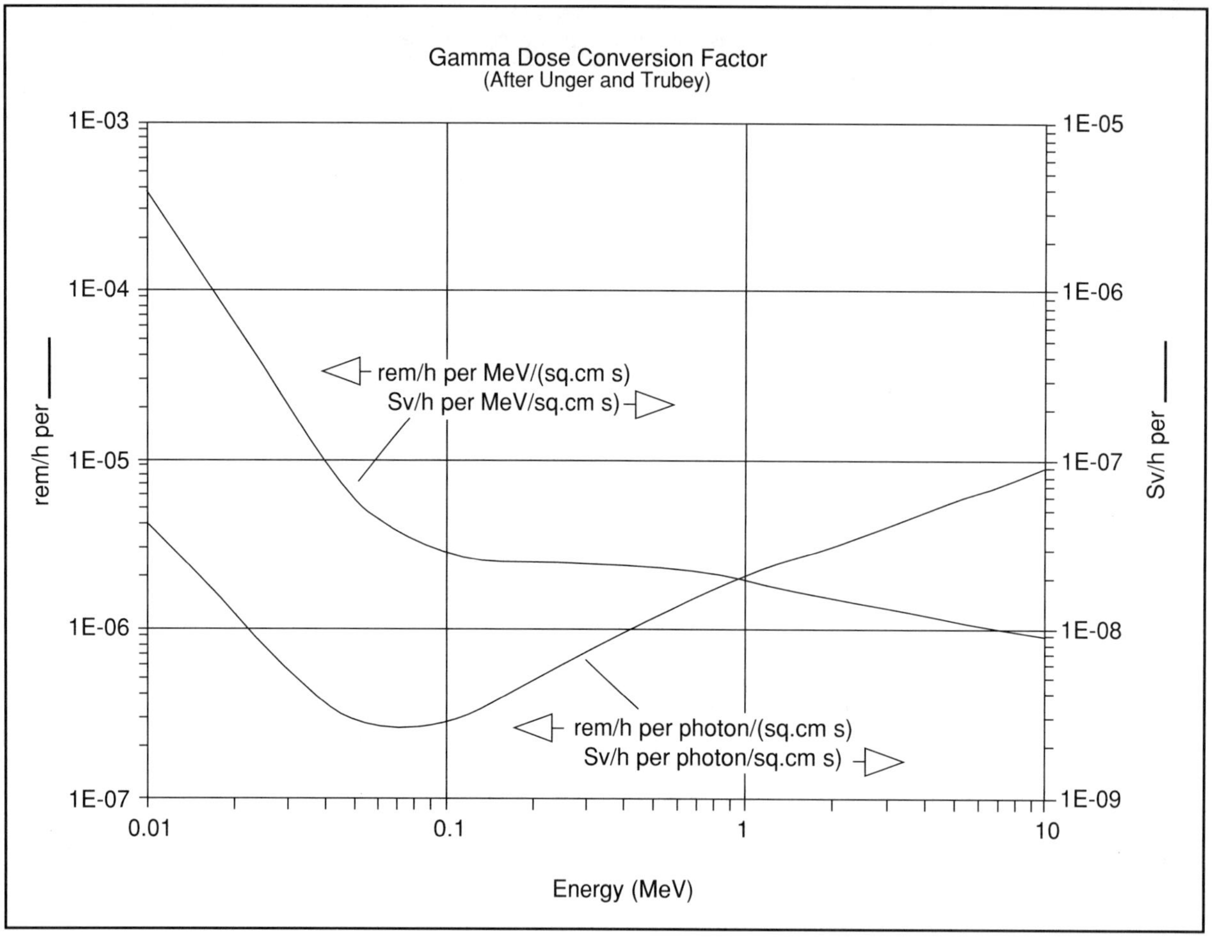

Figure 6.1 Gamma Dose Conversion Curves

Table 6.2.2 Specific Gamma-Ray Dose Constants at 1 Meter
Units: Γ in mSv h^{-1} per MBq, μ in cm^{-1}[a] (After Unger and Trubey ORNL/RSIC-45, 1981)

Nuclide	Half-Life	Γ	μ
^{7}Be	53.4 d	9.292 E −6	1.879
^{11}C	20.5 m	1.937 E −4	1.695
^{13}N	10.0 m	1.938 E −4	1.695
^{16}C	7.1 s	3.984 E −4	0.495
^{15}O	2.0 m	1.940 E −4	1.695
^{18}F	1.8 h	1.879 E −4	1.695
^{22}Na	2.6 y	3.620 E −4	0.852
^{24}Na	15.0 h	5.237 E −4	0.528
^{27}Mg	9.5 m	1.449 E −4	0.869
^{28}Mg	20.9 h	2.375 E −4	0.763
^{26}Al	7.2 E + 5 *y*	4.047 E −4	0.652
^{28}Al	2.2 m	2.384 E −4	0.548
^{31}Si	2.6 h	1.306 E −7	0.676
^{38}Cl	37.2 m	1.942 E −4	0.527
^{41}Ar	1.8 h	1.881 E −4	0.667
^{40}K	1.28 E + 9 *y*	2.208 E −5	0.619
^{42}K	12.4 h	3.869 E −5	0.604
^{43}K	22.6 h	1.811 E −4	1.546
^{45}Ca	162.7 d	8.072 E −12	823.3
^{47}Ca	4.5 d	1.581 E −4	0.686
^{49}Ca	8.7 m	3.615 E −4	0.472
^{44}Sc	3.9 h	3.602 E −4	0.915
^{46}Sc	83.8 d	3.155 E −4	0.787
^{46m}Sc	18.7 s	1.809 E −5	24.378
^{47}Sc	3.4 d	2.170 E −5	18.513
^{48}Sc	1.8 d	5.117 E −4	0.728
^{49}Sc	57.4 m	1.407 E −7	0.556
^{44}Ti	47.3 y	3.909 E −5	28.726
^{45}Ti	3.1 h	1.653 E −4	1.687
^{51}Ti	5.8 m	7.130 E −5	2.110
^{48}V	16.0 d	4.598 E −4	0.770
^{52}V	3.7 m	2.057 E −4	0.626
^{49}Cr	42.1 m	2.029 E −4	1.766
^{51}Cr	27.7 d	6.320 E −6	3.833
^{52}Mn	5.6 d	5.430 E −4	0.773
^{52m}Mn	21.4 m	3.903 E −4	0.795
^{54}Mn	312.7 d	1.382 E −4	0.932
^{56}Mn	2.6 h	2.496 E −4	0.662
^{57}Mn	1.5 m	3.031 E −5	1.697
^{52}Fe	8.3 h	1.413 E −4	1.859
^{59}Fe	44.6 d	1.789 E −4	0.705
^{56}Co	78.8 d	5.205 E −4	0.645
^{57}Co	270.9 d	4.087 E −5	39.809
^{58}Co	70.8 d	1.659 E −4	1.008
^{58}mCo	9.1 h	2.637 E −8	528.9
^{60}Co	5.3 y	3.703 E −4	0.679
^{60}mCo	10.5 m	9.057 E −7	0.837
^{61}Co	1.6 h	2.286 E −5	1.706
^{56}Ni	6.1 d	2.941 E −4	1.003
^{57}Ni	1.5 d	2.911 E −4	0.681
^{65}Ni	2.5 h	8.038 E −5	0.655
^{61}Cu	3.4 h	1.536 E −4	1.497
^{62}Cu	9.7 m	1.910 E −4	1.679
^{64}Cu	12.7 h	3.566 E −5	1.614
^{67}Cu	2.58 d	2.363 E −5	13.011
^{62}Zn	9.3 h	8.990 E −5	1.592
^{65}Zn	244.4 d	8.924 E −5	0.738
^{69}Zn	55.6 m	1.168 E −9	2.362
^{69}mZn	13.8 h	7.983 E −5	2.153
^{66}Ga	9.4 h	3.504 E −4	0.615
^{67}Ga	3.3 d	3.004 E −5	4.768
^{68}Ga	1.1 h	1.789 E −4	1.609
^{72}Ga	14.1 h	3.936 E −4	0.643
^{68}Ge	288 d	1.634 E 5	1345
^{71}Ge	11.8 d	1.653 E −5	1345
^{77}Ge	11.3 h	1.934 E −4	1.089
^{72}As	1.1 d	3.148 E −4	1.107
^{73}As	80.3 d	3.784 E −5	662.1
^{74}As	17.8 d	1.472 E −4	1.475
^{76}As	1.1 d	7.408 E −5	1.036
^{77}As	1.6 d	1.699 E −6	2.522
^{73}Se	7.1 h	2.969 E −4	2.212
^{75}Se	119.8 d	2.323 E −4	9.079
^{77}Br	2.4 d	1.923 E −4	3.068
^{80}Br	17.4 m	2.166 E −5	1.625
^{80m}Br	4.4 h	1.900 E −4	698.2
^{82}Br	1.5 d	4.377 E −4	0.906
^{83}Br	2.4 h	1.401 E −6	1.612
^{84}Br	31.8 m	2.392 E −4	0.573
^{85}Br	172 s	1.059 E −5	0.834
^{79}Kr	1.5 d	1.631 E −4	3.139
^{81}Kr	2.1 E + 5 *y*	1.172 E −4	795.2
^{83m}Kr	1.8 h	3.209 E −5	801.4
^{85}Kr	10.7 y	4.232 E −7	1.681
^{85m}Kr	4.5 h	4.328 E −5	9.045

[a] As used in this table, μ is explained on page 165, equation (3). Data are exclusion of decay products except for Cs^{137}.

(continued)

Table 6.2.2 Specific Gamma-Ray Dose Constants at 1 Meter Units: Γ in mSv h^{-1} per MBq, μ in cm^{-1}[a] (Continued)

Nuclide	Half-Life	Γ	μ	Nuclide	Half-Life	Γ	μ
^{87}Kr	1.3 h	1.169 E −4	0.627	^{95}Nb	35.1 d	1.298 E −4	1.023
^{88}Kr	2.8 h	2.769 E −4	0.556	^{95m}Nb	3.6 d	6.390 E −5	16.959
^{89}Kr	3.2 m	2.626 E −4	0.622	^{96}Nb	23.3 h	4.120 E −4	0.926
^{90}Kr	32.3 s	2.073 E −4	0.733	^{97}Nb	1.2 h	1.175 E −4	1.203
^{81}Rb	4.6 h	2.264 E −4	2.452	^{97m}Nb	60 s	1.262 E −4	1.063
^{82}Rb	1.2 m	2.104 E −4	1.572	^{91}Mo	15.5 m	1.898 E −4	1.660
^{83}Rb	86.2 d	2.085 E −4	2.186	^{93}Mo	3500 y	7.963 E −5	1292
^{84}Rb	32.9 d	2.326 E −4	1.176	^{99}Mo	2.8 d	3.052 E −5	1.165
^{86}Rb	18.7 d	1.458 E −5	0.747	^{101}Mo	14.6 m	2.391 E −4	0.736
^{88}Rb	17.8 m	8.701 E −5	0.571	^{95}Tc	20.0 h	2.092 E −4	1.179
^{89}Rb	15.4 m	2.960 E −4	0.630	^{95m}Tc	61 d	1.939 E −4	1.407
^{90}Rb	157 s	2.548 E −4	0.518	^{96}Tc	4.3 d	4.899 E −4	0.994
^{90m}Rb	258.0 s	4.429 E −4	0.585	^{96m}Tc	51.5 m	4.430 E −5	2.427
^{82}Sr	25.0 d	1.065 E −4	842.8	^{97}Tc	2.6 E + 6 y	7.596 E −5	1176
^{85}Sr	64.8 d	2.052 E −4	2.244	^{97m}Tc	89 d	5.233 E −5	1060
^{85m}Sr	1.1 h	6.004 E −5	8.972	^{98}Tc	4.2 E + 6 y	2.430 E −4	1.130
^{87m}Sr	2.8 h	8.010 E −5	2.872	^{99}Tc	2.1 E + 5 y	1.242 E −10	21.144
^{89}Sr	50.6 d	2.205 E −8	0.858	^{99m}Tc	6.0 h	3.317 E −5	27.731
^{91}Sr	9.5 h	1.118 E −4	0.865	^{101}Tc	14.2 m	6.916 E −5	2.913
^{92}Sr	2.7 h	1.946 E −4	0.651	^{97}Ru	2.9 d	1.194 E −4	10.310
^{93}Sr	7.3 m	3.665 E −4	0.780	^{103}Ru	39.4 d	8.970 E −5	1.724
^{86}Y	14.7 h	6.292 E −4	0.782	^{105}Ru	4.4 h	1.397 E −4	1.202
^{87}Y	3.3 d	1.861 E −4	2.486	^{103m}Rh	56.1 m	6.912 E −6	864
^{88}Y	106.6 d	4.819 E −4	0.661	^{105}Rh	1.5 d	1.588 E −5	3.949
^{90m}Y	3.2 h	1.316 E −4	2.213	^{105m}Rh	45 s	4.251 E −5	98.565
^{91}Y	58.5 d	5.403 E −7	0.697	^{106}Rh	29.9 s	3.734 E −5	1.260
^{91m}Y	49.7 m	1.028 E −4	1.527	^{103}Pd	17.0 d	6.219 E −5	871.6
^{92}Y	3.5 h	3.971 E −5	0.784	^{109}Pd	13.5 h	1.310 E −7	1.706
^{93}Y	10.1 h	1.396 E −5	0.696	^{106m}Ag	8.5 d	5.237 E −4	0.948
^{86}Zr	16.5 h	2.383 E −4	11.219	^{108}Ag	2.4 m	4.399 E −6	1.545
^{88}Zr	83.4 d	1.710 E −4	3.559	^{108m}Ag	127 y	3.436 E −4	1.392
^{89}Zr	3.3 d	2.662 E −4	1.046	^{109m}Ag	39.6 s	2.722 E −5	548.6
^{95}Zr	64.0 d	1.258 E −4	1.059	^{110}Ag	24.6 s	5.558 E −6	1.210
^{97}Zr	16.9 h	2.922 E −5	0.803	^{110m}Ag	249.9 d	4.466 E −4	0.876
^{90}Nb	14.6 h	6.597 E −4	0.627	^{111}Ag	7.5 d	5.329 E −6	3.440
^{91}Nb	1.0 E + 4 y	8.832 E −5	1330	^{109}Cd	464 d	4.983 E −5	683.6
^{91m}Nb	61 d	7.160 E −5	3.692	^{111m}Cd	48.7 m	8.463 E −5	8.502
^{92}Nb	3.6 E + 7 y	3.414 E −4	1.097	^{115}Cd	2.2 d	4.068 E −5	1.711
^{92m}Nb	10.1 d	2.413 E −4	0.977	^{115m}Cd	44.6 d	3.433 E −6	0.778
^{93m}Nb	14.6 y	1.421 E −5	1292	^{117}Cd	2.5 h	1.740 E −4	0.733
^{94}Nb	2.0 E + 4 y	2.648 E −4	0.983	^{117m}Cd	3.4 h	2.935 E −4	0.619
^{94m}Nb	6.3 m	5.481 E −5	1180	^{111}Im	2.8 d	1.356 E −4	10.321

[a] As used in this table, μ is explained on page 165, equation (3). Data are exclusion of decay products except for Cs^{137}.

Table 6.2.2 Specific Gamma-Ray Dose Constants at 1 Meter
Units: Γ in mSv h^{-1} per MBq, μ in cm^{-1a} (Continued)

Nuclide	Half-Life	Γ	μ	Nuclide	Half-Life	Γ	μ
^{113m}In	1.7 h	6.567 E −5	2.858	^{129}I	1.6 E + 7 *y*	3.401 E −5	287
^{114}In	1.2 m	6.223 E −6	1.358	^{130}I	12.4 h	3.791 E −4	1.187
^{114m}In	49.5 d	4.074 E −5	2.318	^{131}I	8.0 d	7.647 E −5	2.409
^{115m}In	4.4 h	5.329 E −5	4.220	^{132}I	2.3 h	3.858 E −4	0.972
^{116m}In	54.1 m	3.660 E −4	0.674	^{133}I	20.8 h	1.105 E −4	1.321
^{117}In	43.8 m	1.359 E −4	1.682	^{134}I	52.6 m	4.251 E −4	0.845
^{117m}In	1.9 h	3.060 E −5	5.608	^{135}I	6.6 h	2.327 E −4	0.664
^{113}Sn	115.1 d	4.844 E −5	462.8	^{136}I	83 s	3.417 E −4	0.579
^{117m}Sn	13.6 d	6.796 E −5	26.595	^{122}Xe	20.1 h	4.867 E −5	7.257
^{119m}Sn	293.0 d	2.789 E −5	517.0	^{123}Xe	2.1 h	1.416 E −4	1.147
^{123}Sn	129.2 d	1.062 E −6	0.744	^{125}Xe	16.8 h	9.622 E −5	4.757
^{125}Sn	9.6 d	4.674 E −5	0.735	^{127}Xe	36.4 d	9.331 E −5	7.526
^{126}Sn	1.0 E + 5 *y*	3.408 E −5	31.647	^{129m}Xe	8.9 d	6.165 E −5	235.8
^{117}Sb	2.8 h	8.219 E −5	14.115	^{131m}Xe	11.8 d	2.533 E −5	263.7
^{122}Sb	2.7 d	8.223 E −5	1.400	^{133}Xe	5.2 d	2.783 E −5	39.877
^{124}Sb	60.2 d	2.883 E −4	0.714	^{133m}Xe	2.2 d	3.034 E −5	19.750
^{125}Sb	2.8 y	1.028 E −4	1.764	^{135}Xe	9.1 h	5.121 E −5	5.015
^{126}Sb	12.4 d	4.860 E −4	1.172	^{135m}Xe	15.4 m	8.651 E −5	1.668
^{126m}Sb	19.0 m	2.824 E −4	1.266	^{137}Xe	3.8 m	3.346 E −5	1.247
^{127}Sb	3.9 d	1.200 E −4	1.255	^{138}Xe	14.1 m	1.679 E −4	0.611
^{129}Sb	4.4 h	2.315 E −4	0.840	^{126}Cs	1.6 m	2.166 E −4	1.581
^{121}Te	16.8 d	1.455 E −4	1.683	^{129}Cs	1.3 d	9.725 E −5	3.213
^{121m}Te	154 d	6.703 E −5	5.779	^{131}Cs	9.7 d	3.363 E −5	310.3
^{123}Te	1.0 E + 13 *y*	2.687 E −5	429.8	^{132}Cs	6.5 d	1.556 E −4	1.295
^{123m}Te	119.7 d	5.261 E −5	24.041	^{134}Cs	2.1 y	2.701 E −4	1.095
^{125m}Te	58 d	6.168 E −5	368.9	^{134m}Cs	2.9 h	1.904 E −5	75.989
^{127}Te	9.4 h	9.428 E −7	2.419	^{136}Cs	13.2 d	3.632 E −4	0.872
^{127m}Te	109 d	1.977 E −5	373.5	^{137}Cs	30.17 y	$\Gamma = 1.032 \times 10^{-4}$	
^{129}Te	1.2 h	1.833 E −5	2.063			from 137 mBa	
^{129m}Te	33.6 d	1.997 E −5	2.000	^{138}Cs	32.2 m	3.422 E −4	0.634
^{131}Te	25.0 m	8.073 E −5	1.203	^{139}Cs	9.4 m	4.260 E −5	0.596
^{131m}Te	30 h	2.452 E −4	0.895	^{131}Ba	11.8 d	1.244 E −4	2.239
^{132}Te	3.3 d	7.549 E −5	10.115	^{133}Ba	10.5 y	1.231 E −4	4.188
^{133}Te	12.4 m	1.584 E −4	0.898	^{133m}Ba	1.6 d	3.372 E −5	8.792
^{133m}Te	55.4 m	3.689 E −4	0.851	^{135m}Ba	1.2 d	2.974 E −5	9.494
^{134}Te	41.8 m	1.731 E −4	1.365	^{137m}Ba	2.6 m	1.081 E −4	1.224
^{122}I	3.6 m	1.901 E −4	1.555	^{139}Ba	1.4 h	7.717 E −6	2.807
^{123}I	13.1 h	7.478 E −5	19.341	^{140}Ba	12.8 d	4.446 E −5	1.889
^{124}I	4.2 d	2.050 E −4	0.968	^{141}Ba	18.3 m	1.562 E −4	0.981
^{125}I	60.1 d	7.432 E −5	373.1	^{142}Ba	10.7 m	1.537 E −4	0.841
^{126}I	12.9 d	1.055 E −4	1.452	^{141}La	3.9 h	6.112 E −6	0.633
^{128}I	25.0 m	1.616 E −5	1.988	^{142}La	1.6 h	3.656 E −4	0.558

[a] As used in this table, μ is explained on page 165, equation (3). Data are exclusion of decay products except for Cs^{137}.

(continued)

Table 6.2.2 Specific Gamma-Ray Dose Constants at 1 Meter
Units: Γ in mSv h^{-1} per MBq, μ in cm^{-1a} (Continued)

Nuclide	Half-Life	Γ	μ	Nuclide	Half-Life	Γ	μ
^{139}Ce	137.7 d	5.554 E −5	22.320	^{175}Yb	4.2 d	8.233 E −6	2.998
^{141}Ce	32.5 d	1.979 E −5	26.056	^{177}Lu	6.7 d	7.636 E −6	10.935
^{143}Ce	1.4 d	6.893 E −5	2.109	^{177m}Lu	160.1 d	2.112 E −4	3.983
^{144}Ce	284.3 d	6.302 E −6	35.806	^{181}Hf	42.4 d	1.061 E −4	2.078
^{142}Pr	19.1 h	8.106 E −6	0.591	^{182}Ta	114.7 d	2.086 E −4	0.751
^{143}Pr	13.6 d	1.524 E −12	1.061	^{181}W	120.9 d	1.389 E −5	52.038
^{144}Pr	17.3 m	4.600 E −6	0.619	^{185}W	75.1 d	5.465 E −9	33.602
^{144m}Pr	7.2 m	9.933 E −6	184.2	^{187}W	23.8 h	8.886 E −5	1.353
^{147}Nd	11.0 d	3.769 E −5	2.234	^{188}W	69.4 d	3.615 E −7	5.327
^{149}Nd	1.7 h	8.112 E −5	2.200	^{182}Re	2.7 d	3.078 E −4	0.853
^{143}Pm	265 d	7.216 E −5	1.222	^{182m}Re	12.7 h	1.994 E −4	0.761
^{144}Pm	363 d	2.958 E −4	1.299	^{183}Re	70 d	4.257 E −5	17.021
^{145}Pm	17.7 y	2.418 E −5	152.1	^{184}Re	38.0 d	1.573 E −4	0.963
^{146}Pm	2020 d	1.462 E −4	1.316	^{184m}Re	169 d	7.678 E −5	1.211
^{147}Pm	2.6 d	7.232 E −10	36.526	^{186}Re	3.8 d	4.909 E −6	28.571
^{148}Pm	5.4 d	8.937 E −5	0.741	^{188}Re	17.0 h	1.094 E −5	1.324
^{148m}Pm	41.3 d	3.567 E −4	1.210	185Os	93.6 d	1.310 E −4	1.219
^{149}Pm	2.2 d	2.317 E −6	2.479	^{190m}Os	9.9 m	3.018 E −4	1.684
^{151}Pm	1.2 d	7.086 E −5	1.966	^{191}Os	15.4 d	1.837 E −5	34.767
^{151}Sm	90 y	2.442 E −8	776.6	^{191m}Os	13.0 h	1.449 E −6	40.828
^{153}Sm	1.9 d	2.440 E −5	69.799	^{193}Os	1.2 d	1.414 E −5	2.450
^{152}Eu	13.6 y	2.012 E −4	0.831	^{190}Ir	11.8 d	2.681 E −4	1.580
^{152m}Eu	9.3 h	5.746 E −5	0.911	^{190m}Ir	1.2 h	6.120 E −11	456.9
^{154}Eu	8.8 y	2.042 E −4	0.802	^{190m}Ir	3.2 h	1.499 E −5	40.962
^{155}Eu	5.0 y	1.804 E −5	28.563	^{192}Ir	74.0 d	1.599 E −4	2.331
^{156}Eu	15.2 d	1.992 E −4	0.647	^{193m}Ir	11.9 d	1.017 E −7	37.618
^{153}Gd	241.6 d	4.659 E −5	79.273	^{194}Ir	19.1 h	1.673 E −5	1.248
^{159}Gd	18.6 h	1.059 E −5	3.622	^{194m}Ir	171 d	4.372 E −4	1.587
^{162}Gd	9.7 m	8.341 E −5	2.282	^{191}Pt	2.7 d	6.588 E −5	2.483
^{157}Tb	150 y	2.426 E −6	114.4	^{193m}Pt	4.3 d	4.649 E −6	40.629
^{160}Tb	72.3 d	1.788 E −4	0.834	^{195m}Pt	4.0 d	2.029 E −5	36.632
^{162}Tb	7.8 m	1.924 E −4	1.018	^{197}Pt	18.3 h	5.647 E −6	17.673
^{157}Dy	8.1 h	8.357 E −5	4.052	^{197m}Pt	1.6 h	1.931 E −5	4.581
^{165}Dy	2.3 h	6.193 E −6	1.817	^{194}Au	1.6 d	1.784 E −4	0.753
^{166}Dy	3.4 d	1.550 E −5	23.196	^{195}Au	183 d	2.362 E −5	36.236
^{166}Ho	1.1 d	6.270 E −6	0.879	^{195m}Au	30.6 s	4.132 E −5	6.174
^{166m}Ho	1200 y	2.870 E −4	1.140	^{196}Au	6.2 d	9.922 E −5	3.261
^{169}Er	9.4 d	3.406 E −10	46.160	^{198}Au	2.7 d	7.882 E −5	2.317
^{171}Er	7.5 h	8.010 E −5	3.957	^{199}Au	3.1 d	1.866 E −5	16.121
^{170}Tm	128.6 d	1.673 E −6	29.074	^{197}Hg	2.7 d	1.874 E −5	29.898
^{171}Tm	1.9 y	2.597 E −7	60.086	^{197m}Hg	23.8 h	2.059 E −5	14.537
^{169}Yb	32.0 d	8.837 E −5	13.301	^{203}Hg	46.6 d	6.841 E −5	6.007

[a] As used in this table, μ is explained on page 165, equation (3). Data are exclusion of decay products except for Cs^{137}.

Table 6.2.2 Specific Gamma-Ray Dose Constants at 1 Meter
Units: Γ in mSv h^{-1} per MBq, μ in cm^{-1}[a] (Continued)

Nuclide	Half-Life	Γ	μ	Nuclide	Half-Life	Γ	μ
^{200}Tl	1.1 d	2.253 E −4	0.886	^{225}Ac	10.0 d	5.172 E −5	472.6
^{201}Tl	3.0 d	2.372 E −5	26.211	^{227}Ac	21.8 y	2.364 E −6	690.1
^{202}Tl	12.2 d	9.438 E −5	2.272	^{228}Ac	6.1 h	2.281 E −4	0.985
^{204}Tl	3.8 y	3.014 E −7	30.056	^{216}Th	30.9 m	1.818 E −5	138.9
^{207}Tl	4.8 m	3.524 E −7	0.870	^{227}Th	18.7 d	1.145 E −4	14.730
^{208}Tl	3.1 m	4.605 E −4	0.554	^{228}Th	1.9 y	2.142 E −5	731.9
^{209}Tl	2.2 m	3.496 E −4	0.705	^{229}Th	7340.0 y	1.989 E −4	103.7
^{210}Tl	1.3 m	4.601 E −4	0.736	^{230}Th	7.7 E + 4 d	1.861 E −5	815.2
^{203}Pb	2.2 d	1.828 E −4	8.722	^{231}Th	1.1 d	1.473 E −4	679.1
^{204m}Pb	1.1 h	3.650 E −4	0.946	^{232}Th	1.4 E + 10 y	1.848 E −5	828.7
^{205}Pb	1.5 E + 7 y	6.789 E −5	1345	^{233}Th	22.3 m	2.587 E −5	3.684
^{210}Pb	22.3 y	6.801 E −5	1098	^{234}Th	24.1 d	2.038 E −5	148.5
^{211}Pb	36.1 m	9.836 E −6	1.211	^{230}Pa	17.4 d	2.387 E −4	1.322
^{212}Pb	10.6 h	7.389 E −5	11.112	^{231}Pa	3.3 + 4 d	1.011 E −4	131.7
^{214}Pb	26.8 m	8.742 E −5	4.027	^{233}Pa	27.0 d	1.335 E −4	7.024
^{206}Bi	6.2 d	6.820 E −4	0.945	^{234}Pa	6.7 h	5.356 E −4	1.107
^{207}Bi	33.4 y	3.603 E −4	1.015	^{234m}Pa	1.2 m	2.776 E −6	0.978
^{208}Bi	3.7 E + 5 y	4.110 E −4	0.532	^{230}U	20.8 d	2.463 E −5	683.5
^{211}Bi	2.1 m	1.274 E −5	3.617	^{231}U	4.2 d	2.120 E −4	293.4
^{212}Bi	1 h	5.264 E −5	1.042	^{232}U	72.0 y	2.403 E −5	716.7
^{213}Bi	45.6 m	3.140 E −5	2.094	^{233}U	159 E + 7 y	7.866 E −6	705.0
^{214}Bi	19.9 m	2.268 E −4	0.672	^{234}U	2.44 E + 5 y	2.097 E −5	720.7
^{209}Po	102 y	9.811 E −7	1.288	^{235}U	7.04 E + 8 y	9.159 E −5	22.675
^{210}Po	138 d	1.424 E −9	0.967	^{236}U	2.34 E + 7 y	1.992 E −5	722.4
^{211}Po	0.5 s	1.328 E −6	1.016	^{237}U	6.7 d	1.589 E −4	54.239
^{213}Po	4.2 − 6 s	5.146 E −9	1.002	^{238}U	4.47 E + 9 y	1.763 E −5	722.5
^{214}Po	1.6 − 4 s	1.398 E −8	0.975	^{239}U	23.4 m	3.630 E −5	23.988
^{215}Po	1.8 − 3 s	2.861 E −8	2.152	^{240}U	14.1 h	7.686 E −5	921.3
^{216}Po	0.1 s	2.424 E −9	0.965	^{235}Np	1.1 y	6.979 E −5	840.5
^{211}At	7.2 h	6.120 E −5	61.088	^{236}Np	1.15 E + 5 y	2.833 E −4	161.6
^{217}At	0.032 s	4.331 E −8	1.378	^{236m}Np	22.5 h	6.390 E −5	69.674
^{218}Rn	0.035 s	1.367 E −7	1.337	^{237}Np	2.1 E + 6 y	1.251 E −4	512.0
^{219}Rn	4 s	1.419 E −5	3.555	^{238}Np	2.1 d	1.497 E −4	0.965
^{220}Rn	55.6 s	9.723 E −8	1.534	^{239}Np	2.4 d	1.386 E −4	19.449
^{222}Rn	3.8 d	7.390 E −8	1.690	^{240}Np	65 m	3.826 E −4	1.342
^{221}Fr	4.8 m	1.193 E −5	11.522	^{240m}Np	7.4 m	1.144 E −4	1.489
^{223}Fr	21.8 m	8.930 E −5	67.566	^{236}Pu	2.9 y	2.405 E −5	863.6
^{222}Ra	38.0 s	2.115 E −6	3.912	^{237}Pu	45.3 d	1.039 E −4	212.7
^{223}Ra	11.4 d	8.789 E −5	10.794	^{238}Pu	87.8 y	2.135 E −5	864.8
^{224}Ra	3.6 d	2.967 E −6	8.124	^{239}Pu	2.41 E + 4 y	8.145 E −6	860.3
^{225}Ra	14.8 d	4.164 E −5	304.4	^{240}Pu	6569 y	2.030 E −5	864.4
^{226}Ra	1600.0 y	3.274 E −6	18.693	^{242}Pu	3.76 E + 5 y	1.684 E −5	864.4

[a] As used in this table, μ is explained on page 165, equation (3). Data are exclusion of decay products except for Cs^{137}.

(continued)

Table 6.2.2 Specific Gamma-Ray Dose Constants at 1 Meter Units: Γ in mSv h^{-1} per MBq, μ in cm^{-1a} (Continued)

Nuclide	Half-Life	Γ	μ	Nuclide	Half-Life	Γ	μ
^{243}Pu	5 h	2.509 E −5	35.548	^{248}Cm	3.4 E + 5 y	1.227 E −5	1054
^{244}Pu	8.3 E + 7 y	1.462 E −5	865.1	^{249}Cm	1.1 h	4.007 E −6	1.478
^{245}Pu	10.6 h	1.046 E −4	1.432	^{250}Bk	3.2 h	1.834 E −4	0.862
^{246}Pu	10.9 d	2.727 E −5	10.771	^{248}Cf	333.5 d	1.229 E −5	1271
^{241}Am	432.2 y	8.479 E −5	260.7	^{249}Cf	350.6 y	1.119 E −4	3.459
^{242}Am	16.0 h	5.476 E −5	720.7	^{250}Cf	13.1 y	1.212 E −5	1269
^{242m}Am	152 y	4.950 E −5	1132	^{251}Cf	900 y	1.162 E −4	43.960
^{243}Am	7380 y	8.456 E −5	71.213	^{252}Cf	2.6 y	1.131 E −5	1269
^{244}Am	10.1 h	3.168 E −4	1.420	^{253}Cf	17.8 d	2.080 E −7	1272
^{245}Am	2 h	2.341 E −5	17.710	^{254}Cf	60.5 d	1.311 E −11	122.5
^{246}Am	25 m	2.149 E −4	0.899	^{253}Es	20.5 d	6.921 E −6	1196
^{242}Cm	163.2 d	1.949 E −5	1054	^{254}Es	275.7 d	1.490 E −4	1229
^{243}Cm	28.5 y	1.286 E −4	23.268	^{254m}Es	1.6 d	1.519 E −4	1.404
^{244}Cm	18.1 y	1.741 E −5	1054	^{255}Es	39.8 d	8.529 E −7	1263
^{245}Cm	8500 y	1.220 E −4	140.0	^{254}Fm	3.2 h	1.121 E −5	1375
^{246}Cm	4750 y	1.551 E −5	1054	^{255}Fm	20.1 h	8.721 E −5	1334
^{247}Cm	1.6 E + 7 y	7.217 E −5	2.675				

[a] As used in this table, μ is explained on page 165, equation (3). Data are exclusion of decay products except for Cs^{137}.

Table 6.3 Thickness of Lead Required to Reduce Useful Beam to Five Percent (Courtesy ICRP, from Publication 33, 1982)

	Type of Source	Half-Value Layer (cm)	Required Lead[a] (cm)
X-rays	50 kV	0.005	0.02
	70 kV	0.010	0.04
	100 kV	0.025	0.11
	125 kV	0.027	0.12
	150 kV	0.029	0.13
	200 kV	0.042	0.18
	250 kV	0.086	0.37
	300 kV	0.17	0.73
	2 MV	1.15	4.97
	4 MV	1.48	6.40
	6 MV	1.54	6.66
	8 MV	1.62	7.00
	10 MV	1.69	7.31
	15 MV	1.66	7.18
	20 MV	1.63	7.05
	25 MV	1.60	6.92
	30 MV	1.57	6.79
	40 MV	1.50	6.48
	50 MV	1.43	6.18
Radionuclides	^{60}Co	1.20	5.19
	^{137}Cs	0.65	2.81

[a] Approximate values for broad beams calculated from half-value layers which were obtained or derived from data in ICRP, 1982.

Table 6.4 Half- and Tenth-Value Layers for Selected Gamma-Ray Sources (Courtesy NCRP, from Report 49, 1976)

				Half-Value Layers			Tenth-Value Layers[a]		
Radionuclide	Atomic Number	Half-Life	Gamma Energy (MeV)	Concrete (cm)	Steel (cm)	Lead (cm)	Concrete (cm)	Steel (cm)	Lead (cm)
Cesium-137	55	27 y	0.66	4.8	1.6	0.65	15.7	5.3	2.1
Cobalt-60	27	5.24 y	1.17, 1.33	6.2	2.1	1.20	20.6	6.9	4.0
Gold-198	79	2.7 d	0.41	4.1	—	0.33	13.5	—	1.1
Iridium-192	77	74 d	0.13 to 1.06	4.3	1.3	0.60	14.7	4.3	2.0
Radium-226	88	1622 y	0.047 to 2.4	6.9	2.2	1.66	23.4	7.4	5.5

[a] Approximate values obtained with large attenuation.

Table 6.5 Gamma-Ray Buildup Factors[a] for Selected Materials: Data for Point Kernel Calculations: ANS-6.4.3 Standard Reference Data (After NUREG/CR-5740, 1991)

Notes on development of data:

1. The American Nuclear Society Standards Committee Working Group, ANS-6.4.3, developed a set of evaluated gamma ray isotropic point-source buildup factors (ANSI/ANS-6.4.3).
2. Buildup factors (largely unpublished) calculated with moments method have been evaluated by recalculating values with Monte Carlo, integral transport, and discrete ordinate methods. The Monte Carlo calculations employing the MCMP code (Radiation Shielding Information Center) validated a large National Institute of Standards and Technology (NIST) database. The NIST[b] moments method calculated buildup factors for Al, Fe, water, air and concrete presented in the following tables. Buildup factors for other elements were also evaluated.
3. Data for Sn, W, Pb and U in these tables were evaluated with the PALLAS[c] computer code which solves the energy and annular-dependent Boltzmann transport equation with general anisotropic scattering in plane and spherical geometries. Not all the elements evaluated by this code which appear in ANSI (ANSI/ANS-6.4.3) standard are presented here.
4. Integral transport calculations employed the ASFIT code.[d]
5. A number of functional forms have been used in parameterize attenuation data. Available forms presented in the ANSI standard are the Taylor and Berger forms and geometric progression (G-P) form. Accuracy is a problem for low-Z material and low energies for the usual Taylor form and Berger form. Tables for these forms will be presented in the ANSI standard, but are not reproduced here.
6. The moments methods calculations for evaluating buildup factors does not account for coherent scattering. NUREG/CR-5740 presents data which tends to confirm that coherent scattering may be neglected for most shielding calculations if the total attenuation coefficient used in the calculations does not include it.
7. Secondary sources (annihilation, fluorescence, and bremsstrahlung) are included in the ASFIT and PALLAS code, but the NIST moment method does not include bremsstrahlung. Such data are important for high-Z materials and for higher source energies.
8. Air has been, traditionally, the response medium. This implies exposure as an endpoint. Hence, exposure buildup factors are presented in Table 6.5.1 (buildup factor, exposure, BD where the energy response function is air).
9. Buildup factor, energy absorption, B_A is the photon buildup factor in which the quantity of interest is the absorbed or deposited energy in the shield medium. The energy response function is that of absorption in the material. These buildup factors are presented in Table 6.5.2.
10. In evaluating the energy deposition in tissue exposed to gamma radiation, it should be noted that the radiation field itself may be altered by the presence of the tissue. In particular, the spectrum at the shield-tissue interface can be quite different from that of an infinite shield medium due to the backscattering of the tissue. Furthermore, the maximum radiation dose to the tissue may not be located at its surface but somewhere inside, due to the buildup of degraded photons by multiple scattering within the tissue. The buildup factors presented in the tables are for an infinite medium of shielding material, and must be corrected, if more realistic dose values are to be obtained for radiation protection purposes.

    Calculations have been performed at the Indira Gandhi Centre for Atomic Energy Research which allow such corrections to be made. These calculations determine the dose and buildup factor at a shield-tissue interface and within the tissue near the interface. The source is a plane parallel beam (1 photon cm^{-2} s^{-1}) normally incident on the shield. The calculation took into account the scattering in both the shield and tissue phantom in slab geometry and determined the peak energy deposition in the tissue. The factors, shown in Table 6.5.3 are independent of shield thickness and source angular distribution to a satisfactory degree.

[a] The ratio of the value total quantity at any point to the contribution to reaching that point without having undergone a collision.

[b] Radiation Shielding Information Center (RSIC) Code Package CCC-200/MCNP, MCMP-A "General Monte Carlo Code for Neutrons and Photon Transport," contributed by Los Alamos National Laboratory.

[c] Tabeuchi, K; and Tanaka, S. PALLAS-PL, SP-Br: A Code for Direct Integration of Transport Equation in One-Dimensional Plane and Spherical Geometries JAERI-M 9695 Japan Atomic Energy Research Institute 1981.

[d] RSIC Code Package CCC-336/ASFIT-VARI Gamma Transport Code for One-Dimensional Finite Systems Contributed by Indira Gandhi Centre for Atomic Energy Research, Kalpakkam, India and Oak Ridge National Laboratory.

Table 6.5.1 Exposure Buildup Factors (After Trubey ORNL/RSIC-49/R1, 1991)

	Energy (MeV)									
R(mfp)[a]	10	8	6	5	4	3	2	1	0.5	0.1
Aluminum										
0.5	1.19	1.22	1.26	1.28	1.32	1.33	1.37	1.45	1.57	1.91
1.0	1.35	1.41	1.49	1.54	1.62	1.68	1.78	1.99	2.28	2.86
2.0	1.64	1.76	1.94	2.04	2.19	2.38	2.66	3.26	4.07	4.87
3.0	1.93	2.11	2.37	2.54	2.78	3.11	3.62	4.76	6.35	7.07
4.0	2.22	2.46	2.81	3.04	3.38	3.86	4.64	6.48	9.14	9.47
5.0	2.52	2.82	3.26	3.55	3.99	4.64	5.72	8.41	1.24E1	1.21E1
6.0	2.83	3.18	3.72	4.08	4.61	5.44	6.86	1.05E1	1.63E1	1.49E1
7.0	3.14	3.55	4.19	4.61	5.24	6.26	8.05	1.29E1	2.07E1	1.80E1
8.0	3.46	3.92	4.66	5.14	5.88	7.10	9.28	1.54E1	2.57E1	2.13E1
10.0	4.12	4.68	5.61	6.23	7.18	8.83	1.19E1	2.10E1	3.76E1	2.87E1
15.0	5.87	6.64	8.09	9.03	1.05E1	1.34E1	1.89E1	3.77E1	7.86E1	5.17E1
20.0	7.74	8.68	1.07E1	1.19E1	1.40E1	1.81E1	2.66E1	5.79E1	1.37E2	8.11E1
25.0	9.74	1.08E1	1.33E1	1.49E1	1.75E1	2.30E1	3.49E1	8.13E1	2.13E2	1.17E2
30.0	1.18E1	1.30E1	1.60E1	1.80E1	2.10E1	2.81E1	4.36E1	1.07E2	3.07E2	1.59E2
35.0	1.41E1	1.52E1	1.89E1	2.15E1	2.47E1	3.33E1	5.27E1	1.36E2	4.21E2	2.08E2
40.0	1.66E1	1.74E1	2.21E1	2.55E1	2.86E1	3.85E1	6.20E1	1.67E2	5.54E2	2.65E2
Iron										
0.5	1.19	1.22	1.25	1.27	1.30	1.32	1.35	1.41	1.48	1.26
1.0	1.33	1.39	1.47	1.51	1.57	1.64	1.71	1.85	1.99	1.40
2.0	1.59	1.71	1.87	1.97	2.12	2.28	2.49	2.85	3.12	1.61
3.0	1.86	2.04	2.30	2.46	2.68	2.96	3.34	4.00	4.44	1.78
4.0	2.16	2.41	2.76	2.98	3.29	3.68	4.25	5.30	5.96	1.94
5.0	2.50	2.81	3.25	3.53	3.93	4.45	5.22	6.74	7.68	2.07
6.0	2.87	3.24	3.78	4.11	4.60	5.25	6.25	8.31	9.58	2.20
7.0	3.27	3.71	4.33	4.73	5.31	6.09	7.33	1.00E1	1.17E1	2.31
8.0	3.71	4.20	4.92	5.38	6.05	6.96	8.45	1.18E1	1.40E1	2.41
10.0	4.69	5.30	6.18	6.75	7.60	8.80	1.08E1	1.58E1	1.91E1	2.61
15.0	7.88	8.64	9.85	1.07E1	1.19E1	1.38E1	1.74E1	2.75E1	3.51E1	3.01
20.0	1.23E1	1.29E1	1.42E1	1.52E1	1.68E1	1.94E1	2.46E1	4.13E1	5.54E1	3.33
25.0	1.81E1	1.82E1	1.93E1	2.03E1	2.21E1	2.54E1	3.25E1	5.70E1	7.99E1	3.61
30.0	2.57E1	2.45E1	2.51E1	2.59E1	2.79E1	3.17E1	4.09E1	7.45E1	1.08E2	3.86
35.0	3.53E1	3.20E1	3.15E1	3.20E1	3.40E1	3.84E1	4.98E1	9.35E1	1.41E2	4.07
40.0	4.76E1	4.09E1	3.88E1	3.88E1	4.06E1	4.55E1	5.91E1	1.14E2	1.77E2	4.23

[a] *Mean free path.* The average distance that photons of a given energy travel before an interaction in a given medium occurs. It is equal to the reciprocal of the attenuation coefficient. Thus, the distance x in ordinary units can be converted into the dimensionless distance μx, the number of *mean free path* lengths (mfp).

(continued)

Table 6.5.1 Exposure Buildup Factors (Continued)

	Energy (MeV)									
R(mfp)[a]	**10**	**8**	**6**	**5**	**4**	**3**	**2**	**1**	**0.5**	**0.1**
Tin										
0.5	1.31	1.33	1.31	1.31	1.28	1.29	1.27	1.33	1.32	1.35
1.0	1.57	1.60	1.54	1.55	1.51	1.56	1.57	1.69	1.61	1.38
2.0	2.05	2.04	1.94	1.97	1.96	2.07	2.17	2.40	2.15	1.41
3.0	2.61	2.51	2.38	2.43	2.45	2.64	2.82	3.14	2.68	1.43
4.0	3.27	3.05	2.87	2.54	3.00	3.25	3.51	3.86	3.16	1.45
5.0	4.09	3.69	3.43	3.52	3.60	3.92	4.23	4.60	3.63	1.47
6.0	5.07	4.45	4.09	4.19	4.29	4.68	5.03	5.43	4.14	1.49
7.0	6.26	5.34	4.83	4.93	5.04	5.48	5.87	6.27	4.64	1.50
8.0	7.69	6.36	5.65	5.74	5.84	6.32	6.74	7.11	5.13	1.52
10.0	1.15E1	8.94	7.63	7.63	7.65	8.19	8.61	8.88	6.13	1.54
15.0	2.96E1	1.97E1	1.49E1	1.41E1	1.35E1	1.38E1	1.40E1	1.38E1	8.74	1.58
20.0	7.21E1	4.07E1	2.64E1	2.35E1	2.11E1	2.05E1	2.01E1	1.91E1	1.14E1	1.61
25.0	1.68E2	7.97E1	4.39E1	3.62E1	3.06E1	2.81E1	2.69E1	2.45E1	1.40E1	1.64
30.0	3.77E2	1.50E2	6.93E1	5.30E1	4.21E1	3.66E1	3.42E1	3.00E1	1.65E1	1.66
35.0	8.20E2	2.71E2	1.05E2	7.44E1	5.54E1	4.57E1	4.19E1	3.56E1	1.90E1	1.68
40.0	1.74E3	4.77E2	1.54E2	1.01E2	7.06E1	5.54E1	4.98E1	4.11E1	2.14E1	1.69
Tungsten										
0.5	1.29	1.31	1.27	1.27	1.23	1.24	1.23	1.23	1.17	1.44
1.0	1.53	1.54	1.46	1.45	1.40	1.44	1.44	1.44	1.30	1.81
2.0	2.04	1.95	1.79	1.78	1.74	1.81	1.86	1.82	1.50	2.52
3.0	2.67	2.43	2.17	2.16	2.13	2.23	2.30	2.17	1.67	3.31
4.0	3.49	3.01	2.61	2.59	2.56	2.69	2.75	2.49	1.81	4.32
5.0	4.53	3.73	3.13	3.08	3.03	3.18	3.22	2.81	1.95	5.71
6.0	5.85	4.59	3.73	3.65	3.57	3.73	3.72	3.13	2.08	7.62
7.0	7.54	5.63	4.43	4.28	4.17	4.32	4.24	3.44	2.20	1.04E1
8.0	9.67	6.89	5.23	5.00	4.81	4.93	4.77	3.75	2.31	1.41E1
10.0	1.58E1	1.03E1	7.22	6.71	6.30	6.30	5.89	4.34	2.52	2.65E1
15.0	5.20E1	2.67E1	1.53E1	1.30E1	1.13E1	1.04E1	8.94	5.77	2.99	1.60E2
20.0	1.64E2	6.64E1	3.03E1	2.33E1	1.83E1	1.54E1	1.23E1	7.06	3.39	1.22E3
25.0	4.99E2	1.59E2	5.71E1	3.93E1	2.77E1	2.12E1	1.59E1	8.24	3.72	1.02E4
30.0	1.47E3	3.67E2	1.03E2	6.30E1	3.98E1	2.77E1	1.96E1	9.34	4.02	8.79E4
35.0	4.21E3	8.27E2	1.80E2	9.76E1	5.52E1	3.50E1	2.35E1	1.04E1	4.28	7.73E5
40.0	1.18E4	1.82E3	3.07E2	1.46E2	7.40E1	4.28E1	2.74E1	1.13E1	4.52	6.88E6

[a] *Mean free path.* The average distance that photons of a given energy travel before an interaction in a given medium occurs. It is equal to the reciprocal of the attenuation coefficient. Thus, the distance x in ordinary units can be converted into the dimensionless distance μx, the number of *mean free path* lengths (mfp).

Table 6.5.1 Exposure Buildup Factors (Continued)

	Energy (MeV)									
R(mfp)[a]	10	8	6	5	4	3	2	1	0.5	0.1
Lead										
0.5	1.28	1.30	1.26	1.25	1.21	1.23	1.21	1.20	1.14	1.51
1.0	1.51	1.51	1.42	1.41	1.36	1.40	1.40	1.38	1.24	2.04
2.0	2.01	1.90	1.73	1.71	1.67	1.73	1.76	1.68	1.39	3.39
3.0	2.63	2.36	2.08	2.05	2.02	2.10	2.14	1.95	1.52	5.60
4.0	3.42	2.91	2.49	2.44	2.40	2.50	2.52	2.19	1.62	9.59
5.0	4.45	3.59	2.96	2.88	2.82	2.93	2.91	2.43	1.71	1.70E1
6.0	5.73	4.41	3.51	3.38	3.28	3.40	3.32	2.66	1.80	3.06E1
7.0	7.37	5.39	4.13	3.93	3.79	3.89	3.74	2.89	1.88	5.49E1
8.0	9.44	6.58	4.84	4.56	4.35	4.41	4.17	3.10	1.95	9.47E1
10.0	1.54E1	9.73	6.61	6.03	5.61	5.56	5.07	3.51	2.10	2.94E2
15.0	5.08E1	2.51E1	1.37E1	1.14E1	9.73	8.91	7.44	4.45	2.39	5.80E3
20.0	1.61E2	6.20E1	2.66E1	1.99E1	1.54E1	1.29E1	9.98	5.27	2.64	1.33E5
25.0	4.95E2	1.48E2	4.96E1	3.29E1	2.30E1	1.75E1	1.26E1	5.98	2.85	3.34E6
30.0	1.47E3	3.44E2	8.89E1	5.22E1	3.26E1	2.25E1	1.54E1	6.64	3.02	8.77E7
35.0	4.28E3	7.79E2	1.55E2	7.99E1	4.46E1	2.81E1	1.82E1	7.23	3.18	2.36E9
40.0	1.22E4	1.72E3	2.62E2	1.19E2	5.92E1	3.40E1	2.10E1	7.79	3.31	6.43E10
Uranium										
0.5	1.27	1.28	1.24	1.23	1.19	1.20	1.19	1.17	1.11	1.04
1.0	1.49	1.48	1.38	1.37	1.32	1.35	1.35	1.31	1.19	1.06
2.0	1.97	1.85	1.66	1.64	1.60	1.64	1.65	1.53	1.30	1.08
3.0	2.56	2.27	1.98	1.94	1.89	1.95	1.95	1.73	1.39	1.10
4.0	3.31	2.78	2.33	2.27	2.21	2.28	2.25	1.90	1.45	1.11
5.0	4.26	3.39	2.74	2.63	2.55	2.62	2.56	2.07	1.52	1.12
6.0	5.43	4.11	3.19	3.04	2.93	2.99	2.88	2.23	1.58	1.13
7.0	6.90	4.96	3.71	3.49	3.33	3.38	3.19	2.38	1.63	1.14
8.0	8.73	5.97	4.28	3.99	3.76	3.78	3.51	2.52	1.68	1.14
10.0	1.39E1	8.61	5.68	5.14	4.72	4.64	4.17	2.78	1.77	1.16
15.0	4.34E1	2.08E1	1.10E1	9.10	7.72	7.06	5.84	3.35	1.96	1.18
20.0	1.31E2	4.86E1	2.01E1	1.51E1	1.16E1	9.80	7.54	3.82	2.11	1.20
25.0	3.85E1	1.10E2	3.54E1	2.37E1	1.65E1	1.28E1	9.27	4.23	2.23	1.22
30.0	1.10E3	2.44E2	6.04E1	3.60E1	2.25E1	1.60E1	1.10E1	4.59	2.33	1.23
35.0	3.08E3	5.27E2	1.00E2	5.29E1	2.97E1	1.94E1	1.27E1	4.91	2.42	1.24
40.0	8.46E3	1.12E3	1.63E2	7.57E1	3.82E1	2.29E1	1.44E1	5.21	2.50	1.25

[a] *Mean free path.* The average distance that photons of a given energy travel before an interaction in a given medium occurs. It is equal to the reciprocal of the attenuation coefficient. Thus, the distance x in ordinary units can be converted into the dimensionless distance μx, the number of *mean free path* lengths (mfp).

(continued)

Table 6.5.1 Exposure Buildup Factors (Continued)

	Energy (MeV)									
R(mfp)[a]	10	8	6	5	4	3	2	1	0.5	0.1
Water										
0.5	1.20	1.23	1.27	1.28	1.31	1.34	1.38	1.47	1.60	2.37
1.0	1.37	1.43	1.51	1.56	1.63	1.71	1.83	2.08	2.44	4.55
2.0	1.68	1.80	1.97	2.08	2.24	2.46	2.81	3.62	4.88	1.18E1
3.0	1.97	2.15	2.41	2.58	2.85	3.23	3.87	5.50	8.35	2.38E1
4.0	2.25	2.46	2.84	3.08	3.46	4.00	4.98	7.68	1.28E1	4.13E1
5.0	2.53	2.82	3.27	3.58	4.07	4.80	6.15	1.01E1	1.84E1	6.52E1
6.0	2.80	3.15	3.70	4.08	4.68	5.61	7.38	1.28E1	2.50E1	9.67E1
7.0	3.07	3.48	4.12	4.58	5.30	6.43	8.65	1.58E1	3.27E1	1.37E2
8.0	3.34	3.80	4.54	5.07	5.92	7.27	9.97	1.90E1	4.15E1	1.87E2
10.0	3.86	4.44	5.37	6.05	7.16	8.97	12.7	2.61E1	6.29E1	3.21E2
15.0	5.14	5.99	7.41	8.49	10.3	13.3	20.1	4.77E1	1.39E2	9.38E2
20.0	6.38	7.49	9.42	10.9	13.4	17.8	28.0	7.40E1	2.52E2	2.17E3
25.0	7.59	8.96	11.4	13.3	16.5	22.4	36.5	1.04E2	4.03E2	4.36E3
30.0	8.78	10.4	13.3	15.7	19.7	27.1	45.2	1.39E2	5.94E2	7.97E3
35.0	9.96	11.9	15.5	18.0	22.8	31.8	54.4	1.77E2	8.28E2	1.35E4
40.0	11.2	13.4	16.4	20.4	25.9	36.5	63.7	2.18E2	1.11E3	2.11E4
Air										
0.5	1.20	1.23	1.27	1.29	1.31	1.34	1.38	1.47	1.60	2.35
1.0	1.37	1.43	1.52	1.57	1.63	1.71	1.83	2.08	2.44	4.46
2.0	1.68	1.80	1.97	2.09	2.25	2.46	2.81	3.60	4.84	1.14E1
3.0	1.97	2.15	2.41	2.60	2.85	3.22	3.86	5.46	8.21	2.25E1
4.0	2.26	2.50	2.85	3.11	3.46	4.00	4.96	7.60	1.26E1	3.84E1
5.0	2.54	2.84	3.28	3.61	4.07	4.79	6.13	1.00E1	1.79E1	5.99E1
6.0	2.82	3.17	3.71	4.12	4.69	5.60	7.35	1.27E1	2.42E1	8.78E1
7.0	3.10	3.51	4.14	4.62	5.31	6.43	8.61	1.56E1	3.16E1	1.23E2
8.0	3.37	3.84	4.57	5.12	5.94	7.26	9.92	1.88E1	4.01E1	1.66E2
10.0	3.92	4.49	5.42	6.13	7.19	8.97	12.6	2.58E1	6.06E1	2.82E2
15.0	5.25	6.08	7.51	8.63	10.3	13.4	20.0	4.70E1	1.34E2	8.00E2
20.0	6.55	7.64	9.58	11.1	13.5	17.9	27.9	7.28E1	2.41E2	1.81E3
25.0	7.84	9.17	11.6	13.6	16.7	22.5	36.2	1.03E2	3.85E2	3.57E3
30.0	9.11	10.7	13.6	16.1	19.9	27.2	45.0	1.36E2	5.67E2	6.43E3
35.0	10.4	12.3	15.4	18.5	23.1	32.0	54.0	1.73E2	7.88E2	1.06E4
40.0	11.6	14.1	16.9	21.0	26.3	36.7	63.2	2.12E2	1.05E3	1.57E4

[a] *Mean free path.* The average distance that photons of a given energy travel before an interaction in a given medium occurs. It is equal to the reciprocal of the attenuation coefficient. Thus, the distance x in ordinary units can be converted into the dimensionless distance μx, the number of *mean free path* lengths (mfp).

Table 6.5.1 Exposure Buildup Factors (Continued)

	Energy (MeV)									
R(mfp)[a]	**10**	**8**	**6**	**5**	**4**	**3**	**2**	**1**	**0.5**	**0.1**
Concrete										
0.5	1.19	1.22	1.26	1.27	1.31	1.33	1.37	1.45	1.57	1.89
1.0	1.35	1.41	1.49	1.53	1.61	1.67	1.77	1.98	2.27	2.78
2.0	1.64	1.76	1.93	2.04	2.18	2.38	2.65	3.24	4.03	4.63
3.0	1.93	2.11	2.37	2.53	2.77	3.09	3.60	4.72	6.26	6.63
4.0	2.22	2.45	2.80	3.03	3.37	3.84	4.61	6.42	8.97	8.80
5.0	2.51	2.81	3.25	3.54	3.98	4.61	5.68	8.33	1.22E1	1.11E1
6.0	2.80	3.16	3.69	4.05	4.60	5.40	6.80	1.04E1	1.59E1	1.36E1
7.0	3.10	3.51	4.14	4.57	5.23	6.20	7.97	1.27E1	2.02E1	1.63E1
8.0	3.40	3.87	4.60	5.09	5.86	7.03	9.18	1.52E1	2.50E1	1.92E1
10.0	4.01	4.59	5.52	6.15	7.15	8.71	1.17E1	2.07E1	3.64E1	2.56E1
15.0	5.57	6.43	7.86	8.85	1.05E1	1.31E1	1.86E1	3.72E1	7.56E1	4.49E1
20.0	7.19	8.31	1.02E1	1.16E1	1.39E1	1.77E1	2.60E1	5.71E1	1.31E2	6.91E1
25.0	8.86	1.02E1	1.27E1	1.44E1	1.74E1	2.25E1	3.39E1	8.01E1	2.03E2	9.79E1
30.0	1.06E1	1.22E1	1.52E1	1.73E1	2.09E1	2.74E1	4.22E1	1.06E2	2.90E2	1.31E2
35.0	1.23E1	1.41E1	1.78E1	2.05E1	2.46E1	3.24E1	5.09E1	1.34E2	3.99E2	1.70E2
40.0	1.45E1	1.62E1	2.05E1	2.48E1	2.84E1	3.74E1	5.98E1	1.64E2	5.23E2	2.14E2

[a] *Mean free path.* The average distance that photons of a given energy travel before an interaction in a given medium occurs. It is equal to the reciprocal of the attenuation coefficient. Thus, the distance x in ordinary units can be converted into the dimensionless distance μx, the number of *mean free path* lengths (mfp).

Table 6.5.2 Energy Absorption Buildup Factors (After Trubey ORNL/RSIC-49/R1, 1991)

	Energy (MeV)									
R(mfp)[a]	**10**	**8**	**6**	**5**	**4**	**3**	**2**	**1**	**0.5**	**0.1**
Aluminum										
0.5	1.18	1.21	1.25	1.28	1.31	1.34	1.39	1.49	1.75	2.43
1.0	1.32	1.39	1.48	1.57	1.62	1.70	1.83	2.10	2.57	4.00
2.0	1.59	1.72	1.91	2.03	2.21	2.43	2.79	3.59	4.87	7.44
3.0	1.85	2.05	2.33	2.53	2.80	3.18	3.82	5.35	7.91	1.12E1
4.0	2.12	2.37	2.75	3.03	3.40	3.95	4.92	7.37	1.16E1	1.52E1
5.0	2.40	2.71	3.18	3.53	4.02	4.75	6.08	9.64	1.61E1	1.96E1
6.0	2.68	3.04	3.62	4.04	4.64	5.57	7.30	1.21E1	2.13E1	2.44E1
7.0	2.97	3.39	4.06	4.56	5.28	6.42	8.57	1.49E1	2.73E1	2.96E1
8.0	3.26	3.74	4.51	5.09	5.92	7.28	9.90	1.79E1	3.42E1	3.52E1
10.0	3.86	4.44	5.43	6.16	7.22	9.05	1.27E1	2.45E1	5.05E1	4.77E1
15.0	5.45	6.27	7.79	8.91	1.06E1	1.37E1	2.03E1	4.43E1	1.07E2	8.67E1
20.0	7.15	8.18	1.03E1	1.18E1	1.40E1	1.86E1	2.85E1	6.84E1	1.89E2	1.37E2
25.0	8.96	1.01E1	1.28E1	1.47E1	1.75E1	2.36E1	3.74E1	9.62E1	2.96E2	1.98E2
30.0	1.09E1	1.22E1	1.52E1	1.76E1	2.11E1	2.88E1	4.68E1	1.27E2	4.30E2	2.71E2
35.0	1.28E1	1.42E1	1.75E1	2.06E1	2.48E1	3.41E1	5.66E1	1.62E2	5.91E2	3.56E2
40.0	1.48E1	1.62E1	1.95E1	2.33E1	2.84E1	3.94E1	6.66E1	1.99E2	7.80E2	4.51E2
Iron										
0.5	1.15	1.18	1.22	1.26	1.31	1.35	1.40	1.53	1.79	1.38
1.0	1.27	1.33	1.42	1.49	1.59	1.70	1.84	2.14	2.66	1.60
2.0	1.48	1.60	1.79	1.93	2.12	2.39	2.76	3.50	4.57	1.94
3.0	1.69	1.88	2.17	2.39	2.68	3.10	3.74	5.04	6.75	2.13
4.0	1.93	2.17	2.57	2.86	3.27	3.86	4.80	6.79	9.25	2.31
5.0	2.19	2.50	2.99	3.37	3.89	4.66	5.93	8.74	1.21E1	2.48
6.0	2.47	2.85	3.45	3.91	4.55	5.51	7.12	1.09E1	1.53E1	2.63
7.0	2.78	3.22	3.93	4.47	5.23	6.39	8.37	1.32E1	1.88E1	2.77
8.0	3.12	3.62	4.44	5.07	5.95	7.30	9.67	1.57E1	2.27E1	2.90
10.0	3.87	4.50	5.54	6.33	7.46	9.23	1.24E1	2.11E1	3.14E1	3.13
15.0	6.29	7.18	8.72	9.92	1.17E1	1.45E1	2.00E1	3.71E1	5.88E1	3.61
20.0	9.59	1.06E1	1.25E1	1.41E1	1.64E1	2.04E1	2.85E1	5.62E1	9.39E1	4.00
25.0	1.40E1	1.48E1	1.69E1	1.87E1	2.16E1	2.67E1	3.77E1	7.79E1	1.36E2	4.34
30.0	1.96E1	1.98E1	2.17E1	2.37E1	2.70E1	3.33E1	4.74E1	1.02E2	1.86E2	4.63
35.0	2.67E1	2.56E1	2.68E1	2.89E1	3.25E1	4.04E1	5.77E1	1.28E2	2.42E2	4.85
40.0	3.54E1	3.24E1	3.21E1	3.40E1	3.79E1	4.78E1	6.84E1	1.56E2	3.05E2	4.98

[a] *Mean free path.* The average distance that photons of a given energy travel before an interaction in a given medium occurs. It is equal to the reciprocal of the attenuation coefficient. Thus, the distance x in ordinary units can be converted into the dimensionless distance μx, the number of *mean free path* lengths (mfp).

Table 6.5.2 Energy Absorption Buildup Factors (Continued)

	Energy (MeV)									
R(mfp)[a]	**10**	**8**	**6**	**5**	**4**	**3**	**2**	**1**	**0.5**	**0.1**
Tin										
0.5	1.29	1.33	1.36	1.39	1.39	1.43	1.45	1.68	1.81	1.30
1.0	1.50	1.57	1.60	1.65	1.66	1.78	1.88	2.28	2.39	1.32
2.0	1.84	1.92	1.95	2.05	2.11	2.37	2.68	3.42	3.35	1.35
3.0	2.21	2.27	2.31	2.46	2.60	3.01	3.55	4.58	4.26	1.38
4.0	2.66	2.66	2.72	2.92	3.14	3.69	4.43	5.70	5.06	1.40
5.0	3.20	3.13	3.19	3.44	3.74	4.43	5.36	6.82	5.83	1.42
6.0	3.86	3.70	3.74	4.05	4.43	5.28	6.43	8.12	6.70	1.44
7.0	4.65	4.35	4.37	4.73	5.18	6.20	7.53	9.43	7.54	1.45
8.0	5.59	5.10	5.05	5.46	5.97	7.14	8.66	1.07E1	8.34	1.46
10.0	8.07	6.98	6.70	7.17	7.77	9.24	1.11E1	1.34E1	9.99	1.49
15.0	1.98E1	1.48E1	1.27E1	1.30E1	1.36E1	1.56E1	1.82E1	2.11E1	1.44E1	1.53
20.0	4.70E1	2.99E1	2.22E1	2.14E1	2.12E1	2.32E1	2.63E1	2.93E1	1.87E1	1.56
25.0	1.08E2	5.76E1	3.65E1	3.29E1	3.07E1	3.18E1	3.52E1	3.78E1	2.31E1	1.58
30.0	2.40E2	1.07E2	5.73E1	4.79E1	4.21E1	4.14E1	4.48E1	4.64E1	2.74E1	1.60
35.0	5.20E2	1.93E2	8.65E1	6.71E1	5.54E1	5.18E1	5.50E1	5.52E1	3.16E1	1.62
40.0	1.10E3	3.38E2	1.27E2	9.10E1	7.06E1	6.28E1	6.55E1	6.39E1	3.56E1	1.63
Tungsten										
0.5	1.34	1.38	1.40	1.43	1.43	1.48	1.48	1.52	1.55	1.46
1.0	1.53	1.60	1.59	1.64	1.62	1.74	1.81	1.89	1.80	1.84
2.0	1.88	1.91	1.87	1.94	1.96	2.18	2.39	2.49	2.14	2.56
3.0	2.30	2.26	2.20	2.29	2.36	2.67	3.01	3.04	2.42	3.33
4.0	2.84	2.69	2.57	2.69	2.81	3.20	3.62	3.52	2.63	4.32
5.0	3.53	3.22	3.02	3.15	3.30	3.79	4.27	3.98	2.83	5.65
6.0	4.40	3.86	3.54	3.68	3.86	4.44	4.98	4.47	3.03	7.44
7.0	5.51	4.62	4.13	4.28	4.48	5.14	5.70	4.94	3.21	9.99
8.0	6.88	5.54	4.81	4.94	5.14	5.87	6.44	5.39	3.38	1.34E1
10.0	1.08E1	7.99	6.49	6.53	6.68	7.49	8.00	6.28	3.71	2.46E1
15.0	3.38E1	1.98E1	1.32E1	1.24E1	1.18E1	1.24E1	1.23E1	8.42	4.42	1.40E2
20.0	1.04E2	4.80E1	2.57E1	2.19E1	1.91E1	1.83E1	1.69E1	1.04E1	5.02	1.04E3
25.0	3.14E2	1.13E2	4.79E1	3.65E1	2.87E1	2.53E1	2.19E1	1.21E1	5.53	8.62E3
30.0	9.18E2	2.60E2	8.59E1	5.83E1	4.13E1	3.31E1	2.72E1	1.38E1	5.98	7.42E4
35.0	2.62E3	5.83E2	1.50E2	8.99E1	5.71E1	4.17E1	3.26E1	1.53E1	6.37	6.50E5
40.0	7.32E3	1.28E3	2.53E2	1.34E2	7.66E1	5.11E1	3.81E1	1.67E1	6.73	5.77E6

[a] *Mean free path.* The average distance that photons of a given energy travel before an interaction in a given medium occurs. It is equal to the reciprocal of the attenuation coefficient. Thus, the distance x in ordinary units can be converted into the dimensionless distance μx, the number of *mean free path* lengths (mfp).

(continued)

Table 6.5.2 Energy Absorption Buildup Factors (Continued)

	Energy (MeV)									
R(mfp)[a]	10	8	6	5	4	3	2	1	0.5	0.1
Lead										
0.5	1.35	1.40	1.41	1.44	1.43	1.49	1.48	1.46	1.48	1.44
1.0	1.54	1.59	1.58	1.62	1.60	1.71	1.78	1.76	1.67	1.89
2.0	1.88	1.89	1.84	1.89	1.91	2.11	2.28	2.23	1.92	3.05
3.0	2.30	2.24	2.15	2.22	2.28	2.56	2.82	2.64	2.11	4.92
4.0	2.85	2.66	2.50	2.59	2.68	3.03	3.35	2.99	2.26	8.25
5.0	3.54	3.17	2.91	3.00	3.12	3.55	3.90	3.32	2.40	1.44E1
6.0	4.40	3.79	3.40	3.48	3.61	4.12	4.50	3.68	2.53	2.54E1
7.0	5.50	4.53	3.94	4.02	4.15	4.72	5.08	4.00	2.65	4.50E1
8.0	6.87	5.41	4.56	4.60	4.73	5.34	5.68	4.30	2.76	7.67E1
10.0	1.08E1	7.76	6.08	6.01	6.06	6.73	6.95	4.90	2.97	2.32E2
15.0	3.38E1	1.90E1	1.21E1	1.11E1	1.04E1	1.08E1	1.03E1	6.26	3.41	4.33E3
20.0	1.05E2	4.59E1	2.31E1	1.91E1	1.64E1	1.57E1	1.39E1	7.44	3.77	9.54E4
25.0	3.19E2	1.08E2	4.26E1	3.13E1	2.43E1	2.12E1	1.77E1	8.48	4.07	2.33E6
30.0	9.44E2	2.49E2	7.57E1	4.03E1	3.44E1	2.74E1	2.15E1	9.41	4.33	6.02E7
35.0	2.73E3	5.62E2	1.31E2	7.51E1	4.70E1	3.41E1	2.55E1	1.03E1	4.56	1.61E9
40.0	7.75E3	1.24E3	2.21E2	1.11E2	6.24E1	4.14E1	2.94E1	1.11E1	4.76	4.35E10
Uranium										
0.5	1.37	1.42	1.43	1.46	1.44	1.49	1.47	1.37	1.45	1.06
1.0	1.56	1.60	1.58	1.61	1.58	1.68	1.72	1.61	1.58	1.08
2.0	1.90	1.89	1.82	1.86	1.87	2.02	2.14	1.94	1.76	1.11
3.0	2.33	2.23	2.11	2.16	2.19	2.41	2.58	2.23	1.89	1.12
4.0	2.87	2.64	2.44	2.49	2.54	2.81	3.01	2.47	1.99	1.14
5.0	3.54	3.12	2.80	2.85	2.91	3.24	3.45	2.69	2.07	1.15
6.0	4.36	3.69	3.22	3.27	3.33	3.70	3.90	2.92	2.17	1.15
7.0	5.40	4.36	3.69	3.72	3.77	4.18	4.35	3.12	2.24	1.16
8.0	6.67	5.16	4.22	4.21	4.24	4.68	4.80	3.31	2.31	1.17
10.0	1.03E1	7.22	5.48	5.35	5.29	5.75	5.74	3.68	2.44	1.18
15.0	3.04E1	1.66E1	1.02E1	9.27	8.57	8.76	8.12	4.47	2.71	1.21
20.0	9.00E1	3.79E1	1.84E1	1.51E1	1.28E1	1.22E1	1.05E1	5.11	2.93	1.23
25.0	2.61E2	8.48E1	3.20E1	2.37E1	1.82E1	1.59E1	1.30E1	5.67	3.10	1.24
30.0	7.43E2	1.86E2	5.40E1	3.56E1	2.47E1	1.99E1	1.54E1	6.15	3.25	1.26
35.0	2.07E3	4.01E2	8.92E1	5.22E1	3.26E1	2.42E1	1.79E1	6.59	3.38	1.27
40.0	5.68E3	8.50E2	1.44E2	7.45E1	4.18E1	2.86E1	2.03E1	6.99	3.49	1.28

[a] *Mean free path.* The average distance that photons of a given energy travel before an interaction in a given medium occurs. It is equal to the reciprocal of the attenuation coefficient. Thus, the distance x in ordinary units can be converted into the dimensionless distance μx, the number of *mean free path* lengths (mfp).

Table 6.5.2 Energy Absorption Buildup Factors (Continued)

	Energy (MeV)									
R(mfp)[a]	10	8	6	5	4	3	2	1	0.5	0.1
Water										
0.5	1.21	1.23	1.27	1.29	1.31	1.34	1.38	1.47	1.61	2.36
1.0	1.38	1.44	1.55	1.57	1.63	1.71	1.83	2.08	2.45	4.52
2.0	1.70	1.82	1.98	2.10	2.26	2.47	2.82	3.62	4.87	1.17E1
3.0	2.00	2.17	2.43	2.62	2.87	3.24	3.87	5.50	8.29	2.35E1
4.0	2.29	2.52	2.87	3.12	3.48	4.01	4.99	7.66	1.27E1	4.06E1
5.0	2.57	2.86	3.31	3.63	4.09	4.81	6.16	1.01E1	1.81E1	6.40E1
6.0	2.85	3.20	3.74	4.14	4.71	5.62	7.38	1.28E1	2.46E1	9.48E1
7.0	3.13	3.53	4.16	4.64	5.33	6.45	8.66	1.57E1	3.22E1	1.34E2
8.0	3.40	3.86	4.59	5.14	5.95	7.28	9.97	1.89E1	4.08E1	1.83E2
10.0	3.94	4.51	5.43	6.14	7.20	8.98	12.7	2.60E1	6.18E1	3.14E2
15.0	5.24	6.08	7.49	8.62	10.3	13.4	20.1	4.74E1	1.37E2	9.17E2
20.0	6.51	7.61	9.52	11.1	13.5	17.8	28.0	7.35E1	2.47E2	2.12E3
25.0	7.75	9.10	11.5	13.5	16.6	22.4	36.4	1.04E2	3.95E2	4.26E3
30.0	8.97	10.6	13.5	15.9	19.8	27.1	45.2	1.38E2	5.82E2	7.78E3
35.0	10.2	12.2	15.5	18.3	23.0	31.8	54.3	1.75E2	8.09E2	1.31E4
40.0	11.3	14.1	17.9	20.7	26.1	36.5	63.6	2.14E2	1.08E3	2.03E4
Air										
0.5	1.20	1.23	1.27	1.29	1.31	1.34	1.38	1.47	1.60	2.35
1.0	1.37	1.43	1.52	1.57	1.63	1.71	1.83	2.08	2.44	4.46
2.0	1.68	1.80	1.97	2.09	2.25	2.46	2.81	3.60	4.84	1.14E1
3.0	1.97	2.15	2.41	2.60	2.85	3.22	3.86	5.46	8.21	2.25E1
4.0	2.26	2.50	2.85	3.11	3.46	4.00	4.96	7.60	1.26E1	3.84E1
5.0	2.54	2.84	3.28	3.61	4.07	4.79	6.13	1.00E1	1.79E1	5.99E1
6.0	2.82	3.17	3.71	4.12	4.69	5.60	7.35	1.27E1	2.42E1	8.78E1
7.0	3.10	3.51	4.14	4.62	5.31	6.43	8.61	1.56E1	3.16E1	1.23E2
8.0	3.37	3.84	4.57	5.12	5.94	7.26	9.92	1.88E1	4.01E1	1.66E2
10.0	3.92	4.49	5.42	6.13	7.19	8.97	12.6	2.58E1	6.06E1	2.82E2
15.0	5.25	6.08	7.51	8.63	10.3	13.4	20.0	4.70E1	1.34E2	8.00E2
20.0	6.55	7.64	9.58	11.1	13.5	17.9	27.9	7.28E1	2.41E2	1.81E3
25.0	7.84	9.17	11.6	13.6	16.7	22.5	36.2	1.03E2	3.85E2	3.57E3
30.0	9.11	10.7	13.6	16.1	19.9	27.2	45.0	1.36E2	5.67E2	6.43E3
35.0	10.4	12.3	15.4	18.5	23.1	32.0	54.0	1.73E2	7.88E2	1.06E4
40.0	11.6	14.1	16.9	21.0	26.3	36.7	63.2	2.12E2	1.05E3	1.57E4

[a] *Mean free path.* The average distance that photons of a given energy travel before an interaction in a given medium occurs. It is equal to the reciprocal of the attenuation coefficient. Thus, the distance x in ordinary units can be converted into the dimensionless distance μx, the number of *mean free path* lengths (mfp).

(continued)

Table 6.5.2 Energy Absorption Buildup Factors (Continued)

	Energy (MeV)									
R(mfp)[a]	**10**	**8**	**6**	**5**	**4**	**3**	**2**	**1**	**0.5**	**0.1**
Concrete										
0.5	1.18	1.21	1.25	1.32	1.31	1.34	1.39	1.49	1.66	2.39
1.0	1.34	1.40	1.48	1.57	1.62	1.70	1.83	2.11	2.55	3.89
2.0	1.61	1.74	1.92	2.05	2.22	2.44	2.80	3.59	4.89	7.06
3.0	1.88	2.07	2.35	2.54	2.81	3.19	3.82	5.35	7.89	1.04E1
4.0	2.16	2.40	2.77	3.04	3.41	3.96	4.92	7.35	1.16E1	1.41E1
5.0	2.43	2.73	3.20	3.55	4.03	4.76	6.07	9.61	1.60E1	1.79E1
6.0	2.71	3.07	3.64	4.06	4.66	5.58	7.28	1.21E1	2.11E1	2.21E1
7.0	2.99	3.41	4.08	4.58	5.29	6.42	8.55	1.48E1	2.70E1	2.66E1
8.0	3.28	3.76	4.52	5.10	5.94	7.27	9.86	1.78E1	3.37E1	3.15E1
10.0	3.85	4.45	5.42	6.16	7.24	9.02	1.26E1	2.43E1	4.96E1	4.21E1
15.0	5.33	6.21	7.70	8.86	1.06E1	1.36E1	2.00E1	4.40E1	1.05E2	7.47E1
20.0	6.86	8.00	1.00E1	1.16E1	1.41E1	1.84E1	2.81E1	6.79E1	1.83E2	1.16E2
25.0	8.45	9.83	1.24E1	1.44E1	1.76E1	2.33E1	3.67E1	9.55E1	2.86E2	1.65E2
30.0	1.01E1	1.17E1	1.47E1	1.73E1	2.12E1	2.84E1	4.57E1	1.26E2	4.14E2	2.22E2
35.0	1.17E1	1.37E1	1.68E1	2.02E1	2.48E1	3.36E1	5.50E1	1.60E2	5.67E2	2.86E2
40.0	1.34E1	1.60E1	1.86E1	2.39E1	2.85E1	3.88E1	6.46E1	1.97E2	7.47E2	3.58E2

[a] *Mean free path.* The average distance that photons of a given energy travel before an interaction in a given medium occurs. It is equal to the reciprocal of the attenuation coefficient. Thus, the distance x in ordinary units can be converted into the dimensionless distance μx, the number of *mean free path* lengths (mfp).

Table 6.5.3 Correction Factors (Shield-Tissue Interface)[a] (After Trubey ORNL/RSIC-49/R1, 1991)

E	X_m	D_{int}	D_{max}	B_∞	B_{int}	B_c	C
Aluminum Medium							
0.10	0.0	8.573E −9	8.573E −9	6.896	8.105	8.105	1.17
0.15	0.0	1.632E −8	1.632E −8	8.885	9.952	9.952	1.12
0.20	0.0	2.379E −8	2.379E −8	9.390	10.26	10.26	1.09
0.30	0.0	3.601E −8	3.601E −8	9.184	9.757	9.757	1.06
0.40	0.0	4.570E −8	4.570E −8	8.680	9.096	9.096	1.05
0.50	0.0	5.327E −8	5.327E −8	8.137	8.454	8.454	1.04
0.60	0.0	5.996E −8	5.996E −8	7.663	7.916	7.916	1.03
0.80	0.0	6.931E −8	6.391E −8	6.928	7.105	7.105	1.02
1.00	0.0	7.684E −8	7.684E −8	6.389	6.523	6.523	1.02
1.50	0.0	9.138E −8	9.138E −8	5.502	5.578	5.578	1.01
2.00	0.0	1.006E −7	1.006E −7	4.967	5.012	5.012	1.01
3.00	0.0	1.122E −7	1.127E −7	4.253	4.263	4.263	1.00
Iron Medium							
0.10	1.0	2.749E −9	2.837E −9	1.828	2.628	2.712	1.48
0.15	0.5	6.101E −9	6.144E −0	2.870	3.723	3.749	1.31
0.20	0.0	1.093E −8	1.093E −8	3.858	4.709	4.709	1.22
0.30	0.0	1.965E −8	1.965E −8	5.112	5.854	5.854	1.15
0.40	0.0	2.870E −8	2.870E −8	5.641	6.267	6.267	1.11
0.50	0.0	3.622E −8	3.662E −8	5.827	6.347	6.347	1.09
0.60	0.0	4.335E −8	4.335E −8	5.839	6.281	6.281	1.08
0.80	0.0	5.391E −8	5.391E −8	5.667	6.001	6.001	1.06
1.00	0.0	6.222E −8	6.222E −8	5.449	5.753	5.753	1.06
1.50	0.0	8.416E −8	8.416E −8	4.982	5.153	5.153	1.03
2.00	0.0	9.559E −8	9.559E −8	4.665	4.771	4.771	1.02
3.00	0.0	1.120E −7	1.102E −7	4.152	4.191	4.191	1.01

[a] Units

E = source energy (MeV)
X_m = depth in tissue where maximum dose occurs (cm)
D_{int} = dose rate at the interface (cGy h^{-1} cm^2 s)
D_{max} = dose rate maximum in tissue (cGy h cm^2 s)
B_∞ = inifinite medium buildup factor for plane parallel source
B_{int} = interface buildup factor for plane parallel source
B_c = corrected buildup factor
C = correction factor (B_c/B_∞)

(continued)

Table 6.5.3 Correction Factors (Shield-Tissue Interface)[a] (Continued)

E	X_m	D_{int}	D_{max}	B_∞	B_{int}	B_c	C
Tin Medium							
0.10	0.0	2.118E −9	2.118E −9	1.415	1.991	1.991	1.40
0.15	1.0	2.942E −9	3.083E −9	1.275	1.800	1.886	1.48
0.20	1.0	4.635E −9	4.772E −9	1.509	2.003	2.062	1.36
0.30	1.0	9.405E −9	9.521E −9	2.076	2.555	2.570	1.23
0.40	0.5	1.567E −8	1.568E −8	2.625	3.098	3.098	1.18
0.50	0.0	2.233E −8	2.233E −8	3.063	3.519	3.519	1.14
0.60	0.0	2.854E −8	2.854E −8	3.337	3.762	3.792	1.12
0.80	0.0	4.004E −8	4.004E −8	3.687	4.056	4.056	1.10
1.00	0.0	4.971E −8	4.971E −8	3.835	4.161	4.161	1.08
1.50	0.0	6.816E −8	6.816E −8	3.957	4.176	4.176	1.05
2.00	0.0	8.286E −8	8.286E −8	3.977	4.138	4.138	1.04
3.00	0.0	1.003E −7	1.003E −7	3.738	3.816	2.816	1.02
Tungsten Medium							
0.10	0.5	4.295E −9	4.320E −9	2.761	3.943	3.966	1.44
0.15	1.0	2.992E −9	3.067E −9	1.294	1.896	1.851	1.43
0.20	1.0	3.875E −9	3.984E −9	1.233	1.665	1.712	1.39
0.30	1.0	6.465E −9	6.559E −9	1.370	1.743	1.768	1.29
0.40	1.0	9.885E −9	9.965E −9	1.607	1.952	1.967	1.22
0.50	1.0	1.367E −8	1.371E −8	1.845	2.154	2.157	1.17
0.60	0.5	1.791E −8	1.793E −8	2.063	2.360	2.361	1.14
0.80	0.0	2.647E −8	2.647E −8	2.487	2.682	2.682	1.08
1.00	0.0	3.447E −8	3.447E −8	2.633	2.886	2.886	1.10
1.50	0.0	5.205E −8	5.205E −8	2.988	3.189	3.189	1.07
2.00	0.0	6.669E −8	6.669E −8	3.192	3.332	3.332	1.04
3.00	0.0	8.504E −8	8.504E −8	3.168	3.237	3.237	1.02

[a] Units

E = source energy (MeV)
X_m = depth in tissue where maximum dose occurs (cm)
D_{int} = dose rate at the interface (cGy h^{-1} cm^2 s)
D_{max} = dose rate maximum in tissue (cGy h cm^2 s)
B_∞ = inifinite medium buildup factor for plane parallel source
B_{int} = interface buildup factor for plane parallel source
B_c = corrected buildup factor
C = correction factor (B_c/B_∞)

Table 6.5.3 Correction Factors (Shield-Tissue Interface)[a] (Continued)

E	X_m	D_{int}	D_{max}	B_∞	B_{int}	B_c	C
Lead Medium							
0.10	0.5	1.005E −8	1.008E −8	6.475	9.406	9.434	1.46
0.15	1.0	3.389E −9	3.442E −9	1.540	2.078	2.110	1.37
0.20	1.0	3.796E −9	3.886E −9	1.252	1.660	1.699	1.36
0.30	1.0	5.970E −9	6.080E −9	1.300	1.640	1.670	1.29
0.40	1.0	8.796E −9	8.877E −9	1.459	1.765	1.781	1.22
0.50	1.0	1.198E −8	1.202E −8	1.635	1.921	1.927	1.18
0.60	0.5	1.547E −8	1.549E −8	1.801	2.071	2.073	1.15
0.80	0.5	2.251E −8	2.253E −8	2.079	2.326	2.236	1.12
1.00	0.0	2.953E −8	2.953E −8	2.296	2.525	2.525	1.10
1.50	0.0	4.627E −8	4.627E −8	2.656	2.835	2.835	1.07
2.00	0.0	6.022E −8	6.002E −8	2.883	3.011	3.011	1.04
3.00	0.0	7.805E −8	7.805E −8	2.906	2.971	2.971	1.02
Water Medium							
0.10	0.0	2.074E −8	2.074E −8	19.47	18.92	18.92	0.97
0.15	0.0	2.929E −8	2.929E −8	17.61	17.27	17.27	0.98
0.20	0.0	3.658E −8	3.658E −8	15.58	15.35	15.35	0.98
0.30	0.0	4.712E −8	4.712E −8	12.64	12.52	12.52	0.99
0.40	0.0	5.546E −8	5.546E −8	10.96	10.88	10.88	0.99
0.50	0.0	6.185E −8	6.185E −8	9.760	9.703	9.703	0.99
0.60	0.0	6.735E −8	6.735E −8	8.911	8.866	8.866	0.99
0.80	0.0	7.565E −8	7.565E −8	7.730	7.699	7.699	0.99
1.00	0.0	8.738E −8	8.738E −8	6.976	6.952	6.952	0.99
1.50	0.0	9.512E −8	0.512E −8	5.806	5.791	5.791	1.00
2.00	0.0	1.029E −7	1.029E −7	5.129	5.118	5.118	1.00
3.00	0.0	1.125E −7	1.120E −7	4.276	4.268	4.268	1.00

[a] Units

E = source energy (MeV)
X_m = depth in tissue where maximum dose occurs (cm)
D_{int} = dose rate at the interface (cGy h^{-1} cm^2 s)
D_{max} = dose rate maximum in tissue (cGy h cm^2 s)
B_∞ = inifinite medium buildup factor for plane parallel source
B_{int} = interface buildup factor for plane parallel source
B_c = corrected buildup factor
C = correction factor (B_c/B_∞)

(continued)

Table 6.5.3 Correction Factors (Shield-Tissue Interface)[a] (Continued)

E	X_m	D_{int}	D_{max}	B_∞	B_{int}	B_c	C
Concrete Medium							
0.10	0.0	7.196E −9	7.196E −9	5.752	6.881	6.881	1.20
0.15	0.0	1.446E −8	1.446E −8	7.703	8.778	8.778	1.14
0.20	0.0	2.159E −8	2.159E −8	8.327	9.244	9.244	1.11
0.30	0.0	3.329E −8	3.329E −8	8.277	8.917	8.917	1.08
0.40	0.0	4.238E −8	4.238E −8	7.841	8.325	8.325	1.06
0.50	0.0	4.961E −8	4.961E −8	7.388	7.774	7.774	1.05
0.60	0.0	5.549E −8	5.549E −8	6.960	7.323	7.323	1.05
0.80	0.0	6.412E −8	6.412E −8	6.243	6.475	6.475	1.04
1.00	0.0	7.064E −8	7.064E −8	5.715	5.899	5.899	1.03
1.50	0.0	8.025E −8	8.025E −8	4.793	4.907	4.907	1.02
2.00	0.0	8.580E −8	8.580E −8	4.205	4.286	4.286	1.02
3.00	0.0	9.233E −8	9.233E −8	3.473	3.515	3.515	1.01

[a] Units
E = source energy (MeV)
X_m = depth in tissue where maximum dose occurs (cm)
D_{int} = dose rate at the interface (cGy h^{-1} cm^2 s)
D_{max} = dose rate maximum in tissue (cGy h cm^2 s)
B_∞ = inifinite medium buildup factor for plane parallel source
B_{int} = interface buildup factor for plane parallel source
B_c = corrected buildup factor
C = correction factor (B_c/B_∞)

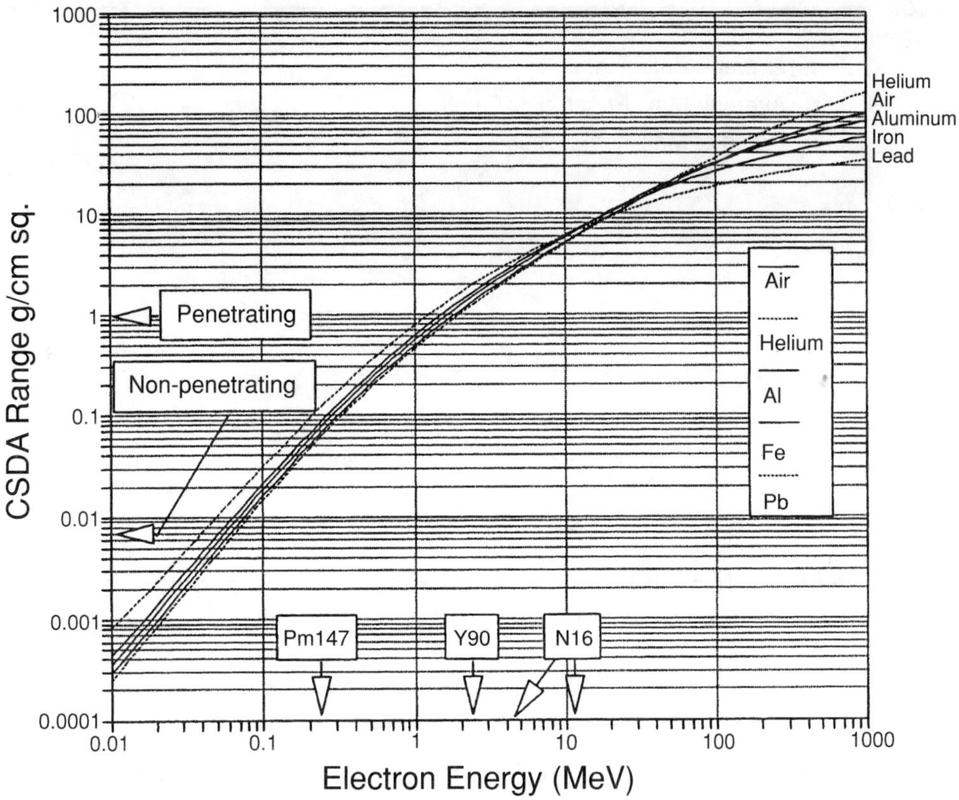

Figure 6.2 Electron Range in Selected Substances. Penetrating (density 1.0) and non-penetrating (density 1.127) refer to skin penetration (7 mg cm^{-2}). CSDA Range represents the average path length traveled by an electron as it slows down from its initial energy to its final energy. (After ICRU Report 37, 1988 as generated by Slaback, 1996)

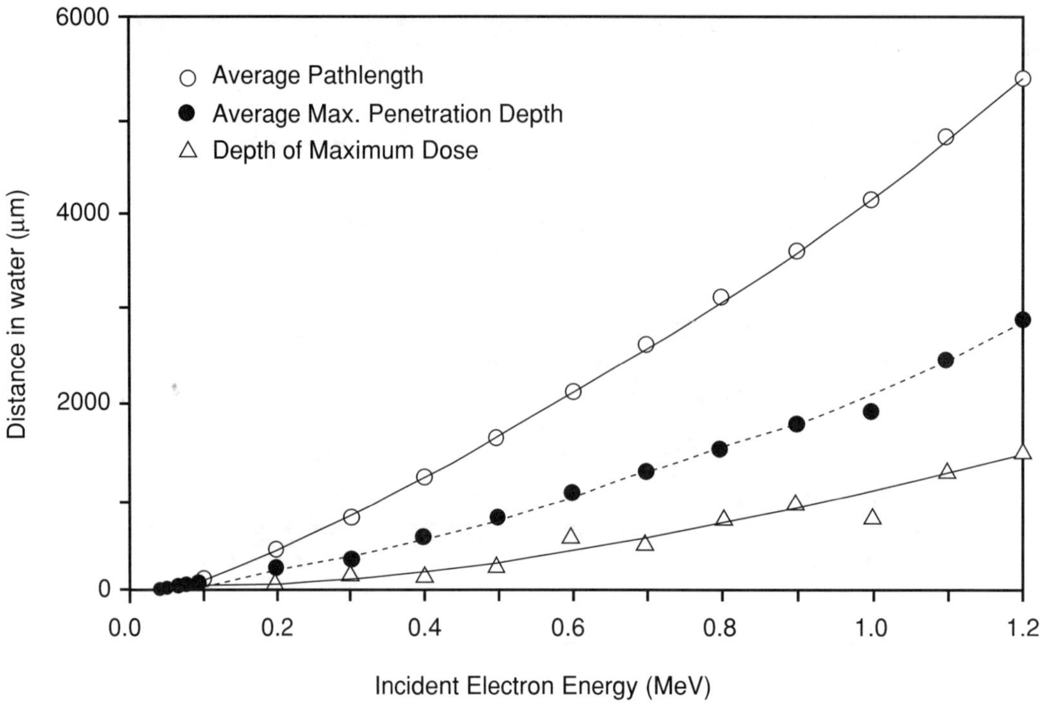

Figure 6.3 Average Path Length, Average Maximum Penetration Depth and Depth of Maximum Dose as Functions of Energy for 100 Electrons Normally Incident on Water Surface at Each Incident Energy Shown. (Reproduced from the journal *Health Physics* with permission from the Health Physics Society from Turner *et al.*, 1988)

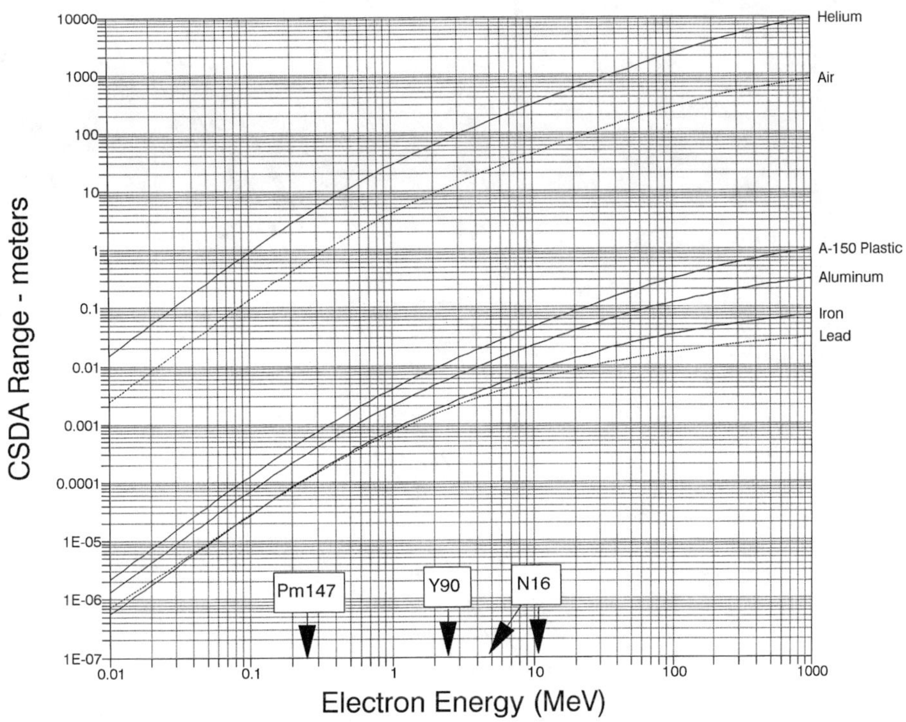

Figure 6.4 The Range of Electrons as a Function of Energy in the Various Materials Indicated. Penetration refers to skin. (After ICRU Report 37, 1988)

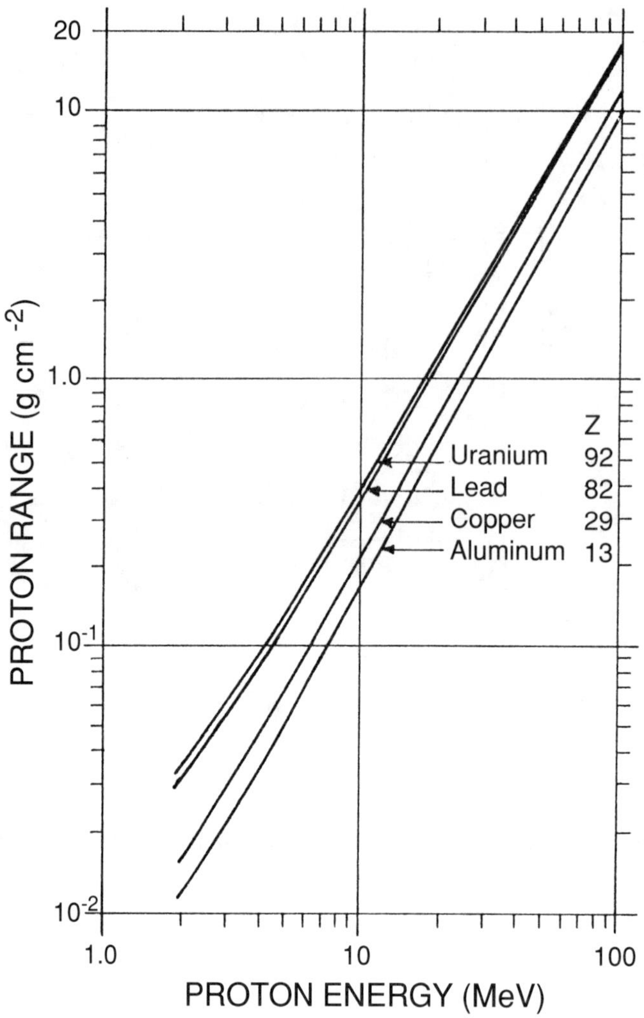

Figure 6.5 Range of Protons. (Courtesy NCRP from Report No. 51, 1977)

Range of protons (R_p) in several materials, as a function of incident proton energy. Data were obtained from Barkas and Berger (1964). Ranges of other light ions of a given energy, E, can be estimated from the following relationships.

Deuterons	(^{2}He + +):	$2R_p$ (at E/2)
Tritons	(^{3}H +):	$3R_p$ (at E/3)
Helium-3	(^{3}He +):	$3R_p$ (at E/3)
	(^{3}He + +):	(3/4)R_p (at E/3)
Helium-4	(^{4}He +):	$4R_p$ (at E/4)
	(^{4}He + +):	R_p (at E/4)

These relationships were derived from Spinks and Woods (1964).
Example: A 4 MeV deuteron has a range of 2 times the range of a 2 MeV proton, i.e., $2 \times 1.2 \times 10^{-2} = 2.4 \times 10^{-2}$ g cm^{-2} in aluminum (density 2.7 g cm^{-3}), or 8.9×10^{-3} cm thickness.

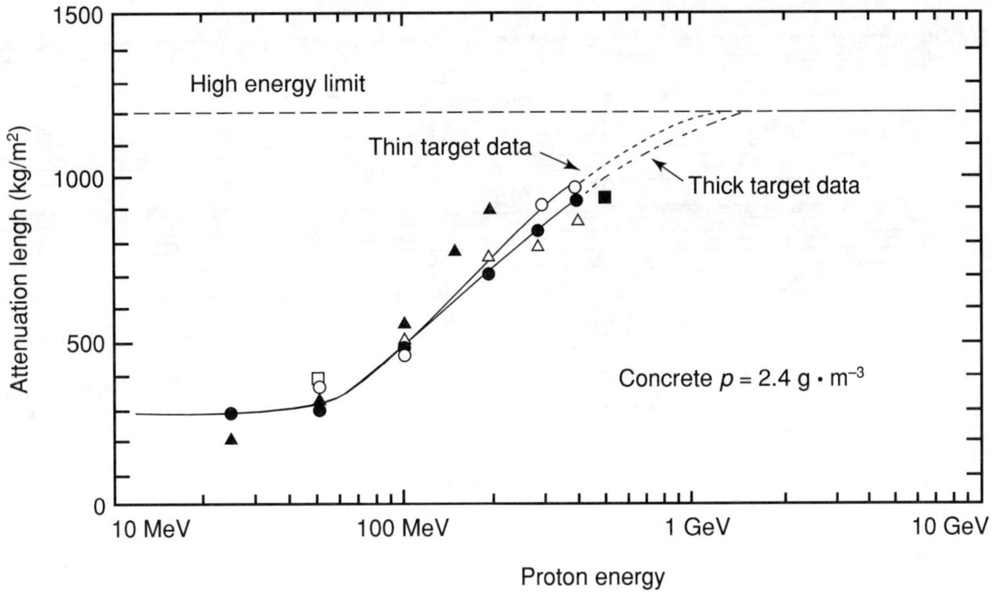

Figure 6.6 Effective Attenuation Length in Concrete as a Function of Proton Energy. (From IAEA 283, 1988)

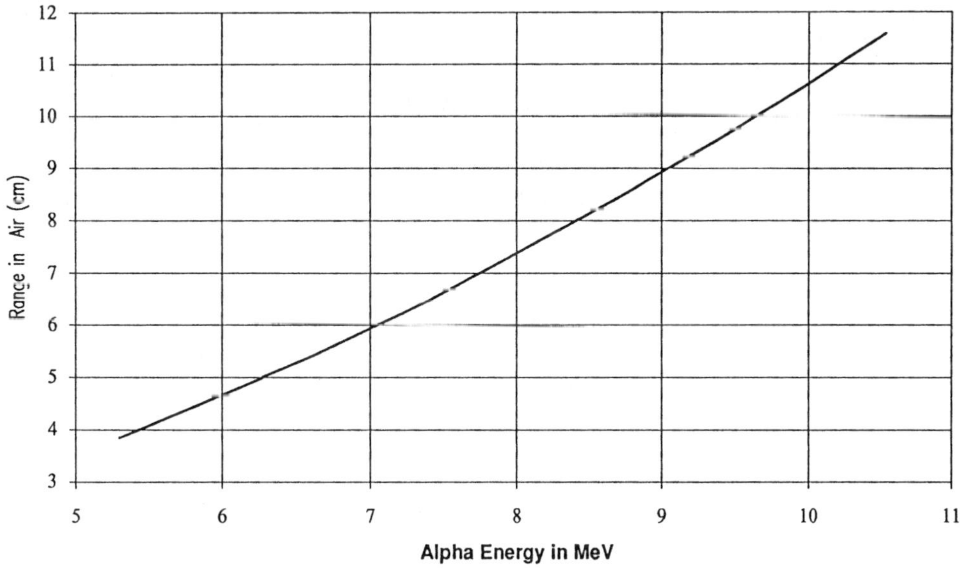

Figure 6.7 Alpha Particle Range in Air. (Courtesy NAS/NRC based on PB-212-907, 1964)

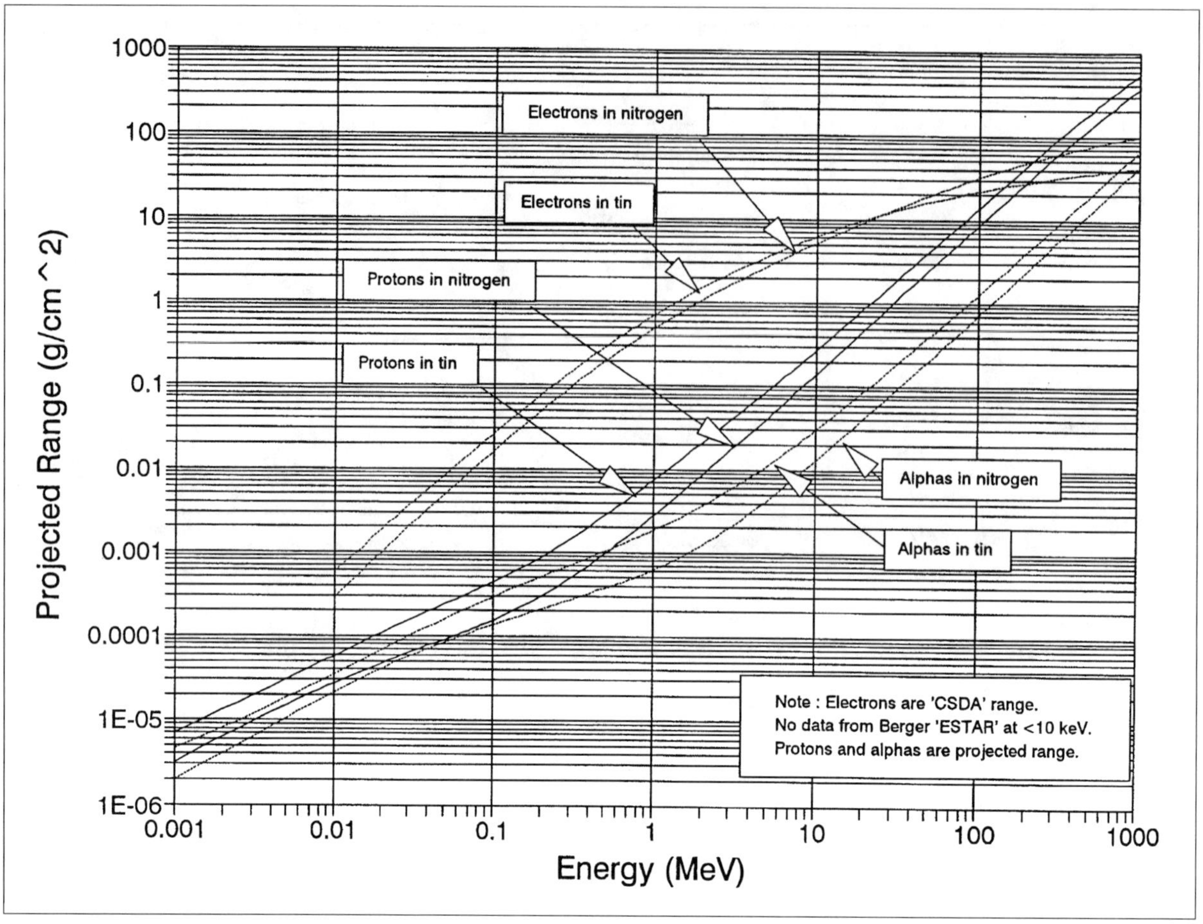

Figure 6.8 Projected Charged Particle Range in Nitrogen and Tin. (From Slaback, personal communication, 1996)

Table 6.6 Protective Barrier Transmission Factor (B) per Curie for 2.5 mR per Hour (Corresponding to 100 mR per 40 hours Weekly Exposure) (Courtesy NCRP from Report No. 49, 1976)

Distance (m)	^{60}Co	^{226}Ra	^{192}Ir	^{137}Cs	^{198}Au
0.5	0.00048	0.00076	0.00114	0.00188	0.0027
1	0.00192	0.00303	0.00455	0.0075	0.0107
1.5	0.0043	0.0068	0.0102	0.0169	0.024
2	0.0077	0.012	0.0182	0.0301	0.043
2.5	0.012	0.019	0.028	0.047	0.067
3	0.0173	0.027	0.404	0.068	0.096

Notes:
1. Applying the appropriate value of B, the necessary thickness of shielding material may be obtained from Figures 6.9, 6.10 and 6.11.
2. If protection is required for non-occupational exposure, add one tenth-value layer thickness for the shielding material chosen.
3. For quantities of material other than a curie, the barrier transmission factor (B) should be adjusted in inverse proportion.

Example:
The required barrier thickness for a radiation worker at a 2-meter distance from a 50 mCi (0.05 Ci) ^{60}Co source is determined from:

$$B = 0.0077 \text{ (from table)} \times \frac{1 \text{ Ci}}{0.05 \text{ Ci}} = 0.154.$$

For concrete, the value of B for ^{60}Co indicates a thickness of 21 cm of concrete. To protect persons other than radiation workers, one tenth-value layer of concrete or 20.6 cm would be added, totaling about 42 cm.

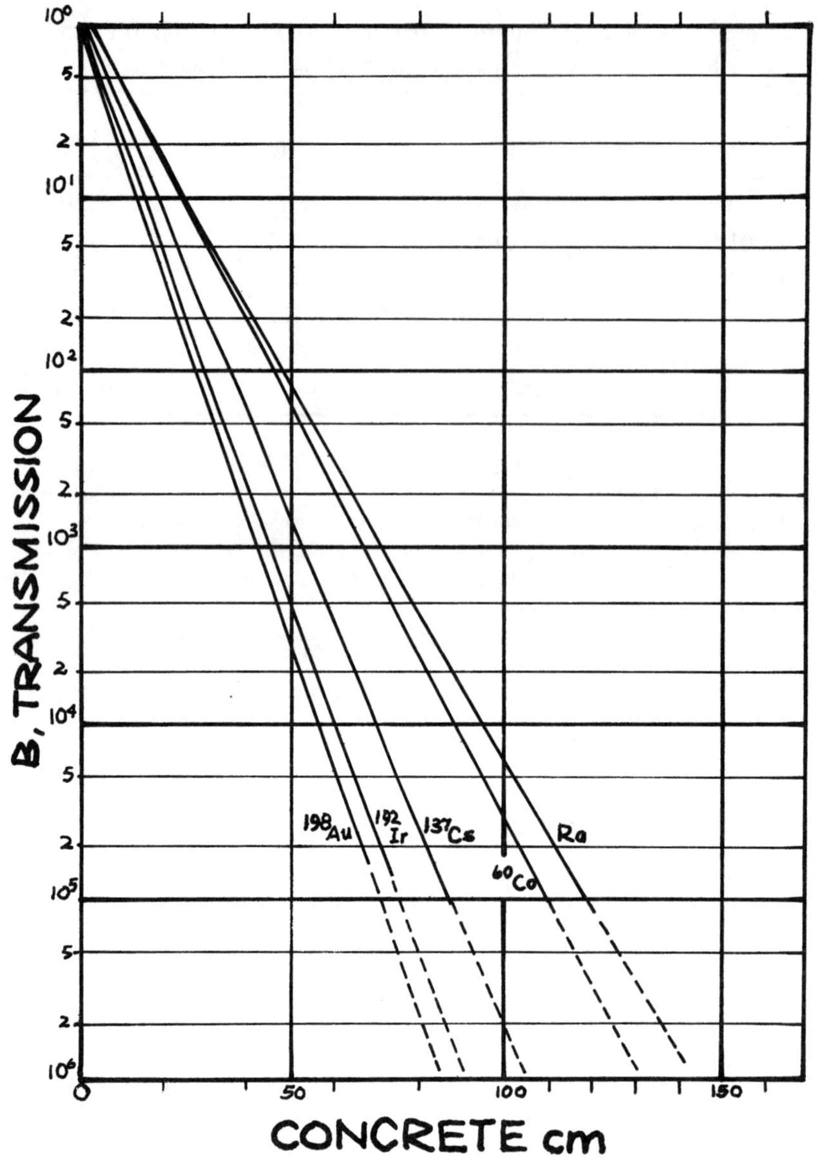

Figure 6.9 Transmission Through Concrete, Density 2.35 g cm^{-3} (147 lb ft^{-3}), of Gamma Rays from Selected Radionuclides. (Courtesy NCRP from Report 49, 1976) Radium (Wyckoff and Kennedy); ^{60}Co, ^{137}Cs, ^{198}Au (Kirn *et al.*); ^{192}Ir (Ritz)

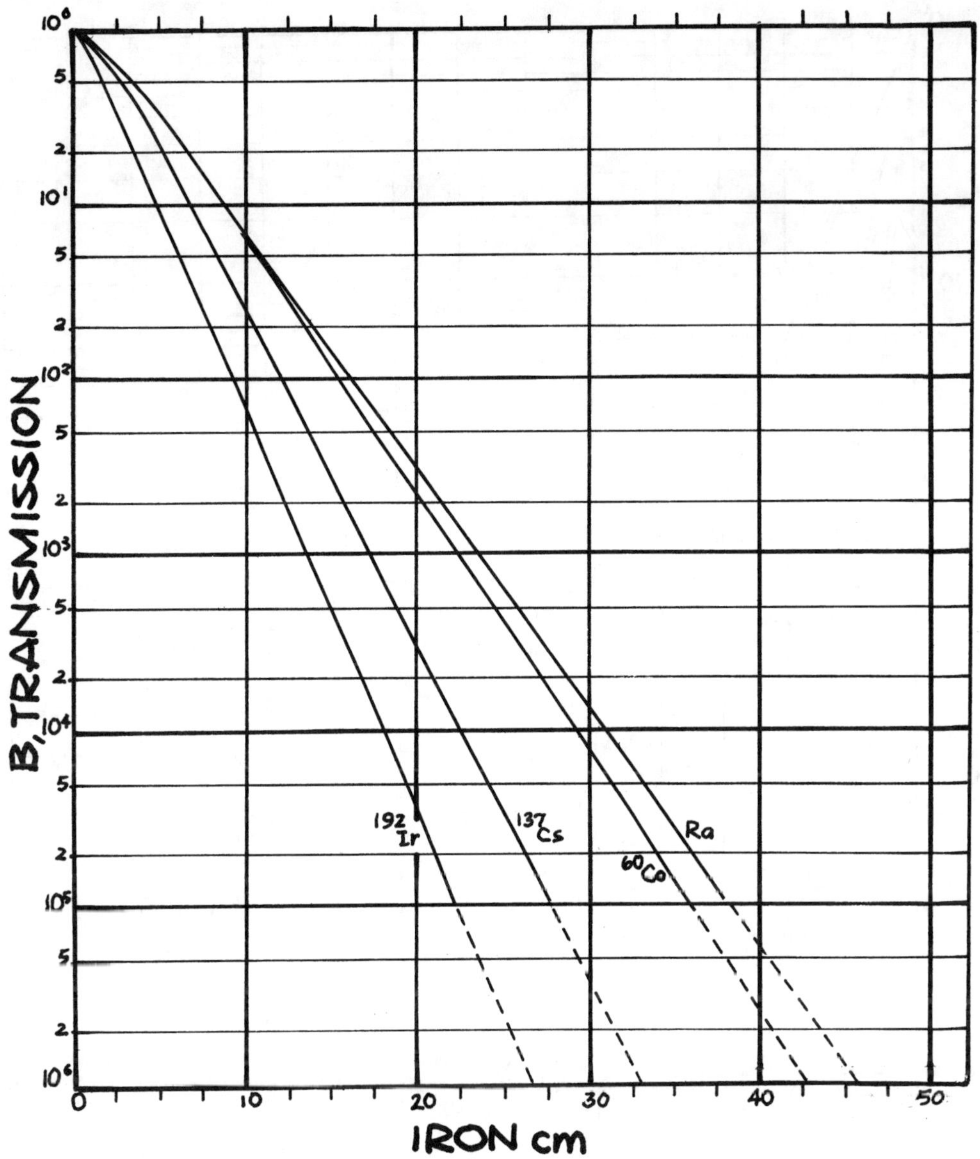

Figure 6.10 Transmission Through Iron of Gamma Rays from Selected Radionuclides. (Courtesy NCRP from Report 49, 1976) Radium (Wyckoff and Kennedy); ^{60}Co, ^{137}Cs (Kirn *et al.*); ^{192}Ir (Ritz)

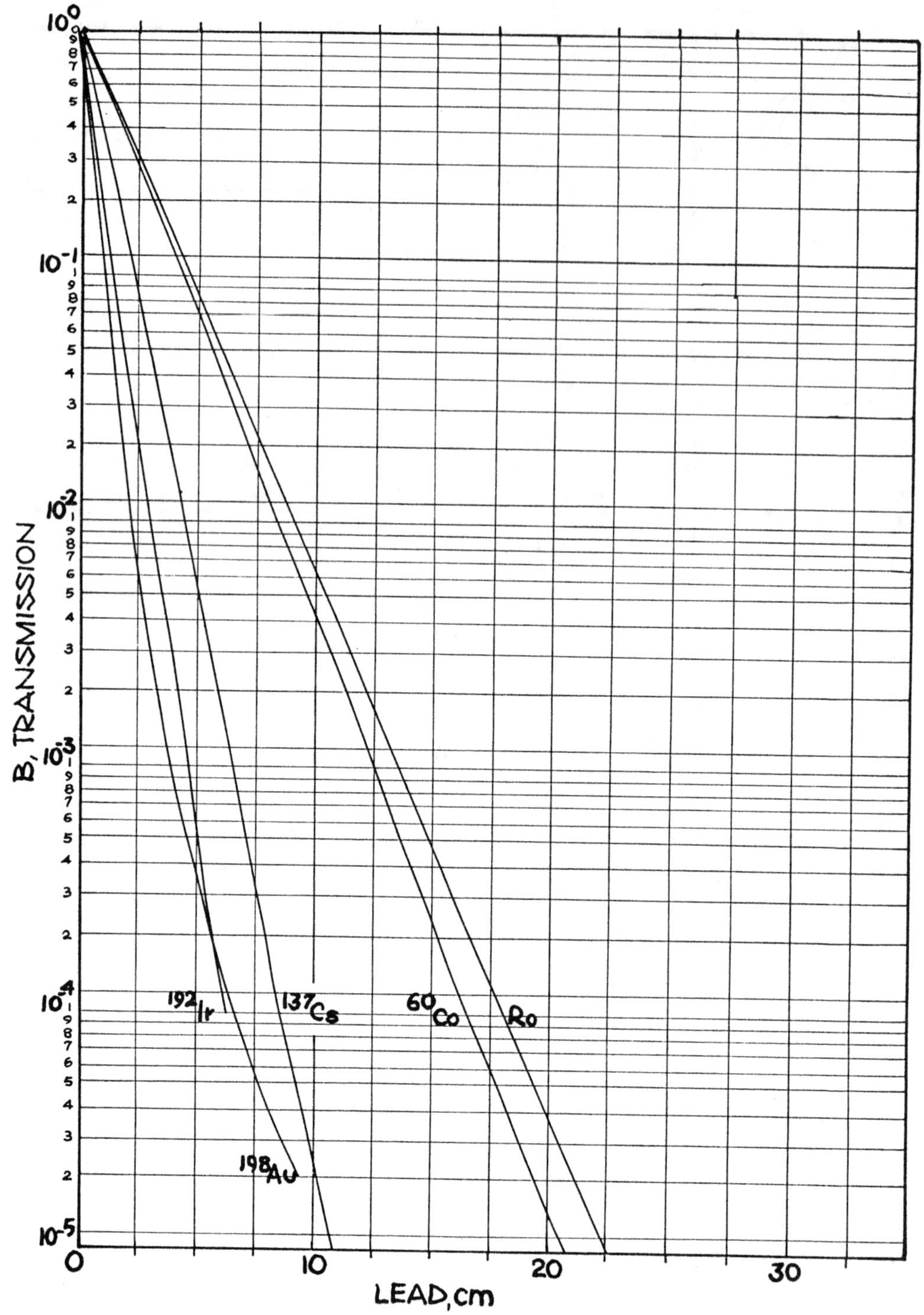

Figure 6.11 Transmission Through Lead of Gamma Rays from Selected Radionuclides (Courtesy NCRP from Report 49, 1976) Radium (Wyckoff and Kennedy); ^{60}Co, ^{137}Cs, ^{198}Au (Kim *et al*); ^{192}Ir (Ritz)

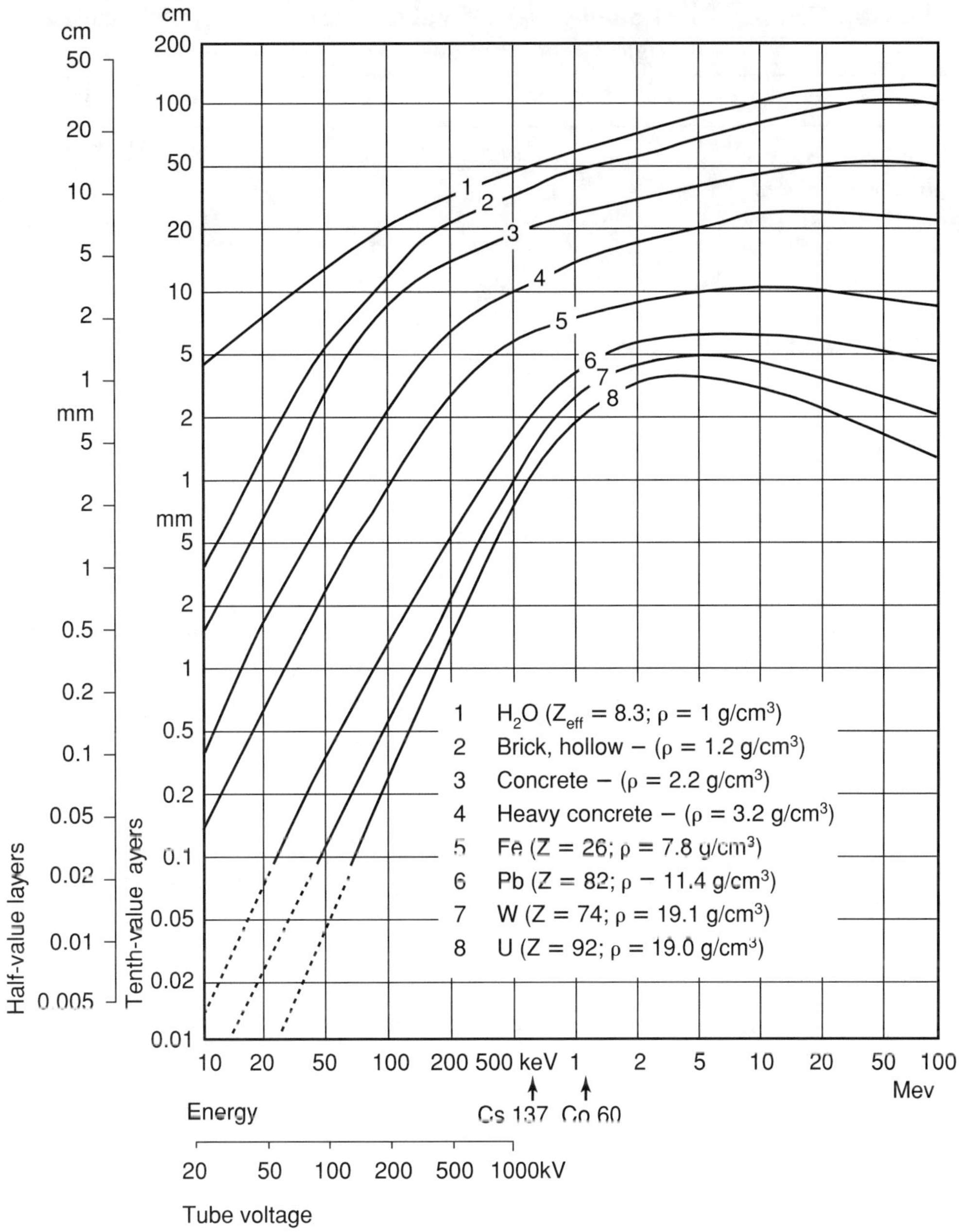

Figure 6.12 Average Half-Value and Tenth-Value Layers of Shielding Materials (Broad Beams).
(Courtesy NBS from Handbook 138, 1982 after Wachsman and Drexler, 1975)

Table 6.7 Tenth-Value Layers of Various Materials at 60 kVp (Reproduced from the journal *Health Physics* with permission from the Health Physics Society from Rajhavendron et al., 1982)

Masonite (g/cm^2)	Concrete (g/cm^2)	Pyrex Glass (g/cm^2)	Water (g/cm^2)	Lead (g/cm^2)	Gypsum (g/cm^2)
17.5	2.1	4.6	13.1	0.96	1.86

Table 6.8 Comparison of Studies of Half-Value Layers and Tenth-Value Layers at High Attenuation (After Rossi *et al.*, 1991)

Material	50 kVp	70 kVp	100 kVp	125 kVp
	HVLs (mm)			
Gypsum wallboard				
Rossi et al., 1991	14.45	26.15	39.29	42.65
Simpkin, 1989[a]	16.86	23.42	33.58	48.63
Glaze et al., 1979	11.00	22.00	46.00	54.00
Steel				
Rossi et al., 1991	0.34	0.78	1.42	2.15
Simpkin, 1989[a]	0.46	0.83	1.80	3.27
Trout et al., 1975	0.30	1.00	2.70	3.60
Plate glass				
Rossi et al., 1991	5.75	9.41	15.83	18.05
Simpkin, 1989[a]	8.47	10.66	15.06	17.54
Trout et al., 1959	5.30	8.90	13.50	16.00
Concrete				
Rossi et al., 1991			12.90	15.66
Simpkin, 1989[a]	9.32	10.36	15.31	18.33
Trout et al., 1959	5.08	12.70	17.78	20.32
NCRP Report No. 49, 1976	4.30	8.40	16.00	20.00
	TVLs (mm)			
Gypsum wallboard				
Rossi et al., 1991	44.30	91.68	128.81	152.10
Glaze et al., 1979	39.00	79.00	112.00	129.00
Steel				
Rossi et al., 1991	0.77	2.37	5.51	7.18
Trout et al., 1975	0.90	3.30	9.00	12.00
Plate glass				
Rossi et al., 1991	16.31	33.71	44.42	51.26
Trout et al., 1974	17.80	29.70	45.00	53.30
Concrete				
Rossi et al., 1991	—	—	42.19	49.57
NCRP Report No. 49, 1976	15.00	28.00	53.00	66.00

[a] HVLs for 50 and 125 kVp obtained by extrapolation and interpolation.

Table 6.9 Computed Broad-Beam Transmission of Constant-Potential Generated X-Rays

(Reproduced from the journal *Health Physics* with permission from the Health Physics Society from Simpkin, 1989)

A Monte Carlo calculation was performed to determine the transmission of broad constant-potential x-ray beams through Pb, concrete, gypsum wallboard, steel and plate glass. The EGS4 code system was used with a simple broad-beam geometric model to generate exposure transmission curves for published 70, 100, 120 and 140 kVcp x-ray spectra. These curves are compared to measured three-phase generated x-ray transmission data in the literature and found to be reasonable. For calculational ease the data are fit to an equation previously shown to describe such curves quite well. These calculated transmission data are then used to create three-phase shielding tables for Pb and concrete, as well as other materials not available in Report No. 49 of the NCRP.

Because SI units are used in the subject paper, a note on their implementation in the methods of NCRP 49 is in order. As in NCRP 49, it is assumed that an x-ray exposure of 2.58×10^{-4} C kg^{-1} will yield to soft tissue an absorbed dose of 0.01 Gy and a dose equivalent of 0.01 Sv. Also, since the design exposure P must be expressed in SI units of dose equivalence, the transmission requirement for leakage radiation (equation 5m of Appendix B, NCRP 49) must be modified. In SI units, this should read:

$$B_{Lx} = \frac{P(d_{\text{sec}})^2(60I)}{WT}, \quad (1)$$

where P is in mSv, d_{sec} is the secondary distance in m, I is the maximum rated continuous tube current in mA, W is the workload in mA-min and T is the occupancy factor.

The beam employed had a half-value layer of 3.00 mm Al at 80 kVcp and a primary output at this potential at 1 m of 3.72 mGy per mA-min (6.2 mR per mAs). This very accurately represents a modern diagnostic x-ray machine. The spectra generated at 70, 100, 120 and 140 kVcp from this tube were investigated. It is described below in Table 6.9.1.

Table 6.9.1 Useful Beam Data for Constant-Potential Generation, GE Maxiray-125B X-Ray Tube (After Fewell *et al.*, 1981)

Potential (kVcp)	Normalized Output (mSv/mA-min at 1 m)	First HVL (mm Al)
70	2.88	2.64
100	5.64	3.77
120	7.62	4.51
140	9.66	5.26

The characteristics of the barrier materials appear in Table 6.9.2.

Table 6.9.2 Density and Elemental Composition Assumed for Concrete, Plate Glass and Steel

	ρ g cm^{-3}	H	C	O	Na	Mg	Al	Si	S	K	Ca	Fe
Concrete[a]	2.35	.0056		.4983	.0171	.0024	.0454	.3152	.0012	.0192	.0826	.0122
Glass[b]	2.5			.4890	.0990	.0146	.0004	.3382	.0015	.0001	.0555	.0020
Steel	7.83		.01									.990

[a] Data for concrete taken from Table 1-3 of Hubbell, 1969.
[b] Data for plate glass corresponds to the mixture listed in Table 1 of Simpkin, 1987b.

For computational ease, the curves for each potential and shielding material were fit to the model of Archer et al. (1983) using a non-linear least-squares fitting routine. This equation has the form

$$K_{\mu x} = K_0 \left[\left(1 + \frac{\beta}{\alpha}\right) e^{\alpha \gamma x} - \frac{\beta}{\alpha} \right]^{-1/\gamma}, \qquad (2)$$

where x is the material thickness and K_0 is the value of $K_{\mu x}$ with no shielding material. K_0 is the radiation output (mSv/mA-min at 1 m) of the primary x-ray beam. The values α, β and γ are the parameters of the fit and are given in Table 6.9.3. These fitting parameters are taken from a compilation of published transmission curves (Simpkin, 1995). Also given in this table is the reduced χ^2 of the fit. Note that the transmission B is simply $K_{\mu x}/K_0$. The solid curves shown in Figure 6.13 through 6.18 are the fits to this equation.

Table 6.9.3 Fitting Parameters of Computed Constant-Potential Transmission Data to Eqn (2)

(From Simpkin, 1995)

	Lead			Concrete			Gypsum		
kVp	α (mm^{-1})	β (mm^{-1})	γ	α (mm^{-1})	β (mm^{-1})	γ	α (mm^{-1})	β (mm^{-1})	γ
25	49.52	194	0.3037	0.3904	1.645	0.2757	0.1576	0.7175	0.3048
30	38.8	178	0.3473	0.3173	1.698	0.3593	0.1208	0.7043	0.3613
35	29.55	164.7	0.3948	0.2528	1.807	0.4648	0.08878	0.6988	0.4245
40				0.1297	0.178	0.2189			
45				0.1095	0.1741	0.2269			
50	8.801	27.28	0.2957	0.09032	0.1712	0.2324	0.03883	0.0873	0.5105
55	7.839	25.92	0.3499	0.07422	0.1697	0.2454	0.03419	0.08315	0.5606
60	6.951	24.89	0.4198	0.06251	0.1692	0.2733	0.02985	0.07961	0.6169
65	6.13	24.09	0.5019	0.05528	0.1696	0.3217	0.02609	0.07597	0.6756
70	5.369	23.49	0.5881	0.05087	0.1696	0.3847	0.02302	0.07163	0.7299
75	4.666	22.69	0.6618	0.04797	0.1663	0.4492	0.02066	0.06649	0.775
80	4.04	21.69	0.7187	0.04583	0.1549	0.4926	0.01886	0.06093	0.8103
85	3.504	20.37	0.755	0.04398	0.1348	0.4943	0.01746	0.05558	0.8392
90	3.067	18.83	0.7726	0.04228	0.1137	0.469	0.01633	0.05039	0.8585
95	2.731	17.07	0.7714	0.04068	0.09705	0.4406	0.01543	0.04571	0.8763
100	2.5	15.28	0.7557	0.03925	0.08567	0.4273	0.01466	0.04171	0.8939
105	2.364	13.41	0.7239	0.03808	0.07862	0.4394	0.01397	0.03815	0.908
110	2.296	11.7	0.6827	0.03715	0.07436	0.4752	0.01336	0.03521	0.9244
115	2.265	10.21	0.6363	0.03636	0.07201	0.5319	0.01283	0.03271	0.9423
120	2.246	8.95	0.5873	0.03566	0.07109	0.6073	0.01235	0.03047	0.9566
125	2.219	7.923	0.5386	0.03502	0.07113	0.6974	0.01192	0.02863	0.9684
130	2.17	7.094	0.4909	0.03445	0.0716	0.7969	0.01155	0.02702	0.9802
135	2.102	6.45	0.4469	0.03394	0.07263	0.9099	0.01122	0.02561	0.9901
140	2.009	5.916	0.4018	0.03345	0.07476	1.047	0.01088	0.02436	0.9964
145	1.895	5.498	0.358	0.03296	0.07875	1.224	0.01056	0.02313	0.9987
150	1.757	5.177	0.3156	0.03243	0.08599	1.467	0.0103	0.02198	1.013

Table 6.9.3 Fitting Parameters of Computed Constant-Potential Transmission Data to Eqn (2) (Continued)

	Steel			Plate Glass			Wood		
kVp	α (mm^{-1})	β (mm^{-1})	γ	α (mm^{-1})	β (mm^{-1})	γ	α (mm^{-1})	β (mm^{-1})	γ
25	9.364	0.4125	0.3202	0.3804	1.543	0.2869	0.0223	0.0434	0.1937
30	7.406	0.4193	0.3959	0.3061	1.599	0.3693	0.02166	0.03966	0.2843
35	5.716	0.4341	0.4857	0.2396	1.694	0.4683	0.01901	0.03873	0.3732
40									
45									
50	1.187	4.84	0.4021	0.09721	0.1799	0.4912	0.01076	0.001862	1.17
55	1.493	4.515	0.4293	0.08552	0.1661	0.5112	0.01012	0.001404	1.269
60	1.183	4.219	0.4571	0.07452	0.1539	0.5304	0.009512	0.0009672	1.333
65	0.9172	3.982	0.4922	0.06514	0.1443	0.5582	0.00899	0.000647	1.353
70	0.7149	3.798	0.5378	0.05791	0.1357	0.5967	0.00855	0.000539	1.194
75	0.5793	3.629	0.5908	0.05291	0.128	0.6478	0.008203	0.0006421	1.062
80	0.4921	3.428	0.6427	0.04955	0.1208	0.7097	0.007903	0.000864	0.9703
85	0.4355	3.178	0.6861	0.04721	0.114	0.7786	0.007686	0.001056	1.015
90	0.3971	2.913	0.7204	0.0455	0.1077	0.8522	0.007511	0.001159	1.081
95	0.3681	2.654	0.7461	0.0441	0.1013	0.9222	0.007345	0.001133	1.116
100	0.3415	2.42	0.7645	0.04278	0.09466	0.9791	0.00723	0.0009343	1.309
105	0.3135	2.227	0.7788	0.04143	0.08751	1.014	0.00705	0.0006199	1.365
110	0.2849	2.061	0.7897	0.04008	0.08047	1.030	0.006921	0.0001976	3.309
115	0.2579	1.922	0.8008	0.03878	0.07394	1.033	0.006864	−0.0003908	0.6469
120	0.2336	1.797	0.8116	0.03758	0.06808	1.031	0.006726	−0.0008308	1.006
125	0.213	1.677	0.8217	0.03652	0.06304	1.031	0.006584	−0.001214	1.192
130	0.1969	1.557	0.8309	0.03561	0.05874	1.037	0.006472	−0.001539	1.285
135	0.1838	1.44	0.8391	0.03481	0.05519	1.049	0.006306	−0.001731	1.465
140	0.1724	1.328	0.8458	0.03407	0.05145	1.057	0.006191	−0.001849	1.53
145	0.1616	1.225	0.8519	0.03336	0.04795	1.063	0.006115	−0.001869	1.498
150	0.1501	1.132	0.8566	0.03266	0.04491	1.073	0.00602	−0.001752	1.483

[a] The 25–35 kVp data are for molybdenum-anode x-ray tubes. All other data are for tungsten-anode tubes.

The equation of Archer et al. deserves further discussion. One can calculate in closed form the HVL of the broad x-ray beam as a function of penetrated material thickness x. Explicitly,

$$\mathrm{HVL}(x) = \left(\frac{1}{\alpha\gamma}\ln\left[\frac{2^{\gamma}\left[\left(1+\frac{\beta}{\alpha}\right)e^{\alpha\gamma x}-\frac{\beta}{\alpha}\right]+\frac{\beta}{\alpha}}{1+\frac{\beta}{\alpha}}\right]\right) - x. \tag{3}$$

The values calculated from eqn (3) for the HVL at the greatest material thickness plotted for Simpkin's computed data from 1989 are given in Table 6.9.4. These are the HVLs at high attenuation required for adequate shielding of leakage radiation. The Monte Carlo calculation yields half-value layers somewhat less conservative than those compiled in NCRP 49. Values in parentheses are calculated using the 1995 compiled data set and a transmission of 1E-04 instead of the greatest material thickness.

Table 6.9.4 Half-Value Layers at High Attenuation Calculated from Eqn (3) Original values calculated using fits from Simpkin, 1989. New values (in parentheses) calculated using fits from Table 6.9.3 (Simpkin, 1995) for values of x determined for a transmission of 1E-04.

	Half-Value Layers at High Attenuation (mm)			
Material	**70 kVcp**	**100 kVcp**	**120 kVcp**	**140 kVcp**
Lead	0.134 (0.129)	0.245 (0.277)	0.253 (0.309)	0.250 (0.345)
Concrete	10.4 (13.6)	15.3 (17.7)	17.7 (19.4)	20.3 (20.7)
Gypsum	23.6 (30.1)	33.6 (47.3)	46.0 (56.1)	51.1 (63.7)
Steel	0.825 (0.970)	1.81 (2.03)	3.25 (2.97)	3.40 (4.02)
Plate Glass	10.7 (12.0)	15.1 (16.2)	17.1 (18.4)	19.1 (20.3)
Wood	(81.1)	(95.9)	(103)	(112)

Shielding Requirements

The constant-potential transmission data generated above can be used to produce radiation shielding tables using the methods outlines in a previous work (Simpkin 1987a)[a]. This technique accounts for all radiation types and sources in an installation, discarding the ''add one HVL'' rule imposed by NCRP 49 for secondary barriers. Using the modification to the leakage requirement in SI units [eqn (1) above], the minimum barrier thicknesses surrounding radiographic and fluoroscopic installations operated at various workloads are given in Tables 6.9.5 and 6.9.6 respectively. The assumptions used to complete these tables follow those made in NCRP 49 and are listed at the bottom of each table.

It is difficult to compare the calculated constant-potential shielding requirements in Tables 6.9.5 and 6.9.6 for lead and concrete to the corresponding single-phase requirements in Tables 5 and 7 in Appendix C, NCRP 49. Firstly, it must be appreciated that the requirements listed in these NCRP 49 tables were calculated using 150 kVp single-phase data. Despite a correction for workload, the published 100 and 125 kVp requirements are artificial. Secondly, the secondary barrier requirements in NCRP 49 were generated using the ''add one HVL'' rule which has been proven to be overly conservative (Archer, 1983; Simpkin, 1987a). The NCRP 49 tables generally err on the side of safety.

For 140 kVcp the requirements at these distances are 1.89, 1.64, 1.39, 1.15, 0.89 and 0.68 mm Pb. These and the corresponding concrete requirements support the general conclusion that barrier thicknesses found for three-phase equipment will nearly match those for single-phase generation of somewhat higher potential. For the x-ray spectra and radiation output selected here, this work indicates that the difference in the high potential range is 10 kVp.

---

[a] $$\sum_{i=1}\left(\frac{K_{ux}(S)_i}{K_{ux_i}}+\frac{K_{ux}(S)_i}{K_{ux_{s_i}}}+\frac{\exp(-\ln 2S/\mathrm{HVL}_i)}{B_{Lx_i}}\right)=1.$$

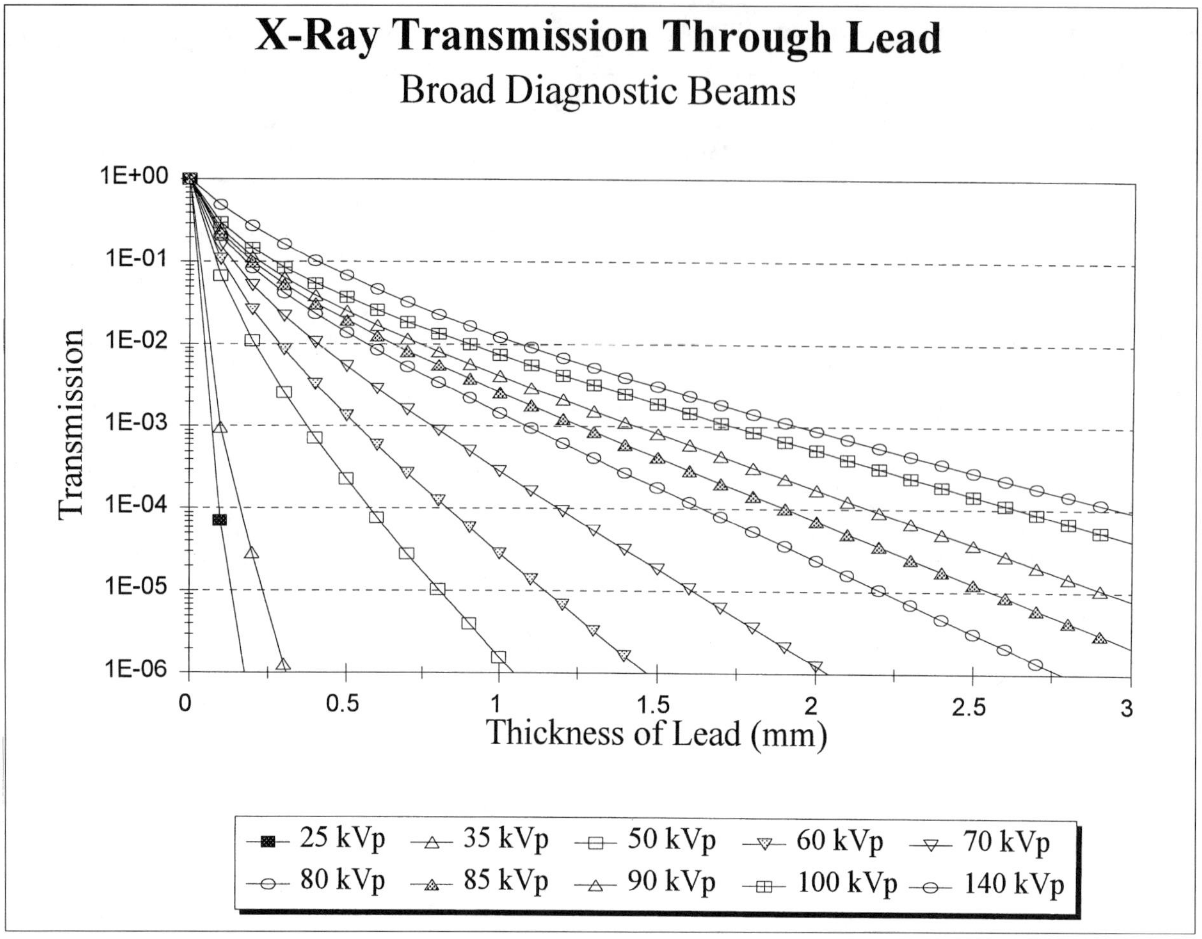

Figure 6.13 Computed Broad-Beam Transmission ($K_{\mu x}/K_0$) of Constant-Potential-Generated X-Rays Through Lead.

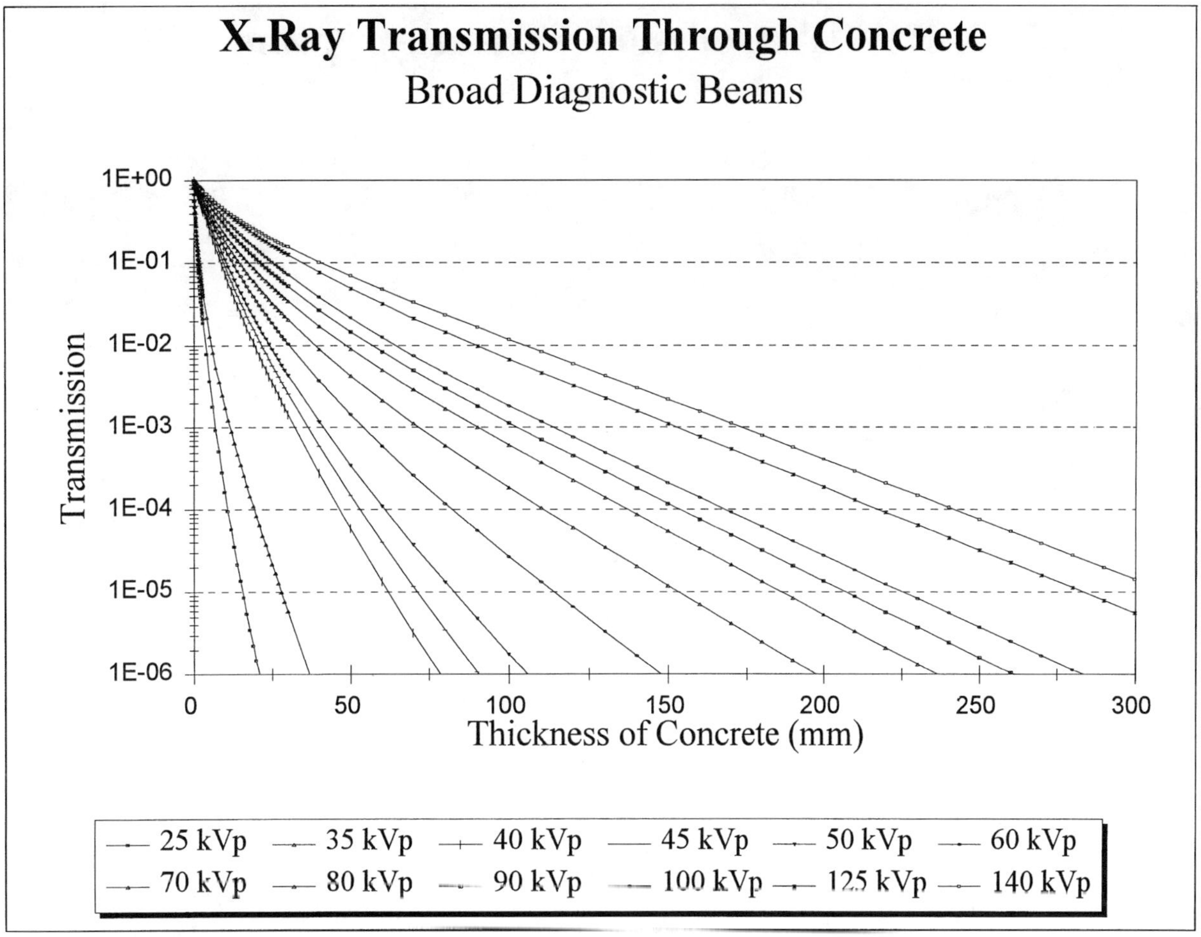

Figure 6.14 Computed Broad-Beam Transmission ($K_{\mu\lambda}$) of Constant-Potential-Generated X-Rays Through Concrete. Error bars indicate one standard deviation in the Monte Carlo calculation. Solid curves are the fit of the data to eqn (2). The transmission curves are for 25kVp (leftmost) to 140kVp (rightmost).

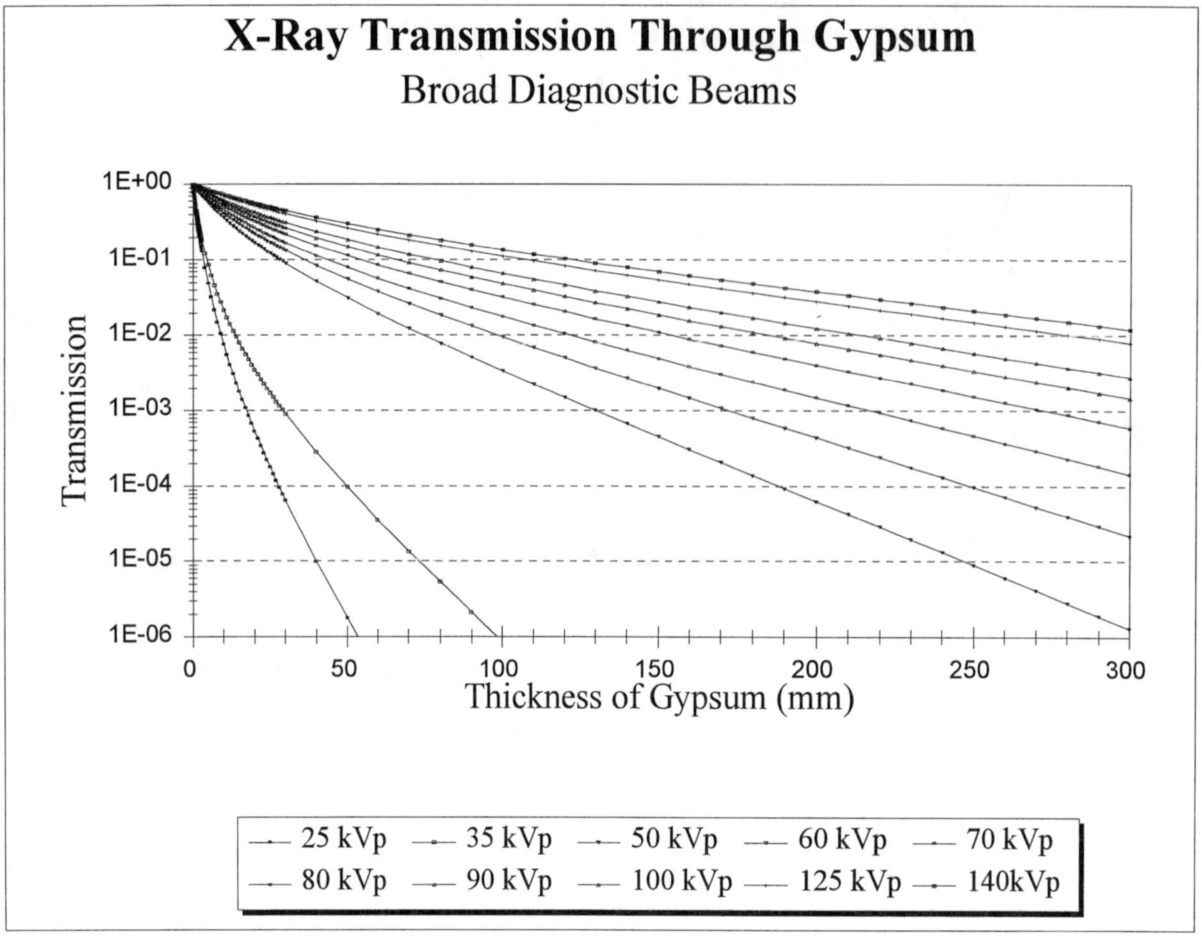

Figure 6.15 Computed Broad-Beam Transmission ($K_{\mu x}/k_0$) of Constant-Potential-Generated X-Rays Through Gypsum Wallboard.

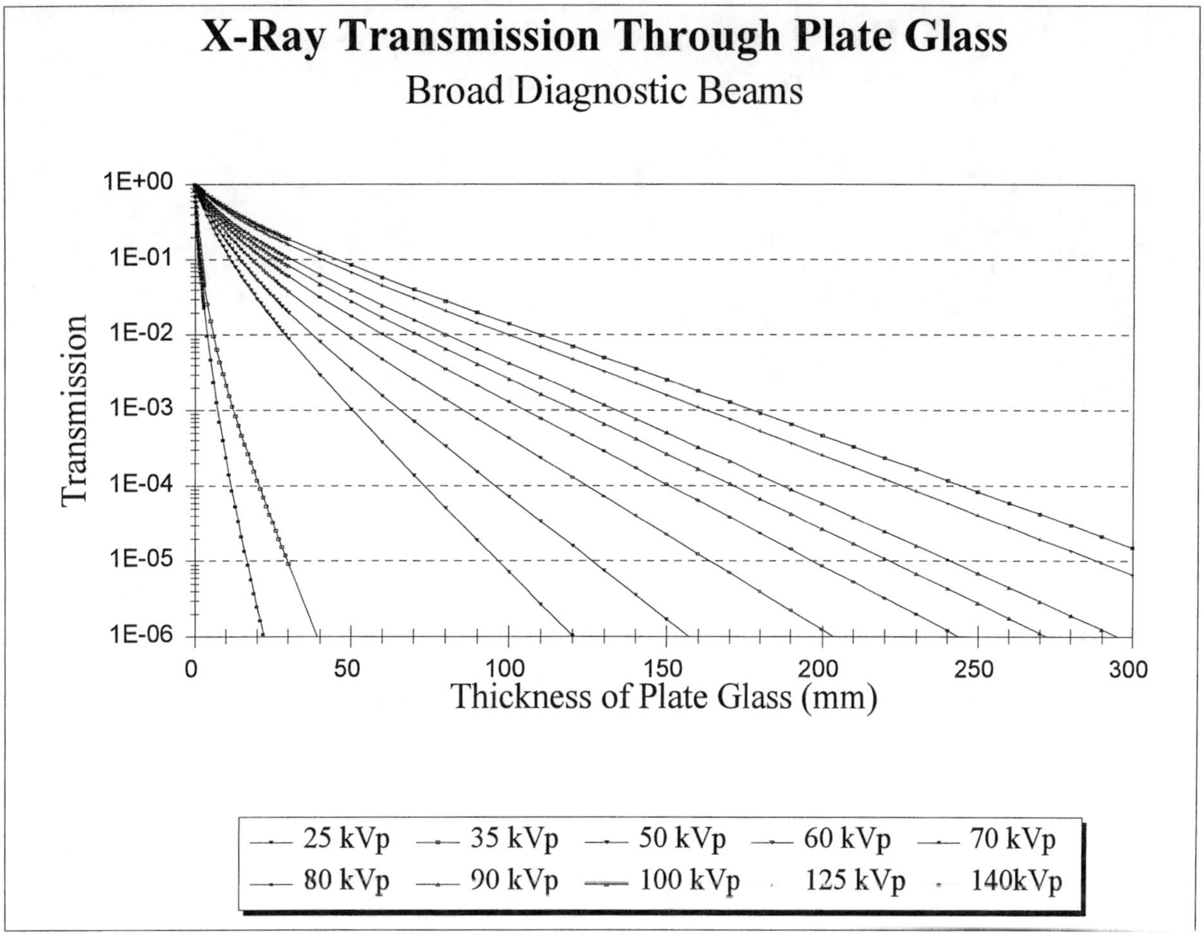

Figure 6.16 Computed Broad-Beam Transmission ($K_{\mu x}$) of Constant Potential-Generated X-Rays Through Plate Glass.

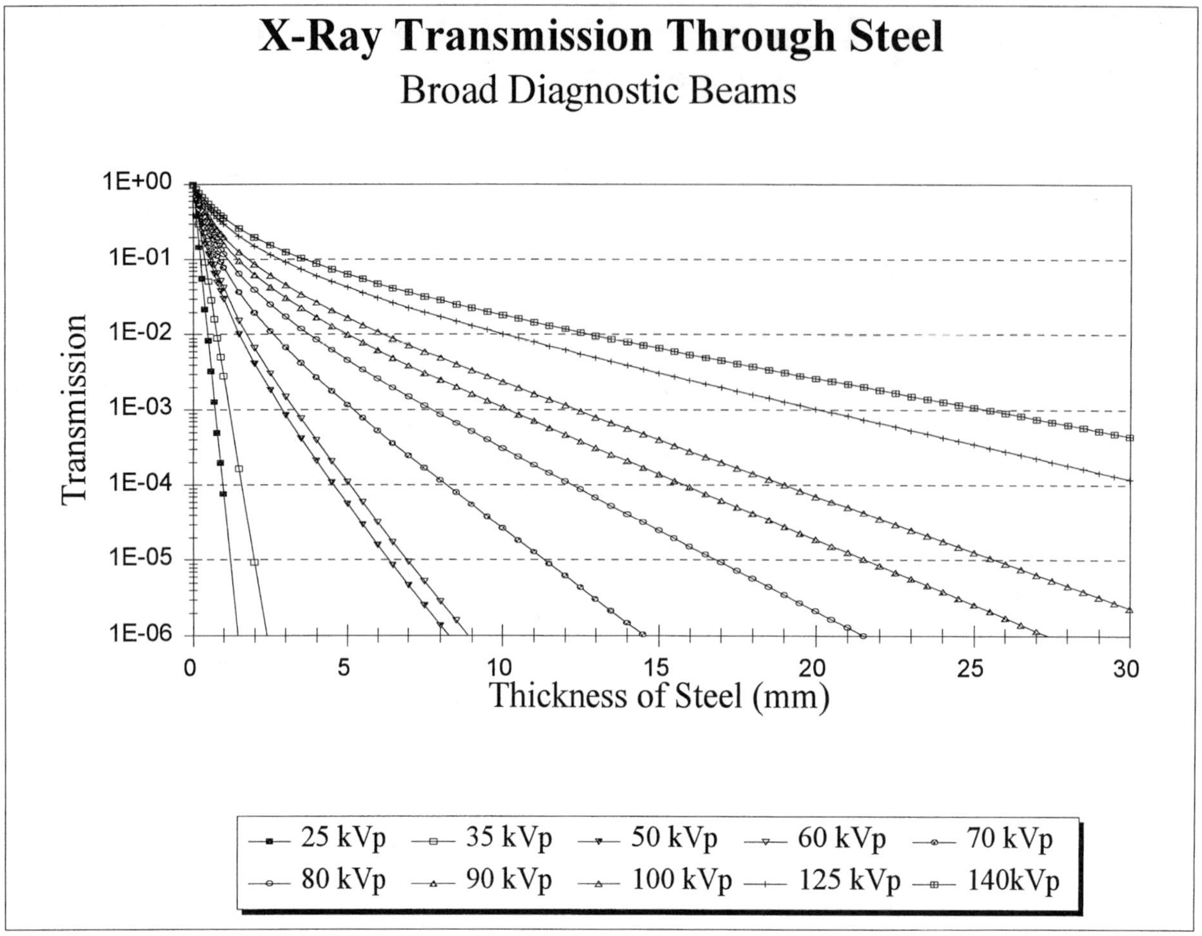

Figure 6.17 Computed Broad-Beam Transmission ($K_{\mu x}$) of Constant-Potential-Generated X-Rays Through Steel.

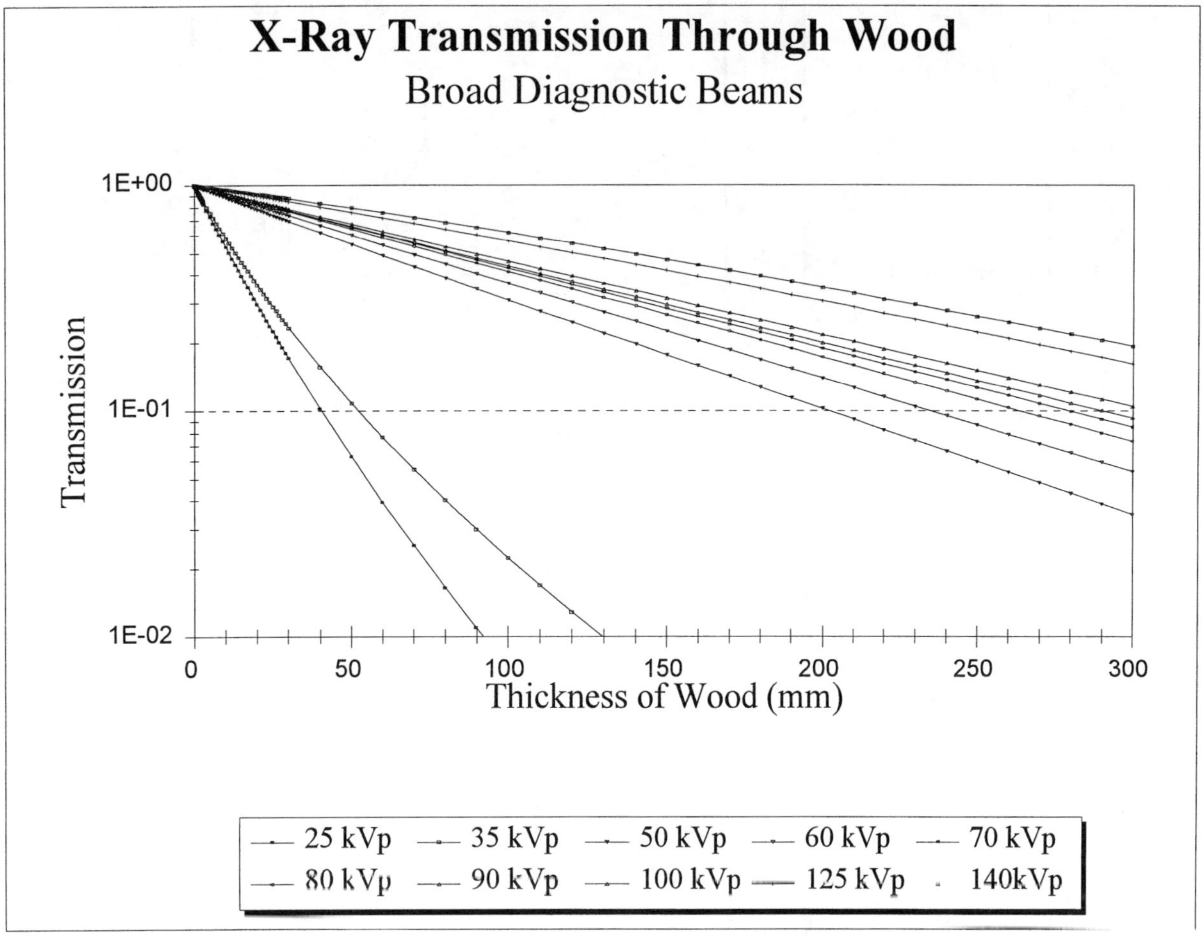

Figure 6.18 Computed Broad-Beam Transmission ($K_{\mu x}$) of Constant Potential-Generated X-Rays Through Wood.

Table 6.9.5 X-Radiation Shielding Requirements for Radiographic Installations Using Constant-Potential Generation (Required Barrier Thicknesses Indicated in mm. WUT is the Product of Workload, Use Factor and Occupancy Factor)

WUT in mA-min				Distance (m)						
70 kV	100 kVcp	120 kVcp	140 kVcp							
1000	1000	400	200	1.5	2.1	3.0	4.2	6.1	8.4	12.2
500	500	200	100		1.5	2.1	3.0	4.2	6.1	8.4
250	250	100	50			1.5	2.1	3.0	4.2	6.1
125	125	50	25				1.5	2.1	3.0	4.2
62.5	62.5	25	12.5					1.5	2.1	3.0

Material	Potential (kVcp) 70	100	120	140	70	100	120	140	70	100	120	140	70	100	120	140	70	100	120	140	70	100	120	140	70	100	120	140
Primary Controlled area																												
Pb	0.93	2.02	1.96	1.89	0.80	1.79	1.71	1.64	0.67	1.54	1.46	1.39	0.55	1.30	1.22	1.15	0.42	1.05	0.96	0.89	0.32	0.84	0.75	0.68	0.22	0.61	0.52	0.46
concrete	87.7	151	164	176	77.7	136	146	157	67.1	121	128	136	57.2	106	111	116	46.4	89.7	92.4	94.6	37.3	75.7	76.2	76.2	27.2	59.7	57.7	55.4
gypsum wallboard	205	345	441	473	182	312	394	418	157	278	344	362	134	245	297	308	108	209	245	249	86.6	177	201	198	62.5	141	150	141
steel	5.66	14.4	20.5	24.1	4.88	12.7	17.5	20.8	4.08	10.8	14.4	17.3	3.34	9.13	11.6	14.0	2.56	7.30	8.70	10.5	1.95	5.80	6.50	7.64	1.32	4.18	4.34	4.66
plate glass	94	156	164	174	83.6	142	148	155	72.6	126	130	136	62.3	111	114	117	50.9	94.7	95.2	96.5	41.4	80.7	79.4	79.0	30.6	64.5	61.1	58.6
Primary Uncontrolled area																												
Pb	1.37	2.84	2.79	2.72	1.24	2.60	2.55	2.47	1.10	2.35	2.29	2.22	0.98	2.11	2.04	1.97	0.84	1.85	1.77	1.71	0.72	1.62	1.54	1.48	0.58	1.36	1.28	1.21
concrete	122	202	223	244	112	188	205	224	101	172	187	203	91.4	157	170	183	80.3	140	151	162	70.7	126	135	143	59.7	110	116	121
gypsum wallboard	285	457	601	656	262	425	554	603	237	390	505	546	214	357	458	492	188	321	406	432	165	289	361	381	140	253	309	322
steel	8.38	20.4	31.2	35.4	7.58	18.6	28.0	32.1	6.74	16.8	24.7	28.6	5.95	15.0	21.6	25.3	5.08	13.1	18.2	21.6	4.35	11.5	15.4	18.5	3.52	9.56	12.3	14.9
plate glass	130	206	221	237	119	191	205	219	108	176	187	199	97.7	161	170	181	86.2	145	152	160	76.4	131	136	142	64.9	115	118	122
Secondary Controlled area																												
Pb	0.14	0.46	0.35	0.28	0.05	0.28	0.19	0.14	0.00	0.13	0.07	0.03	0.00	0.04	0.01	0.00	0.00	0.00	0.00	0.00	0.00	0.00	0.00	0.00	0.00	0.00	0.00	0.00
concrete	13.6	42.0	39.1	35.6	5.80	28.6	24.1	19.4	0.00	15.8	10.5	5.52	0.00	6.13	1.10	0.00	0.00	0.00	0.00	0.00	0.00	0.00	0.00	0.00	0.00	0.00	0.00	0.00
gypsum wallboard	30.6	98.4	98.4	87.1	12.5	66.3	57.2	44.5	0.00	34.3	22.0	11.3	0.00	10.9	1.95	0.00	0.00	0.00	0.00	0.00	0.00	0.00	0.00	0.00	0.00	0.00	0.00	0.00
steel	0.83	3.17	3.18	2.77	0.30	1.89	1.66	1.12	0.00	0.88	0.64	0.23	0.00	0.30	0.06	0.00	0.00	0.00	0.00	0.00	0.00	0.00	0.00	0.00	0.00	0.00	0.00	0.00
plate glass	14.8	45.4	41.6	38.1	6.39	31.3	26.2	21.2	0.00	17.5	11.5	6.02	0.00	6.68	1.17	0.00	0.00	0.00	0.00	0.00	0.00	0.00	0.00	0.00	0.00	0.00	0.00	0.00
Secondary Uncontrolled area																												
Pb	0.55	1.21	1.10	1.01	0.43	0.98	0.86	0.78	0.29	0.74	0.63	0.55	0.18	0.53	0.42	0.35	0.07	0.32	0.23	0.17	0.01	0.17	0.11	0.06	0.00	0.06	0.02	0.00
concrete	46.2	91.6	96.1	99.9	36.3	76.9	79.1	80.5	26.1	61.4	61.2	60.3	16.8	47.1	44.8	41.9	7.60	31.9	27.7	23.2	1.61	20.0	14.8	9.77	0.00	8.33	3.13	0.00
gypsum wallboard	106	210	255	262	83.2	177	208	209	59.5	143	159	154	37.9	110	114	104	16.6	74.2	67.0	54.5	3.28	44.8	32.7	20.9	0.00	15.8	5.78	0.00
steel	3.39	8.68	11.9	12.6	2.61	6.99	9.02	9.41	1.80	5.24	6.18	6.21	1.07	3.69	3.88	3.57	0.41	2.18	1.98	1.45	0.07	1.18	0.93	0.46	0.00	0.42	0.18	0.00
plate glass	48.8	95.2	97.9	101	38.5	80.6	81.3	82.2	27.8	65.1	63.8	62.6	18.1	50.6	47.5	44.5	8.36	34.8	29.9	25.3	1.80	22.0	16.1	10.7	0.00	9.14	3.36	0.00

Notes:
WUT is the product of the workload (mA-min), the use factor and the occupancy factor.
D_{scat} is 0.8 m.
Field size is 1000 cm^2.
Scattered to incident ratio, a, is 0.0005, 0.0013, 0.0015, 0.0016 at 70, 100, 120, 140 kVcp, respectively.
Maximum continuous rated tube current is 5, 5, 4, 3 mA at 70, 100, 120, 140 kVcp, respectively.

Table 6.9.6 X-Radiation Shielding Requirements for Fluoroscopic Installations Using Constant-Potential Generation (Required Barrier Thicknesses Indicated in mm. WUT is the product of workload, use factor and occupancy factor)

WUT in mA-min				Distance (m)						
70 kV	100 kVcp	120 kVcp	140 kVcp							
2000	2000	800	800	1.5	2.1	3.0	4.2	6.1	8.4	12.2
1000	1000	400	200		1.5	2.1	3.0	4.2	6.1	8.4
500	500	200	100			1.5	2.1	3.0	4.2	6.1
250	250	100	100				1.5	2.1	3.0	4.2
125	125	50	25					1.5	2.1	3.0

Material	Potential (kVcp)																											
	70	100	120	140	70	100	120	140	70	100	120	140	70	100	120	140	70	100	120	140	70	100	120	140	70	100	120	140
Secondary Controlled area																												
Pb	0.26	0.71	0.61	0.53	0.15	0.50	0.40	0.34	0.06	0.31	0.23	0.17	0.01	0.16	0.10	0.06	0.00	0.06	0.02	0.00	0.00	0.01	0.00	0.00	0.00	0.00	0.00	0.00
concrete	24.2	60.6	60.6	59.8	15.2	46.3	44.3	41.5	6.81	31.9	28.0	23.7	1.05	19.4	14.5	9.59	0.00	8.03	3.00	0.00	0.00	0.98	0.00	0.00	0.00	0.00	0.00	0.00
gypsum wallboard	55.2	141	158	153	34.1	109	113	103	14.7	74.4	67.7	55.5	2.11	43.4	31.7	20.5	0.00	15.1	5.51	0.00	0.00	1.35	0.00	0.00	0.00	0.00	0.00	0.00
steel	1.60	5.01	5.82	5.97	0.91	3.50	3.65	3.40	0.35	2.11	1.95	1.45	0.05	1.11	0.89	0.44	0.00	0.40	0.17	0.00	0.00	0.05	0.00	0.00	0.00	0.00	0.00	0.00
plate glass	26.0	64.5	63.4	62.3	16.5	50.0	47.0	44.1	7.54	35.0	30.3	25.8	1.17	21.6	15.8	10.6	0.00	8.83	3.22	0.00	0.00	1.04	0.00	0.00	0.00	0.00	0.00	0.00
Secondary Uncontrolled area																												
Pb	0.69	1.50	1.40	1.32	0.56	1.26	1.16	1.08	0.43	1.02	0.91	0.83	0.31	0.79	0.68	0.61	0.18	0.55	0.45	0.38	0.09	0.37	0.28	0.22	0.02	0.20	0.13	0.09
concrete	57.7	111	119	126	47.7	96.1	102	106	37.3	80.4	83.5	85.8	27.6	65.8	66.7	66.6	17.4	49.9	48.3	46.0	9.45	36.7	33.4	29.5	2.27	22.4	17.7	12.8
gypsum wallboard	133	253	316	333	110	221	270	280	85.5	186	221	224	63.1	153	174	171	39.2	117	124	115	20.8	85.9	82.5	70.8	4.65	51.0	39.9	28.1
steel	4.25	10.8	15.5	16.7	3.46	9.04	12.5	13.5	2.63	7.24	9.40	10.1	1.87	5.59	6.71	7.01	1.08	3.87	4.15	4.00	0.51	2.55	2.46	2.01	0.10	1.33	1.11	0.63
plate glass	60.8	115	120	126	50.5	99.9	103	107	40.0	84.4	85.9	87.3	29.6	69.8	69.3	68.9	18.8	53.6	51.1	48.7	10.4	40.0	35.9	31.9	2.54	24.8	19.3	14.1

Notes:
WUT is the product of the workload (mA-min), the use factor and the occupancy factor.
D_{scat} is 0.45 m.
Field size is 400 cm^2.
Scattered to incident ratio, a, is 0.0005, 0.0013, 0.0015, 0.0016 at 70, 100, 120, 140 kVcp, respectively.
Maximum continuous rated tube current is 5, 5, 4, 3 mA at 70, 100, 120, 140 kVcp, respectively.

Table 6.10 Shielding Requirements for Mammography (Reproduced from the journal *Health Physics* with permission from the Health Physics Society from Simpkin, 1987b)

Shielding requirements for mammography installations have been investigated. To apply the methodologies of NCRP Report No. 49, the scatter-to-incident ratio of a typical mammography beam was measured, and the broad beam transmission was calculated for several representative beam spectra. These calculations were found to compare favorably with published low kVp tungsten-targeted x-ray transmission through a variety of shielding materials. Radiation shielding tables were developed from the calculated transmissions through Pb, concrete, gypsum, steel, plate glass, and water, using a technique which eliminates the ''add one HVL'' rule. It is concluded that Mo-targeted x-ray beams operated at 35 kVp require half the shielding of W-targeted beams operated at 50 kVp, and that adequate, cost effective shielding calculations will consider alternatives to Pb.

Table 6.10.1 Primary Mammography Shielding Requirements for Pb, Concrete, Gypsum, Steel, Plate Glass and Water for Three Beam Qualities WUT is the product of the workload, use factor and occupancy factor (From Simpkin, 1987b)

WUT (mA-min per week)	Distance (m)						
2000	1.5	2.1	3.0	4.2	6.1	8.4	12.2
1000		1.5	2.1	3.0	4.2	6.1	8.4
500			1.5	2.1	3.0	4.2	6.1
250				1.5	2.1	3.0	4.2
125					1.5	2.1	3.0

	W[a]	Mo/Be[b]	Mo/g[c]	W[a]	Mo/Be[b]	Mo/g[c]	W[a]	Mo/Be[b]	Mo/g[c]	W[a]	Mo/Be[b]	Mo/g[c]	W[a]	Mo/Be[b]	Mo/g[c]	W[a]	Mo/Be[b]	Mo/g[c]	W[a]	Mo/Be[b]	Mo/g[c]
Controlled Area																					
Lead (mm)	.39	.14	.11	.33	.12	.09	.28	.10	.08	.23	.09	.07	.18	.07	.06	.15	.07	.05	.10	.06	.04
Concrete (mm)	41	16	12	36	14	9.8	30	11	7.7	25	9.1	5.9	20	7.0	4.3	16	5.5	3.3	12	4.0	2.4
Gypsum (mm)	103	41	31	92	35	26	79	29	20	68	24	15	55	18	11	43	14	8.3	31	10	5.9
Steel (mm)	2.2	0.7	.55	1.9	0.5	.45	1.6	.5	.35	1.3	.4	.27	1.0	.31	.19	.8	.25	.15	.56	.18	.10
Plate Glass (mm)	42	17	13	37	14	11	31	12	8.2	26	10	6.3	21	7.5	4.6	17	5.8	3.5	12	4.3	2.5
Water (mm)	285	156	124	258	139	107	231	120	89	204	103	74	175	85	58	149	70	46	120	55	34
Uncontrolled Area																					
Lead (mm)	.57	.21	.18	.51	.19	.16	.46	.16	.13	.40	.14	.11	.34	.12	.09	.30	.10	.08	.24	.09	.07
Concrete (mm)	59	24	20	54	21	18	48	19	15	43	17	13	37	14	10	32	12	8.4	27	9.6	6.3
Gypsum (mm)	143	62	51	131	56	45	119	50	39	107	44	33	94	37	27	83	31	22	70	26	16
Steel (mm)	3.3	1.1	.94	2.9	1.0	.82	2.6	.9	7	2.3	.8	.59	2.0	.63	.47	1.7	.54	.38	1.4	.43	.28
Plate Glass (mm)	61	26	21	55	23	19	50	20	16	44	18	14	38	15	11	33	13	8.9	28	10	6.7
Water (mm)	377	217	184	350	199	166	322	180	148	295	163	131	265	143	111	240	127	95	211	108	77

[a] W anode, 50 kVp, 2.03 mm Al filter, HVL = 2.01 mm Al (spectrum MW18 (FDA)79-8071). Radiation output $\dot{x}_n$ = .00052 C kg^{-1} As^{-1} (2.0 mR mAs^{-1}).

[b] Mo anode, 35 kVp, 0.03 mm Mo filter, HVL = 0.53 mm Al (spectrum MO29 (FDA)79-8071). Radiation output $\dot{x}_n$ = .0015 C kg^{-1} As^{-1} (6.0 mR mAs^{-1}).

[c] Mo anode, 35 kVp, 0.03 mm Mo filter, HVL = 0.53 mm Al (spectrum MO29 (FDA)79-8071). Radiation output $\dot{x}_n$ = .00044 C kg^{-1} As^{-1} (1.7 mR mAs^{-1}). (glass window tube).

Table 6.10.2 Secondary Mammography Shielding Requirements for Pb, Concrete, Gypsum, Steel, Plate Glass and Water for Three Beam Qualities WUT is the product of the workload, use factor and occupancy factor (From Simpkin, 1987b)

WUT (mA-min per week)	Distance (m)						
2000	1.5	2.1	3.0	4.2	6.1	8.4	12.2
1000		1.5	2.1	3.0	4.2	6.1	8.4
500			1.5	2.1	3.0	4.2	6.1
250				1.5	2.1	3.0	4.2
125					1.5	2.1	3.0

	W[a]	Mo/Be[b]	Mo/g[c]	W[a]	Mo/Be[b]	Mo/g[c]	W[a]	Mo/Be[b]	Mo/g[c]	W[a]	Mo/Be[b]	Mo/g[c]	W[a]	Mo/Be[b]	Mo/g[c]	W[a]	Mo/Be[b]	Mo/g[c]	W[a]	Mo/Be[b]	Mo/g[c]
Controlled Area																					
Lead (mm)	.12	.05	.048	.05	.03	.02	0	.006	0	0	0	0	0	0	0	0	0	0	0	0	0
Concrete (mm)	9.4	4.5	4.5	4.4	2.1	1.8	0	.4	0	0	0	0	0	0	0	0	0	0	0	0	0
Gypsum (mm)	21	10	10	10	4.8	4.1	0	.9	0	0	0	0	0	0	0	0	0	0	0	0	0
Steel (mm)	.60	.24	.24	.3	.11	.1	0	.02	0	0	0	0	0	0	0	0	0	0	0	0	0
Plate Glass (mm)	9.6	4.8	4.7	4.5	2.2	2.0	0	.4	0	0	0	0	0	0	0	0	0	0	0	0	0
Water (mm)	57	34	31	30	19	14	0	5.4	0	0	0	0	0	0	0	0	0	0	0	0	0
Uncontrolled Area																					
Lead (mm)	.36	.15	.15	.29	.12	.12	.21	.09	.09	.14	.06	.06	.07	.03	.03	.02	.01	.004	0	0	0
Concrete (mm)	28	14	14	22	11	11	17	8.2	8.2	11	5.5	5.4	5.6	0.7	2.5	1.3	.8	.3	0	0	0
Gypsum (mm)	61	31	31	49	25	25	37	18	18	25	12	12	13	6.0	5.5	2.9	2.0	.72	0	0	0
Steel (mm)	1.8	.74	.74	1.4	.59	.59	1.1	.44	.44	.71	.29	.29	.35	.14	.13	.07	.04	.02	0	0	0
Plate Glass (mm)	28	15	15	22	12	12	17	8.7	8.6	12	5.8	5.8	5.7	2.8	2.6	1.3	.9	.4	0	0	0
Water (mm)	148	93	92	121	75	74	93	57	55	67	40	37	37	22	18	11	10	3.2	0	0	0

[a] W anode, 50 kVp, 2.03 mm Al filter, HVL = 2.01 mm Al (spectrum MW18 (FDA)79-8071). Radiation output $\dot{x}_n$ = .00052 C kg^{-1} As^{-1} (2.0 mR mAs^{-1}).
[b] Mo anode, 35 kVp, 0.03 mm Mo filter, HVL = 0.53 mm Al (spectrum MO29 (FDA)79-8071). Radiation output $\dot{x}_n$ = .0015 C kg^{-1} As^{-1} (6.0 mR mAs^{-1}). (Be window tube).
[c] Mo anode, 35 kVp, 0.03 mm Mo filter, HVL = 0.53 mm Al (spectrum MO29 (FDA)79-8071). Radiation output $\dot{x}_n$ = .00044 C kg^{-1} As^{-1} (1.7 mR mAs^{-1}). (glass window tube).

Table 6.10.3 Primary and Secondary Mammography Shielding Requirements for 30 kVp Radiation Filtered with 0.03 mm Mo. WUT is the Product of the Workload, Use Factor and Occupancy Factor. (Reproduced from the journal *Health Physics* with permission from the Health Physics Society from Simpkin, 1987b)

WUT (mA-min per week)	Distance (m)						
2000	1.5	2.1	3.0	4.2	6.1	8.4	12.2
1000		1.5	2.1	3.0	4.2	6.1	8.4
500			1.5	2.1	3.0	4.2	6.1
250				1.5	2.1	3.0	4.2
125					1.5	2.1	3.0

	Pri	Sec	Pri	Sec	Pri	Sec	Pri	Sec	Pri	Sec	Pri	Sec	Pri	Sec
Controlled Area														
Lead (mm)	.095	.032	.087	.017	.078	.002	.069	0	.06	0	.052	0	.043	0
Concrete (mm)	11	3.5	9.2	1.6	7.6	.13	6.2	0	4.9	0	3.9	0	3.0	0
Gypsum (mm)	29	8.1	24	3.7	20	.3	16	0	13	0	10	0	7.5	0
Steel (mm)	.48	.16	.41	.07	.34	.006	.28	0	.22	0	.18	0	.13	0
Plate Glass (mm)	12	3.7	9.8	1.7	8.1	.13	6.6	0	5.2	0	4.2	0	3.2	0
Water (mm)	120	29	105	15	92	1.6	77	0	64	0	53	0	42	0
Uncontrolled Area														
Lead (mm)	.15	.091	.13	.073	.11	.055	.10	.038	.089	.021	.081	.007	.071	0
Concrete (mm)	17	11	15	8.5	13	6.3	11	4.2	9.6	2.0	8.1	.52	6.5	0
Gypsum (mm)	45	25	40	20	35	15	30	9.8	25	4.7	21	1.2	17	0
Steel (mm)	.8	.5	.67	.4	.59	.29	.51	.19	.43	.09	.37	.03	.3	0
Plate Glass (mm)	18	11	16	9.0	14	6.6	12	4.4	10	2.1	8.6	.56	7.0	0
Water (mm)	171	80	155	65	140	49	125	34	109	18	95	5.9	80	0

Mo anode 30 kVp, 0.03 mm Mo filter, Be window tube, HVL = 0.36 mm Al. Radiation output at 1 m, X $\bar{X}_n$ = .001 C kg^{-1} As^{-1} (4.0 mR mAs^{-1}).

Table 6.11 Calculated Exposure Rates from Patients (Point Sources) at Various Distances Containing Selected Radionuclides[a] (Reproduced with permission from Frost, D. and Jammet, H. *Manual on Radiation Protection in Hospitals and General Practice,* Vol. 2. Unsealed Sources. Geneva, WHO, 1975, Annex 5, p. 108)

	Calculated Exposure Rate in mR/h at Following Distances from Sources or Patient Containing 100 mCi				Time in Hours:Minutes to Achieve the Maximum Permissible Dose for One Week (100 mrem)			
Radionuclide	500 cm	1 m	2 m	3 m	50 cm	1 m	2 m	3 m
^{22}Na	480	120	30	13.0	0:13	0.50	3:20	7:40
^{24}Na	740	180	45	20.0	0:08	0:33	2:15	5:00
^{47}Ca	230	57	14	6.3	0:26	1:45	7:10	15:55
^{51}Cr	6	1.5	0.4	0.2	16:40	67:00	—	—
^{58}Co	220	55	14	6.1	0:27	1:50	7:10	16:25
^{60}Co	520	130	33	14.0	0:12	0:46	3:00	7:10
^{59}Fe	250	64	16	8.0	0:23	1:35	6:15	12:30
^{75}Se	80	20	5	2.2	1:15	5:00	20:00	45:00
^{85}Sr + ^{85m}Rb	120	30	7.5	3.3	0:50	3:20	13:20	30:00
^{99m}Tc + ^{99}Mo	22	5.5	1.4	0.6	4:35	18:00	—	—
^{125}I	12	3	0.8	0.3	8:20	33:00	—	—
^{131}I	88	22	5.5	2.4	1:10	4:30	18:00	42:00
^{137}Cs	130	33	8.3	3.8	0:46	3:00	12:00	26:00
^{182}Ta	270	68	17	8.4	0:22	1:30	5:55	11:55
^{192}Ir	190	48	12	5.3	0:32	2:05	8:20	19:00
^{198}Au	92	23	5.8	2.6	1:05	4:20	17:00	38:00
^{203}Hg	52	13	3.3	1.5	1:55	7:45	30:00	67:00
^{222}Rn	330	83	21	9.2	0:18	1:10	4:45	10:50

[a] The exposure rate is calculated for point sources without considering the attenuation within the patient's body. Depending on the distribution of the nuclide within the body and the radiation energy, the actual exposure rate when individually measured will be somewhat smaller than the quoted values, which are upper limits. For ^{125}I the values entered here are the maximum values obtained from measurements on average patients at Memorial Hospital, New York City. The values for ^{222}Rn are valid for its equilibrium with short-lived daughters and when using a 0.5 mm platinum filter. Sources within patients will, of course, decay according to the effective half-life, which depends on the physical half-life and the biological half-life.

Table 6.12 Shielding Data for Radionuclides Used in Nuclear Medicine

Radionuclide	Major X- and Gamma-Ray Energies, keV[a]	Half-Value Layer in mm of Lead[b]
^{123}I	27 (71%), 159 (83%)[c]	0.04
^{133}Xe	30 (38%), 81 (37%)	0.2
^{201}Tl	71 (47%), 167 (11%)	0.23
^{99m}Tc	140 (89%)	0.3
^{67}Ga	93 (38%), 184 (21%), 300 (17%)	0.66
^{131}I	364 (81%)	3.0
^{111}In	23 (68%), 171 (91%), 245 (94%)	1.3
^{82}Rb	511 (192%), 777 (13%)	6.0
^{15}O	511 (200%)	5.5
^{11}C	511 (200%)	5.5
^{18}F	511 (194%)	5.5
^{13}N	511 (200%)	5.5

[a] Emission data abstracted from NCRP, a Handbook of Radioactivity Measurements Procedures, 2nd edition, 1985.
[b] In general, the use of 10 half-value layers will reduce the intensity to 1,000th the unshielded value.
[c] Percent (%) indicates number of gamma rays per 100 disintegrations.

Table 6.13 Equilibrium Tenth-Value Layer for High-Energy Broad-Beam Bremsstrahlung Attenuation (Courtesy IAEA from No. 188, 1979)

	TVL Values ($g\ cm^{-2}$)						
			Energy (E_o)				
Material	From[a] $(\mu_{tot}/\rho)_{min}$	Highest Values for $E_o < 100$[b] MeV	4.8 GeV[c]	6.3 GeV[d]	6 GeV[e]	3–7GeV[f]	1 GeV[g]
Sand (SiO_2)	114	—	—	—	—	119	—
Concrete	114	115	—	—	—	101	—
Heavy concrete	—	—	100–122 100–131	122	—	106	—
Aluminum	107	—	—	—	146	—	—
Iron (or steel)	78	85	—	—	—	78	—
Copper	76	—	—	82	89	—	91
Lead	55	55–65	—	52	56	55	56

[a] From Figure 6.19.6 for 0° bremsstrahlung.
[b] Based on values of the minimum photon attenuation coefficient.
[c] Bathow et al., E_o = 4.8 GeV. This paper gives TVL values of 100 to 122 or 100 to 131 $g\ cm^{-2}$ (increasing from 0° to 90°), depending on instrumentation.
[d] Bathow et al., E_o = 6.3 GeV.
[e] Bathow et al., E_o = 6 GeV.
[f] Dinter and Tesch, E_o = 3–7 GeV, 0 = 30 − 90°.
[g] Nelson et al., E_o = 1 GeV.

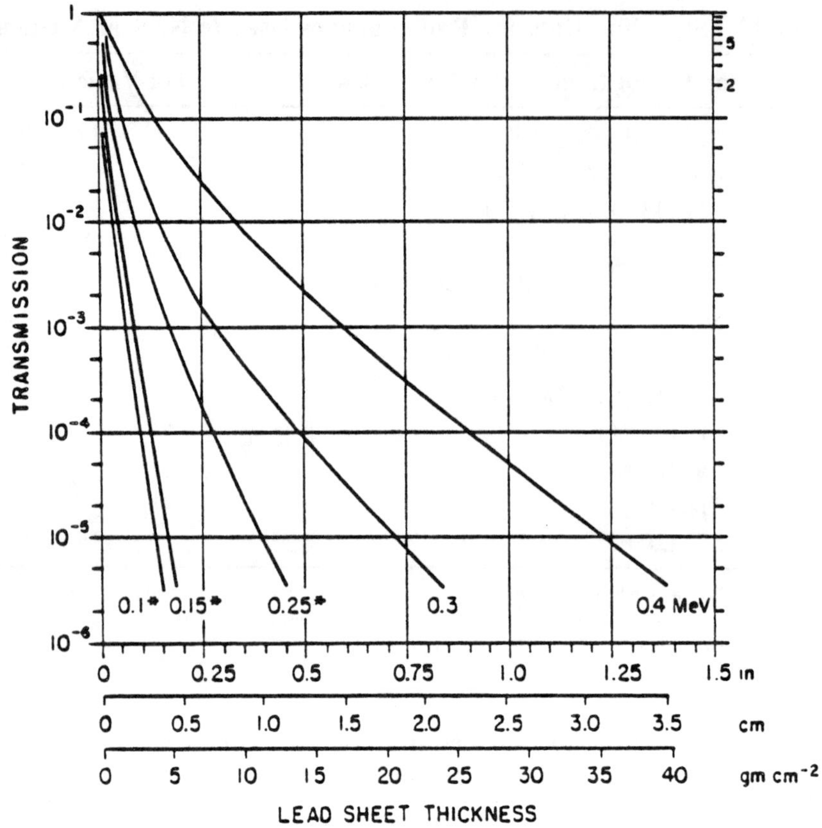

Figure 6.19.1 Shielding for Accelerator Facilities Broad-Beam Transmission Through Lead of X-Rays Produced by 0.1- to 0.4-MeV Electrons. (Courtesy NCRP from Report No. 51, 1977)

Transmission through lead (density 11.3 g cm^{-3}) of x-rays produced by 0.1- to 0.4-MeV electrons, under broad beam conditions. Electron energies designated by an asterisk (*) were accelerated by voltages with pulsed wave form, unmarked electron energies were accelerated by a constant potential generator. Curves represent transmission in dose equivalent index ratio. Curves were derived from NCRP Report No. 34, 1970.

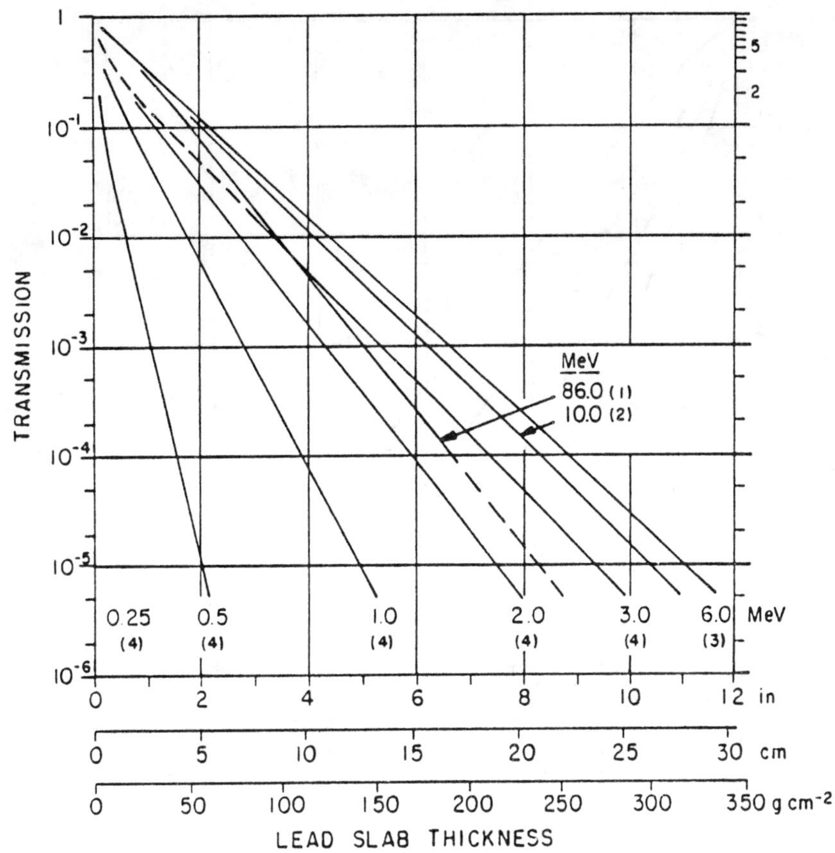

Figure 6.19.2 Shielding for Accelerator Facilities Broad-Beam Transmission Through Lead of X-Rays Produced by 0.5- to 86-MeV Electrons. (Courtesy NRCP from Report No. 51, 1977)

Transmission of thick target x-rays through lead (density 11.3 g cm^{-3}), under broad beam conditions. Energy designations on each curve (0.5- to 86-MeV) refer to the monoenergetic electron energy incident on the thick x-ray producing target. Curves represent transmission in dose equivalent index ratio. Curves were derived from: 1) Miller and Kennedy, 1956; 2) ICRP Publication No. 4, 1964; 3) Karzmark and Capone, 1968, and 4) NCRP Report No. 34, 1970 and NCRP Report No. 49, 1976

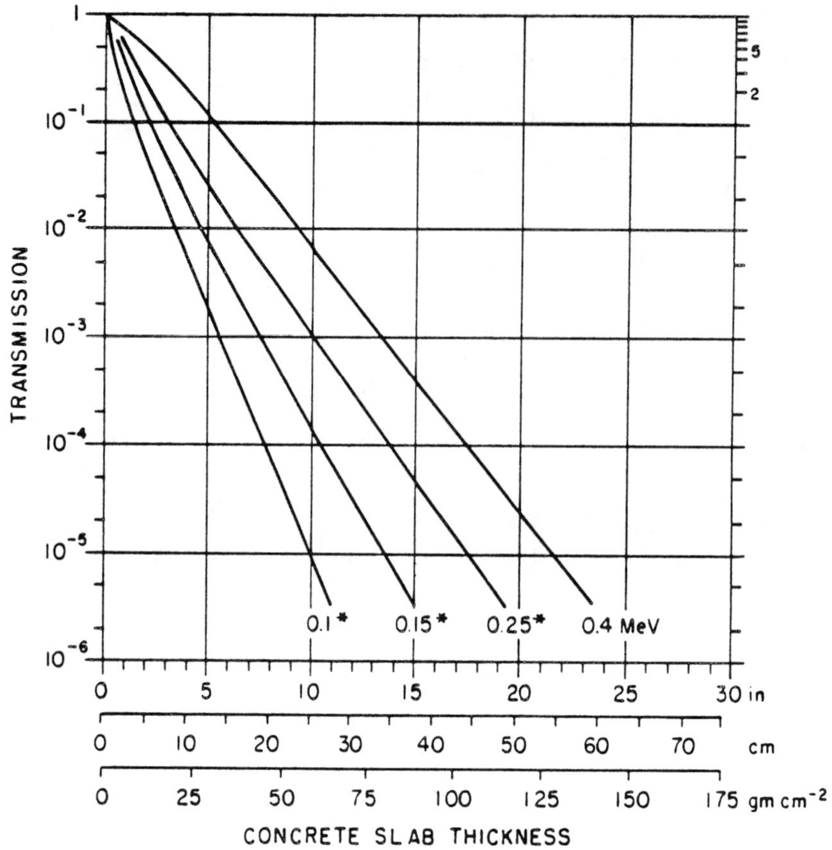

Figure 6.19.3 Shielding for Accelerator Facilities Broad-Beam Transmission Through Concrete of X-Rays Produced by 0.1- to 0.4-MeV Electrons. (Courtesy NCRP from Report No. 51, 1977)

Transmission through concrete (density 2.35 g cm^{-3}) of x-rays produced by 0.1- to 0.4-MeV electrons, under broad beam conditions. Electron energies designated by an asterisk (*) were accelerated by voltages with pulsed wave form; unmarked electron energies were accelerated by a constant potential generator. Curves represent transmission in dose equivalent index ratio. Curves were derived from NCRP Report No. 34, 1970.

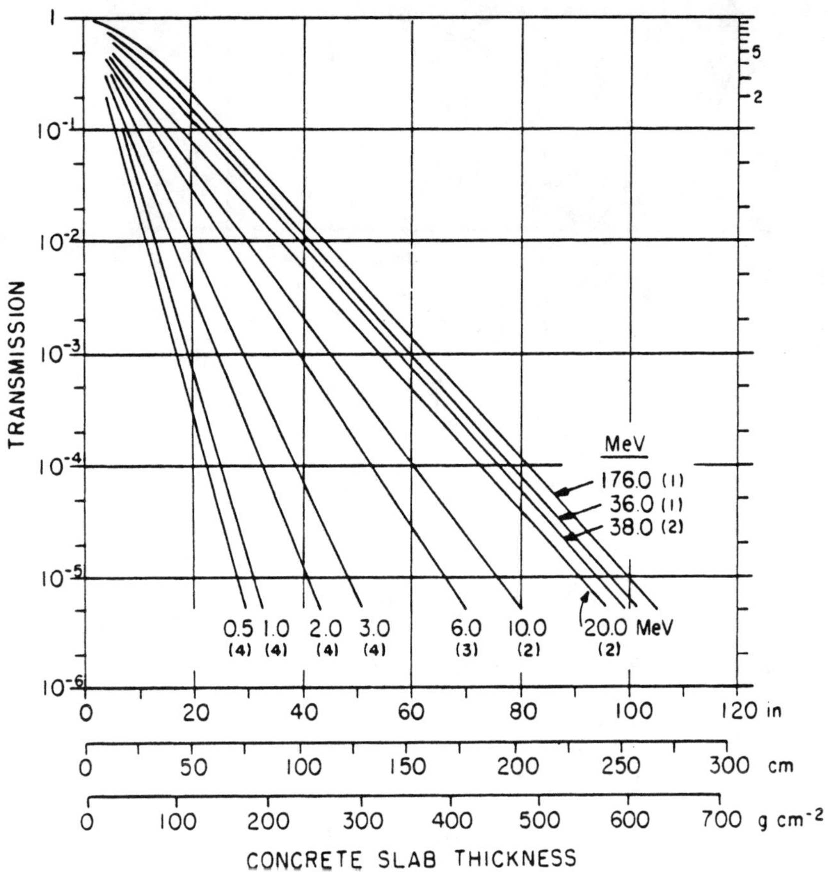

Figure 6.19.4 Shielding for Accelerator Facilities Broad-Beam Transmission Through Concrete of X-Rays Produced by 0.50- to 176-MeV Electrons. (Courtesy NCRP from Report No. 51, 1977)

Tranmission of thick target x-rays through ordinary concrete (density 2.35 g cm^{-3}), under broad beam conditions. Energy designations on each curve (0.5- to 176-MeV) refer to the monoenergetic electron energy incident on the thick x-ray producing target. Curves represent transmission in dose equivalent index ratio. Curves derived from: 1) Miller and Kennedy, 1956; 2) Kirn and Kennedy, 1954; 3) Karzmark and Capone, 1968; and 4) NCRP Report No. 34, 1970 and NCRP Report No. 49, 1976.

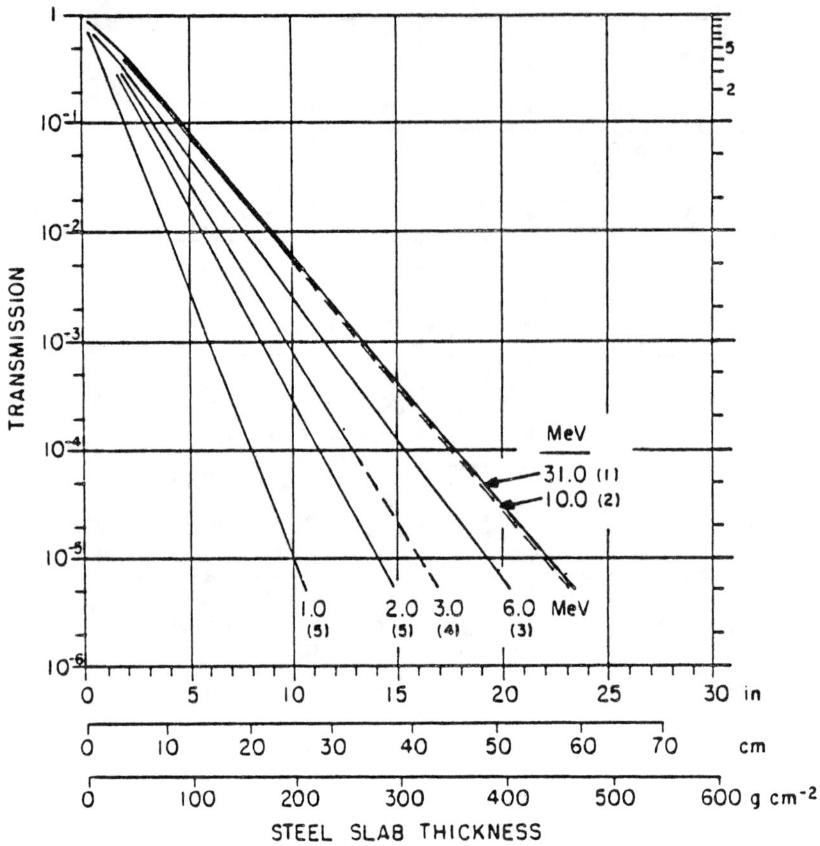

Figure 6.19.5 Shielding for Accelerator Facilities Broad Beam Transmission Through Steel of X-Rays Produced by 1- to 31-MeV Electrons. (Courtesy NCRP from Report No. 51, 1977)

Transmission of thick target x-rays through steel (density 7.8 g cm^{-3}) under broad beam conditions. Energy designations on each curve refer to the monoenergetic electron energy incident on the thick x-ray producing target. Curves represent transmission in dose equivalent index ratio. Curves were derived from: 1) Wideroe, 1953; 2) O'Connor et al., 1949; 3) Karzmark and Capone, 1968; 4) Goldie et al., 1954; and 5) Buechner et al., 1948.

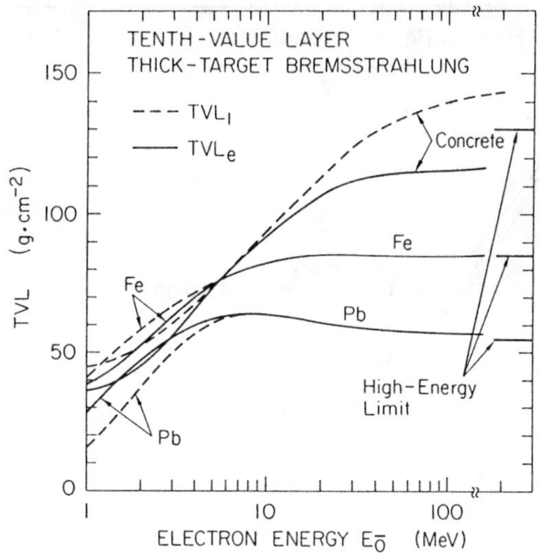

Figure 6.19.6 Values of Dose-Equivalent Tenth-Value Layers (TVLs) in Ordinary Concrete, Iron (Steel) and Lead (Courtesy IAEA from No. 188, 1979) for thick target bremsstrahlung under broad beam conditions at 0°, as a function of the energy $E_{\bar{o}}$ of electrons incident on a high Z target. The solid curves show the 'equilibrium' tenth-value layer, TVL_e, the dashed curves the ''first'' tenth-value layer, TVL_1, or the thickness closest to the radiation source needed to reduce the dose equivalent by a factor of ten. The TVLs are plotted in units of g cm^{-2} to facilitate comparison and interpolation to other materials. Presumed high energy values are indicated at the right. The smoothed curves are adapted from several sources, taking into account the behavior at both lower and higher energies.

The curves shown represent a subjective average of data from several sources and are believed accurate enough for most room shielding calculations. There is a surprising lack of consistency among the reported shielding measurements (for iron and lead, up to 15–20% deviation from the curves shown). These variations may indicate that the effective TVL for these materials is very geometry and/or spectrum dependent. In critical applications, it is suggested that the chosen shielding thickness be based on measurements for the specific radiation source and geometry at hand. Sources of original data are:

DIN-6847: Concrete, steel, lead: 1 MeV
NCRP 34: Concrete, lead: <1, 1, 2, 3, 4 MeV
NCRP34: Steel: <1, 4, 6 MeV
EMI Therapy Systems. Concrete, steel, copper, tungesten, lead: 4 MeV
Varian Associates: Concrete, steel, lead: 4, 8, 15 MeV
Maruyama et al.: Concrete, heavy concrete, steel, lead: 4, 6, 10, 20, 30, 32 MeV
Coleman: Concrete, steel, lead: 5, 8, 16 MeV
Karzmark and Capone: Concrete, steel, lead: 6 MeV
Kirn and Kennedy: Concrete: 6, 10, 20, 30 38 MeV
Miller and Kennedy: Concrete, lead: 86, 178 MeV
Buechner et al: Steel: 1, 2 MeV
Goldie et al.: Steel: 3 MeV
Goldie et al.: Steel: 3 MeV
Scag: Steel: 6-90 MeV
O'Connor et al.: Steel: 10 MeV

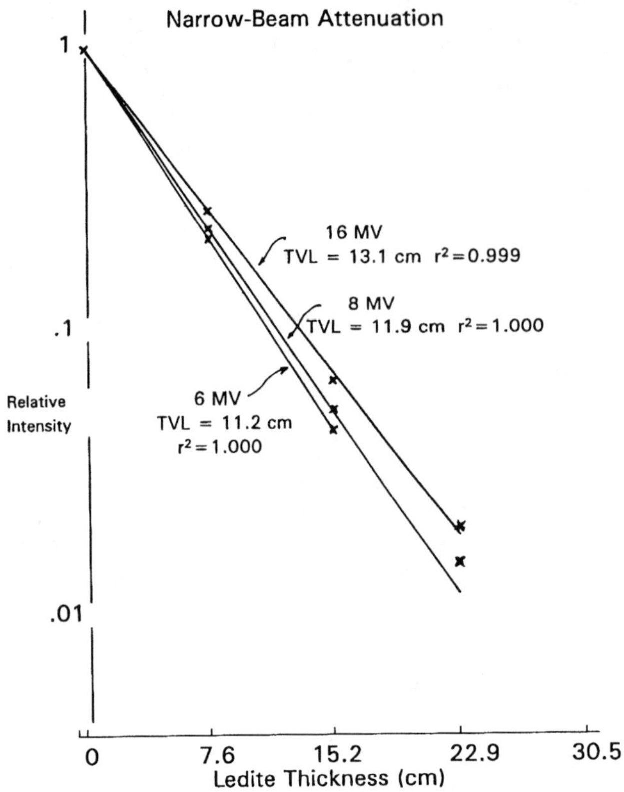

Narrow-beam attenuation in "good geometry" for three photon energies.

Figure 6.20 Narrow Beam Photon Attenuation in Ledite. Ledite is a new high-density shielding material supplied by Atomic Industries, Inc. of Telford, PA in the form of pre-cast interlocking blocks. These blocks contain steel scrap as the aggregate in a matrix of Portland cement resulting in a density of about 4.7 grams per cubic centimeter. This yields a reduction in shielding dimensions compared to ordinary concrete. Ledite is useful for shielding at medical radiation therapy facilities, and provides the neutron absorption required for high-energy linear accelerators. (From Barish, 1993)

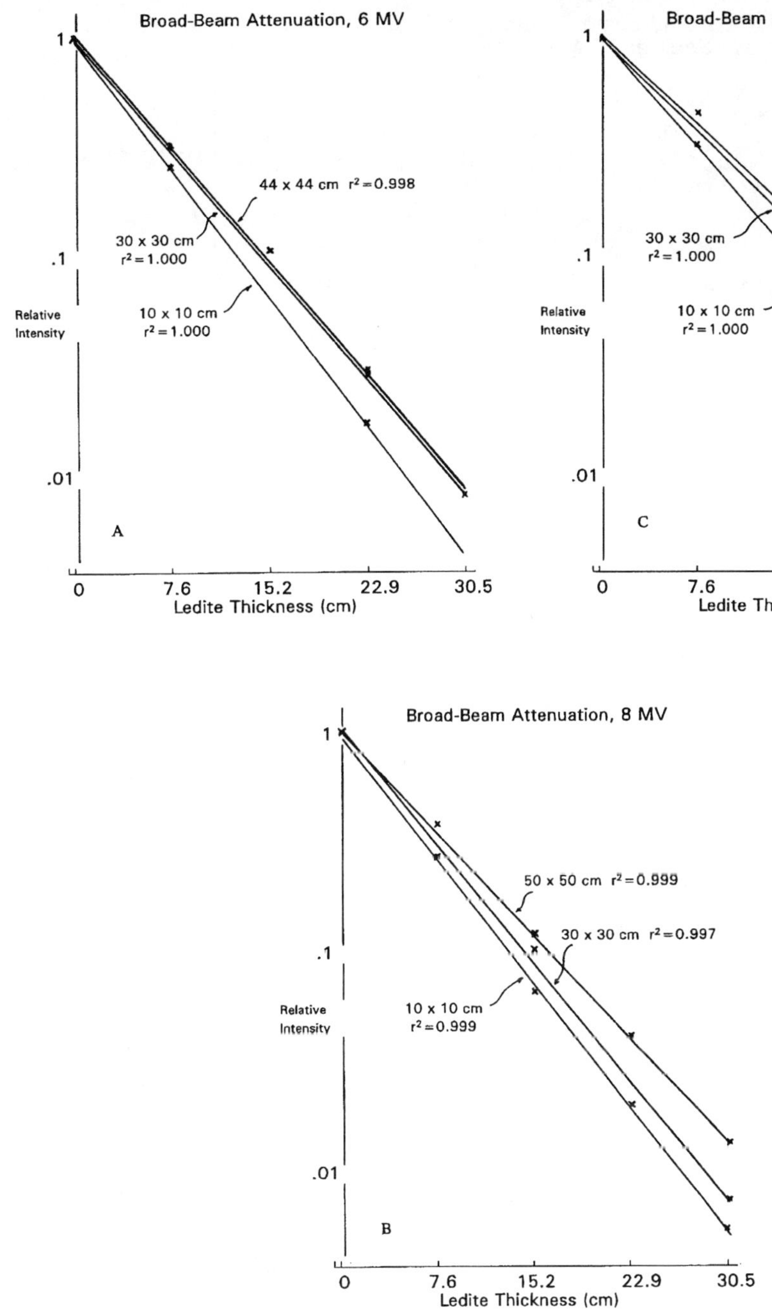

Broad-beam attenuation for three photon energies.

Figure 6.21 Broad-Bean Attenuation in Ledite for Three Photon Energies (From Barish, 1993)

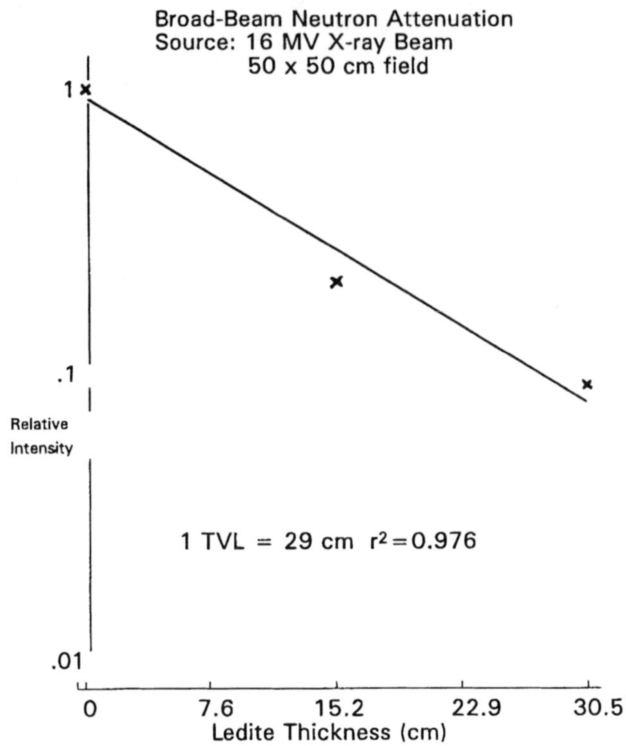

Broad-beam neutron attenuation. Neutrons are secondary to the production of 16 MV x rays.

Figure 6.22 Broad-Beam Secondary Neutron Attenuation in Ledite (From Barish, 1993)

Table 6.14 Specific Gravities, Weight Ratios and Compressive Strengths of Selected Aggregates

(From Abdul-Majid and Othman, 1994)

Type	SG[a] (ore)	SG (concrete)	Weight ratio C:FA:CA	Compressive Strength[b] (Mpa)	Relative Compressive Strength (%)
Ordinary concrete	2.77	2.4	1:1.5:3	31.07	100.0
Barite concrete	4.04	2.9	1:1.5:4.49	33.40	107.5
Pyrite concrete	3.97	2.85	1:1.5:4.4	42.33	136.2
Basalt concrete	2.97	2.5	1:1.5:3.85	45.15	145.3
Marble concrete	2.75	2.4	1:1.5:3	31.08	102.5
Hematite concrete	2.41	2.1	1:1.5:3.18	15.34	49.4
Polyethylene mortar	0.95	1.55	1:1.5:1.07	15.15	48.8
PVC mortar	1.4	1.8	1:1.5:1.72	22.62	72.8

[a] Specific gravities (SG) of ores and of the different types of concrete and their weight ratios at a volume ratio of 1:1.85:3.5 of cement (C), fine aggregates (FA), and coarse aggregates (CA), respectively.

[b] Compressive strength for the different types of concrete or mortar used in narrow-beam geometry after 28 d of curing under water, and their values relative to ordinary concrete.

Table 6.15 Gamma and Neutron Attenuation Coefficients of Selected Aggregates (From Abdul-Majid and Othman, 1994)

	Gamma-Ray (MeV)						Neutron ^{241}Am-Be Spectrum	
	0.662		1.172		1.332			
Type	Linear (cm^{-1})	Mass ($cm^2\ g^{-1}$)	Linear (cm^{-1})	Mass ($cm^2\ g^{-1}$)	Linear (cm^{-1})	Mass ($cm^2\ g^{-1}$)	Linear (cm^{-1})	Mass ($cm^2\ g^{-1}$)
Ordinary concrete	0.168	0.070	0.141	0.059	0.132	0.055	0.085	0.035
Barite concrete	0.203	0.071	0.155	0.055	0.145	0.051	0.080	0.028
Pyrite concrete	0.203	0.070	0.157	0.054	0.149	0.051	0.085	0.029
Basalt concrete	0.174	0.070	0.142	0.057	0.131	0.053	0.083	0.033
Marble concrete	0.166	0.069	0.138	0.058	0.129	0.054	0.088	0.037
Hematite concrete	0.148	0.070	0.128	0.061	0.122	0.058	0.080	0.038
Polyethylene mortar	0.110	0.071	0.096	0.062	0.090	0.058	0.095	0.061
PVC mortar	0.123	0.069	0.099	0.055	0.096	0.053	0.085	0.047

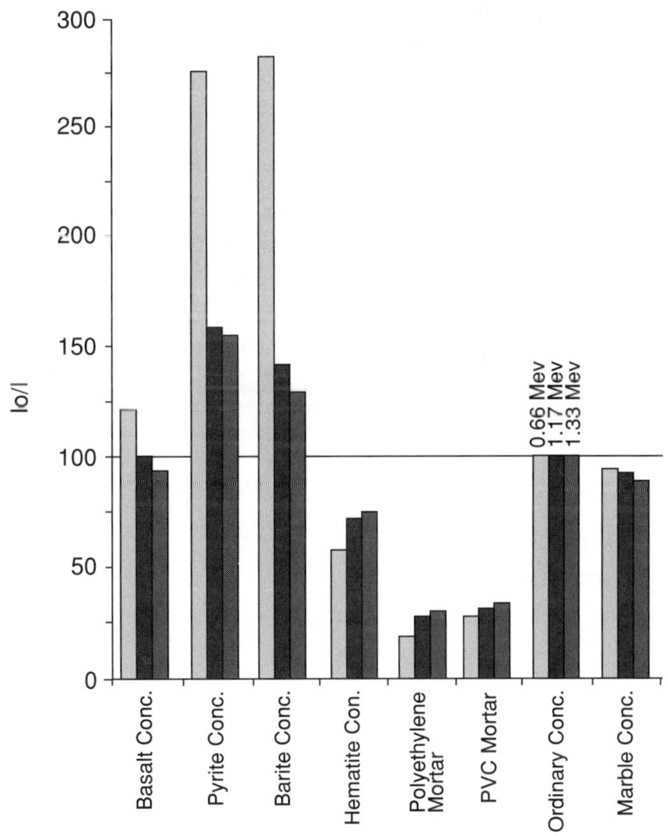

Gamma-ray intensities at different energies and 30-cm thickness for all types of materials tested in narrow-beam geometry relative to ordinary concrete (in %).

Figure 6.23 Relative Gamma Shielding Abilities (i.e., unattenuated to attenuated (Io/I), of Indicated Materials. (After Abdul-Mahid and Othman, 1994)

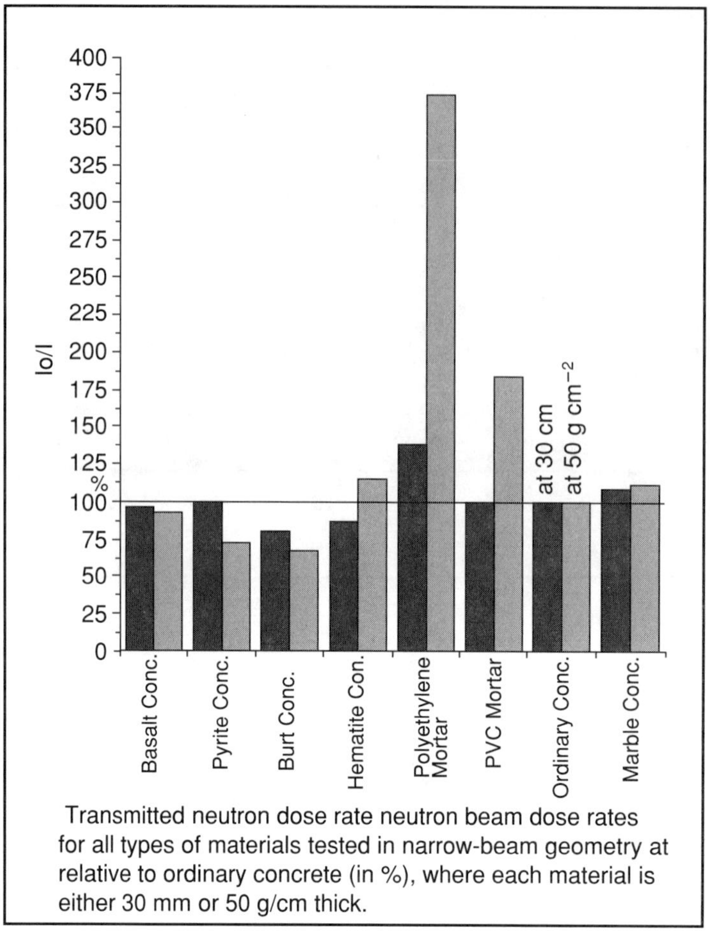

Figure 6.24 Relative Neutron Shielding Abilities (i.e., unattenuated to attenuated (Io/I), of Indicated Materials.

References

Abdul-Majid, S., Othman, F. ''Neutron attenuation characteristics of polyethylene, polyvinyl chloride, and heavy aggregate concrete and mortars,'' *Health Phys* **66:**327–338; 1994.

American National Standards Institute (ANSI). *Neutron and Gamma-Ray Flux-to-Dose-Rate Factors.* ANSI/ANS-6.1.1-1977, American Nuclear Society; La Grange Park, IL.

Archer, B.R., Thornby, J.I., Bushong, S.C. ''Diagnostic x-ray shielding design based on an empirical model of photon attenuation.'' *Health Phys* **44:**507–517; 1983.

Barish, R.J. ''Evaluation of a new high-density shielding material,'' *Health Phys* **64:**412–416; 1993.

Barkas, W.H., Berger, M.J. *Tables of Energy Losses and Ranges of Heavy Charged Particles.* NASA Report No. SP-3013; Washington, DC; 1964.

Bathow, G., Freytag, E., Tesch, K. ''Measurements on 6.3 GeV electromagnetic cascades and cascade-produced neutrons,'' *Nucl Phys* **B2:** 669; 1967.

Bathow, G., Freytag, E., Kobberling, M., Tesch, K., Kajikawa, R. ''Measurements of the longitudinal and lateral development of electromagnetic cascades in lead, copper and aluminum at 6 GeV,'' *Nucl Phys* **B20:** 592; 1970.

Buechner, W.W., Van de Graaff, R.J., Feshback, H., Burrill, E.A., Sperduto, A., McIntosh, L.R. ''An investigation of radiography in the range from 0.5 to 2.5 million volts,'' *ASTM Bulletin* **54;** 1948.

Coleman, G.J. *A Review of Shielding Data for the SL75-20 Linear Accelerator.* M.E.L. Equipment Co., Particle Accelerator Division, Publication No. 1013-10-75; Manor Royal, Crawley, Sussex; 1975.

Deutscher Normenausschuss (DNA), Medizinische Elektronen-Beschleuniger Anlagen, Draft Rep. No. DIN-6847, Part 2: Radiation Protection Rules for Installation, Beuth-Vertrieb, Berlin; 1975.

Dinter, H., Tesch, K. ''Measurements of dose and shielding parameters of electron-photon stray radiation from a high energy electron beam,'' *Deutsches Elektronen-Synchrotron,* Report DESY 76/19; Hamburg; 1976.

DO-88 (From EPA 520/1-75-001-A)

EMI Therapy Systems. Private communication; Sunnyvale, California; 1977.

Fewell, T.R., Shuping, E.R., Hawkins, K.R. *Handbook of Computed Tomography X-Ray Spectra.* U.S. Food and Drug Administration, Center for Devices and Radiological Health; HHS Publication (FDA) 81-8162; Rockville, MD 1981.

Frost, D., Jammet, H. *Manual on Radiation Protection in Hospitals and General Practice,* Vol. 2. World Health Organization; Geneva; 1975.

Glaze, S.A., Schnieders, N.J., Bushong, S.C. ''Use of gypsum wallboard for diagnostic x-ray protective barriers,'' *Health Phys* **36:**587–593; 1979.

Goldie, C.H., Wright, K.A., Anson, J.H., Cloud, R.W., Trump, J.G. ''Radiographic properties of x-rays in the two to six million volt range,'' *ASTM Bulletin* **49;** 1954.

Hubbell, J.H. *Photon Cross Sections, Attenuation Coefficients, and Energy Absorption Coefficients from 10 keV to 100 GeV.* NSRDS-NBS 29, National Bureau of Standards; Washington, DC; 1969.

International Atomic Energy Agency, IAEA No. 188; 1979.

International Atomic Energy Agency, IAEA No. 283; 1988.

International Commission on Radiation Protection (ICRP). Publication No. 4; 1964.

International Commission on Radiation Protection (ICRP). *Protection Against Ionizing Radiation from External Sources Used in Medicine.* ICRP Publication 33; Pergamon Press; Elmsford, NY; 1982.

International Commission on Radiation Units (ICRU). *Stopping Pavers for Electrons and Positrons.* ICRU Report 37; Bethesda, MD; 1984.

Karzmark, C.J., Capone, T. ''Measurements of 6 MV X-rays, I. Primary radiation absorption in lead, steel and concrete,'' *Br J Radiol* **41**:33; 1968.

Kirn, F.S., Kennedy, R.J. ''How much concrete for shielding?,'' *Nucleonics* **12**:44; 1954.

Kirn, F.S., Kennedy, R.J., Wycoff, O. ''Attenuation of gamma rays at oblique incidence,'' *Radiology* **63**:94; 1954.

Kocher, D.C. *Radioactive Decay Data Tables: A Handbook of Decay Data for Application to Radiation Dosimetry and Radiological Assessments.* U.S. Department of Energy; DOE/TIC-11026; 1981.

Maruyama, T., Kumamoto, Y., Kato, Y., Hashizume, T., Uamamoto, M. ''Attenuation of 4-32 MV X-rays in ordinary concrete, heavy concrete, iron and lead,'' *Health Phys* **20**:277; 1977.

Miller, W., Kennedy, R.J. Attenuation of 86 and 176 MeV synchroton X-rays in concrete and lead, *Radiat Res* **4**:360; 1956.

Nachtigall, D. *Table of Specific Gamma—Ray Constants.* Verlag, Karl Thiemig KG; Munich; 1969.

National Academy of Sciences—National Research Council (NAS/NRC). *Studies on Penetration of Charged Particles.* PB-212-907; Washington, DC; 1964.

National Bureau of Standards (NBS). *Medical Physics Data Book.* NBS Handbook 138; Washington, DC; 1982.

National Bureau of Standards (NBS). *Medical X-Ray Protection up to Three Million Volts.* Handbook 76; 1962.

National Council on Radiation Protection and Measurements (NCRP). *Medical X-Ray and Gamma Ray Protection for Energies Up to 10 MeV—Equipment Design and Use.* NCRP Report No. 33; Bethesda, MD; 1968.

National Council on Radiation Protection and Measurements (NCRP). *Medical X-Ray and Gamma-Ray Protection for Energies up to 10 MeV—Structural Shielding Design and Evaluation.* NCRP Report No. 34; Washington, DC; 1970.

National Council on Radiation Protection and Measurements (NCRP). *Structural Shielding Design and Evaluation for Medical Use of X-Rays and Gamma Rays of Energies Up to 10 MeV.* NCRP Report No. 49; Bethesda, MD; 1976.

National Council on Radiation Protection and Measurements (NCRP). *Radiation Protection Design Guidelines for 0.1–100 MeV Particle Accelerator Facilities.* NCRP Report No. 51; Bethesda, MD; 1977.

Nuclear Regulatory Commission ''New gamma ray build-up factor data point kernel calculations: ANS-6.4.3 standard reference data'' NUREG/CR-5740; Oak Ridge National Laboratory; Oak Ridge, TN; 1991.

O'Connor, D.T., Criscuolo, E.L., Pace, A.L. ''10 MeV X-ray technique,'' *Papers on Radiography Am Soc Test Mater* **10**; and ASTM Spec. Tech. Publ. No. 96;1949.

Radiological Health Handbook; 1970.

Rajhavendron, C.P., Nagarajan, P.S., Venkataraman, G. ''Shielding Calculations Below 100 kVp,'' *Health Phys* **42**:717–723, 1982.

Rich, B. Personal communication; 1991.

Ritz, H. ''Broad and narrow beam attenuation of Ir^{192} gamma rays in concrete, steel and lead,'' *Nondestr Test* **16**: 269; 1958.

Rossi, R.P., Ritenour, R., Christodoulou, E. ''Broad beam transmission properties of some common shielding materials for use in diagnostic radiology,'' *Health Phys* **61**:601–608; 1991.

Scag, D.A. ''Discussion of radiographic characteristics of high energy X-rays,'' *Nondestr Test* **12**:47; 1954.

Simpkin, D.J. ''A general solution to the shielding of medical x and gamma rays by the NCRP 49 methods,'' *Health Phys* 52: 431–436; 1987a.

Simpkin, D.J. ''Shielding requirements for mammography,'' *Health Phys* **53**:267–279; 1987b.

Simpkin, D.J. ''Shielding requirement for constant potential diagnostic x-ray beams determined by a Monte Carlo calculation,'' *Health Phys* **56**:151–164; 1989.

Simpkin, D.J. ''Transmission data for shielding diagnostic x-ray facilities,'' *Health Phys* **68**:704–709; 1995.

Spinks, J.W.T., Woods, R.J. *An Introduction to Radiation Chemistry,* John Wiley & Sons; New York; 1964.

Trubey, D.K. *New Gamma-Ray Buildup Factor Data for Point Kernel Calculations. ANS-6.4.3,* Standard Reference Data; NUREG/CR-5740 ORNL/RSIC-49/R1; Oak Ridge National Laboratory; Oak Ridge, TN; 1991.

Turner, J.E., Hanson, R.N., Souleyrette, M., Martz, D.E., Rhea, T.A., Schmidt, D.W. ''Calculations for beta dosimetry using Monte Carlo Code (OREC) for electron transport in water,'' *Health Phys* **55:**741–750; 1988.

Unger, L.M., Trubey, D.K. *Specific Gamma-Ray Dose Constants for Nuclides Important to Dosimetry and Radiological Assessment.* ORNL/RSIC-45; Oak Ridge National Laboratory; Oak Ridge, TN; 1981.

Varian Associates, *Linatron High Energy X-Ray Applications.* Varian Associates, Radiation Division; Palo Alto, CA; 1975.

Wachsmann, F., Drexler, G. *Graphs and Tables for Use in Radiology,* Springer-Verlag; New York; 1975.

Wideroe, R. ''The Brown Boveri 31 million volt dual beam betatron,'' *Nondestr Test* **11:**23; 1953.

Wyckoff, H.O., Kennedy, R.J. ''Concrete as a protective barrier for gamma rays from radium,'' *J Research NBS* **42:**431; 1949.

CHAPTER 7

NEUTRON PRODUCTION, SHIELDING AND ACTIVATION

This chapter contains information on neutron cross-sections, production, spectra and yields; detection and detectors; shielding with various materials, particularly with ordinary concrete; and neutron activation products of interest to health physicists. Neutron dosimetry is covered in Chapter 13.

TABLE OF CONTENTS

Table 7.1 Neutron Energy Terminology

Term	Derivation than	Range of Energies
Cold	Neutrons produced by a thermal environment much less than 20°C	Typically those with a wavelength >4 Å, i.e., <0.005 eV
Thermal	Neutrons in thermal equilibrium with surrounding	Most probable energy for the number density distribution at 20°C is 0.025 eV. Maxwellian distribution of 20°C extends to about 0.1 eV
Epithermal	Neutrons of energy greater than thermal	Energies above about 0.2 eV
Cadmium	Neutrons which are strongly absorbed by cadmium	Energies below about 0.4 eV
Epicadmium	Neutrons which are not strongly absorbed by cadmium	Energies above about 0.6 eV
Slow	Neutrons of energy slightly greater than thermal	Usually means less thna 1–10 eV Occasionally means less than 1 keV
Resonance	In pile neutron physics usually refers to neutrons which are strongly captured in the resonance of U-238, and of a few commonly used detectors, e.g., In, Au	A broad band of energies from about 1 eV to about 300 eV Termed ''intermediate'' in NCRP 38
Intermediate	Neutrons between slow and fast	From a few hundred eV to about 0.5 MeV
Fast		Neutrons of energy greater than about 0.5 MeV
Ultra Fast (relativistic)	Inelastic and nuclear reactions become comparable in frequency to elastic reactions	Neutrons of energy greater than about 20 MeV
Pile	Neutrons of all energies present in nuclear reactors	About 0.001 eV to approximately 15 MeV
Fission	Neutrons formed directly in fission	About 100 keV to approximately 15 MeV Most probable energy 0.8 MeV Average energy 2.0 MeV

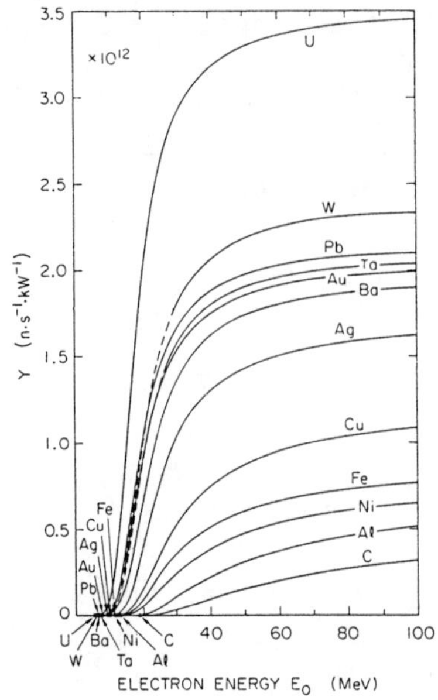

Figure 7.1 Yield of Photoneutrons Produced in Electromagnetic Cascades Initiated by Electrons Incident on Thick Targets Per Unit Beam Power, as a Function of Incident Energy (From IAEA Technical Report Series 188, 1979)

Table 7.2 Sources of Neutrons

Source	Reaction	Average Neutron Energy (MeV)	Yield[a] (Gy/C)	Characteristic Problems
Accelerators	H^3(p,n) He^3	0.7, 3.2[b]	0.75	
	H^2(d,n) He^3	2.45[c]	1.3	γ, Tritium
	H^3(d,n) He^4	14.1[c]	1.3	
			0.5–2 × 10^8 ns^{-1}/ μA[d]	γ, Tritium
	Li^7(d,n) Be^8	13.3[c]		γ, f.p., α
Critical Assemblies & Reactors	Fission	Fission Spectrum		
			(n/sec/per Ci)[a]	
Mock Fission (Po + Be + B + Li + F)	α, n	Fission Spectrum	4 × 10^5	α
Na^{24} + Be	γ, n	0.83	1.3 × 10^5	γ
Na^{24} + D_2O	γ, n	0.22	2.7 × 10^5	γ
Mn^{56} + Be	γ, n	0.1 (90%), 0.3 (10%)	2.9 × 10^4	γ
Mn^{56} + D_2O	γ, n	0.22	3.1 × 10^3	γ
Ga^{72} + Be	γ, n	0.78	5 × 10^4	γ
Ga^{72} + D_2O	γ, n	0.13	6 × 10^4	γ
Y^{88} + Be	γ, n	0.16	1 × 10^5	γ
Y^{88} + D	γ, n	0.31	3 × 10^3	γ
In^{116} + Be	γ, n	0.30	8.2 × 10^3	γ
Sb^{124} + Be	γ, n	0.024	1.9 × 10^5	γ
La^{140} + Be	γ, n	0.62	3 × 10^3	γ
La^{140} + D_2O	γ, n	0.15	8 × 10^3	γ
Ra^{228} + Be	γ, n	0.83	3.5 × 10^4	γ
Ra^{228} + D_2O	γ, n	0.20	9.5 × 10^4	γ
Ra + Be	α, n	Spectrum	3.0 × 10^4	α, γ, Rn
Ra + Be	α, n	5.0	1.7 × 10^7	α, γ, Rn
Ra + B	γ, n	3.0	6.8 × 10^6	α, γ, Rn
Ra + D_2O	α, n	0.12	1 × 10^3	α, γ, Rn
Rn^{222} + Be	α, n	5	1.5 × 10^7	α, γ, Rn
Po^{210} + Be	α, n	4	3 × 10^6	α
Po^{210} + B	α, n	2.5	9 × 10^5	α
Po^{210} + F	α, n	1.4	4 × 10^5	α
Po^{210} + Li	α, n	0.42	9 × 10^4	α
Ac^{227} + Be	α, n			α
Pu^{239} + Be	α, n	4	10^6	α
Cf^{252}	Spon. Fission	Fission Spectrum	10^6	α

[a] For photoneutron sources (γ, n reactions) "Standard Yield" is given, i.e., 1 gram of target material at 1 cm from 1 Ci of γ emitter. Higher yields are possible. For (α, n) reactions, yields are an indefinite function of target material and emitter mixing.
[b] Forward direction energies with 1.5 and 4 MeV protons respectively.
[c] Energies are for low (a few hundred keV) projectile energies. Higher energy projectiles will produce higher energy neutrons.
[d] For a new target over the range of 100–500 keV.

Table 7.3 Data on Neutron Production[a] (Courtesy NCRP after Report 38, 1971)

Target	Residual Nucleus	Q/MeV	Reaction Yields: Thick Target Yield (n/μC) or Nominal Cross Section (barns)	Corresponding Incident Particle Energy (MeV)	Degree of Gamma-Ray Contamination	Gamma-Ray Energies (MeV)	Residual Activity or Comparative Dosage
				(p,n) Reactions			
^{3}H	^{3}He	−0.76	0.50 barn	3.0 (peak)	Considerable ≃ 10^{-8} γ/proton	20	None
^{7}Li	^{7}Be	−1.65	0.50 barn	2.2 (peak)	Considerable ≃ 2×10^{-8} γ/proton	17	Considerable (^{7}Be)
^{9}Be	^{9}B	−1.85			Considerable ≃ 10^{-9} γ/proton		None
				(d,n) Reactions			
^{2}H	^{3}He	3.26	2.5×10^{6} n/μC 0.05 barn	0.25 0.25	None	None	None
^{3}H	^{4}He	17.6	~108 n/μC 5 barn	0.20 0.10	Slight		None
^{6}Li	^{7}Be	3.38			0.3 γ/n	0.4	Moderate (^{7}Be)
^{6}Li	$^{3}He + ^{4}He$	1.79	1.7×10^{7} n/μC	0.6		0.4	None
^{7}Li	$^{4}He + ^{4}He$	15.1	0.06 barn	0.2	0.3 γ/n	4.9	None
^{9}Be	^{10}B	4.36	4×10^{6} n/μC	0.4		3.6; 2.2; 1.7; 1.0; 0.7; 0.4	Small (^{10}Be)
			0.4 barn	5.0			
^{10}B	^{11}C	6.47				8.9; 6.7; 6.4; 4.5	Small (^{11}C)
^{11}B	^{12}C	13.7					None
^{12}C	^{13}N	0.28	35×10^{-3} barn/ster (0°)	2.2–3	4.45 γ/n		Slight (^{13}N)
^{13}C	^{14}N	5.3				6.1; 5.0; 3.3; 2.3; 1.6; 0.7	None
^{14}N	^{15}O	5.12			None		Slight (^{15}O)
^{19}F	^{20}Ne	10.65				10.6; 9.1; 8.4; 6.4; 5.2; 3.5; 2.8; 1.6; 0.5	
				(γ,n) Reactions			
^{2}H	^{1}H	−2.226	2.7×10^{-3} barn	4.0 (max)			
^{9}Be	^{8}Be (2α)	−1.666	1×10^{-3} barn	1.7 (max)			

(continued)

Table 7.3 Data on Neutron Production[a] (Continued)

(α,n) Reactions

Target	Residual Nucleus	Q/MeV	Yield n s^{-1} Ci^{-1}	Reaction	Degree of Gamma-Ray Contamination	Gamma-Ray Energies (MeV)	Residual Activity or Comparative Dosage
^{7}Li	^{10}B	−2.78	5×10^4	Po-Li		0.8; 0.48	$n/\gamma \simeq 0.25$
^{9}Be	^{12}C		2.3×10^6	Po-Be		0.8; 4.45	$n/\gamma \simeq 4.0$
^{9}Be	^{12}C	5.7	1.7×10^7	Ra-Be	Considerable		$n/\gamma < 0.01$
^{10}B	^{13}N	1.07	6×10^5	Po-B		0.8; 3.7; 2.4	$n/\gamma \simeq 5.0$
^{11}B	^{14}N	0.15	7×10^6	Ra-B	Considerable		$n/\gamma < 0.01$
			2×10^5	Po-F		0.8; 1.3; 1.5	$n/\gamma \simeq 1.0$
^{19}F	^{22}Na	−2.3	2.5×10^6	Ra-BeF_4	Considerable		$n/\gamma < 0.01$
^{23}Na	^{26}Al	−3.88	4×10^4	Po-Na		0.8; 0.4; 1.1; 1.8; 2.6	$n/\gamma \simeq 0.03$
^{25}Mg	^{28}Si	2.67	3×10^4	Po-Mg		0.8; 1.8; 4.0	$n/\gamma \simeq 0.15$
^{26}Mg	^{29}Si	0.04					
^{27}Al	^{30}P	−2.92	2×10^4	Po-Al		0.8; 1.3; 2.3; 3.6	$n/\gamma \simeq 0.1$

[a] Information in the last two columns is qualitative only.

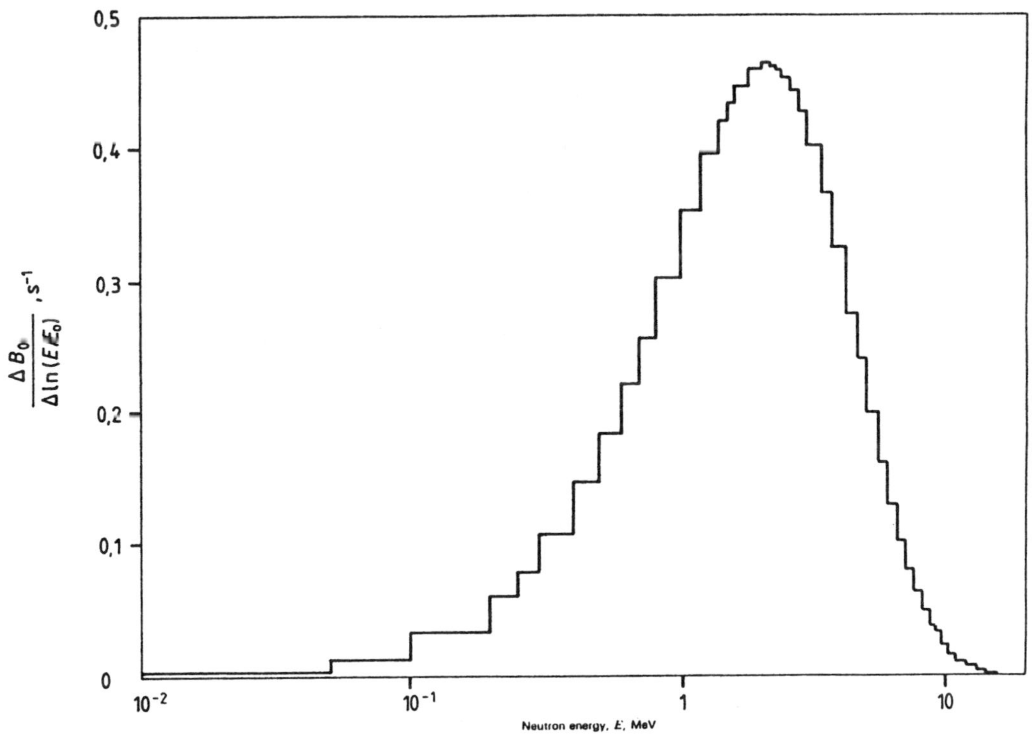

Figure 7.2 Neutron Spectrum from a ^{252}Cf Spontaneous Fission Source (From Eisenhauer, 1992, personal communication)

Note: This is a "lethargy" plot. Y-axis is sometimes labeled Eϕ(E) or ϕ(u). The x-axis is logarithm in E. The relative area under the histogram is proportional to the number of neutrons.

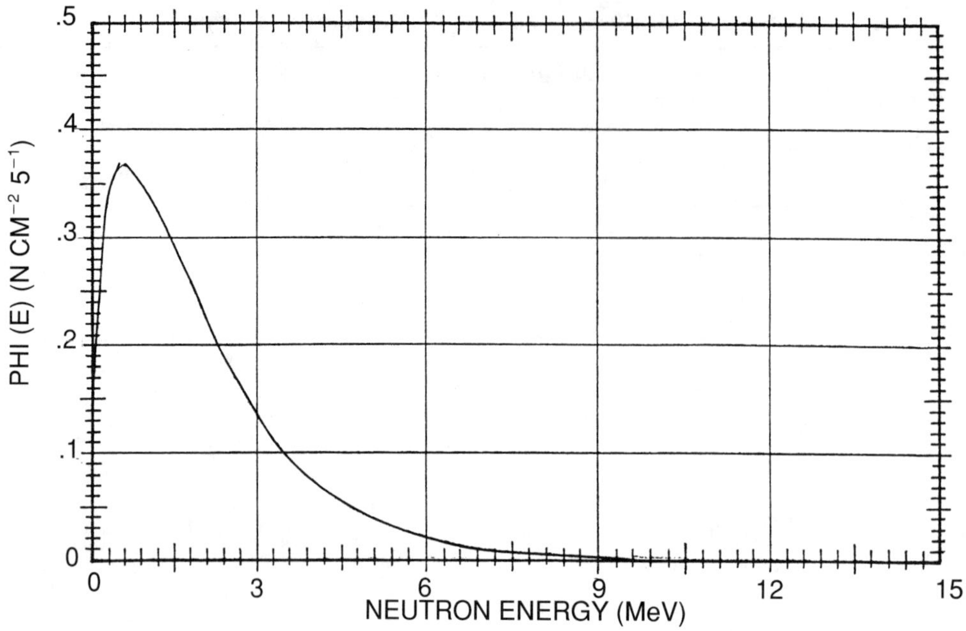

Figure 7.3 ^{235}**U Fission Neutron Spectrum** (After Grundl and Lamaze, 1988)

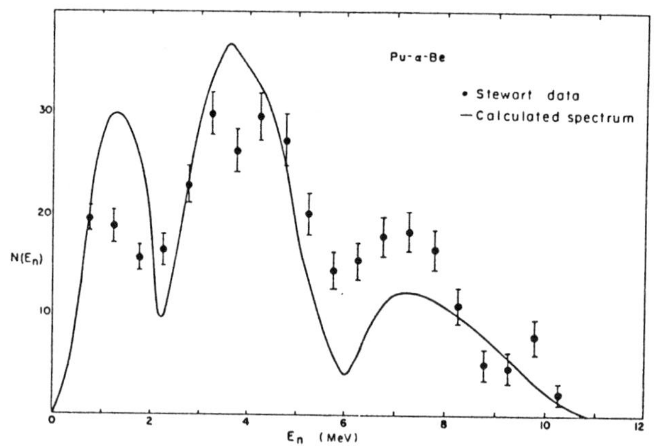

Figure 7.4 **Pu-α-Be Neutron Spectra** (Courtesy Academic Press. From *Accelerator Health Physics,* Patterson and Thomas, 1973)

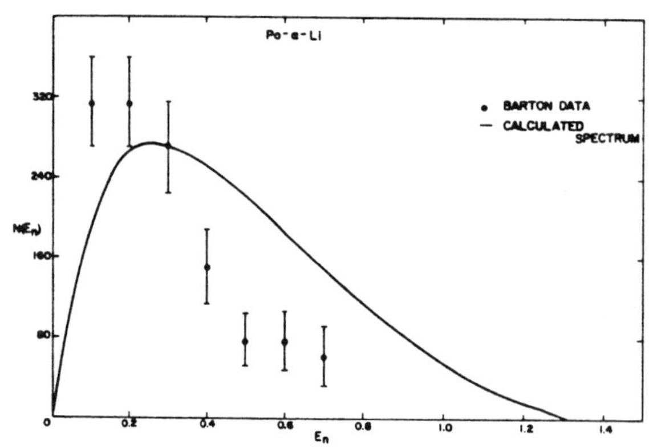

Figure 7.5 **Calculated and Measured Neutron Energy Spectra of a Po-Li Neutron Source** (Courtesy Academic Press. From *Accelerator Health Physics*, Patterson and Thomas, 1973)

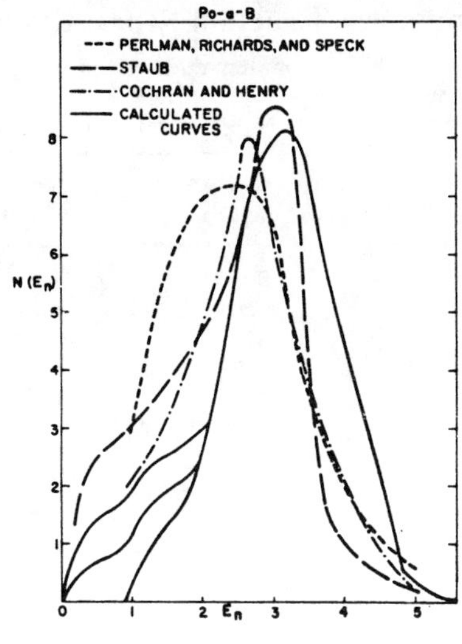

Figure 7.6 Neutron Energy Spectrum Calculated for a Po-Natural B Neutron Source Compared with Several Experimental Spectra (Courtesy Academic Press. From *Accelerator Health Physics*, Patterson and Thomas, 1973)

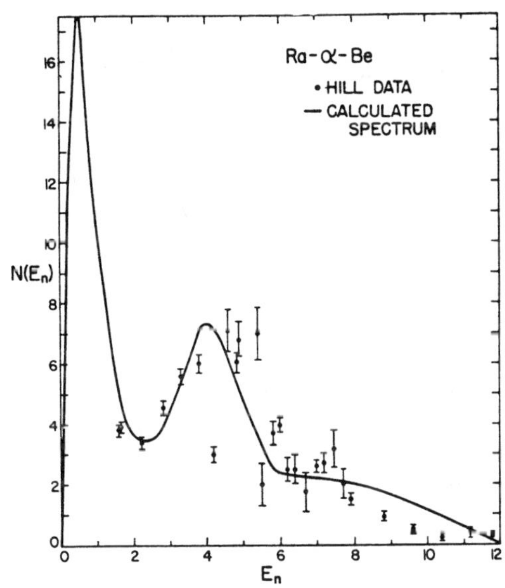

Figure 7.7 Calculated Neutron Energy Spectrum for a Ra-Be Source. The experiments of Hill are shown for comparison (Courtesy Academic Press. From *Accelerator Health Physics*, Patterson and Thomas, 1973)

Table 7.4 Relative Isotopic Abundances, Reaction Separation Energies and Decay Data (Courtesy NCRP From Report 79, 1987)

Nuclide			(γ,n) Reaction				(γ,pn) Reaction				(γ,2n) Reaction			
Chem. Symb.	Mass No.	Rel. Abund.	S_n[a] (MeV)	$t_{1/2}$	Decay	Q (MeV)	S_{pn}[a] (MeV)	$t_{1/2}$	Decay	Q (MeV)	S_{2n} (MeV)	$t_{1/2}$	Decay	Q (MeV)
H	2	0.02	2.23	s			—				—			
Be	9	100	1.67	s			18.92	s			20.56	53 d	EC	0.86
C	12	98.89	18.72	20.4 min	β+	1.98	27.41	s			31.84	19 s	β+	2.89
	13	1.11	4.95	s			20.90	s			23.66	20.4 m	β+	1.98
N	14	99.63	10.55	10 min	β+	2.21	12.49	s			30.62	11 ms	β+	17.3
	15	0.36	10.83	s			18.38	s			21.39	9.96 m	β+	2.21
O	16	99.75	15.66	122 s	β+	2.75	22.96	s			28.89	71 s	β+	5.15
	17	0.03	4.14	s			16.27	s			19.81	122 s	β+	2.76
	18	0.20	8.05	s			12.83	7.1 s	β−	10.4	12.19	s		
Mg	24	78.99	16.53	11.3 s	β+	4.06	24.11	2.6 y	β+	2.8	29.68	2.86 s	β+	4.79
	25	10.00	7.33	s			19.02	s			23.86	11.3 s	β+	4.06
	26	11.01	11.09	s			23.16	15 h	β−	5.5	18.43	s		
Al	27	100	13.06	>10^5 y	β+	4.00	19.36	s			24.42	7.18 s	β+	4.28
				6.4 s	β+	4.23								
Si	28	92.23	17.18	4.13s	β+	4.81	24.64	10^5y	β+	4.0	30.49	2.21 s	β+	5.06
	29	4.67	8.74	s			20.06	s			25.65	4.13 s	β+	4.81
	30	3.10	10.61	s			22.94	2.24 min	β−	4.6	19.08	s		
Cr	50	4.4	13.00	42 min	β+	2.63	21.14	16 d	EC	4.0	23.58	21 h	EC	1.7
	52	83.8	12.04	28 d	EC	0.75	21.56	s			21.30	s		
	53	9.5	7.94	s			18.44	s			19.98	28 d	EC	0.8
	54	2.4	9.72	s			20.85	3.8 min	β−	4.0	17.66	s		
Fe	54	5.8	13.38	8.5 min	β+	3.74	20.91	21 min	β+	4.71	24.10	8.3 h	β+	2.37
								5.6 d	EC	5.08				
	56	91.7	11.19	2.7 y	EC	0.23	20.41	312 d	EC	1.38	20.50	s		0.23
	57	2.1	7.65	s			17.83	s			18.84	27 y	EC	
	58	0.2	10.04	s			20.60	2.6 h	β−	3.70	17.69	s		
Co	59	100	10.45	71 d	β+	2.31	17.41	s			19.03	271 d	EC	0.84
Ni	58	68.2	12.20	36 h	β+	3.27	19.55	79 d	β+	4.6	22.47	6.1 d	EC	2.13
	60	26.1	11.34	10^5 y	EC	1.07	19.99	71 d	EC	2.3	20.39	s		
	61	1.1	7.82	s			17.35	s			12.21	10^5 y	EC	1.10
	62	3.5	10.60	s			20.46	5.3 y	β−	2.8	18.42	s		
	64	0.9	9.66	100 y	β−	0.07	20.95	1.5 min	β−	5.3	16.50	s		
Cu	63	69.2	10.85	9.7 m	β+	3.95	16.72	s			19.74	3.4 h	β+	2.24
	65	30.8	9.91	12.7 h	β+	1.68	17.11	100 y	β−	0.07	17.83	s		
					β−	0.58								
Zn	64	48.6	11.86	38 min	β+	5.5	14.04	9.7 min	β+	3.95	20.98	9.2 h	EC	1.63
	66	27.9	11.06	244 d	EC	1.4	18.84	13 h	EC	1.67	19.04	s		
									β−	0.58				
	67	4.1	7.05	s			16.33	s			18.11	244 d	EC	1.32
	68	18.7	10.20	s			19.11	5.1 min	β−	2.64	17.25	s		
	70	0.6	9.21	56 min	β−	0.90	19.5	31 s	β−	4.62	15.70	s		

(continued)

Table 7.4 Relative Isotopic Abundances, Reaction Separation Energies and Decay Data (Continued)

Nuclide			(γ,n) Reaction				(γ,pn) Reaction				(γ,2n) Reaction			
Chem. Symb.	Mass No.	Rel. Abund.	S_n[a] (MeV)	$t_{1/2}$	Decay	Q (MeV)	S_{pn}[a] (MeV)	$t_{1/2}$	Decay	Q (MeV)	S_{2n} (MeV)	$t_{1/2}$	Decay	Q (MeV)
W	180	0.1	8.41	38 min	EC	1.06	14.5	2.4 h	EC	1.91	15.3	21 d	EC	0.09
	182	26.3	8.06	121 d	EC	0.19	14.67	8.1 h	EC	0.86	14.75	s		
									β−	0.71				
	183	14.3	6.19	s			13.28	s			14.25	121 d	EC	0.19
	184	30.6	7.41	s			14.63	115 d	β−	1.81	13.60	s		
	186	28.6	7.20	75 d	β−	0.43	15.0	8.7 h	β−	2.87	12.95	s		
Pt	190	0.1	8.8	11 h	EC	1.91	14.4	41 h	EC	2.8	15.7	10 d	EC	0.54
	192	0.8	8.7	2.9 d	EC	1.00	15.0	12 d	EC	2.0	15.1	s		
	194	32.9	8.38	4.3 d	EC	0.06	15.30	74 d	β−	1.5	14.63	s		
									EC	1.1				
	195	33.8	6.11	s			13.47	s			14.49	4.3 d	EC	0.06
	196	25.3	7.92	s			15.50	19 h	β−	2.3	14.03	s		
	198	7.2	7.5	18 h	β−	0.72	15.8	52 s	β−	3.2	13.4	s		
								1.4 h	β−	1.2				
Au	197	100	8.06	6.2 d	EC	1.49	13.71	s			14.72	183 d	EC	0.23
					β−	0.68								
Pb	204	1.4	8.4	52 h	EC	0.97	14.5	12 d	EC	1.37	15.3	10^5 y	EC	0.05
	206	24.1	8.09	10^7 y	EC	0.06	14.80	3.8 y	β−	0.76	14.82	s		
									EC	0.35				
	207	22.1	6.74	s			13.99	s			14.82	10^7 y	EC	0.06
	208	52.4	7.37	s			14.85	4.2 min	β−	1.53	14.11	s		
U	234	0.01	6.84	10^5 y		4.91	13.15	1.3 d	β−	1.34	12.60	72 y		5.41
	235	0.72	5.30	10^5 y		4.86	11.93	27 d	β−	0.57	12.14	10^5 y		4.91
	238	99.27	6.15	6.8 d	β−	0.52	13.6	9.1 min	β−	3.1	11.28	10^5 y		4.57

Note. Q values give the total energy available for the decay processes indicated. For positron decay the maximum positron energy is: $E_{\beta+} = Q - 2mc^2$, where $mc^2 = 0.511$ MeV. No attempt has been made to give the energies of gamma rays that often follow decay by electron capture (EC) or beta decay. The energies of gamma rays following electron capture can approach the Q values listed above. 's' indicates a stable reaction product. See Figure 7.1 for the total photoneutron production yield.

Source of data: Relative abundances (Holden, 1977), Separation Energies (Wapstra and Bos, 1977), Decay Data (Lederer and Shirley, 1977).

[a] Separation energy associated with the specified neutron production reaction.

Table 7.4.1 Photoneutron Production Features

Cross-section	$2.25\ 10^{-3}\ A^{5/3}$ mb MeV^{-1}	Giant resonance neutron yield from very thick targets, for photons up to 30 MeV. Some light Z nuclides are up to one-fourth of this value.
Energy of giant resonance	15–18 MeV for A > 60 18–25 MeV for A < 60	
Threshold	generally >7 MeV	notable exceptions: Be, ^2H

Table 7.5 Characteristics of Selected Radioactive Neutron Sources (Courtesy IAEA From Tech. Rept. Series 188, 1979)

Source	Reaction	Half-life	Average Neutron Energy (MeV)	Yield per Bq (neutrons s^{-1})[a]	Yield per Ci (neutrons s^{-1})[a]
^{210}Po-Be	α,n	138.4 d	4.2	68×10^{-6}	2.5×10^{6}
^{226}Ra-Be	α,n	1620 yr	4.0	351×10^{-6}	1.3×10^{7}
^{238}Pu-Be	α,n	86.4 yr	4.5	62×10^{-6}	2.3×10^{6}
^{241}Am-Be	α,n	458 yr	4.5	59×10^{-6}	2.2×10^{6}
^{210}Po-B	α,n	138.4 d	^{10}B: 6.3 ^{11}B: 4.5	16×10^{-6} [b]	6.0×10^{5} [b]
^{124}Sb-Be	γ,n	60 d	0.024	35×10^{-6} [b,c]	1.3×10^{6} [b,c]
^{252}Cf	spontaneous fission	2.65 yr	2.35 (fission spectrum)	62 (from 1 g)[d]	2.3×10^{12} (from 1 g)[d]

[a] Compacted mixtures.
[b] Relatively monoenergetic.
[c] Yield can be increased about four times by encasing in beryllium.
[d] Specific activity: 19.7×10^{12}Bq g^{-1} (532 Ci g^{-1}).

Table 7.6 Z-Dependence of Cross-Section per Atom ($\sigma \propto Z^m$) (Courtesy IAEA From Tech. Rept Series 188, 1979)

Particle Type	Physical Effect	Exponent m[a]
Photon	Photoelectric effect	4.6
	Coherent scattering	2.6
	Incoherent (Compton) scattering	1
	Pair production	2[b]
Electron	Collision (ionization)	1
	Radiation (bremsstrahlung)	2[b]
	Angular scattering power	2[b]
Hadron (proton, neutron, meson, etc.)	Nuclear scattering	2/3

[a] Values of m are both Z- and energy dependent. These should be taken as nominal values.
[b] $Z(Z+1)$ is a better representation of the Z-dependence than is Z^2.

Table 7.7 Half-Thicknesses of Materials for Neutrons from Po-Be Sources Using Plate Absorbers (From USAEC Isotopes, 1953)

Material	Half Thickness, cm
Paraffin	6.6
Water	5.4
12% Borax in water	5.3
Brass	4.9
Steel (cold roll)	4.9
Lead	6.8
Aluminum	7.8

Table 7.8 Data on Source Strength and Size of Shielding Spheres for Po-Be Sources (From USAEC Isotopes, 1953)

Source Strength		Neutrons/sec/cm² at Surface of Paraffin Sphere of Indicated Diameter			
Curies	Neutrons per sec	14 in.	18 in.	22 in.	25 in.
1	2.5×10^6	80			
2	5.0×10^6	161			
3	7.5×10^6	242			
4	1.0×10^7	322	108		
5	1.25×10^7	402	135		
6	1.50×10^7	483	162		
7	1.75×10^7	564	189		
8	2.0×10^7	644	216		
10	2.5×10^7		270		
12	3.0×10^7		324		
14	3.5×10^7		378		
15	3.75×10^7		405	150	
20	5.0×10^7			200	
24	6.0×10^7			240	
28	7.0×10^7			280	140
30	7.5×10^7				150
35	8.75×10^7				175
40	1.0×10^8				200

Table 7.9 Radioactive and Spontaneous Fission Half-Lives of Selected Isotopes (After Denham, 1968)[b]

Isotope	Radioactive Half-Life (Years)	Specific Activity (Ci/g)	Spontaneous Fission Half-Life (Years)	Fission Fraction (%)	Neutrons per Fission	Calculated Neutron Emission Rate (n/sec/g)
^{238}U	4.468×10^9	3.36×10^{-7}		5.45×10^{-5}%	1.98	0.013
^{238}Pu	87.7	17.1		1.85×10^{-7}%	2.24	2.6×10^3
^{239}Pu	24,110	0.062	5.5×10^{15}	3.1×10^{-10}%	2.877	0.0204
^{240}Pu	6564	0.227		5.75×10^{-6}%	2.21	1.07×10^3
^{242}Pu	3.76×10^5	0.00393		5.54×10^{-5}%	2.153	173
^{244}Pu	8.08×10^7	1.8×10^{-5}		0.123%	2.3	1900
^{241}Am	432.2	3.43	2×10^{14}	4.3×10^{-10}%		0.6
^{244}Cm	18.1	80.9	1.3×10^7	1.347×10^{-4}%	2.696	1.09×10^7
^{246}Cm	4730	0.307		0.0263 %	2.95	8.8×10^6
^{248}Cm	3.4×10^5	0.0042		8.39 %	3.157	4.2×10^7
^{250}Cm	9000	0.16		86%	3.17	1.6×10^{10}
^{250}Cf	13.08	109		0.077	3.51	1.1×10^{10}
^{252}Cf	2.645	536.4	85	3.09%	3.767	2.3×10^{12}
^{254}Cf	0.166	8480		99.7%	3.83	1.2×10^{15}
^{249}Bk[a]	0.877	1637	6×10^8	4.76×10^{-8}%	3.395	9.8×10^4
^{257}Fm	0.275	5060		0.2%	3.796	1.4×10^{12}

[a] Beta emitter; all others decay by alpha emission.

[b] Data partially from Mughabghab (1984), Dillman (1975), Firestone (1996), and Brookhaven National Data Center.

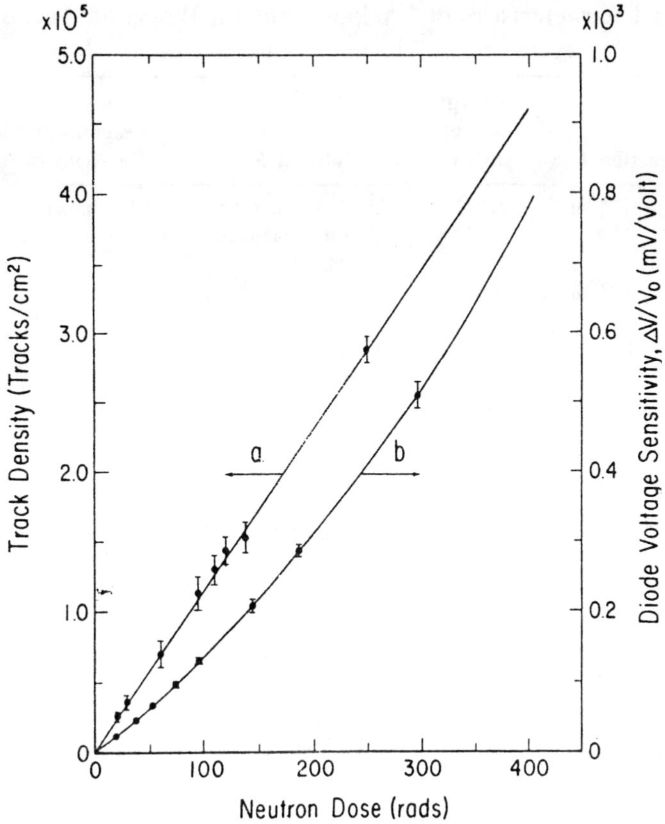

Figure 7.8 Comparison of Calibration Curves for Track Detectors (a) and Silicon (b), as Measured with a ^{252}Cf Neutron Source in Air. The diode voltage sensitivity, $\Delta V/V_0$, is the change in diode forward voltage before and after irradiation, divided by the pre-irradiation voltage. (From NCRP Report 79, 1987 after Wilenzick *et al.*, 1973)

Table 7.10 Important Characteristics of Various Neutron Detection Techniques (Courtesy IAEA; from Technical Reports Series 188, 1979)

Detector	Reaction	Energy Range (MeV)	Detector Size[a]	Response to Flux of 1 Neutron cm^{2a}	Background Response[a]
Gold foils moderated	$^{197}Au(n,\gamma)^{198}Au$	0.02 to 20	2.54 cm dia., 0.5 g foil in paraffin cylinder	2.1 counts/min[b]	10 counts/min
Gold foils bare	$^{197}Au(n,\gamma)^{198}Au$	thermal	2.54 cm dia., 0.5 g foil	1.8 counts/min[b]	10 counts/min
Sulphur	$^{32}S(n,p)^{32}P$	>3	2.54 cm dia., 4 g disk	0.049 counts/min[c]	10 counts/min
Plastic scintillator	$^{12}C\ (n,2n)^{11}C$	>20	13 to 2700 g	88 counts/min at 85% efficiency[c], 1700 g scintillator	165 counts/min 1700 g scintillator
Mercury	Hg( )^{149}Tb[d]	>600	up to 500 g	0.03 counts/min[b]	0.1 counts/min
Gold foils	^{197}Au( )^{149}Tb[d]	>600	2.54 cm dia., 0.5 g	2.7×10^{-6} counts/min[b]	0.1 counts/min
BF_3 proportional counter moderator	$^{10}B(n,\alpha)^7Li$	0.02 to 20	400 cm^3 at 20 cm Hg, 96% enriched	400 counts/min, 6 cm thick moderator	2 to 3 counts/min
Polyethylene-lined prop. counter	Proton recoil	0.05 to 20	800 cm^2 PE radiator, Ar-CO_2 filled	1 count = 15 MeV/cm^2 at zero bias	<1 count/min
Large bismuth fission counter	$^{209}Bi(n,f)$	>50	30 cm dia. parallel plates 60 g Bi	1.05 counts/min at zero bias, E_n = 220 MeV	<1 count/h
Small bismuth fission counter	$^{209}Bi(n,f)$	>50	5 cm dia parallel plates	0.02 counts/min at zero bias	<1 count/h
Thorium fission counter	$^{232}Th(n,f)$	>2	5 cm dia parallel plates	0.017 counts/min at zero bias (PuBe spectrum)	<1 count/min
Gold foil, moderated	$^{197}Au(n,\gamma)^{198}Au$	0.02 to 20	5.08 cm dia., 2.0 g foil	10.1 counts/min[c]	48 counts/min NaI(Tl)
Gold foil, bare	$^{197}Au(n,\gamma)^{198}Au$	thermal	5.08 cm dia., 2.0 g foil	13.4 counts/min[c]	48 counts/min NaI(Tl)
Large indium foil, bare	$^{115}In(n,\gamma)^{116m}In$	thermal	7.6 cm by 15.2 cm foils (four) 46 g total	300 counts/min (estimated)	75 counts/min NaI(Tl)
Aluminum	$^{27}Al(n,\alpha)^{24}Na$	>6	16.9 to 6600 g	101 counts/min, 6600 g[c], E_n = 14 MeV	111 counts/min, 16.9 g, 118 counts/min, 6600 g NaI(Tl)
Aluminum	^{27}Al( )^{22}Na[d]	>25	16.9 g	0.21 counts/min[c]	67 counts/min NaI(Tl)
Plastic scintillator	^{12}C( )^{7}Be[d]	>30	2.54 cm dia. by 2.54 cm high	0.0114 counts/min[c]	59 counts/min NaI(Tl)
Emulsion (Ilford)	Proton recoil	2 to 20	600 μm thick		
Emulsion (Ilford)	Star production	>20	600 μm thick		
Neutron film Kodak Type-B	Proton recoil	0.5 to 25	~30 μm thick	0.00083 track per normally incident neutron	
Mica fission-track plates	Fission in Bi, Pb, Au	>50 in Bi	>1 cm^2	1.79×10^{-6} tracks per neutron for Bi	

[a] Typical values.
[b] At saturation, zero decay time and zero bias.
[c] Saturation and zero decay time.
[d] ( ) are "empty" in original table.

Table 7.10.1 Characteristics of Selected Neutron Detectors[a] (Reproduced from the journal *Health Physics* with permission from the Health Physics Society from Auman et al., 1992)

Detector	Measured Dose Equivalent Rates (μSv h^{-1}) 25 keV	144 keV	800 keV	D_2O ^{252}Cf
TEPC	3	26	680	220
Proton recoil	3	63	950	210
Bonner spheres	5	45	770	250
^{3}He	3	28	1600	410
PRS-2 remball	5	38	620	N[b]
Film badge	3	74	930	210
TLD	6	94	770	N[b]

[a] Results from the four neutron spectra. *Note:* There is no normalization between sources in terms of source strength, but the responses can be compared to those of the PRS-2 and the TLD which were previously calibrated.

[b] No measurements reported because these systems were previously calibrated to this source.

Table 7.11 Sensitivities of Some Fission Reactions Used in Neutron Dosimetry (Courtesy IAEA from Tech. Rept. Series 188, 1979, Adapted from Becker, 1972)

Fissionable Material	Sensitivity (Tracks/Neutron) — Neutron Energy, E_n: Thermal	Fission	~4 (Pu-Be)	14 MeV	230 MeV	5500 MeV
U (nat)	3.5×10^{-5}	4.2×10^{-6}	4.5×10^{-6}	1.4×10^{-5}		3.6×10^{-6}
U-235	3.5×10^{-3}	1.6×10^{-4}				
Th		4.0×10^{-7}	1.2×10^{-6}	4.5×10^{-6}		
Np-237		1.8×10^{-6}		1.8×10^{-6}		
Ta					5.0×10^{-8}	6.1×10^{-7}
Be					2.0×10^{-6}	
Au					1.5×10^{-7}	9.3×10^{-7}
Bi						1.1×10^{-6}

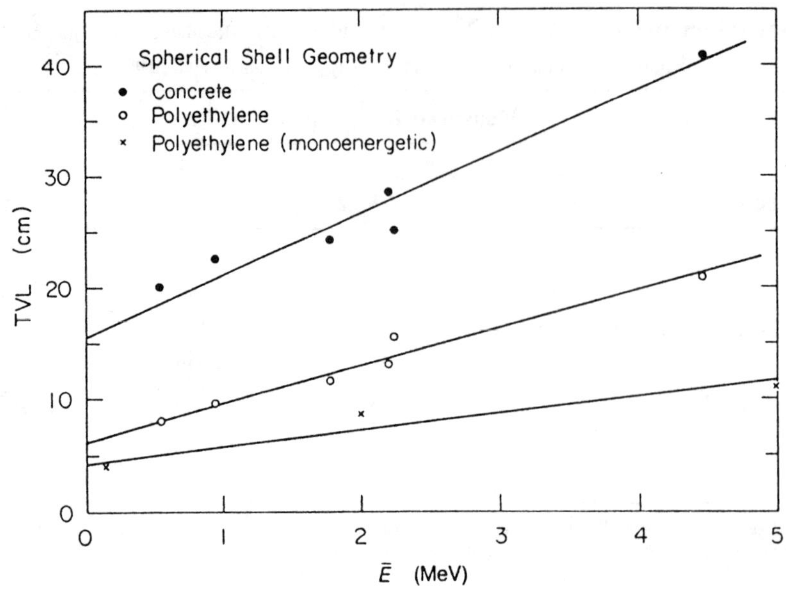

Figure 7.9 Dose-Equivalent Tenth-Value Layer (TVL) for Spherical Shell Shielding as a Function of the Average Energy of the Neutron Source. The lines are least-squares fits to the calculated points. (Courtesy NCRP from Report 79, 1987 based on data from McCall, 1979)

Table 7.12.1 Thermal-Neutron Capture Prompt Gamma-Ray Data by Element (After Lone, 1981)

Z	Number of Lines	Total gammas per Neutron Capture[b]	Average Energy[b] (keV)	Maximum Energy (keV)	Elemental Cross-Section (barns)
1 H	1	1.000	2223	2223	0.332
3 Li	6	1.118	2094	7247	0.0363
4 Be	11	1.608	4239	6809	0.0092
5 B	4	1.975	5573	7005	0.103
5 B(n,a)[a]	1	0.937	478	478	767
6 C	3	1.293	3791	4945	0.00337
7 N	50	2.634	4386	10829	0.0747
8 O	4	2.820	1469	3271	0.00027
9 F	35	1.787	3692	6601	0.0095
10 Ne	119	3.451	2158	6760	0.038
11 Na	64	2.831	2457	6395	0.4
12 Mg	99	3.264	2785	9282	0.063
13 Al	172	1.826	3937	7724	0.23
14 Si	89	2.598	3699	10608	0.16
15 P	130	2.671	2971	7938	0.18
16 S	18	2.771	3118	8641	0.52
17 Cl	449	2.886	3293	8578	33.2
18 Ar	49	3.081	1988	8787	0.678
19 K	286	3.183	2660	7770	2.1
20 Ca	113	2.681	3134	7306	0.43
21 Sc	244	3.127	2805	8760	0.43
22 Ti	121	2.277	3096	10646	6.1
23 V	109	1.820	4015	7311	5.04
24 Cr	63	1.868	4953	9720	3.1
25 Mn	314	2.364	3173	7270	13.3
26 Fe	187	1.717	4620	10046	2.55
27 Co	132	2.081	2904	7491	37.2
28 Ni	120	1.436	5930	8999	4.43
29 Cu	130	1.987	3901	7915	3.79
30 Zn	104	1.130	3418	9118	1.1
31 Ga	144	2.019	3453	7003	2.9
32 Ge	126	1.837	2047	8733	2.3
33 As	192	0.917	2757	7283	4.3
34 Se	167	0.722	2800	9182	11.7
35 Br	129	0.792	1090	7894	6.8
36 Kr	150	3.175	2281	9636	25
37 Rb	201	0.609	2216	8651	0.37
38 Sr	250	2.167	2463	8379	1.21
39 Y	76	2.107	3261	6751	1.28

(continued)

Table 7.12.1 Thermal-Neutron Capture Prompt Gamma-Ray Data by Element (Continued)

Z	Number of Lines	Total gammas per Neutron Capture[b]	Average Energy[b] (keV)	Maximum Energy (keV)	Elemental Cross-Section (barns)
40 Zr	94	1.815	2227	8635	0.185
41 Nb	182	1.016	1912	7229	1.15
42 Mo	154	1.320	1737	8374	2.65
43 Tc	26	0.998	182	299.48	19
44 Ru	87	0.708	1893	9135.2	2.56
45 Rh	89	0.482	2019	6997.9	150
46 Pd	111	0.845	1246	8331.2	6.9
47 Ag	97	0.877	1300	7268.4	63.6
48 Cd	181	1.690	1522	9043.4	2450
49 In	158	0.931	1474	6411.4	193.5
50 Sn	231	0.786	2016	9326.1	0.63
51 Sb	82	0.341	1778	6804.8	5.4
52 Te	122	0.495	2612	8817.1	4.7
53 I	275	0.677	1673	6740.15	6.2
54 Xe	141	3.328	1413	9301.4	24.5
55 Cs	203	1.353	797	6715.6	29
56 Ba	130	1.564	2493	9120	1.2
57 La	274	2.090	1679	5160.9	9.14
58 Ce	61	4.085	1015	5403.5	0.63
59 Pr	164	1.019	2128	5842.9	11.5
60 Nd	130	2.195	1552	7111	50.5
61 Pm					
62 Sm	81	2.504	631	7214.2	5800
63 Eu	31	0.129	678	6418.7	4600
64 Gd	102	1.032	1440	7286.7	49000
65 Tb	361	1.337	731	6375.86	25.5
66 Dy	169	1.225	1529	5879.9	930
67 Ho	83	0.433	1203	6051.5	66.5
68 Er	91	1.228	1031	6951.4	162
69 Tm	93	0.425	1624	6552.6	103
70 Yb	179	1.040	1814	8017.6	36.6
71 Lu	71	0.366	965	6803.6	77.3
72 Hf	122	1.260	1196	6356.9	102
73 Ta	110	0.603	1526	6062.85	21.08
74 W	119	1.280	1758	7410.7	18.5
75 Re	71	0.450	824	6119.2	88
76 Os	151	1.353	1063	7990.5	15.3
77 Ir	77	0.427	2429	6081.3	426
78 Pt	190	0.999	2040	7920.9	10
79 Au	123	1.254	2675	6511.9	98.8
80 Hg	84	2.241	2360	6457.5	375.5
81 Tl	102	0.612	2957	6654.4	3.4
82 Pb	2	0.991	7336	7367.7	0.17
83 Bi	3	1.117	4118	4171.1	0.033
90 Th	112	0.656	3205	4769.6	7.4
94 Pu	20	0.027	5408	6535.4	268.8

[a] Not a 'prompt gamma', but included because boron is commonly used in shielding materials.

[b] The energy total represented by these average is deficient for many nuclides (Molár, 1995), particularly above Z = 29 where the deficiency frequently >80%.

Table 7.12.2 Thermal-Neutron Capture Prompt Gamma-Ray Data by Energy

Energy[a] (keV)	Element	Intensity[a] (γ/100 captures)	Thermal Cross-Section[b] (barns)	Parent Nuclide[b] % Abundance	Energy[a] (keV)	Element	Intensity[a] (γ/100 captures)	Thermal Cross-Section[b] (barns)	Parent Nuclide[b] % Abundance
93.7	Zr	37.3	0.19	100.0	627.5	Ba	12.3	1.2	100.0
145.1	Ga	50.0	4.86	40.0	636.2	P	12.2	0.18	100.0
159.3	Cu	10.0	4.5	69.1	645.9	V	11.2	4.88	99.8
162.4	In	14.7	202	95.7	651.2	Cd	13.9	250.0	100.0
165.0	As	20.0	4.3	100.0	737.6	Sm	11.0	5.8E + 3	100.0
175.1	Ge	11.4	2.3	100.0	749.2	Cr	11.0	3.1	100.0
181.9	Gd	18.3	4.9E + 4	15.7	770.3	K	55.2	1.96	93.3
186.2	In	13.8	202	95.7	778.3	Mo	62.0	14.5	15.7
192.0	Ga	19.5	4.86	40.0	835.1	Cr	26.9	3.1	100.0
194.6	Ga	10.6	4.86	40.0	841.1	S	79.5	0.53	95.0
197.9	Ga	13.7	4.86	40.0	847.7	Mo	10.6	14.5	15.7
198.4	Ag	23.9	63.6	100.0	850.0	Mo	13.3	14.5	15.7
199.4	Gd	9.5	4.9E4	100.0	868.4	Ge	14.8	2.3	100.0
212.0	Mn	10.6	13.3	100.0	870.6	Na	21.9	0.40	100.0
214.8	Au	14.1	99.0	100.0	898.0	Sr	27.8	1.21	100.0
229.8	Co	21.0	37.2	100.0	944.0	Gd	8.6	2.5E + 5	15.7
238.9	Se	27.2	85.0	9.0	944.0	Gd	10.6	4.9E + 4	100.0
245.7	Br	11.4	6.8	100.0	1070.6	P	8.6	0.18	100.0
273.0	In	20.4	202	95.7	1077.4	Zn	18.9	1.1	100.0
277.1	Co	12.0	37.2	100.0	1164.7	Cl	19.9	3.2	100.0
278.2	Cu	19.0	4.5	69.1	1171.3	Sn	7.9	0.63	100.0
282.6	Sb	4.8	6.3	57.3	1186.5	Gd	10.8	4.9E + 4	100.0
333.3	Pt	15.9	10.0	100.0	1261.7	C	29.9	3.4E − 3	98.9
333.4	Sm	98.9	5.8E + 3	100.0	1273.3	Si	17.3	0.17	92.2
341.7	Ti	35.6	7.8	73.7	1293.3	Sn	12.8	0.63	100.0
352.3	Fe	11.2	2.55	100.0	1381.5	Ti	93.7	7.8	73.7
356.1	Pt	27.6	10.0	100.0	1413.1	P	14.0	0.18	100.0
368.1	Hg	81.4	375	100.0	1434.1[c]	V	100.0	4.88	99.8
439.4	Sm	55.5	5.8E3	100.0	1435.3	Ba	14.1	1.2	100.0
465.1	Ni	13.0	4.43	100.0	1633.1[d]	F	100.0	9.5E − 3	100.0
472.4	Na	59.8	0.40	100.0	1693.9	Hg	14.1	375	100.0
505.9	Sm	17.9	5.8E3	100.0	1778.8[e]	Al	100.0	0.23	100.0
516.7	Cl	18.5	33.2	100.0	1808.9	Mg	30.0	6.3E − 2	100.0
558.5	Cd	72.7	250.0	100.0	1836.1	Sr	57.8	1.21	100.0
584.5	Sm	10.1	5.8E + 3	100.0	1884.8	N	21.7	7.5E − 2	99.6
585.2	Mg	25.6	6.3E − 2	100.0	1942.0	Ca	74.8	0.40	96.9
596.4	Ge	33.1	2.3	100.0	2032.5	Li	96.6	3.6E − 2	92.5

[a] Data are primarily derived from Lone et al., 1981.
[b] Data are primarily derived from Erdtmann, 1976.
[c] $T_{1/2}$ = 3.746 minutes.
[d] $T_{1/2}$ = 11.0 seconds.
[e] $T_{1/2}$ = 2.31 minutes.

(continued)

Table 7.12.2 Thermal-Neutron Capture Prompt Gamma-Ray Data by Energy (Continued)

Energy[a] (keV)	Element	Intensity[a] (γ/100 captures)	Thermal Cross-Section[b] (barns)	Parent Nuclide[b] % Abundance	Energy[a] (keV)	Element	Intensity[a] (γ/100 captures)	Thermal Cross-Section[b] (barns)	Parent Nuclide[b] % Abundance
2073.7	K	11.5	1.96	93.3	6380.7	Si	13.4	0.17	92.2
2092.9	Si	23.3	0.17	92.2	6395.4	Na	22.2	0.40	100.0
2154.2	P	15.2	0.18	100.0	6418.3	Ti	40.9	7.8	73.7
2223.2	H	100.0	5.3E − 4	100.0	6517.2	V	17.9	4.88	99.8
2238.9	Cr	8.3	3.1	100.0	6705.8	Co	8.5	37.2	100.0
2379.7	S	46.8	0.53	95.0	6759.3	B	39.5	0.10	100.0
2828.1	Mg	42.5	6.3E − 2	100.0	6761.7	Ti	32.8	7.8	73.7
3028.0	Ge	39.0	2.3	100.0	6837.0	Ni	10.8	4.43	100.0
3539.1	Si	73.8	0.17	92.2	6876.8	Co	8.5	37.2	100.0
3683.9	C	32.5	3.4E − 3	98.9	7005.1	B	47.9	0.10	100.0
3900.3	P	16.0	0.18	100.0	7162.7	V	13.2	4.88	99.8
4443.0	B	76.0	0.10	100.0	7367.7	Pb	94.1	0.17	100.0
4710.2	B	34.2	0.10	100.0	7631.1	Fe	27.7	2.55	100.0
4934.4	Si	68.0	0.17	92.2	7637.0	Cu	15.0	4.5	69.1
4945.3	C	68.4	3.4E − 3	98.9	7645.5	Fe	24.4	2.55	100.0
5269.2	N	29.8	7.5E − 2	99.6	7723.9	Al	25.9	0.23	100.0
5298.0	N	21.1	7.5E − 2	99.6	7863.3	Zn	10.6	1.1	100.0
5420.5	S	62.2	0.53	95.0	7916.0	Cu	27.0	4.5	69.1
5975.1	Co	7.3	37.2	100.0	8884.1	Cr	27.0	3.1	100.0
6111.0	Cl	20.0	33.2	100.0	8998.8	Ni	37.7	4.43	100.0

[a] Data are primarily derived from Lone et al., 1981.
[b] Data are primarily derived from Erdtmann, 1976.
[c] $T_{1/2}$ = 3.746 minutes.
[d] $T_{1/2}$ = 11.0 seconds.
[e] $T_{1/2}$ = 2.31 minutes.

Table 7.13 Gamma Rays from Spontaneous Fission of ^{252}Cf (Courtesy ICRU from Report 26, 1977)

Energy (MeV)	Photon Abundance/($s^{-1}g^{-1}$ or Bq g^{-1})		
	Prompt Gamma Rays	Equilibrium Fission Product Gamma Rays	Total
0–0.5	3.3×10^{12}	1.3×10^{12}	4.6×10^{12}
0.5–1.0	1.7×10^{12}	4.0×10^{12}	5.7×10^{12}
1.0–1.5	7.7×10^{11}	9.1×10^{11}	1.7×10^{12}
1.5–2.0	4.2×10^{11}	3.5×10^{11}	7.7×10^{11}
2.0–2.5	2.2×10^{11}		2.2×10^{11}
2.5–3.0	1.1×10^{11}		1.1×10^{11}
3.0–3.5	5.6×10^{10}		5.6×10^{10}
3.5–4.0	3.0×10^{10}		3.0×10^{10}
4.0–4.5	1.7×10^{10}		1.7×10^{10}
4.5–5.0	8.2×10^{9}		8.2×10^{9}
5.0–5.5	4.9×10^{9}		4.9×10^{9}
5.5–6.0	1.8×10^{9}		1.8×10^{9}
6.0–6.5	1.0×10^{9}		1.0×10^{9}

Table 7.14 Fast Neutron Threshold Reactions (From Slaback, 1991, personal communication)

Reaction	Half-Life (Nuclide Produced)	σ(mb)[a] at Effective Threshold	σ(mb)[a] max	Effective Threshold (MeV)[b]	First Non-Zero Cross Section (MeV)[c]
$^{19}F(n,2n)^{18}F$	110 min	9.98	111	12.1	11
$^{24}Mg(n,p)^{24}Na$	15.0 h	41.5	225	7.0	5.6
$^{27}Al(n,p)^{27}Mg$	9.46 min	19.3	104	4.5	2.6
$^{27}Al(n,\alpha)^{24}Na$	15.0 h	19.0	129	7.1	5.3
$^{31}P(n,p)^{31}Si$	2.62 h	53.1	148	2.4	2.0
$^{32}S(n,p)^{32}P$	14.3 d	97.5	385	2.7	1.2
$^{46}Ti(n,p)^{46}Sc$	83.3 d	15.6	280	3.8	2.1
$^{54}Fe(n,p)^{54}Mn$	313 d	187	590	3.3	1.4
$^{55}Mn(n,2n)^{54}Mn$	313 d	259	900	11.5	10.3
$^{56}Fe(n,p)^{56}Mn$	2.59 h	15.6	114	6.1	4.5
$^{58}Ni(n,p)^{58}Co$, ^{58m}Co	71.3 d, 9.15 h	163	662	2.8	0.8
$^{58}Ni(n,2n)^{57}Ni$	36.0 h	8.5	54.3	13.2[d]	12.4
$^{63}Cu(n,2n)^{62}Cu$	9.76 min	174	693	12.4	11.6
$^{64}Zn(n,p)^{64}Cu$	12.7 h	127	301	4.0	1
$^{65}Cu(n,2n)^{64}Cu$	12.7 h	234	1100	11.2	10
$^{103}Rh(n,n')^{103m}Rh$	56.1 min	252	1090	0.7	0.2
$^{107}Ag(n,2n)^{106}Ag$	24.1 min	662	1520	10.7	9.6
$^{115}In(n,n')^{115m}In$	4.50 h	152	321	1.4	0.4
$^{127}I(n,2n)^{126}I$	12.8 d	1070	1750	11.5	9.1
$^{232}Th(n,f)$ fission products		66.7	364	1.4	1.2
$^{237}Np(n,f)$ fission products		1080	2680	0.7	<0.1
$^{238}U(n,f)$ fission products		226	1350	1.4	0.7

[a] After Schott et al., 1974 and ICRU 26, 1977.
[b] After NCRP 79, 1984; from ICRU 26, 1977.
[c] Schott et al., 1974.
[d] (Personal Communication, L. Slaback, 1991), References give value as 12.3.

Table 7.15 Useful Thermal Neutron Detectors (Courtesy NCRP After Report 79, 1984)

Nuclide or Element	Reaction	Half-Life of Nuclide Produced	$\sigma_o \times 10^{24}$ for Production (cm^2)
^{3}He	$(n,p)^{3}H$	12.3 y	5327
^{6}Li	$(n,t)^{4}He$	stable[b]	945
^{10}B	$(n,\alpha)^{7}Li$	stable	3837
^{23}Na(IS)[a]	$(n,\gamma)^{24}Na$	15.0 h	0.534
^{45}Sc(IS)[a]	$(n,\gamma)^{46}Sc$	85 d	22.3
^{51}V	$(n,\gamma)^{52}V$	3.8 min	4.9
^{55}Mn(IS)[a]	$(n,\gamma)^{56}Mn$	2.58 h	13.3
^{59}Co(IS)[a]	$(n,\gamma)^{60}Co$	5.24 y	36.6
^{63}Cu	$(n,\gamma)^{64}Cu$	12.8 h	4.5
^{115}In	$(n,\gamma)^{116m}In$	54 min	157
^{157}Gd	$(n,\gamma)^{158}Gd$	stable	242000
^{197}Au(IS)[a]	$(n,\gamma)^{198}Au$	2.70 d	98.8
^{236}U	fission	many	577

[a] (IS) denotes natural monoisotopic element.
[b] ^{4}He stable, tritium (t) is radioactive.

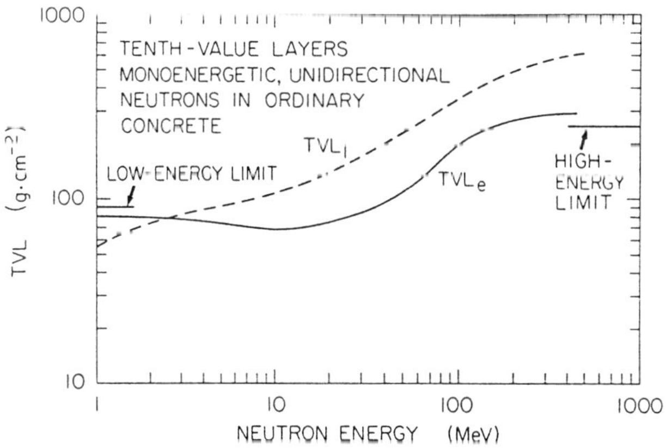

Figure 7.10 Dose-Equivalent Tenth-Value Layer, TVL, for Broad Beams of Monoenergetic, Unidirectional Neutrons Incident on Ordinary Concrete, as a Function of Neutron Energy E_n. The dashed curve represents TVL_1 (the ''first'' TVL) and the solid curve is the TVL_e, corresponding to the nearly exponential attenuation of subsequent layers. The dose equivalent from n-capture gamma rays is implicitly taken into account. The curves are based on discrete-ordinate calculations of Roussin and Schmidt (1971), Roussin *et al.* (1973), and Alsmiller *et al.* (1969), using in part the smoothed data of Wyckoff and Chilton (1973). The low-energy limit is to indicate that the TVL_e does not vary greatly below the energy range shown. The high-energy limit is based on semi-empirical considerations. (Courtesy IAEA from Technical Report Series 188, 1979)

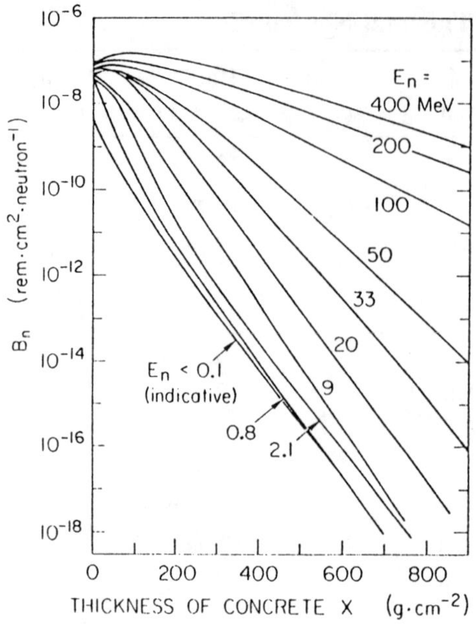

Figure 7.11 Attenuation of Broad Beams of Monoenergetic, Unidirectional Neutrons Perpendicularly Incident on Ordinary Concrete. The abscissa is the thickness of concrete, x, in g cm^{-3}, the ordinate is the ratio B_n of dose equivalent in rem at shielding thickness x to unshielded neutron fluence in n cm^{-2}. The dose equivalent contribution of gamma rays is implicitly included (References as for Fig. 7.10.)
(Courtesy IAEA from Technical Report Series 188, 1979)

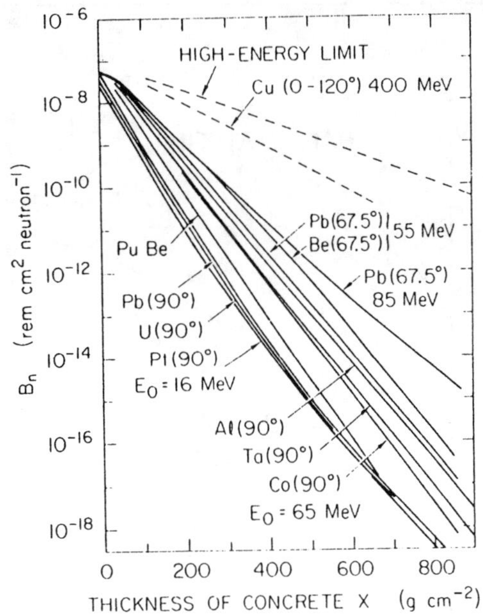

Figure 7.12 Attenuation of Unidirectional Broad Beams of Neutrons, for Representative Photoneutron Spectra, Perpendicularly Incident on Ordinary Concrete. The abscissa is the thickness of concrete, x, in g cm^{-2}, and the ordinate is the ratio B_n of dose equivalent to unshielded neutron fluence. The labels indicate target material, laboratory angle of neutron emission and endpoint energy E_o of the bremsstrahlung beam. The dose equivalent from gamma rays is implicitly included. The curves are derived by folding the monoenergetic neutron shielding data cited for Figure 7.11 together with measured photoneutron spectra (adapted from Wyckoff and Chilton, 1973). Also shown for comparison are curves for neutrons from a Pu-Be source (Ibid.), for photoneutrons produced in Cu at E_o = 400 MeV (unnormalized, from Alsmiller and Barish, 1973), as well as the presumed high-energy limit (unnormalized). (Courtesy IAEA from Technical Report Series 188, 1979)

Table 7.16 Neutron Dose-Equivalent TVL Values for Representative Low-Energy Spectra

(Courtesy IAEA from Technical Report Series 188, 1979)

Material	Spectrum	TVL (g cm^{-2})
Paraffin (solid)	Am-Be	23
Wood	Am-Be	28
Water	Fission	22
Sand (S$_i$O)	Am-Be	74
Ordinary concrete	Am-Be	96
Heavy concrete	Am-Be	110
Iron (steel)	Fission	280–330
Lead	Fission	900–1070

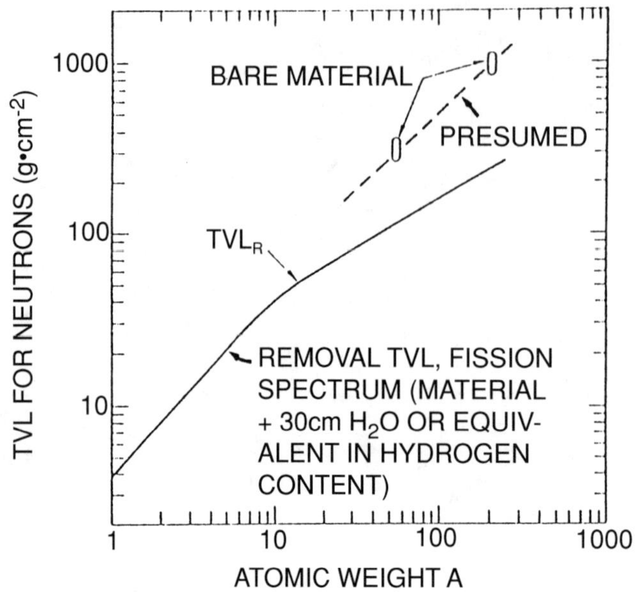

Figure 7.13 Neutron Removal Tenth-Value Layer (TVL_R) as a Function of Atomic Weight (A) of Shielding Material. The solid curve is for a fission spectrum, assuming a backing of 30 cm of water or the equivalent in hydrogen content (derived from Chapman and Storrs, 1955). The points above show TVLs for the fission spectrum on iron and lead, without hydrogenous backing, for comparison (adapted from Shure *et al.*, 1969). The dashed curve is an interpolation. (Courtesy IAEA from Technical Report Series 188, 1979)

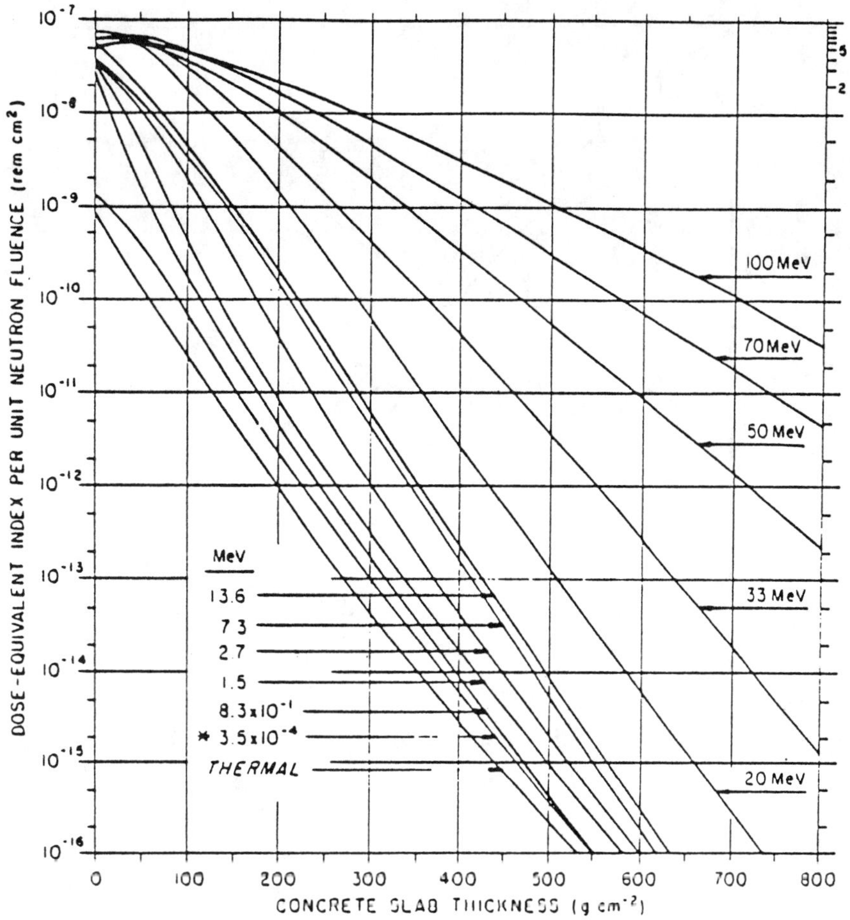

Figure 7.14 Dose-Equivalent Index Transmission Through Concrete from Monoenergetic Neutrons
(Courtesy NCRP from Report 51, 1977)

Dose-equivalent index transmission per unit fluence (rem/cm^2) of monoenergetic neutrons incident normally on slabs of ordinary concrete. Multi-collision dose equivalent index per unit fluence is calculated to include the dose equivalent index contribution by capture gamma rays produced within the slab. Energies noted on the curves refer to the average energies of neutrons in the energy bins chosen for the discrete-ordinate calculations, as follows:

Energy Bin (MeV)	Average Energy (MeV)
$0–4.14 \times 10^{-7}$	"thermal"
$1.01 \times 10^{-4}–5.38 \times 10^{-4}$	3.5×10^{-4} [a]
$5.50 \times 10^{-1}–1.11$	8.3×10^{-1}
1.11–1.83	1.5
2.46–3.01	2.7
6.36–8.19	7.3
12.2–15.0	13.6
15.0–25.0	20
25.0–40.0	33
40.0–60.0	50
60.0–80.0	70
80.0–125.0	100

[a] The transmission curve for this average energy is typical of transmission curves in the energy range 1×10^{-4} to 5×10^{-1}.
These calculations were prepared by Wyckoff and Chilton (1973), based on Roussin and Schmidt (1971) and Roussin et al. (1973).

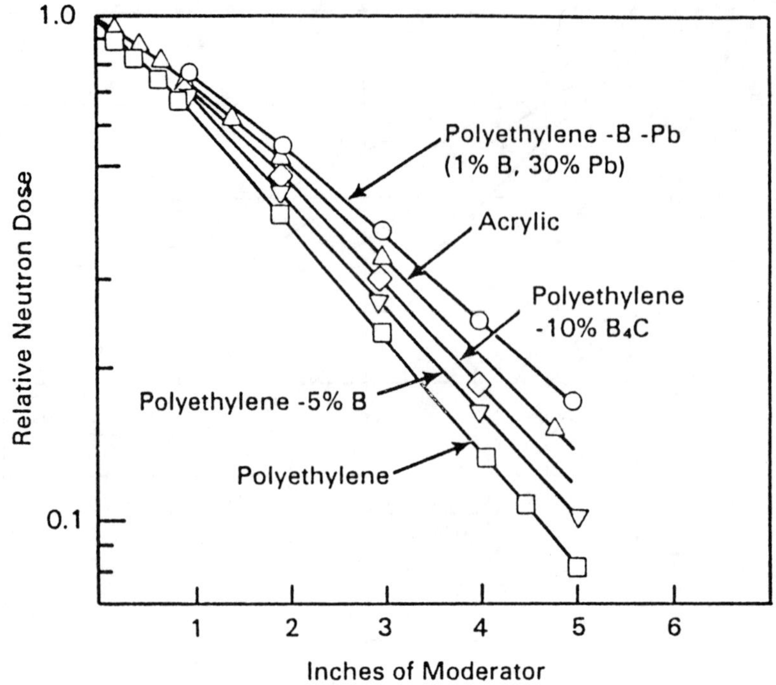

Figure 7.15 Shielding Effectiveness of Various Slab Shields for a PuF_4 Neutron Source (From PNL 6534, 1988)

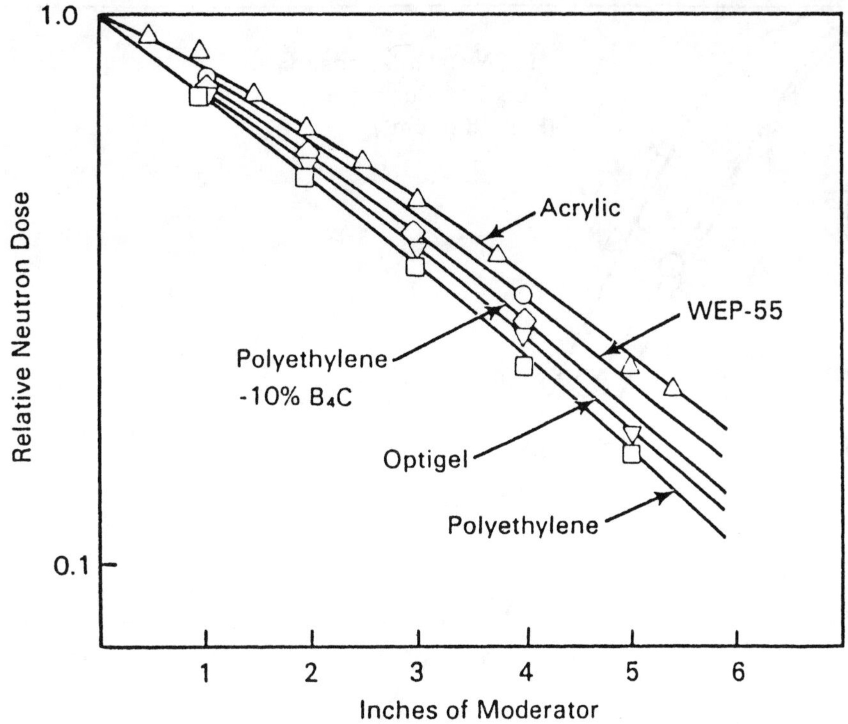

Figure 7.16 Shielding Effectiveness of Various Slab Shields for a ^{252}Cf Fission Neutron Source
(From Engle, 1967)

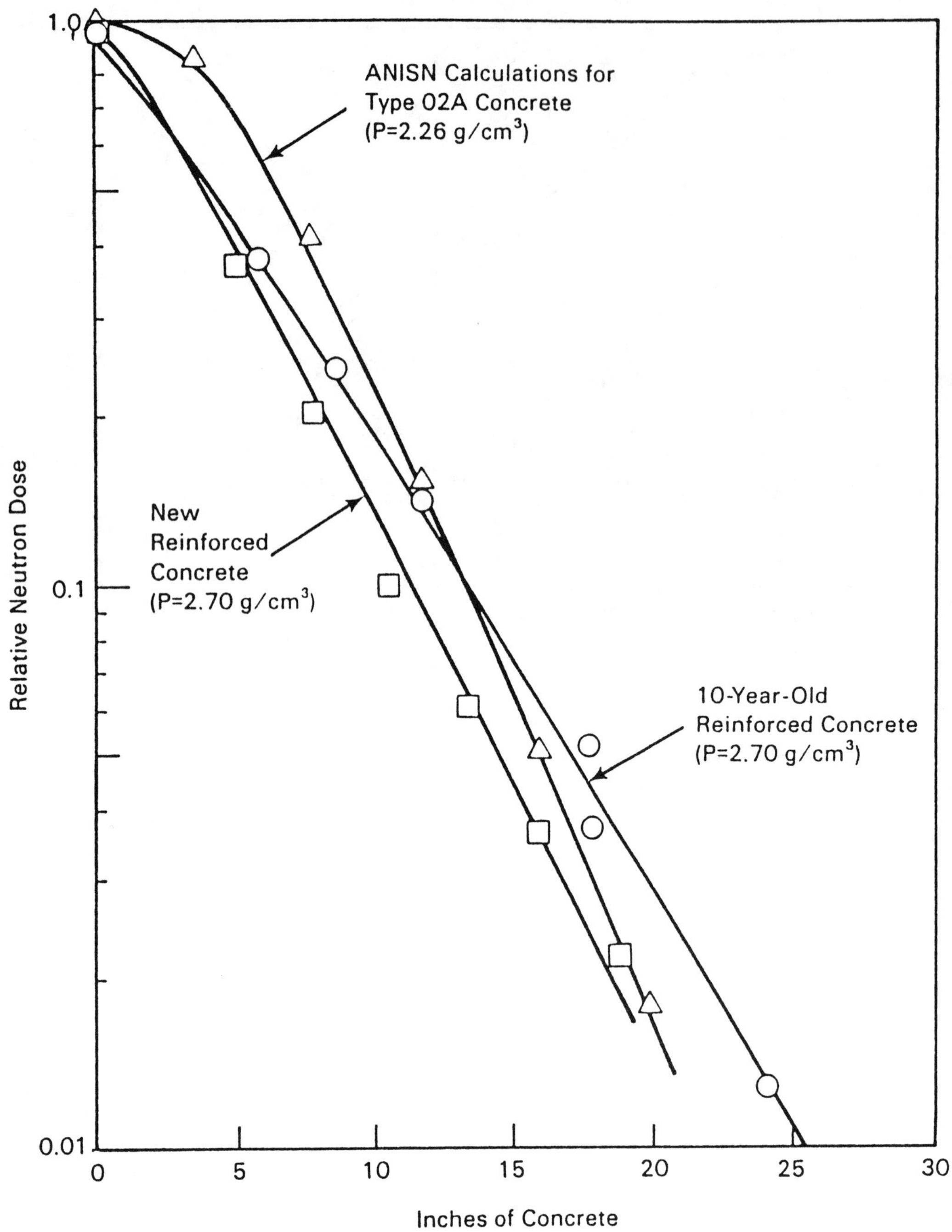

Figure 7.17 Shielding Effectiveness of Concrete for ^{252}Cf Fission Neutrons. Figure shows the shielding effectiveness of concrete using a ^{252}Cf source and ANISN calculation. Measurements were made using relatively new concrete ($<$2 years old) and concrete that was approximately 10 years old. (From Engle, 1967)

Table 7.17 Maxwellian Distribution for Neutrons[a]

Maxwellian Number Density Distribution n

Energy distribution	$n(E)\,dE = (2/\sqrt{\pi})\,(E^{1/2}/E_T^{3/2})\,\exp(-E/E_T)\,dE$	(in neutrons cm^{-3})
Velocity distribution	$n(v)\,dv = (4/\sqrt{\pi})(v^2/v_T^3)\,\exp(-v^2/v_T^2)\,dv$	(in neutrons cm^{-3})
Wavelength distribution	$n(\lambda)\,d\lambda = (4/\sqrt{\pi})\,(\lambda_T^3/\lambda^4)\,\exp(-\lambda_T^2/\lambda^2)\,d\lambda$	(in neutrons cm^{-3})

	In Energy	**In Velocity**	**In Wavelength**
Most probable* energy	$\mathbf{(1/2)\,E_T}$	$(1/\sqrt{2})\,v_T = 0.707\,v_T$	$\sqrt{2}\,\lambda_T = 1.414\,\lambda_T$
Most probable* velocity	E_T	$\mathbf{v_T}$	λ_T
Most prob* wavelength	$2\,E_T$	$\sqrt{2}\,v_T = 1.414\,v_T$	$\mathbf{(1/\sqrt{2})\,\lambda_T = 0.707\,\lambda_T}$
Mean energy	$\mathbf{(3/2)\,E_T = 1.5\,E_T}$	$\sqrt{(3/2)}\,v_T = 1.225\,v_T$	$\sqrt{(2/3)}\,\lambda_T = 0.816\,\lambda_T$
Mean velocity	$(4/\pi)\,E_T = 1.273\,E_T$	$\mathbf{(2/\sqrt{\pi})\,v_T = 1.128\,v_T}$	$(\sqrt{\pi}/2)\,\lambda_T = 0.886\,\lambda_T$
Mean wavelength	$(\pi/4)\,E_T = 0.785\,E_T$	$(\sqrt{\pi}/2)\,v_T = 0.886\,v_T$	$\mathbf{(2/\sqrt{\pi})\,\lambda_T = 1.128\,\lambda_T}$

Maxwellian Flux Density Distribution Φ = nv**

Energy distribution	$\Phi(E)\,dE = (E/E_T^2)\,\exp(-E/E_T)\,dE$	(in neutrons $cm^{-2}s^{-1}$)
Velocity distribution	$\Phi(v)\,dv = 2\,(v^3/v_T^4)\,\exp(-v^2/v_T^2)\,dv$	(in neutrons $cm^{-2}s^{-1}$)
Velocity distribution	$\Phi(\lambda)\,d\lambda = 2\,(\lambda_T^4/\lambda^5)\,\exp(-\lambda_T^2/\lambda^2)\,d\lambda$	(in neutrons $cm^{-2}s^{-1}$)

	In Energy	**In Velocity**	**In Wavelength**
Most probable* energy	$\mathbf{E_T}$	v_T	λ_T
Most probable* velocity	$(3/2)\,E_T$	$\mathbf{\sqrt{(3/2)}\,v_T = 1.225\,v_T}$	$\sqrt{(2/3)}\,\lambda_T = 0.816\,\lambda_T$
Most prob* wavelength	$(5/2)\,E_T$	$\sqrt{(5/2)}\,v_T = 1.581\,v_T$	$\sqrt{(2/5)}\,\lambda_T = \mathbf{0.632\,\lambda_T}$
Mean energy	$\mathbf{2\,E_T}$	$\sqrt{(2)}\,v_T = 1.414\,v_T$	$(1/\sqrt{2})\,\lambda_T = 0.707\,\lambda_T$
Mean velocity	$(9\pi/16)\,E_T = 1.767\,E_T$	$(3\sqrt{\pi}/4)\,v_T = \mathbf{1.329\,v_T}$	$[4/(3\sqrt{\pi})]\,\lambda_T = 0.752\,\lambda_T$
Mean wavelength	$(4/\pi)\,E_T = 1.273\,E_T$	$(2/\sqrt{\pi})\,v_T = 1.128\,v_T$	$(\sqrt{\pi}/2)\,\lambda_T = \mathbf{0.886\,\lambda_T}$

* the 'most probable' value is the maximum of the distribution. **Called Fluence Rate by ICRU.
$E_T = k\,T = 8.61\,10^{-5}\,T$ (E = eV, T = °K, (v in cm s^{-1}); 1 Å = 10^{-8} cm = 10^{-10} m)
$v_T = 1.38\,10^6\,\sqrt{E} = 1.28\,10^4\,\sqrt{T}$, $\lambda_T = h/(2\,mE_T)^{1/2}$, $\lambda_T(Å) = 0.286/\sqrt{E_T}$

Most probable neutron velocity for neutrons at equilibrium at the following temperatures:

	For a Temperature of 60 K			**For a Temperature of 295 K(22°C)**		
Distribution	**Energy**	**Velocity**	**Wavelength**	**Energy**	**Velocity**	**Wavelength**
Number density	5.17 meV	992 m/s	3.98 Å	25.4 meV	2199 m/s	1.79 Å
Flux density	7.75 meV	1215 m/s	3.25 Å	38.1 meV	2694 m/s	1.46 Å

[a] After D. Milner (internal NBSR note).

Note: The maxwellian distribution can be significantly distorted by the 1/v neutron capture process. Also note that the above energy units are millielectron volts.

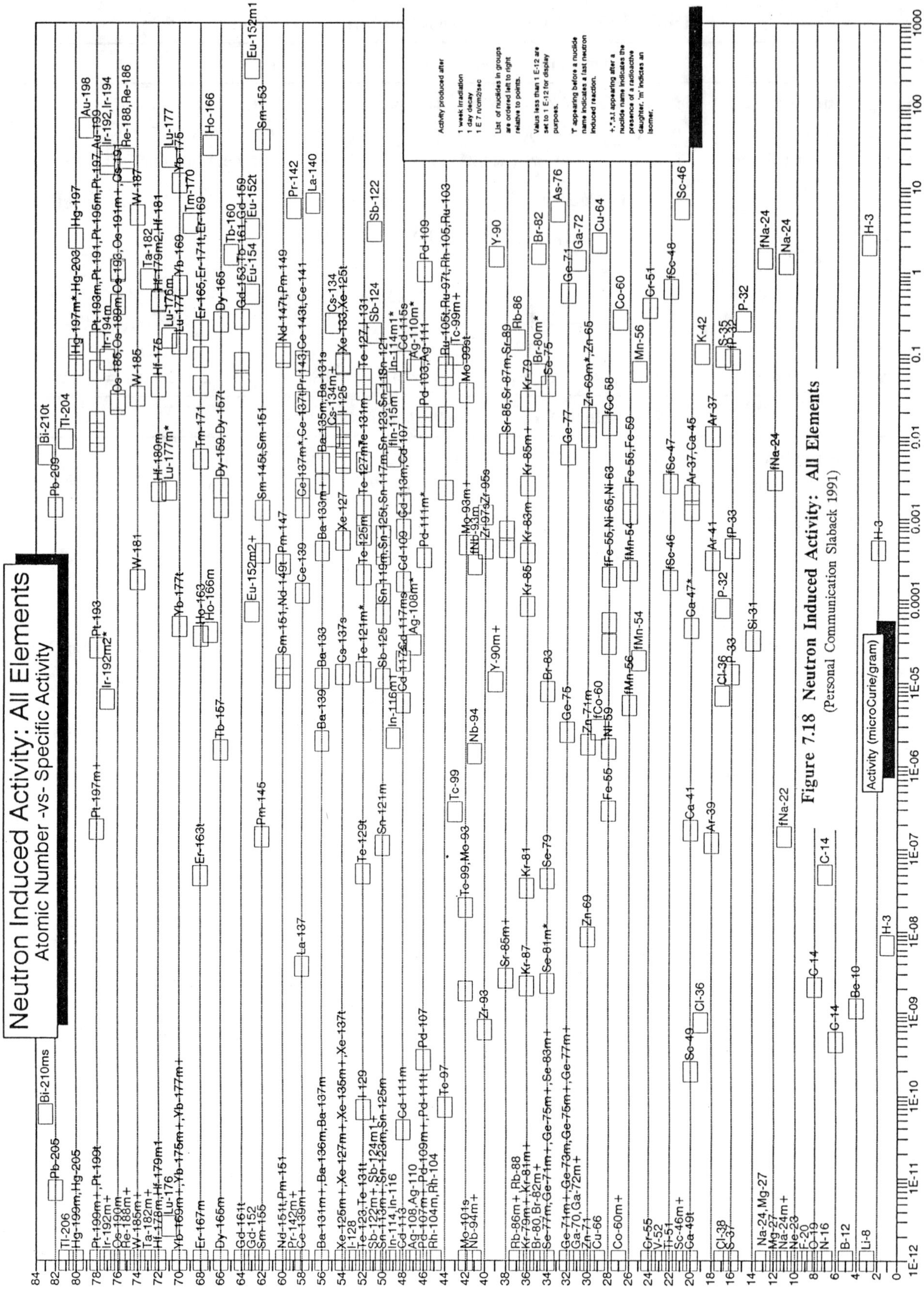

Figure 7.18 Neutron-Induced Activity: All Elements (From Slaback, 1991, personal communication)

Table 7.18 Neutron Activation Database (From Slaback, 1991, personal communication)

A personal computer based database in a spreadsheet format was prepared for the evaluation of the activation characteristics of experimental samples. Cross-section data from the IAEA[a] were used. By convention these cross-sections are for 2200 ms^{-1} neutrons. The effective cross-section for spectrally distributed neutrons other than 'thermal' neutrons will need to be adjusted. The fast neutron reaction data were weighted assuming a fission spectrum. Provision for production via epithermal reactions and radioactive daughters is included in the code.

Notes related to Figure 7.18: Not all the reactions in Table 7.18.1 are shown in the figure. Typically only the small cross-section reactions, e.g., <1 barn, are excluded. For display purposes results of less than 10^{-12} μCi g^{-1} are shown as that value. All points are labeled except for several xenon, cadmium, and tellurium nuclides. Where the labels are grouped the left-to-right order of the labels correspond to the unlabeled points on a left to right order. Those reactions produced by fast neutrons are identified by an ''f'' in front of the nuclide label. Several radioactive daughters that result only from the decay of an induced parent are included in these results, primarily when the daughter is longer lived than the parent.

[a] IAEA, Handbook on Nuclear Activation Data, Tech. Rept. Series No. 273, IAEA, 1987. Note that the entry for ^{88}Sr of 0.058 b in IAEA is in error.

Table 7.18.1 Health Physics Neutron Activation Database

Notation on nuclide name:

m, m1, m2 indicate metastable states. Decay may be to the ground state or another nuclide.

+ indicates radioactive daughter production already included in daughter listing, several parent $t_{1/2}$'s required to achieve calculated daughter activity. In most cases the added activity to the daughter is small.

* indicates radioactive daughter production NOT calculated, approximate secular equilibrium exists.
s indicates radioactive daughter of this nuclide in secular equilibrium after several daughter $t_{1/2}$'s

t indicates transient equilibrium via beta decay. Accumulation of that nuclide during irradiation is separately calculated.

Reaction = b indicates production via decay from an activation produced parent (the preceeding line in this table)

Notes relating to Table 7.18.1:

- Calculational parameters:
  1 gram total sample size (assumed to be 100% of the natural element)
  1×10^7 n cm^{-2} s^{-1} equivalent thermal neutron fluence
  0 = cadmium ratio (*i.e.*, no epithermal neutrons)
  1 = thermal/fast neutron ratio (*i.e.*, for reactions indicated as fast, f = Y)
- Typically, for a decay chain where the daughter is also produced (isomers) the activity of the parent has been added to that of the daughter when the daughter $t_{1/2}$ is much longer (true for most cases) and the parent $t_{1/2}$ is relatively short, *e.g.*, less than 1 day, so that all the daughter will be made relatively promptly.
- In cases where the above condition is not met an * is put next to the nuclide name to warn that the daughter production has not been accounted for. In most cases the daughter is in a simple decay equilibrium.
- Where the decay product is a new nuclide a line has been added to the database to account for this. This production mode is indicated in the reaction column by 'b'. Where both m and g state contribute to daughter production it is simplified to a single parent, that with the greater cross-section or that with the longer half-life together with the sum of the cross-sections.
- In a few cases where the parent nuclide $t_{1/2}$ is very short all production is assigned to the daughter and no entry is made for the parent.
- No correction for neutron burn up has been made.
- Most cross-section data is from IAEA 273.
- Fast neutron data from NBSIR 85-3151, Compendium of Benchmark Neutron Fields is for reaction above the Cd cutoff, 0.4 eV.
- Fast neutron reaction data from IAEA 273 has been weighted by a unit fluence fast maxwellian spectrum as described in NBSIR 85-3151, but no further weighting for a 1/v or thermal component has been made.
- Not all n,2n fast neutron reactions are listed in this table.

Table 7.18.1 Health Physics Thermal Neutron Activation Database (Continued)

Target Nucleus	Target Isotopic Abund %	Nuclide Made	Half-life	Cross-sect'n (b)	Reaction	f ?	Activity (μCi) After Specified Irradiation Time: 1 minute	1 hour	1 day	1 year	Saturated Activity (μCi)
H-2	0.015	H-3	12.346 y	5e − 04	act	n	6.77E − 13	4.06E − 11	9.74E − 10	3.46E − 07	6.34E − 06
He-3	0.00013	H-3	12.346 y	5333	n,p	n	4.02E − 08	2.41E − 06	5.78E − 05	2.05E − 02	3.76E − 01
Li-7	92.5	Li-8	0.844 s	0.045	act	n	9.77E − 01	9.77E − 01	9.77E − 01	9.77E − 01	9.77E − 01
Li-6	7.5	H-3	12.346 y	940	n,a	n	2.04E − 04	1.23E − 02	2.94E − 01	1.04E + 02	1.91E + 03
Be-9	100	Be-10	1.6 My	0.008	act	n	1.13E − 13	6.80E − 12	1.63E − 10	5.95E − 08	1.37E − 01
Be-9	100	He-6	0.805 s	0.033	n,a	y	5.93E − 01	5.93E − 01	5.93E − 01	5.93E − 01	5.93E − 01
B-11	80	B-12	0.020 s	0.006	act	n	6.51E − 02	6.51E − 02	6.51E − 02	6.51E − 02	6.51E − 02
B-11	80	Li-8	0.844 s	1e − 04	n,a	y	1.66E − 03	1.66E − 03	1.66E − 03	1.66E − 03	1.66E − 03
C-12	98.9	C-11	20.30 m	4e − 10	n,2n	y	1.89E − 10	4.91E − 09	5.63E − 09	5.63E − 09	5.63E − 09
C-13	1.11	C-14	5736 y	0.001	act	n	4.38E − 14	2.63E − 12	6.30E − 11	2.30E − 08	1.90E − 04
N-14	99.64	C-14	5736 y	0.002	n,p	n	4.87E − 12	2.92E − 10	7.02E − 09	2.56E − 06	2.12E − 02
N-15	0.36	N-16	7.14 s	2e − 05	act	n	9.35E − 07	9.38E − 07	9.38E − 07	9.38E − 07	9.38E − 07
O-16	99.75	N-16	7.14 s	2e − 05	n,p	y	1.92E − 04	1.93E − 04	1.93E − 04	1.93E − 04	1.93E − 04
O-16	99.75	O-15	122.00 s	5e − 10	n,2n	y	1.55E − 09	5.38E − 09	5.38E − 09	5.38E − 09	5.38E − 09
O-17	0.039	C-14	5736 y	0.235	n,a	n	2.02E − 13	1.21E − 11	2.90E − 10	1.06E − 07	8.78E − 04
O-17	0.039	N-17	4.2 s	9e − 06	n,p	y	3.21E − 08	3.21E − 08	3.21E − 08	3.21E − 08	3.21E − 08
O-18	0.205	O-19	2.71 s	2e − 04	act	n	2.33E − 06	2.97E − 06	2.97E − 06	2.97E − 06	2.97E − 06
F-19	100	F-20	11.0 s	0.01	act	n	8.04E − 02	8.22E − 02	8.22E − 02	8.22E − 02	8.22E − 02
F-19	100	O-19	26.9s	0.001	n,p	y	9.10E − 03	1.16E − 02	1.16E − 02	1.16E − 02	1.16E − 02
F-19	100	N-16	7.1 s	0.008	n,a	y	6.71E − 02	6.73E − 02	6.73E − 02	6.73E − 02	6.73E − 02
F-19	100	F-18	109.80 m	7e − 06	n,2n	y	3.93E − 07	1.97E − 05	6.25E − 05	6.25E − 05	6.25E − 05
Ne-22	9.23	Ne-23	38.0 s	0.046	act	n	2.07E − 02	3.11E − 02	3.11E − 02	3.11E − 02	3.11E − 02
Na 23	100	Na 24m+	0.020 s	0.4	act	n	2.83E + 00	2.83E + 00	2.83E + 00	2.83E + 00	2.83E + 00
Na-23	100	Na-24	15.0 h	0.53	act	n	2.88E − 03	1.69E − 01	2.51E + 00	3.75E + 00	3.75E + 00
Na-23	100	Na-22	2.602 y	2e − 06	n,2n	y	7.89E − 12	4.73E − 10	1.14E − 08	3.64E − 06	1.56E − 05
Na-23	100	Ne-23	37.200 s	0.002	n,p	y	7.14E − 03	1.06E − 02	1.06E − 02	1.06E − 02	1.06E − 02
Na-23	100	F-20	11.000 s	8e − 04	n,a	y	5.29E − 03	5.41E − 03	5.41E − 03	5.41E − 03	5.41E − 03
Mg-25	10	Na-25	59.300 s	0.003	n,p	y	1.05E − 03	2.08E − 03	2.08E − 03	2.08E − 03	2.08E − 03
Mg-26	11.01	Mg-27	9.46 m	0.035	act	n	1.70E − 03	2.38E − 02	2.41E − 02	2.41E − 02	2.41E − 02
Mg-24	78.99	Na-24	15.03 h	0.002	n,p	y	6.03E − 06	3.69E − 04	5.49E − 03	8.20E − 03	8.20E − 03
Al-27	100	Al-28	2.25 m	0.232	act	n	3.71E − 01	1.40E + 00	1.40E + 00	1.40E + 00	1.40E + 00
Al-27	100	Na-24	15.03 h	7e − 04	n,a	y	3.36E − 06	1.97E − 04	2.93E − 03	4.37E − 03	4.37E − 03
Al-27	100	Mg-27	9.458 m	0.004	n,p	y	1.70E − 03	2.38E − 02	2.41E − 02	2.41E − 02	2.41E − 02
Si-28	92.23	Al-28	2.250 m	0.006	n,p	y	9.10E − 03	3.43E − 02	3.43E − 02	3.43E − 02	3.43E − 02
Si-29	4.67	Al-29	6.500 m	0.003	n,p	y	8.75E − 05	8.64E − 04	8.65E − 04	8.65E − 04	8.65E − 04
Si-30	3.1	Si-31	2.62 h	0.107	act	n	7.92E − 05	4.18E − 03	1.80E − 02	1.80E − 02	1.80E − 02
Si-30	3.1	Mg-27	9.458 m	2e − 04	n,a	y	1.84E − 06	2.58E − 05	2.61E − 05	2.61E − 05	2.61E − 05
P-31	100	P-32	14.3 d	0.172	act	n	3.04E − 05	1.82E − 03	4.27E − 02	9.03E − 01	9.03E − 01
P-31	100	Si-31	2.62 h	0.036	n,p	y	8.32E − 04	4.39E − 02	1.89E − 01	1.89E − 01	1.89E − 01
S-32	95.02	P-32	14.3 d	0.069	n,p	y	1.09E − 05	6.52E − 04	1.53E − 02	3.23E − 01	3.23E − 01
S-33	0.75	P-33	25.3 d	0.002	n,p	n	1.41E − 09	8.44E − 08	2.00E − 06	7.40E − 05	7.40E − 05
S-33	0.75	P-33	25.3 d	0.076	n,p	y	5.35E − 08	3.21E − 06	7.60E − 05	2.81E − 03	2.81E − 03
S-34	4.2	S-35	87.2 d	0.24	act	n	2.66E − 07	1.60E − 05	3.82E − 04	4.56E − 02	4.83E − 02
S-34	4.2	P-34	12.40 s	4e − 04	n,p	y	8.34E − 05	8.65E − 05	8.65E − 05	8.65E − 05	8.65E − 05
S-36	0.015	S-37	5.10 m	0.15	act	n	1.29E − 05	1.02E − 04	1.02E − 04	1.02E − 04	1.02E − 04

[a] My, million years.

(continued)

Table 7.18.1 Health Physics Thermal Neutron Activation Database (Continued)

Target Nucleus	Target Isotopic Abund %	Nuclide Made	Half-life	Cross-sect'n (b)	Reaction	f ?	Activity (μCi) After Specified Irradiation Time: 1 minute	1 hour	1 day	1 year	Saturated Activity (μCi)
Cl-35	75.77	Cl-36	0.3 My[a]	43.6	act	n	6.75E − 10	4.05E − 08	9.72E − 07	3.55E − 04	1.54E + 02
Cl-35	75.77	S-35	87.2 d	0.078	n,p	y	1.52E − 06	9.10E − 05	2.18E − 03	2.60E − 01	2.75E − 01
Cl-35	75.77	P-32	14.3 d	0.009	n,a	y	1.04E − 06	6.26E − 05	1.47E − 03	3.10E − 02	3.10E − 02
Cl-37	24.23	Cl-38m+	1.00 s	0.047	act	n	5.01E − 02	5.01E − 02	5.01E − 02	5.01E − 02	5.01E − 02
Cl-37	24.23	Cl-38	37.2 m	0.423	act	n	8.33E − 03	3.04E − 01	4.51E − 01	4.51E − 01	4.51E − 01
Cl-37	24.23	S-37	5.1 m	4e − 04	n,p	y	5.19E − 05	4.05E − 04	4.05E − 04	4.05E − 04	4.05E − 04
Ar-36	0.34	Ar-37	34.8 d	5.2	act	n	1.11E − 06	6.63E − 05	1.58E − 03	7.99E − 02	7.99E − 02
Ar-38	0.07	Ar-39	269 y	0.8	act	n	1.18E − 11	7.05E − 10	1.69E − 08	6.17E − 06	2.40E − 03
Ar-40	99.59	Ar-41	1.83 h	0.66	act	n	1.68E − 02	8.43E − 01	2.67E + 00	2.67E + 00	2.67E + 00
K-39	93.3	Cl-36	0.3 My	0.008	n,a	y	1.37E − 13	8.22E − 12	1.97E − 10	7.20E − 08	3.12E − 02
K-41	6.7	K-42	12.36 h	1.46	act	n	3.63E − 04	2.12E − 02	2.87E − 01	3.88E − 01	3.88E − 01
K-41	6.7	Ar-41	1.83 h	0.002	n,p	y	3.51E − 06	1.76E − 04	5.59E − 04	5.59E − 04	5.59E − 04
K-41	6.7	Cl-38	37.2 m	8e − 04	n,a	y	3.73E − 06	1.36E − 04	2.02E − 04	2.02E − 04	2.02E − 04
Ca-40	96.94	Ca-41	0.13 My	0.41	act	n	1.64E − 11	9.84E − 10	2.36E − 08	8.62E − 06	1.62E + 00
Ca-40	96.94	Ar-37	34.8 d	0.013	n,a	y	7.09E − 07	4.25E − 05	1.01E − 03	5.12E − 02	5.13E − 02
Ca-43	0.135	K-43	22.30 h	3e − 04	n,p	y	7.94E − 10	4.69E − 08	8.06E − 07	1.53E − 06	1.53E − 06
Ca-44	2.08	Ca-45	165 d	0.88	act	n	1.98E − 07	1.18E − 05	2.84E − 04	5.31E − 02	6.77E − 02
C1-44	21.08	Ar-41	1.83 h	6e − 05	n,a	y	2.96E − 08	1.48E − 06	4.70E − 06	4.70E − 06	4.70E − 06
Ca-46	0.003	Ca-47*	4.54 d	0.74	act	n	8.33E − 09	4.98E − 07	1.11E − 05	7.86E − 05	7.86E − 05
Ca-48	0.19	Ca-49t	8.72 m	1.09	act	n	5.37E − 04	6.96E − 03	7.02E − 03	7.02E − 03	7.02E − 03
Ca-48	0.19	Sc-49	57.3 m	1.09	b	n	3.27E − 06	3.02E − 03	7.02E − 03	7.02E − 03	7.02E − 03
Ca-48	0.19	Ca-47*	4.54 d	4e − 04	n,2n	y	2.46E − 10	1.47E − 08	3.28E − 07	2.32E − 06	2.32E − 06
Sc-45	100	Sc-46m+	18.7 s	9.8	act	n	3.16E + 01	3.54E + 01	3.54E + 01	3.54E + 01	3.54E + 01
Sc-45	100	Sc-46	84.0 d	27.2	act	n	5.64E − 04	3.38E − 02	8.08E − 01	9.35E + 01	9.84E + 01
Sc-45	100	Ca-45	165.0 d	0.015	n,p	y	1.58E − 07	9.49E − 06	2.27E − 04	4.25E − 02	5.43E − 02
Sc-45	100	K-42	12.36 h	2e − 04	n,a	y	6.15E − 07	3.59E − 05	4.87E − 04	6.58E − 04	6.58E − 04
Ti-46	8	Sc-46	84 d	0.012	n,p	y	1.91E − 08	1.15E − 06	2.74E − 05	3.18E − 03	3.34E − 03
Ti-46	8	Ti-45	3.08 h	8e − 06	n,2n	y	8.27E − 09	4.45E − 07	2.20E − 06	2.21E − 06	2.21E − 06
Ti-47	7.3	Sc-47	3.422 d	0.018	n,p	y	6.40E − 07	3.82E − 05	8.34E − 04	4.55E − 03	4.55E − 03
Ti-48	73.8	Sc-48	43.67 h	4e − 04	n,p	y	2.63E − 07	1.56E − 05	3.15E − 04	9.94E − 04	9.94E − 04
Ti-48	73.8	Ca-45	165.0 d	le − 05	n,a	y	9.49E − 11	5.59E − 09	1.36E − 07	2.55E − 05	3.25E − 05
Ti-50	5.3	Ti-51	4.80 m	0.179	act	n	3.48E − 03	3.09E − 02	3.09E − 02	3.09E − 02	3.09E − 02
Ti-50	5.3	Ca-47*	4.5 d	5e − 07	n,a	y	8.41E − 12	5.03E − 10	1.12E − 08	7.94E − 08	7.94E − 08
V-51	99.75	V-52	3.75 m	4.93	act	n	2.65E + 00	1.57E + 01	1.57E + 01	1.57E + 01	1.57E + 01
V-51	99.75	Ti-51	5.76 m	9e − 04	n,p	y	3.14E − 04	2.77E − 03	2.77E − 03	2.77E − 03	2.77E − 03
V-51	99.75	Sc-48	43.67 h	2e − 05	n,a	y	1.85E − 08	1.10E − 06	2.22E − 05	7.00E − 05	7.00E − 05
Cr-50	4.35	Cr-51	27.7 d	15.9	act	n	3.91E − 05	2.35E − 03	5.56E − 02	2.25E + 00	2.25E + 00
Cr-50	4.35	Cr-49	42.10 m	6e − 06	n,2n	y	1.39E − 08	5.33E − 07	8.50E − 07	8.50E − 07	8.50E − 07
Cr-52	83.79	V-52	3.75 m	0.001	n,p	y	4.82E − 04	2.86E − 03	2.86E − 03	2.86E − 03	2.86E − 03
Cr-53	9.5	V-53	1.61 m	4e − 04	n,p	y	4.49E − 05	1.28E − 04	1.28E − 04	1.28E − 04	1.28E − 04
Cr-54	2.36	Cr-55	3.60 m	0.36	act	n	4.48E − 03	2.56E − 02	2.56E − 02	2.56E − 02	2.56E − 02
Mn-55	100	Mn-56	2.58 h	13.3	act	n	1.76E − 01	9.27E + 00	3.93E + 01	3.94E + 01	3.94E + 01
Mn-55	100	Mn-54	312.7 d	3e − 04	n,2n	y	1.18E − 09	7.05E − 08	1.69E − 06	4.24E − 04	7.64E − 04
Mn-55	100	V-52	3.75 m	le − 04	n,a	y	5.49E − 05	3.26E − 04	3.26E − 04	3.26E − 04	3.26E − 04

[a] My, million years.

Table 7.18.1 Health Physics Thermal Neutron Activation Database (Continued)

Target Nucleus	Target Isotopic Abund %	Nuclide Made	Half-life	Cross-sect'n (b)	Reaction	f ?	Activity (μCi) After Specified Irradiation Time: 1 minute	1 hour	1 day	1 year	Saturated Activity (μCi)
Fe-54	5.8	Fe-55	2.70 y	2.25	act	n	1.92E − 07	1.15E − 05	2.77E − 04	8.91E − 02	3.93E − 01
Fe-54	5.8	Mn-54	312.7 d	0.082	n,p	y	2.20E − 08	1.32E − 06	3.16E − 05	7.92E − 03	1.43E − 02
Fe-54	5.8	Cr-51	27.7 d	6e − 04	n,a	y	1.82E − 09	1.09E − 07	2.59E − 06	1.05E − 04	1.05E − 04
Fe-54	5.8	Fe-53	8.51 m	5e − 06	n,2n	y	6.84E − 08	8.68E − 07	8.74E − 07	8.74E − 07	8.74E − 07
Fe-56	91.72	Mn-56	2.58 h	0.001	n,p	y	1.27E − 05	6.72E − 04	2.85E − 03	2.85E − 03	2.85E − 03
Fe-58	0.31	Fe-59	44.6 d	1.28	act	n	1.20E − 07	7.21E − 06	1.72E − 04	1.11E − 02	1.11E − 02
Co-59	100	Co-60m+	10.5 m	18.8	act	n	3.31E + 00	5.09E + 01	5.19E + 01	5.19E + 01	5.19E + 01
Co-59	100	Co-60	5.27 y	37.45	act	n	2.58E − 05	1.55E − 03	3.72E − 02	1.27E + 01	1.03E + 02
Co-59	100	Fe-59	44.6 d	0.001	n,p	y	4.23E − 08	2.54E − 06	6.04E − 05	3.90E − 03	3.92E − 03
Co-59	100	Mn-56	2.58 h	2e − 04	n,a	y	1.92E − 06	1.01E − 04	4.30E − 04	4.30E − 04	4.30E − 04
Co-59	100	Co-58	70.8 d	4e − 04	n,2n	y	7.50E − 09	4.50E − 07	1.07E − 05	1.07E − 03	1.10E − 03
Ni-58	67.76	Ni-57	36.10 h	5e − 06	n,2n	y	2.98E − 09	1.77E − 07	3.44E − 06	9.32E − 06	9.32E − 06
Ni-58	67.76	Ni-59	75000 y	4.6	act	n	1.54E − 10	9.23E − 09	2.21E − 07	8.08E − 05	8.75E + 00
Ni-58	67.76	Fe-55	2.70 y	3e − 05	n,a	n	2.79E − 11	1.67E − 09	4.01E − 08	1.29E − 05	5.71E − 05
Ni-58	67.76	Fe-55	2.7 y	0.003	n,a	y	2.79E − 09	1.67E − 07	4.01E − 06	1.29E − 03	5.71E − 03
Ni-58	67.76	Co-58	70.8 d	0.111	n,p	y	1.43E − 06	8.61E − 05	2.06E − 03	2.05E − 01	2.11E − 01
Ni-58	67.76	Co-58m+	9.10 h	0.035	n,p	y	8.54E − 05	4.94E − 03	5.65E − 02	6.73E − 02	6.73E − 02
Ni-60	26.1	Co-60	5.272 y	0.002	n,p	y	4.07E − 10	2.44E − 08	5.86E − 07	2.01E − 04	1.63E − 03
Ni-60	26.1	Co-60m+	10.48 m	0.002	n,p	y	9.51E − 05	1.46E − 03	1.49E − 03	1.49E − 03	1.49E − 03
Ni-61	1.13	Co-61	1.65 h	0.001	n,p	y	2.94E − 07	1.45E − 05	4.22E − 05	4.22E − 05	4.22E − 05
Ni-62	3.71	Ni-63	100 y	14.5	act	n	1.86E − 08	1.12E − 06	2.68E − 05	9.75E − 03	1.41E + 00
Ni-62	3.71	Fe-59	44.6 d	9e − 05	n,a	y	9.46E − 11	5.67E − 09	1.35E − 07	8.74E − 06	8.77E − 06
Ni-64	0.95	Ni-65	2.52 h	1.58	act	n	1.75E − 04	9.18E − 03	3.81E − 02	3.82E − 02	3.82E − 02
Cu-63	69.1	Cu-62	9.74 m	le − 04	n,2n	y	1.52E − 05	2.18E − 04	2.21E − 04	2.21E − 04	2.21E − 04
Cu-63	69.1	Cu-64	12.7 h	4.5	act	n	7.30E − 03	4.27E − 01	5.87E + 00	8.03E + 00	8.03E + 00
Cu-63	69.1	Co-60	5.272 y	6e − 04	n,a	y	2.68E − 10	1.61E − 08	3.86E − 07	1.32E − 04	1.07E − 03
Cu-65	30.9	Cu-66	5.10 m	2.17	act	n	2.13E − 01	1.68E + 00	1.68E + 00	1.68E + 00	1.68E + 00
Cu-65	30.9	Ni-65	2.5 h	5e − 04	n,p	y	1.70E − 06	8.93E − 05	3.71E − 04	3.71E − 04	3.71E − 04
Zn-64	48.9	Zn-65	265 d	0.76	act	n	1.72E − 06	1.03E − 04	2.47E − 03	5.81E − 01	9.45E − 01
Zn-64	48.9	Cu-64	12.7 h	0.031	n,p	y	3.50E − 05	2.05E − 03	2.81E − 02	3.86E − 02	3.86E − 02
Zn-66	27.9	Zn-65	265 d	0.005	n,2n	y	6.25E − 09	3.75E − 07	8.99E − 06	2.12E − 03	3.44E − 03
Zn-66	27.9	Cu-66	5.1 m	6e − 04	n,p	y	5.42E − 05	4.27E − 04	4.27E − 04	4.27E − 04	4.27E − 04
Zn-67	4.1	Cu-67	61.9 h	0.001	n,p	y	1.99E − 08	1.19E − 06	2.51E − 05	1.07E − 04	1.07E − 04
Zn-68	18.6	Zn-69m*	13.9 h	0.072	act	n	2.66E − 05	1.56E − 03	2.24E − 02	3.21E − 02	3.21E − 02
Zn-68	18.6	Zn-69	56.0 m	1	act	n	5.48E − 03	2.33E − 01	4.45E − 01	4.45E − 01	4.45E − 01
Zn-68	18.6	Ni-65	2.5 h	7e − 05	n,a	y	1.51E − 07	7.92E − 06	3.29E − 05	3.29E − 05	3.29E − 05
Zn-70	0.62	Zn-71m	3.90 h	0.009	act	n	3.71E − 07	2.04E − 05	1.24E − 04	1.25E − 04	1.25E − 04
Zn-70	0.62	Zn-71	2.40 m	0.083	act	n	3.00E − 04	1.20E − 03	1.20E − 03	1.20E − 03	1.20E − 03
Ga-69	60	Ga-70	21.1 m	1.68	act	n	7.68E − 02	2.05E + 00	2.38E + 00	2.38E + 00	2.38E + 00
Ga-69	60	Zn-69ms	13.8 h	5e − 04	n,p	y	5.87E − 07	3.44E − 05	4.92E − 04	7.02E − 04	7.02E − 04
Ga-71	40	Ga-72m+	0.036 s	0.15	act	n	1.38E − 01	1.38E − 01	1.38E − 01	1.38E − 01	1.38E − 01
Ga-71	40	Ga-72	14.1 h	4.71	act	n	3.54E − 03	2.07E − 01	2.99E + 00	4.32E + 00	4.32E + 00
Ge-70	20.7	Ge-69	39.1 h	0.002	n,2n	y	2.56E − 07	1.52E − 05	3.00E − 04	8.66E − 04	8.66E − 04
Ge-70	20.7	Ge-71m+	0.020 s	0.28	act	n	1.35E − 01	1.35E − 01	1.35E − 01	1.35E − 01	1.35E − 01

[a] My, million years.

(continued)

Table 7.18.1 Health Physics Thermal Neutron Activation Database (Continued)

Target Nucleus	Target Isotopic Abund %	Nuclide Made	Half-life	Cross-sect'n (b)	Reaction	f ?	Activity (μCi) After Specified Irradiation Time: 1 minute	1 hour	1 day	1 year	Saturated Activity (μCi)
Ge-70	20.7	Ge-71	11.2 d	3.43	act	n	7.09E − 05	4.25E − 03	9.91E − 02	1.65E + 00	1.65E + 00
Ge-72	27.5	Ge-73m	0.530 s	0.98	act	n	6.09E − 01	6.09E − 01	6.09E − 01	6.09E − 01	6.09E − 01
Ge-72	27.5	Ga-72	14.1 h	2e − 05	n,p	y	1.12E − 08	6.56E − 07	9.47E − 06	1.37E − 05	1.37E − 05
Ge-72	27.5	Zn-69ms	13.8 h	3e − 05	n,a	y	1.30E − 08	7.61E − 07	1.09E − 05	1.55E − 05	1.55E − 05
Ge-74	36.4	Ge-75m+	48.0 s	0.17	act	n	7.89E − 02	1.36E − 01	1.36E − 01	1.36E − 01	1.36E − 01
Ge-74	36.4	Ge-75	83.0 m	0.51	act	n	3.40E − 03	1.61E − 01	4.08E − 01	4.08E − 01	4.08E − 01
Ge-74	36.4	Zn-71ms	3.9 h	3e − 06	n,a	y	5.92E − 09	3.26E − 07	1.97E − 06	2.00E − 06	2.00E − 06
Ge-76	7.7	Ge-77m+	54.0 s	0.1	qct	n	8.86E − 03	1.65E − 02	1.65E − 02	1.65E − 02	1.65E − 02
Ge-76	7.7	Ge-77	11.3 h	0.16	act	n	2.70E − 05	1.57E − 03	2.03E − 02	2.64E − 02	2.64E − 02
As-75	100	As-74	17.8 d	3e − 04	n,2n	y	1.94E − 08	1.16E − 06	2.74E − 05	7.16E − 04	7.16E − 04
As-75	100	As-76	26.4 h	4.48	act	n	4.25E − 03	2.52E − 01	4.54E + 00	9.72E + 00	9.72E + 00
As-75	100	Ge-75	83.00 m	5e − 04	n,p	y	8.12E − 06	3.85E − 04	9.77E − 04	9.77E − 04	9.77E − 04
Se-74	0.9	Se-75	120 d	51.8	act	n	4.11E − 06	2.47E − 04	5.91E − 03	9.01E − 01	1.03E + 00
Se-74	0.9	As-74	18 d	0.007	n,p	y	3.54E − 09	2.12E − 07	4.99E − 06	1.31E − 04	1.31E − 04
Se-76	9	Se-77m	17.5 s	22	act	n	3.85E + 00	4.24E + 00	4.24E + 00	4.24E + 00	4.24E + 00
Se-77	7.6	Se-77m	17.5 s	0.733	n,n′	y	1.07E − 01	1.18E − 01	1.18E − 01	1.18E − 01	1.18E − 01
Se-78	23.5	Se-77m	17.5 s	0.001	n,2n	y	4.45E − 04	4.90E − 04	4.90E − 04	4.90E − 04	4.90E − 04
Se-78	23.5	Se-79m+	3.90 m	0.38	act	n	3.03E − 02	1.86E − 01	1.86E − 01	1.86E − 01	1.86E − 01
Se-78	23.5	Se-79	65000 y	0.43	act	n	4.28E − 12	2.57E − 10	6.16E − 09	2.25E − 06	2.11E − 01
Se-80	50	Se-79m	3.9 m	0.01	n,2n	y	1.66E − 03	1.02E − 02	1.02E − 02	1.02E − 02	1.02E − 02
Se-80	50	Se-81m*	57.3 m	0.08	act	n	9.78 − 04	4.20E − 02	8.14E − 02	8.14E − 02	8.14E − 02
Se-80	50	Se-81	18.0 m	0.53	act	n	2.04E − 02	4.86E − 01	5.39E − 01	5.39E − 01	5.39E − 01
Se-82	9.1	Se-83m+	69.0 s	0.039	act	n	3.19E − 03	7.05E − 03	7.05E − 03	7.05E − 03	7.05E − 03
Se-82	9.1	Se-83t	22.4 m	0.044	act	n	2.42E − 04	6.71E − 03	7.95E − 03	7.95E − 03	7.95E − 03
Se-82	9.1	Br-83	2.39 h	0.044	b	n	5.87E − 07	1.13E − 03	7.94E − 03	7.95E − 03	7.95E − 03
Br-79	50.69	Br-80m*	4.42 h	2.4	act	n	6.54E − 03	3.64E − 01	2.45E + 00	2.51E + 00	2.51E + 00
Br-79	50.69	Br-80	18.0 m	8.6	act	n	3.39E − 01	8.09E + 00	8.98E + 00	8.98E + 00	8.98E + 00
Br-79	50.69	As-76	26.40 h	2e − 05	n,a	y	9.14E − 09	5.41E − 07	9.76E − 06	2.09E − 05	2.09E − 05
Br-81	49.31	Br-82m+	6.10 m	2.43	act	n	2.59E − 01	2.41E + 00	2.41E + 00	2.41E + 00	2.41E + 00
Br-81	49.31	Br-82	35.3 h	2.7	act	n	8.74E − 04	5.20E − 02	1.00E + 00	2.68E + 00	2.68E + 00
Br-81	49.31	Se-81mt	57.30 m	1e − 05	n,p	y	1.73E − 07	7.41E − 06	1.44E − 05	1.44E − 05	1.44E − 05
Kr-78	0.35	Kr-79m+	50.0 s	0.17	act	n	7.01E − 04	1.24E − 03	1.24E − 03	1.24E − 03	1.24E − 03
Kr-78	0.35	Kr-79	34.9 h	6.2	act	n	1.50E − 05	8.90E − 04	1.72E − 02	4.53E − 02	4.53E − 02
Kr-80	2.25	Kr-81m+	13.3 s	4.55	act	n	1.99E − 01	2.08E − 01	2.08E − 01	2.08E − 01	2.08E − 01
Kr-80	2.25	Kr-81	0.21 My	11.5	act	n	3.31E − 12	1.98E − 10	4.76E − 09	1.74E − 06	5.26E − 01
Kr-82	11.6	Kr-83m	1.83 h	14	act	n	2.03E − 02	1.02E + 00	3.22E + 00	3.22E + 00	3.22E + 00
Kr-84	57	Kr-85m+	4.48 h	0.09	act	n	2.56E − 04	1.42E − 02	9.70E − 02	9.94E − 02	9.94E − 02
Kr-84	57	Kr-85	10.76 y	0.059	act	n	7.97E − 09	4.78E − 07	1.15E − 05	4.06E − 03	6.51E − 02
Kr-86	17.3	Kr-87	76.3 m	0.003	act	n	8.88E − 06	4.13E − 04	9.82E − 04	9.82E − 04	9.82E − 04
Rb-85	72.17	Rb-84	32.9 d	2e − 04	n,2n	y	4.04E − 09	2.42E − 07	5.76E − 06	2.76E − 04	2.76E − 04
Rb-85	72.17	Rb-86m+	1.02 m	0.053	act	n	3.61E − 02	7.33E − 02	7.33E − 02	7.33E − 02	7.33E − 02
Rb-85	72.17	Rb-86	18.7 d	0.48	act	n	1.71E − 05	1.02E − 03	2.41E − 02	6.63E − 01	6.63E − 01
Rb-87	27.83	Rb-88	17.8 m	0.12	act	n	2.39E − 03	5.64E − 02	6.25E − 02	6.25E − 02	6.25E − 02
Sr-84	0.56	Sr-85m+	67.7 m	0.6	act	n	6.63E − 05	2.99E − 03	6.51E − 03	6.51E − 03	6.51E − 03

[a] My, million years.

Table 7.18.1 Health Physics Thermal Neutron Activation Database (Continued)

Target Nucleus	Target Isotopic Abund %	Nuclide Made	Half-life	Cross-sect'n (b)	Reaction	f ?	Activity (μCi) After Specified Irradiation Time: 1 minute	1 hour	1 day	1 year	Saturated Activity (μCi)
Sr-84	0.56	Sr-85	64.9 d	0.87	act	n	7.00E − 08	4.20E − 06	1.00E − 04	9.25E − 03	9.44E − 03
Sr-86	9.9	Sr-87m	2.81 h	0.84	act	n	6.46E − 04	3.44E − 02	1.57E − 01	1.57E − 01	1.57E − 01
Sr-87	7	Sr-87m	2.81 h	0.112	n,n′	y	6.02E − 05	3.21E − 03	1.46E − 02	1.47E − 02	1.47E − 02
Sr-88	82.6	Sr-87m	2.81 h	0.01	n,2n	y	6.27E − 05	3.34E − 03	1.52E − 02	1.53E − 02	1.53E − 02
Sr-88	82.6	Sr-89	50.5 d	0.006	act	n	8.45E − 08	5.07E − 06	1.21E − 04	8.80E − 03	8.86E − 03
Sr-88	82.6	Rb-88	15.2 m	1e − 05	n,p	y	6.81E − 07	1.43E − 05	1.53E − 05	1.53E − 05	1.53E − 05
Y-89	100	Y-88	106.6 d	2e − 04	n,2n	y	1.29E − 09	7.73E − 08	1.85E − 06	2.59E − 04	2.85E − 04
Y-89	100	Y-89m	15.7 s	0.128	n,n′	y	2.18E − 01	2.34E − 01	2.34E − 01	2.34E − 01	2.34E − 01
Y-89	100	Y-90m +	3.19 h	0.001	act	n	6.61E − 06	3.57E − 04	1.82E − 03	1.83E − 03	1.83E − 03
Y-89	100	Y-90	64.1 h	1.28	act	n	4.22E − 04	2.52E − 02	5.35E − 01	2.34E + 00	2.34E + 00
Y-89	100	Sr-89	50.5 d	3e − 04	n,p	y	5.40E − 09	3.24E − 08	7.73E − 06	5.63E − 04	5.67E − 04
Y-89	100	Rb-86	18.7 d	2e − 06	n,a	y	9.41E − 11	5.64E − 09	1.33E − 07	3.66E − 06	3.66E − 06
Zr-90	51.45	Zr-89	78.4 h	8e − 05	n,2n	y	1.04E − 08	6.22E − 07	1.35E − 05	7.07E − 05	7.07E − 05
Zr-90	51.45	Y-90	64.1 h	2e − 04	n,p	y	3.02E − 08	1.80E − 06	3.83E − 05	1.68E − 04	1.68E − 04
Zr-92	17.1	Zr-93	1.5 My	0.22	act	n	5.85E − 14	3.51E − 12	8.43E − 11	3.08E − 08	6.66E − 02
Zr-92	17.1	Sr-89	50.5 d	1e − 05	n,a	y	4.04E − 11	2.42E − 09	5.77E − 08	4.21E − 06	4.24E − 06
Zr-94	17.5	Zr-95s	64.0 d	0.05	act	n	1.14E − 07	6.82E − 06	1.63E − 04	1.48E − 02	1.51E − 02
Zr-96	2.8	Zr-97s	16.8 h	0.023	act	n	7.50E − 07	4.41E − 05	6.86E − 04	1.09E − 03	1.09E − 03
Nb-93	100	Nb-92mt	10.1 d	5e − 04	n,2n	y	3.99E − 08	2.39E − 06	5.56E − 05	8.40E − 04	8.40E − 04
Nb-93	100	Nb-92	37 My	5e − 04	b	y	6.36E − 22	2.56E − 18	1.44E − 15	1.51E − 11	8.40E − 04
Nb-93	100	Nb-94m +	6.20 m	1.15	act	n	2.13E − 01	2.01E + 00	2.01E + 00	2.01E + 00	2.01E + 00
Nb-93	100	Nb-94	20000 y	1.15	act	n	1.33E − 10	7.96E − 09	1.91E − 07	6.97E − 05	2.01E + 00
Nb-93	100	Nb-93m	14.6 y	0.164	n,n′	y	2.59E − 08	1.56E − 06	3.73E − 05	1.33E − 02	2.87E − 01
Nb-93	100	Y-90	64.1 h	7e − 05	n,a	y	2.23E − 08	1.33E − 06	2.83E − 05	1.24E − 04	1.24E − 04
Mo-92	14.8	Mo-93m +	6.90 h	0.019	act	n	8.32E − 06	4.75E − 04	4.53E − 03	4.98E − 03	4.98E − 03
Mo-92	14.8	Mo-93	3500 y	0.019	act	n	1.87E − 12	1.12E − 10	2.70E − 09	9.85E − 07	4.98E − 03
Mo-92	14.8	Nb-92mt	10.13 d	0.007	n,p	y	8.71E − 08	5.22E − 06	1.21E − 04	1.83E − 03	1.83E − 03
Mo-92	14.8	Nb-92	37 My	0.007	b	y	1.39E − 21	5.58E − 18	3.15E − 15	3.30E − 11	1.83E − 03
Mo-92	14.8	Zr-89	78.40 h	4e − 05	n,a	y	1.54E − 09	9.22E − 08	2.00E − 06	1.05E − 05	1.05E − 05
Mo-95	15.92	Nb-95	34.98 d	1e − 04	n,p	y	5.25E − 10	3.15E − 08	7.49E − 07	3.82E − 05	3.82E − 05
Mo-96	23.4	Nb-96	23.40 h	2e − 04	n,p	y	4.50E − 08	2.66E − 06	4.64E − 05	9.13E − 05	9.13E − 05
Mo-98	24.4	Mo-99st	66.00 h	0.13	act	n	9.22E − 06	5.50E − 04	1.17E − 02	5.27E − 02	5.27E − 02
Mo-98	24.4	Tc-99	0.21 My	0.13	b	n	2.89E − 17	1.04E − 13	5.53E − 11	1.72E − 07	5.27E − 02
Mo-98	24.4	Zr-95	64.00 d	1e − 05	n,a	y	4.24E − 11	2.54E − 09	6.07E − 08	5.53E − 06	5.63E − 06
Mo-100	9.6	Mo-101s	14.6 m	0.199	act	n	1.44E − 03	2.93E − 02	3.11E − 02	3.11E − 02	3.11E − 02
Tc-98	100	Tc-99m +	6.00 h	0.93	act	n	2.97E − 03	1.69E − 01	1.45E + 00	1.54E + 00	1.54E + 00
Tc-98	100	Tc-99	0.21 My	2.6	act	n	2.71E − 11	1.63E − 09	3.90E − 08	1.43E − 05	4.32E + 00
Ru-96	5.5	Ru-97t	2.90 d	0.29	act	n	4.49E − 06	2.68E − 04	5.75E − 03	2.70E − 02	2.70E − 02
Ru-96	5.5	Tc-97	3 My	0.29	b	n	1.14E − 18	4.08E − 15	2.18E − 12	7.13E − 09	2.70E − 02
Ru-102	31.6	Ru-103	39.4 d	1.21	act	n	7.46E − 06	4.48E − 04	1.07E − 02	6.09E − 01	6.10E − 01
Ru-104	18.6	Ru-105t	4.44 h	0.32	act	n	2.42E − 04	1.35E − 02	9.10E − 02	9.32E − 02	9.32E − 02
Ru-104	18.6	Rh-105	35.4 h	0.32	b	n	3.95E − 08	1.34E − 04	2.69E − 02	9.32E − 02	9.32E − 02
Rh-103	100	Rh-103m	56.12 m	0.533	n,n′	y	1.03E − 02	4.41E − 01	8.42E − 01	8.42E − 01	8.42E − 01
Rh-103	100	Rh-104m	4.40 m	10	act	n	2.30E + 00	1.58E + 01	1.58E + 01	1.58E + 01	1.58E + 01

[a] My, million years.

(continued)

Table 7.18.1 Health Physics Thermal Neutron Activation Database (Continued)

Target Nucleus	Target Isotopic Abund %	Nuclide Made	Half-life	Cross-sect'n (b)	Reaction	f ?	Activity (μCi) After Specified Irradiation Time: 1 minute	1 hour	1 day	1 year	Saturated Activity (μCi)
Rh-103	100	Rh-104	42.0 s	135	act	n	1.34E + 02	2.13E + 02	2.13E + 02	2.13E + 02	2.13E + 02
Rh-103	100	Ru-103	39.4 d	1e − 04	n,p	y	2.07E − 09	1.24E − 07	2.95E − 06	1.69E − 04	1.69E − 04
Pd-102	1	Pd-103	17.0 d	3.4	act	n	1.54E − 06	9.21E − 05	2.17E − 03	5.43E − 02	5.43E − 02
Pd-106	27.3	Pd-107m+	2.13 s	0.013	act	n	4.68E − 03	5.45E − 03	5.45E − 03	5.45E − 03	5.45E − 03
Pd-106	27.3	Pd-107	6.5 My	0.305	act	n	2.59E − 14	1.56E − 12	3.73E − 11	1.36E − 08	1.28E − 01
Pd-108	26.7	Pd-109m+	4.69 m	0.183	act	n	1.01E − 02	7.36E − 02	7.36E − 02	7.36E − 02	7.36E − 02
Pd-108	26.7	Pd-109	13.5 h	8.483	act	n	2.93E − 03	1.71E − 01	2.42E + 00	3.41E + 00	3.41E + 00
Pd-110	11.8	Pd-111m*	5.50 h	0.037	act	n	1.36E − 05	7.65E − 04	6.15E − 03	6.46E − 03	6.46E − 03
Pd-110	11.8	Pd-111t	22.0m	0.19	act	n	1.03E − 03	2.82E − 02	3.32E − 02	3.32E − 02	3.32E − 02
Pd-110	11.8	Ag-111	7.47 d	0.227	b	n	3.98E − 08	8.43E − 05	3.44E − 03	3.96E − 02	3.96E − 02
Ag-107	51.83	Ag-106ms	8.50 d	5e − 04	n,2n	y	2.05E − 08	1.23E − 06	2.84E − 05	3.63E − 04	3.63E − 04
Ag-107	51.83	Ag-108m*	127 y	0.33	act	n	2.70E − 09	1.62E − 07	3.89E − 06	1.42E − 03	2.60E − 01
Ag-107	51.83	Ag-108	2.41 m	37.27	act	n	7.34E + 00	2.94E + 01	2.94E + 01	2.94E + 01	2.94E + 01
Ag-109	48.17	Ag-110m*	250 d	4.7	act	n	6.50E − 06	3.90E − 04	9.34E − 03	2.15E + 00	3.38E + 00
Ag-109	48.17	Ag-110	24.6 s	86.3	act	n	5.06E + 01	6.21E + 01	6.21E + 01	6.21E + 01	6.21E + 01
Ag-109	48.17	Pd-109	13.46 h	6e − 05	n,p	y	3.70E − 08	2.17E − 06	3.06E − 05	4.32E − 05	4.32E − 05
Cd-106	1.2	Cd-107	6.50 h	1	act	n	3.27E − 05	1.86E − 03	1.70E − 02	1.84E − 02	1.84E − 02
Cd-106	1.2	Ag-106	24.00 m	0.003	n,p	y	1.73E − 06	5.01E − 05	6.08E − 05	6.08E − 05	6.08E − 05
Cd-108	0.9	Cd-109	453 d	1.1	act	n	1.59E − 08	9.51E − 07	2.28E − 05	6.38E − 03	1.49E − 02
Cd-110	12.4	Cd-111m	49.0 m	0.14	act	n	3.61E − 04	1.47E − 02	2.57E − 02	2.57E − 02	2.57E − 02
Cd-110	12.4	Ag-110	24.6 s	0.003	n,p	y	4.94E − 04	6.06E − 04	6.06E − 04	6.06E − 04	6.06E − 04
Cd-111	12.8	Cd-111m	49.00 m	0.288	n,n′	y	7.59E − 04	3.09E − 02	5.41E − 02	5.41E − 02	5.41E − 02
Cd-112	24	Cd-111m	49.00 m	4e − 04	n,2n	y	2.06E − 06	8.38E − 05	1.47E − 04	1.47E − 04	1.47E − 04
Cd-112	24	Cd-113m	14.6 y	2.2	act	n	6.93E − 08	4.16E − 06	9.98E − 05	3.56E − 02	7.67E − 01
Cd-112	24	Cd-113	9000 Ty	2.2	act	n	1.12E − 22	6.75E − 21	1.62E − 19	5.91E − 17	4.49E − 01
Cd-114	28.8	Cd-115ms	44.8d	0.036	act	n	1.59E − 07	9.54E − 06	2.27E − 04	1.48E − 02	1.48E − 02
Cd-114	28.8	Cd-115s	53.38 h	0.3	act	n	2.67E − 05	1.59E − 03	3.30E − 02	1.23E − 01	1.23E − 01
Cd-116	7.6	Cd-117ms	3.31 h	0.025	act	n	9.29E − 06	5.04E − 04	2.65E − 03	2.67E − 03	2.67E − 03
Cd-116	7.6	Cd-117s	2.42 h	0.05	act	n	2.54E − 05	1.33E − 03	5.33E − 03	5.33E − 03	5.33E − 03
In-113	4.3	In-114m2+	0.042 s	3.1	act	n	1.92E − 01	1.92E − 01	1.92E − 01	1.92E − 01	1.92E − 01
In-113	4.3	In-114m1*	49.5 d	8.1	act	n	4.88E − 06	2.93E − 04	6.98E − 03	4.99E − 01	5.02E − 01
In-113	4.3	In-114	71.9 s	3.9	act	n	1.06E − 01	2.42E − 01	2.42E − 01	2.42E − 01	2.42E − 01
In-115	95.7	In-116m2+	2.20 s	81	act	n	1.10E + 02	1.10E + 02	1.10E + 02	1.10E + 02	1.10E + 02
In-115	95.7	In-116m1	54.0 m	162.3	act	n	2.80E + 00	1.18E + 02	2.20E + 02	2.20E + 02	2.20E + 02
In-115	95.7	In-116	14.0 s	40	act	n	5.14E + 01	5.42E + 01	5.42E + 01	5.42E + 01	5.42E + 01
In-115	95.7	In-115m	4.36 h	0.19	n,n′	y	6.81E − 04	3.78E − 02	2.52E − 01	2.57E − 01	2.57E − 01
Sn-112	1	Sn-113m+	20.0 m	0.3	act	n	1.48E − 04	3.81E − 03	4.36E − 03	4.36E − 03	4.36E − 03
Sn-112	1	Sn-113	115 d	0.98	act	n	5.96E − 08	3.58E − 06	8.56E − 05	1.27E − 02	1.42E − 02
Sn-116	14.4	Sn-117m	14.0 d	0.006	act	n	4.17E − 08	2.50E − 06	5.86E − 05	1.21E − 03	1.21E − 03
Sn-118	24.1	Sn-119m	245 d	0.01	act	n	6.53E − 09	3.92E − 07	9.39E − 06	2.14E − 03	3.32E − 03
Sn-120	32.8	Sn-121m	55.0 y	0.001	act	n	1.07E − 11	6.40E − 10	1.54E − 08	5.57E − 06	4.45E − 04
Sn-120	32.8	Sn-121	27.0 h	0.14	act	n	2.66E − 05	1.58E − 03	2.86E − 02	6.23E − 02	6.23E − 02
Sn-122	4.7	Sn-123m	40.1 m	0.001	act	n	1.07E − 06	4.05E − 05	6.27E − 05	6.27E − 05	6.27E − 05
Sn-122	4.7	Sn-123	129 d	0.18	act	n	4.20E − 08	2.52E − 06	6.04E − 05	9.69E − 03	1.13E − 02

[a] My, million years.

(continued)

Table 7.18.1 Health Physics Thermal Neutron Activation Database (Continued)

Target Nucleus	Target Isotopic Abund %	Nuclide Made	Half-life	Cross-sect'n (b)	Reaction	f ?	Activity (μCi) After Specified Irradiation Time: 1 minute	1 hour	1 day	1 year	Saturated Activity (μCi)
Sn-124	5.8	Sn-125t	9.64 d	0.004	act	n	1.52E − 08	9.11E − 07	2.11E − 05	3.05E − 04	3.05E − 04
Sn-124	5.8	Sn-125m	9.50 m	0.134	act	n	6.96E − 04	9.77E − 03	9.90E − 03	9.90E − 03	9.90E − 03
Sn-124	5.8	Sb-125	2.76 y	0.134	b	n	1.74E − 10	2.26E − 07	6.95E − 06	2.27E − 03	1.02E − 02
Sb-121	57.3	Sb-122m +	4.20 m	0.06	act	n	7.04E − 03	4.62E − 02	4.63E − 02	4.63E − 02	4.63E − 02
Sb-121	57.3	Sb-122	2.70 d	5.9	act	n	8.11E − 04	4.84E − 02	1.03E + 00	4.55E + 00	4.55E + 00
Sb-123	42.7	Sb-124m2*	20.0 m	0.019	act	n	3.66E − 04	9.39E − 03	1.07E − 02	1.07E − 02	1.07E − 02
Sb-123	42.7	Sb-124m1 +	1.60 m	0.037	act	n	7.35E − 03	2.09E − 02	2.09E − 02	2.09E − 02	2.09E − 02
Sb-123	42.7	Sb-124	60.3 d	4.145	act	n	1.87E − 05	1.12E − 03	2.68E − 02	2.31E + 00	2.34E + 00
Te-120	0.09	Te-121m*	154 d	0.34	act	n	1.30E − 09	7.78E − 08	1.86E − 06	3.35E − 04	4.15E − 04
Te-120	0.09	Te-121	16.8 d	2	act	n	6.99E − 08	4.19E − 06	9.87E − 05	2.44E − 03	2.44E − 03
Te-122	2.4	Te-123m*	119.7 d	1.1	act	n	1.42E − 07	8.50E − 06	2.03E − 04	3.10E − 02	3.52E − 02
Te-122	2.4	Te-123	12 Ty	2.3	act	n	8.09E − 21	4.86E − 19	1.17E − 17	4.25E − 15	7.37E − 02
Te-124	4.6	Te-125m	58.0 d	0.04	act	n	2.00E − 08	1.20E − 06	2.87E − 05	2.38E − 03	2.42E − 03
Te-126	18.7	Te-127m*	109 d	0.135	act	n	1.44E − 07	8.64E − 06	2.07E − 04	2.94E − 02	3.26E − 02
Te-126	18.7	Te-127	9.35 h	0.9	act	n	2.68E − 04	1.55E − 02	1.81E − 01	2.17E − 01	2.17E − 01
Te-128	31.8	Te-129ms	33.6 d	0.015	act	n	8.69E − 08	5.21E − 06	1.24E − 04	6.06E − 03	6.07E − 03
Te-128	31.8	Te-129t	69.6 m	0.2	act	n	8.00E − 04	3.63E − 02	8.08E − 02	8.08E − 02	8.08E − 02
Te-128	31.8	I-129	16 My	0.2	b	n	3.30E − 17	9.87E − 14	8.91E − 12	3.50E − 09	8.08E − 02
Te-130	34.5	Te-131m	30.0 h	0.02	act	n	3.33E − 06	1.97E − 04	3.68E − 03	8.64E − 03	8.64E − 03
Te-130	34.5	Te-131t	25.0 m	0.27	act	n	3.19E − 03	9.45E − 02	1.17E − 01	1.17E − 01	1.17E − 01
Te-130	34.5	I-131	8.04 d	0.27	b	n	9.59E − 08	2.14E − 04	9.40E − 03	1.17E − 01	1.17E − 01
I-127	100	I-126	13.00 d	9e − 04	n,2n	y	4.27E − 08	2.56E − 06	5.99E − 05	1.15E − 03	1.15E − 03
I-127	100	I-128	25.0 m	6.2	act	n	2.17E − 01	6.44E + 00	7.95E + 00	7.95E + 00	7.95E + 00
I-127	100	Te-127m*	109.00 d	1e − 05	n,p	y	7.24E − 11	4.35E − 09	1.04E − 07	1.48E − 05	1.64E − 05
I-127	100	Te-127	9.5 h	9e − 06	n,p	y	1.37E − 08	7.93E − 07	9.32E − 06	1.13E − 05	1.13E − 05
Xe-124	0.096	Xe-125m +	55.0 s	28	act	n	1.87E 02	3.53E 02	3.53E 02	3.53E 02	3.53E 02
Xe-124	0.096	Xe-125t	16.8 h	165	act	n	1.43E − 04	8.40E − 03	1.31E − 01	2.08E − 01	2.08E − 01
Xe-124	0.096	I-125	59.9 d	165	b	n	5.74E − 10	2.04E − 06	8.75E − 04	2.05E − 01	2.08E − 01
Xe-126	0.09	Xe-127m +	75.0 s	0.45	act	n	2.23E − 04	5.23E − 04	5.23E − 04	5.23E − 04	5.23E − 04
Xe-126	0.09	Xe-127	36.4 d	3.5	act	n	5.38E − 08	3.23E − 06	7.67E − 05	4.07E − 03	4.07E − 03
Xe-128	1.919	Xe-129m	8.90 d	0.48	act	n	6.33E − 07	3.79E − 05	8.78E − 04	1.17E − 02	1.17E − 02
Xe-130	4.08	Xe-131m	11.8 d	0.45	act	n	9.38E 07	5.62E 05	1.31E − 03	2.30E − 02	2.30E − 02
Xe-132	26.89	Xe-133m +	2.26 d	0.05	act	n	3.53E − 06	2.10E − 04	4.38E − 03	1.66E − 02	1.66E − 02
Xe-132	26.89	Xe-133	5.72 d	0.45	act	n	1.26E − 05	7.51E − 04	1.70E − 02	1.49E − 01	1.49E − 01
Xe-134	10.4	Xe-135m +	15.6 m	0.003	act	n	1.65E − 05	3.53E − 04	3.79E − 04	3.79E − 04	3.79E − 04
Xe-134	10.4	Xe-135	9.14 h	0.265	act	n	4.23E − 05	2.44E − 03	2.81E − 02	3.35E − 02	3.35E − 02
Xe-136	8.87	Xe-137t	3.90 m	0.26	act	n	4.49E − 03	2.76E − 02	2.76E − 02	2.76E − 02	2.76E − 02
Xe-136	8.87	Cs-137s	30.17 y	0.26	b	n	1.01E − 10	6.56E − 08	1.73E − 06	6.27E − 04	2.76E − 02
Cs-133	100	Cs-134m +	2.89 h	2.5	act	n	1.22E − 02	6.52E − 01	3.05E + 00	3.06E + 00	3.06E + 00
Cs-133	100	Cs-134	2.05 y	29	act	n	2.28E − 05	1.37E − 03	3.29E − 02	1.02E + 01	3.55E + 01
Cs-133	100	I-130	12.36 h	3e − 06	n,a	y	3.77E − 09	2.20E − 07	2.99E − 06	4.04E − 06	4.04E − 06
Ba-130	0.101	Ba-131m +	14.5 m	2.5	act	n	1.48E − 04	2.98E − 03	3.16E − 03	3.16E − 03	3.16E − 03
Ba-130	0.101	Ba-131s	11.6 d	11.3	act	n	5.93E − 07	3.55E − 05	8.29E − 04	1.43E − 02	1.43E − 02
Ba-132	0.097	Ba-133m +	39.0 h	0.5	act	n	1.77E − 07	1.05E − 05	2.08E − 04	5.98E − 04	5.98E − 04

[a] My, million years.

(continued)

Table 7.18.1 Health Physics Thermal Neutron Activation Database (Continued)

Target Nucleus	Target Isotopic Abund %	Nuclide Made	Half-life	Cross-sect'n (b)	Reaction	f ?	Activity (μCi) After Specified Irradiation Time: 1 minute	1 hour	1 day	1 year	Saturated Activity (μCi)
Ba-132	0.097	Ba-133	10.5 y	7	act	n	1.05E − 09	6.31E − 08	1.51E − 06	5.35E − 04	8.37E − 03
Ba-132	0.097	Cs-132	6.5 d	0.012	n,p	y	1.07E − 09	6.39E − 08	1.46E − 06	1.44E − 05	1.44E − 05
Ba-134	2.42	Ba-135m	29.0 h	0.158	act	n	1.85E − 06	1.10E − 04	2.03E − 03	4.64E − 03	4.64E − 03
Ba-135	6.59	Ba-136m	0.320 s	0.014	act	n	1.10E − 03	1.10E − 03	1.10E − 03	1.10E − 03	1.10E − 03
Ba-136	7.81	Ba-137m	2.60 m	0.01	act	n	2.19E − 04	9.35E − 04	9.35E − 04	9.35E − 04	9.35E − 04
Ba-136	7.81	Cs-136	13.1 d	4e − 06	n,p	y	1.20E − 11	7.20E − 10	1.69E − 08	3.27E − 07	3.27E − 07
Ba-137	11.23	Ba-137m	2.6 m	0.225	n,n′	y	7.14E − 03	3.00E − 02	3.00E − 02	3.00E − 02	3.00E − 02
Ba-138	71.66	Ba-137m	2.6 m	0.002	n,2n	y	4.82E − 04	2.03E − 03	2.03E − 03	2.03E − 03	2.03E − 03
Ba-138	71.66	Ba-139	83.3 m	0.36	act	n	2.52E − 03	1.20E − 01	3.04E − 01	3.04E − 01	3.04E − 01
Ba-138	71.66	Xe-135	9.1 h	2e − 06	n,a	y	2.03E − 09	1.17E − 07	1.35E − 06	1.61E − 06	1.61E − 06
La-139	99.911	La-140	40.2 h	8.93	act	n	3.00E − 03	1.78E − 01	3.54E + 00	1.04E + 01	1.04E + 01
Ce-136	0.193	Ce-137m*	34.4 h	0.95	act	n	7.37E − 07	4.38E − 05	8.41E − 04	2.19E − 03	2.19E − 03
Ce-136	0.193	Ce-137t	9.00 h	6.3	act	n	1.87E − 05	1.08E − 03	1.23E − 02	1.46E − 02	1.46E − 02
Ce-136	0.193	La-137	60000 y	7.25	b	n	2.36E − 16	8.29E − 13	2.88E − 10	1.93E − 07	1.67E − 02
Ce-138	0.25	Ce-139m+	55.0 s	0.015	act	n	2.35E − 05	4.42E − 05	4.42E − 05	4.42E − 05	4.42E − 05
Ce-138	0.25	Ce-139	137 d	1.115	act	n	1.15E − 08	6.92E − 07	1.66E − 05	2.77E − 03	3.29E − 03
Ce-140	88.48	Ce-141	32.5 d	0.57	act	n	8.68E − 06	5.21E − 04	1.24E − 02	5.86E − 01	5.86E − 01
Ce-140	88.48	La-140	40.22 h	0.004	n,p	y	1.27E − 06	7.56E − 05	1.50E − 03	4.42E − 03	4.42E − 03
Ce-142	11.07	Ce-143t	33.0 h	0.95	act	n	4.22E − 05	2.51E − 03	4.77E − 02	1.21E − 01	1.21E − 01
Ce-142	11.07	Pr-143	13.58 d	0.95	b	n	7.48E − 10	2.67E − 06	1.30E − 03	1.21E − 01	1.21E − 01
Pr-141	100	Pr-142m+	14.6 m	3.9	act	n	2.09E − 01	4.24E + 00	4.50E + 00	4.50E + 00	4.50E + 00
Pr-141	100	Pr-142	19.2 h	11.5	act	n	7.98E − 03	4.71E − 01	7.69E + 00	1.33E + 01	1.33E + 01
Pr-141	100	Cr-141	32.50 d	1e − 04	n,p	y	2.05E − 09	1.23E − 07	2.92E − 06	1.38E − 04	1.39E − 04
Nd-146	17.18	Nd-147t	11.06 d	1.4	act	n	1.17E − 05	6.99E − 04	1.63E − 02	2.68E − 01	2.68E − 01
Nd-146	17.18	Pm-147	2.62 y	1.4	b	n	2.93E − 12	1.05E − 08	5.95E − 06	5.98E − 02	2.68E − 01
Nd-148	5.72	Nd-149t	1.80 h	2.5	act	n	1.01E − 03	5.03E − 02	1.57E − 01	1.57E − 01	1.57E − 01
Nd-148	5.72	Pm-149	53.1 h	2.5	b	n	1.10E − 07	3.47E − 04	3.83E − 02	1.57E − 01	1.57E − 01
Nd-150	5.6	Nd-151t	12.0 m	1.2	act	n	4.09E − 03	7.06E − 02	7.29E − 02	7.29E − 02	7.29E − 02
Nd-150	5.6	Pm-151	28.4 h	1.2	b	n	8.40E − 07	1.27E − 03	3.20E − 02	7.29E − 02	7.29E − 02
Sm-144	3.16	Sm-145t	340 d	0.7	act	n	3.54E − 08	2.12E − 06	5.09E − 05	1.31E − 02	2.50E − 02
Sm-144	3.16	Pm-145	17.7 y	0.7	b	n	1.32E − 15	4.75E − 12	2.73E − 09	2.84E − 04	2.50E − 02
Sm-150	7.47	Sm-151	93.0 y	102	act	n	1.17E − 07	7.03E − 06	1.69E − 04	6.14E − 02	8.27E + 00
Sm-152	26.63	Sm-153	46.8 h	206	act	n	1.45E − 02	8.64E − 01	1.76E + 01	5.87E + 01	5.87E + 01
Sm-154	22.53	Sm-155	23.5 m	5.5	act	n	3.81E − 02	1.09E + 00	1.31E + 00	1.31E + 00	1.31E + 00
Eu-151	47.77	Eu-152m2+	96.0 m	4.2	act	n	1.56E − 02	7.60E − 01	2.16E + 00	2.16E + 00	2.16E + 00
Eu-151	47.77	Eu-152m1	9.30 h	3215	act	n	2.05E + 00	1.19E + 02	1.38E + 03	1.66E + 03	1.66E + 03
Eu-151	47.77	Gd-152	110 Ty	3215	b	n	1.67E − 17	1.12E − 16	1.52E − 14	1.04E − 11	1.66E + 03
Eu-151	47.77	Eu-152t	12.7 y	5935	act	n	3.17E − 04	1.90E − 02	4.57E − 01	1.62E + 02	3.06E + 03
Eu-151	47.77	Gd-152	110 Ty	5935	b	n	3.83E − 17	1.96E − 16	1.33E − 17	5.16E − 13	3.06E + 03
Eu-153	52.23	Eu-154	8.50 y	603	act	n	5.20E − 05	3.12E − 03	7.48E − 02	2.62E + 01	3.35E + 02
Gd-152	0.2	Gd-153	242 d	1100	act	n	4.69E − 06	2.81E − 04	6.74E − 03	1.53E + 00	2.36E + 00
Gd-158	24.9	Gd-159	18.0 h	2.5	act	n	4.11E − 04	2.42E − 02	3.87E − 01	6.41E − 01	6.41E − 01
Gd-160	21.9	Gd-161t	3.70 m	0.77	act	n	2.93E − 02	1.72E − 01	1.72E − 01	1.72E − 01	1.72E − 01

[a] My, million years.

Table 7.18.1 Health Physics Thermal Neutron Activation Database (Continued)

Target Nucleus	Target Isotopic Abund %	Nuclide Made	Half-life	Cross-sect'n (b)	Reaction	f ?	Activity (μCi) After Specified Irradiation Time: 1 minute	1 hour	1 day	1 year	Saturated Activity (μCi)
Gd-160	21.9	Tb-161	6.91 d	0.77	b	n	1.05E − 06	6.52E − 04	1.63E − 02	1.72E − 01	1.72E − 01
Tb-159	100	Tb-160	72.1 d	23.2	act	n	1.59E − 04	9.51E − 03	2.27E − 01	2.30E + 01	2.38E + 01
Dy-156	0.0524	Dy-157t	8.10 h	33	act	n	2.57E − 05	1.48E − 03	1.57E − 02	1.80E − 02	1.80E − 02
Dy-156	0.0524	Tb-157	150 y	33	b	n	1.13E − 13	3.96E − 10	1.31E − 07	8.31E − 05	1.80E − 02
Dy-158	0.0902	Dy-159	144 d	43	act	n	1.34E − 07	8.01E − 06	1.92E − 04	3.31E − 02	4.00E − 02
Dy-164	28.18	Dy-165m	1.15 m	1700	act	n	2.15E + 02	4.75E + 02	4.75E + 02	4.75E + 02	4.75E + 02
Dy-164	28.18	Dy-165	2.35 h	1000	act	n	1.37E + 00	7.14E + 01	2.79E + 02	2.80E + 02	2.80E + 02
Ho-165	100	Ho-165m	1200 y	3.5	act	n	3.79E − 09	2.28E − 07	5.46E − 06	1.99E − 03	3.45E + 00
Ho-165	100	Ho-166	27.2 h	61.2	act	n	2.56E − 02	1.52E + 00	2.76E + 01	6.04E + 01	6.04E + 01
Er-162	0.136	Er-163t	75.1 m	19	act	n	2.38E − 04	1.10E − 02	2.60E − 02	2.60E − 02	2.60E − 02
Er-162	0.136	Ho-163	10 y	19	b	n	1.57E − 11	4.77E − 08	4.56E − 06	1.74E − 03	2.60E − 02
Er-164	1.56	Er-165	10.34 h	13	act	n	2.25E − 04	1.30E − 02	1.61E − 01	2.01E − 01	2.01E − 01
Er-166	33.41	Er-167m	2.35 s	15	act	n	4.91E + 00	4.91E + 00	4.91E + 00	4.91E + 00	4.91E + 00
Er-168	27.07	Er-169	9.60 d	1.95	act	n	2.56E − 05	1.54E − 03	3.56E − 02	5.11E − 01	5.11E − 01
Er-170	14.88	Er-171t	7.52 h	5.7	act	n	1.25E − 03	7.15E − 02	7.23E − 01	8.12E − 01	8.12E − 01
Er-170	14.88	Tm-171	1.92 y	5.7	b	n	4.28E − 10	1.50E − 06	4.80E − 04	2.46E − 01	8.12E − 01
Tm-169	100	Tm-170	130 d	103	act	n	3.67E − 04	2.20E − 02	5.27E − 01	8.50E + 01	9.92E + 01
Yb-168	0.14	Yb-169m+	46.0 s	3470	act	n	2.80E + 00	4.71E + 00	4.71E + 00	4.71E + 00	4.71E + 00
Yb-168	0.14	Yb-169	31.8 d	3470	act	n	7.12E − 05	4.27E − 03	1.01E − 01	4.71E + 00	4.71E + 00
Yb-174	31.84	Yb-175m+	0.067 s	46	act	n	1.37E + 01	1.37E + 01	1.37E + 01	1.37E + 01	1.37E + 01
Yb-174	31.84	Yb-175	4.20 d	65	act	n	2.22E − 03	1.33E − 01	2.95E + 00	1.94E + 01	1.94E + 01
Yb-176	12.73	Yb-177m+	6.50 s	2.4	act	n	2.82E − 01	2.83E − 01	2.83E − 01	2.83E − 01	2.83E − 01
Yb-176	12.73	Yb-177t	1.90 h	2.4	act	n	1.71E − 03	8.64E − 02	2.83E − 01	2.83E − 01	2.83E − 01
Yb-176	12.73	Lu-177	6.74 d	2.4	b	n	6.12E − 08	1.96E − 04	2.46E − 02	2.83E − 01	2.83E − 01
Lu-175	97.4	Lu-176m	3.69 h	15.1	act	n	4.28E − 02	2.34E + 00	1.35E + 01	1.37E + 01	1.37E + 01
Lu-175	97.4	Lu-176	33 Gy	7	act	n	2.53E − 16	1.52E − 14	3.65E − 13	1.33E − 10	6.34E + 00
Lu-176	2.6	Lu-177m*	115 d	2.1	act	n	2.11E − 07	1.27E − 05	3.03E − 04	4.49E − 02	5.05E − 02
Lu-176	2.6	Lu-177	6.74 d	2100	act	n	3.61E − 03	2.16E − 01	4.93E + 00	5.05E + 00	5.05E + 01
Hf-174	0.163	Hf-175	70.0 d	390	act	n	4.09E − 06	2.45E − 04	5.86E − 03	5.79E − 01	5.95E − 01
Hf-177	18.56	Hf-178m	4.30 s	1.1	act	n	1.88E − 01	1.88E − 01	1.88E − 01	1.88E − 01	1.88E − 01
Hf-178	27.1	Hf-179m2	25.1 d	10	act	n	4.75E − 05	2.85E − 03	6.75E − 02	2.48E + 00	2.48E + 00
Hf-178	27.1	Hf-179m1	18.6 s	53	act	n	1.17E + 01	1.31E + 01	1.31E + 01	1.31E + 01	1.31E + 01
Hf-179	13.75	Hf-180m	5.50 h	0.34	act	n	8.92E − 05	5.03E − 03	4.04E − 02	4.25E − 02	4.25E − 02
Hf-180	35.22	Hf-181	42.5 d	12.6	act	n	4.54E − 05	2.73E − 03	6.49E − 02	4.00E + 00	4.01E + 00
Ta-181	99.9877	Ta-182m+	16.5 m	0.012	act	n	4.44E − 04	9.92E − 03	1.08E − 02	1.08E − 02	1.08E − 02
Ta-181	99.9877	Ta-182	115.1 d	21.5	act	n	8.08E − 05	4.85E − 03	1.16E − 01	1.72E + 01	1.93E + 01
Ta-181	99.9877	Lu-178	28.5 m	2e − 07	n,a	y	3.46E − 09	1.10E − 07	1.44E − 07	1.44E − 07	1.44E − 07
W-180	0.135	W-181	121 d	3.5	act	n	1.70E − 08	1.02E − 06	2.44E − 05	3.74E − 03	4.27E − 03
W-182	26.3	Ta-182	115 d	4e − 06	n,p	y	3.93E − 12	2.36E − 10	5.65E − 09	8.36E − 07	9.41E − 07
W-183	14.3	Ta-183	5 d	3e − 06	n,p	y	3.60E − 11	2.15E − 09	4.85E − 08	3.82E − 07	3.82E − 07
W-184	30.6	W-185m+	1.62 m	0.002	act	n	1.88E − 04	5.41E − 04	5.41E − 04	5.41E − 04	5.41E − 04
W-184	30.6	W-185	75.0 d	1.8	act	n	3.13E − 06	1.88E − 04	4.48E − 03	4.71E − 01	4.87E − 01
W-184	30.6	Hf-181	42.5 d	2e − 07	n,a	y	6.13E − 13	3.68E − 11	8.76E − 10	5.40E − 08	5.41E − 08
W-186	28.4	W-185	75.0 d	0.01	n,2n	y	1.59E − 08	9.57E − 07	2.29E − 05	2.40E − 03	2.49E − 03

[a] My, million years.

(continued)

Table 7.18.1 Health Physics Thermal Neutron Activation Database (Continued)

Target Nucleus	Target Isotopic Abund %	Nuclide Made	Half-life	Cross-sect'n (b)	Reaction	f ?	Activity (μCi) After Specified Irradiation Time: 1 minute	1 hour	1 day	1 year	Saturated Activity (μCi)
W-186	28.4	W-187	23.9 h	37	act	n	4.44E − 03	2.63E − 01	4.61E + 00	9.20E + 00	9.20E + 00
Re-185	37.07	Re-184ms	165.0 d	6e − 04	n,2n	y	5.90E − 10	3.54E − 08	8.48E − 07	1.59E − 04	2.02E − 04
Re-185	37.07	Re-184	38.0 d	0.005	n,2n	y	1.90E − 08	1.14E − 06	2.71E − 05	1.50E − 03	1.50E − 03
Re-185	37.07	Re-186	88.9 h	112	act	n	4.75E − 03	2.84E − 01	6.23E + 00	3.65E + 01	3.65E + 01
Re-187	62.93	Re-186	88.9 h	0.01	n,2n	y	7.12E − 07	4.25E − 05	9.35E − 04	5.48E − 03	5.48E − 03
Re-187	62.93	Re-188m+	18.7 m	73	act	n	1.45E + 00	3.57E + 01	4.00E + 01	4.00E + 01	4.00E + 01
Re-187	62.93	Re-188	16.7 h	75	act	n	2.84E − 02	1.67E + 00	2.59E + 01	4.11E + 01	4.11E + 01
Os-184	0.018	Os-185	94 d	3005	act	n	2.46E − 06	1.48E − 04	3.53E − 03	4.46E − 01	4.79E − 01
Os-188	13.3	Os-189m	5.70 h	4.3	act	n	1.00E − 03	5.67E − 02	4.68E − 01	4.95E − 01	4.95E − 01
Os-189	16.1	Os-190m	10.00 m	0.26	act	n	2.41E − 03	3.55E − 02	3.16E − 02	3.62E − 02	3.61E − 02
Os-190	26.4	Os-191m+	15.0 h	13.2	act	n	2.30E − 03	1.35E − 01	2.00E + 00	2.99E + 00	2.99E + 00
Os-190	26.4	Os-191	15.0 d	17.1	act	n	1.24E − 04	7.44E − 03	1.75E − 01	3.87E + 00	3.87E + 00
Os-192	41	Os-193	31.5 h	1.97	act	n	2.51E − 04	1.49E − 02	2.81E − 01	6.85E − 01	6.85E − 01
Ir-191	38.5	Ir-192m2*	241 y	0.32	act	n	5.74E − 10	3.45E − 08	8.27E − 07	3.01E − 04	1.05E − 01
Ir-191	38.5	Ir-192m+	1.40 m	300	act	n	3.84E + 01	9.84E + 01	9.84E + 01	9.84E + 01	9.84E + 01
Ir-191	38.5	Ir-192	74.2 d	924	act	n	1.97E − 03	1.18E − 01	2.82E + 00	2.93E + 02	3.03E + 02
Ir-193	61.5	Ir-194m	171 d	5.8	act	n	8.47E − 06	5.08E − 04	1.22E − 02	2.32E + 00	3.01E + 00
Ir-193	61.5	Ir-194	19.0 h	110	act	n	3.47E − 02	2.04E + 00	3.33E + 01	5.71E + 01	5.71E + 01
Pr-190	0.0127	Pt-191	3.00 d	150	act	n	2.62E − 06	1.56E − 04	3.37E − 03	1.63E − 02	1.63E − 02
Pt-192	0.78	Pt-193m	4.40 d	2.2	act	n	1.59E − 06	9.52E − 05	2.12E − 03	1.45E − 02	1.45E − 02
Pt-192	0.78	Pt-193	50.0 y	14	act	n	2.44E − 09	1.46E − 07	3.25E − 06	1.27E − 03	9.26E − 02
Pt-194	32.9	Pt-195m	4.10 d	0.09	act	n	2.92E − 06	1.74E − 04	3.86E − 03	2.48E − 02	2.48E − 02
Pt-196	25.2	Pt-197m+	1.50 h	0.05	act	n	8.03E − 05	3.87E − 03	1.05E − 02	1.05E − 02	1.05E − 02
Pt-196	25.2	Pt-197	18.0 h	0.74	act	n	9.93E − 05	5.85E − 03	9.34E − 02	1.55E − 01	1.55E − 01
Pt-198	7.19	Pt-199m+	14.0 s	0.027	act	n	1.51E − 03	1.60E − 03	1.60E − 03	1.60E − 03	1.60E − 03
Pt-198	7.19	Pt-199t	31.0 m	3.7	act	n	4.83E − 03	1.62E − 01	2.19E − 01	2.19E − 01	2.19E − 01
Pt-198	7.19	Au-199	3.14 d	3.7	b	n	3.72E − 07	9.01E − 04	4.21E − 02	2.19E − 01	2.19E − 01
Au-197	100	Au-196	6.18 d	0.003	n,2n	y	1.93E − 07	1.16E − 05	2.63E − 04	2.48E − 03	2.48E − 03
Au-197	100	Au-197m	7.8 s	0.38	n,n′	y	3.12E − 01	3.14E − 01	3.14E − 01	3.14E − 01	3.14E − 01
Au-197	100	Au-198	2.70 d	98.8	act	n	1.45E − 02	8.68E − 01	1.85E + 01	8.16E + 01	8.16E + 01
Hg-196	0.146	Hg-197m*	24.0 h	120	act	n	7.00E − 05	4.14E − 03	7.27E − 02	1.46E − 01	1.46E − 01
Hg-196	0.146	Hg-197	65.0 h	3080	act	n	6.64E − 04	3.96E − 02	8.43E − 01	3.73E + 00	3.73E + 00
Hg-198	10.02	Hg-199m	43.0 m	0.018	act	n	2.37E − 05	9.19E − 04	1.48E − 03	1.48E − 03	1.48E − 03
Hg-202	29.8	Hg-203	46.9 d	4.9	act	n	1.21E − 05	7.24E − 04	1.73E − 02	1.17E + 00	1.18E + 00
Hg-204	6.85	Hg-205	5.50 m	0.43	act	n	2.78E − 03	2.35E − 02	2.35E − 02	2.35E − 02	2.35E − 02
Tl-203	29.5	Tl-202	12.2 d	0.003	n,2n	y	2.79E − 08	1.67E − 06	3.91E − 05	7.10E − 04	7.10E − 04
Tl-203	29.5	Tl-204	3.78 y	11	act	n	9.08E − 07	5.45E − 05	1.31E − 03	4.36E − 01	2.60E + 00
Tl-203	29.5	Hg-203	46.9 d	9e − 06	n,p	y	2.18E − 11	1.31E − 09	3.12E − 08	2.12E − 06	2.13E − 06
Tl-205	70.5	Tl-206	4.19 m	0.1	act	n	8.53E − 03	5.60E − 02	5.60E − 02	5.60E − 02	5.60E − 02
Pb-204	1.4	Pb-203	51.88 h	0.002	n,2n	y	6.09E − 09	3.63E − 07	7.51E − 06	2.74E − 05	2.74E − 05
Pb-204	1.4	Pb-204m	66.90 m	0.38	n,n′	y	4.37E − 05	1.96E − 03	4.25E − 03	4.25E − 03	4.25E − 03
Pb-204	1.4	Pb-205	14.0 My	0.661	act	n	6.95E − 16	4.17E − 14	1.00E − 12	3.66E − 10	7.38E − 03
Pb-208	52.3	Pb-209	3.30 h	0.487	act	n	6.96E − 04	3.78E − 02	1.98E − 01	1.99E − 01	1.99E − 01
Bi-209	100	Bi-210ms	3.5 My	0.019	act	n	5.57E − 15	3.34E − 13	8.03E − 12	2.93E − 09	1.48E − 02
Bi-209	100	Bi-210t	5.01 d	0.014	act	n	1.05E − 06	6.27E − 05	1.41E − 03	1.09E − 02	1.09E − 02
Bi-209	100	Po-210	138.4 d	0.014	b	n	1.82E − 12	6.54E − 09	3.60E − 06	9.09E − 03	1.09E − 02

[a] My, million years.

References

Alsmiller, R.G., Jr., Mynatt, F.R., Barish, J., Engle, W.W., Jr. ''Shielding against neutrons in the energy range 50 to 400 MeV,'' *Nucl Instrum Meth* **72:**213;1969; also ORNL-TM-2554.

Alsmiller, R.G., Jr., Barish, J. ''Shielding against the neutrons produced when 400 MeV electrons are incident on a thick copper target,'' *Part Accel* **5:**155; 1973.

Auman, L.E., Miller, W.H., Graham, C.C., Stretch, C.D., Welty, T.J., West, L., Jr. ''An intercomparison of neutron dosimeters and detectors for in-containment dosimetry,'' *Health Physics* **62**(2):190–193; 1982.

Becker, K. ''Dosimetric applications of track etching,'' in Attix, F.H., ed. *Topics in Radiation Dosimetry* Suppl. 1, Chapter 2 Academic Press; New York; 1972.

Chapman, G.T., Storrs, C.L. *Effective Neutron Removal Cross Sections for Shielding.* Oak Ridge National Laboratory, Rep. AECD-3978; 1955.

Dillman, L.T., T.D. Jones. ''Internal Dosimetry of Spontaneously Fissioning Nuclides,'' Health Physics **29**:111–123, July 1975.

Engle, W.W., Jr. *A User's Manual for ANISN,* K-1693. Oak Ridge National Laboratory; Oak Ridge, TN; 1967.

Firestone, R.B. *Table of Isotopes.* John Wiley & Sons, 1996.

Grundl, J.A., Eisenhauer, C.M. *Compendium of Benchmark Neutron Fields for Reactor Dosimetry—Standard Neutron Field Entries.* NBSIR 85-3151; National Bureau of Standards; Gaithersburg, MD; 1986.

Grundl, J.A., Lamaze, G.P. *Activation Foil Irradiation By Reactor Cavity Fission Sources.* NBS Special Publication 250-14; National Bureau of Standards; Gaithersburg, MD; 1988.

Hess, W.N. *Ann Phys* **6**(2):115; 1959.

Holden, N.E. *Isotopic Composition of the Elements and their Variation in Nature; A Preliminary Report.* Report BNL-NCS-50605; Brookhaven National Laboratory; 1977.

International Atomic Energy Agency (IAEA). *Radiological Safety Aspects of the Operation of Electron Linear Accelerators,* Technical Reports Series No. 188, IAEA; Vienna; 1979.

International Atomic Energy Agency (IAEA). *Handbook on Nuclear Activation Data.* Technical Report Series No. 273, IAEA; Vienna; 1987.

International Commission on Radiation Units (ICRU). *Neutron Dosimetry for Biology and Medicine.* ICRU Report 26; Bethesda, MD; 1977.

Lederer, C.M., Shirley, V.S. *Table of Isotopes, 7th ed.,* John Wiley & Sons; New York; 1978.

Lone, M.A., Leavitt, R.A., Harrison, D.A. *Prompt Gamma Rays from Thermal Neutron Capture.* Atomic Data Nucl Data Tables **26**(1981)511.

McCall, R.C. Unpublished data (from NCRP Report No. 79); 1979.

Molnár, G., Lindstrom, R. *Status of Cold Neutron Capture Gamma-Ray Data for Analytic Chemistry.* NEA/NSC/DOC (95) 1, p 351, 1995.

Mughabghab, S.F. *Neutron Cross-sections.* Vol II, Part B, Academic Press; 1984.

National Council on Radiation Protection and Measurements (NCRP). *Radiation Protection Design Guidelines for 0.1–100 MeV Particle Accelerator Facilities.* Report No. 51, NCRP; Bethesda, MD; 1977.

National Council on Radiation Protection and Measurements (NCRP). *Neutron Contamination from Medical Electron Accelerators.* Report No. 79, NCRP; Bethesda, MD; 1987.

National Council on Radiation Protection and Measurements (NCRP). *Protection Against Neutron Radiation.* Report No. 38; NCRP; Bethesda, MD; 1971.

Patterson, H.W., Thomas, R.H. *Accelerator Health Physics,* Academic Press, New York, NY; 1973.

PNL. *Health Physics Manual of Good Practices for Plutonium Facilities,* PNL-6534; Pacific Northwest Laboratory; Richland, WA; 1988.

Roussin, R.W., Schmidt, F.A.R. ''Adjoint S_N calculations of coupled neutron and gamma-ray transport through concrete slabs,'' *Nucl Eng Des* **15**:319; 1971.

Roussin, R.W., Alsmiller, R.G., Jr., Barish, J. ''Calculations of the transport of neutrons and secondary gamma rays through concrete for incident neutrons in the energy range 15 to 75 MeV.'' *Nucl Eng Des* **24:**250; 1973.

Schott, A. et al. *Compilation of Threshold Reaction Neutron Cross-Sections for Neutron Dosimetry and Other Applications.* EANDC 95 ''U''; 1974.

Shure, K., O'Brien, J.A., Rothberg, D.M. ''Neutron dose rate attenuation by iron and lead,'' *Nucl Sci Eng* **35:**371; 1969.

Slaback, L. Personal communications; National Institute of Standards and Technology; Gaithersburg, MD; 1991.

Stoddard, D.H. *Radiation Protection Properties of Californium-252.* USAEC Report DP-986; 1965.

U.S. Atomic Energy Commission ''Isotopes'' **3**:11–12; Now U.S. Department of Energy; Washington, DC; July 1953.

Wapstra, A.H., Bos, K. ''The 1977 atomic mass evaluation,'' *At Data Nucl Data Tables* **19:**177; 1977.

Wilenzick, R.M., Almond, P.R., Oliver, G.D., DeAlmeida, C.E. ''Measurement of fast neutrons produced by high energy x-ray beams of medical electron accelerators,'' *Phys Med Biol* **18:**396; 1973.

Wyckoff, J.M., Chilton, A.B. ''Dose due to practical neutron energy incident on concrete shielding walls,'' in *Proceedings of the Third International Congress of the International Radiation Protection Association.* Snyder, W.S., Ed., Report No. CONF-730907; page 694 National Technical Information Service; Springfield, VA; 1973.

CHAPTER 8

RADIONUCLIDE DATA

Chapter 8 presents tables on selected alpha, beta, gamma and x-ray emitters by increasing energy; information on specific activity for selected radionuclides; naturally occurring radionuclides; the natural decay series and the artificially produced neptunium series.

A table of alpha emitters is listed by increasing atomic number and by energy.

The table of β emitters presented is useful in identifying unknown β emitters whose energies have been determined by standard laboratory techniques. It is also a handy guide to β-emitting nuclides for applications requiring specific energies.

Gamma rays for radionuclides of importance to radiological assessments and radiation protection are listed by increasing energy. The energies and branching ratios are important for radionuclide determinations with gamma spectrometry detectors.

This section also presents a table of x-ray energies which are useful for radiochemical analyses. A number of nuclides emit x-rays as part of their decay scheme. These x-rays may be counted with Ar proportional counters, Ge planar or n-type Ge co-axial detectors, or thin crystal NaI(TI) scintillation counters. In both cases, spectral measurements can be made and both qualitative and quantitative information obtained on the sample.

Nuclear decay data (energy and probability by radiation type) for more than 100 radionuclides that are important to health physicists are presented in a schematic manner after the International Commission on Radiation Protection Publication 38 (updated by Eckerman 1991) and from Kocher 1981. These nuclides are produced by reactors or accelerators, or are used in medicine or industry.

TABLE OF CONTENTS

Table 8.1 Selected Alpha Emitters by Atomic Number[a] (After HASL-300 1990 from Brown 1986 and *Physik Datem*, 1985)

Radionuclide	Half Life	Isotopic Abundance (%)	α Emission (when not 100%)	Energy (MeV)
^{144}Nd	2.4×10^{15} y	23.8		1.83
^{146}Sm	1.03×10^{8} y			2.46
^{147}Sm	1.06×10^{11} y	15.0		2.233
^{148}Gd	74.6 y			3.183
^{150}Gd	1.79×10^{6} y			2.726
^{152}Gd	1.08×10^{14} y	0.20		2.14
^{154}Dy	1.0×10^{9} y			2.872
^{174}Hf	2.0×10^{15} y	0.162		2.50
^{186}Os	2.0×10^{15} y	1.58		2.76
^{190}Pt	6.0×10^{11} y	<0.02		3.175
^{210m}Bi	3.00×10^{6} y			4.946(57%), 4.908(38%), 4.569(4%)
^{211}Bi(AcC)	2.14 min			6.623(84%), 6.279(16%)
^{212}Bi(ThC′)[b]	60.55 min		3.954%	6.090(26.8%), 6.051(70.2%), 5.768(1.7%), 5.607(1.1%)
^{206}Po	8.80 d		5.45%	5.223
^{208}Po	2.898 y			5.116
^{209}Po	102.0 y			4.862
^{210}Po(RaF)	138.378 d			5.304
^{212}Po(ThC′)	298.0 ns			8.784
^{213}Po	4.2 μs			8.375
^{214}Po(RaC′)	164.3 μs			7.687
^{215}Po(AcC)	1.780 ms			7.386
^{216}Po(ThA)	150.0 ms			6.779
^{218}Po(RaA)	3.11 min			6.002
^{211}At	7.214 h		41.7%	5.868
^{217}At	32.3 ms			7.067
^{219}Rn(^{219}Em)	3.96 s			6.819(80.9%), 6.553(12.2%), 6.425(7.5%)
^{220}Rn(^{220}Em,Tn)	55.6 s			6.288
^{222}Rn(^{222}Em,Rn)	3.823 d			5.490
^{221}Fr	4.9 min			6.341(83.4%), 6.243(1.3%), 6.127(15.1%)
^{223}Ra(AcX)	11.43 d			5.747(9.5%), 5.716(52.5%), 5.607(24.2%), 5.540(9.2%), others
^{224}Ra(ThX)	3.66 d			5.686(95.1%), 5.449(5%)
^{226}Ra	1600.0 y			4.784(94.5%), 4.601(5.6%)

(continued)

Table 8.1 Selected Alpha Emitters by Atomic Number[a] (Continued)

Radionuclide	Half Life	Isotopic Abundance (%)	α Emission (when not 100%)	Energy (MeV)
^{225}Ac	10.0 d			5.829(51.6%), 5.793(18.1%), 5.791(8.6%), 5.731(10%), 5.637(4.5%), others
^{227}Th(Rd Ac)	18.718 d			6.038%(24.5%), 5.978(23.4%), 5.757(20.3%), 5.714(4.9%), 5.710(8.2%), others
^{228}Th(Rd Th)	1.913 y			5.423(72.4%), 5.339(27%)
^{229}Th	7340.0 y			5.050(5.2%), 4.968(6.0%), 4.901(10.2%), 4.845(56.2%), 4.814(9.3%), others
^{230}Th(Io)	7.54×10^4 y			4.688(76.3%), 4.621(23.4%)
^{232}Th(Th)	1.405×10^{10} y	100.		4.010(77%), 3.952(23%)
^{231}Pa(Pa)	3.276×10^4 y			5.057(11%), 5.028(20%), 5.011(25.4%), 4.950(22.8%), 4.736(8.4%), others
^{230}U	20.8 d			5.889(67.4%), 5.818(32%), others
^{232}U	68.9 y			5.320(68.6%), 5.264(31.7%)
^{223}U	1.592×10^5 y			4.824(82.7%), 4.783(14.9%), others
^{234}U(UII)	2.454×10^5 y	0.0055		4.775(72.5%), 4.724(28.4%)
^{235}U(AcU)	7.037×10^8 y	0.7200		4.599(5%), 4.556(4.2%), 4.400(55%), 4.365(17%), 4.218(5.7%), others
^{236}U	2.342×10^7 y			4.494(74%), 4.445(26%)
^{238}U(UI)	4.468×10^9 y	99.2745		4.196(77%), 4.147(23%)
^{237}Np	2.14×10^6 y			4.873(2.6%), 4.788(47%), 4.771(25%), 4.766(8%), 4.640(6.2%), others
^{236}Pu	2.851 y			5.768(68.1%), 5.721(30.6%)
^{238}Pu	87.74 y			5.499(70.9%), 5.456(29%)
^{239}Pu	2.409×10^4 y			5.156(73.1%), 5.143(15%), 5.105(11.8%)
^{240}Pu	6563.0 y			5.168(73%), 5.124(27%)
^{242}Pu	3.763×10^5 y			4.901(78%), 4.856(22.4%)
^{244}Pu	8.26×10^7 y			4.589(80.5%), 4.546(19.4%)

Table 8.1 Selected Alpha Emitters by Atomic Number[a] (Continued)

Radionuclide	Half Life	Isotopic Abundance (%)	α Emission (when not 100%)	Energy (MeV)
^{241}Am	432.2 y			5.486(84%), 5.443(13%), 5.388(1.6%)
^{243}Am	7380.0 y			5.275(88%), 5.234(11%), 5.180(1.1%)
^{240}Cm	27.0 d			6.291(71.1%), 6.248(28.9%)
^{242}Cm	162.94 d			6.113(74%), 6.070(26%)
^{243}Cm	28.5 y			6.067(1.5%), 6.058(4.7%), 5.992(6.5%), 5.785(73.5%), 5.742(10.6%), others
^{244}Cm	18.099 y			5.805(76.4%), 5.763(23.6%), others
^{245}Cm	8500.0 y			5.362(93.2%), 5.304(5.0%), others
^{246}Cm	4730.0 y			5.386(79%), 5.343(21%)
^{247}Cm	1.56×10^7 y			5.265(13.8%), 5.210(5.7%), 4.868(71%), 4.818(4.7%), others
^{248}Cm[b]	3.40×10^5 y		91.7%	5.078(81.9%), 5.035(18%)
^{247}Bk	1380.0 y			5.795(5.5%), 5.709(17%), 5.687(13%), 5.530(45%), 5.500(7%), others
^{246}Cf	35.7 h			6.750(78.0%), 6.708(21.8%)
^{248}Cf	334.0 d			6.258(80.0%), 6.217(19.6%)
^{249}Cf	350.6 y			6.194(2.2%), 6.140(1.1%), 5.945(4%), 5.903(2.8%), 5.812(84.4%), others
^{250}Cf	13.08 y			6.031(84.6%), 5.989(15.1%)
^{251}Cf	898.0 y			6.074(2.7%), 6.014(11.6%), 5.852(27%), 5.814(4.2%), 5.677(35%), others
^{252}Cf[b]	2.645 y		96.9%	6.118(84%), 6.076(15.8%)
^{252}Es[b]	1.291 y		76.0%	6.632(80.2%), 6.562(13.6%), 6.482(2.2%), others
^{253}Es	20.47 d			6.633(89.8%), 6.592(6.6%), others
^{254}Es	275.7 d			6.429(93.1%), 6.416(1.8%), 6.359(2.6%)

(continued)

Table 8.1 Selected Alpha Emitters by Atomic Number[a] (Continued)

Radionuclide	Half Life	Isotopic Abundance (%)	α Emission (when not 100%)	Energy (MeV)
^{255}Es[b]	39.8 d		8.0%	6.300(87.7%), 6.260(9.8%), 6.213(2.5%)
^{252}Fm	25.39 h			7.04(84%), 6.998(15%)
^{253}Fm[b]	3.00 d		12.0%	7.024(6.7%), 6.943(42.7%), 6.901(9.8%), 6.847(8.4%), 6.674(23.2%), others
^{255}Fm	20.07 h			7.022(93.4%), 6.963(5.0%), others
^{257}Fm	100.5 d			6.695(3.5%), 6.520(93.6%), 6.441(2.0%)
^{258}Md	55 d			6.790(28%), 6.716(72%)

[a] Most short-lived nuclides are included as principal members of the natural decay series (see Tables 8.7–8.10). Other isotopes listed are of importance in environmental analysis. Half lives and energies after *Physiks Datem* if discrepancies exist.
[b] Relative α-intensity normalized to 100 α decays.

Table 8.2 Selected Alpha Emitters by Energy (MeV)[a] (From HASL 300, 1990, after Brown et al. 1986)

Series	3.8–4.0	4.0–4.2	4.2–4.4	4.4–4.6	4.6–4.8	4.8–5.0	5.0–5.2	5.2–5.4	5.4–5.6	5.6–5.8	5.8–6.0	6.0–6.2	6.2–6.4
Uranium Series:		^{238}U			^{234}U ^{230}Th ^{226}Ra			^{210}Po	^{222}Rn			^{218}Po	
Thorium Series:	^{232}Th	^{232}Th						^{228}Th	^{228}Th ^{224}Ra	^{212}Bi ^{224}Ra		^{212}Bi	^{220}Rn
Actinium Series:			^{235}U	^{235}U	^{231}Pa	^{231}Pa	^{231}Pa			^{223}Ra ^{227}Th	^{227}Th	^{227}Th	
Neptunium Series:[b]					^{237}Np ^{233}U	^{233}U ^{229}Th	^{229}Th	^{241}Am	^{241}Am	^{225}Ac	^{225}Ac	^{221}Fr	^{221}Fr
All Emitters:	^{232}Th	^{232}Th ^{238}U	^{235}U	^{210m}Bi ^{235}U ^{236}U ^{244}Pu	^{226}Ra ^{230}Th ^{231}Pa ^{233}U ^{234}U ^{237}Np	^{209}Po ^{210m}Bi ^{229}Th ^{231}Pa ^{233}U ^{237}Np ^{242}Pu ^{247}Cm	^{208}Po ^{229}Th ^{231}Pa ^{239}Pu ^{240}Pu ^{243}Am ^{248}Cm	^{206}Po ^{210}Po ^{228}Th ^{232}U ^{241}Am ^{243}Am ^{245}Cm ^{246}Cm ^{247}Cm	^{222}Rn ^{223}Ra ^{224}Ra ^{228}Th ^{238}Pu ^{241}Am ^{247}Bk	^{212}Bi ^{223}Ra ^{224}Ra ^{225}Ac ^{227}Th ^{236}Pu ^{243}Cm ^{244}Cm ^{247}Bk ^{251}Cf	^{211}At ^{225}Ac ^{227}Th ^{230}U ^{243}Cm ^{244}Cm ^{249}Cf ^{250}Cf ^{251}Cf	^{212}Bi ^{218}Po ^{221}Fr ^{227}Th ^{242}Cm ^{243}Cm ^{249}Cf ^{250}Cf ^{251}Cf ^{252}Cf	^{211}Bi ^{220}Rn ^{221}Fr ^{240}Cm ^{248}Cf ^{254}Es ^{255}Es

Series	6.4–6.6	6.6–6.8	6.8–7.0	7.0–7.2	7.2–7.4	7.4–7.6	7.6–7.8	7.8–8.0	8.0–8.2	8.2–8.4	8.4–8.6	8.6–8.8
Uranium Series:							^{214}Po					
Thorium Series:		^{216}Po										^{212}Po
Actinium Series:	^{219}Rn	^{211}Bi	^{219}Rn		^{215}Po							
Neptunium Series:[b]				^{217}At						^{213}Po		
All Emitters:	^{210}Rn ^{252}Es ^{253}Es ^{254}Es ^{257}Fm	^{211}Bi ^{216}Po ^{246}Cf ^{252}Es ^{253}Es ^{253}Fm ^{257}Fm ^{258}Md	^{219}Rn ^{252}Fm ^{253}Fm ^{255}Fm	^{217}At ^{252}Fm ^{253}Fm ^{255}Fm	^{215}Po		^{214}Po			^{213}Po		^{212}Po

[a] A listing may denote more than one energy. Other isotopes listed are of importance in environmental analysis.

[b] Also called the Americium Series.

Table 8.3 Selected Beta Emitters by Maximum Energy (keV) (Data from Radioactive Decay Tables, D. Kocher, DoE/TIC-11026)

Element Symbol	Z	A	Max. Energy (keV)	Average Energy (keV)	Intensity %	Rank by Abund. 1 = high	Other Most Energetic Beta Energy (keV)	Other Most Abundant Beta: Energy (keV)	Other Most Abundant Beta: Intensity %	Number of Betas
Re	75	187	2.64	0.7	100.0	1				1
Pb	82	210	16.5	4.1	80.2	1	63	63	19.8	2
H	1	3	18.6	5.7	100.0	1				1
Pu	94	241	20.81	5.2	100.0	1				1
Pd	46	107	33	9.3	100.0	1				1
Cm	96	250	37	9.0	14.0	1				1
Ra	88	228	38.9	9.9	100.0	1				1
Ru	44	106	39.4	10.0	100.0	1				1
Ac	89	227	43.7	11.1	54.0	1	34	34	35.0	3
Zr	40	93	61.5	19.5	100.0	1				1
Ni	28	63	65.87	17.1	100.0	1				1
Ho	67	166m	72	18.7	73.4	1	1314	32	17.2	7
Sm	62	151	76.1	19.7	99.1	1	55	55	0.9	2
Ag	47	110	83.9	21.8	67.3	1	531	531	30.5	3
Tm	69	171	96.7	25.2	97.8	1	30	30	2.2	2
Bk	97	249	126.4	33.0	100.0	1				1
Os	76	191	139	36.7	100.0	1				1
Eu	63	155	141	37.4	46.0	1	246	159	26.0	6
Se	34	79	149	52.2	100.0	1				1
Pu	94	246	150	40.0	73.0	1	330	330	27.0	3
Lu	71	177m	151.8	40.5	78.5	1				1
I	53	129	152	40.9	100.0	1				1
C	6	14	156.478	49.5	100.0	1				1
Nb	41	95m	159.8	43.4	100.0	1				
S	16	35	167.47	48.8	100.0	1				1
Th	90	234	188.6	50.6	72.5	1	96	96	18.5	4
Np	93	236	195	52.3	5.0	1	355	355	5.0	2
Cs	55	135	205	56.3	100.0	1				1
Hg	80	203	212.2	57.7	100.0	1				1
Si	14	32	213	64.7	100.0	1				1
Te	52	132	215	59.4	100.0	1				1
Pm	61	147	224.7	62.0	100.0	1				1
Ru	44	103	226	63.2	90.0	1	723	113	6.4	4
Nb	41	91	234	108.7+	0.2	1				1
U	92	237	238	64.8	53.1	1	252	252	43.7	5
P	15	33	249	76.6	100.0	1				1
Sn	50	126	250	70.0	100.0	1				1
Ir	77	194m	252.5	69.7	100.0	1				1
Ca	20	45	256.9	77.2	100.0	1				1
Au	79	196	258	71.3	6.9	1				1
Pa	91	233	260.4	71.4	33.0	1	232	232	28.0	4
Rb	37	87	273.3	78.8	100.0	1				1
Es	99	255	280	76.7	92.0	1				1
Cf	98	253	287	97.0	99.7	1				1
Th	90	231	287.6	79.6	49.0	1	311	305	35.0	7
Tc	43	99	293.6	84.6	100.0	1				1

+ indicates positron emission

Table 8.3 Selected Beta Emitters by Maximum Energy (keV) (Continued)

Element Symbol	Z	A	Max. Energy (keV)	Average Energy (keV)	Intensity %	Rank by Abund. 1 = high	Other Most Energetic Beta Energy (keV)	Other Most Abundant Beta Energy (keV)	Other Most Abundant Beta Intensity %	Number of Betas
Au	79	199	294.6	82.4	66.2	1	453	245	20.5	3
Sb	51	125	303.4	87.0	39.9	1	622	131	18.1	7
Co	27	60	317.9	95.8	100.0	1	1550	1550	0.2	2
Ce	58	144	318.2	91.1	77.2	1	238	185	19.6	3
Cd	48	113	322	93.3	100.0	1				1
Ra	88	225	322	90.0	72.0	1	362	362	28.0	2
Zn	30	65	329.9	143.0+	1.4	1				1
Pb	82	212	334	94.4	85.1	1	573	573	9.9	3
Cs	55	136	341	98.8	95.1	1	682	174	2.5	4
Br	35	77	343	151.7+	0.7	1				1
Xe	54	133	346	100.3	99.3	1	267	267	0.7	2
W	74	188	349	99.7	99.0	1	285	58	0.8	3
Er	68	169	350.2	100.6	55.0	1	342	342	45.0	2
Sc	21	46	357.3	112.0	100.0	1				1
Zr	40	95	366	109.3	55.4	1	1123	399	43.7	4
Sb	51	126	370	109.0	29.0	1	1790	1790	19.0	14
Te	52	134	376.568	110.8	42.9	1	453	453	41.1	3
Am	95	244	387	109.6	100.0	1				1
Cu	29	67	390	121.0	57.0	1	575	482	22.0	4
Tc	43	98	394	118.0	100.0	1				1
Dy	66	166	402	117.5	92.0	1	484	484	7.0	3
Hf	72	181	407	118.7	93.0	1	403	403	7.0	2
Pm	61	148m	407	120.0	54.0	1	1007	695	22.0	4
W	74	185	432.4	126.8	99.9	1				1
Ce	58	141	434.6	129.6	70.5	1	580	580	29.5	2
Np	93	239	435.9	125.3	52.0	1	714	330	35.0	5
U	92	240	440	125.0	100.0	1				1
Sc	21	47	441.1	142.7	68.0	1	601	601	32.0	2
Br	35	82	444.3	137.8	97.9	1	265	265	1.4	2
Te	52	131m	451	136.2	36.9	1	2431	532	16.6	18
Y	39	87	451.3	200.5+	0.2	1				1
Mg	12	28	458.9	155.9	95.1	1	860	212	4.7	3
Fe	26	59	465.8	149.2	53.1	1	1565	273	45.2	4
Yb	70	175	467.9	139.2	86.5	1	354	72	10.3	3
Nb	41	94	471	145.8	100.0	1				1
Co	27	58	475	201.2+	14.9	1				1
Es	99	254	477	137.3	67.0	1	1126	437	19.0	3
Pa	91	234	484	141.0	24.0	1	1259	654	16.0	18
Eu	63	156	487	147.0	32.0	1	2453	2453	27.0	14
In	49	115	495	152.0	100.0	1				1
Lu	71	177	497.1	148.9	78.7	1	384	176	12.3	3
Pa	91	230	507	148.7	9.3	1	192	192	0.2	2
Cs	55	137	511.6	156.8	94.6	1	1173	1173	5.4	2
Kr	36	88	521	165.0	67.0	1	2913	2913	14.0	15
Ta	73	182	522	157.2	40.8	1	590	258	28.9	8
Np	93	236m	536	158.0	39.7	1	491	491	8.3	2

+ indicates positron emission

(continued)

Table 8.3 Selected Beta Emitters by Maximum Energy (keV) (Continued)

Element Symbol	Z	A	Max. Energy (keV)	Average Energy (keV)	Intensity %	Rank by Abund. 1 = high	Other Most Energetic Beta Energy (keV)	Other Most Abundant Beta Energy (keV)	Other Most Abundant Beta Intensity %	Number of Betas
Na	11	22	545.5	215.5+	89.8	1				1
Sr	38	90	546	195.8	100.0	1				1
Sr	38	92	550	174.0	96.0	1	1930	1930	4.0	4
Be	4	10	555.8	202.5	100.0	1				1
Sb	51	117	564	258.0+	1.7	1				1
Ar	18	39	565	218.8	100.0	1				1
Rh	45	105	567	179.4	75.0	1	261	248	19.7	3
Tb	65	160	568.7	175.0	45.6	1	1747	867	24.6	11
Eu	63	154	569.4	175.7	36.5	1	1844	247	27.9	15
Mn	25	52a	575.3	241.6+	29.4	1				1
Cu	29	64	578.2	190.2	37.2	1	653	653	17.9	2
Bi	83	211	579	174.6	0.3	1				1
Pu	94	243	582	172.7	59.0	1	590	498	29.0	6
Cd	48	113m	586	185.4	100.0	1				1
I	53	131	606.3	191.6	89.3	1	807	334	7.4	5
Kr	36	79	609	265.0+	6.9	1	348	348	0.2	2
Sb	51	124	611.3	194.0	52.8	1	2302	2302	21.9	12
Am	95	242	619	184.8	42.0	1	661	661	41.0	2
W	74	187	626.7	193.5	58.7	1	1313	1313	25.1	10
F	9	18	633.5	249.8+	96.7	1				1
Cd	48	117	636	204.0	32.2	1	2213	2213	21.0	22
Pt	78	197	641.6	197.7	82.0	1	719	719	11.0	3
Pb	82	209	644.6	197.6	100.0	1				1
Sb	51	129	650	208.0	26.6	1	2271	534	22.5	22
Sc	21	48	657	226.5	89.0	1	482	482	10.0	2
Cs	55	134	657.9	210.1	70.1	1	415	89	27.4	3
Cd	48	117a	667	216.0	46.9	1	1916	569	21.6	16
Ir	77	192	672	208.9	48.3	1	845	536	41.4	4
Pb	82	214	672	207.0	48.0	1	1024	729	42.5	5
Kr	36	85b	687	251.4	99.6	1	173	173	0.4	2
As	33	77	690	231.8	97.1	1	451	451	1.5	4
Ca	20	47	690	240.9	81.7	1	1988	1988	18.0	2
Te	52	127	694	224.7	98.8	1	276	276	1.2	2
Eu	63	152	696	221.8	13.6	1	1475	1475	8.4	7
V	23	48	697	291.4+	50.1	1				1
Sm	62	153	702	224.4	44.1	1	805	632	34.1	4
Pt	78	197m	709	221.8	3.3	1				1
Cl	17	36	709.6	251.3	99.0	1				1
Xe	54	138	710	231.0	32.6	1	2730	2290	20.1	15
Tc	43	95	717	341.0+	0.3	1	513	513	0.2	2
Te	52	127m	725	252.9	1.8	1				1
In	49	117	743	245.0	99.8	1	1140	1140	0.2	2
Bk	97	250	748	228.0	83.1	1	1780	709	5.9	4
Nb	41	96	749	250.6	95.9	1	746	746	2.8	4
Y	39	88	755	355.2+	0.2	1				1
Mo	42	101	763	256.0	20.7	1	2603	849	11.7	38

+ indicates positron emission

Table 8.3 Selected Beta Emitters by Maximum Energy (keV) (Continued)

Element Symbol	Z	A	Max. Energy (keV)	Average Energy (keV)	Intensity %	Rank by Abund. 1=high	Other Most Energetic Beta Energy (keV)	Other Most Abundant Beta Energy (keV)	Other Most Abundant Beta Intensity %	Number of Betas
Tl	80	204	763.4	243.9	97.4	1				1
Rb	37	84	777	338.5+	13.7	1	1658	1658	13.5	3
Np	93	240m	780	241.0	100.0	1				1
Pm	61	146	795	259.9	34.1	1	162	162	2.2	2
Fe	26	52	804	340.0+	56.0	1				1
Nd	60	147	804.7	264.0	81.1	1	485	365	15.3	5
Cs	55	132	814	270.0	1.6	1	421	247	0.4	3
K	19	43	827	298.0	92.2	1	1817	1224	3.6	4
Kr	36	85a	840.7	290.4	78.6	1	711	711	0.3	2
Pm	61	151	843	278.0	42.7	1	1188	1188	10.0	22
Ni	28	57	843	359.0+	33.1	1	716	716	5.7	4
In	49	115m	861	291.0	3.6	1				1
I	53	126	862	289.7	27.2	1	1251	1251	9.0	5
Cm	96	249	891	279.0	96.3	1	522	257	1.8	5
Sb	51	127	896	304.1	34.9	1	1493	1108	22.8	13
Am	95	245	896.1	281.0	77.4	1	643	643	15.6	3
Zr	40	89	904.7	396.9+	22.9	1				1
Zn	30	69	905	320.9	100.0	1				1
Xe	54	135	909	308.0	96.1	1	751	551	3.1	4
Br	35	83	918	323.0	98.6	1	389	389	1.3	2
Pu	94	245	930	295.0	57.0	1	1210	370	15.0	10
Pr	59	143	935.3	315.6	100.0	1				1
As	33	74	944.5	408.0+	26.6	1	1540	1353	18.8	4
Ga	31	72	956	341.8	27.9	1	3158	667	21.5	16
Gd	64	162	960	320.0	100.0	1				1
C	6	11	960.1	385.6+	99.8	1				1
Au	79	198	960.7	314.6	98.7	1	285	285	1.3	2
Tm	69	170	967.9	323.1	76.0	1	884	884	24.0	2
Gd	64	159	974.7	328.6	70.0	1	917	917	21.0	4
Ba	56	140	991	340.0	37.0	1	1005	454	26.0	5
Ba	56	142	1000	340.0	40.0	1	2120	1120	18.0	13
In	49	116	1009	351.0	50.8	1	871	871	32.8	6
Pd	46	109	1027.9	361.0	99.9	1				1
Ag	47	111	1028	360.4	91.9	1	783	686	7.0	3
I	53	130	1040	361.0	47.5	1	1176	622	46.7	9
Ti	22	45	1040.6	439.1	84.8	1				1
Rb	37	81	1050	458.0	31.4	1	600	600	1.7	2
Tl	81	200	1064	495.0	0.3	1				1
Er	68	171	1065.5	362.2	94.0	1	1485	1485	2.3	6
Pm	61	149	1071	369.0	96.2	1	785	785	3.4	3
Re	75	186	1076.6	362.0	71.0	1	939	939	22.0	2
Fr	87	223	1097	361.1	57.0	1	1068	1017	17.0	9
Ce	58	143	1104	384.6	48.0	1	1398	1398	38.0	7
Sr	38	91	1104	398.9	33.9	1	2684	2684	30.8	11
Cd	48	115	1111.3	394.4	60.1	1	850	583	35.2	4
Bk	97	251	1120	360.5	100.0	1				1
Os	76	193	1132	383.1	53.0	1	1059	1059	19.4	11
Bi	83	210	1161.4	389.0	100.0	1				1
Ac	89	228	1168	386.0	32.0	1	2079	1741	12.0	31
Al	13	26	1174.2	543.9+	81.8	1				1

+ indicates positron emission

(continued)

Table 8.3 Selected Beta Emitters by Maximum Energy (keV) (Continued)

Element Symbol	Z	A	Max. Energy (keV)	Average Energy (keV)	Intensity %	Rank by Abund. 1 = high	Other Most Energetic Beta Energy (keV)	Other Most Abundant Beta Energy (keV)	Other Most Abundant Beta Intensity %	Number of Betas
I	53	132	1185	422.0	18.9	1	2140	2140	16.9	23
U	92	239	1191	392.0	68.0	1	1266	1266	28.0	7
Ru	44	105	1193	432.2	49.9	1	1525	1112	20.0	13
Ar	18	41	1198.3	459.3	99.2	1	2492	2492	0.8	2
N	7	13	1198.5	491.8+	99.8	1				1
Mo	42	99	1214	442.7	82.7	1	848	436	17.3	5
Nb	41	94m	1215	444.0	0.5	1				1
Cu	29	61	1216.4	524.2+	51.3	1	1149	933	5.6	4
Am	95	246	1220	400.0	37.6	1	2260	1460	16.3	23
I	53	133	1230	441.0	83.5	1	1530	880	4.2	10
Th	90	233	1238.6	412.1	51.0	1	1245	1245	30.0	11
Np	93	238	1247.8	412.4	45.0	1	329	263	42.4	7
Y	39	86	1254	550.0+	12.4	1	3174	1578	5.6	14
Co	27	61	1254.7	474.4	96.3	1	414	414	3.7	2
Nb	41	97	1274.9	469.8	98.3	1	908	908	1.1	5
I	53	134	1280	460.0	32.5	1	2420	1560	16.3	14
Dy	66	165	1285	453.1	83.4	1	1190	1190	14.6	4
Se	34	73	1290	562.0+	64.6	1	1651	1651	0.7	3
K	19	40	1311.6	508.5	89.3	1				1
Tc	43	101	1318	487.0	89.0	1	1080	1080	6.5	7
La	57	140	1348.2	487.4	44.5	1	2164	1677	20.7	9
Pb	82	211	1373	473.3	93.0	1	968	541	5.0	4
Tb	65	162	1380	490.0	96.0	1	2530	2530	0.4	6
Na	11	24	1390.2	553.9	99.9	1				1
Sn	50	123	1397	523.1	99.4	1	308	308	0.6	2
Sb	51	122	1417	522.4	67.3	1	1981	1981	25.7	3
Bi	83	213	1420	491.0	64.0	1	1127	980	32.0	4
Tl	81	207	1422	494.1	99.8	1	524	524	0.3	2
I	53	135	1450	535.0	23.6	1	2180	1030	21.8	20
Cr	24	49	1453	625.5+	46.3	1	1606	1515	34.6	3
Co	27	56	1460.5	631.9+	18.7	1	423	423	1.1	2
Te	52	129	1470	544.5	90.0	1	1220	1011	8.6	6
Sc	21	44	1476.3	632.9+	94.4	1				1
Nd	60	149	1478	539.8	26.4	1	1500	1151	24.0	10
Au	79	194	1487	679.0+	1.0	1	1159	1159	0.6	2
Si	14	31	1490.8	595.6	100.0	1				1
Sr	38	89	1491	583.0	100.0	1				1
Nb	41	90	1500	662.2+	53.0	1				1
Xe	54	123	1505	674.0+	17.2	1	1476	1476	3.9	3
Bi	83	214	1540	539.0	17.9	1	3270	1505	17.7	30
Y	39	91	1543	603.8	99.7	1	338	338	0.3	2
Te	52	129m	1604	607.3	32.8	1	908	908	3.3	4
Cd	48	115m	1621	615.0	98.0	1	687	687	1.1	4

+ indicates positron emission

Table 8.3 Selected Beta Emitters by Maximum Energy (keV) (Continued)

Element Symbol	Z	A	Max. Energy (keV)	Average Energy (keV)	Intensity %	Rank by Abund. 1 = high	Other Most Energetic Beta Energy (keV)	Other Most Abundant Beta Energy (keV)	Other Most Abundant Beta Intensity %	Number of Betas
Ag	47	108	1650	629.0	95.9	1	1017	1017	1.8	3
Sr	38	93	1690	660.0	17.9	1	3620	2730	15.5	29
P	15	32	1710.4	694.9	100.0	1				1
O	8	15	1731.9	735.2 +	99.9	1				1
Re	75	182	1738	789.0 +	1.8	1				1
Mg	12	27	1765.5	724.4	71.0	1	1595	1595	29.0	2
In	49	117a	1770	680.0	34.5	1	1612	1612	18.3	2
Rb	37	86	1774.4	709.3	91.2	1	698	698	8.8	2
Tl	81	208	1794	646.5	49.3	1	1517	1283	23.2	7
Sb	51	126m	1810	694.0	81.0	1	1190	1190	3.3	4
Tl	81	209	1825	659.0	100.0	1				1
Ho	67	166	1854.3	693.8	51.0	1	1774	1774	48.0	4
Eu	63	152m	1865	704.1	67.3	1	1521	1521	1.8	4
Tl	81	210	1870	680.0	56.0	1	2340	1320	25.0	3
Ga	31	68	1899.1	836.0 +	87.7	1	822	822	1.2	2
Zr	40	97	1914.1	756.6	86.0	1	1406	552	5.5	10
In	49	114	1985	776.9	99.3	1	685	685	0.2	2
Sc	21	49	2004	823.1	99.9	1				1
Br	35	80	2006	805.0	85.0	1	1390	1390	6.2	5
Np	93	240	2070	733.0	52.0	1	1510	1510	31.9	14
Ge	32	77	2070	838.9	20.6	1	2486	1512	19.2	26
Te	52	131	2099	825.0	59.2	1	1756	1647	21.8	11
La	57	142	2119	826.0	21.5	1	4517	1974	20.1	25
Re	75	188	2119.7	795.1	71.4	1	1965	1965	25.3	7
I	53	128	2127	835.7	80.2	1	1684	1684	13.0	3
I	53	124	2135	973.6 +	12.0	1	1532	1532	11.0	3
Ni	28	65	2137	875.7	60.7	1	1022	655	28.1	5
Ti	22	51	2146	888.2	91.9	1	1537	1537	8.1	2
Pr	59	142	2159	832.8	96.3	1	583	583	3.7	2
Ca	20	49	2184	908.6	91.5	1	2896	1196	7.1	6
Rb	37	89	2223	903.1	34.0	1	4503	1275	33.0	10
Bi	83	212	2246	831.6	48.4	1	1519	1519	8.0	6
Te	52	133	2250	890.0	33.3	1	2660	2660	28.6	11
Ir	77	194	2251	847.5	85.4	1	1923	1923	9.2	9
Pa	91	234m	2281	825.4	98.6	1	1471	1236	0.7	3
Y	39	90	2283.9	934.8	100.0	1				1
Ba	56	139	2306	912.0	78.0	1	2140	2140	22.0	3
Sn	50	125	2350	938.0	83.0	1	1261	460	5.9	11
Ba	56	141	2380	947.0	24.5	1	2840	2560	19.0	24
Te	52	133m	2390	960.0	38.2	1	1740	1740	29.3	3
La	57	141	2430	967.0	97.0	1	1080	1080	2.6	3
Pm	61	148	2464	975.0	55.5	1	1914	999	33.3	5
As	33	72	2495	1115.0 +	64.7	1	3329	3329	16.6	6
Rb	37	85	2500	1030.0	95.7	1	1690	770	2.2	6
Rb	37	90m	2511	1038.0	16.2	1	5828	5828	15.0	30

+ indicates positron emission

(continued)

Table 8.3 Selected Beta Emitters by Maximum Energy (keV) (Continued)

Element Symbol	Z	A	Max. Energy (keV)	Average Energy (keV)	Intensity %	Rank by Abund. 1 = high	Other Most Energetic Beta Energy (keV)	Other Most Abundant Beta Energy (keV)	Other Most Abundant Beta Intensity %	Number of Betas
V	23	52	2542.42	1074.0	99.2	1	1209	1209	0.6	3
Kr	36	90	2610	1086.0	62.0	1	4390	4390	29.0	19
Mn	25	52b	2632.8	1173.8+	96.4	1	905	905	0.2	2
Mn	25	57	2678	1135.0	80.8	1	2556	2556	11.5	7
Mn	25	56	2848.6	1216.7	56.2	1	1038	1038	27.8	4
Al	13	28	2864.2	1242.3	100.0	1				1
Cs	55	138	2880	1179.0	44.1	1	3890	3430	13.8	26
Y	39	93	2890	1214.0	90.2	1	2623	2623	4.6	8
Ag	47	110m	2892.8	1199.3	95.2	1	2235	2235	4.4	2
Cu	29	62	2927	1316.0+	97.6	1	1754	1754	0.1	2
As	33	76	2968.6	1266.9	51.0	1	2410	2410	34.7	8
Pr	59	144	2996	1221.4	97.7	1	2300	2300	1.2	3
I	53	122	3120	1414.0+	63.0	1	2550	2550	12.0	5
Rb	37	82	3356	1524.0+	83.3	1	2580	2580	11.7	4
Mo	42	91	3416	1553.0+	93.4	1	1835	1779	0.2	3
Kr	36	87	3486	1502.0	40.7	1	3889	3889	30.4	13
K	19	42	3521.1	1563.9	82.1	1	1996	1996	17.5	3
Rh	45	106	3541	1509.0	78.7	1	3029	2407	9.8	6
Y	39	92	3634	1563.0	85.7	1	2700	1294	6.5	8
Cs	55	126	3810	1740.0+	51.0	1	3420	3420	24.0	6
Ga	31	66	4153	1904.1+	49.3	1	1780	924	3.7	6
Cs	55	139	4204	1794.0	84.0	1	2921	2921	6.3	30
N	7	16	4288.3	1941.2	68.0	1	10419	10419	26.0	4
Xe	54	137	4344	1862.0	67.0	1	3889	3889	30.0	7
I	53	136	4370	1880.0	35.4	1	5690	5690	30.4	26
Br	35	84	4670	2072.0	32.0	1	3790	3790	13.7	18
Cl	17	38	4917	2244.1	56.0	1	2749	1107	32.5	3
Kr	36	89	4970	2210.0	23.0	1	4470	2370	14.4	47
Rb	37	88	5315	2372.4	78.0	1	3479	2581	13.3	9
Rb	37	90	6553	2976.0	37.0	1	5721	5721	14.3	21
Tm	69	171	30	7.6	2.2	2	97	97	97.8	2
Ho	67	166m	32	8.0	17.2	2	1314	72	73.4	7
Ac	89	227	34.4	8.7	35.0	2	44	44	54.0	3
Sm	62	151	54.6	14.0	0.9	2	76	76	99.1	2
W	74	188	58	14.9	0.8	2	349	349	99.0	3
Pb	82	210	63	16.1	19.8	2	17	17	80.2	2
Yb	70	175	71.6	18.4	10.3	2	468	468	86.5	3
Cs	55	134	88.5	23.1	27.4	2	658	658	70.1	3
Th	90	234	96.2	24.9	18.5	2	189	189	72.5	4
Ru	44	103	113	29.8	6.4	2	723	226	90.0	4
Sb	51	125	130.8	34.8	18.1	2	622	303	39.9	7
Eu	63	155	159	42.8	26.0	2	246	141	46.0	6
Pm	61	146	162	43.5	2.2	2	795	795	34.1	2
Kr	36	85b	173	47.5	0.4	2	687	687	99.6	2

+ indicates positron emission

Table 8.3 Selected Beta Emitters by Maximum Energy (keV) (Continued)

Element Symbol	Z	A	Max. Energy (keV)	Average Energy (keV)	Intensity %	Rank by Abund. 1=high	Other Most Energetic Beta Energy (keV)	Other Most Abundant Beta Energy (keV)	Other Most Abundant Beta Intensity %	Number of Betas
Cs	55	136	174.4	47.2	2.5	2	682	341	95.1	4
Lu	71	177	175.8	47.3	12.3	2	497	497	78.7	3
Ce	58	144	184.7	50.2	19.6	2	318	318	77.2	3
Pa	91	230	192	51.6	0.2	2	507	507	9.3	2
Mg	12	28	211.8	65.2	4.7	2	860	459	95.1	3
Pa	91	233	231.8	63.0	28.0	2	260	260	33.0	4
Au	79	199	244.8	67.3	20.5	2	453	295	66.2	3
Cs	55	132	247	69.0	0.4	2	814	814	1.6	3
Eu	63	154	247.4	68.8	27.9	2	1844	569	36.5	15
Rh	45	105	248	69.9	19.7	2	567	567	75.0	3
U	92	237	251.9	68.8	43.7	2	238	238	53.1	5
Cm	96	249	257	70.0	1.8	2	891	891	96.3	5
Ta	73	182	258	71.6	28.9	2	590	522	40.8	8
Np	93	238	263.4	72.2	42.4	2	1248	1248	45.0	7
Br	35	82	264.6	76.2	1.4	2	444	444	97.9	2
Xe	54	133	267	75.1	0.7	2	346	346	99.3	2
Fe	26	59	273.4	81.0	45.2	2	1565	466	53.1	4
Te	52	127	276	78.2	1.2	2	694	694	98.8	2
Au	79	198	284.8	79.4	1.3	2	961	961	98.7	2
Th	90	231	304.8	84.8	35.0	2	311	288	49.0	7
Sn	50	123	308	88.6	0.6	2	1397	1397	99.4	2
Np	93	239	329.8	92.1	35.0	2	714	436	52.0	5
Pu	94	246	330	92.0	27.0	2	150	150	73.0	3
I	53	131	333.8	96.6	7.4	2	807	606	89.3	5
Y	39	91	338.1	99.9	0.3	2	1543	1543	99.7	2
Er	68	169	341.8	97.9	45.0	2	350	350	55.0	2
Kr	36	79	348	154.0+	0.2	2	609	609	6.9	2
Np	93	236	355	105.6	5.0	2	195	195	5.0	2
Ra	88	225	362	103.0	28.0	2	322	322	72.0	2
Nd	60	147	364.8	106.1	15.3	2	805	805	81.1	5
Pu	94	245	370	105.0	15.0	2	1210	930	57.0	10
Br	35	83	389	118.0	1.3	2	918	918	98.6	2
Zr	40	95	399	120.4	43.7	2	1123	366	55.4	4
Hf	72	181	403	117.5	7.0	2	407	407	93.0	2
Co	27	61	413.5	129.6	3.7	2	1255	1255	96.3	2
Co	27	56	422.6	179.4+	1.1	2	1461	1461	18.7	2
Mo	42	99	436	133.0	17.3	2	1214	1214	82.7	5
Es	99	254	437	124.7	19.0	2	1126	477	67.0	3
As	33	77	451	141.0	1.5	2	690	690	97.1	4
Te	52	134	453.312	137.0	41.1	2	377	377	42.9	3
Ba	56	140	454	136.0	26.0	2	1005	991	37.0	5
Sn	50	125	460	139.8	5.9	2	2350	2350	83.0	11
Cu	29	67	482	154.0	22.0	2	575	390	57.0	4

+ indicates positron emission

(continued)

Table 8.3 Selected Beta Emitters by Maximum Energy (keV) (Continued)

Element Symbol	Z	A	Max. Energy (keV)	Average Energy (keV)	Intensity %	Rank by Abund. 1=high	Other Most Energetic Beta Energy (keV)	Other Most Abundant Beta Energy (keV)	Other Most Abundant Beta Intensity %	Number of Betas
Sc	21	48	482	157.9	10.0	2	657	657	89.0	2
Dy	66	166	484	145.3	7.0	2	402	402	92.0	3
Np	93	236m	491	143.0	8.3	2	536	536	39.7	2
Pu	94	243	498	145.1	29.0	2	582	582	59.0	6
Tc	43	95	513	230.0+	0.2	2	717	717	0.3	2
Tl	81	207	524	156.3	0.3	2	1422	1422	99.8	2
Ag	47	110	530.7	165.6	30.5	2	134	84	67.3	3
Te	52	131m	532	164.8	16.6	2	2431	451	36.9	18
Sb	51	129	534	166.0	22.5	2	2271	650	26.6	22
Ir	77	192	536	161.2	41.4	2	845	672	48.3	4
Pb	82	211	541	161.9	5.0	2	1373	1373	93.0	4
Xe	54	135	551	171.0	3.1	2	909	909	96.1	4
Zr	40	97	551.5	175.3	5.5	2	1914	1914	86.0	10
Cd	48	117a	569	179.0	21.6	2	1916	667	46.9	16
Pb	82	212	573	172.7	9.9	2	334	334	85.1	3
Ce	58	141	580	180.7	29.5	2	435	435	70.5	2
Pr	59	142	583	181.5	3.7	2	2159	2159	96.3	2
Cd	48	115	583.4	184.6	35.2	2	1111	1111	60.1	4
Rb	37	81	600	264.0+	1.7	2	1050	1050	31.4	2
Sc	21	47	600.5	204.0	32.0	2	441	441	68.0	2
I	53	130	622	197.0	46.7	2	1176	1040	47.5	9
Sm	62	153	632	198.6	34.1	2	805	702	44.1	4
Am	95	245	643.2	192.9	15.6	2	896	896	77.4	3
Cu	29	64	652.9	278.1+	17.9	2	578	578	37.2	2
Pa	91	234	654	198.1	16.0	2	1259	484	24.0	18
Ni	28	65	655.2	220.9	28.1	2	2137	2137	60.7	5
Am	95	242	661.2	199.0	41.0	2	619	619	42.0	2
Ga	31	72	667	223.5	21.5	2	3158	956	27.9	16
In	49	114	685	222.3	0.2	2	1985	1985	99.3	2
Ag	47	111	686	223.5	7.0	2	1028	1028	91.9	3
Cd	48	115m	687.2	241.7	1.1	2	1621	1621	98.0	4
Pm	61	148m	695	222.0	22.0	2	1007	407	54.0	4
Rb	37	86	697.6	232.5	8.8	2	1774	1774	91.2	2
Bk	97	250	709	214.4	5.9	2	1780	748	83.1	4
Kr	36	85a	710.8	238.2	0.3	2	841	841	78.6	2
Ni	28	57	716	304.0+	5.7	2	843	843	33.1	4
Pt	78	197	719	225.3	11.0	2	642	642	82.0	3
Pb	82	214	729	227.0	42.5	2	1024	672	48.0	5
Nb	41	96	746	249.7	2.8	2	749	749	95.9	4
Rb	37	85	770	260.0	2.2	2	2500	2500	95.7	6
Pm	61	149	785	256.1	3.4	2	1071	1071	96.2	3
Ga	31	68	821.7	352.6+	1.2	2	1899	1899	87.7	2
Mo	42	101	849	290.0	11.7	2	2603	763	20.7	38
Tb	65	160	867.3	286.0	24.6	2	1747	569	45.6	11

+ indicates positron emission

Table 8.3 Selected Beta Emitters by Maximum Energy (keV) (Continued)

Element Symbol	Z	A	Max. Energy (keV)	Average Energy (keV)	Intensity %	Rank by Abund. 1=high	Other Most Energetic Beta Energy (keV)	Other Most Abundant Beta Energy (keV)	Other Most Abundant Beta Intensity %	Number of Betas
In	49	116	871	295.0	32.8	2	1009	1009	50.8	6
I	53	133	880	299.0	4.2	2	1530	1230	83.5	10
Tm	69	170	883.6	290.4	24.0	2	968	968	76.0	2
Mn	25	52b	905.1	382.9+	0.2	2	2633	2633	96.4	2
Te	52	129m	908	308.3	3.3	2	1604	1604	32.8	4
Nb	41	97	908.4	314.9	1.1	2	1275	1275	98.3	5
Gd	64	159	916.7	305.7	21.0	2	975	975	70.0	4
Ga	31	66	924	397.0+	3.7	2	4153	4153	49.3	6
Cu	29	61	933.4	399.3+	5.6	2	1216	1216	51.3	4
Re	75	186	939.4	308.8	22.0	2	1077	1077	71.0	2
Bi	83	213	980	319.0	32.0	2	1420	1420	64.0	4
Pm	61	148	999	340.0	33.3	2	2464	2464	55.5	5
Te	52	129	1011	350.0	8.6	2	1470	1470	90.0	6
Fr	87	223	1017	330.9	17.0	2	1097	1097	57.0	9
Ag	47	108	1017	356.0	1.8	2	1650	1650	95.9	3
I	53	135	1030	359.0	21.8	2	2180	1450	23.6	20
Mn	25	56	1037.9	381.9	27.8	2	2849	2849	56.2	4
Os	76	193	1059	354.4	19.4	2	1132	1132	53.0	11
Tc	43	101	1080	385.0	6.5	2	1318	1318	89.0	7
La	57	141	1080	373.0	2.6	2	2430	2430	97.0	3
Cl	17	38	1107	420.3	32.5	2	4917	4917	56.0	3
Sb	51	127	1108	390.9	22.8	2	1493	896	34.9	13
Ru	44	105	1112	397.5	20.0	2	1525	1193	49.9	13
Ba	56	142	1120	390.0	18.0	2	2120	1000	40.0	13
In	49	117	1140	406.0	0.2	2	743	743	99.8	2
Nd	60	149	1151	402.4	24.0	2	1500	1478	26.4	10
Au	79	194	1159	535.0+	0.6	2	1487	1487	1.0	2
Nb	41	95	1161.3	437.8	5.4	2	957	160	100.0	3
Cs	55	137	1173.2	415.2	5.4	2	512	512	94.6	2
Pm	61	151	1188	417.0	10.0	2	1118	843	42.7	22
Dy	66	165	1190	414.1	14.6	2	1285	1285	83.4	4
Sb	51	126m	1190	424.0	3.3	2	1810	1810	81.0	4
Ca	20	49	1196	456.1	7.1	2	2896	2184	91.5	6
V	23	52	1208.78	458.4	0.6	2	2542	2542	99.2	3
K	19	43	1224	469.0	3.6	2	1817	827	92.2	4
Pa	91	234m	1236	410.2	0.7	2	2281	2281	98.6	3
Th	90	233	1245.2	414.6	30.0	2	1239	1239	51.0	11
I	53	126	1251	458.6	9.0	2	1134	862	27.2	5
U	92	239	1265.8	420.3	28.0	2	1191	1191	68.0	7
Rb	37	89	1275	473.6	33.0	2	4503	2223	34.0	10
Tl	81	208	1283	438.7	23.2	2	1794	1794	49.3	7
Y	39	92	1294	480.0	6.5	2	3634	3634	85.7	8
W	74	187	1312.5	457.1	25.1	2	1178	627	58.7	10

+ indicates positron emission

(continued)

Table 8.3 Selected Beta Emitters by Maximum Energy (keV) (Continued)

Element Symbol	Z	A	Max. Energy (keV)	Average Energy (keV)	Intensity %	Rank by Abund. 1 = high	Other Most Energetic Beta Energy (keV)	Other Most Abundant Beta Energy (keV)	Other Most Abundant Beta Intensity %	Number of Betas
Tl	81	210	1320	450.0	25.0	2	2340	1870	56.0	3
As	33	74	1353	530.9	18.8	2	1540	945	26.6	4
Br	35	80	1390	526.0	6.2	2	2006	2006	85.0	5
Ce	58	143	1398	507.5	38.0	2	1104	1104	48.0	7
Am	95	246	1460	490.0	16.3	2	2260	1220	37.6	23
Eu	63	152	1475	535.6	8.4	2	1064	696	13.6	7
Xe	54	123	1476	661.0+	3.9	2	1505	1505	17.2	3
Er	68	171	1485.4	534.7	2.3	2	1066	1066	94.0	6
Bi	83	214	1505	525.0	17.7	2	3270	1540	17.9	30
Np	93	240	1510	514.0	31.9	2	2070	2070	52.0	14
Ge	32	77	1512	583.5	19.2	2	2486	2070	20.6	26
Cr	24	49	1515	653.7+	34.6	2	1606	1453	46.3	3
Bi	83	212	1519	530.7	8.0	2	2246	2246	48.4	6
Eu	63	152m	1521	554.1	1.8	2	1865	1865	67.3	4
I	53	124	1532	685.9+	11.0	2	2135	2135	12.0	3
Ti	22	51	1537	606.7	8.1	2	2146	2146	91.9	2
Co	27	60	1549.73	606.4	0.2	2	318	318	100.0	2
I	53	134	1560	580.0	16.3	2	2420	1280	32.5	14
Y	39	86	1578	696.0+	5.6	2	3174	1254	12.4	14
Mg	12	27	1594.8	645.7	29.0	2	1766	1766	71.0	2
In	49	117a	1612	610.0	18.3	2	1770	1770	34.5	2
Te	52	131	1647	622.0	21.8	2	2099	2099	59.2	11
Se	34	73	1651	725.0+	0.7	2	1290	1290	64.6	3
Rb	37	84	1658	756.3+	13.5	2	890	777	13.7	3
La	57	140	1677	629.5	20.7	2	2164	1348	44.5	9
I	53	128	1684	637.3	13.0	2	2127	2127	80.2	3
Te	52	133m	1740	670.0	29.3	2	2390	2390	38.2	3
Ac	89	228	1741	611.0	12.0	2	2079	1168	32.0	31
Cu	29	62	1754	767.5+	0.1	2	2927	2927	97.6	2
Ho	67	166	1773.7	651.1	48.0	2	1854	1854	51.0	4
Mo	42	91	1779	790.0	0.2	2	3416	3416	93.4	3
Sb	51	126	1790	689.0	19.0	2	1170	370	29.0	14
Ir	77	194	1922.6	707.2	9.2	2	2251	2251	85.4	9
Sr	38	92	1930	777.0	4.0	2	1040	550	96.0	4
Re	75	188	1964.7	728.6	25.3	2	2120	2120	71.4	7
La	57	142	1974	761.0	20.1	2	4517	2119	21.5	25
Sb	51	122	1981	772.1	25.7	2	1417	1417	67.3	3
Ca	20	47	1988	816.8	18.0	2	690	690	81.7	2
K	19	42	1996.4	822.3	17.5	2	3521	3521	82.1	3
Ba	56	139	2140	837.0	22.0	2	2306	2306	78.0	3
I	53	132	2140	841.0	16.9	2	1617	1185	18.9	23
Cd	48	117	2213	882.0	21.0	2	1939	636	32.2	22
Ag	47	110m	2235	894.1	4.4	2	2893	2893	95.2	2

+ indicates positron emission

Table 8.3 Selected Beta Emitters by Maximum Energy (keV) (Continued)

Element Symbol	Z	A	Max. Energy (keV)	Average Energy (keV)	Intensity %	Rank by Abund. 1=high	Other Most Energetic Beta Energy (keV)	Other Most Abundant Beta Energy (keV)	Other Most Abundant Beta Intensity %	Number of Betas
Xe	54	138	2290	908.0	20.1	2	2730	710	32.6	15
Pr	59	144	2300	894.4	1.2	2	2996	2996	97.7	3
Sb	51	124	2302.3	918.6	21.9	2	1656	611	52.8	12
Kr	36	89	2370	970.0	14.4	2	4970	4970	23.0	47
Rh	45	106	2407	977.0	9.8	2	3541	3541	78.7	6
As	33	76	2409.5	996.3	34.7	2	2969	2969	51.0	8
Eu	63	156	2453	966.0	27.0	2	1404	487	32.0	14
Ar	18	41	4292	1076.7	0.8	2	1198	1198	99.2	2
Tb	65	162	2530	980.0	0.4	2	1380	1380	96.0	6
I	53	122	2550	1152.0+	12.0	2	3120	3120	63.0	5
Mn	25	57	2556	1077.0	11.5	2	2678	2678	80.8	7
Ba	56	141	2560	1029.0	19.0	2	2840	2380	24.5	24
Rb	37	82	2580	1157.0+	11.7	2	3356	3356	83.3	4
Rb	37	88	2581	1070.6	13.3	2	5315	5315	78.0	9
Y	39	93	2623	1087.0	4.6	2	2890	2890	90.2	8
Te	52	133	2660	1080.0	28.6	2	2250	2250	33.3	11
Sr	38	91	2684	1121.2	30.8	2	2031	1104	33.9	11
Sr	38	93	2730	1140.0	15.5	2	3620	1690	17.9	29
Kr	36	88	2913	1233.0	14.0	2	2717	521	67.0	15
Cs	55	139	2921	1196.0	6.3	2	4204	4204	84.0	30
As	33	72	3329	1526.0+	16.6	2	2638	2495	64.7	6
Cs	55	126	3420	1560.0+	24.0	2	3810	3810	51.0	6
Cs	55	138	3430	1433.0	13.8	2	3890	2880	44.1	26
Br	35	84	3790	1650.0	13.7	2	4670	4670	32.0	18
Kr	36	87	3889	1694.8	30.4	2	3486	3486	40.7	13
Xe	54	137	3889	1649.0	30.0	2	4344	4344	67.0	7
Kr	36	90	4390	1935.0	29.0	2	3780	2610	62.0	19
I	53	136	5690	2500.0	30.4	2	4710	4370	35.4	26
Rb	37	90	5721	2574.0	14.3	2	6553	6553	37.0	21
Rb	37	90m	5828	2620.0	15.0	2	5004	2511	16.2	30
N	7	16	10418.7	4979.2	26.0	2	4288	4288	68.0	4

+ indicates positron emission

Table 8.4 Calculation of Specific Activity (From Cember, 1983)

Note that the becquerel (or curie), although used as a unit of quantity, does not mention anything about the mass or volume of the radioactive material in which the specified number of transformations occur. The concentration of radioactivity, or the relationship between the mass of radioactive material and the activity is called the specific activity. Specific activity is the number of becquerels (or curies) per unit mass or volume. The specific activity of a carrier-free radioisotope, that is a radioisotope that is not mixed with any other isotope of the same element, may be calculated as follows:

If λ is the *transformation constant* in units of reciprocal seconds, then the number of transformations per second (tps), and hence the number of becquerels in an aggregation of N atoms, is simply given by λN.

If the radioisotope under consideration weighs 1 gram, then, the number of atoms is given by

$$N = \frac{6.022 \times 10^{23} \; atoms/mole}{A \; g/mole}, \tag{1}$$

where A *is the atomic weight of the isotope*. The activity per unit weight, or the specific activity, therefore is:

$$SA = \lambda N = \frac{\lambda \times 6.022 \times 10^{23}}{A} \; Bq/g. \tag{2}$$

Equation (2) gives the desired relationship between the specific activity and weight of an isotope, and can be calculated in terms of the isotope's *half-life* by substituting 0.693/T for λ in equation (2):

$$\lambda N = \frac{0.693}{T} \times \frac{6.022 \times 10^{23}}{A} \; Bq/g,$$

$$SA = \frac{4.17 \times 10^{23}}{A \times T} \; Bq/g. \tag{3}$$

Note that equations (2) and (3) are valid only if λ and T are given in *time units of seconds*.

Table 8.4.1 Values for Specific Activity of Selected Radionuclides[a,b]

At. Wt. (A)	Isotope	Half-Life (T)		Sp. Act. (TBq/g)[c]	At. Wt. (A)	Isotope	Half-Life (T)		Sp. Act. (TBq/g)[c]
3	^{3}H	12.350	y	3.57E + 02	133	Te-133	12.450	m	4.20E + 06
11	^{11}C	20.380	m	3.10E + 07	135	I-135	6.610	h	1.30E + 05
14	^{14}C	5730.000	y	1.65E − 01	133	Ba-133	10.500	y	9.48E + 00
7	^{7}Be	53.440	d	1.29E + 04	134	Cs-134	2.062	y	4.79E + 01
13	^{13}N	9.970	m	5.37E + 07	136	Cs-136	13.100	d	2.71E + 03
16	^{16}N	7.200	s	3.62E + 09	137	Cs-137	30.000	y	3.22E + 00
18	^{18}F	109.740	m	3.52E + 06	137	Ba-137m	2.552	m	1.99E + 07
22	^{22}Na	2.602	y	2.31E + 02	140	Ba-140	12.740	d	2.71E + 03
24	^{24}Na	15.000	h	3.22E + 05	140	La-140	40.272	h	2.06E + 04
32	^{32}P	14.290	d	1.06E + 04	141	Ce-141	32.501	d	1.05E + 03
35	^{35}S	87.440	d	1.58E + 03	143	Ce-143	33.000	h	2.46E + 04
36	^{36}Cl	3.01×10^5	y	1.22E − 03	143	Pr-143	13.560	d	2.49E + 03
41	^{41}Ar	1.827	h	1.55E + 06	144	Ce-144	284.300	d	1.18E + 02
42	^{42}K	12.36	h	2.23E + 05	144	Pr-144	17.280	m	2.80E + 06
45	^{45}Ca	163.000	d	6.58E + 02	147	Pm-147	2.623	y	3.43E + 01
46	^{46}Sc	83.830	d	1.25E + 03	181	W-181	121.200	d	2.20E + 02
51	^{51}Cr	27.704	d	3.42E + 03	182	Ta-182	115.000	d	2.31E + 02
54	^{54}Mn	312.500	d	2.86E + 02	185	W-185	75.100	d	3.48E + 02
56	^{56}Mn	2.579	h	8.03E + 05	192	Ir-192	74.020	d	3.40E + 02
55	^{55}Fe	2.700	y	8.91E + 01	198	Au-198	2.696	d	9.05E + 03
59	^{59}Fe	44.529	d	1.84E + 03	199	Au-199	3.139	d	7.73E + 03
57	^{57}Co	270.900	d	3.13E + 02	203	Hg-203	46.600	d	5.11E + 02
59	^{59}Ni	7.5×10^4	y	2.99E − 03	204	Tl-204	3.779	y	1.72E + 01
60	^{60}Co	5.271	y	4.18E + 01	207	Tl-207	4.770	m	7.04E + 06
63	^{63}Ni	96.000	y	2.19E + 00	210	Pb-210	22.300	y	2.83E + 00
65	^{65}Ni	2.520	h	7.08E + 05	210	Bi-210	5.012	d	4.59E + 03
64	^{64}Cu	12.701	h	1.43E + 05	210	Po-210	138.380	d	1.66E + 02
65	^{65}Zn	243.900	d	3.05E + 02	212	Po-212	0.305	μs	6.45E + 15
72	^{72}Ga	14.100	h	1.14E + 05	224	Ra-224	3.660	d	5.89E + 03
76	^{76}As	26.320	h	5.79E + 04	226	Ra-226	1600.000	y	3.66E − 02
82	^{82}Br	35.300	h	4.00E + 04	228	Ra-228	5.750	y	1.01E + 01
86	^{86}Rb	18.660	d	3.01E + 03	228	Ac-228	6.130	h	8.29E + 04
89	^{89}Sr	50.500	d	1.07E + 03	228	Th-228	1.913	y	3.03E + 01
90	^{90}Sr	29.120	y	5.05E + 00	227	Th-227	18.718	d	1.14E + 03
90	^{90}Y	64.000	h	2.01E + 04	229	Th-229	7340.000	y	7.87E − 03
92	^{92}Sr	2.710	h	4.65E + 05	230	Th-230	7.7×10^4	y	7.47E − 04
92	^{92}Y	3.540	h	3.56E + 05	231	Th-231	25.520	h	1.97E + 04
95	^{95}Zr	63.980	d	7.95E + 02	232	Th-232	1.41×10^{10}	y	4.05E − 09
95	^{95}Nb	35.150	d	1.45E + 03	234	Th-234	24.100	d	8.56E + 02
99	^{99}Mo	66.000	h	1.77E + 04	232	U-232	72.000	y	7.92E − 01
99	^{99m}Tc	6.020	h	1.94E + 05	233	U-233	1.59×10^5	y	3.57E − 04
103	^{103}Ru	39.280	d	1.19E + 03	234	U-234	2.45×10^5	y	2.31E − 04
106	^{106}Ru	368.200	d	1.24E + 02	235	U-235	7.04×10^8	y	8.00E − 08
110	^{110m}Ag	249.900	d	1.76E + 02	236	U-236	2.34×10^7	y	2.40E − 06
110	^{110}Ag	24.600	s	1.54E + 08	237	U-237	6.750	d	3.02E + 03
123	^{123}I	13.200	h	7.14E + 04	238	U-238	4.47×10^9	y	1.24E − 08
125	^{125}I	60.140	d	6.42E + 02	238	Pu-238	87.740	y	6.34E − 01
129	^{129}I	1.57×10^7	y	6.53E − 06	239	Np-239	2.355	d	8.58E + 03
131	^{131}I	8.040	d	4.59E + 03	239	Pu-239	24065.000	y	2.30E − 03
132	^{132}Te	78.200	h	1.12E + 04	240	Pu-240	6537.000	y	8.43E − 03
132	^{132}I	2.300	h	3.82E + 05	241	Pu-241	14.400	y	3.81E + 00
133	^{133}I	20.800	h	4.19E + 04	241	Am-241	432.200	y	1.27E − 01
133	^{133}Xe	5.245	d	6.92E + 03	252	Cf-252	2.638	y	1.99E + 01

[a] Half-lives after ICRP 38 1983, may differ from Kocher 1981.
[b] To obtain specific activity in Ci/g multiply table entry by 27.03.
[c] 1 TBq = 10^{12} Bq

Table 8.5 X-Ray Energies Useful for Radiochemical Analyses[a] (From HASL 300, 1990 after Browne et al. 1986, Wapstra et al. 1959, and Siegbøhn 1965)

		Energy (keV)		
Z	**Element**	**K_α**	**$K'_{\beta1}$**	**$K'_{\beta2}$**
3	Li	0.05		
4	Be	0.11		
5	B	0.18		
6	C	0.28		
7	N	0.40		
8	O	0.53		
9	F	0.68		
10	Ne	0.85		
11	Na	1.04		
12	Mg	1.25		
13	Al	1.49		
14	Si	1.74		
15	P	2.01		
16	S	2.31		
17	Cl	2.62		
18	Ar	2.96	3.19	
19	K	3.31	3.59	
20	Ca	3.69	4.01	
21	Sc	4.09	4.46	
22	Ti	4.51	4.93	
23	V	4.95	5.43	
24	Cr	5.42	5.95	
25	Mn	5.90	6.49	
26	Fe	6.40	7.06	
27	Co	6.93	7.65	
28	Ni	7.47	8.26	
29	Cu	8.03	8.91	
30	Zn	8.63	9.57	
31	Ga	9.24	10.3	
32	Ge	9.88	11.1	
33	As	10.5	11.7	
34	Si	11.2	12.5	
35	Br	11.9	13.3	
36	Kr	12.6	14.1	
37	Rb	13.4	15.0	
38	Sr	14.1	15.8	16.1
39	Y	14.9	16.7	17.0
40	Zr	15.7	17.7	18.0
41	Nb	16.6	18.6	19.0
42	Mo	17.4	19.6	20.0
43	Te	18.3	20.6	21.0
44	Ru	19.2	21.6	22.1
45	Rh	20.2	22.7	23.2

Table 8.5 X-Ray Energies Useful for Radiochemical Analyses[a] (Continued)

		Energy (keV)		
Z	Element	K_α	$K'_{\beta 1}$	$K'_{\beta 2}$
46	Pd	21.1	23.8	24.3
47	Ag	22.1	24.9	25.5
48	Cd	23.1	26.1	26.6
49	In	24.1	27.3	27.9
50	Sn	25.1	28.4	29.1
51	Sb	26.3	29.7	30.4
52	Te	27.3	31.0	31.7
53	I	28.5	32.3	33.0
54	Xe	29.6	33.6	34.4
55	Cs	30.8	34.9	35.8
56	Ba	32.0	36.4	37.2
57	La	33.3	37.8	38.7
58	Ce	34.5	39.3	40.2
59	Pr	35.9	40.7	41.8
60	Nd	37.2	42.3	43.3
61	Pm	38.5	43.8	44.9
62	Sm	39.8	45.4	46.6
63	Eu	41.3	47.0	48.2
64	Cd	42.7	48.7	49.9
65	Tb	44.1	50.4	51.7
66	Dy	45.6	52.1	53.4
67	Ho	47.1	53.8	55.3
68	Er	48.7	55.6	57.1
69	Tm	50.3	57.5	59.0
70	Yb	51.9	59.4	60.9
71	Lu	53.5	61.3	62.9
72	Hf	55.2	63.2	64.9
73	Ta	57.1	65.2	67.0
74	W	58.8	67.2	69.1
75	Re	60.6	69.3	71.2
76	Os	62.4	71.4	73.4
77	Ir	64.3	73.6	75.6
78	Pt	66.2	75.7	77.8
79	Au	68.2	78.0	80.1
80	Hg	70.1	80.1	82.5
81	Tl	72.1	82.4	84.9
82	Pb	74.2	84.7	87.3
83	Bi	76.3	87.1	89.8
84	Po	78.4	89.6	92.3
85	At	80.5	92.7	95.0
86	Rn	82.8	94.7	97.5
87	Fr	85.0	97.3	100.2
88	Ra	87.3	99.9	103.0

(continued)

Table 8.5 X-Ray Energies Useful for Radiochemical Analyses[a] (Continued)

		Energy (keV)		
Z	Element	K_α	$K'_{\beta 1}$	$K'_{\beta 2}$
89	Ac	89.7	102.6	105.7
90	Th	92.1	105.3	108.6
91	Pa	94.5	108.1	111.4
92	U	97.0	111.0	114.5
93	Np	99.5	113.9	117.5
94	Pu	102.1	116.9	120.5
95	Am	104.7	119.9	123.6
96	Cm	107.5	123.0	126.9
97	Bk	110.2	126.2	130.2
98	Cf	113.0	129.4	133.5
99	Es	115.9	132.7	136.9
100	Fm	118.8	136.0	140.4
101	Md	122.8	139.4	144.9
102	No	124.8	142.7	147.5
103	Lw	127.9	146.2	151.2
104		130.5	149.7	154.5

[a] K Shell vacancies are filled by a higher shell electron. In the process an energy E_K-E_x is liberated either as an x-ray or an Auger electron. The most important x-ray transitions are designated as,

$K_{\alpha 1} = K - L_{III}$ $\quad K_{\beta 1} = K - M_{III}$ $\quad K_{\beta 4} = K - N_{II}$

$K_{\alpha 2} = K - L_{III}$ $\quad K_{\beta 2} = K - N_{III}$ $\quad K_{\beta 5} = K - M_{IV}$

$K_{\beta 3} = K - M_{II}$

With moderate resolution only $K'_{\beta 1}$ and $K'_{\beta 2}$ can be resolved.

$$K'_{\beta 1} = K_{\beta 1} + K_{\beta 3} + K_{\beta 5}$$

$$K'_{\beta 2} = K_{\beta 2} + K_{\beta 4}$$

The same is true for K_α

$$K_\alpha = K_{\alpha 1} + K_{\alpha 2}$$

The present table lists the values for K_α, $K_{\beta' 1}$ and $K_{\beta' 2}$. Electron binding energies used in this table were based on the tabulations of Wapstra et al 1959 and Siegbahn 1965.

Table 8.6 Gamma (& X-Ray) Energies of Radionuclides of Interest to Health Physicists by Increasing Energy[a]

Energy (MeV)	Radio-nuclide	Probability per Decay	Energy (MeV)	Radio-nuclide	Probability per Decay	Energy (MeV)	Radio-nuclide	Probability per Decay
.001690	^{85}Sr	.016470	.005405	^{54}Mn	.074288	.008616	^{67}Ga	.164720
.002170	^{95m}Nb	.020584	.005415	^{52}Mn	.103070	.008639	^{67}Ga	.322970
.002170	^{93m}Nb	.024555	.005415	^{54}Mn	.147110	.008650	^{187}W	.086825
.002170	^{93}Mo	.030352	.005430	^{51}Cr	.026172	.008910	^{192}Ir	.014625
.002420	^{97}Ru	.045772	.005430	^{147}Nd	.079239	.008910	^{65}Zn	.046052
.002700	^{103m}Rh	.040315	.005640	^{148m}Pm	.010736	.009440	^{192}Ir	.040934
.003130	^{111}In	.070853	.005640	^{151}Pm	.056243	.009570	^{67}Ga	.065838
.003290	^{113m}In	.023351	.005640	^{152}Eu	.150290	.009710	^{197}Hg	.501240
.003314	^{41}Ca	.123320	.005850	^{153}Sm	.118660	.009990	^{198}Au	.012732
.003600	^{126}Sn	.111590	.005888	^{55}Fe	.082372	.009990	^{201}Tl	.444390
.003770	^{131m}Te	.016695	.005899	^{55}Fe	.162790	.010300	^{211}Bi	.010471
.003770	^{125}I	.154380	.005950	^{52}Mn	.020631	.010300	^{212}Bi	.076864
.003770	^{125}Sb	.049470	.005950	^{54}Mn	.029445	.010300	^{203}Hg	.072156
.003770	^{123}I	.093039	.006060	^{155}Eu	.080104	.010508	^{75}Se	.161090
.003770	^{125m}Te	.150900	.006060	^{156}Eu	.054406	.010544	^{75}Se	.314010
.003770	^{129m}Te	.047537	.006060	^{154}Eu	.076319	.010600	^{208}Tl	.028851
.003770	^{127m}Te	.073215	.006391	^{56}Co	.073316	.010600	^{209}Tl	.087179
.003940	^{134}Te	.035433	.006391	^{57}Co	.166290	.010800	^{212}Pb	.154930
.003940	^{131}Te	.014449	.006391	^{58}Co	.077827	.010800	^{210}Pb	.243240
.003940	^{131m}Te	.011091	.006404	^{58}Co	.153500	.010800	^{214}Pb	.135050
.003940	^{133m}Te	.016721	.006404	^{56}Co	.144610	.011100	^{213}Bi	.018304
.003940	^{132}Te	.072597	.006404	^{57}Co	.327990	.011100	^{219}Rn	.010405
.003940	^{129}Te	.061630	.006490	^{55}Fe	.032852	.011400	^{221}Fr	.022661
.004110	^{135m}Xe	.016569	.006500	^{160}Tb	.106810	.011700	^{223}Ra	.247410
.004110	^{133m}Xe	.077570	.006930	^{59}Ni	.197620	.011700	^{75}Se	.072690
.004110	^{131m}Xe	.083680	.006950	^{166m}Ho	.211800	.012000	^{225}Ac	.212950
.004110	^{129}I	.081710	.006915	^{57}Ni	.061315	.012300	^{228}Th	.095590
.004290	^{134m}Cs	.164140	.006915	^{59}Ni	.100190	.012300	^{227}Th	.418000
.004290	^{133}Xe	.061419	.006930	^{57}Ni	.120940	.012300	^{230}Th	.084298
.004290	^{138}Xe	.060694	.007060	^{56}Co	.029202	.012300	^{232}Th	.083904
.004470	^{137m}Ba	.010381	.007060	^{58}Co	.030998	.012300	^{223}Fr	.336810
.004470	^{136}Cs	.028180	.007060	^{57}Co	.066234	.012300	^{229}Th	.810550
.004505	^{48}V	.028901	.007180	^{169}Yb	.505260	.012598	^{85m}Kr	.011162
.004511	^{48}V	.057344	.007461	^{61}Cu	.042708	.012649	^{85m}Kr	.021631
.004650	^{142}Ba	.038376	.007461	^{64}Cu	.048943	.012700	^{225}Ra	.157630
.004650	^{140}Ba	.147130	.007478	^{64}Cu	.096344	.012700	^{231}Pa	.432100
.004930	^{48}V	.011471	.007478	^{61}Cu	.084070	.013000	^{227}Ac	.011523
.004945	^{51}Cr	.065943	.007650	^{57}Ni	.024604	.013000	^{233}U	.039226
.004952	^{51}Cr	.130840	.007650	^{59}Ni	.040205	.013000	^{235}U	.309130
.005030	^{144}Ce	.015785	.008028	^{65}Zn	.115060	.013000	^{232}U	.120160
.005030	^{141}Ce	.026505	.008048	^{65}Zn	.226060	.013000	^{234}U	.105030
.005030	^{144m}Pr	.110890	.008150	^{181}W	.223010	.013000	^{236}U	.099792
.005030	^{143}Ce	.096319	.008260	^{61}Cu	.017115	.013000	^{238}U	.088313
.005405	^{52}Mn	.052050	.008260	^{64}Cu	.019614	.013000	^{228}Ac	.391080

(continued)

Table 8.6 Gamma (& X-Ray) Energies of Radionuclides of Interest to Health Physicists by Increasing Energy (Continued)

Energy (MeV)	Radio-nuclide	Probability per Decay	Energy (MeV)	Radio-nuclide	Probability per Decay	Energy (MeV)	Radio-nuclide	Probability per Decay
.013300	^{234}Th	.095655	.018251	^{99m}Tc	.021021	.028317	^{132}Te	.183060
.013300	^{231}Th	.707750	.018251	^{97}Ru	.200280	.028317	^{134}Te	.087667
.013300	^{237}Np	.591930	.018367	^{99m}Tc	.040194	.028612	^{133}Te	.011696
.013336	^{85}Sr	.170690	.018367	^{99}Mo	.017297	.028612	^{131}Te	.068516
.013336	^{88}Kr	.023716	.018367	^{97}Ru	.382940	.028612	^{133m}Te	.066455
.013395	^{85m}Kr	.011830	.018600	^{93m}Nb	.017835	.028612	^{132}Te	.340900
.013395	^{88}Kr	.045873	.018600	^{95m}Nb	.065281	.028612	^{131m}Te	.052738
.013395	^{85}Sr	.330150	.018600	^{93}Mo	.099947	.028612	^{134}Te	.163250
.013600	^{239}Pu	.044141	.020074	^{103m}Rh	.021995	.029373	^{237}Np	.139860
.013600	^{238}Pu	.115750	.020216	^{103m}Rh	.041815	.029458	^{131}I	.013468
.013600	^{244}Pu	.079317	.020600	^{99m}Tc	.012059	.029458	^{135m}Xe	.038443
.013600	^{233}Pu	.489200	.020600	^{97}Ru	.114890	.029458	^{131m}Xe	.154790
.013600	^{242}Pu	.091325	.021650	^{126}Sn	.012395	.029458	^{133m}Xe	.160100
.013600	^{240}Pu	.110120	.022700	^{103m}Rh	.013017	.029458	^{129}I	.199560
.013600	^{234}Pa	1.136300	.022984	^{111}In	.236280	.029700	^{126}Sn	.053387
.013850	^{140}Ba	.011730	.023174	^{111}In	.445810	.029779	^{131}I	.024987
.013900	^{241}Am	.427000	.023280	^{126}Sn	.064010	.029779	^{129}I	.370240
.013900	^{243}Am	.390500	.024002	^{113m}In	.068312	.029779	^{135m}Xe	.071324
.013900	^{240}U	.430940	.024210	^{113m}In	.128650	.029779	^{131m}Xe	.287180
.013900	^{237}U	.711390	.025640	^{231}Th	.146520	.029779	^{133m}Xe	.297040
.014098	^{87m}Sr	.029161	.026111	^{126}Sn	.083339	.029970	^{140}Ba	.140250
.014165	^{87m}Sr	.056296	.026100	^{111}In	.145970	.030625	^{135}Xe	.014461
.014300	^{246}Cm	.091830	.026345	^{237}U	.022774	.030625	^{138}Xe	.010265
.014300	^{244}Cm	.103070	.026345	^{241}Am	.024000	.030625	^{133}Xe	.136410
.014300	^{242}Cm	.115430	.026359	^{126}Sn	.156070	.030625	^{134m}Cs	.089498
.014300	^{242}Am	.126620	.027202	^{131m}Te	.035883	.030973	^{135}Xe	.026780
.014300	^{247}Cm	.059275	.027202	^{133m}Te	.014570	.030973	^{138}Xe	.019009
.014300	^{238}Np	.373890	.027202	^{125}Sb	.127890	.030973	^{133}Xe	.222620
.014300	^{248}Cm	.072670	.027202	^{127}Te	.104150	.030973	^{134m}Cs	.165740
.014300	^{243}Cm	.608090	.027202	^{129m}Te	.078797	.031000	^{131m}Te	.023239
.014300	^{239}Np	.617880	.027202	^{125}I	.392330	.031000	^{125m}Te	.209330
.014300	^{245}Cm	.636130	.027202	^{125m}Te	.323220	.031000	^{125}Sb	.082825
.014300	^{240}Np	1.094400	.027202	^{123}I	.246310	.031000	^{129m}Te	.051032
.014413	^{57}Co	.095429	.027300	^{113m}In	.042740	.031000	^{127m}Te	.067455
.014600	^{243}Pu	.118840	.027360	^{231}Pa	.093000	.031000	^{123}I	.159520
.014600	^{242m}Am	.299270	.027472	^{133m}Te	.027182	.031000	^{125}I	.254090
.014958	^{91m}Y	.016527	.027472	^{131m}Te	.066946	.031300	^{229}Th	.040800
.015000	^{88}Kr	.012039	.027472	^{127m}Te	.194320	.031817	^{137m}Ba	.020703
.015000	^{85}Sr	.086645	.027472	^{129m}Te	.147010	.031817	^{136}Cs	.049454
.015000	^{242}Am	.196510	.027472	^{125}Sb	.238600	.032194	^{137m}Ba	.038197
.015000	^{252}Cr	.072804	.027472	^{123}I	.459540	.032194	^{136}Cs	.091244
.015800	^{87m}Sr	.015126	.027472	^{125m}Te	.603020	.032300	^{133m}Te	.023288
.016521	^{93m}Nb	.032324	.027472	^{125}I	.731960	.032300	^{131m}Te	.018481
.016521	^{95m}Nb	.118310	.027513	^{88}Kr	.020622	.032300	^{131}Te	.024011
.016521	^{93}Mo	.181140	.027770	^{129}Te	.162590	.032300	^{134}Te	.057210
.016615	^{93m}Nb	.062041	.028317	^{131m}Te	.028320	.032300	^{132}Te	.119460
.016615	^{95m}Nb	.227090	.028317	^{131}Te	.036793	.033034	^{141}Ba	.019526
.016615	^{93}Mo	.347680	.028317	^{133m}Te	.035686	.033034	^{142}Ba	.055450

Table 8.6 Gamma (& X-Ray) Energies of Radionuclides of Interest to Health Physicists by Increasing Energy (Continued)

Energy (MeV)	Radio-nuclide	Probability per Decay	Energy (MeV)	Radio-nuclide	Probability per Decay	Energy (MeV)	Radio-nuclide	Probability per Decay
.033442	^{139}Ba	.017208	.043534	^{243}Am	.055440	.067412	^{61}Cu	.038745
.033442	^{141}Ba	.035959	.043800	^{147}Nd	.090554	.068804	^{197}Hg	.353600
.033442	^{142}Ba	.102120	.044100	^{240}U	.016500	.068895	^{201}Tl	.273570
.033600	^{135m}Xe	.025356	.045208	^{160}Tb	.060309	.069300	^{187}W	.056307
.033600	^{131m}Xe	.102100	.045297	^{155}Eu	.012916	.069672	^{153}Sm	.051700
.033600	^{133m}Xe	.105600	.045400	^{148m}Pm	.011745	.070819	^{198}Au	.013695
.033600	^{129}I	.131620	.045400	^{152}Eu	.146390	.070832	^{203}Hg	.047450
.035000	^{133}Xe	.090644	.045400	^{151}Pm	.056722	.070819	^{201}Tl	.465250
.035000	^{134m}Cs	.059470	.045998	^{160}Tb	.107890	.072060	^{187}W	.119070
.035492	^{125}Sb	.041649	.046503	^{210}Pb	.040500	.072804	^{208}Tl	.020311
.035492	^{125m}Te	.064900	.047000	^{153}Sm	.122170	.072804	^{209}Tl	.058804
.035492	^{125}I	.064900	.048221	^{166m}Ho	.108890	.072871	^{211}Bi	.012663
.035550	^{144}Ce	.024311	.048700	^{156}Eu	.027282	.072871	^{203}Hg	.080424
.035550	^{143}Ce	.176840	.048700	^{155}Eu	.046042	.074100	^{133m}Te	.013050
.035550	^{141}Ce	.048821	.048700	^{154}Eu	.051694	.074670	^{243}Am	.660000
.035550	^{144m}Pr	.086780	.049128	^{166m}Ho	.193410	.074815	^{212}Pb	.106940
.036026	^{144}Ce	.044525	.049720	^{132}Te	.131120	.074815	^{214}Pb	.062130
.036026	^{141}Ce	.089416	.049773	^{169}Yb	.527770	.074969	^{208}Tl	.034310
.036026	^{142}Ce	.323880	.050100	^{227}Th	.084000	.074969	^{209}Tl	.099331
.036026	^{144m}Pr	.158940	.050100	^{223}Fr	.316980	.075280	^{233}Pa	.012584
.036400	^{137m}Ba	.013900	.050742	^{169}Yb	.934110	.075700	^{192}Ir	.019675
.036400	^{136}Cs	.033205	.052100	^{160}Tb	.043227	.076862	^{213}Bi	.012519
.037800	^{141}Ba	.013205	.053226	^{214}Pb	.011054	.077108	^{214}Pb	.104600
.037800	^{142}Ba	.037501	.055700	^{166m}Ho	.078899	.077108	^{212}Pb	.180030
.038171	^{147}Nd	.129560	.056277	^{181}W	.186950	.077352	^{197}Hg	.185000
.038725	^{148m}Pm	.013241	.057365	^{143}Ce	.117600	.077600	^{142}Ba	.096120
.038725	^{147}Nd	.235570	.057500	^{169}Yb	.383010	.078000	^{197}Hg	.154690
.039522	^{148m}Pm	.016710	.057532	^{181}W	.326270	.079290	^{213}Bi	.020970
.039522	^{151}Pm	.080698	.059537	^{241}Am	.359000	.079445	^{134}Te	.210000
.039522	^{152}Eu	.208260	.059537	^{237}U	.340200	.079800	^{227}Th	.020000
.039581	^{129}I	.075200	.059718	^{187}W	.076022	.079800	^{223}Fr	.076075
.039857	^{212}Bi	.010225	.060010	^{155}Eu	.011124	.080106	^{144}Ce	.015984
.040000	^{225}Ra	.310000	.061140	^{187}W	.131750	.080183	^{121}I	.026182
.040118	^{148}Pm	.030271	.061487	^{192}Ir	.011323	.080300	^{201}Tl	.204650
.040118	^{152}Eu	.377280	.063000	^{234}Pa	.032640	.080589	^{166m}Ho	.127050
.040118	^{151}Pm	.146190	.063001	^{192}Ir	.019555	.080997	^{133}Xe	.364830
.040700	^{144}Ce	.016727	.063119	^{169}Yb	.437470	.081070	^{223}Ra	.148700
.040700	^{141}Ce	.033592	.063290	^{234}Th	.038116	.081140	^{131m}Te	.040682
.040700	^{144m}Pr	.059709	.064280	^{126}Sn	.095830	.081520	^{221}Fr	.012865
.040700	^{143}Ce	.121670	.064830	^{237}U	.011813	.082600	^{203}Hg	.035549
.040902	^{153}Sm	.172630	.064887	^{151}Pm	.019694	.083230	^{225}Ac	.010156
.041542	^{153}Sm	.312180	.065122	^{192}Ir	.026350	.083780	^{223}Ra	.247000
.042309	^{156}Eu	.038335	.065200	^{181}W	.137540	.084000	^{243}Pu	.230000
.042309	^{154}Eu	.072639	.065834	^{151}Pm	.011679	.084210	^{231}Th	.064350
.042309	^{155}Eu	.064697	.066050	^{75}Se	.010226	.084371	^{228}Th	.012100
.042996	^{154}Eu	.130880	.066832	^{192}Ir	.045197	.084900	^{209}Tl	.044120
.042996	^{155}Eu	.116570	.066910	^{136}Cs	.124630	.084900	^{208}Tl	.015239
.042996	^{156}Eu	.069073	.066989	^{197}Hg	.206860	.085430	^{223}Fr	.014713

(continued)

Table 8.6 Gamma (& X-Ray) Energies of Radionuclides of Interest to Health Physicists by Increasing Energy (Continued)

Energy (MeV)	Radio-nuclide	Probability per Decay	Energy (MeV)	Radio-nuclide	Probability per Decay	Energy (MeV)	Radio-nuclide	Probability per Decay
.085430	^{227}Th	.014069	.099550	^{243}Cm	.142860	.130520	^{169}Yb	.110580
.085430	^{229}Th	.164740	.099800	^{225}Ac	.017000	.131200	^{234}Pa	.204000
.086100	^{225}Ac	.016815	.099860	^{234}Pa	.048960	.133000	^{245}Cm	.062720
.086290	^{136}Cs	.062811	.100000	^{227}Th	.010615	.133540	^{144}Ce	.108000
.086440	^{229}Th	.030600	.100000	^{223}Fr	.011101	.134220	^{187}W	.094608
.086503	^{237}Np	.126000	.100000	^{229}Th	.124300	.135340	^{201}Tl	.026500
.086545	^{155}Eu	.309000	.100020	^{151}Pm	.025648	.135400	^{134}I	.037592
.086590	^{233}Pa	.018914	.101070	^{237}U	.263160	.136000	^{75}Se	.592020
.086788	^{160}Tb	.133000	.101930	^{151}Pm	.013053	.136480	^{57}Co	.106030
.086940	^{126}Sn	.089170	.102060	^{131m}Te	.079426	.137030	^{229}Th	.016320
.087300	^{214}Pb	.046683	.103180	^{153}Sm	.283000	.138100	^{138}Cs	.014879
.087300	^{212}Pb	.080351	.103760	^{247}Cm	.019318	.140510	^{99}Mo	.037888
.087570	^{126}Sn	.370000	.103760	^{239}Np	.236540	.140510	^{99m}Tc	.890700
.088000	^{133m}Te	.020880	.103760	^{240}Np	.137020	.142650	^{59}Fe	.010300
.088470	^{227}Th	.023178	.103760	^{242}Am	.058888	.143760	^{235}U	.105000
.088470	^{233}Fr	.024239	.103760	^{245}Cm	.218820	.144240	^{223}Ra	.032400
.088470	^{229}Th	.271400	.103760	^{243}Cm	.229680	.145440	^{141}Ce	.484000
.088964	^{156}Eu	.090480	.104840	^{151}Pm	.035495	.147200	^{240}Np	.013905
.089953	^{228}Ac	.021326	.105000	^{228}Ac	.016121	.148300	^{229}Th	.013872
.089953	^{235}U	.027289	.105000	^{235}U	.020629	.149200	^{105}Ru	.016700
.090884	^{231}Pa	.010186	.105310	^{155}Eu	.206720	.149720	^{131m}Te	.050755
.091106	^{147}Nd	.280000	.106130	^{239}Np	.227010	.149720	^{131}Te	.689000
.091266	^{67}Ga	.028560	.108000	^{237}Np	.011951	.151180	^{85m}Kr	.752780
.092287	^{237}Np	.015841	.109140	^{235}U	.015000	.152200	^{240}Np	.083430
.092380	^{234}Th	.027248	.109780	^{169}Yb	.173630	.152700	^{234}Pa	.068340
.092800	^{234}Th	.026884	.111000	^{234}Pa	.118480	.153220	^{136}Cs	.074576
.093311	^{67}Ga	.357000	.111000	^{233}Pa	.081809	.153750	^{138}Xe	.059535
.093350	^{228}Ac	.034846	.111760	^{132}Te	.018480	.154210	^{223}Ra	.055800
.093350	^{235}U	.044590	.114000	^{237}U	.123130	.156480	^{229}Th	.011220
.093613	^{169}Yb	.026578	.116300	^{132}Te	.019360	.159000	^{123}I	.834000
.094000	^{227}Th	.014000	.117000	^{242}Am	.027700	.159390	^{47}Sc	.680000
.094665	^{234}Pa	.156970	.117000	^{243}Cm	.108040	.162640	^{140}Ba	.067320
.094665	^{233}Pa	.108390	.117000	^{239}Np	.111270	.163350	^{235}U	.047000
.094900	^{223}Ra	.111980	.117000	^{245}Cm	.102930	.163590	^{151}Pm	.016259
.094900	^{133m}Te	.087000	.117000	^{240}Np	.064454	.163630	^{237}Np	.010470
.095868	^{237}Np	.025800	.117210	^{209}Tl	.770000	.163890	^{136}Cs	.046061
.096733	^{75}Se	.034086	.118190	^{169}Yb	.018818	.163930	^{131m}Xe	.019600
.097080	^{237}U	.162900	.121120	^{75}Se	.167440	.164340	^{133m}Te	.023490
.098439	^{233}Pa	.175670	.121780	^{152}Eu	.284320	.164610	^{237}U	.018617
.098439	^{234}Pa	.254420	.122060	^{57}Co	.855100	.165520	^{231}Pa	.014489
.098480	^{148m}Pm	.024741	.122320	^{223}Ra	.011900	.165850	^{139}Ba	.173600
.098860	^{240}Np	.050985	.123070	^{154}Eu	.404640	.165980	^{88}Kr	.031036
.099450	^{228}Ac	.013019	.124500	^{229}Th	.012240	.167430	^{201}Tl	.100000
.099550	^{242}Am	.036628	.125400	^{234}Pa	.010200	.167770	^{151}Pm	.087936
.099550	^{247}Cm	.012016	.127190	^{57}Ni	.129310	.168870	^{133m}Te	.114840
.099550	^{239}Np	.147130	.127240	^{101}Tc	.028168	.171280	^{111}In	.902400
.099550	^{240}Np	.085229	.127420	^{134m}Cs	.129000	.174000	^{245}Cm	.064000
.099550	^{245}Cm	.136110	.129080	^{228}Ac	.027700	.175000	^{240}Np	.060255

Table 8.6 Gamma (& X-Ray) Energies of Radionuclides of Interest to Health Physicists by Increasing Energy (Continued)

Energy (MeV)	Radio-nuclide	Probability per Decay	Energy (MeV)	Radio-nuclide	Probability per Decay	Energy (MeV)	Radio-nuclide	Probability per Decay
.175360	^{48}Sc	.074700	.220610	^{43}K	.041052	.274700	^{91}Sr	.010043
.176330	^{125}Sb	.068926	.221450	^{82}Br	.022577	.275210	^{151}Pm	.071677
.176550	^{136}Cs	.135590	.223800	^{126}Sb	.013947	.276990	^{141}Ba	.245920
.176820	^{142}Ba	.014774	.226400	^{234}Pa	.060180	.277350	^{208}Tl	.067864
.177100	^{133m}Te	.014790	.227200	^{234}Pa	.056100	.277600	^{239}Np	.141000
.177160	^{151}Pm	.038701	.227760	^{138}Cs	.015107	.277600	^{243}Cm	.139660
.177210	^{169}Yb	.214370	.228180	^{243}Cm	.105750	.277950	^{134}Te	.213000
.180890	^{134}Te	.180000	.228180	^{239}Np	.107160	.278000	^{247}Cm	.034000
.181060	^{99}Mo	.062336	.228160	^{132}Te	.880000	.278560	^{131m}Te	.017822
.183715	^{235}U	.540000	.231520	^{142}Ba	.101460	.278600	^{126}Sb	.023909
.184110	^{101}Tc	.016159	.231560	^{143}Ce	.020160	.279190	^{203}Hg	.773000
.184420	^{166m}Ho	.726000	.232420	^{151}Pm	.010534	.279530	^{75}Se	.252360
.184580	^{67}Ga	.197060	.233220	^{133m}Xe	.103000	.280450	^{166m}Ho	.296210
.184970	^{227}Th	.017273	.234900	^{223}Fr	.028211	.282960	^{61}Cu	.123000
.186000	^{234}Pa	.020400	.235470	^{134}I	.019845	.283670	^{231}Pa	.016000
.186210	^{226}Ra	.032800	.235690	^{95m}Np	.250430	.284300	^{131}I	.060521
.189630	^{148m}Pm	.011036	.236000	^{227}Th	.115000	.285900	^{149}Pm	.031000
.190220	^{141}Ba	.486000	.238630	^{212}Pb	.446460	.286100	^{227}Th	.016000
.192340	^{59}Fe	.031100	.240090	^{151}Pm	.038930	.287400	^{247}Cm	.020000
.192700	^{240}Np	.067671	.249930	^{131m}Te	.075939	.288110	^{148m}Pm	.125580
.193630	^{229}Th	.045900	.240980	^{224}Ra	.039500	.288450	^{135}I	.030899
.196320	^{88}Kr	.259850	.241520	^{92}Sr	.029700	.292050	^{223}Ra	.013533
.197040	^{160}Tb	.049020	.241980	^{214}Pb	.074913	.293260	^{143}Ce	.420000
.197950	^{169}Yb	.349200	.242560	^{138}Xe	.034965	.293700	^{234}Pa	.039780
.198600	^{75}Se	.014472	.244690	^{152}Eu	.074935	.295210	^{214}Pb	.192470
.200630	^{131m}Te	.075552	.245390	^{111}Ag	.012291	.295960	^{192}Ir	.290150
.200980	^{234}Pa	.011220	.245390	^{111}In	.940000	.296500	^{126}Sb	.044829
.201240	^{134}Te	.087000	.247940	^{154}Eu	.066021	.298570	^{169}Tb	.270750
.202120	^{235}U	.010000	.248900	^{234}Pa	.028560	.299800	^{227}Th	.018400
.203000	^{234}Pa	.012240	.249790	^{135}Xe	.899000	.300080	^{231}Pa	.023000
.205000	^{223}Fr	.010777	.254150	^{97}Zr	.012533	.300090	^{212}Pb	.034067
.205310	^{235}U	.047000	.255120	^{142}Ba	.178000	.300120	^{233}Pa	.066392
.205800	^{192}Ir	.032873	.256200	^{227}Th	.063000	.300220	^{67}Ga	.159940
.208010	^{237}U	.220190	.258310	^{138}Xe	.315000	.300740	^{166m}Ho	.037171
.208950	^{67}Ga	.022420	.259720	^{166m}Ho	.010527	.302670	^{231}Pa	.023000
.209010	^{151}Pm	.017862	.261070	^{169}Yb	.017654	.303910	^{75}Se	.013216
.209280	^{228}Ac	.044320	.261550	^{133m}Te	.156600	.304240	^{141}Ba	.265840
.209750	^{239}Np	.032430	.262700	^{132}I	.014410	.304400	^{227}Th	.013500
.209750	^{243}Cm	.032921	.262900	^{105}Ru	.072000	.304840	^{140}Ba	.045058
.210470	^{134}Te	.219000	.264650	^{75}Se	.598000	.304870	^{85m}Kr	.139890
.210600	^{227}Th	.012600	.266900	^{93}Y	.068502	.306100	^{105}Rh	.051264
.210970	^{229}Th	.032640	.269460	^{223}Ra	.136000	.306810	^{101}Tc	.883000
.213360	^{133m}Te	.028710	.270230	^{228}Ac	.036010	.307000	^{240}Np	.013905
.215650	^{160}Tb	.037145	.270800	^{240}Np	.083430	.307730	^{169}Yb	.108060
.215680	^{97}Ru	.855000	.271230	^{219}Rn	.106000	.308460	^{192}Ir	.296780
.215880	^{166m}Ho	.025700	.272100	^{234}Pa	.010200	.309020	^{142}Ba	.022606
.217600	^{221}Fr	.125000	.272450	^{89}Rb	.014152	.311630	^{148m}Pm	.039159
.220500	^{135}I	.017452	.273650	^{136}Cs	.126620	.311980	^{233}Pa	.386000

(continued)

Table 8.6 Gamma (& X-Ray) Energies of Radionuclides of Interest to Health Physicists by Increasing Energy (Continued)

Energy (MeV)	Radio-nuclide	Probability per Decay	Energy (MeV)	Radio-nuclide	Probability per Decay	Energy (MeV)	Radio-nuclide	Probability per Decay
.311990	^{133}Te	.708000	.372400	^{234}Pa	.013260	.439900	^{147}Nd	.012040
.315880	^{239}Np	.015933	.372760	^{43}K	.872730	.440420	^{213}Bi	.279670
.316500	^{105}Ru	.117000	.373050	^{61}Cu	.021156	.440880	^{151}Pm	.015343
.316510	^{192}Ir	.828530	.377740	^{52m}Mn	.016828	.443980	^{152}Eu	.028114
.318900	^{105}Rh	.192000	.380440	^{125}Sb	.014958	.444900	^{133m}Te	.022620
.319410	^{147}Nd	.019600	.388400	^{87m}Sr	.822530	.445030	^{223}Ra	.011800
.320080	^{51}Cr	.098300	.389780	^{141}Ba	.013948	.445690	^{151}Pm	.040762
.323870	^{223}Ra	.038800	.391690	^{113m}In	.649000	.446800	^{110m}Ag	.036434
.323950	^{151}Pm	.012137	.392490	^{160}Tb	.012825	.448200	^{240}Np	.166860
.324480	^{97}Ru	.108590	.393400	^{105}Ru	.042000	.448500	^{92}Y	.023352
.326100	^{105}Ru	.011800	.393530	^{67}Ga	.044768	.451520	^{166m}Ho	.029185
.327640	^{228}Ac	.032132	.396430	^{138}Xe	.063000	.452320	^{131m}Te	.015498
.328770	^{140}La	.205300	.396870	^{43}K	.114310	.452320	^{131}Te	.182240
.329700	^{227}Th	.029000	.396960	^{133m}Te	.014790	.457580	^{141}Ba	.050544
.330070	^{231}Pa	.013000	.398620	^{233}Pa	.012738	.458800	^{234}Pa	.015300
.331900	^{125}Sn	.012900	.400650	^{75}Se	.114220	.458920	^{134}I	.012976
.332350	^{237}U	.012191	.401360	^{138}Xe	.021735	.459600	^{129}Te	.071000
.334140	^{133m}Te	.054340	.401810	^{219}Rn	.065000	.461000	^{134}Te	.108000
.334200	^{227}Th	.011500	.402580	^{87}Kr	.495000	.462110	^{133m}Te	.020010
.334270	^{131m}Te	.095699	.402600	^{247}Cm	.720000	.462150	^{141}Ba	.050544
.334300	^{239}Np	.020304	.404840	^{21}Pb	.029400	.462200	^{240}Np	.013905
.334800	^{142}Ba	.012460	.405450	^{134}I	.073466	.462790	^{138}Cs	.307490
.338280	^{223}Ra	.027300	.407630	^{133}Te	.300900	.462920	^{131m}Te	.018210
.338320	^{228}Ac	.113570	.408980	^{138}Cs	.046619	.463000	^{228}Ac	.044320
.340080	^{151}Pm	.229000	.409510	^{228}Ac	.021329	.463380	^{125}Sb	.103530
.340500	^{233}Pa	.045162	.410940	^{166m}Ho	.111080	.464640	^{134}Te	.051000
.340570	^{136}Cs	.484540	.411110	^{152}Eu	.022144	.464830	^{166m}Ho	.011979
.342130	^{111}Ag	.066800	.411800	^{198}Au	.955100	.465070	^{209}Tl	.965800
.343710	^{141}Ba	.150170	.413500	^{105}Ru	.024800	.467260	^{141}Ba	.057834
.344270	^{152}Eu	.264880	.414070	^{148m}Pm	.186630	.467400	^{240}Np	.020394
.344500	^{133m}Te	.022620	.414700	^{126}Sb	.832810	.468070	^{192}Ir	.480550
.344910	^{151}Pm	.021755	.415760	^{233}Pa	.016212	.469400	^{105}Ru	.175000
.346000	^{247}Cm	.013000	.417630	^{135}I	.035190	.469700	^{125}Sn	.012900
.347200	^{133m}Te	.011310	.418010	^{130}I	.341550	.470000	^{105}Ru	.013000
.350200	^{105}Ru	.011000	.423700	^{140}Ba	.032461	.471850	^{133m}Te	.020010
.350590	^{143}Ce	.033600	.425030	^{142}Ba	.049840	.474720	^{133}Te	.012036
.351070	^{211}Bi	.129450	.427080	^{211}Pb	.013230	.475350	^{134}Cs	.014600
.351920	^{214}Pb	.372100	.427890	^{125}Sb	.293300	.477590	^{7}Be	.104200
.355390	^{97}Zr	.022746	.428810	^{151}Pm	.043579	.478590	^{133m}Te	.015660
.355570	^{133m}Te	.014790	.429020	^{133m}Te	.012180	.479530	^{187}W	.233520
.362230	^{88}Kr	.022490	.430560	^{92}Sr	.033300	.482030	^{223}Fr	.012278
.363800	^{142}Ba	.039160	.432530	^{140}La	.029411	.484580	^{192}Ir	.031628
.364480	^{131}I	.811640	.432780	^{148m}Pm	.053488	.487030	^{140}La	.455490
.364980	^{131m}Te	.012011	.433350	^{134}I	.041885	.487390	^{129}Te	.013064
.365780	^{166m}Ho	.024176	.434490	^{138}Xe	.203180	.488880	^{134}I	.014121
.366270	^{65}Ni	.046060	.435060	^{134}Te	.186000	.489230	^{47}Ca	.067410
.366430	^{99}Mo	.013696	.435400	^{133m}Te	.010440	.490360	^{143}Ce	.019740
.369800	^{234}Pa	.029580	.437550	^{140}Ba	.019941	.492660	^{131}Te	.048368

Table 8.6 Gamma (& X-Ray) Energies of Radionuclides of Interest to Health Physicists by Increasing Energy (Continued)

Energy (MeV)	Radio-nuclide	Probability per Decay	Energy (MeV)	Radio-nuclide	Probability per Decay	Energy (MeV)	Radio-nuclide	Probability per Decay
.497080	^{103}Ru	.889000	.555200	^{126}Sb	.016935	.619070	^{82}Br	.430710
.499200	^{105}Ru	.024000	.557570	^{91m}Y	.950800	.620100	^{91}Sr	.017225
.501260	^{148m}Pm	.067461	.561100	^{92}Y	.024047	.620350	^{110m}Ag	.027656
.505900	^{132}I	.050337	.563230	^{134}Cs	.083800	.621200	^{132}I	.015792
.506800	^{234}Pa	.016320	.565900	^{234}Pa	.014280	.621790	^{134}I	.105910
.507200	^{240}Np	.018540	.565990	^{134}Te	.189000	.621840	^{106}Rh	.098056
.507630	^{97}Zr	.052919	.566400	^{240}Np	.268830	.622030	^{133m}Te	.013920
.510530	^{133}I	.018127	.568700	^{234}Pa	.030600	.625230	^{141}Ba	.034506
.510840	^{208}Tl	.215570	.569320	^{134}Cs	.154300	.625520	^{187}W	.011630
.511000	^{65}Zn	.028300	.569500	^{234}Pa	.109140	.627960	^{134}I	.023662
.511000	^{56}Co	.395000	.571000	^{166m}Ho	.054668	.629970	^{148m}Pm	.889980
.511000	^{58}Co	.298600	.573800	^{126}Sb	.066745	.630220	^{132}I	.137190
.511000	^{64}Cu	.357400	.574000	^{234}Pa	.020400	.631940	^{131m}Te	.035532
.511000	^{13}N	1.996100	.574040	^{133m}Te	.023490	.635890	^{125}Sb	.113210
.511000	^{18}F	1.934600	.575300	^{105}Ru	.010700	.636230	^{151}Pm	.014656
.511000	^{22}Na	1.798000	.578090	^{142}La	.013650	.636260	^{134}Te	.017100
.511000	^{61}Cu	1.229100	.583140	^{208}Tl	.842310	.636970	^{131}I	.072605
.511000	^{44}Sc	1.887400	.586050	^{130}I	.016929	.641170	^{142}La	.525000
.511000	^{52m}Mn	1.932300	.586300	^{131m}Te	.019760	.645850	^{124}Sb	.072620
.511000	^{48}V	1.002000	.588580	^{192}Ir	.045735	.646290	^{156}Eu	.070928
.511000	^{11}C	1.995300	.588600	^{61}Cu	.011808	.647400	^{133m}Te	.293190
.511000	^{15}O	1.998000	.591810	^{154}Eu	.048273	.647880	^{141}Ba	.059292
.511000	^{57}Ni	.801600	.593000	^{126}Sb	.074714	.650600	^{132}I	.026649
.511000	^{52}Mn	.588000	.593400	^{43}K	.110330	.652300	^{91}Sr	.028925
.511850	^{206}Rh	.206000	.595360	^{134}I	.113540	.652900	^{91}Sr	.078000
.513700	^{234}Pa	.013260	.599470	^{156}Eu	.023088	.654260	^{131}Te	.015296
.513990	^{85}Sr	.992700	.599740	^{148m}Pm	.125400	.656010	^{61}Cu	.104920
.514400	^{134}I	.023375	.599840	^{142}Ba	.016020	.656100	^{105}Ru	.024000
.522650	^{132}I	.160880	.600560	^{125}Sb	.177740	.656300	^{126}Sb	.021916
.526560	^{135m}Xe	.809970	.601100	^{240}Np	.203940	.657710	^{89}Rb	.099760
.528960	^{123}I	.013928	.602040	^{131}Te	.041960	.657750	^{110}Ag	.044865
.529810	^{166m}Ho	.095106	.602520	^{97}Zr	.013926	.657750	^{110m}Ag	.943880
.529870	^{133}I	.863200	.602710	^{124}Sb	.978700	.657900	^{97}Nb	.980900
.531020	^{147}Nd	.131320	.604410	^{192}Ir	.082024	.661650	^{137m}Ba	.899800
.531490	^{101}Tc	.010243	.604700	^{134}Cs	.976000	.664550	^{143}Ce	.052500
.534850	^{133m}Te	.017400	.604800	^{84}Br	.017724	.664800	^{234}Pa	.013260
.536090	^{130}I	.990000	.606100	^{240}Np	.015759	.665050	^{131m}Te	.043394
.537320	^{140}Ba	.255000	.606300	^{82}Br	.011663	.665450	^{214}Bi	.015690
.539100	^{130}I	.013959	.606640	^{125}Sb	.050213	.665850	^{134}Te	.012000
.540830	^{134}I	.078236	.608190	^{135}Xe	.028948	.666330	^{126}Sb	.996190
.545140	^{101}Tc	.060044	.609310	^{214}Bi	.462810	.666700	^{234}Pa	.016320
.546560	^{135}I	.071239	.610330	^{103}Ru	.056007	.667690	^{132}I	.987000
.546940	^{138}Cs	.107580	.611260	^{148}Pm	.010212	.668540	^{130}I	.961290
.547100	^{132}I	.012535	.611260	^{148m}Pm	.054823	.669800	^{132}I	.049350
.550270	^{148}Pm	.220000	.611520	^{166m}Ho	.014157	.669900	^{234}Pa	.014280
.550270	^{148m}Pm	.948720	.612460	^{192}Ir	.053357	.670510	^{166m}Ho	.053506
.551550	^{187}W	.054365	.617490	^{43}K	.805140	.671410	^{125}Sb	.018126
.554320	^{82}Br	.705640	.618370	^{187}W	.067102	.671600	^{132}I	.052311

(continued)

Table 8.6 Gamma (& X-Ray) Energies of Radionuclides of Interest to Health Physicists by Increasing Energy (Continued)

Energy (MeV)	Radio-nuclide	Probability per Decay	Energy (MeV)	Radio-nuclide	Probability per Decay	Energy (MeV)	Radio-nuclide	Probability per Decay
.673870	^{87}Kr	.019058	.733000	^{234}Pa	.087720	.795840	^{134}Cs	.854000
.675000	^{126}Sb	.036859	.733890	^{133m}Te	.028710	.796300	^{234}Pa	.038760
.675890	^{198}Au	.010602	.736500	^{84}Br	.013082	.800510	^{133m}Te	.019140
.676400	^{105}Ru	.167000	.738000	^{234}Pa	.010200	.801930	^{134}Cs	.087300
.677340	^{134}I	.084915	.739100	^{141}Ba	.045198	.802200	^{84}Br	.060768
.677610	^{110m}Ag	.106750	.739480	^{130}I	.822690	.805600	^{234}Pa	.033660
.685810	^{187}W	.291670	.739580	^{99}Mo	.128000	.806170	^{214}Bi	.012335
.685990	^{130}I	.010692	.742590	^{134}Te	.147000	.807860	^{47}Ca	.068908
.686990	^{110m}Ag	.064656	.742810	^{234}Pa	.024480	.809800	^{132}I	.028623
.691210	^{166m}Ho	.013576	.743360	^{97m}Nb	.979600	.810310	^{166m}Ho	.571360
.692410	^{154}Eu	.016931	.744200	^{131m}Te	.015885	.810760	^{58}Co	.994300
.692700	^{234}Pa	.015300	.744210	^{52}Mn	.900000	.811770	^{156}Eu	.104000
.694700	^{101}Tc	.011479	.744260	^{110m}Ag	.046439	.812200	^{132}I	.056259
.695000	^{126}Sb	.996190	.749800	^{91}Sr	.229780	.815850	^{140}La	.234910
.695880	^{129m}Te	.032716	.751790	^{140}La	.044021	.818020	^{110m}Ag	.072773
.696010	^{131}Te	.011932	.752270	^{166m}Ho	.120520	.818500	^{136}Cs	.997000
.696490	^{144}Pr	.014800	.752830	^{151}Pm	.013282	.819600	^{234}Pa	.026520
.697000	^{126}Sb	.288900	.755180	^{228}Ac	.010526	.822600	^{125}Sn	.037840
.698330	^{82}Br	.281590	.755600	^{234}Pa	.014280	.822780	^{131m}Te	.061216
.699000	^{234}Pa	.046920	.756710	^{95}Zr	.553450	.826300	^{234}Pa	.040800
.702750	^{133m}Te	.037410	.756870	^{154}Eu	.043304	.827810	^{82}Br	.241600
.706100	^{234}Pa	.031620	.763130	^{208}Tl	.016367	.830560	^{166m}Ho	.096558
.706580	^{133}I	.014933	.763930	^{110m}Ag	.222760	.831600	^{234}Pa	.056100
.706670	^{110m}Ag	.166780	.765280	^{160}Tb	.019285	.831720	^{141}Ba	.015989
.707360	^{105}Ru	.012810	.766680	^{134}I	.041026	.831960	^{211}Pb	.028616
.709310	^{124}Sb	.014191	.767200	^{134}Te	.300000	.834830	^{88}Kr	.129750
.710540	^{154}Eu	.015850	.768360	^{214}Bi	.050425	.834830	^{54}Mn	.999760
.711690	^{166m}Ho	.540870	.772170	^{228}Ac	.015512	.835500	^{228}Ac	.017451
.712970	^{134}Te	.042000	.772610	^{132}I	.761960	.836800	^{135}I	.066661
.713100	^{131m}Te	.014335	.772870	^{187}W	.044027	.840230	^{142}Ba	.030260
.713820	^{124}Sb	.023782	.773670	^{131m}Te	.382020	.844060	^{134}Te	.012000
.717750	^{151}Pm	.041220	.776340	^{91}Sr	.011908	.844300	^{92}Y	.012510
.719650	^{133}Te	.066552	.776490	^{82}Br	.833100	.844390	^{133}Te	.032568
.720500	^{126}Sb	.537940	.778000	^{99}Mo	.044800	.845430	^{87}Kr	.072765
.721960	^{143}Ce	.051240	.778820	^{166m}Ho	.030274	.846750	^{56}Co	.999580
.722780	^{124}Sb	.110980	.778890	^{152}Eu	.127410	.846750	^{56}Mn	.988700
.722890	^{131}I	.018025	.779750	^{133m}Te	.033930	.847000	^{240}Np	.046350
.723300	^{154}Eu	.197000	.780200	^{132}I	.012338	.847020	^{134}I	.954100
.723470	^{156}Eu	.060216	.780700	^{234}Pa	.011220	.848130	^{52}Mn	.033200
.724180	^{95}Zr	.436560	.782490	^{131m}Te	.077876	.852210	^{131m}Te	.206510
.724500	^{105}Ru	.490000	.785460	^{212}Bi	.019694	.856280	^{133}I	.012344
.725700	^{148m}Pm	.328400	.785910	^{214}Pb	.010956	.856800	^{126}Sb	.176330
.727000	^{132}I	.031584	.786270	^{234}Pa	.014280	.857290	^{134}I	.069649
.727170	^{212}Bi	.118290	.786770	^{133}Te	.055932	.860370	^{208}Tl	.124550
.727200	^{132}I	.021714	.793600	^{234}Pa	.015300	.861570	^{142}La	.019950
.728500	^{132}I	.010857	.793750	^{131m}Te	.138700	.863910	^{133m}Te	.194880
.730740	^{134}I	.019082	.794700	^{228}Ac	.046259	.867010	^{156}Eu	.014040
.731690	^{133m}Te	.014790	.795700	^{133m}Te	.013050	.867320	^{152}Eu	.041601

Table 8.6 Gamma (& X-Ray) Energies of Radionuclides of Interest to Health Physicists by Increasing Energy (Continued)

Energy (MeV)	Radio-nuclide	Probability per Decay	Energy (MeV)	Radio-nuclide	Probability per Decay	Energy (MeV)	Radio-nuclide	Probability per Decay
.867400	^{240}Np	.083430	.935520	^{52}Mn	.945000	1.004800	^{154}Eu	.178890
.867820	^{140}La	.056339	.937480	^{110m}Ag	.341870	1.007500	^{133m}Te	.010440
.871800	^{138}Cs	.051121	.944100	^{48}V	.077600	1.007600	^{82}Br	.012680
.873190	^{154}Eu	.115000	.944350	^{156}Eu	.013936	1.009800	^{138}Cs	.298330
.875330	^{133}I	.044714	.946000	^{234}Pa	.122400	1.011400	^{142}La	.043575
.875800	^{105}Ru	.034000	.947100	^{93}Y	.019502	1.013800	^{148m}Pm	.202830
.876290	^{141}Ba	.035964	.947690	^{89}Rb	.092220	1.014600	^{132}I	.031946
.876400	^{234}Pa	.040800	.947770	^{228}Ac	.041168	1.015900	^{84}Br	.062456
.876800	^{132}I	.010758	.947860	^{134}I	.040358	1.021100	^{133}Te	.026904
.879360	^{160}Tb	.285000	.948540	^{131}Te	.022599	1.021300	^{97}Zr	.012069
.880500	^{234}Pa	.010200	.948750	^{142}Ba	.089000	1.021800	^{43}K	.018787
.880510	^{234}Pa	.122400	.949000	^{234}Pa	.081600	1.024300	^{91}Sr	.325000
.881500	^{84}Br	.422000	.950940	^{166m}Ho	.026935	1.024500	^{97}Nb	.010790
.882830	^{133m}Te	.056550	.953320	^{92}Sr	.036000	1.025900	^{238}Np	.082110
.883240	^{234}Pa	.122400	.954000	^{126}Sb	.011954	1.028500	^{238}Np	.173740
.884090	^{134}I	.652600	.954550	^{132}I	.180620	1.029800	^{133m}Te	.013050
.884670	^{110m}Ag	.725840	.955590	^{234}Pa	.010099	1.031900	^{89}Rb	.580000
.884900	^{240}Np	.037080	.959100	^{240}Np	.023175	1.037500	^{48}Sc	.975000
.888800	^{240}Np	.011124	.960500	^{156}Eu	.016224	1.037800	^{56}Co	.140340
.889250	^{46}Sc	.999840	.962290	^{160}Tb	.090250	1.038600	^{134}Cs	.010000
.894850	^{142}La	.093975	.964010	^{152}Eu	.144410	1.038800	^{135}I	.079250
.894900	^{142}Ba	.110360	.964600	^{228}Ac	.052076	1.040300	^{134}I	.019082
.896500	^{240}Np	.129780	.966150	^{160}Tb	.242250	1.043700	^{142}La	.030450
.898020	^{88}Rb	.140380	.968200	^{124}Sb	.019183	1.044000	^{82}Br	.273260
.899000	^{234}Pa	.041820	.969110	^{228}Ac	.166200	1.045200	^{124}Sb	.018595
.908630	^{61}Cu	.011931	.969400	^{105}Ru	.023400	1.048100	^{136}Cs	.795610
.910000	^{131m}Te	.032933	.972610	^{135}I	.012016	1.050500	^{106}Rh	.017304
.911070	^{228}Ac	.277000	.973900	^{240}Np	.213210	1.059700	^{131m}Te	.015498
.912580	^{133m}Te	.870000	.974670	^{134}I	.046751	1.061800	^{133}Te	.012744
.914720	^{133m}Te	.165300	.977420	^{56}Co	.014254	1.065100	^{156}Eu	.052416
.914850	^{148}Pm	.114550	.978190	^{133m}Te	.094830	1.066600	^{125}Sn	.086000
.915330	^{148m}Pm	.171680	.978800	^{234}Pa	.014280	1.072600	^{134}I	.152660
.915500	^{125}Sn	.037840	.980400	^{133m}Te	.023490	1.073400	^{135}I	.014948
.915980	^{240}Np	.013905	.980500	^{234}Pa	.030600	1.078500	^{142}Ba	.092560
.919630	^{140}La	.028838	.980500	^{234}Pa	.020400	1.079200	^{156}Eu	.048880
.920620	^{131m}Te	.012011	.982900	^{133m}Te	.011310	1.085800	^{152}Eu	.099630
.923980	^{238}Np	.024752	.983500	^{48}Sc	1.000000	1.088900	^{125}Sn	.040420
.925000	^{234}Pa	.029580	.983500	^{48}V	1.000000	1.089700	^{152}Eu	.016793
.925240	^{140}La	.070854	.984000	^{234}Pa	.019380	1.093600	^{142}Ba	.022072
.925550	^{134}Te	.016500	.984450	^{238}Np	.238000	1.099200	^{59}Fe	.565000
.925800	^{91}Sr	.037375	.985780	^{88}Kr	.013148	1.101600	^{135}I	.016022
.926000	^{234}Pa	.112200	.987760	^{240}Np	.046350	1.102700	^{156}Eu	.015851
.926720	^{234}Pa	.091800	.989300	^{126}Sb	.067741	1.112000	^{152}Eu	.133020
.930670	^{133}Te	.044604	.996320	^{154}Eu	.102940	1.114300	^{138}Xe	.014742
.933840	^{115m}Cd	.013300	.997250	^{131}Te	.033416	1.115100	^{160}Tb	.015010
.934060	^{214}Bi	.032071	1.000100	^{88}Kr	.018892	1.115500	^{65}Zn	.507500
.934400	^{133m}Te	.013050	1.000800	^{133}Te	.062304	1.115500	^{65}Ni	.148290
.934460	^{92}Y	.139000	1.000900	^{142}Ba	.078320	1.118600	^{138}Xe	.026586

(continued)

Table 8.6 Gamma (& X-Ray) Energies of Radionuclides of Interest to Health Physicists by Increasing Energy (Continued)

Energy (MeV)	Radio-nuclide	Probability per Decay	Energy (MeV)	Radio-nuclide	Probability per Decay	Energy (MeV)	Radio-nuclide	Probability per Decay
1.120300	^{214}Bi	.151470	1.248100	^{89}Rb	.423400	1.408000	^{152}Eu	.207470
1.120500	^{46}Sc	.999870	1.250700	^{88}Kr	.011210	1.434100	^{52}Mn	1.000000
1.124000	^{135}I	.036049	1.252000	^{141}Ba	.017302	1.434100	^{52m}Mn	.982230
1.125500	^{131m}Te	.114300	1.252200	^{133}Te	.011328	1.435900	^{138}Cs	.763000
1.126500	^{142}Ba	.015308	1.260400	^{135}I	.286100	1.436600	^{124}Sb	.011353
1.131500	^{135}I	.225160	1.271900	^{160}Tb	.070300	1.442600	^{132}I	.014213
1.136000	^{132}I	.029610	1.274500	^{154}Eu	.354950	1.452700	^{234}Pa	.010200
1.136200	^{134}I	.097318	1.274500	^{22}Na	.999400	1.455200	^{134}I	.022898
1.141300	^{88}Kr	.012837	1.277400	^{156}Eu	.032136	1.457600	^{135}I	.086402
1.142300	^{92}Sr	.028800	1.281000	^{214}Bi	.014802	1.459100	^{133m}Te	.021750
1.143400	^{132}I	.013522	1.290700	^{132}I	.011351	1.463800	^{84}Br	.019834
1.147000	^{131}Te	.049608	1.291600	^{59}Fe	.432000	1.465100	^{148}Pm	.222000
1.147200	^{138}Cs	.012437	1.293600	^{41}Ar	.991600	1.474800	^{82}Br	.165790
1.148000	^{97}Zr	.026459	1.295300	^{132}I	.019740	1.475800	^{110m}Ag	.040020
1.148900	^{131m}Te	.015110	1.297100	^{47}Ca	.749000	1.481800	^{65}Ni	.235000
1.153500	^{156}Eu	.071760	1.298200	^{133}I	.023306	1.502800	^{135}I	.010729
1.154100	^{156}Eu	.053040	1.299000	^{152}Eu	.016052	1.505000	^{110m}Ag	.130630
1.155200	^{214}Bi	.016973	1.312100	^{48}V	.975000	1.509200	^{214}Bi	.022203
1.157000	^{44}Sc	.998810	1.312100	^{48}Sc	1.000000	1.518400	^{88}Kr	.021521
1.157500	^{130}I	.113060	1.312200	^{160}Tb	.028500	1.524700	^{42}K	.179000
1.158000	^{214}Bi	.035073	1.317500	^{82}Br	.269090	1.529800	^{88}Kr	.109340
1.160200	^{142}La	.019425	1.325500	^{124}Sb	.014974	1.538100	^{89}Rb	.025520
1.167600	^{240}Np	.046350	1.332500	^{60}Co	1.000000	1.545800	^{142}La	.033075
1.167900	^{134}Cs	.018000	1.333200	^{133}Te	.099120	1.562300	^{110m}Ag	.011798
1.173200	^{132}I	.010857	1.333600	^{52}Mn	.050700	1.566400	^{135}I	.012875
1.173200	^{60}Co	1.000000	1.343600	^{138}Cs	.011445	1.567000	^{209}Tl	.996890
1.175100	^{56}Co	.022790	1.348900	^{133m}Te	.025230	1.588000	^{228}Ac	.035456
1.175400	^{87}Kr	.011237	1.353300	^{234}Pa	.017340	1.593000	^{154}Eu	.010294
1.177900	^{160}Tb	.144400	1.354500	^{141}La	.026200	1.596500	^{154}Eu	.018457
1.185200	^{61}Cu	.036285	1.360200	^{56}Co	.042882	1.596500	^{140}La	.954900
1.197500	^{141}Ba	.048600	1.362700	^{97}Zr	.013462	1.613200	^{138}Cs	.016214
1.199900	^{160}Tb	.023560	1.363000	^{142}La	.023625	1.613800	^{134}I	.043602
1.202200	^{142}Ba	.053400	1.365200	^{134}Cs	.030400	1.620600	^{212}Bi	.027495
1.204100	^{142}Ba	.137060	1.366400	^{156}Eu	.017576	1.630400	^{228}Ac	.018614
1.206600	^{131m}Te	.097636	1.368200	^{124}Sb	.025055	1.646000	^{131m}Te	.012398
1.208300	^{124}Sb	.013366	1.368500	^{24}Na	.999990	1.661300	^{214}Bi	.011545
1.212800	^{48}Sc	.023800	1.369500	^{88}Kr	.014774	1.668500	^{234}Pa	.012240
1.212800	^{152}Eu	.013805	1.372100	^{132}I	.024675	1.678000	^{135}I	.095271
1.213000	^{126}Sb	.023909	1.377600	^{57}Ni	.779000	1.682400	^{141}Ba	.014143
1.213300	^{84}Br	.026164	1.377700	^{214}Bi	.041051	1.683300	^{133m}Te	.057420
1.230700	^{156}Eu	.089440	1.379900	^{142}Ba	.033998	1.691000	^{124}Sb	.490330
1.233100	^{142}La	.020475	1.383900	^{92}Sr	.900000	1.694600	^{234}Pa	.012240
1.235300	^{136}Cs	.197410	1.384300	^{110m}Ag	.242580	1.706500	^{135}I	.040912
1.236400	^{133}I	.014933	1.394100	^{234}Pa	.030600	1.717700	^{133}Te	.033984
1.238100	^{214}Bi	.059405	1.398600	^{132}I	.071064	1.722900	^{142}La	.016800
1.238300	^{56}Co	.669720	1.401500	^{214}Bi	.013914	1.729600	^{214}Bi	.029702
1.242400	^{156}Eu	.067600	1.405400	^{92}Y	.047816	1.740500	^{87}Kr	.020493
1.246200	^{52}Mn	.042100	1.408000	^{214}Bi	.024867	1.741200	^{84}Br	.016458

Table 8.6 Gamma (& X-Ray) Energies of Radionuclides of Interest to Health Physicists by Increasing Energy (Continued)

Energy (MeV)	Radio-nuclide	Probability per Decay	Energy (MeV)	Radio-nuclide	Probability per Decay	Energy (MeV)	Radio-nuclide	Probability per Decay
1.741500	^{134}I	.026715	2.004900	^{133m}Te	.033060	2.269900	^{156}Eu	.011232
1.750500	^{97}Zr	.013462	2.007500	^{89}Rb	.023780	2.392100	^{88}Kr	.346000
1.756400	^{142}La	.033075	2.011900	^{87}Kr	.028957	2.397000	^{142}La	.162750
1.757500	^{57}Ni	.070889	2.015400	^{56}Co	.030287	2.447900	^{214}Bi	.015591
1.764500	^{214}Bi	.158380	2.015800	^{138}Xe	.122540	2.484100	^{84}Br	.067520
1.768300	^{138}Xe	.167270	2.025500	^{142}La	.013650	2.521700	^{140}La	.034567
1.771400	^{56}Co	.155130	2.026600	^{156}Eu	.035360	2.542700	^{142}La	.112350
1.787200	^{134}I	.013348	2.027700	^{133m}Te	.020880	2.554800	^{87}Kr	.093060
1.791200	^{135}I	.076961	2.029600	^{84}Br	.021100	2.558100	^{87}K	.039105
1.806800	^{134}I	.057246	2.029800	^{88}Kr	.045291	2.570100	^{89}Rb	.098600
1.810700	^{56}Mn	.271890	2.034900	^{56}Co	.077767	2.598500	^{56}Co	.168930
1.836000	^{88}Rb	.214000	2.035400	^{88}Kr	.037368	2.614700	^{208}Tl	.998000
1.847400	^{214}Bi	.020920	2.038700	^{142}La	.011025	2.639600	^{138}Cs	.076300
1.850900	^{138}Xe	.014238	2.049200	^{133m}Te	.010440	2.666800	^{142}La	.018900
1.877000	^{156}Eu	.017264	2.055200	^{142}La	.029400	2.677900	^{88}Rb	.019581
1.877500	^{84}Br	.011394	2.079200	^{138}Xe	.014427	2.707200	^{89}Rb	.020300
1.881500	^{133}Te	.014160	2.091000	^{124}Sb	.057254	2.754100	^{24}Na	.998620
1.885700	^{133m}Te	.011310	2.097700	^{156}Eu	.042744	2.824100	^{84}Br	.011394
1.887700	^{131m}Te	.013561	2.100400	^{142}La	.010500	2.972000	^{142}La	.033075
1.897300	^{84}Br	.149390	2.113100	^{56}Mn	.143360	3.009700	^{56}Co	.010596
1.901300	^{142}La	.087150	2.118600	^{214}Bi	.011743	3.045400	^{84}Br	.025320
1.917800	^{93}Y	.014050	2.180900	^{156}Eu	.024336	3.202200	^{56}Co	.031787
1.919400	^{57}Ni	.147230	2.186700	^{156}Eu	.039520	3.235300	^{84}Br	.020678
1.921100	^{132}I	.011844	2.187200	^{142}La	.058275	3.253500	^{56}Co	.077867
1.937700	^{156}Eu	.021424	2.195800	^{88}Kr	.131830	3.273200	^{56}Co	.018492
1.950300	^{89}Rb	.011832	2.196000	^{89}Rb	.133400	3.314700	^{142}La	.013650
1.966000	^{156}Eu	.042016	2.200700	^{84}Br	.011816	3.365800	^{84}Br	.029118
2.000900	^{131m}Te	.020147	2.204200	^{214}Bi	.049833	3.508800	^{89}Rb	.011484
2.001700	^{125}Sn	.020640	2.218000	^{138}Cs	.151840	3.632700	^{142}La	.011550
2.002200	^{132}I	.010857	2.231800	^{88}Kr	.033908	3.927500	^{84}Br	.068786
2.004200	^{142}La	.010500	2.240300	^{48}V	.024100	6.129200	^{16}N	.690000
2.004800	^{138}Xe	.053550	2.252300	^{138}Xe	.022869	7.115100	^{16}N	.050000

[a] This table contains the same radionuclides as those listed in Table 8.13.

Table 8.7 Thorium Series (4n)[a] (Personal communication L. Slaback after Kocher 1981 and ICRP Report No. 38, 1983. In case of discrepancy, ICRP value given)

			Major Radiation Energies (MeV) and Intensities[b]					
			α		β		γ	
Nuclide	Historical Name	Half-Life	MeV	%	MeV	%	MeV	%
$^{232}_{90}Th$	Thorium	1.405×10^{10} y	3.83	0.2			.059	.19
↓			3.95	23			.126	.04
			4.01	76.8				
$^{228}_{88}Ra$	Mesothorium I	5.75 y			.0389	100	.0067	6×10^{-5}
↓								
$^{228}_{89}Ac$	Mesothorium II	6.13 h			.983	7	.338	11.4
↓					1.014	6.6	.911	27.7
					1.115	3.4	.969	16.6
					1.17	32	1.588	3.5
					1.74	12		
					2.08	8		
					(+33 more βs)			
$^{228}_{90}Th$	Radiothorium	1.913 y	5.34	26.7			0.084	1.19
↓			5.42	72.4			.132	.11
							.166	.08
							.216	.27
$^{224}_{88}Ra$	Thorium X	3.66 d	5.45	4.9			.241	3.9
↓			5.686	95.1				
$^{220}_{86}Rn$	Emanation	55.6 s	6.288	99.9			.55	.07
↓	Thoron (Tn)							
$^{216}_{84}Po$	Thorium A	.15 s	6.78	100			.128	.002
↓								
$^{212}_{82}Pb$	Thorium B	10.64 h			.158	5.2	.239	44.6
↓					.334	85.1	.300	3.4
					.573	9.9		
$^{212}_{83}Bi$	Thorium C	60.55 m	6.05	25	1.59	8	.040	1.0
↓			6.09	9.6	2.246	48.4	.727	11.8
							1.620	2.75
64.07% ↓ / 35.93% ↓								
$^{212}_{84}Po$	Thorium C′	305 ns	8.785	100				
$^{208}_{81}Tl$	Thorium C″	3.07 m			1.28	25	.277	6.8
↓					1.52	21	.5108	21.6
					1.80	50	.583	85.8
↓							.860	12
$^{208}_{82}Pb$							2.614	100
	Thorium D	Stable						

[a] This expression describes the mass number of any member in this series, where n is an integer. For example: $^{232}_{90}Th$ (4n).....4(58) = 232

[b] Intensities refer to percentage of disintegrations of the nuclide itself, not to original parent of series. Gamma percents are given in terms of observable emissions, not transitions.

Table 8.8 Neptunium Series (4n + 1)[a,b] (Personal communication L. Slaback after Kocher 1981 and ICRP Report No. 38, 1983. In case of discrepancy, ICRP value given)

Nuclide	Historical Name	Half-Life	Major Radiation Energies (MeV) and Intensities[c]					
			α		β		γ	
			MeV	%	MeV	%	MeV	%
$^{241}_{94}Pu$	Plutonium	14.4 y	4.85	.0003	.021	~100	.149	00019
~100% , .0023%			4.90	.0020			.0263	2.4
↓							.0595	35.7
							.099	.02
$^{241}_{95}Am$	Americium	432.2 y	5.43	12.8			.103	.02
↓			5.486	85.2				
$^{237}_{92}U$	Uranium	6.75 d			.238	53.1	.060	33.5
					.252	43.7	.208	21.7
							.030	14
↓							.0865	12.6
$^{237}_{93}Np$	Neptunium	2.14×10^6 y	4.64	6.2			.143	.4
↓			4.766	8				
			4.772	25				
			4.789	47.1				
$^{233}_{91}Pa$	Protactinium	27.0 d			.156	22.6	.300	6.2
↓					.173	14.6	.312	36
					.231	26.9	.340	4.2
					.260	30.9		
$^{233}_{92}U$	Uranium	1.585×10^5 y	4.78	13.2			.0424	.088
↓			4.825	84.4			.097	.028
$^{229}_{90}Th$	Thorium	7340 y	4.846	56.3			.031	4.1
↓			4.902	10.2			.086	3.1
			4.969	6			.124	1.2
			4.979	3.2			.137	1.6
			5.05	6.8			.148	1.4
							.156	1.1
							.194	4
							.211	3
$^{225}_{88}Ra$	Radium	14.8 d			.322	67.3	.040	29
↓					.362	32.7		
$^{225}_{89}Ac$	Actinium	10.0 d	5.73	10			.0996	4.1
↓			5.79	27			.157	.35
			5.83	50.9			.1877	.55
$^{221}_{89}Fr$	Francium	4.8 m	6.127	15			.2176	12.5
↓			6.341	82.7			.4095	0.12
$^{217}_{85}As$	Astatine	.032 s	7.07	~100			.594	.04
↓								
$^{213}_{83}Bi$	Bismuth	45.65 m	5.87	2.0	.98	32	.292	.49
			5.55	.16	1.42	65	.324	.16
97.84% , 2.16%							.4397	27.3
↓							1.101	.39
$^{213}_{84}Po$	Polonium	4.2 μs	8.785	~100				
↓								
$^{208}_{81}Tl$	Thallium	2.2 m			1.825	100	.117	81.1
↓							.467	81.1
							1.586	98.4
$^{208}_{82}Pb$								
$^{209}_{82}Pb$	Lead	3.253 h			.645	100		
↓								
$^{209}_{83}Bi$	Bismuth	stable ($>2 \times 10^{18}$ y)						

[a] This expression describes the mass number of any member in this series, where n is an integer. For example: $^{229}_{90}Th$ (4n + 1) = 229.

[b] Also referred to as the Americium Series.

[c] Intensities refer to percentage of disintegrations of the nuclide itself, not to original parent of series. Gamma percents are given in terms of observable emissions, not transitions.

Table 8.9 Uranium Series (4n + 2)[a] (Personal communication L. Slaback after Kocher 1981 and ICRP Report No. 38, 1983. In case of discrepancy, ICRP value given)

			Major Radiation Energies (MeV) and Intensities[b]					
			α		β		γ	
Nuclide	Historical Name	Half-Life	MeV	%	MeV	%	MeV	%
$^{238}_{92}U$ ↓	Uranium I	4.468×10^9 y	4.15 4.20	22.9 76.8			.0496	.07
$^{234}_{90}Th$ ↓	Uranium X_1	24.1 d			.076 .095 .096 .1886	2.7 6.2 18.6 72.5	.0633 .0924 .0928 .1128	3.8 2.7 2.7 .24
$^{234m}_{91}Pa$ 99.87% , 0.13% ↓ $^{234}_{91}Pa$ ↓	Uranium X_2	1.17 m			2.28	98.6	.766 1.001	.207 .59
↓ $^{234}_{91}Pa$ IT ↓ ↓	Uranium Z	6.7 h			22 βs $E_{Avg} = 0.224$ $E_{max} = 1.26$		.132 .570 .883 .926 .946	19.7 10.7 11.8 10.9 12
$^{234}_{92}U$ ↓	Uranium II	244,500 y	4.72 4.77	27.4 72.3			.053 .121	.12 .04
$^{230}_{90}Th$ ↓	Ionium	7.7×10^4 y	4.621 4.688	23.4 76.2			.0677 .142 .144	.37 .07 .045
$^{226}_{88}Ra$ ↓	Radium	1600 ± 7 y	4.60 4.78	5.55 94.4			.186	3.28
$^{222}_{86}Rn$ ↓	Emanation Radon (Rn)	3.823 d	5.49	99.9			.510	.078
$^{218}_{84}Po$ ↓	Radium A	3.05 m	6.00	~100	.33	.02	.837	.0011

(continued)

Table 8.9 Uranium Series (4n + 2)[a] (Continued)

Nuclide	Historical Name	Half-Life	Major Radiation Energies (MeV) and Intensities[b]					
			α		β		γ	
			MeV	%	MeV	%	MeV	%
99.98%, 0.02%								
$^{214}_{82}$Pb	Radium B	26.8 m			.67	48	.2419	7.5
					.73	42.5	.295	19.2
					1.03	6.3	.352	37.1
$^{218}_{85}$At	Astatine	2 s	6.66	6.4			.786	1.1
			6.7	89.9			.053	6.6
			6.757	3.6				
$^{214}_{83}$Bi	Radium C	19.9 m	5.45	.012	1.42	8.3	.609	46.1
			5.51	.008	1.505	17.6	1.12	15.0
					1.54	17.9	1.765	15.9
					3.27	17.7	2.204	5.0
99.979%, 0.021%								
$^{214}_{84}$Po	Radium C′	164 μs	7.687	100			.7997	.010
$^{210}_{81}$Tl	Radium C″	1.3 m			1.32	25	.2918	79.1
					1.87	56	.7997	99
					2.34	29	.860	6.9
							1.110	6.9
							1.21	17
							1.310	21
							1.410	4.9
							2.010	6.9
							2.090	4.9
$^{210}_{82}$Pb	Radium D	22.3 y	3.72	.000002	.016	80	.0465	4
					.063	20		
$^{210}_{83}$Bi	Radium E	5.01 d	4.65	.00007	1.161	~100		
			4.69	.00005				
– 100%, .00013%								
$^{210}_{84}$Po	Radium F	138.378 d	5.305	100			.802	.0011
$^{206}_{81}$Tl	Radium E	4.20 m			1.571	100	.803	.0055
$^{206}_{82}$Pb	Radium G	stable						

[a] This expression describes the mass number of any member in this series, where n is an integer. For example: $^{206}{}_{82}$Pb (4n + 2)...4(51) + 2 = 206.

[b] Intensities refer to percentage of disintegrations of the nuclide itself, not to original parent of series. Gamma percents are given: in terms of observable emissions, not transitions.

Table 8.10 Actinium Series (4n + 3)[a]

(Personal communication L. Slaback after Kocher 1981 and ICRP Report No. 38, 1983. In case of discrepancy, ICRP value given)

			Major Radiation Energies (MeV) and Intensities[b]					
			α		β		γ	
Nuclide	Historical Name	Half-Life	MeV	%	MeV	%	MeV	%
$^{235}_{92}U$ ↓	Actinouranium	7.038×10^{8} y	4.2–4.32 4.366 4.398 4.5–4.6	10.3 17.6 56 11.3			.1438 .163 .1857 .205	10.5 4.7 54 4.7
$^{231}_{90}Th$ ↓	Uranium Y	25.5 h			.205 .287 .304	15 49 35	.0256 .0842	14.8 6.5
$^{231}_{91}Pa$ ↓	Protactinium	3.276×10^{4} y	4.95 5.01 5.029 5.058	23 25.6 20.2 11.1			.0274 .2837 .300 .3027 .330	9.3 1.6 2.3 4.6 1.3
$^{227}_{89}Ac$ ↓	Actinium	21.77 y	4.94 4.95	.53 .66	.019 .034 .044	10 35 54	.070 .100 .160	.017 .032 .019
98.87% ↓ $^{227}_{90}Th$, 1.38% ↓ $^{223}_{87}Fr$								
$^{227}_{90}Th$ ↓	Radioactinium	18.718 d	5.757 5.978 6.038	20.2 23.3 24.4			.050 .236 .300 .304 .330	8.5 11.2 2.0 1.1 2.7
$^{223}_{87}Fr$ ↓	Actinium K	21.8 m	5.44	~.006	1.15 25 betas Eavg. = 0.343 E_{max} = 1.097	~100	.050 .0798 .2349	34 9.2 3.4
$^{223}_{88}Ra$ ↓	Actinium X	11.43 d	5.607 5.716 5.747	24.1 52.2 9.45			.144 .154 .269 .324 .338	3.3 5.6 13.6 3.9 2.8
$^{219}_{86}Rn$ ↓	Emanation Actinon (An)	3.96 s	6.425 6.55 6.819	7.4 12.1 80.3			.271 .4018	9.9 6.6
$^{215}_{84}Po$ ↓	Actinium A	1.78 ms	7.386	~100	.74	~.00023	.4388	.04
~100% ↓ $^{211}_{82}Pb$, .00023% ↓ $^{215}_{85}At$								
$^{211}_{82}Pb$ ↓	Actinium B	36.1 m			.26 .97 1.37	4.8 1.4 92.9	.405 .427 .832	3.0 1.38 2.8
$^{215}_{85}At$ ↓	Astatine	~0.1 ms	8.026	~100			.404	.047
$^{211}_{83}Bi$ ↓	Actinium C	2.14 m	6.28 6.62	16 84	.579	.27	.351	12.7
0.273% ↓ $^{211}_{84}Po$, 99.73% ↓ $^{207}_{81}Tl$								
$^{211}_{84}Po$ ↓	Actinium C′	.516 s	7.42	98.9			.570 .898	.54 .52
$^{207}_{81}Tl$ ↓	Actinium C″	4.77 m			1.42	99.8	.897	0.24
$^{207}_{82}Pb$	Actinium D	stable						

[a] This expression describes the mass number of any member in this series, where n is an integer. For example: $^{207}_{82}Pb$ (4n + 3)...4(51) + 3 = 207

[b] Intensities refer to percentage of disintegrations of the nuclide itself, not to original parent of series. Gamma percents are given in terms of observable emissions, not transitions.

Table 8.11 Naturally-Occurring Radionuclides
(In addition to the four decay series Table 8.7–8.10) (Personal Communication Peterson, 1991)

Radionuclide (Half-Life)	Abundance (%)	Decay Energy (MeV)		Specific Activity	Internal Dose (mSv/yr)	
Primordial Radionuclides						
^{40}K	0.0118	β, EC	1.31	30.7 Bq (g K)$^{-1}$	β	0.17
(1.3×10^9 y)		γ	1.46		γ	0.02
					Total	0.19
^{87}Rb	27.8	β	0.27	925 Bq (g Rb)$^{-1}$	β	0.003
(4.8×10^{10} y)						
Cosmogenic Radionuclides						
^{3}H		β	0.018	~555 Bq (L H_2O)$^{-1}$		0.015
(12.3 y)				(pretesting)		
^{7}Be		EC, γ	0.477	0.01 Bq (kg air)$^{-1}$		<0.001
(53 d)						
^{14}C		β	0.156	0.22 Bq (g C)$^{-1}$ [a]		
(5,730 y)				(19th century)		
				0.17 Bq (g C)$^{-1}$		
				(Est. year 2000)		

[a] The decrease in the specific activity of is due to dilution by old carbon (low ^{14}C content) from burning fossil fuels. This dilution effect is known as the ''Seuss effect.''

Table 8.12 Typical Uranium Isotopic Abundances (g of isotope per 100 g of uranium) (From DOE Report DE88-013620, 1988)

Isotope	Natural	Typical Commercial Feed Enrichment	Typical Depleted
^{238}U	99.2739 ± 0.0007	97.01	99.75
^{235}U	0.7204 ± 0.0007	2.96	0.25
^{234}U	0.0057 ± 0.0002	0.03	0.0005

Table 8.13 Half Life, Decay Modes and Radioactive Decay Products of Selected Radionuclides of Interest to Health Physicists (After Eckeman 1991)

The table contains the half-life, decay modes and identification of radioactive decay products and their fractional yield (branching fraction) for the radionuclides of interest to health physicists. The presentation includes data for all nuclides (and their radioactive decay products) which were contained in the dose coefficient tabulations. All the data presented here are contained in ICRP Publication 38.

Table 8.13 contains the complete information necessary to assemble the full decay chain for the radionuclide. For example, consider ^{99}Mo, the parent nuclide of the ^{99m}Tc generator used widely in nuclear medicine. From Table 8.13 the following entries are relevant.

Nuclide	Half Life		Decay Modes	Decay Products			
				Nuclide/Fraction		Nuclide/Fraction	
^{99}Mo	66.0	h	B−	^{99m}Tc	8.760^{-e01}	^{99}Tc	1.240^{-e01}
^{99m}Tc	6.02	h	IT	^{99}Tc	1.000^{e+00}		
^{99}Tc	2.13E5	y	B−				

The first entry indicates that ^{99}Mo decays by beta minus decay with half life of 66.0 h. Beta decay forms the ^{99}Tc nucleus in a metastable state 87.6% of the ^{99}Mo transformations form ^{99m}Tc) and in the ground state (12.4% of the ^{99}Mo transformations form ^{99}Tc). The decay characteristics of ^{99m}Tc are given in the second entry; it decays by isomeric transition with a half life of 6.02 h to ^{99}Tc. The next entry indicates that ^{99}Tc decays by beta minus decay with a half life of 2.13×10^5 y. No radioactive decay products are formed by nuclear transformations of ^{99}Tc, the ^{99}Ru nucleus formed is stable.

The abbreviations of time units are:

Time Units	
Symbol	**Definition**
y	year
d	day
h	hour
m	minute
s	second
μs	micro second

The decay modes are abbreviated as:

Definition of Decay modes	
Symbol	**Definition**
A	Alpha decay
B−	Beta minus decay
B+	Beta plus decay
EC	Electron capture
IT	Isomeric transition
SF	Spontaneous fission

Table 8.13 Half-Life, Decay Modes and Radioactive Decay Products of Selected Radionuclides of Interest to Health Physicists

			Decay Products and Fractional Yield			
Nuclide	$T_{1/2}$	Decay Mode	Nuclide	Fraction	Nuclide	Fraction
Hydrogen						
^{3}H	12.35 y	B−				
Beryllium						
^{10}Be	1.6E6 y	B−				
Carbon						
^{11}C	20.38 m	EC B+				
^{14}C	5730 y	B−				
Sodium						
^{22}Na	2.602 y	EC B+				
^{24}Na	15.00 h	B−				
Phosphorus						
^{32}P	14.29 d	B−				
Argon						
^{37}Ar	35.02 d	EC				
^{39}Ar	269 y	B−				
^{41}Ar	1.827 h	B−				
Calcium						
^{41}Ca	1.4E5 y	EC				
^{45}Ca	163 d	B−				
Scandium						
^{46}Sc	83.83 d	B−				
Chromium						
^{51}Cr	27.70 d	EC				
Manganese						
^{54}Mn	312.5 d	EC				
^{56}Mn	2.5785 h	B−				
Iron						
^{55}Fe	2.7 y	EC				
^{59}Fe	44.529 d	B−				
Cobalt						
^{57}Co	270.9 d	EC				
^{60}Co	5.271 y	B−				
Nickel						
^{59}Ni	7.5E4 6	EC				
^{63}Ni	96 y	B−				
^{65}Ni	2.520 h	B−				
Copper						
^{64}Cu	12.701 h	B− EC B+				
Zinc						
^{65}Zn	243.9 d	EC B+				
^{69}Zn	57 m	B−				

(continued)

Table 8.13 Half-Life, Decay Modes and Radioactive Decay Products of Selected Radionuclides of Interest to Health Physicists (Continued)

			Decay Products and Fractional Yield			
Nuclide	$T_{1/2}$	Decay Mode	Nuclide	Fraction	Nuclide	Fraction
Selenium						
^{79}Se	65000 y	B−				
Bromine						
^{82}Br	35.30 h	B−				
^{83}Br	2.39 h	B−	^{83m}Kr	1.000 E + 00		
^{84}Br	31.80 m	B−				
Krypton						
^{83m}Kr	1.83 h	IT				
^{85m}Kr	4.48 h	IT B−	^{85}Kr	2.110 E − 01		
^{85}Kr	10.72 y	B−				
^{87}Kr	76.3 m	B−	^{87}Rb	1.000 E + 00		
^{88}Kr	2.84 h	B−	^{88}Rb	1.000 E + 00		
Rubidium						
^{86}Rb	18.66 d	B−				
^{88}Rb	17.8 m	B−				
^{89}Rb	15.2 m	B−	^{89}Sr	1.000 E + 00		
Strontium						
^{89}Sr	50.5 d	B−				
^{90}Sr	29.12 y	B−	^{90}Y	1.000 E + 00		
^{91}Sr	9.5 h	B−	^{91m}Y	5.780 E − 01	^{91}Y	4.220 E − 01
Yttrium						
^{90}Y	64.0 h	B−				
^{91m}Y	49.71 m	IT	^{91}Y	1.000 E + 00		
^{91}Y	58.51 d	B−				
^{92}Y	3.54 h	B−				
^{93}Y	10.1 h	B−	^{93}Zr	1.000 E + 00		
Zirconium						
^{93}Zr	1.53E6 y	B−	^{93m}Nb	1.000 E + 00		
^{95}Zr	63.98 d	B−	^{95m}Nb	7.000 E − 03	^{95}Nb	9.930 E − 01
^{97}Zr	16.90 h	B−	^{97m}Nb	9.470 E − 01	^{97}Nb	5.300 E − 02
Niobium						
^{93m}Nb	13.6 y	IT				
^{94}Nb	2.03E4 y	B−				
^{95m}Nb	86.6 h	IT	^{95}Nb	1.000 E + 00		
^{95}Nb	35.15 d	B−				
^{97m}Nb	60 s	IT	^{97}Nb	1.000 E + 00		
^{97}Nb	72.1 m	B−				
Molybdenum						
^{93}Mo	3.5E3 y	EC	^{93m}Nb	1.000 E + 00		
^{99}Mo	66.0 h	B−	^{99m}Tc	8.760 E − 01	^{99}Tc	1.240 E − 01

Table 8.13 Half-Life, Decay Modes and Radioactive Decay Products of Selected Radionuclides of Interest to Health Physicists (Continued)

			Decay Products and Fractional Yield			
Nuclide	**$T_{1/2}$**	**Decay Mode**	**Nuclide**	**Fraction**	**Nuclide**	**Fraction**
Technetium						
^{99m}Tc	6.02 h	IT	^{99}Tc	1.000 E + 00		
^{99}Tc	2.13E5 y	B−				
^{101}Tc	14.2 m	B−				
Ruthenium						
^{103}Ru	39.28 d	B−	^{103m}Rh	9.970 E − 01		
^{105}Ru	4.44 h	B−	^{105}Rh	1.000 E + 00		
^{106}Ru	368.2 d	B−	^{106}Rh	1.000 E + 00		
Rhodium						
^{103m}Rh	56.12 m	IT				
^{105}Rh	35.36 h	B−				
^{106m}Rh	132 m	B−				
^{106}Rh	29.9 s	B−				
Palladium						
^{107}Pd	6.5E6 y	B−				
^{109}Pd	13.427 h	B−				
Silver						
^{110m}Ag	249.9 d	IT B−	^{110}Ag	1.330 E − 02		
^{110}Ag	24.6 s	B− EC				
^{111}Ag	7.45 d	B−				
Cadmium						
^{113m}Cd	13.6 y	B−				
^{113}Cd	9.3E15 y	B−				
^{115m}Cd	44.6 d	B	^{115}In	1.000 E + 00		
Tin						
^{123}Sn	129.2 d	B−				
^{125}Sn	9.64 d	B−	^{125}Sb	1.000 E + 00		
^{126}Sn	1.0E5 y	B−	^{126m}Sb	1.000 E + 00		
Antimony						
^{124}Sb	60.20 d	B−				
^{125}Sb	2.77 y	B−	^{125m}Te	2.280 E − 01		
^{126m}Sb	19.0 m	IT B−	^{126}Sb	1.400 E − 01		
^{126}Sb	12.4 d	B−				
^{127}Sb	3.85 d	B−	^{127m}Te	1.760 E − 01	^{127}Te	8.240 E − 01
Tellurium						
^{125m}Te	58 d	IT				
^{127m}Te	109 d	IT B−	^{127}Te	9.760 E − 01		
^{127}Te	9.35 h	B−				
^{129m}Te	33.6 d	IT B−	^{129}I	3.500 E − 01	^{129}Te	6.500 E − 01
^{129}Te	69.6 m	B−	^{129}I	1.000 E + 00		
^{131m}Te	30 h	IT B−	^{131}I	7.780 E − 01	^{131}Te	2.220 E − 01
^{131}Te	25.0 m	B−	^{131}I	1.000 E + 00		
^{132}Te	78.2 h	B−	^{132}I	1.000 E + 00		
^{133m}Te	55.4 m	IT B−	^{133}I	8.700 E − 01	^{133}Te	1.300 E − 01
^{133}Te	12.45 m	B−	^{133}I	1.000 E + 00		
^{134}Te	41.8 m	B−	^{134}I	1.000 E + 00		

(continued)

Table 8.13 Half-Life, Decay Modes and Radioactive Decay Products of Selected Radionuclides of Interest to Health Physicists (Continued)

			Decay Products and Fractional Yield			
Nuclide	$T_{1/2}$	Decay Mode	Nuclide	Fraction	Nuclide	Fraction
Iodine						
^{129}I	1.57E7 y	B−				
^{130}I	12.36 h	B−				
^{131}I	8.04 d	B−	^{131m}Xe	1.110 E − 02		
^{132}I	2.30 h	B−				
^{133}I	20.8 h	B−	^{133m}Xe	2.900 E − 02	^{133}Xe	9.710 E − 01
^{134}I	52.6 m	B−				
^{135}I	6.61 h	B−	^{135m}Xe	1.540 E − 01	^{135}Xe	8.460 E − 01
Xenon						
^{131m}Xe	11.9 d	IT				
^{133m}Xe	2.188 d	IT	^{133}Xe	1.000 E + 00		
^{133}Xe	5.245 d	B−				
^{135m}Xe	15.29 m	IT B−	^{135}Cs	4.500 E − 05	^{135}Xe	9.999 E − 01
^{135}Xe	9.09 h	B−	^{135}Cs	1.000 E + 00		
Cesium						
^{134m}Cs	2.90 h	IT	^{134}Cs	1.000 E + 00		
^{134}Cs	2.062 y	EC B−				
^{135m}Cs	53 m	IT	^{135}Cs	1.000 E + 00		
^{135}Cs	2.3E6 y	B−				
^{136}Cs	13.1 d	B−				
^{137}Cs	30.0 y	B−	^{137m}Ba	9.460 E − 01		
^{138}Cs	32.2 m	B−				
Barium						
^{37m}Ba	2.552 m	IT				
^{139}Ba	82.7 m	B−				
^{140}Ba	12.74 d	B−	^{140}La	1.000 E + 00		
^{141}Ba	18.27 m	B−	^{141}La	1.000 E + 00		
^{142}Ba	10.6 m	B−	^{142}La	1.000 E + 00		
Lanthanum						
^{140}La	40.272 h	B−				
^{141}La	3.93 h	B−	^{141}Ce	1.000 E + 00		
^{142}La	92.5 m	B−				
Cerium						
^{141}Ce	32.501 d	B−				
^{143}Ce	33.0 h	B−	^{143}Pr	1.000 E + 00		
^{144}Ce	284.3 d	B−	^{144m}Pr	1.780 E − 02	^{144}Pr	9.822 E − 01
Praseodymium						
^{143}Pr	13.56 d	B−				
^{144m}Pr	7.2 m	IT B−	^{144}Pr	9.990 E − 01		
^{144}Pr	17.28 m	B−				

Table 8.13 Half-Life, Decay Modes and Radioactive Decay Products of Selected Radionuclides of Interest to Health Physicists (Continued)

Nuclide	$T_{1/2}$	Decay Mode	Decay Products and Fractional Yield			
			Nuclide	Fraction	Nuclide	Fraction
Neodymium						
^{147}Nd	10.98 d	B−	^{147}Pm	1.000 E + 00		
Promethium						
^{147}Pm	2.6234 y	B−	^{147}Sm	1.000 E + 00		
^{148m}Pm	41.3 d	B− IT	^{148}Pm	4.600 E − 02		
^{148}Pm	5.37 d	B−				
^{149}Pm	53.08 h	B−				
Samarium						
^{151}Sm	90 y	B−				
^{153}Sm	46.7 h	B−				
Europium						
^{152}Eu	13.33 y	B− EC B+	^{152}Gd	2.792 E − 01		
^{154}Eu	8.8 y	EC B−				
^{155}Eu	4.96 y	B−				
^{156}Eu	15.19 d	B−				
Terbium						
^{160}Tb	72.3 d	B−				
Holmium						
^{166m}Ho	1.20E3 y	B−				
Tungsten						
^{181}W	121.2 d	EC				
^{185}W	75.1 d	B−				
^{187}W	23.9 h	B−	^{187}Re	1.000 E + 00		
Thallium						
^{207}Tl	4.77 m	B−				
^{208}Tl	3.07 m	B−				
^{209}Tl	2.20 m	B−	^{209}Pb	1.000 E + 00		
Lead						
^{209}Pb	3.253 h	B−				
^{210}Pb	22.3 y	B−	^{210}Bi	1.000 E + 00		
^{211}Pb	36.1 m	B−	^{211}Bi	1.000 E + 00		
^{212}Pb	10.64 h	B−	^{212}Bi	1.000 E + 00		
^{214}Pb	26.8 m	B−	^{214}Bi	1.000 E + 00		
Bismuth						
^{210}Bi	5.012 d	B−	^{210}Po	1.000 E + 00		
^{211}Bi	2.14 m	A B−	^{207}Tl	9.972 E − 01	^{211}Po	2.800 E − 03
^{212}Bi	60.55 m	B− A	^{208}Tl	3.593 E − 01	^{212}Po	6.407 E − 01
^{213}Bi	45.65 m	B− A	^{209}Tl	2.160 E − 02	^{213}Po	9.784 E − 01
^{214}Bi	19.9 m	B−	^{214}Po	9.998 E − 01		

(continued)

Table 8.13 Half-Life, Decay Modes and Radioactive Decay Products of Selected Radionuclides of Interest to Health Physicists (Continued)

			Decay Products and Fractional Yield			
Nuclide	$T_{1/2}$	Decay Mode	Nuclide	Fraction	Nuclide	Fraction
Polonium						
^{210}Po	138.38 d	A				
^{211}Po	0.516 s	A				
^{212}Po	0.305 μs	A				
^{213}Po	4.2 μs	A	^{209}Pb	1.000 E + 00		
^{214}Po	164.3 μs	A	^{210}Pb	1.000 E + 00		
^{216}Po	0.15 s	A	^{212}Pb	1.000 E + 00		
^{218}Po	3.05 m	A B−	^{214}Pb	9.998 E − 01	^{218}At	2.000 E − 04
Astatine						
^{217}At	0.0323 s	A	^{213}Bi	1.000 E + 00		
^{218}At	2 s	A	^{214}Bi	9.990 E − 01		
Radon						
^{219}Rn	3.96 s	A	^{215}Po	1.000 E + 00		
^{220}Rn	55.6 s	A	^{216}Po	1.000 E + 00		
^{222}Rn	3.8235 d	A	^{218}Po	1.000 E + 00		
Francium						
^{221}Fr	4.8 m	A	^{217}At	1.000 E + 00		
^{223}Fr	21.8 m	B−	^{223}Ra	9.999 E − 01		
Radium						
^{223}Ra	11.434 d	A	^{219}Rn	1.000 E + 00		
^{224}Ra	3.66 d	A	^{220}Rn	1.000 E + 00		
^{225}Ra	14.8 d	B−	^{225}Ac	1.000 E + 00		
^{226}Ra	1600 y	A	^{222}Rn	1.000 E + 00		
^{228}Ra	5.75 y	B−	^{228}Ac	1.000 E + 00		
Actinium						
^{225}Ac	10.0 d	A	^{221}Fr	1.000 E + 00		
^{227}Ac	21.773 y	B− A	^{223}Fr	1.380 E − 02	^{227}Th	9.862 E − 01
^{228}Ac	6.13 h	B−	^{228}Th	1.000 E + 00		
Thorium						
^{227}Th	18.718 d	A	^{223}Ra	1.000 E + 00		
^{228}Th	1.9131 y	A	^{224}Ra	1.000 E + 00		
^{229}Th	7340 y	A	^{225}Ra	1.000 E + 00		
^{230}Th	7.7E4 y	A	^{226}Ra	1.000 E + 00		
^{231}Th	25.52 h	B−	^{231}Pa	1.000 E + 00		
^{232}Th	1.405E10 y	A	^{228}Ra	1.000 E + 00		
^{234}Th	24.10 d	B−	^{234m}Pa	9.980 E − 01	^{234}Pa	2.000 E − 03
Protactinium						
^{231}Pa	3.276E4 y	A	^{227}Ac	1.000 E + 00		
^{233}Pa	27.0 d	B−	^{233}U	1.000 E + 00		
^{234m}Pa	1.17 m	B− IT	^{234}U	9.987 E − 01	^{234}Pa	1.300 E − 03
^{234}Pa	6.70 h	B−	^{234}U	1.000 E + 00		

Table 8.13 Half-Life, Decay Modes and Radioactive Decay Products of Selected Radionuclides of Interest to Health Physicists (Continued)

			Decay Products and Fractional Yield			
Nuclide	$T_{1/2}$	Decay Mode	Nuclide	Fraction	Nuclide	Fraction
Uranium						
^{232}U	72 y	A	^{228}Th	1.000 E + 00		
^{233}U	1.585E5 y	A	^{229}Th	1.000 E + 00		
^{234}U	2.445E5 y	A	^{230}Th	1.000 E + 00		
^{235}U	703.8E6 y	A	^{231}Th	1.000 E + 00		
^{236}U	2.3415E7 y	A	^{232}Th	1.000 E + 00		
^{238}U	4.468E9 y	SF A	^{234}Th	1.000 E + 00	SF	5.400 E − 05
^{240}U	14.1 h	B−	^{240m}Np	1.000 E + 00		
Neptunium						
^{237}Np	2.14E6 y	A	^{233}Pa	1.000 E + 00		
^{239}Np	2.355 d	B−	^{239}Pu	1.000 E + 00		
^{240m}Np	7.4 m	B−	^{240}Pu	9.989 E − 01		
Plutonium						
^{238}Pu	87.74 y	SF A	^{234}U	1.000 E + 00	SF	1.840 E − 09
^{239}Pu	24065 y	A	^{235}U	1.000 E + 00		
^{240}Pu	6537 y	SF A	^{236}U	1.000 E + 00	SF	4.950 E − 08
^{241}Pu	14.4 y	A B−	^{237}U	2.450 E − 05	^{241}Am	1.000 E + 00
^{242}Pu	3.763E5 y	SF A	^{238}U	1.000 E + 00	SF	5.500 E − 06
^{243}Pu	4.956 h	B−	^{243}Am	1.000 E + 00		
^{244}Pu	8.26E7 y	SF A	^{240}U	1.000 E + 00	SF	1.250 E − 03
Americium						
^{241}Am	432.2 y	A	^{237}Np	1.000 E + 00		
^{242}Am	16.02 h	EC B−	^{242}Cm	8.270E − 01	^{242}Pu	1.730 E − 01
^{243}Am	7380 y	A	^{239}Np	1.000 E + 00		
Curium						
^{242}Cm	162.8 d	SF A	^{238}Pu	1.000 E + 00	SF	6.800 E − 08
^{243}Cm	28.5 y	A EC	^{239}Pu	9.980 E − 01	^{243}Am	2.400 E − 03
^{244}Cm	18.11 y	SF A	^{240}Pu	1.000 E + 00	SF	1.350 E − 06
^{245}Cm	8500 y	A	^{241}Pu	1.000 E + 00		
^{247}Cm	1.56E7 y	A	^{243}Pu	1.000 E + 00		
^{248}Cm	3.39E5 y	SF A	^{244}Pu	9.174 E − 01	SF	8.260 E − 02
Californium						
^{242}Cf	2.638 y	SF A	^{248}Cm	9.691 E − 01	SF	3.092 E − 02

Table 8.14 Energy and Probability by Radiation Type for Selected Radionuclides of Interest to Health Physicists (After Kocher, 1981)[a]

Nuclide	Probability per Decay	Energy[b] (MeV)	Average Energy (MeV)
H-3	Half-life: 12.28 years		
	Betas:		
	1.000000	.018601	.005685
Be-7	Half-life: 53.44 days		
	Gammas & X-rays:		
	.104200	.477590	
Be-10	Half-life: 1600000 years		
	Betas:		
	1.000000	.555800	.202500
C-11	Half-life: 20.48 minutes		
	Positrons:		
	.997670	.960100	.385600
	Electrons:		
	.002218	.000170	
	Gammas & X-rays:		
	.000002	.000183	
	1.995300	.511000	
N-13	Half-life: 9.97 minutes		
	Positrons:		
	.998040	1.198500	.491800
	Electrons:		
	.001856	.000260	
	Gammas & X-rays:		
	.000004	.000277	
	1.996100	.511000	
C-14	Half-life: 5730 years		
	Betas:		
	1.000000	.156480	.049470
O-15	Half-life: 122.24 seconds		
	Positrons:		
	.999000	1.731900	.735200
	Gammas & X-rays:		
	1.998000	.511000	
N-16	Half-life: 7.13 seconds		
	Betas:		
	.010000	1.546800	.630400
	.049000	3.301900	1.461500
	.680000	4.288300	1.941200
	.260000	10.419000	4.979200
	.000110	4.369300	1.998800
	Gammas & X-rays:		
	.001300	1.754800	
	.007600	2.741200	
	.690000	6.129200	
	.050000	7.115100	
	.001607	6.334200	
F-18	Half-life: 109.74 minutes		
	Positrons:		
	.967300	.633500	.249800
	Electrons:		
	.030691	.000520	
	Gammas & X-rays:		
	.000179	.000525	
	1.934600	.511000	
Na-22	Half-life: 2.602 years		
	Positrons:		
	.898400	.545520	.215540
	.000600	2.842100	.834800
	Electrons:		
	.092004	.000820	
	Gammas & X-rays:		
	.001250	.000849	
	.999400	1.274500	
	1.798000	.511000	
Na-24	Half-life: 15 hours		
	Betas:		
	.999350	1.390200	.553900
	.000620	.276700	.088600
	Gammas & X-rays:		
	.999990	1.368500	
	.998620	2.754100	
	.000641	3.823600	
P-32	Half-life: 14.29 days		
	Betas:		
	1.000000	1.710400	.694900
S-35	Half-life: 87.44 days		
	Betas:		
	1.000000	.167470	.048830
K-40	Half-life: 1277000000 years		
	Betas:		
	.893300	1.311600	.508540
	Electrons:		
	.072154	.002660	
	Gammas & X-rays:		
	.009376	.002958	
	.106700	1.460800	
Ar-41	Half-life: 1.827 hours		
	Betas:		
	.991700	1.198300	.459300
	.007800	2.492000	1.076700
	.000520	.815000	.294000
	Gammas & X-rays:		
	.991600	1.293600	
	.000520	1.677000	
Ca-41	Half-life: 103000 years		
	Electrons:		
	.770280	.002970	
	Gammas & X-rays:		
	.123320	.003314	
K-42	Half-life: 12.36 hours		
	Betas:		
	.003190	1.683700	.700900
	.175000	1.996400	.822300
	.821000	3.521100	1.563900
	.001170	.520000	.191500
	Gammas & X-rays:		
	.003186	.312750	
	.179000	1.524700	
	.001409	1.446400	
K-43	Half-life: 22.6 hours		
	Betas:		
	.022400	.422430	.137000
	.922000	.826740	.298000
	.036000	1.223600	.469000
	.013000	1.817000	.762000
	Gammas & X-rays:		
	.002684	.184000	
	.041052	.220610	
	.872730	.372760	
	.114310	.396870	
	.001093	.404300	
	.110330	.593400	
	.805140	.617490	
	.001471	.800800	
	.003280	.990250	
	.001590	1.015100	
	.018787	1.021800	
	.001024	1.394200	
Sc-44	Half-life: 3.927 hours		
	Positrons:		
	.943700	1.476300	.632900
	Electrons:		
	.085509	.000310	
	.042196	.003300	
	Gammas & X-rays:		
	.000154	.000340	
	.002438	.003688	
	.004847	.003692	
	.000932	.004010	
	.998810	1.157000	
	.009120	1.499500	
	.001123	2.656400	
	.000033	2.375000	
	1.887400	.511000	
Sc-46	Half-life: 83.8 days		
	Betas:		
	.999960	.357340	.112000
	.000036	1.477800	.580900

[a] RSIC computer data file (DLC-80) contains x ray and photon data not in Kocher 1981. They are included in this table.

[b] Maximum energy for betas and positrons.

Table 8.14 Energy and Probability by Radiation Type for Selected Radionuclides of Interest to Health Physicists (Continued)

	Probability per Decay	Energy[b] (MeV)	Average Energy (MeV)
	Gammas & X-rays:		
	.999840	.889250	
	.999870	1.120500	
	.000000	2.009800	
Ca-47	Half-life: 4.536 days		
	Betas:		
	.817000	.690480	.240900
	.180000	1.987600	.816800
	.001090	.935400	.373990
	Gammas & X-rays:		
	.067410	.489230	
	.001049	.530400	
	.001947	.767000	
	.068908	.807860	
	.749000	1.297100	
	.000348	1.542200	
Sc-47	Half-life 3.422 days		
	Betas:		
	.680000	.441110	.142700
	.320000	.600500	.204000
	Electrons:		
	.005943	.000420	
	.003001	.004000	
	.003842	.154420	
	Gammas & X rays:		
	.000013	.000450	
	.000249	.004505	
	.000494	.004511	
	.000099	.004930	
	.680000	.159390	
Sc-48	Half life: 43.67 hours		
	Betas:		
	.100100	.481520	.157900
	.899900	.656870	.226500
	Electrons:		
	.002311	.000420	
	.001167	.004000	
	.001494	.170390	
	Gammas & X-rays:		
	.000005	.000450	
	.000097	.004505	
	.000192	.004511	
	.000038	.004930	
	.074700	.175360	
	1.000000	.983500	
	.975000	1.037500	
	.023800	1.212800	
	1.000000	1.312100	
V-48	Half-life: 15.971 days		
	Positrons:		
	.501000	.697380	.291400
	Electrons:		
	.735540	.000420	
	.348470	.004000	
	Gammas & X-rays:		
	.001548	.000450	
	.028901	.004505	
	.057344	.004511	
	.011471	.004930	
	.001500	.803230	
	.007700	.928320	
	.077600	.944100	
	1.000000	.983500	
	.975000	1.312100	
	.001200	1.437300	
	.024100	2.240300	
	.000270	2.361500	
	1.002000	.511000	
Cr-51	Half-life: 27.704 days		
	Electrons:		
	1.446800	.000470	
	.668860	.004380	
	Gammas & X-rays:		
	.003335	.000510	
	.065943	.004945	
	.130840	.004952	
	.026172	.005430	
	.098300	.320080	
Mn-52m	Half-life: 21.4 minutes		
	Positrons:		
	.001640	.905110	.382900
	.964000	2.632800	1.173800
	.000504	.965300	.410230
	Electrons:		
	.023708	.000540	
	.010672	.004780	
	Gammas & X-rays:		
	.016828	.377740	
	.000062	.000570	
	.001241	.005405	
	.002458	.005415	
	.000492	.005950	
	.982230	1.434100	
	.002161	1.727500	
	.001722	1.643900	
	1.932300	.511000	
Mn-52	Half-life: 5.591 days		
	Positrons:		
	.294000	.575310	.241600
	Electrons:		
	.994270	.000540	
	.447470	.004780	
	Gammas:		
	.002592	.000570	
	.052050	.005405	
	.103070	.005415	
	.020631	.005950	
	.009800	.346030	
	.001830	.399560	
	.002100	.502050	
	.003900	.600180	
	.004000	.647450	
	.900000	.744210	
	.033200	.848130	
	.945000	.935520	
	.042100	1.246200	
	.003800	1.247900	
	.050700	1.333600	
	1.000000	1.434100	
	.003707	.884480	
	.588000	.511000	
Mn-54	Half-life: 312.7 days		
	Electrons:		
	1.420300	.000540	
	.638660	.004780	
	Gammas & X-rays:		
	.003702	.000570	
	.074288	.005405	
	.147110	.005415	
	.029445	.005950	
	.999760	.834830	
Fe-55	Half-life: 2.7 years		
	Electrons:		
	1.394800	.000610	
	.607380	.005190	
	Gammas & X-rays:		
	.004197	.000640	
	.082372	.005888	
	.162790	.005899	
	.032852	.006490	
Mn-56	Half-life: 2.5785 hours		
	Betas:		
	.011600	.325630	.099100
	.146000	.735530	.255200
	.278000	1.037900	.381900
	.562000	2.848600	1.216700
	.001189	.987800	.373140
	Gammas & X-rays:		
	.988700	.846750	
	.271890	1.810700	
	.143360	2.113100	
	.009887	2.522900	
	.006525	2.657500	

[a] RSIC computer data file (DLC-80) contains x ray and photon data not in Kocher 1981. They are included in this table.
[b] Maximum energy for betas and positrons.

(continued)

Table 8.14 Energy and Probability by Radiation Type for Selected Radionuclides of Interest to Health Physicists (Continued)

	Probability per Decay	Energy[b] (MeV)	Average Energy (MeV)
	.003065	2.959800	
	.001681	3.369600	
	.001626	1.351400	
Co-56	Half-life: 78.76 days		
	Positrons:		
	.010500	.422630	.179400
	.187000	1.460500	.631900
	Electrons:		
	1.098200	.000670	
	.465050	.005620	
	Gammas & X-rays:		
	.003415	.000700	
	.073316	.006391	
	.144610	.006404	
	.029202	.007060	
	.001919	.733630	
	.003069	.787840	
	.999580	.846750	
	.014254	.977420	
	.001399	.996900	
	.140340	1.037800	
	.001260	1.140300	
	.022790	1.175100	
	.669720	1.238300	
	.001210	1.335500	
	.042882	1.360200	
	.001739	1.442700	
	.155130	1.771400	
	.006497	1.810700	
	.007127	1.963800	
	.030287	2.015400	
	.077767	2.034900	
	.003758	2.113100	
	.003878	2.213000	
	.001200	2.276100	
	.168930	2.598500	
	.010596	3.009700	
	.031787	3.202200	
	.077867	3.253500	
	.018492	3.273200	
	.009296	3.451400	
	.001899	3.548100	
	.007074	1.452800	
	.395000	.511000	
Ni-57	Half-life: 36.08 hours		
	Positrons:		
	.004100	.301540	.130000
	.008700	.463480	.197000
	.057000	.716200	.304000
	.331000	.843390	.359000
	Electrons:		
	.821250	.000750	
	.336070	.006070	
	.012931	.119480	
	.001422	.126260	
	Gammas & X-rays:		
	.002884	.000780	
	.061315	.006915	
	.120940	.006930	
	.024604	.007650	
	.129310	.127190	
	.001246	1.046400	
	.779000	1.377600	
	.070889	1.757500	
	.147230	1.919400	
	.001324	2.803900	
	.004962	1.192500	
	.801600	.511000	
Co-57	Half-life: 270.9 days		
	Electrons:		
	2.493400	.000670	
	1.054800	.005620	
	.695050	.007301	
	.077842	.013567	
	.011496	.014320	
	.018385	.114950	
	.001830	.121220	
	.014208	.129360	
	.001474	.135630	
	Gammas & X-rays:		
	.007754	.000700	
	.166290	.006391	
	.327990	.006404	
	.066234	.007060	
	.095429	.014413	
	.855100	.122060	
	.106030	.136480	
	.001599	.692000	
	.000287	.536020	
Co-58	Half-life: 70.8 days		
	Positrons:		
	.149300	.475040	.201200
	Electrons:		
	1.164900	.000670	
	.493660	.005620	
	Gammas & X-rays:		
	.003622	.000700	
	.077827	.006391	
	.153500	.006404	
	.030998	.007060	
	.994300	.810760	
	.007358	.863940	
	.005369	1.674700	
	.298600	.511000	
Fe-59	Half-life: 44.63 days		
	Betas:		
	.013700	.130790	.035700
	.452000	.273440	.081000
	.531000	.465780	.149200
	.001800	1.565000	.614500
	.000910	.084100	.022200
	Gammas & X-rays:		
	.010300	.142650	
	.031100	.192340	
	.002600	.334800	
	.565000	1.099200	
	.432000	1.291600	
	.000910	1.227900	
Ni-59	Half-life: 75000 years		
	Electrons:		
	1.342300	.000750	
	.549180	.006070	
	Gammas & X-rays:		
	.004715	.000780	
	.100190	.006915	
	.197620	.006930	
	.040205	.007650	
Co-60	Half-life: 5.271 years		
	Betas:		
	1.000000	.317900	.095790
	Gammas & X-rays:		
	1.000000	1.173200	
	1.000000	1.332500	
	.000163	.693820	
Cu-61	Half-life: 3.408 hours		
	Positrons:		
	.025400	.560390	.238800
	.056000	.933440	.399300
	.019800	1.149000	.494200
	.513000	1.216400	.524200
	.000368	.307800	.133100
	Electrons:		
	.514960	.000840	
	.203670	.006540	
	.004766	.059079	
	Gammas & X-rays:		
	.001964	.000850	
	.042708	.007461	
	.084070	.007478	

[a] RSIC computer data file (DLC-80) contains x ray and photon data not in Kocher 1981. They are included in this table.
[b] Maximum energy for betas and positrons.

Table 8.14 Energy and Probability by Radiation Type for Selected Radionuclides of Interest to Health Physicists (Continued)

	Probability per Decay	Energy[b] (MeV)	Average Energy (MeV)
	.017115	.008260	
	.038745	.067412	
	.123000	.282960	
	.021156	.373050	
	.004059	.529170	
	.011808	.588600	
	.104920	.656010	
	.003555	.816690	
	.002435	.841210	
	.011931	.908630	
	.002792	1.099600	
	.036285	1.185200	
	.008216	1.198200	
	1.229100	.511000	
Ni-63	Half-life: 100.1 years		
	Betas:		
	1.000000	.065870	.017130
Cu-64	Half-life: 12.701 hours		
	Betas:		
	.372000	.578200	.190200
	Positrons:		
	.178700	.652900	.278100
	Electrons:		
	.590750	.000840	
	.233410	.006540	
	Gammas & X-rays:		
	.002253	.000850	
	.048943	.007461	
	.096344	.007478	
	.019614	.008260	
	.004898	1.345900	
	.357400	.511000	
Ni-65	Half-life: 2.52 hours		
	Betas:		
	.005400	.412060	.128700
	.008400	.513560	.166100
	.281000	.655170	.220900
	.098000	1.021500	.372000
	.607000	2.137000	.875700
	Gammas & X-rays:		
	.046060	.366270	
	.002867	.507800	
	.001410	.609300	
	.148290	1.115500	
	.235000	1.481800	
	.004747	1.623400	
	.003877	1.724900	
	.001701	.814830	
Zn-65	Half-life: 244.4 days		
	Positrons:		
	.014150	.329900	.143000
	Electrons:		
	1.267300	.000920	
	.482880	.007030	
	Gammas & X-rays:		
	.005729	.000930	
	.115060	.008028	
	.226060	.008048	
	.046052	.008910	
	.507500	1.115500	
	.000060	.557750	
	.028300	.511000	
Zn-69	Half-life: 55.6 minutes		
	Betas:		
	.999990	.904500	.320900
	.000014	.490600	.160910
	Gammas & X-rays:		
	.000014	.413900	
Ga-67	Half-life: 3.261 days		
	Electrons:		
	1.648900	.000990	
	.602060	.007530	
	.002085	.081607	
	.268110	.083652	
	.032844	.092117	
	.010853	.093175	
	.003330	.174920	
	Gammas & X-rays:		
	.008286	.001010	
	.164720	.008616	
	.322970	.008639	
	.065838	.009570	
	.028560	.091266	
	.357000	.093311	
	.197060	.184580	
	.022420	.208950	
	.159940	.300220	
	.044768	.393530	
	.001385	.887690	
	.001247	.629410	
Se-75	Half-life: 119.78 days		
	Electrons:		
	1.295000	.001240	
	.418330	.009110	
	.050232	.012533	
	.009807	.022874	
	.002093	.024196	
	.003599	.054183	
	.026451	.084866	
	.003545	.095206	
	.006246	.109250	
	.015570	.124130	
	.001610	.134470	
	.003809	.252780	
	.001792	.267660	
	Gammas & X-rays:		
	.009129	.001280	
	.161090	.010508	
	.314010	.010544	
	.072690	.011700	
	.010226	.066050	
	.034086	.096733	
	.167440	.121120	
	.592020	.136000	
	.014472	.198600	
	.598000	.264650	
	.252360	.279530	
	.013216	.303910	
	.114220	.400650	
	.000972	.332650	
Se-79	Half-life: 65000 years		
	Betas:		
	1.000000	.149000	.052200
Br-82	Half-life: 35.3 hours		
	Betas:		
	.013590	.264580	.076200
	.979000	.444340	.137800
	.000900	.536500	.171600
	Gammas & X-rays:		
	.007165	.092184	
	.001416	.137400	
	.022577	.221450	
	.007998	.273450	
	.705640	.554320	
	.011663	.606300	
	.430710	.619070	
	.281590	.698330	
	.833100	.776490	
	.241600	.827810	
	.003666	.952100	
	.012680	1.007600	
	.273260	1.044000	
	.006248	1.081400	
	.269090	1.317500	
	.001083	1.426000	
	.165790	1.474800	
	.007406	1.650300	
	.001133	1.779600	
	.007588	.743580	
Br-84	Half-life: 31.8 minutes		
	Betas:		
	.002200	.483900	.152000
	.021000	.556500	.179000

[a] RSIC computer data file (DLC-80) contains x ray and photon data not in Kocher 1981. They are included in this table.

[b] Maximum energy for betas and positrons.

(continued)

Table 8.14 Energy and Probability by Radiation Type for Selected Radionuclides of Interest to Health Physicists (Continued)

	Probability per Decay	Energy[b] (MeV)	Average Energy (MeV)
	.004900	.588800	.191000
	.117000	.745800	.253000
	.002900	.794300	.272000
	.001800	.802700	.276000
	.025000	.967300	.343000
	.004900	1.197500	.442000
	.095000	1.307300	.490000
	.039000	1.590800	.616000
	.011300	1.914100	.763000
	.074000	1.973100	.790000
	.019000	2.050200	.826000
	.003400	2.183800	.888000
	.016000	2.327600	.955000
	.121000	2.775900	1.166000
	.137000	3.791500	1.650000
	.320000	4.673000	2.072000
	.000630	2.836000	1.194000
	Gammas & X-rays:		
	.003081	.230200	
	.003081	.354700	
	.005697	.382000	
	.017724	.604800	
	.013082	.736500	
	.060768	.802200	
	.422000	.881500	
	.003587	.947500	
	.007807	.987300	
	.004600	1.005700	
	.062456	1.015900	
	.001435	1.082600	
	.001435	1.119100	
	.001097	1.185000	
	.026164	1.213300	
	.019834	1.463800	
	.001013	1.534700	
	.006583	1.578100	
	.004009	1.607600	
	.016458	1.741200	
	.002448	1.818700	
	.011394	1.877500	
	.149390	1.897300	
	.021100	2.029600	
	.002152	2.094200	
	.011816	2.200700	
	.067520	2.484100	
	.001393	2.593700	
	.003038	2.622900	
	.004937	2.758700	
	.011394	2.824100	
	.001772	2.988700	
	.025320	3.045400	
	.002110	3.202100	
	.020678	3.235300	
	.029118	3.365800	
	.068786	3.927500	
	.002785	4.084600	
	.006749	1.122900	
Kr-85m[c]	Half-life: 4.48 hours		
	Betas:		
	.002900	.710840	.238200
	.786000	.840690	.290400
	.000210	.260000	.074600
	Electrons:		
	.076149	.001500	
	.020989	.010800	
	.059291	.290540	
	.008967	.302950	
	.002954	.304580	
	.038472	.001680	
	.010415	.011400	
	.031466	.135980	
	.003500	.149110	
	.001152	.150860	
	Gammas & X-rays:		
	.001003	.001590	
	.011162	.012598	
	.021631	.012649	
	.005509	.014100	
	.139890	.304870	
	.000586	.001690	
	.006116	.013336	
	.011830	.013395	
	.003105	.015000	
	.003011	.129850	
	.752780	.151180	
	.000211	.581280	
Kr-85	Half-life: 10.72 years		
	Betas:		
	.004370	.173020	.047500
	.995631	.687020	.251400
	Gammas & X-rays:		
	0.004340	.513990	
Sr-85	Half-life: 64.84 days		
	Electrons:		
	1.081500	.001680	
	.290670	.011400	
	.006254	.498790	
	Gammas & X-rays:		
	.016470	.001690	
	.170690	.013336	
	.330150	.013395	
	.086645	.015000	
	.992700	.513990	
	.000139	.868500	
Kr-87[c]	Half-life: 76.3 minutes		
	Betas:		
	.005000	.580480	.187800
	.001080	.833660	.287500
	.044000	.928400	.326400
	.005800	1.077800	.389300
	.095000	1.334200	.500400
	.055100	1.474600	.562600
	.004200	1.510600	.578700
	.006200	2.148500	.870000
	.001600	2.311000	.945600
	.001240	2.499100	1.033700
	.069000	3.043600	1.294200
	.407000	3.486400	1.502000
	.304000	3.889000	1.694800
	Electrons:		
	.001939	.001680	
	.000577	.011400	
	.001742	.387380	
	Gammas & X-rays:		
	.000030	.001690	
	.000339	.013336	
	.000655	.013395	
	.000172	.015000	
	.495000	.402580	
	.019058	.673870	
	.001683	.814250	
	.007524	.836370	
	.072765	.845430	
	.001386	.946640	
	.011237	1.175400	
	.006484	1.338000	
	.002871	1.382500	
	.001237	1.389900	
	.003564	1.531200	
	.001287	1.578000	
	.001040	1.611200	
	.020493	1.740500	
	.001386	1.842600	
	.028957	2.011900	
	.002129	2.408500	
	.093060	2.554800	
	.039105	2.558100	
	.003168	2.811400	
	.004504	3.308500	
	.006499	1.620100	
Sr-87m	Half-life: 2.805 hours		
	Electrons:		
	.178550	.001790	
	.044979	.012100	
	.145560	.372300	
	.021336	.386180	

[a] RSIC computer data file (DLC-80) contains x ray and photon data not in Kocher 1981. They are included in this table.

[b] Maximum energy for betas and positrons.

[c] Branching to radioactive daughter(s) shown in Table 8.13.

Table 8.14 Energy and Probability by Radiation Type for Selected Radionuclides of Interest to Health Physicists (Continued)

	Probability per Decay	Energy[b] (MeV)	Average Energy (MeV)
	.007039	.388040	
	.003200	.001680	
	.000842	.011400	
	Gammas & X-rays:		
	.002903	.001810	
	.029161	.014098	
	.056296	.014165	
	.015126	.015800	
	.822530	.388400	
	.000049	.001690	
	.000494	.013336	
	.000956	.013395	
	.000251	.015000	
Kr-88[c]	Half-life: 2.84 hours		
	Betas:		
	.003530	.141890	.038000
	.026500	.364580	.109000
	.670000	.520850	.165000
	.091000	.681240	.227000
	.001400	.823920	.284000
	.002040	.997480	.355000
	.019200	1.198300	.441000
	.002300	1.251900	.464000
	.002200	1.471500	.561000
	.009000	1.730900	.678000
	.001000	1.771600	.697000
	.013000	2.050700	.825000
	.002600	2.522500	1.052000
	.018000	2.716700	1.136000
	.140000	2.913000	1.233000
	.001010	.687000	.233830
	Electrons:		
	.149310	.001680	
	.040387	.011400	
	.107170	.012313	
	.001329	.013060	
	.012332	.025448	
	.002729	.027191	
	.002079	.150780	
	.011433	.181120	
	.001377	.194250	
	Gammas & X-rays:		
	.002274	.001690	
	.023716	.013336	
	.045873	.013395	
	.012039	.015000	
	.020622	.027513	
	.001972	.122270	
	.031036	.165980	
	.259850	.196320	
	.002526	.240710	
	.001073	.311690	
	.001453	.334710	
	.022490	.362230	
	.006436	.390540	
	.001280	.421700	
	.007266	.471800	
	.002353	.677340	
	.005328	.788280	
	.001246	.790320	
	.129750	.834830	
	.001730	.850340	
	.006712	.862330	
	.002941	.944920	
	.013148	.985780	
	.001419	.990090	
	.018892	1.000100	
	.004844	1.039600	
	.001419	1.049500	
	.012837	1.141300	
	.009965	1.179500	
	.006885	1.185000	
	.001419	1.209800	
	.001384	1.212700	
	.003633	1.245200	
	.011210	1.250700	
	.001592	1.325000	
	.001592	1.352300	
	.014774	1.369500	
	.002180	1.406900	
	.001142	1.464800	
	.021521	1.518400	
	.109340	1.529800	
	.004567	1.603800	
	.006643	1.685600	
	.001384	1.892800	
	.001003	1.908700	
	.045291	2.029800	
	.037368	2.035400	
	.002872	2.186500	
	.131830	2.195800	
	.033908	2.231800	
	.007301	2.352100	
	.346000	2.392100	
	.001038	2.408900	
	.006228	2.548400	
	.001488	2.771000	
Rb-88	Half-life: 17.8 minutes		
	Betas:		
	.006600	.462100	.143600
	.003620	.469630	.146300
	.001430	.572310	.184300
	.021300	.801140	.273700
	.002100	.901290	.314500
	.009800	2.096500	.844500
	.133000	2.580900	1.070600
	.041000	3.479000	1.496500
	.780000	5.315000	2.372400
	.000627	1.390000	.526380
	Gammas & X-rays:		
	.140380	.898020	
	.001027	1.366300	
	.007426	1.382400	
	.002161	1.779800	
	.214000	1.836000	
	.001177	2.111200	
	.004216	2.118900	
	.001798	2.577700	
	.019581	2.677900	
	.001091	2.734000	
	.002440	3.009400	
	.002140	3.218500	
	.001305	3.486500	
	.001434	4.742700	
	.003330	1.474600	
Rb-89[c]	Half-life: 15.44 minutes		
	Betas:		
	.015200	.994340	.353200
	.330000	1.275100	.473600
	.021900	1.795800	.706400
	.030000	1.932900	.769100
	.340000	2.222900	.903100
	.004600	2.445600	1.007100
	.004900	2.495400	1.030400
	.002200	2.562800	1.062000
	.002400	3.029600	1.284800
	.250000	4.503000	1.987400
	.003690	.776000	.272390
	Gammas & X-rays:		
	.014152	.272450	
	.005394	.289760	
	.099760	.657710	
	.001624	.766790	
	.092220	.947690	
	.002262	1.025300	
	.580000	1.031900	
	.002204	1.220300	
	.001218	1.228400	
	.423400	1.248100	
	.003538	1.473200	
	.001972	1.501100	
	.025520	1.538100	
	.003306	1.940200	
	.023780	2.007500	
	.002320	2.058000	
	.133400	2.196000	

[a] RSIC computer data file (DLC-80) contains x ray and photon data not in Kocher 1981. They are included in this table.
[b] Maximum energy for betas and positrons.
[c] Branching to radioactive daughter(s) shown in Table 8.13.

(continued)

Table 8.14 Energy and Probability by Radiation Type for Selected Radionuclides of Interest to Health Physicists (Continued)

	Probability per Decay	Energy[b] (MeV)	Average Energy (MeV)
	.001798	2.280100	
	.098600	2.570100	
	.020300	2.707200	
	.011484	3.508800	
	.011832	1.950300	
Sr-89	Half-life: 50.55 days		
	Betas:		
	.999850	1.491300	.583000
	.000150	.582200	.187600
	Gammas & X-rays:		
	.000150	.909100	
Sr-90[c]	Half-life: 28.6 years		
	Betas:		
	1.000000	.546000	.195800
Y-90	Half-life: 64.1 hours		
	Betas:		
	.999890	2.283900	.934800
	.000115	.523200	.186500
Sr-91[c]	Half-life: 9.5 hours		
	Betas:		
	.002310	.404660	.122900
	.014400	.477270	.148800
	.020200	.617370	.200900
	.003610	.703580	.234300
	.339000	1.104100	.398900
	.017700	1.138100	.413400
	.001850	1.210300	.444500
	.244000	1.378600	.518000
	.006430	1.497100	.570500
	.033000	2.031000	.812900
	.308000	2.684000	1.121200
	.001270	.355000	.110210
	Gammas & X-rays:		
	.004355	.261200	
	.002535	.272700	
	.010043	.274700	
	.001430	.379900	
	.017225	.620100	
	.005395	.631300	
	.028925	.652300	
	.078000	.652900	
	.004550	.653000	
	.229780	.749800	
	.005590	.761400	
	.001560	.820800	
	.001820	.879700	
	.037375	.925800	
	.325000	1.024300	
	.002178	1.054600	
	.001235	1.140800	
	.009067	1.280900	
	.009522	1.413400	
	.001625	1.473800	
	.002828	1.651400	
	.001560	1.724000	
	.011908	.776340	
Y-91m[c]	Half-life: 49.71 minutes		
	Electrons:		
	.049532	.001910	
	.012051	.012700	
	.041700	.540530	
	.005610	.555200	
	.001850	.557180	
	Gammas & X-rays:		
	.001114	.001920	
	.008578	.014883	
	.016527	.014958	
	.004544	.016700	
	.950800	.557570	
Y-91	Half-life: 58.51 days		
	Betas:		
	.003000	.338100	.099900
	.997000	1.543000	.603800
	Gammas & X-rays:		
	.003000	1.204900	
Sr-92	Half-life: 2.71 hours		
	Betas:		
	.960000	.546100	.174000
	.003000	.976660	.345000
	.002100	1.037600	.371000
	.040000	1.930000	.777000
	Gammas & X-rays:		
	.029700	.241520	
	.033300	.430560	
	.002610	.491300	
	.003690	.650700	
	.036000	.953320	
	.028800	1.142300	
	.900000	1.383900	
	.001710	.664620	
Y-92	Half-life: 3.54 hours		
	Betas:		
	.001000	.814400	.278000
	.065000	1.294100	.480000
	.002400	1.567100	.601000
	.004300	1.786700	.700000
	.011600	2.138400	.869000
	.023000	2.251000	.920000
	.034000	2.699500	1.123000
	.857000	3.634000	1.563000
	.000372	.558000	.183400
	Gammas & X-rays:		
	.023352	.448500	
	.004851	.492600	
	.024047	.561100	
	.012510	.844300	
	.006255	.912600	
	.139000	.934460	
	.002433	1.132400	
	.047816	1.405400	
	.003600	1.847300	
	.001519	1.647200	
Y-93[c]	Half-life: 10.1 hours		
	Betas:		
	.001870	.432320	.132000
	.016000	.705380	.235000
	.001450	1.419900	.535000
	.003770	1.439600	.544000
	.002660	1.464600	.555000
	.025100	1.942900	.771000
	.046000	2.623100	1.087000
	.902000	2.890000	1.214000
	.001192	.890000	.310460
	Electrons:		
	.001554	.002020	
	.000407	.013400	
	.001507	.248900	
	Gammas & X-rays:		
	.000043	.002040	
	.000318	.015691	
	.000611	.015775	
	.000172	.017700	
	.068502	.266900	
	.006081	.680200	
	.019502	.947100	
	.001028	1.203300	
	.002377	1.425400	
	.003355	1.450500	
	.014050	1.917800	
	.001552	2.184600	
	.001713	2.190800	
	.003257	1.413300	
Zr-93[c]	Half-life: 1530000 years		
	Betas:		
	1.000000	.061531	.019500
Mo-93[c]	Half-life: 3500 years		
	Electrons:		
	.981380	.002150	
	.211830	.014000	
	Gammas & X-rays:		
	.030352	.002170	
	.181140	.016521	

[a] RSIC computer data file (DLC-80) contains x ray and photon data not in Kocher 1981. They are included in this table.
[b] Maximum energy for betas and positrons.
[c] Branching to radioactive daughter(s) shown in Table 8.13.

Table 8.14 Energy and Probability by Radiation Type for Selected Radionuclides of Interest to Health Physicists (Continued)

	Probability per Decay	Energy[b] (MeV)	Average Energy (MeV)
	.347680	.016615	
	.099947	.018600	
Nb-93m	Half-life: 14.6 years		
	Electrons:		
	.793940	.002150	
	.150000	.011784	
	.037800	.014000	
	.661000	.028072	
	.142000	.030302	
	.046900	.030712	
	Gammas & X-rays:		
	.024555	.002170	
	.032324	.016521	
	.062041	.016615	
	.017835	.018600	
Zr-95[c]	Half-life: 64.02 days		
	Betas:		
	.554000	.366380	.109300
	.437000	.398910	.120400
	.007800	.887410	.327000
	.001000	1.123100	.405400
	Gammas & X-rays:		
	.436560	.724180	
	.553450	.756710	
Nb-95m[c]	Half-life: 86.6 hours		
	Betas:		
	.001340	.957170	.334970
	.054000	1.161300	.437800
	.000039	.374900	.111960
	Electrons:		
	.665530	.002150	
	.138360	.014000	
	.549050	.216700	
	.109620	.232990	
	.036193	.235220	
	Gammas & X-rays:		
	.020584	.002170	
	.118310	.016521	
	.227090	.016615	
	.065281	.018600	
	.250430	.235690	
	.001297	.204120	
	.000039	.629070	
Zr-97[c]	Half-life: 16.9 hours		
	Betas:		
	.004900	.409900	.124300
	.055000	.551500	.175300
	.018800	.892950	.309200
	.005000	.906910	.314900
	.001800	1.004700	.355400
	.003800	1.109100	.399400
	.006500	1.109600	.399600
	.002100	1.381300	.517200
	.044000	1.406400	.528300
	.860000	1.914100	.756600
	Gammas & X-rays:		
	.001021	.202200	
	.002321	.218680	
	.012533	.254150	
	.002507	.272270	
	.001114	.330430	
	.022746	.355390	
	.003249	.400390	
	.052919	.507630	
	.005106	.513470	
	.013926	.602520	
	.002507	.690630	
	.001207	.699200	
	.009284	.703800	
	.001207	.795700	
	.006499	.804530	
	.002228	.829800	
	.003342	.854900	
	.002878	.971390	
	.012069	1.021300	
	.001114	1.119100	
	.026459	1.148000	
	.009748	1.276100	
	.013462	1.362700	
	.013462	1.750500	
	.003528	1.851600	
	.002135	.344090	
Nb-97m[c]	Half-life: 60 seconds		
	Electrons:		
	.019904	.002150	
	.004385	.014000	
	.017400	.724370	
	.002250	.740660	
	Gammas & X-rays:		
	.000616	.002170	
	.003750	.016521	
	.007197	.016615	
	.002069	.018600	
	.979600	.743360	
Nb-97	Half-life: 72.1 minutes		
	Betas:		
	.001180	.303810	.088200
	.001670	.417340	.126600
	.002060	.664260	.217600
	.010800	.908400	.314900
	.983000	1.274900	.469800
	.000880	.815900	.277300
	Electrons:		
	.001746	.002270	
	.000417	.014800	
	.001766	.637900	
	Gammas & X-rays:		
	.000073	.002290	
	.000388	.017374	
	.000743	.017479	
	.000218	.019600	
	.001471	.480900	
	.980900	.657900	
	.010790	1.024500	
	.001569	1.268600	
	.001177	1.515600	
	.004904	.798260	
Ru-97	Half-life: 2.9 days		
	Electrons:		
	.971390	.002170	
	.198050	.015500	
	.028300	.194640	
	.003403	.212640	
	.001846	.303440	
	Gammas & X-rays:		
	.045772	.002420	
	.200280	.018251	
	.382940	.018367	
	.114890	.020600	
	.001077	.108800	
	.855000	.215680	
	.108590	.324480	
	.001171	.460550	
	.008721	.569270	
	.003054	.713310	
Mo-99[c]	Half-life: 66.02 hours		
	Betas:		
	.001130	.214590	.059800
	.001360	.352650	.104200
	.173000	.436040	.133000
	.013600	.847600	.289600
	.827000	1.214000	.442700
	.000578	.559300	.180890
	Electrons:		
	.043503	.002170	
	.008946	.015500	
	.028881	.019540	
	.003498	.037542	
	.003743	.119460	
	.007854	.160020	
	.001172	.178020	
	Gammas & X-rays:		
	.002050	.002420	

[a] RSIC computer data file (DLC-80) contains x ray and photon data not in Kocher 1981. They are included in this table.

[b] Maximum energy for betas and positrons.

[c] Branching to radioactive daughter(s) shown in Table 8.13.

(continued)

Table 8.14 Energy and Probability by Radiation Type for Selected Radionuclides of Interest to Health Physicists (Continued)

	Probability per Decay	Energy[b] (MeV)	Average Energy (MeV)
	.009046	.018251	
	.017297	.018367	
	.005190	.020600	
	.008832	.040584	
	.037888	.140510	
	.062336	.181060	
	.013696	.366430	
	.128000	.739580	
	.044800	.778000	
	.001331	.822900	
	.002584	.680130	
Tc-99m[c]	Half-life: 6.02 hours		
	Electrons:		
	.745460	.001626	
	.245840	.002102	
	.102680	.002170	
	.020788	.015500	
	.087928	.119460	
	.006134	.121590	
	.010607	.137470	
	.001905	.139590	
	.002300	.139960	
	Gammas & X-rays:		
	.004838	.002420	
	.021021	.018251	
	.040194	.018367	
	.012059	.020600	
	.890700	.140510	
	.000214	.142630	
Tc-99	Half-life: 213000 years		
	Betas:		
	.999990	.293600	.084600
	.000015	.204200	.056500
	Gammas & X-rays:		
	.000006	.089360	
Tc-101	Half-life: 14.2 minutes		
	Betas:		
	.012000	.623500	.201000
	.008200	.686580	.225000
	.003090	.696030	.229000
	.019400	.782170	.263000
	.001600	.905000	.312000
	.065000	1.079900	.385000
	.890000	1.318200	.487000
	Electrons:		
	.019192	.002530	
	.003891	.016200	
	.005577	.105120	
	.001212	.161990	
	.012009	.284690	
	.001404	.303590	
	Gammas & X-rays:		
	.001010	.002560	
	.004273	.019150	
	.008139	.019279	
	.002495	.021700	
	.028168	.127240	
	.005828	.179570	
	.016159	.184110	
	.002746	.233710	
	.003073	.238260	
	.883000	.306810	
	.001395	.311500	
	.001121	.393330	
	.001086	.515950	
	.010243	.531490	
	.060044	.545140	
	.004150	.627050	
	.011479	.694700	
	.006887	.715520	
	.001854	.720000	
	.002305	.842790	
	.001272	.928710	
	.004780	.617830	
Ru-103[c]	Half-life: 39.35 days		
	Betas:		
	.064000	.112820	.029800
	.900000	.226070	.063200
	.002380	.467920	.143800
	.035000	.723150	.239200
	.001023	.140900	.038725
	Electrons:		
	.010117	.002390	
	.002097	.017000	
	.006795	.030055	
	.004072	.473860	
	Gammas & X-rays:		
	.000532	.002700	
	.002511	.020074	
	.004773	.020216	
	.001486	.022700	
	.003734	.053275	
	.002489	.294980	
	.003200	.443800	
	.889000	.497080	
	.008268	.557040	
	.056007	.610330	
	.001249	.486930	
Rh-103m	Half-life: 56.119 minutes		
	Electrons:		
	.765980	.002390	
	.095200	.016528	
	.018374	.017000	
	.713000	.036336	
	.144000	.039121	
	.047500	.039667	
	Gammas & X-rays:		
	.040315	.002700	
	.021995	.020074	
	.041815	.020216	
	.013017	.022700	
	.000704	.039748	
Rh-105m	Half-life: 4.44 hours		
	Betas:		
	.001080	.220170	.061300
	.003400	.431180	.130800
	.002000	.475700	.147000
	.013200	.540720	.170100
	.044700	.572510	.181800
	.005000	.596490	.190700
	.001130	.702540	.231100
	.052200	.948220	.329300
	.200000	1.111700	.397500
	.181000	1.131900	.406000
	.002900	1.155900	.416200
	.499000	1.193300	.432200
	.005000	1.525200	.576800
	.001630	.447000	.140310
	Electrons:		
	.006662	.002390	
	.001381	.017000	
	.003520	.062680	
	.002037	.125980	
	.001598	.239680	
	Gammas & X-rays:		
	.000351	.002700	
	.001653	.020074	
	.003143	.020216	
	.000978	.022700	
	.003200	.085900	
	.016700	.149200	
	.001400	.163600	
	.001000	.183600	
	.001500	.225000	
	.072000	.262900	
	.117000	.316500	
	.011800	.326100	
	.007900	.330900	
	.003000	.350000	
	.011000	.350200	
	.042000	.393400	
	.001800	.407500	

[a] RSIC computer data file (DLC-80) contains x ray and photon data not in Kocher 1981. They are included in this table.
[b] Maximum energy for betas and positrons.
[c] Branching to radioactive daughter(s) shown in Table 8.13.

Table 8.14 Energy and Probability by Radiation Type for Selected Radionuclides of Interest to Health Physicists (Continued)

	Probability per Decay	Energy[b] (MeV)	Average Energy (MeV)
	.024800	.413500	
	.175000	.469400	
	.013000	.470000	
	.005900	.489600	
	.024000	.499200	
	.003000	.500400	
	.003600	.513700	
	.001300	.539200	
	.001300	.575000	
	.010700	.575300	
	.002300	.632300	
	.002800	.638600	
	.003500	.652600	
	.002000	.656000	
	.024000	.656100	
	.167000	.676400	
	.490000	.724500	
	.001900	.822100	
	.007300	.845900	
	.034000	.875800	
	.005900	.907700	
	.023400	.969400	
	.003400	1.017200	
	.002300	1.321100	
	.012810	.707360	
Rh-105	Half-life: 35.36 hours		
	Betas:		
	.197000	.248000	.069900
	.052200	.260800	.073900
	.750000	.566900	.179400
	.000403	.124200	.033000
	Electrons:		
	.003842	.002500	
	.001359	.014420	
	.000767	.017700	
	.002880	.294550	
	Gammas & X-rays:		
	.000228	.002840	
	.000992	.021020	
	.001882	.021177	
	.000598	.023800	
	.001670	.280100	
	.051264	.306100	
	.192000	.318900	
	.000630	.294920	
Ru-106[c]	Half-life: 368.2 days		
	Betas:		
	1.000000	.039401	.010030
Rh-106	**Half-life: 29.92 seconds**		
	Betas:		
	.004270	1.539500	.582000
	.019200	1.978800	.780000
	.098000	2.407300	.977000
	.005800	2.413000	.979000
	.082000	3.029200	1.267000
	.787000	3.541000	1.509000
	.004167	1.118000	.404710
	Gammas & X-rays:		
	.206000	.511850	
	.007004	.616170	
	.098056	.621840	
	.004161	.873600	
	.017304	1.050500	
	.003955	1.128000	
	.001566	1.562200	
	.005797	1.357000	
Pd-107	Half-life: 6500000 years		
	Betas:		
	1.000000	.033101	.009300
Pd-109	Half-life: 13.453 hours		
	Betas:		
	.998790	1.027900	.361000
	.001130	.450100	.139880
	Gammas & X-rays:		
	.001354	.508600	
Ag-110m[c]	Half-life: 249.85 days		
	Betas:		
	.673000	.083866	.021800
	.004070	.133810	.035700
	.305000	.530670	.165600
	.001863	.315300	.092836
	Electrons:		
	.013287	.000563	
	.011118	.002610	
	.001404	.018500	
	.008259	.090966	
	.003937	.112670	
	.002278	.002720	
	.000411	.019300	
	.002567	.631040	
	Gammas		
	.000748	.002980	
	.001956	.021990	
	.003705	.022163	
	.001194	.024900	
	.000096	.098856	
	.000161	.003130	
	.000615	.022984	
	.001161	.023174	
	.000380	.026100	
	.001057	.365440	
	.036434	.446800	
	.027656	.620350	
	.002341	.626250	
	.943880	.657750	
	.001416	.676600	
	.106750	.677610	
	.064656	.686990	
	.166780	.706670	
	.002832	.708120	
	.0091	.7345	
	.046439	.744260	
	.222760	.763930	
	.072773	.818020	
	.725840	.884670	
	.341870	.937480	
	.001246	.997230	
	.001321	1.334300	
	.242580	1.384300	
	.040020	1.475800	
	.130630	1.505000	
	.011798	1.562300	
Ag-110	Half-life: 24.57 seconds		
	Betas:		
	.044200	2.235000	.894100
	.951900	2.892800	1.199300
	.000866	1.124800	.406850
	Electrons:		
	.002658	.002500	
	.000468	.017700	
	Gammas & X-rays:		
	.000158	.002840	
	.000605	.021020	
	.001148	.021177	
	.000365	.023800	
	.044865	.657750	
	.000969	1.046000	
In-111	Half-life: 2.83 days		
	Electrons:		
	1.002700	.002720	
	.157720	.019300	
	.084090	.144570	
	.010499	.167260	
	.002450	.170510	
	.050384	.218680	
	.007849	.241370	
	.001814	.244620	
	Gammas & X-rays:		
	.070853	.003130	
	.236280	.022984	
	.445810	.023174	
	.145970	.026100	
	.902400	.171280	

[a] RSIC computer data file (DLC-80) contains x ray and photon data not in Kocher 1981. They are included in this table.
[b] Maximum energy for betas and positrons.
[c] Branching to radioactive daughter(s) shown in Table 8.13.

(continued)

Table 8.14 Energy and Probability by Radiation Type for Selected Radionuclides of Interest to Health Physicists (Continued)

Nuclide	Probability per Decay	Energy[b] (MeV)	Average Energy (MeV)
	.940000	.245390	
	.000028	.150810	
Ag-111	Half-life: 7.46 days		
	Betas:		
	.07000	.685900	.223500
	.011000	.782610	.278900
	.919000	1.028000	.360400
	.000560	.237000	.067793
	Electrons:		
	.000907	.002720	
	.000164	.019300	
	.001022	.315420	
	Gammas		
	.000064	.003130	
	.000245	.022984	
	.000462	.023174	
	.000151	.026100	
	.001202	.096750	
	.012291	.245390	
	.066800	.342130	
	.000559	.654720	
Cd-113m	Half-life: 13.7 years		
	Betas:		
	.999770	.585700	.185400
In-113m	Half-life: 1.658 hours		
	Electrons:		
	.296530	.002840	
	.042300	.020100	
	.282000	.363750	
	.054800	.387450	
	.011100	.390860	
	.002450	.391570	
	Gammas & X-rays:		
	.023351	.003290	
	.068312	.024002	
	.128650	.024210	
	.042740	.027300	
	.649000	.391690	
Cd-115m[c]	Half-life: 44.6 days		
	Betas:		
	.001960	.202730	.055800
	.006050	.330400	.096000
	.011450	.687160	.241700
	.980000	1.621000	.615000
	.000559	.410600	.124710
	Gammas & X-rays:		
	.001929	.484470	
	.013300	.933840	
	.005918	1.290600	
	.000972	.932730	
In-115	Half-life: 4.6e + 15 years		
	Betas:		
	1.000000	.495000	.152000
Sn-123	Half-life: 129.2 days		
	Betas:		
	.006000	.308350	.088600
	.994000	1.397000	.523100
	.000343	.347000	.101760
	Gammas & X-rays:		
	.006000	1.088600	
	.000363	.992900	
I-123	Half-life: 13.13 hours		
	Electrons:		
	.940730	.003190	
	.123630	.022700	
	.135940	.127190	
	.017597	.154060	
	.004329	.157990	
	Gammas & X-rays:		
	.093039	.003770	
	.246310	.027202	
	.459540	.027472	
	.159520	.031000	
	.834000	.159000	
	.001259	.346350	
	.004287	.440020	
	.003161	.505330	
	.013928	.528960	
	.003820	.538540	
	.004763	.494440	
Sb-124	Half-life: 60.2 days		
	Betas:		
	.005200	.130080	.034600
	.005020	.203200	.055900
	.087600	.211290	.058300
	.003700	.421640	.126200
	.528000	.611270	.194000
	.002580	.722440	.236000
	.006400	.813240	.271300
	.040900	.865660	.292000
	.021300	.947060	.324700
	.051400	1.579500	.593400
	.025300	1.656400	.627300
	.219000	2.302300	.918600
	.003890	.447600	.138780
	Electrons:		
	.003404	.003190	
	.000514	.022700	
	.004110	.570890	
	Gammas & X-rays:		
	.000337	.003770	
	.001024	.027202	
	.001910	.027472	
	.000663	.031000	
	.001292	.400030	
	.002055	.443990	
	.001664	.525500	
	.978700	.602710	
	.001468	.632360	
	.072620	.645850	
	.014191	.709310	
	.023782	.713820	
	.110980	.722780	
	.001272	.735670	
	.007438	.790740	
	.019183	.968200	
	.018595	1.045200	
	.014974	1.325500	
	.009983	1.355200	
	.025055	1.368200	
	.004404	1.376300	
	.011353	1.436600	
	.002153	1.445200	
	.006264	1.489100	
	.004013	1.526400	
	.001957	1.579900	
	.490330	1.691000	
	.057254	2.091000	
	.013366	1.208300	
Sn-125[c]	Half-life: 9.64 days		
	Betas:		
	.002200	.062200	.016000
	.001900	.075101	.019500
	.001100	.096300	.025200
	.005300	.109600	.028900
	.022000	.348400	.101700
	.039000	.367300	.108000
	.059000	.460390	.139800
	.001300	.544000	.169600
	.003100	1.001000	.347300
	.027000	1.260500	.456000
	.830000	2.350000	.938000
	.000787	.366000	.114860
	Gammas & X-rays:		
	.012900	.331900	
	.002236	.350900	
	.012900	.469700	
	.009460	.800500	
	.037840	.822600	
	.002322	.893700	

[a] RSIC computer data file (DLC-80) contains x ray and photon data not in Kocher 1981. They are included in this table.
[b] Maximum energy for betas and positrons.
[c] Branching to radioactive daughter(s) shown in Table 8.13.

Table 8.14 Energy and Probability by Radiation Type for Selected Radionuclides of Interest to Health Physicists (Continued)

	Probability per Decay	Energy[b] (MeV)	Average Energy (MeV)
	.037840	.915500	
	.001462	.934700	
	.002580	1.017100	
	.086000	1.066600	
	.009460	1.087400	
	.040420	1.088900	
	.001032	1.151300	
	.001892	1.173200	
	.002150	1.221000	
	.004644	1.419500	
	.001462	1.805700	
	.020640	2.001700	
	.001806	2.275200	
	.007031	.833210	
Sb-125[c]	Half-life: 2.77 years		
	Betas:		
	.136000	.095387	.024900
	.058100	.124650	.033100
	.181000	.130780	.034800
	.015900	.241600	.067500
	.399000	.303420	.087000
	.074000	.445710	.134500
	.135000	.622040	.215500
	Electrons:		
	.500200	.003190	
	.499780	.003678	
	.001809	.014941	
	.064187	.022700	
	.078716	.030553	
	.015826	.034486	
	.005206	.035324	
	.010339	.144520	
	.001861	.171390	
	.003373	.396080	
	Gammas & X-rays:		
	.049470	.003770	
	.127890	.027202	
	.238600	.027472	
	.082825	.031000	
	.041649	.035492	
	.002610	.116950	
	.001813	.172620	
	.068926	.176330	
	.003226	.204130	
	.002432	.208090	
	.001314	.227910	
	.004171	.321030	
	.014958	.380440	
	.001819	.408010	
	.293300	.427890	
	.003021	.443500	
	.103530	.463380	
	.177740	.600560	
	.050213	.606640	
	.113210	.635890	
	.018126	.671410	
	.000697	.159030	
Te-125m	Half-life: 58 days		
	Electrons:		
	.884440	.003190	
	.070498	.022700	
	.426990	.056646	
	.122660	.030553	
	.024662	.034486	
	.008113	.035324	
	.518990	.077462	
	.373000	.104340	
	.085899	.108270	
	.022500	.109110	
	Gammas & X-rays:		
	.150900	.003770	
	.323220	.027202	
	.603020	.027472	
	.209330	.031000	
	.064900	.035492	
	.002830	.109280	
	.000000	.144780	
I-125	Half-life: 60.14 days		
	Electrons:		
	1.561000	.003190	
	.778800	.003678	
	.196910	.022700	
	.122660	.030553	
	.024662	.034486	
	.008113	.035324	
	Gammas & X-rays:		
	.154380	.003770	
	.392330	.027202	
	.731960	.027472	
	.254090	.031000	
	.064900	.035492	
Sn-126[c]	Half-life: 100000 years		
	Betas:		
	1.000000	.250100	.070000
	Electrons:		
	1.201300	.003070	
	.031718	.012149	
	.021071	.016952	
	.578220	.018002	
	.316850	.018582	
	.004115	.020706	
	.001363	.021498	
	.123780	.021756	
	.044915	.021800	
	.062538	.022336	
	.040859	.022548	
	.020611	.023128	
	.053856	.033789	
	.004116	.037942	
	.001079	.041696	
	.164070	.056449	
	.088060	.057079	
	.007187	.059582	
	.001706	.063336	
	.063400	.082242	
	.011322	.082872	
	.013019	.085996	
	.002701	.086626	
	.002800	.086788	
	Gammas & X-rays:		
	.111590	.003600	
	.012395	.021650	
	.064010	.023280	
	.083339	.026111	
	.156070	.026359	
	.053387	.029700	
	.004995	.042640	
	.095830	.064280	
	.089170	.086940	
	.370000	.087570	
	.000999	.022700	
Sb-126	Half-life: 12.4 days		
	Betas:		
	.005000	.090401	.024000
	.020900	.114300	.030000
	.290000	.371400	.109000
	.059000	.393500	.117000
	.084000	.494700	.152000
	.042000	.575900	.181000
	.005600	.591000	.204000
	.005000	.725100	.237000
	.004800	.727500	.238000
	.081000	.753900	.248000
	.048000	.799600	.266000
	.160000	1.068400	.374000
	.009000	1.168800	.416000
	.190000	1.788900	.689000
	Electrons:		
	.015803	.003190	
	.002186	.022700	
	.001435	.264690	
	.009910	.382890	

[a] RSIC computer data file (DLC-80) contains x ray and photon data not in Kocher 1981. They are included in this table.
[b] Maximum energy for betas and positrons.
[c] Branching to radioactive daughter(s) shown in Table 8.13.

(continued)

Table 8.14 Energy and Probability by Radiation Type for Selected Radionuclides of Interest to Health Physicists (Continued)

	Probability per Decay	Energy[b] (MeV)	Average Energy (MeV)
	.001449	.409760	
	.003238	.634520	
	.002909	.663190	
	Gammas & X-rays:		
	.001563	.003770	
	.004356	.027202	
	.008127	.027472	
	.002821	.031000	
	.003985	.149300	
	.004981	.208600	
	.013947	.223800	
	.023909	.278600	
	.044829	.296500	
	.004981	.297100	
	.832810	.414700	
	.009962	.415300	
	.016935	.555200	
	.066745	.573800	
	.074714	.593000	
	.008966	.620200	
	.008966	.639700	
	.021916	.656300	
	.996190	.666330	
	.036859	.675000	
	.996190	.695000	
	.288900	.697000	
	.537940	.720500	
	.176330	.856800	
	.011954	.954000	
	.004981	.959600	
	.067741	.989300	
	.009962	1.034800	
	.001992	1.061300	
	.008966	1.063900	
	.023909	1.213000	
	.002789	1.476200	
Te-127m[c]	Half-life: 109 days		
	Betas:		
	.018200	.724650	.252900
	.000113	.077000	.020075
	Electrons:		
	.740280	.003190	
	.052276	.022700	
	.418200	.056446	
	.432930	.083321	
	.102100	.087254	
	.027193	.088092	
	.011564	.003310	
	.001433	.023600	
	.012142	.024431	
	.001729	.052412	
	Gammas & X-rays:		
	.073215	.003770	
	.104150	.027202	
	.194320	.027472	
	.067455	.031000	
	.000867	.088260	
	.001214	.003940	
	.003047	.028317	
	.005674	.028612	
	.001988	.032300	
	.003783	.057600	
	.000113	.648610	
Te-127	Half-life: 9.35 hours		
	Betas:		
	.011840	.276090	.078200
	.987890	.694000	.224700
	.000267	.485000	.148270
	Gammas & X-rays:		
	.001344	.360300	
	.009880	.417900	
	.001301	.172690	
Te-129[c]	Half-life: 69.6 minutes		
	Betas:		
	.008100	.386320	.114100
	.001960	.668070	.214900
	.002300	.938350	.320600
	.086000	1.010600	.350000
	.005200	1.219600	.437000
	.900000	1.470200	.544500
	.000565	.262000	.074546
	Electrons:		
	.587100	.003310	
	.648730	.022582	
	.130070	.026698	
	.043086	.027584	
	Gammas & X-rays:		
	.061630	.003940	
	.162590	.027770	
	.001661	.208960	
	.003529	.250620	
	.005226	.278430	
	.001519	.281260	
	.071000	.459600	
	.013064	.487390	
	.001768	.802100	
	.004544	1.083900	
	.001761	1.111600	
	.003779	.656880	
Te-129m	Half-life: 33.6 days		
	Betas:		
	.001660	.202110	.055500
	.007600	.873940	.294800
	.033000	.907630	.308300
	.328000	1.603500	.607300
	.000839	.674000	.232540
	Electrons:		
	.480650	.003190	
	.039548	.022700	
	.316390	.073686	
	.240280	.100560	
	.055604	.104490	
	.014593	.105330	
	.001054	.003310	
	.001164	.022582	
	Gammas & X-rays:		
	.047537	.003770	
	.078797	.027202	
	.147010	.027472	
	.051032	.031000	
	.001472	.105500	
	.000111	.003940	
	.001290	.556650	
	.032716	.695880	
	.007629	.729570	
	.003084	.742520	
I-129	Half-life: 15700000 years		
	Betas:		
	1.000000	.152420	.040900
	Electrons:		
	.735390	.003430	
	.789000	.005020	
	.087579	.024600	
	.107000	.034128	
	.021600	.038439	
	.007140	.039373	
	Gammas & X-rays:		
	.081710	.004110	
	.199560	.029458	
	.370240	.029779	
	.131620	.033600	
	.075200	.039581	
I-130	Half-life: 12.36 hours		
	Betas:		
	.003160	.231620	.064000
	.003280	.354650	.103000
	.004920	.375500	.110000
	.001840	.556810	.173000
	.467000	.621910	.197000
	.021400	.812360	.270000
	.001730	.902030	.306000
	.475000	1.039900	.361000
	.014300	1.175800	.418000

[a] RSIC computer data file (DLC-80) contains x ray and photon data not in Kocher 1981. They are included in this table.
[b] Maximum energy for betas and positrons.
[c] Branching to radioactive daughter(s) shown in Table 8.13.

Table 8.14 Energy and Probability by Radiation Type for Selected Radionuclides of Interest to Health Physicists (Continued)

	Probability per Decay	Energy[b] (MeV)	Average Energy (MeV)
	.002700	.308000	.091433
	Electrons:		
	.013506	.003430	
	.001851	.024600	
	.004748	.383450	
	.006227	.501530	
	.003413	.633980	
	.002287	.704920	
	Gammas & X-rays:		
	.001501	.004110	
	.004217	.029458	
	.007824	.029779	
	.002782	.033600	
	.341550	.418010	
	.002366	.457720	
	.008524	.510350	
	.990000	.536090	
	.013959	.539100	
	.006623	.553900	
	.016929	.586050	
	.006148	.603530	
	.961290	.668540	
	.010692	.685990	
	.822690	.739480	
	.001010	.800230	
	.002356	.808290	
	.001911	.877350	
	.008771	.967020	
	.005524	1.096500	
	.002534	1.122200	
	.113060	1.157500	
	.001792	1.222600	
	.007484	1.272100	
	.003445	1.403900	
	.008538	.809940	
Te-131[c]	Half-life: 25 minutes		
	Betas:		
	.011990	.748380	.245600
	.011860	.804950	.267600
	.013400	.821850	.274200
	.001190	.902520	.306200
	.005400	.950780	.325600
	.099900	1.102100	.387700
	.025900	1.150700	.408000
	.011780	1.372300	.502000
	.218000	1.647000	.622000
	.007800	1.756300	.670000
	.592000	2.099300	.825000
	.002090	.446000	.136040
	Electrons:		
	.137650	.003310	
	.017301	.023600	
	.144690	.116550	
	.018672	.144530	
	.004671	.148640	
	.001932	.419150	
	Gammas & X-rays:		
	.014449	.003940	
	.036793	.028317	
	.068516	.028612	
	.024011	.032300	
	.689000	.149720	
	.001723	.151100	
	.007028	.342950	
	.008957	.384060	
	.182240	.452320	
	.048368	.492660	
	.004272	.544880	
	.001027	.567330	
	.041960	.602040	
	.001171	.605550	
	.015296	.654260	
	.001791	.696190	
	.004685	.727000	
	.001998	.841990	
	.001309	.856080	
	.001378	.898540	
	.008750	.934480	
	.022599	.948540	
	.003307	.951390	
	.033416	.997250	
	.007992	1.008000	
	.001723	1.098300	
	.049608	1.147000	
	.001102	1.148500	
	.001178	1.277400	
	.004823	1.294300	
	.001054	1.427100	
	.001151	1.500600	
	.011932	.696010	
I-131[c]	Half-life: 8.04 days		
	Betas:		
	.021200	.247910	.069360
	.006270	.303880	.086950
	.073600	.333830	.096620
	.893000	.606320	.191580
	.003930	.806870	.283250
	.000690	.629700	.200220
	Electrons:		
	.049501	.003430	
	.005911	.024600	
	.035346	.045622	
	.004634	.074730	
	.001176	.079041	
	.002481	.249740	
	.015421	.329920	
	.002443	.359030	
	Gammas & X-rays:		
	.005500	.004110	
	.013468	.029458	
	.024987	.029779	
	.008883	.033600	
	.026182	.080183	
	.002648	.177210	
	.060521	.284300	
	.002507	.325780	
	.811640	.364480	
	.003605	.502990	
	.072605	.636970	
	.002195	.642700	
	.018025	.722890	
	.002304	.329390	
Xe-131m	Half-life: 11.84 days		
	Electrons:		
	.753120	.003430	
	.067932	.024600	
	.612000	.129370	
	.286000	.158480	
	.065000	.162790	
	.017800	.163720	
	Gammas & X-rays:		
	.083680	.004110	
	.154790	.029458	
	.287180	.029779	
	.102100	.033600	
	.019600	.163930	
Te-131m[c]	Half-life: 30 hours		
	Betas:		
	.005600	.160610	.043300
	.003100	.189570	.051800
	.002000	.254620	.071500
	.004500	.260520	.073300
	.009500	.262800	.074000
	.016500	.317030	.091300
	.003410	.367930	.108000
	.022700	.420210	.125600
	.054000	.430240	.129000
	.369000	.450980	.136200
	.001000	.457050	.138300
	.021400	.506680	.155700
	.166000	.532110	.164800
	.015000	.543600	.169000
	.025000	.785250	.259900
	.002200	1.116100	.394000
	.003700	1.371500	.502000

[a] RSIC computer data file (DLC-80) contains x ray and photon data not in Kocher 1981. They are included in this table.
[b] Maximum energy for betas and positrons.
[c] Branching to radioactive daughter(s) shown in Table 8.13.

(continued)

Table 8.14 Energy and Probability by Radiation Type for Selected Radionuclides of Interest to Health Physicists (Continued)

	Probability per Decay	Energy[b] (MeV)	Average Energy (MeV)
	.002000	1.425500	.525000
	.038000	2.431300	.970000
	.001817	.800000	.269130
	Electrons:		
	.168810	.003190	
	.018010	.022700	
	.144080	.150440	
	.054390	.177310	
	.011966	.181240	
	.003041	.182080	
	.105650	.003310	
	.013317	.023600	
	.048004	.047971	
	.048768	.068891	
	.006306	.075952	
	.001570	.080068	
	.006362	.096872	
	.001588	.100990	
	.010659	.116550	
	.001376	.144530	
	.001911	.167460	
	.001169	.207760	
	.002345	.301100	
	Gammas & X-rays:		
	.016695	.003770	
	.035883	.027202	
	.066946	.027472	
	.023239	.031000	
	.008547	.182250	
	.011091	.003940	
	.028320	.028317	
	.052738	.028612	
	.018481	.032300	
	.001279	.079190	
	.040682	.081140	
	.001472	.086430	
	.001705	.101600	
	.079426	.102060	
	.007090	.134860	
	.050755	.149720	
	.001279	.159660	
	.007361	.182250	
	.001550	.183110	
	.002131	.188130	
	.005037	.189760	
	.001162	.190520	
	.075552	.200630	
	.004262	.213980	
	.001937	.230650	
	.075939	.240930	
	.006509	.253170	
	.003100	.255440	
	.001085	.269200	
	.017822	.278560	
	.003874	.283200	
	.003758	.309470	
	.095699	.334270	
	.001356	.335440	
	.003874	.342920	
	.002092	.351300	
	.002286	.354700	
	.012011	.364980	
	.002015	.383900	
	.002790	.417400	
	.006625	.432400	
	.015498	.452320	
	.018210	.462920	
	.003138	.468160	
	.002325	.492660	
	.001356	.524800	
	.001046	.530700	
	.001124	.541400	
	.019760	.586300	
	.003100	.602040	
	.001395	.609400	
	.043394	.665050	
	.001550	.685900	
	.003991	.695620	
	.003913	.702500	
	.014335	.713100	
	.015885	.744200	
	.382020	.773670	
	.005424	.774100	
	.077876	.782490	
	.138700	.793750	
	.061216	.822780	
	.001550	.844900	
	.003874	.852210	
	.206510	.852210	
	.006199	.856080	
	.001937	.865100	
	.001007	.872300	
	.032933	.910000	
	.012011	.920620	
	.001162	.923400	
	.007826	.941270	
	.001550	.987800	
	.001705	.999260	
	.001046	1.035400	
	.015498	1.059700	
	.114300	1.125500	
	.009686	1.128000	
	.015110	1.148900	
	.003836	1.148900	
	.006587	1.150900	
	.001395	1.165500	
	.097636	1.206600	
	.006587	1.237300	
	.006974	1.315200	
	.001007	1.340600	
	.001085	1.394800	
	.012398	1.646000	
	.013561	1.887700	
	.020147	2.000900	
	.003487	2.168500	
	.003836	2.270700	
	.035532	.631940	
Te-132[c]	Half-life: 78.2 hours		
	Betas:		
	1.000000	.215140	.059400
	Electrons:		
	.691590	.003310	
	.641520	.016551	
	.086081	.023600	
	.084744	.044532	
	.016984	.048648	
	.005606	.049534	
	.008760	.078591	
	.008209	.083131	
	.001144	.106570	
	.001071	.111110	
	.071016	.194990	
	.013376	.222970	
	.003379	.227090	
	Gammas & X-rays:		
	.072597	.003940	
	.183060	.028317	
	.340900	.028612	
	.119460	.032300	
	.131120	.049720	
	.018480	.111760	
	.019360	.116300	
	.880000	.228160	
I-132	Half-life: 2.3 hours		
	Betas:		
	.002600	.319100	.092000
	.001200	.353200	.103000
	.001900	.424400	.127000
	.005300	.503320	.154000
	.003300	.521760	.161000
	.007600	.689190	.223000
	.124000	.741140	.242000
	.019000	.739740	.242000
	.003200	.825570	.275000
	.035500	.909990	.309000

[a] RSIC computer data file (DLC-80) contains x ray and photon data not in Kocher 1981. They are included in this table.

[b] Maximum energy for betas and positrons.

[c] Branching to radioactive daughter(s) shown in Table 8.13.

Table 8.14 Energy and Probability by Radiation Type for Selected Radionuclides of Interest to Health Physicists (Continued)

Probability per Decay	Energy[b] (MeV)	Average Energy (MeV)
.081000	.966400	.331000
.027500	.991320	.342000
.033600	.996070	.343000
.024900	1.155100	.409000
.189000	1.185100	.422000
.009500	1.229100	.440000
.001130	1.392700	.510000
.017000	1.412600	.519000
.101000	1.469800	.543000
.020000	1.468000	.543000
.001400	1.539600	.574000
.124000	1.616900	.608000
.169000	2.139600	.841000
.004954	.440000	.134480
Electrons:		
.005510	.003430	
.000755	.024600	
.001384	.488090	
.003514	.633130	
.001905	.738050	
Gammas & X-rays:		
.000612	.004110	
.001720	.029458	
.003192	.029779	
.001135	.033600	
.002369	.147200	
.001382	.183300	
.001875	.254800	
.014410	.262700	
.007205	.284800	
.001382	.316500	
.004935	.363500	
.002961	.387800	
.004738	.416800	
.004836	.431900	
.006021	.446000	
.001777	.473900	
.001481	.478500	
.004145	.488200	
.050337	.505900	
.160880	.522650	
.005231	.535500	
.001086	.540000	
.012535	.547100	
.001382	.600000	
.003948	.620800	
.015792	.621200	
.137190	.630220	
.026649	.650600	
.003948	.659000	
.987000	.667690	
.049350	.669800	

	Probability per Decay	Energy[b] (MeV)	Average Energy (MeV)
	.052311	.671600	
	.031584	.727000	
	.021714	.727200	
	.010857	.728500	
	.003948	.764500	
	.761960	.772610	
	.012338	.780200	
	.004244	.784500	
	.028623	.809800	
	.056259	.812200	
	.005823	.863300	
	.010758	.876800	
	.009179	.910300	
	.004145	.927600	
	.180620	.954550	
	.005626	.983700	
	.004738	1.034700	
	.029610	1.136000	
	.013522	1.143400	
	.002764	1.147400	
	.010857	1.173200	
	.001777	1.272700	
	.011351	1.290700	
	.019740	1.295300	
	.008883	1.297600	
	.001184	1.317800	
	.024675	1.372100	
	.071064	1.398600	
	.014213	1.442600	
	.001352	1.476800	
	.002961	1.757500	
	.011844	1.921100	
	.010857	2.002200	
	.002369	2.086800	
	.001974	2.172700	
	.001184	2.223200	
	.001678	2.390500	
	.031946	1.014600	
Te-133m[c]	Half-life: 55.4 minutes		
	Betas:		
	.195000	1.527600	.570000
	.293000	1.744200	.670000
	.382000	2.391600	.960000
	Electrons:		
	.060865	.003190	
	.007313	.022700	
	.058500	.302330	
	.013650	.329200	
	.003562	.333130	
	.159290	.003310	
	.016781	.023600	

Probability per Decay	Energy[b] (MeV)	Average Energy (MeV)
.079605	.040931	
.004802	.048331	
.016913	.054831	
.040890	.061731	
.023490	.068912	
.003967	.082812	
.019140	.089712	
Gammas & X-rays:		
.006020	.003770	
.014570	.027202	
.027182	.027472	
.009436	.031000	
.054340	.334140	
.016721	.003940	
.035686	.028317	
.066455	.028612	
.023288	.032300	
.013050	.074100	
.006960	.081500	
.020880	.088000	
.087000	.094900	
.023490	.164340	
.114840	.168870	
.014790	.177100	
.008700	.178200	
.003480	.184450	
.006090	.193220	
.005220	.198200	
.028710	.213360	
.004350	.220940	
.003480	.224030	
.006090	.244280	
.005220	.251490	
.008700	.257640	
.156600	.261550	
.008700	.285700	
.022620	.344500	
.011310	.347220	
.014790	.355570	
.009570	.362810	
.005220	.376830	
.014790	.396960	
.012180	.429020	
.010440	.435400	
.022620	.444900	
.020010	.462110	
.020010	.471850	
.015660	.478590	
.004350	.519600	
.017400	.534850	
.023490	.574040	
.013920	.622030	

[a] RSIC computer data file (DLC-80) contains x ray and photon data not in Kocher 1981. They are included in this table.
[b] Maximum energy for betas and positrons.
[c] Branching to radioactive daughter(s) shown in Table 8.13.

(continued)

Table 8.14 Energy and Probability by Radiation Type for Selected Radionuclides of Interest to Health Physicists (Continued)

Radionuclide	Probability per Decay	Energy[b] (MeV)	Average Energy (MeV)
	.293190	.647400	
	.037410	.702750	
	.014790	.731690	
	.028710	.733890	
	.033930	.779750	
	.013050	.795700	
	.019140	.800510	
	.194880	.863910	
	.056550	.882830	
	.004350	.897700	
	.870000	.912580	
	.165300	.914720	
	.013050	.934400	
	.094830	.978190	
	.023490	.980400	
	.011310	.982900	
	.010440	1.007500	
	.013050	1.029800	
	.025230	1.348900	
	.021750	1.459100	
	.009570	1.516100	
	.008700	1.531600	
	.057420	1.683300	
	.009570	1.704400	
	.011310	1.885700	
	.033060	2.004900	
	.020880	2.027700	
	.010440	2.049200	
I-133[c]	Half-life: 20.8 hours		
	Betas:		
	.004100	.169980	.046000
	.012400	.373850	.110000
	.003970	.409620	.122000
	.037500	.461760	.140000
	.031300	.523570	.162000
	.005420	.707700	.230000
	.041600	.884670	.299000
	.018100	1.016200	.352000
	.835000	1.230100	.441000
	.010700	1.526800	.573000
	.000270	.850000	.284000
	Electrons:		
	.004845	.003430	
	.000664	.024600	
	.005982	.495310	
	Gammas & X-rays:		
	.000538	.004110	
	.001513	.029458	
	.002807	.029779	
	.000998	.033600	
	.003565	.262700	
	.001165	.267170	
	.001036	.345430	
	.001122	.361080	
	.001528	.418050	
	.003090	.422910	
	.018127	.510530	
	.863200	.529870	
	.005395	.617970	
	.006448	.680250	
	.014933	.706580	
	.004566	.768380	
	.001537	.820510	
	.012344	.856280	
	.044714	.875330	
	.002124	.909670	
	.005516	1.052300	
	.001373	1.060100	
	.014933	1.236400	
	.023306	1.298200	
	.001485	1.350400	
	.006072	.535240	
Xe-133m[c]	Half-life: 2.19 days		
	Electrons:		
	.698130	.003430	
	.070263	.024600	
	.633000	.198660	
	.206000	.227770	
	.045600	.232080	
	.012200	.233010	
	Gammas & X-rays:		
	.077570	.004110	
	.160100	.029458	
	.297040	.029779	
	.105600	.033600	
	.103000	.233220	
Xe-133	Half-life: 5.245 days		
	Betas:		
	.006900	.266680	.075100
	.993000	.346300	.100600
	.000076	.043500	.011100
	Electrons:		
	.496930	.003550	
	.056275	.025500	
	.003291	.043636	
	.532660	.045012	
	.081358	.075283	
	.016709	.079780	
	.004341	.080766	
	Gammas & X-rays:		
	.061419	.004290	
	.136410	.030625	
	.252620	.030973	
	.090644	.035000	
	.002165	.079621	
	.364830	.080997	
	.000712	.177700	
Te-133[c]	Half-life: 12.45 minutes		
	Betas:		
	.003500	.429700	.129000
	.018000	.776400	.256000
	.008500	.833100	.279000
	.087000	1.252400	.450000
	.044000	1.405900	.520000
	.005000	1.596100	.600000
	.132000	1.636800	.620000
	.070000	1.657200	.630000
	.013000	2.183200	.860000
	.333000	2.250300	.890000
	.286000	2.658000	1.080000
	Electrons:		
	.023367	.003310	
	.002953	.023600	
	.020815	.278820	
	.003044	.306800	
	.004213	.374460	
	Gammas & X-rays:		
	.002453	.003940	
	.006280	.028317	
	.011696	.028612	
	.004098	.032300	
	.708000	.311990	
	.002832	.384600	
	.005664	.392900	
	.300900	.407630	
	.012036	.474720	
	.005664	.546400	
	.004956	.587100	
	.002832	.613600	
	.066552	.719650	
	.055932	.786770	
	.032568	.844390	
	.044604	.930670	
	.062304	1.000800	
	.026904	1.021100	
	.012744	1.061800	
	.011328	1.252200	
	.009204	1.307700	
	.007788	1.313500	
	.099120	1.333200	
	.005664	1.405700	
	.003540	1.474000	
	.004956	1.518600	
	.002832	1.588200	
	.033984	1.717700	

[a] RSIC computer data file (DLC-80) contains x ray and photon data not in Kocher 1981. They are included in this table.

[b] Maximum energy for betas and positrons.

[c] Branching to radioactive daughter(s) shown in Table 8.13.

Table 8.14 Energy and Probability by Radiation Type for Selected Radionuclides of Interest to Health Physicists (Continued)

	Probability per Decay	Energy[b] (MeV)	Average Energy (MeV)
	.005664	1.825100	
	.014160	1.881500	
	.002832	2.136500	
	.002832	2.228000	
	.000708	2.540600	
Te-134[c]	Half-life: 41.8 minutes		
	Betas:		
	.147000	.193530	.052941
	.429000	.376570	.110830
	.411000	.453310	.136990
	Electrons:		
	.337540	.003310	
	.041224	.023600	
	.005580	.043661	
	.270900	.046276	
	.002937	.068251	
	.002232	.071642	
	.041580	.074257	
	.008400	.078373	
	.002037	.079259	
	.026820	.147720	
	.009396	.168070	
	.004860	.175700	
	.020586	.177300	
	.001224	.179820	
	.001566	.196050	
	.003504	.205280	
	.008754	.244780	
	.001321	.272760	
	.002176	.401890	
	.001091	.427830	
	.001115	.532820	
	Gammas & X-rays:		
	.035433	.003940	
	.087667	.028317	
	.163250	.028612	
	.057210	.032300	
	.0013	.0439	
	.002790	.076830	
	.210000	.079445	
	.003300	.101420	
	.001800	.131050	
	.180000	.180890	
	.006000	.183050	
	.087000	.201240	
	.219000	.210470	
	.004800	.259800	
	.213000	.277950	
	.186000	.435060	
	.108000	.461000	
	.051000	.464640	
	.189000	.565990	
	.017100	.636260	
	.009000	.645400	
	.012000	.665850	
	.042000	.712970	
	.147000	.742590	
	.300000	.767200	
	.012000	.844060	
	.004500	.896020	
	.016500	.925550	
	.004500	1.027000	
	.001200	.110140	
I-134	Half-life: 52.6 minutes		
	Betas:		
	.014800	.774580	.255000
	.003300	.789560	.261000
	.001530	.835500	.279000
	.012200	1.066200	.372000
	.325000	1.282600	.460000
	.005300	1.377100	.500000
	.081000	1.496200	.550000
	.163000	1.561500	.580000
	.036700	1.602400	.600000
	.076000	1.741500	.660000
	.112000	1.797000	.690000
	.011200	1.847900	.710000
	.037000	2.230400	.880000
	.115000	2.418800	.970000
	.002260	.795000	.263550
	Electrons:		
	.015183	.003430	
	.001896	.024600	
	.011428	.100840	
	.001496	.129950	
	.001409	.200910	
	.001124	.370890	
	.001927	.812460	
	.001194	.849530	
	Gammas & X-rays:		
	.001687	.004110	
	.004321	.029458	
	.008016	.029779	
	.002850	.033600	
	.037592	.135400	
	.006869	.139030	
	.001059	.151980	
	.002576	.162480	
	.006965	.188470	
	.002481	.217000	
	.019845	.235470	
	.001307	.278800	
	.005152	.319810	
	.004961	.351080	
	.073466	.405450	
	.006106	.411000	
	.041885	.433350	
	.012976	.458920	
	.003626	.465500	
	.014121	.488880	
	.023375	.514400	
	.078236	.540830	
	.008778	.565520	
	.002099	.570750	
	.113540	.595360	
	.105910	.621790	
	.023662	.627960	
	.084915	.677340	
	.008301	.706650	
	.019082	.730740	
	.007633	.739180	
	.041026	.766680	
	.005248	.816380	
	.954100	.847020	
	.069649	.857290	
	.001908	.864000	
	.652600	.884090	
	.001431	.922600	
	.040358	.947860	
	.003530	.966900	
	.046751	.974670	
	.019082	1.040300	
	.152660	1.072600	
	.006869	1.100100	
	.007251	1.103200	
	.097318	1.136200	
	.003530	1.159100	
	.001336	1.164000	
	.003530	1.190000	
	.002099	1.239000	
	.005629	1.269500	
	.001050	1.322400	
	.001431	1.336000	
	.004484	1.352600	
	.002194	1.414300	
	.001717	1.428200	
	.001717	1.431400	
	.022898	1.455200	
	.007728	1.470000	
	.001145	1.505500	
	.005057	1.541500	
	.043602	1.613800	
	.002576	1.629200	
	.004007	1.644300	
	.002290	1.655200	
	.026715	1.741500	

[a] RSIC computer data file (DLC-80) contains x ray and photon data not in Kocher 1981. They are included in this table.
[b] Maximum energy for betas and positrons.
[c] Branching to radioactive daughter(s) shown in Table 8.13.

(continued)

Table 8.14 Energy and Probability by Radiation Type for Selected Radionuclides of Interest to Health Physicists (Continued)

	Probability per Decay	Energy[b] (MeV)	Average Energy (MeV)
	.057246	1.806800	
	.001813	1.925900	
	.001717	2.020600	
	.002099	2.159900	
	.002385	2.312400	
	.001527	2.467400	
	.013348	1.787200	
Cs-134m	Half-life: 2.9 hours		
	Electrons:		
	1.328000	.003550	
	.772770	.005546	
	.158720	.010043	
Cs-134	Half-life: 2.062 years		
	Betas:		
	.274000	.088543	.023060
	.024800	.415090	.123400
	.701000	.657860	.210110
	.000530	.975500	.335290
	Electrons:		
	.006553	.003670	
	.000828	.026400	
	.001255	.531870	
	.004909	.567260	
	.002203	.758400	
	Gammas & X-rays:		
	.000894	.004470	
	.002144	.031817	
	.003955	.032194	
	.001439	.036400	
	.014600	.475350	
	.083800	.563230	
	.154300	.569320	
	.976000	.604700	
	.854000	.795840	
	.087300	.801930	
	.010000	1.038600	
	.018000	1.167900	
	.030400	1.365200	
	.000354	.276880	
I-135[c]	Half-life: 6.61 hours		
	Betas:		
	.001400	.235910	.066000
	.001260	.244890	.068000
	.001400	.263690	.074000
	.010800	.302280	.086000
	.009100	.339010	.098000
	.013900	.353760	.103000
	.047300	.455530	.138000
	.073300	.477960	.145000
	.015700	.618060	.196000
	.011000	.665110	.213000
	.079000	.742680	.243000
	.006100	.816560	.272000
	.087000	.919780	.313000
	.218000	1.032900	.359000
	.079000	1.145700	.405000
	.074000	1.253400	.451000
	.001000	1.262600	.454000
	.236000	1.450600	.535000
	.012000	1.579500	.591000
	.019000	2.184500	.858000
	.001540	.647000	.207220
	Electrons:		
	.002197	.003430	
	.000301	.024600	
	.001501	.185940	
	.001211	.253890	
	Gammas & X-rays:		
	.000244	.004110	
	.000686	.029458	
	.001273	.029779	
	.000452	.033600	
	.017452	.220500	
	.002317	.229720	
	.001840	.264260	
	.030899	.288450	
	.003033	.290270	
	.001860	.361850	
	.002317	.403030	
	.003004	.414830	
	.035190	.417630	
	.003033	.429930	
	.005522	.433740	
	.003147	.451630	
	.071239	.546560	
	.001288	.575970	
	.004549	.649850	
	.001288	.690130	
	.006580	.707920	
	.001516	.785480	
	.001717	.797710	
	.066661	.836800	
	.001459	.961460	
	.008869	.971960	
	.012016	.972610	
	.001545	.995090	
	.079250	1.038800	
	.016022	1.101600	
	.036049	1.124000	
	.225160	1.131500	
	.001030	1.159900	
	.008726	1.169000	
	.009012	1.240500	
	.286100	1.260400	
	.006065	1.367900	
	.003147	1.448400	
	.086402	1.457600	
	.010729	1.502800	
	.012875	1.566400	
	.095271	1.678000	
	.040912	1.706500	
	.076961	1.791200	
	.005779	1.830700	
	.002947	1.927300	
	.008697	2.045900	
	.006123	2.255500	
	.009527	2.408700	
	.014948	1.073400	
Xe-135m[c]	Half-life: 15.36 minutes		
	Electrons:		
	.149120	.003430	
	.016871	.024600	
	.151990	.492000	
	.028899	.521110	
	.009520	.525420	
	Gammas & X-rays:		
	.016569	.004110	
	.038443	.029458	
	.071324	.029779	
	.025356	.033600	
	.809970	.526560	
Cs-135	Half-life: 2300000 years		
	Betas:		
	1.000000	.205000	.056300
Xe-135[c]	Half-life: 9.11 hours		
	Betas:		
	.001230	.096581	.025300
	.031300	.550810	.171000
	.005850	.751010	.246000
	.961000	.909210	.308000
	.000750	.178000	.048000
	Electrons:		
	.053166	.003550	
	.005966	.025500	
	.056817	.213810	
	.009170	.244080	
	.002337	.248580	
	Gammas & X-rays:		
	.006571	.004290	
	.014461	.030625	
	.026780	.030973	
	.009609	.035000	
	.002886	.158200	
	.899000	.249790	
	.002203	.358390	
	.003578	.407990	
	.028948	.608190	
	.002093	.684330	

[a] RSIC computer data file (DLC-80) contains x ray and photon data not in Kocher 1981. They are included in this table.

[b] Maximum energy for betas and positrons.

[c] Branching to radioactive daughter(s) shown in Table 8.13.

Table 8.14 Energy and Probability by Radiation Type for Selected Radionuclides of Interest to Health Physicists (Continued)

Nuclide	Probability per Decay	Energy[b] (MeV)	Average Energy (MeV)
	.052278	.011029	
	.036921	.025500	
	.347200	.091435	
	.004424	.102700	
	.403740	.121710	
	.090074	.126200	
	.022717	.127190	
	.002704	.132970	
	Gammas & X-rays:		
	.164140	.004290	
	.009400	.011260	
	.089498	.030625	
	.165740	.030973	
	.059470	.035000	
	.129000	.127420	
	.000062	.138680	
Cs-136	Half-life: 13.16 days		
	Betas:		
	.024900	.174390	.047200
	.002100	.191550	.052300
	.951000	.341000	.098800
	.022000	.681540	.219000
	Electrons:		
	.206650	.003670	
	.019108	.026400	
	.073155	.029469	
	.018404	.048849	
	.010419	.060921	
	.002667	.065617	
	.003773	.072219	
	.002531	.080301	
	.001541	.103670	
	.023790	.115780	
	.049746	.126450	
	.001407	.129090	
	.005505	.139110	
	.006727	.147230	
	.001812	.151930	
	.039751	.157900	
	.008890	.162600	
	.002326	.163640	
	.001583	.236210	
	.012114	.303130	
	.002083	.334580	
	.002413	.781060	
	.001122	1.010600	
	Gammas & X-rays:		
	.028180	.004470	
	.049454	.031817	
	.091244	.032194	
	.033205	.036400	
	.124630	.066910	
	.062811	.086290	
	.004088	.109660	
	.074576	.153220	
	.046061	.163890	
	.006281	.166530	
	.135590	.176550	
	.005982	.187250	
	.126620	.273650	
	.005982	.319870	
	.484540	.340570	
	.009771	.507210	
	.997000	.818500	
	.795610	1.048100	
	.197410	1.235300	
	.003300	.787240	
Cs-137[c]	Half-life: 30.17 years		
	Betas:		
	.946000	.511550	.156800
	.054000	1.173200	.415200
Ba-137m	Half-life: 2.552 minutes		
	Electrons:		
	.076131	.003670	
	.007999	.026400	
	.080800	.624210	
	.014600	.655660	
	.004800	.660360	
	Gammas & X-rays:		
	.010381	.004470	
	.020703	.031817	
	.038197	.032194	
	.013900	.036400	
	.899800	.661650	
Xe-138	Half-life: 14.13 minutes		
	Betas:		
	.002270	.231620	.064000
	.004600	.249030	.070000
	.030600	.402420	.119000
	.095000	.476940	.145000
	.326000	.713320	.231000
	.002800	.717880	.233000
	.002300	.945990	.323000
	.001600	1.367900	.498000
	.001900	1.534800	.571000
	.002700	1.788000	.682000
	.201000	2.289800	.908000
	.138000	2.327900	.925000
	.051000	2.481600	.996000
	.050000	2.729200	1.099000
	.090000	2.724300	1.107000
	.001680	1.680000	.637170
	Electrons:		
	.491070	.003550	
	.320890	.003633	
	.105870	.004619	
	.509580	.005136	
	.103730	.009633	
	.034251	.010619	
	.004235	.025500	
	.016074	.117770	
	.003393	.148040	
	.002406	.206580	
	.018050	.222330	
	.002898	.252600	
	.001077	.360450	
	.002722	.398510	
	Gammas & X-rays:		
	.060694	.004290	
	.001921	.004850	
	.006961	.010850	
	.010265	.030625	
	.019009	.030973	
	.006821	.035000	
	.059535	.153750	
	.034965	.242560	
	.315000	.258310	
	.004284	.282510	
	.001071	.335280	
	.005009	.371440	
	.063000	.396430	
	.021735	.401360	
	.203180	.434490	
	.003622	.500220	
	.002520	.530070	
	.001166	.537760	
	.001166	.555950	
	.003055	.568530	
	.001228	.588840	
	.001449	.654080	
	.002961	.865820	
	.006206	.869350	
	.001323	.896870	
	.003276	.912510	
	.009198	.917130	
	.001355	.936360	
	.002299	.941250	
	.004095	1.093900	
	.002142	1.098800	
	.001071	1.102200	
	.014742	1.114300	
	.005134	1.141600	
	.001323	1.145400	
	.002646	1.571800	
	.002363	1.614600	
	.167270	1.768300	
	.001796	1.812500	
	.014238	1.850900	

[a] RSIC computer data file (DLC-80) contains x ray and photon data not in Kocher 1981. They are included in this table.
[b] Maximum energy for betas and positrons.
[c] Branching to radioactive daughter(s) shown in Table 8.13.

(continued)

Table 8.14 Energy and Probability by Radiation Type for Selected Radionuclides of Interest to Health Physicists (Continued)

	Probability per Decay	Energy[b] (MeV)	Average Energy (MeV)
	.005639	1.925400	
	.053550	2.004800	
	.122540	2.015800	
	.014427	2.079200	
	.022869	2.252300	
	.006206	2.321900	
	.001733	2.497600	
	.026586	1.118600	
Cs-138	Half-life: 32.2 minutes		
	Betas:		
	.002570	.700120	.226000
	.001630	.821900	.273000
	.001000	1.087500	.380000
	.001900	1.249900	.447000
	.004800	1.394700	.509000
	.002040	1.407400	.514000
	.003000	1.636000	.614000
	.004300	1.682900	.634000
	.002270	1.963000	.759000
	.001710	1.990900	.771000
	.002730	2.087300	.815000
	.003400	2.166400	.850000
	.001690	2.280000	.902000
	.006500	2.338800	.929000
	.002000	2.398500	.956000
	.003700	2.449000	.979000
	.002000	2.478300	.992000
	.016000	2.550500	1.025000
	.088000	2.690400	1.090000
	.016800	2.746800	1.115000
	.441000	2.884300	1.179000
	.006600	2.914500	1.193000
	.073000	3.022300	1.243000
	.128000	3.112000	1.284000
	.138000	3.431300	1.433000
	.044000	3.894100	1.649000
	.002913	1.780000	.679550
	Electrons:		
	.010053	.003670	
	.001117	.026400	
	.005803	.100660	
	.001384	.132110	
	.001326	.190320	
	.003167	.425340	
	.000985	.509500	
	Gammas & X-rays:		
	.001371	.004470	
	.002891	.031817	
	.005333	.032194	
	.001941	.036400	
	.001297	.112600	
	.014879	.138100	
	.005036	.191960	
	.003281	.193890	
	.001747	.212320	
	.015107	.227760	
	.002899	.324900	
	.002442	.363930	
	.001908	.365290	
	.046619	.408980	
	.004273	.421590	
	.307490	.462790	
	.004273	.516740	
	.107580	.546940	
	.001084	.683590	
	.001457	.766100	
	.002327	.773310	
	.003281	.782080	
	.051121	.871800	
	.001144	.880800	
	.001808	.935030	
	.298330	1.009800	
	.001587	1.054300	
	.012437	1.147200	
	.001679	1.199200	
	.003968	1.203700	
	.001373	1.264900	
	.011445	1.343600	
	.003662	1.415700	
	.763000	1.435900	
	.009690	1.445000	
	.001831	1.495600	
	.003662	1.555300	
	.001373	1.614100	
	.001068	1.717100	
	.001114	1.727700	
	.001373	1.778300	
	.001175	2.023900	
	.001106	2.062300	
	.002136	2.210700	
	.151840	2.218000	
	.001679	2.499400	
	.002388	2.583200	
	.076300	2.639600	
	.001198	2.731100	
	.001511	3.339000	
	.002274	3.367000	
	.016214	1.613200	
Ba-139	Half-life: 83.1 minutes		
	Betas:		
	.003200	.885470	.297400
	.220000	2.140100	.837000
	.780000	2.306000	.912000
	.000617	.901000	.304670
	Electrons:		
	.032007	.003800	
	.003410	.027400	
	.036282	.126930	
	.004861	.159590	
	.001285	.164490	
	Gammas & X-rays:		
	.004783	.004650	
	.009344	.033034	
	.017208	.033442	
	.006320	.037800	
	.173600	.165850	
	.002800	1.420500	
	.001053	1.271100	
Ba-140[c]	Half-life: 12.789 days		
	Betas:		
	.260000	.453850	.136000
	.102000	.567470	.177000
	.044000	.872320	.306000
	.370000	.991170	.340000
	.220000	1.005000	.357000
	Electrons:		
	.984640	.003800	
	.505560	.007584	
	.104400	.012489	
	.034486	.013580	
	.605880	.023704	
	.001942	.027400	
	.124820	.028609	
	.041233	.029700	
	.016022	.123720	
	.002154	.156370	
	.001983	.265920	
	.002652	.498400	
	Gammas & X-rays:		
	.147130	.004650	
	.011730	.013850	
	.140250	.029970	
	.005320	.033034	
	.009797	.033442	
	.003598	.037800	
	.002142	.132840	
	.067320	.162640	
	.045058	.304840	
	.032461	.423700	
	.019941	.437550	
	.001530	.467570	
	.255000	.537320	
	.000714	.118840	
La-140	Half-life: 40.22 hours		
	Betas:		
	.006400	1.213100	.438200

[a] RSIC computer data file (DLC-80) contains x ray and photon data not in Kocher 1981. They are included in this table.

[b] Maximum energy for betas and positrons.

[c] Branching to radioactive daughter(s) shown in Table 8.13.

Table 8.14 Energy and Probability by Radiation Type for Selected Radionuclides of Interest to Health Physicists (Continued)

	Probability per Decay	Energy[b] (MeV)	Average Energy (MeV)
	.111100	1.238800	.441100
	.058900	1.244400	.443500
	.011900	1.279300	.458200
	.056300	1.296200	.465300
	.445000	1.348200	.487400
	.050800	1.412300	.514700
	.207000	1.677000	.629500
	.052000	2.164000	.846200
	.001615	.957800	.328890
	Electrons:		
	.017058	.003940	
	.002503	.018046	
	.001621	.028400	
	.001856	.028473	
	.001513	.068974	
	.002382	.090678	
	.008068	.288320	
	.001072	.322220	
	.004400	.446590	
	Gammas & X-rays:		
	.002549	.004840	
	.004718	.034279	
	.008656	.034720	
	.003223	.039300	
	.001910	.109420	
	.005538	.131120	
	.001241	.173550	
	.004297	.241970	
	.004870	.266550	
	.205300	.328770	
	.029411	.432530	
	.455490	.487030	
	.044021	.751790	
	.234910	.815850	
	.056339	.867820	
	.028838	.919630	
	.070854	.925240	
	.005347	.950900	
	.954900	1.596500	
	.008508	2.348800	
	.034567	2.521700	
	.001041	2.547100	
	.004163	1.208000	
Ba-141[c]	Half-life: 18.27 minutes		
	Betas:		
	.006200	.561030	.174000
	.002400	.589200	.184000
	.001700	.644100	.205000
	.008200	.653970	.208000
	.006500	.813090	.269000
	.004800	.849440	.283000
	.022600	1.104100	.386000
	.041000	1.157300	.408000
	.026000	1.185700	.420000
	.025100	1.289100	.463000
	.023200	1.402000	.511000
	.002100	1.463900	.538000
	.067000	1.528300	.566000
	.003900	1.604000	.599000
	.003400	1.840800	.703000
	.015800	1.858000	.711000
	.037000	1.963400	.758000
	.001900	2.038200	.791000
	.126000	2.100600	.819000
	.021300	2.198300	.863000
	.005400	2.203600	.866000
	.245000	2.382100	.947000
	.190000	2.562700	1.029000
	.120000	2.839700	1.156000
	Electrons:		
	.066797	.003800	
	.007127	.027400	
	.075816	.151300	
	.010060	.183950	
	.002658	.188860	
	Gammas & X-rays:		
	.009981	.004650	
	.019526	.033034	
	.035959	.033442	
	.013205	.037800	
	.009866	.112940	
	.004666	.162960	
	.005200	.180500	
	.486000	.190220	
	.245920	.276990	
	.265840	.304240	
	.150170	.343710	
	.003013	.349350	
	.006124	.364380	
	.001215	.381310	
	.013948	.389780	
	.050544	.457580	
	.050544	.462150	
	.057834	.467260	
	.004568	.522190	
	.004277	.524200	
	.003985	.527420	
	.001021	.561900	
	.002673	.572090	
	.002673	.572090	
	.002479	.599280	
	.002576	.608910	
	.034506	.625230	
	.002965	.636050	
	.003839	.641380	
	.059292	.647880	
	.001895	.670040	
	.001118	.674200	
	.002284	.675700	
	.001409	.685700	
	.001069	.687800	
	.002965	.698500	
	.002236	.700000	
	.003159	.704800	
	.045198	.739100	
	.001021	.753900	
	.001458	.762200	
	.001118	.778200	
	.001021	.805400	
	.003451	.826340	
	.015989	.831720	
	.001701	.832600	
	.001555	.867900	
	.035964	.876290	
	.002090	.880600	
	.001312	.908800	
	.007339	.929470	
	.007679	.943250	
	.008213	.981630	
	.001312	.996600	
	.001069	1.012300	
	.003110	1.034500	
	.001021	1.040400	
	.003645	1.046300	
	.002333	1.094000	
	.002527	1.160800	
	.009720	1.160800	
	.048600	1.197500	
	.004325	1.224800	
	.001507	1.235500	
	.008651	1.264200	
	.005443	1.273600	
	.006950	1.278200	
	.002479	1.309100	
	.006318	1.311200	
	.009963	1.323700	
	.002333	1.345300	
	.001652	1.357500	
	.007436	1.377000	
	.002867	1.405600	
	.008699	1.436800	
	.007144	1.458600	
	.003256	1.501800	
	.003256	1.550600	
	.002673	1.568800	
	.007873	1.654000	

[a] RSIC computer data file (DLC-80) contains x ray and photon data not in Kocher 1981. They are included in this table.

[b] Maximum energy for betas and positrons.

[c] Branching to radioactive daughter(s) shown in Table 8.13.

(continued)

Table 8.14 Energy and Probability by Radiation Type for Selected Radionuclides of Interest to Health Physicists (Continued)

	Probability per Decay	Energy[b] (MeV)	Average Energy (MeV)
	.014143	1.682400	
	.001798	1.713200	
	.001944	1.735600	
	.003305	1.740800	
	.005103	1.795900	
	.001361	1.912700	
	.001944	1.990300	
	.003985	2.026600	
	.001166	2.136700	
	.001652	2.164700	
	.001021	2.278900	
	.001944	2.469000	
	.017302	1.252000	
La-141[c]	Half-life: 3.94 hours		
	Betas:		
	.001200	.736680	.239000
	.026100	1.075500	.373000
	.970000	2.430000	.967000
	.002618	.400000	.125450
	Gammas & X-rays:		
	.026200	1.354500	
	.001179	1.693300	
	.003107	1.674300	
Ce-141	Half-life: 32.5 days		
	Betas:		
	.705000	.434560	.129600
	.295000	.580000	.180700
	Electrons:		
	.162820	.004080	
	.015962	.029400	
	.187790	.103450	
	.025942	.138610	
	.005421	.143930	
	.001491	.145140	
	Gammas & X-rays:		
	.026505	.005030	
	.048821	.035550	
	.089416	.036026	
	.033592	.040700	
	.484000	.145440	
Ba-142[c]	Half-life: 10.7 minutes		
	Betas:		
	.126000	.742560	.240000
	.001600	.916600	.310000
	.400000	.996000	.340000
	.180000	1.121600	.390000
	.004400	1.333100	.480000
	.003000	1.391800	.510000
	.007100	1.407800	.510000
	.003700	1.609400	.600000
	.046000	1.775000	.670000
	.031000	1.768000	.670000
	.002700	1.899800	.730000
	.001600	2.045100	.790000
	.180000	2.122400	.830000
	Electrons:		
	.256830	.003800	
	.020239	.027400	
	.215310	.038675	
	.105730	.071334	
	.023069	.076239	
	.006056	.077330	
	Gammas & X-rays:		
	.038376	.004650	
	.055450	.033034	
	.102120	.033442	
	.037501	.037800	
	.003560	.069400	
	.008900	.076800	
	.096120	.077600	
	.009256	.122890	
	.005162	.154220	
	.001068	.162000	
	.014774	.176820	
	.001958	.216300	
	.002670	.222600	
	.101460	.231520	
	.001602	.242700	
	.178000	.255120	
	.006764	.269330	
	.001780	.283900	
	.009256	.286200	
	.022606	.309020	
	.012460	.334800	
	.002492	.337100	
	.001424	.346700	
	.039160	.363800	
	.004628	.379100	
	.003382	.417800	
	.049840	.425030	
	.009790	.432300	
	.003026	.434400	
	.002136	.448100	
	.003916	.457300	
	.003026	.473400	
	.001068	.488300	
	.002314	.513300	
	.001068	.537500	
	.003026	.558300	
	.002492	.590700	
	.016020	.599840	
	.003204	.604200	
	.006052	.769400	
	.002492	.786400	
	.002136	.792200	
	.004094	.823400	
	.030260	.840230	
	.110360	.894900	
	.089000	.948750	
	.078320	1.000900	
	.004806	1.032800	
	.092560	1.078500	
	.022072	1.093600	
	.003026	1.122600	
	.015308	1.126500	
	.003916	1.148300	
	.053400	1.202200	
	.137060	1.204100	
	.001602	1.283400	
	.033998	1.379900	
	.001602	.685100	
La-142	Half-life: 95.4 minutes		
	Betas:		
	.015000	.474130	.143300
	.001000	.541600	.167100
	.002600	.666500	.212700
	.005800	.797880	.262600
	.005800	.799960	.263500
	.012000	.841550	.279600
	.015000	.884170	.296400
	.043000	.903890	.304200
	.017000	.904920	.304600
	.006300	1.047300	.361900
	.018000	1.057700	.366100
	.025000	1.096700	.382100
	.013600	1.517200	.560000
	.013100	1.775400	.673000
	.081000	1.820700	.693000
	.037000	1.850300	.706000
	.201000	1.974400	.761000
	.215000	2.119300	.826000
	.020000	2.152800	.841000
	.069000	2.329800	.921000
	.021000	2.512800	1.004000
	.008000	2.864400	1.165000
	.030000	2.980900	1.219000
	.052000	3.875800	1.634000
	.070000	4.517000	1.910000
	Electrons:		
	.001913	.003940	
	.000222	.028400	
	.002499	.600730	
	Gammas & X-rays:		
	.000286	.004840	

[a] RSIC computer data file (DLC-80) contains x ray and photon data not in Kocher 1981. They are included in this table.
[b] Maximum energy for betas and positrons.
[c] Branching to radioactive daughter(s) shown in Table 8.13.

Table 8.14 Energy and Probability by Radiation Type for Selected Radionuclides of Interest to Health Physicists (Continued)

	Probability per Decay	Energy[b] (MeV)	Average Energy (MeV)
	.000647	.034279	
	.001187	.034720	
	.000442	.039300	
	.001575	.106100	
	.001050	.174100	
	.001050	.367300	
	.001050	.393700	
	.002625	.420800	
	.004200	.433340	
	.001575	.514700	
	.001575	.532000	
	.013650	.578090	
	.001575	.619500	
	.525000	.641170	
	.019950	.861570	
	.002100	.878200	
	.093975	.894850	
	.001050	.946500	
	.004200	.962200	
	.001050	.991200	
	.002625	1.006700	
	.043575	1.011400	
	.001050	1.039200	
	.030450	1.043700	
	.001575	1.061800	
	.001575	1.070300	
	.001050	1.074200	
	.002625	1.088900	
	.001050	1.112600	
	.001050	1.116700	
	.005250	1.130600	
	.001575	1.144500	
	.019425	1.160200	
	.001575	1.174300	
	.004200	1.190900	
	.003150	1.231500	
	.020475	1.233100	
	.002100	1.242300	
	.001050	1.264700	
	.001050	1.270100	
	.001050	1.288000	
	.003675	1.323200	
	.001050	1.332300	
	.001050	1.354600	
	.023625	1.363000	
	.002100	1.373600	
	.004725	1.389300	
	.002100	1.395300	
	.001575	1.402200	
	.001575	1.445500	
	.001050	1.455100	
	.001575	1.493700	
	.004725	1.516300	
	.002625	1.535500	
	.005250	1.540200	
	.033075	1.545800	
	.003150	1.618200	
	.002100	1.651400	
	.002625	1.688100	
	.016800	1.722900	
	.001050	1.752400	
	.033075	1.756400	
	.002100	1.768000	
	.002100	1.771000	
	.001050	1.793800	
	.001575	1.806300	
	.001050	1.817100	
	.005775	1.885400	
	.087150	1.901300	
	.002625	1.923000	
	.001575	1.933500	
	.005250	1.948200	
	.001575	1.960600	
	.010500	2.004200	
	.013650	2.025500	
	.011025	2.038700	
	.005250	2.050400	
	.029400	2.055200	
	.007350	2.076900	
	.004200	2.086100	
	.010500	2.100400	
	.003675	2.126200	
	.005775	2.139300	
	.005775	2.180300	
	.058275	2.187200	
	.003675	2.290500	
	.008400	2.358400	
	.004725	2.364400	
	.162750	2.397700	
	.002100	2.419500	
	.004200	2.459400	
	.001575	2.513200	
	.001050	2.532300	
	.007875	2.539400	
	.112350	2.542700	
	.007875	2.663500	
	.018900	2.666800	
	.002100	2.672600	
	.003150	2.782300	
	.006300	2.800800	
	.008400	2.818100	
	.002625	2.828600	
	.007875	2.970000	
	.033075	2.972000	
	.001050	2.991700	
	.005250	2.999900	
	.002100	3.007100	
	.007350	3.012900	
	.001050	3.022300	
	.005775	3.034300	
	.004200	3.046900	
	.001575	3.075900	
	.002100	3.155000	
	.003150	3.181000	
	.003150	3.236700	
	.002100	3.242400	
	.001575	3.273200	
	.013650	3.314700	
	.003150	3.401900	
	.003675	3.459300	
	.008925	3.612100	
	.011550	3.632700	
	.003150	3.719100	
	.002625	3.850400	
Ce-143[c]	Half-life: 33 hours		
	Betas:		
	.003800	.057301	.014700
	.005100	.294560	.083600
	.014200	.517250	.158200
	.003900	.564400	.175000
	.121000	.733090	.237400
	.480000	1.104400	.384600
	.380000	1.397600	.507500
	.001940	.187000	.051705
	Electrons:		
	.591670	.004080	
	.656210	.015374	
	.057818	.029400	
	.092786	.050530	
	.019522	.055854	
	.005327	.057061	
	.001996	.189570	
	.022008	.251270	
	.003423	.286430	
	Gammas & X-rays:		
	.096319	.005030	
	.176840	.035550	
	.323880	.036026	
	.121670	.040700	
	.117600	.057365	
	.002940	.169000	
	.002058	.216000	
	.020160	.231560	
	.420000	.293260	
	.002856	.338000	
	.033600	.350590	

[a] RSIC computer data file (DLC-80) contains x ray and photon data not in Kocher 1981. They are included in this table.
[b] Maximum energy for betas and positrons.
[c] Branching to radioactive daughter(s) shown in Table 8.13.

(continued)

Table 8.14 Energy and Probability by Radiation Type for Selected Radionuclides of Interest to Health Physicists (Continued)

	Probability per Decay	Energy[b] (MeV)	Average Energy (MeV)
	.001344	.433020	
	.001176	.439000	
	.019740	.490360	
	.002436	.587280	
	.052500	.664550	
	.051240	.721960	
	.009240	.880390	
	.003654	1.103000	
	.008925	.610620	
Pr-143	Half-life: 13.56 days		
	Betas:		
	1.000000	.935300	.315600
	.000000	.193300	.062600
	Gammas & X-rays:		
	.000000	.741980	
Ce-144[c]	Half-life: 284.3 days		
	.196000	.184660	.050200
	.047000	.238090	.066100
	.772000	.318200	.091100
	Electrons:		
	.096963	.004080	
	.006381	.011441	
	.011234	.026785	
	.007948	.029400	
	.003141	.032109	
	.008165	.034095	
	.033886	.038115	
	.002267	.039419	
	.004683	.073271	
	.001250	.078595	
	.053244	.091553	
	.007312	.126710	
	.001955	.132030	
	Gammas & X-rays:		
	.015785	.005030	
	.002830	.033620	
	.024311	.035550	
	.044525	.036026	
	.016727	.040700	
	.003888	.040930	
	.015984	.080106	
	.108000	.133540	
	.001325	.067350	
Pr-144m[c]	Half-life: 7.2 minutes		
	Electrons:		
	.681210	.004080	
	.333800	.017039	
	.028373	.029400	
	.501700	.052195	
	.124930	.057519	
	.038277	.058726	
	Gammas & X-rays:		
	.110890	.005030	
	.086780	.035550	
	.158940	.036026	
	.059709	.040700	
	.000819	.059030	
Pr-144	Half-life: 17.28 minutes		
	Betas:		
	.010800	.810320	.266600
	.011700	2.299500	.894400
	.977400	2.996000	1.221400
	.000113	.104400	.369190
	Gammas & X-rays:		
	.014800	.696490	
	.003004	1.489200	
	.007740	2.185700	
	.000204	1.058600	
Nd-147[c]	Half-life: 10.98 days		
	Betas:		
	.022200	.209910	.057600
	.153000	.364790	.106100
	.008100	.406550	.119900
	.005800	.485290	.146700
	.811000	.804700	.264000
	.000660	.215300	.059200
	Electrons:		
	.416010	.004380	
	.037481	.031500	
	.487200	.045922	
	.003121	.075296	
	.071120	.083678	
	.015204	.089457	
	.004312	.090776	
	.001023	.274230	
	.001825	.485830	
	Gammas & X-rays:		
	.079239	.005430	
	.129560	.038171	
	.235570	.038725	
	.090554	.043800	
	.280000	.091106	
	.003976	.120480	
	.002044	.196640	
	.008036	.275370	
	.019600	.319410	
	.008736	.398160	
	.001400	.410480	
	.012040	.439900	
	.001540	.489240	
	.131320	.531020	
	.002660	.594800	
	.008148	.685900	
	.000655	.616620	
Pm-147[c]	Half-life: 2.6234 years		
	Betas:		
	.999940	.224700	.061960
	.000057	.103500	.027098
	Gammas & X-rays:		
	.000029	.121260	
Sm-147	Half-life: 106000000000 years		
	Alphas:		
	1.000000	2.247600	
Pm-148	Half-life: 5.37 days		
	Betas:		
	.013600	.406040	.120000
	.333000	.998870	.340000
	.002350	1.039500	.356000
	.094000	1.913700	.728000
	.555000	2.464000	.975000
	.002299	.585000	.191740
	Electrons:		
	.001297	.004530	
	.000131	.032600	
	.001817	.503440	
	Gammas & X-rays:		
	.000266	.005640	
	.000480	.039522	
	.000869	.040118	
	.000337	.045400	
	.220000	.550270	
	.003530	.592830	
	.010212	.611260	
	.002353	.874180	
	.009812	.896420	
	.114550	.914850	
	.222000	1.465100	
	.003048	1.293900	
Pm-148m[c]	Half-life: 41.3 days		
	Betas:		
	.540000	.407150	.120000
	.186000	.505630	.154000
	.220000	.695260	.222000
	.009200	1.006900	.343000
	Electrons:		
	.049166	.004380	
	.027720	.030516	
	.002107	.031500	
	.030786	.054072	
	.008736	.059851	
	.002373	.061170	
	.003906	.068272	

[a] RSIC computer data file (DLC-80) contains x ray and photon data not in Kocher 1981. They are included in this table.

[b] Maximum energy for betas and positrons.

[c] Branching to radioactive daughter(s) shown in Table 8.13.

Table 8.14 Energy and Probability by Radiation Type for Selected Radionuclides of Interest to Health Physicists (Continued)

Nuclide	Probability per Decay	Energy[b] (MeV)	Average Energy (MeV)
	.001063	.074051	
	.052417	.004530	
	.004556	.032600	
	.037360	.051646	
	.006037	.090743	
	.001680	.096757	
	.002318	.142800	
	.008037	.241280	
	.001394	.280370	
	.001068	.367240	
	.007836	.503440	
	.001300	.542530	
	.005269	.583140	
	.001396	.678870	
	Gammas & X-rays:		
	.009365	.005430	
	.007282	.038171	
	.013241	.038725	
	.005090	.043800	
	.009324	.075700	
	.000003	.061500	
	.010736	.005640	
	.016710	.039522	
	.030271	.040118	
	.011745	.045400	
	.024741	.098480	
	.011036	.189630	
	.125580	.288110	
	.039159	.311630	
	.001780	.362090	
	.186630	.414070	
	.053488	.432780	
	.004183	.460570	
	.067461	.501260	
	.948720	.550270	
	.004005	.553240	
	.002136	.571950	
	.125400	.599740	
	.054823	.611260	
	.889980	.629970	
	.328400	.725700	
	.171680	.915330	
	.202830	1.013800	
	.001931	.714790	
Pm-149	Half-life: 53.08 hours		
	Betas:		
	.001260	.189200	.051400
	.033900	.785100	.256100
	.962300	1.071000	.369000
	.002548	.441000	.133450
	Electrons:		
	.002866	.004530	
	.001352	.014757	
	.000176	.032600	
	.002443	.239070	
	Gammas & X-rays:		
	.000587	.005640	
	.000645	.039522	
	.001169	.040118	
	.000453	.045400	
	.031000	.285900	
	.001023	.859400	
	.002985	.598330	
Pm-151	Half-life: 28.4 hours		
	Betas:		
	.001590	.223660	.062000
	.010400	.234510	.065000
	.003200	.300640	.085000
	.023500	.310340	.088000
	.062000	.365360	.106000
	.011500	.414020	.122000
	.031600	.446930	.133000
	.002050	.524440	.160000
	.007500	.666880	.212000
	.004400	.697680	.223000
	.071000	.742300	.240000
	.019500	.792410	.259000
	.127000	.843090	.278000
	.033300	.864050	.287000
	.018500	.881210	.293000
	.001900	.885360	.295000
	.024200	.979000	.332000
	.014300	1.019600	.348000
	.085000	1.020200	.348000
	.033000	1.083200	.374000
	.027000	1.118300	.388000
	.100000	1.188000	.417000
	.003230	.600000	.191320
	Electrons:		
	.507870	.003098	
	.274600	.004530	
	.001747	.016069	
	.014929	.017943	
	.099849	.018053	
	.056877	.019000	
	.019859	.022884	
	.004253	.023957	
	.006171	.027413	
	.005056	.029385	
	.022004	.032600	
	.001875	.033427	
	.037446	.053183	
	.002898	.055099	
	.015401	.057150	
	.045079	.058005	
	.008164	.058097	
	.003175	.061981	
	.004234	.063164	
	.002231	.064111	
	.006658	.068482	
	.001953	.074496	
	.005283	.092280	
	.002864	.092451	
	.001022	.096337	
	.006496	.097102	
	.001457	.098294	
	.001796	.103120	
	.005886	.116760	
	.005074	.120930	
	.003041	.121550	
	.010952	.130320	
	.003287	.162180	
	.001734	.169420	
	.001454	.185590	
	.001118	.228380	
	.002107	.293250	
	Gammas & X-rays:		
	.056243	.005640	
	.009389	.025680	
	.080698	.039522	
	.146190	.040118	
	.056722	.045400	
	.002175	.062903	
	.019694	.064887	
	.011679	.065834	
	.004832	.069718	
	.002107	.076219	
	.003664	.098040	
	.025648	.100020	
	.013053	.101930	
	.035495	.104840	
	.005061	.139290	
	.002175	.143170	
	.001488	.147550	
	.001511	.156180	
	.008931	.162950	
	.016259	.163590	
	.087936	.167770	
	.009160	.168380	
	.008702	.176540	
	.038701	.177160	
	.001695	.186600	
	.009435	.201960	
	.001305	.204150	
	.017862	.209010	

[a] RSIC computer data file (DLC-80) contains x ray and photon data not in Kocher 1981. They are included in this table.

[b] Maximum energy for betas and positrons.

[c] Branching to radioactive daughter(s) shown in Table 8.13.

(continued)

Table 8.14 Energy and Probability by Radiation Type for Selected Radionuclides of Interest to Health Physicists (Continued)

	Probability per Decay	Energy[b] (MeV)	Average Energy (MeV)
	.003412	.227200	
	.010534	.232420	
	.001626	.236600	
	.001969	.236700	
	.005267	.237020	
	.038930	.240090	
	.001649	.254300	
	.006000	.258130	
	.071677	.275210	
	.002267	.280100	
	.008794	.290760	
	.002359	.306740	
	.012137	.323950	
	.001076	.325800	
	.002107	.329760	
	.229000	.340080	
	.021755	.344910	
	.001351	.349830	
	.001145	.353320	
	.009664	.379870	
	.001878	.407020	
	.015343	.440880	
	.040762	.445690	
	.003000	.451420	
	.001282	.490300	
	.002015	.516250	
	.003618	.565010	
	.001168	.574970	
	.014656	.636230	
	.002496	.654250	
	.003618	.668700	
	.002908	.669200	
	.009274	.671300	
	.003527	.704220	
	.001488	.709290	
	.001053	.712020	
	.041220	.717750	
	.004855	.736130	
	.013282	.752830	
	.001099	.769100	
	.009595	.772800	
	.002290	.785070	
	.005267	.807910	
	.001718	.817650	
	.003000	.848670	
	.001008	.877690	
	.003641	.948710	
	.043579	.428810	
Sm-151	Half-life: 90 years		
	Betas:		
	.008800	.054560	.013960
	.991200	.076100	.019680
	Electrons:		
	.004849	.004690	
	.005914	.013488	
	.002040	.019740	
	Gammas & X-rays:		
	.001064	.005850	
	.000296	.021540	
Sm-153	Half-life: 46.7 hours		
	Betas:		
	.341000	.632350	.198600
	.441000	.702020	.224400
	.005500	.707760	.226500
	.210000	.805200	.263400
	.001494	.262100	.080927
	Electrons:		
	.540580	.004690	
	.003238	.011758	
	.231620	.021153	
	.044986	.033700	
	.004740	.034848	
	.003413	.040965	
	.001852	.048911	
	.410350	.054660	
	.037896	.061620	
	.008272	.067872	
	.002326	.069312	
	.002240	.075314	
	.001334	.081566	
	.061694	.095127	
	.013358	.101380	
	.003849	.102820	
	Gammas & X-rays:		
	.118660	.005850	
	.172630	.040902	
	.312180	.041542	
	.122170	.047000	
	.051700	.069672	
	.001940	.075422	
	.002000	.083366	
	.001580	.089484	
	.007180	.097430	
	.283000	.103180	
	.002775	.422660	
Eu-152[c]	Half-life: 13.6 years		
	Betas:		
	.017800	.175900	.047500
	.024000	.385240	.112500
	.136000	.696060	.221800
	.002300	.710070	.227000
	.002930	.888650	.295300
	.008900	1.063800	.364800
	.084400	1.474900	.535600
	.001855	.256900	.074287
	Electrons:		
	.733780	.004530	
	.056787	.032600	
	.194760	.074945	
	.106330	.114040	
	.024309	.120060	
	.006682	.121430	
	.006092	.197860	
	.001559	.236960	
	.007135	.004840	
	.000544	.034900	
	.008238	.294030	
	.001807	.335900	
	Gammas & X-rays:		
	.150290	.005640	
	.208260	.039522	
	.377280	.040118	
	.146390	.045400	
	.284320	.121780	
	.074935	.244690	
	.004266	.295930	
	.001245	.329350	
	.001007	.415940	
	.028114	.443980	
	.003021	.443980	
	.004134	.488660	
	.004823	.564030	
	.001290	.566410	
	.001418	.656440	
	.001484	.674610	
	.008373	.688630	
	.002650	.719330	
	.003100	.810430	
	.001606	.841540	
	.041601	.867320	
	.004014	.919310	
	.002552	.926250	
	.001139	.963390	
	.144410	.964010	
	.006598	1.005200	
	.002464	1.084900	
	.099630	1.085800	
	.133020	1.112000	
	.013805	1.212800	
	.001783	1.249800	
	.001010	1.292700	
	.207470	1.408000	
	.004875	1.457500	
	.002570	1.528100	
	.008688	.685780	

[a] RSIC computer data file (DLC-80) contains x ray and photon data not in Kocher 1981. They are included in this table.

[b] Maximum energy for betas and positrons.

[c] Branching to radioactive daughter(s) shown in Table 8.13.

Table 8.14 Energy and Probability by Radiation Type for Selected Radionuclides of Interest to Health Physicists (Continued)

	Probability per Decay	Energy[b] (MeV)	Average Energy (MeV)
	.001674	.006060	
	.002190	.042309	
	.003946	.042996	
	.001558	.048700	
	.264880	.344270	
	.008556	.367710	
	.022144	.411110	
	.001507	.503390	
	.004529	.586260	
	.004688	.678580	
	.001685	.764840	
	.127410	.778890	
	.016793	1.089700	
	.001669	1.109100	
	.016052	1.299000	
	.007111	.631380	
Gd-152	Half-life: 1.1e + 14 years		
	Alphas:		
	1.000000	2.149600	
Eu-154	Half-life: 8.8 years		
	Betas:		
	.279000	.247410	.068800
	.007700	.306080	.086900
	.001490	.321210	.091700
	.015800	.349830	.100900
	.001170	.407400	.119800
	.002810	.435660	.129300
	.001880	.548600	.168300
	.365000	.569100	.175700
	.006400	.703180	.224500
	.002450	.715410	.229000
	.174000	.839180	.276000
	.020000	.970720	.327500
	.002900	1.151500	.400400
	.002400	1.596000	.587400
	.114000	1.843900	.695000
	.002139	.412000	.131260
	Electrons:		
	.325360	.004840	
	.018034	.034900	
	.267870	.072831	
	.167930	.114690	
	.039048	.121190	
	.010966	.122690	
	.005374	.197700	
	.001492	.239560	
	Gammas & X-rays:		
	.076319	.006060	
	.072639	.042309	
	.130880	.042996	
	.051694	.048700	
	.404640	.123070	
	.002272	.188250	
	.066021	.247940	
	.002094	.401300	
	.005040	.444500	
	.002165	.478260	
	.002556	.557560	
	.008412	.582000	
	.048273	.591810	
	.003088	.625220	
	.001399	.676590	
	.016931	.692410	
	.001739	.715760	
	.197000	.723300	
	.043304	.756870	
	.004650	.815550	
	.005502	.845390	
	.002307	.850640	
	.115000	.873190	
	.004614	.892730	
	.008235	.904050	
	.102940	.996320	
	.178890	1.004800	
	.001420	1.047400	
	.001029	1.118500	
	.002662	1.128400	
	.002165	1.140900	
	.001313	1.241600	
	.008980	1.246200	
	.354950	1.274500	
	.006496	1.494400	
	.010294	1.593000	
	.018457	1.596500	
	.015850	.710540	
Eu-155	Half-life: 4.96 years		
	Betas:		
	.007200	.099930	.026100
	.022000	.128010	.033900
	.460000	.140690	.037400
	.260000	.159460	.042800
	.077000	.185990	.050400
	.180000	.246000	.068300
	Electrons:		
	.012054	.002024	
	.341500	.004840	
	.003488	.008519	
	.082763	.009771	
	.137630	.010374	
	.009518	.012644	
	.031518	.016869	
	.004933	.018137	
	.010401	.018374	
	.002939	.019139	
	.003838	.023054	
	.001429	.024632	
	.001208	.029549	
	.016063	.034900	
	.003997	.035823	
	.112170	.036306	
	.006200	.036922	
	.001808	.043416	
	.016686	.051634	
	.044445	.055069	
	.003693	.058129	
	.001050	.059634	
	.017242	.078169	
	.003708	.084664	
	.001041	.086169	
	.006636	.096932	
	.001836	.103430	
	Gammas & X-rays:		
	.080104	.006060	
	.003183	.026513	
	.064697	.042309	
	.116570	.042996	
	.012916	.045297	
	.046042	.048700	
	.011124	.060010	
	.001514	.086062	
	.309000	.086545	
	.206720	.105310	
	.001845	.069302	
Eu-156	Half-life: 15.19 days		
	Betas:		
	.046000	.183110	.050000
	.024000	.247520	.069000
	.001600	.249500	.069000
	.113000	.266270	.075000
	.001270	.331580	.095000
	.060000	.426410	.126000
	.320000	.487090	.147000
	.009600	.500630	.152000
	.004400	.506620	.154000
	.024000	1.086600	.374000
	.051000	1.210600	.425000
	.045000	1.284900	.456000
	.014500	1.403600	.505000
	.270000	2.453000	.966000
	.002030	.164000	.044555
	Electrons:		
	.231940	.004840	
	.009518	.034900	
	.142960	.038725	
	.163770	.080588	

[a] RSIC computer data file (DLC-80) contains x ray and photon data not in Kocher 1981. They are included in this table.

[b] Maximum energy for betas and positrons.

[c] Branching to radioactive daughter(s) shown in Table 8.13.

(continued)

Table 8.14 Energy and Probability by Radiation Type for Selected Radionuclides of Interest to Health Physicists (Continued)

	Probability per Decay	Energy[b] (MeV)	Average Energy (MeV)
	.038364	.087083	
	.010677	.088588	
	.001249	.148970	
	Gammas & X-rays:		
	.054406	.006060	
	.038335	.042309	
	.069073	.042996	
	.027282	.048700	
	.090480	.088964	
	.007904	.199210	
	.002205	.434400	
	.001466	.472700	
	.001820	.490340	
	.023088	.599470	
	.070928	.646290	
	.009152	.709860	
	.060216	.723470	
	.001102	.797730	
	.104000	.811770	
	.001602	.820360	
	.002257	.841100	
	.001258	.858360	
	.001560	.865980	
	.014040	.867010	
	.013936	.944350	
	.003120	.947460	
	.016224	.960500	
	.001560	.961000	
	.003869	.969830	
	.003401	1.011900	
	.001196	1.027400	
	.005304	1.040400	
	.052416	1.065100	
	.003744	1.076000	
	.048880	1.079200	
	.001425	1.129500	
	.002964	1.140500	
	.071760	1.153500	
	.053040	1.154100	
	.001404	1.156000	
	.002933	1.169100	
	.089440	1.230700	
	.067600	1.242400	
	.032136	1.277400	
	.017576	1.366400	
	.003016	1.682100	
	.002548	1.857400	
	.017264	1.877000	
	.021424	1.937700	
	.001893	1.946300	
	.042016	1.966000	
	.035360	2.026600	
	.001300	2.032500	
	.042744	2.097700	
	.001258	2.116500	
	.024336	2.180900	
	.039520	2.186700	
	.009984	2.205400	
	.011232	2.269900	
	.015851	1.102700	
Tb-160	Half-life: 72.3 years:		
	Betas:		
	.002180	.299010	.084600
	.044000	.434460	.128600
	.009300	.447030	.132800
	.094000	.474830	.142300
	.033100	.545810	.166900
	.456000	.568730	.175000
	.001700	.677660	.214400
	.058000	.784370	.254300
	.246000	.867300	.286000
	.003800	1.549600	.565200
	.050000	1.746600	.649900
	.000142	.547800	.167600
	Electrons:		
	.401810	.005160	
	.211470	.033000	
	.013495	.037200	
	.316540	.077742	
	.075411	.084741	
	.020748	.086372	
	.008186	.143250	
	.001255	.161860	
	.003152	.187990	
	.004007	.244780	
	Gammas & X-rays:		
	.106810	.006500	
	.060309	.045208	
	.107890	.045998	
	.043227	.052100	
	.133000	.086788	
	.049020	.197040	
	.037145	.215650	
	.270750	.298570	
	.008151	.309560	
	.003325	.337320	
	.012825	.392490	
	.005510	.682330	
	.019285	.765280	
	.001786	.872030	
	.285000	.879360	
	.090250	.962290	
	.242250	.966150	
	.009690	1.002900	
	.005225	1.102600	
	.015010	1.115100	
	.144400	1.177900	
	.023560	1.199900	
	.070300	1.271900	
	.028500	1.312200	
	.005089	.651350	
Ho-166m	Half-life: 1200 years		
	Betas:		
	.172000	.031784	.008000
	.734000	.072373	.018700
	.004040	.303600	.085900
	.009000	.483290	.144900
	.021300	.643360	.201300
	.011200	.948080	.316400
	.034000	1.313800	.464100
	Electrons:		
	.709080	.005500	
	.217260	.023104	
	.003369	.037165	
	.022186	.039700	
	.001773	.061555	
	.002447	.063675	
	.501850	.070838	
	.121590	.078382	
	.033287	.080140	
	.001765	.084899	
	.001003	.111410	
	.150280	.126930	
	.003367	.158390	
	.070640	.174660	
	.016771	.182210	
	.004639	.183970	
	.001311	.206130	
	.018217	.222960	
	.001877	.243260	
	.005480	.270700	
	.001629	.278240	
	.001084	.472320	
	.001217	.654200	
	.002491	.752820	
	Gammas & X-rays:		
	.211800	.006950	
	.108890	.048221	
	.193410	.049128	
	.078899	.055700	
	.127050	.080589	
	.001605	.094650	
	.001612	.119040	
	.002447	.121160	
	.726000	.184420	
	.002207	.190710	

[a] RSIC computer data file (DLC-80) contains x ray and photon data not in Kocher 1981. They are included in this table.

[b] Maximum energy for betas and positrons.

[c] Branching to radioactive daughter(s) shown in Table 8.13.

Table 8.14 Energy and Probability by Radiation Type for Selected Radionuclides of Interest to Health Physicists (Continued)

	Probability per Decay	Energy[b] (MeV)	Average Energy (MeV)
	.004254	.214760	
	.025700	.215880	
	.002062	.231280	
	.010527	.259720	
	.296210	.280450	
	.037171	.300740	
	.001699	.339780	
	.024176	.365780	
	.111080	.410940	
	.002178	.496700	
	.095106	.529810	
	.054668	.571000	
	.005590	.594370	
	.014157	.611520	
	.001546	.644450	
	.053506	.670510	
	.013576	.691210	
	.540870	.711690	
	.002178	.712400	
	.003674	.736670	
	.120520	.752270	
	.030274	.778820	
	.571360	.810310	
	.096558	.830560	
	.007187	.875640	
	.026935	.950940	
	.002374	1.120300	
	.001968	1.146800	
	.008276	1.241400	
	.001786	1.282100	
	.004980	1.400700	
	.004842	1.427100	
	.006286	.416610	
Yb-169	Half-life: 31.97 days		
	Electrons:		
	.399410	.003729	
	1.600000	.005670	
	.946780	.006094	
	.093042	.010634	
	.020721	.018443	
	.006829	.020278	
	.083721	.034223	
	.101200	.040900	
	.349000	.050387	
	.071308	.053003	
	.013342	.058797	
	.015836	.060812	
	.004292	.062647	
	.060487	.071130	
	.014458	.083497	
	.004199	.091306	
	.056430	.099661	
	.012623	.107470	
	.013700	.108070	
	.003681	.109310	
	.004253	.115880	
	.102900	.117820	
	.051641	.120400	
	.012496	.128210	
	.003483	.130050	
	.127460	.138560	
	.018393	.167090	
	.004159	.174900	
	.001188	.176740	
	.020952	.187840	
	.004679	.195650	
	.001341	.197480	
	.005241	.248340	
	.001513	.297610	
	Gammas & X-rays:		
	.505260	.007180	
	.003298	.008401	
	.002134	.020750	
	.527770	.049773	
	.934110	.050742	
	.383010	.057500	
	.437470	.063119	
	.026578	.093613	
	.173630	.109780	
	.018818	.118190	
	.110580	.130520	
	.214370	.177210	
	.349200	.197950	
	.001222	.240300	
	.017654	.261070	
	.108060	.307730	
	.001843	.344060	
W-181	Half-life: 120.95 days		
	Electrons:		
	.848820	.003502	
	.573460	.006350	
	.029952	.046200	
	Gammas & X-rays:		
	.009870	.006210	
	.223010	.008150	
	.186950	.056277	
	.326270	.057532	
	.137540	.065200	
	.001401	.147690	
W-185	Half-life: 75.1 days		
	Betas:		
	.999210	.432400	.126800
	.000790	.307000	.096900
	Gammas & X-rays:		
	.000210	.125360	
W-187[c]	Half-life: 23.83 hours		
	Betas:		
	.004840	.433060	.127000
	.006700	.447950	.131900
	.002000	.495940	.148000
	.043000	.539630	.163000
	.587000	.626700	.193500
	.055000	.686980	.215100
	.035000	.694130	.217600
	.001000	.800730	.256800
	.023000	1.178300	.401700
	.251000	1.312500	.457100
	.000217	.197300	.055688
	Electrons:		
	.086919	.000384	
	.035039	.004168	
	.193260	.006700	
	.001068	.016703	
	.004245	.023703	
	.001311	.031133	
	.001337	.033298	
	.002505	.042074	
	.011290	.047000	
	.016669	.059533	
	.175970	.062544	
	.004941	.069128	
	.029896	.121690	
	.006859	.131290	
	.002100	.133600	
	.003960	.134610	
	.004273	.407850	
	.001086	.467000	
	.001745	.546690	
	Gammas & X-rays:		
	.086825	.008650	
	.076022	.059718	
	.131750	.061140	
	.056307	.069300	
	.119070	.072060	
	.094608	.134220	
	.001523	.206290	
	.001274	.246180	
	.233520	.479530	
	.006895	.511760	
	.054365	.551550	
	.001301	.589090	
	.067102	.618370	
	.011630	.625520	
	.291670	.685810	
	.003184	.745210	

[a] RSIC computer data file (DLC-80) contains x ray and photon data not in Kocher 1981. They are included in this table.
[b] Maximum energy for betas and positrons.
[c] Branching to radioactive daughter(s) shown in Table 8.13.

(continued)

Table 8.14 Energy and Probability by Radiation Type for Selected Radionuclides of Interest to Health Physicists (Continued)

	Probability per Decay	Energy[b] (MeV)	Average Energy (MeV)
	.044027	.772870	
	.003590	.864550	
	.001514	.879430	
	.004230	.276220	
Re-187	Half-life: 47000000000 years		
	Betas:		
	1.000000	.002641	.000661
Ir-192	Half-life: 74.02 days		
	Betas:		
	.056500	.255950	.070800
	.414000	.536080	.161200
	.483000	.672420	.208900
	.004000	.844530	.275900
	.000987	.093000	.024933
	Electrons:		
	.031078	.006880	
	.001594	.048300	
	.005227	.131920	
	.003649	.192830	
	.001180	.202750	
	.076020	.007240	
	.003505	.051000	
	.001192	.057951	
	.001300	.122470	
	.019237	.217560	
	.017896	.230060	
	.044658	.238110	
	.008792	.282080	
	.002867	.292660	
	.007716	.294580	
	.019470	.302630	
	.002511	.305160	
	.004839	.313210	
	.001483	.315790	
	.010236	.389680	
	.002946	.454190	
	.001509	.526020	
	Gammas & X-rays:		
	.014625	.008910	
	.011323	.061487	
	.019555	.063001	
	.008399	.071400	
	.004674	.201310	
	.032873	.205800	
	.002615	.283260	
	.007264	.374480	
	.031628	.484580	
	.003985	.489060	
	.000797	.423070	
	.040934	.009440	
	.026350	.065122	
	.045197	.066832	
	.019675	.075700	
	.001806	.136350	
	.290150	.295960	
	.296780	.308460	
	.828530	.316510	
	.006645	.416460	
	.480550	.468070	
	.045735	.588580	
	.082024	.604410	
	.053357	.612460	
	.003016	.884510	
	.000986	.871730	
Au-198	Half-life: 2.696 days		
	Betas:		
	.013200	.284810	.079410
	.986500	.960700	.314600
	.000250	1.372500	.467200
	Electrons:		
	.020774	.007600	
	.000977	.053800	
	.028749	.328700	
	.010220	.396970	
	.003333	.408240	
	Gammas & X-rays:		
	.012732	.009990	
	.008053	.068895	
	.013695	.070819	
	.006024	.080300	
	.955100	.411800	
	.010602	.675890	
	.002292	1.087700	
Hg-197	Half-life: 64.14 hours		
	Electrons:		
	.891090	.007420	
	.026707	.052400	
	.593850	.062999	
	.143930	.073927	
	.045140	.076593	
	.004782	.110700	
	Gammas & X-rays:		
	.501240	.009710	
	.206860	.066989	
	.353600	.068804	
	.185000	.077352	
	.154690	.078000	
	.004976	.191420	
	.000389	.268730	
Hg-203	Half-life: 46.6 days		
	Betas:		
	1.000000	.212210	.057700
	Electrons:		
	.108230	.007780	
	.005577	.055200	
	.169000	.193660	
	.043500	.263840	
	.010600	.275480	
	.003400	.278340	
	Gammas & X-rays:		
	.072156	.010300	
	.047450	.070832	
	.080424	.072871	
	.035549	.082600	
	.773000	.279190	
Tl-201	Half-life: 73.06 hours		
	Electrons:		
	.113000	.000770	
	.725060	.007600	
	.081400	.015761	
	.070180	.017351	
	.025300	.027038	
	.021736	.028628	
	.074730	.052238	
	.033207	.053800	
	.002400	.082778	
	.154000	.084328	
	.012747	.120500	
	.003922	.131780	
	.026200	.152590	
	.006100	.163870	
	.001960	.166630	
	Gammas & X-rays:		
	.444390	.009990	
	.002200	.030600	
	.002200	.032190	
	.273570	.068895	
	.465250	.070819	
	.204650	.080300	
	.026500	.135340	
	.001600	.165880	
	.100000	.167430	
	.000000	.001570	
Pb-210[c]	Half-life: 22.26 years		
	Betas:		
	.802000	.016498	.004140
	.198000	.063001	.016130
	Electrons:		
	.335910	.008150	
	.579150	.030116	
	.181040	.042504	
	Gammas & X-rays:		
	.243240	.010800	
	.040500	.046503	

[a] RSIC computer data file (DLC-80) contains x ray and photon data not in Kocher 1981. They are included in this table.

[b] Maximum energy for betas and positrons.

[c] Branching to radioactive daughter(s) shown in Table 8.13.

Table 8.14 Energy and Probability by Radiation Type for Selected Radionuclides of Interest to Health Physicists (Continued)

	Probability per Decay	Energy[b] (MeV)	Average Energy (MeV)
Bi-210[c]	Half-life: 5.013 days		
	Betas:		
	1.000000	1.161400	.389000
Po-210	Half-life: 138.378 days		
	Alphas:		
	.999990	5.304500	
	.000011	4.524000	
	Gammas & X-rays:		
	.000011	.803100	
Ra-223[c]	Half-life: 11.434 days		
	Alphas:		
	.001600	5.288000	
	.001300	5.339000	
	.001300	5.367000	
	.022700	5.345000	
	.010000	5.501000	
	.091600	5.537000	
	.242000	5.606000	
	.525000	5.715000	
	.095000	5.745000	
	.003200	5.857500	
	.008500	5.870000	
	.002947	5.348200	
	Electrons:		
	.518000	.003343	
	.126870	.005508	
	.001701	.008376	
	.279000	.008710	
	.126750	.009948	
	.011880	.013551	
	.073661	.023915	
	.004230	.027118	
	.125390	.045831	
	.180790	.055805	
	.019739	.060230	
	.014625	.062700	
	.002366	.081116	
	.001757	.092808	
	.013804	.104270	
	.003296	.117840	
	.001151	.121220	
	.023296	.126190	
	.032922	.136160	
	.005540	.139750	
	.003770	.140590	
	.019343	.143140	
	.007868	.149730	
	.002723	.153110	
	.001216	.154150	
	.090440	.171060	
	.015404	.225470	
	.009500	.239880	
	.016592	.251410	
	.003917	.264980	
	.001345	.268360	
	.001265	.273270	
	.002805	.305820	
	.001739	.320230	
	.002053	.346630	
	Gammas & X-rays:		
	.247410	.011700	
	.002000	.080190	
	.148700	.081070	
	.247000	.083780	
	.111980	.094900	
	.004500	.098234	
	.011900	.122320	
	.032400	.144240	
	.055800	.154210	
	.006830	.158630	
	.001360	.179520	
	.136000	.269460	
	.001510	.288180	
	.038800	.323870	
	.001950	.328380	
	.027300	.338280	
	.002200	.342900	
	.003400	.349800	
	.004720	.371680	
	.011800	.445030	
	.013533	.292050	
Rn-219[c]	Half-life: 3.96 seconds		
	Alphas:		
	.075000	6.424700	
	.001200	6.529000	
	.129000	6.552800	
	.796000	6.819300	
	.000887	6.230700	
	Electrons:		
	.013793	.008330	
	.003967	.037485	
	.000557	.059700	
	.001110	.113650	
	.012296	.178130	
	.007229	.254290	
	.002491	.267080	
	.002301	.308710	
	.001007	.384870	
	Gammas & X-rays:		
	.010405	.011100	
	.005255	.076862	
	.008802	.079290	
	.003950	.089800	
	.001160	.130590	
	.106000	.271230	
	.065000	.401810	
	.001951	.388450	
Po-215[c]	Half-life: .00178 seconds		
	Alphas:		
	.999440	7.386400	
	.000560	6.954100	
	Gammas & X-rays:		
	.000340	.438700	
Pb-211[c]	Half-life: 36.1 minutes		
	Betas:		
	.006600	.263570	.072800
	.050000	.541070	.161900
	.013000	.968160	.315600
	.930000	1.373000	.473300
	.000880	.253000	.070858
	Electrons:		
	.003842	.008150	
	.003087	.049033	
	.000137	.058200	
	.002411	.314320	
	.002011	.336550	
	Gammas & X-rays:		
	.002782	.010800	
	.001247	.074815	
	.002100	.077108	
	.000937	.087300	
	.029400	.404840	
	.013230	.427080	
	.003695	.704590	
	.005390	.766470	
	.028616	.831960	
	.004719	.517630	
Bi-211[c]	Half-life: 2.13 minutes		
	Alphas:		
	.162260	6.278800	
	.835010	6.623100	
	Betas:		
	.002730	.579000	.174600
	Electrons:		
	.015707	.007780	
	.000878	.055200	
	.026610	.265540	
	.004624	.335720	
	.001423	.347370	
	Gammas & X-rays:		
	.010471	.010300	
	.007471	.070832	
	.012663	.072871	

[a] RSIC computer data file (DLC-80) contains x ray and photon data not in Kocher 1981. They are included in this table.

[b] Maximum energy for betas and positrons.

[c] Branching to radioactive daughter(s) shown in Table 8.13.

(continued)

Table 8.14 Energy and Probability by Radiation Type for Selected Radionuclides of Interest to Health Physicists (Continued)

	Probability per Decay	Energy[b] (MeV)	Average Energy (MeV)
	.005597	.082600	
	.129450	.351070	
Tl-207	Half-life: 4.77 minutes		
	Betas:		
	.002500	.524170	.156300
	.997500	1.422000	.494100
	Gammas & X-rays:		
	.002400	.897830	
	.000031	.459070	
Po-211	Half-life: .516 seconds		
	Alphas:		
	.005370	6.570000	
	.005460	6.892800	
	.989160	7.450400	
	Gammas & X-rays:		
	.005380	.569670	
	.005219	.897830	
	.000032	.328200	
Ra-224[c]	Half-life: 3.62 days		
	Alphas:		
	.049000	5.449000	
	.951000	5.685600	
	.000176	5.093600	
	Electrons:		
	.004472	.008710	
	.000124	.062700	
	.004424	.142580	
	.004898	.222930	
	.001742	.236500	
	Gammas & X-rays:		
	.003966	.011700	
	.001260	.081070	
	.002092	.083780	
	.000949	.094900	
	.039500	.240980	
	.000180	.464950	
Rn-220[c]	Half-life: 55.61 seconds		
	Alphas:		
	.999030	6.288300	
	.000970	5.747000	
	Gammas & X-rays:		
	.000950	.549730	
Po-216	Half-life: .146 seconds		
	Alphas:		
	.999980	6.778500	
	.000018	5.985000	
	Gammas & X-rays:		
	.000018	.804900	
Pb-212[c]	Half-life: 10.643 hours		
	Betas:		
	.052200	.157520	.041900
	.851000	.334180	.094400
	.099000	.572800	.172700
	Electrons:		
	.213940	.008150	
	.034821	.024664	
	.011751	.058200	
	.006145	.098802	
	.001922	.111190	
	.330820	.148100	
	.013422	.209560	
	.057146	.222240	
	.013483	.234630	
	.004509	.237690	
	.002323	.283700	
	Gammas & X-rays:		
	.154930	.010800	
	.106940	.074815	
	.180030	.077108	
	.080351	.087300	
	.006025	.115190	
	.446460	.238630	
	.034067	.300090	
	.000520	.176670	
Bi-212[c]	Half-life: 60.55 minutes		
	Alphas:		
	.004024	5.607100	
	.006000	5.768100	
	.252230	6.050800	
	.096292	6.090100	
	.000651	5.612700	
	Betas:		
	.011700	.440150	.128100
	.004300	.566670	.170300
	.034400	.625360	.190600
	.026100	.733300	.228700
	.080000	1.518800	.530700
	.484000	2.246000	.831600
	.000480	.445000	.129700
	Electrons:		
	.115300	.007780	
	.191210	.024510	
	.059203	.036153	
	.000039	.055200	
	.001178	.202540	
	.000572	.008330	
	.000038	.059700	
	.001254	.634060	
	Gammas & X-rays:		
	.076864	.010300	
	.010225	.039857	
	.000331	.070832	
	.000560	.072871	
	.000248	.082600	
	.003174	.288070	
	.001296	.327960	
	.003475	.452830	
	.000946	.379500	
	.000431	.011100	
	.000355	.076862	
	.000595	.079290	
	.000267	.089800	
	.118290	.727170	
	.019694	.785460	
	.006522	.893430	
	.003133	.952100	
	.009527	1.078600	
	.005563	1.512800	
	.027495	1.620600	
	.001215	1.679500	
	.001982	1.806000	
	.000281	1.074000	
Tl-208	**Half-life: 3.053 minutes**		
	Betas:		
	.002220	.811540	.257800
	.001640	.866640	.278200
	.029200	1.031000	.340200
	.005800	1.072100	.356000
	.232000	1.283500	.438700
	.227000	1.516800	.532500
	.493000	1.794200	.646500
	.002040	.712000	.223520
	Electrons:		
	.041518	.007970	
	.002309	.056700	
	.001617	.123400	
	.001299	.145360	
	.002715	.164610	
	.030539	.189350	
	.005239	.261490	
	.001622	.273500	
	.018798	.422840	
	.003169	.494980	
	.012803	.495130	
	.001043	.506990	
	.003504	.567280	
	.001154	.579290	
	.002802	.772370	
	.001597	2.526700	
	Gammas & X-rays:		
	.028851	.010600	
	.020311	.072804	
	.034310	.074969	
	.015239	.084900	
	.001697	.211400	

[a] RSIC computer data file (DLC-80) contains x ray and photon data not in Kocher 1981. They are included in this table.
[b] Maximum energy for betas and positrons.
[c] Branching to radioactive daughter(s) shown in Table 8.13.

Table 8.14 Energy and Probability by Radiation Type for Selected Radionuclides of Interest to Health Physicists (Continued)

	Probability per Decay	Energy[b] (MeV)	Average Energy (MeV)
	.003094	.233360	
	.007984	.252610	
	.067864	.277350	
	.215570	.510840	
	.842310	.583140	
	.002026	.722040	
	.016367	.763130	
	.124550	.860370	
	.001247	.927600	
	.001966	.982700	
	.003693	1.093900	
	.998000	2.614700	
	.003573	.840360	
Po-212	Half-life: 2.98e-7 seconds		
	Alphas:		
	1.000000	8.784900	
Ra-225[c]	Half-life: 14.8 days		
	Betas:		
	.720000	.322000	.090000
	.280000	.362000	.103000
	Electrons:		
	.151440	.009280	
	.309070	.020160	
	.101370	.034998	
	Gammas & X-rays:		
	.157630	.012700	
	.310000	.040000	
Ac-225[c]	Half-life: 10 days		
	Alphas:		
	.002300	5.286000	
	.001300	5.444000	
	.001000	5.553000	
	.012000	5.579000	
	.011000	5.608000	
	.044000	5.636200	
	.014000	5.681000	
	.029000	5.722600	
	.100000	5.731000	
	.086000	5.791000	
	.181000	5.792000	
	.516000	5.829000	
	.003780	5.450400	
	Electrons:		
	.021532	.007263	
	.067200	.007361	
	.221640	.008900	
	.130900	.017961	
	.064380	.019861	
	.023100	.021348	
	.001700	.023663	
	.046410	.031948	
	.022866	.033848	
	.048015	.044261	
	.009420	.045461	
	.001008	.048953	
	.001500	.051161	
	.002900	.053061	
	.004800	.054961	
	.012800	.055761	
	.009672	.056113	
	.006000	.056261	
	.011440	.058248	
	.003240	.059448	
	.004020	.061747	
	.015000	.064261	
	.000961	.064300	
	.001060	.067048	
	.009657	.068741	
	.001760	.068948	
	.003360	.069748	
	.002200	.070248	
	.001200	.073247	
	.004384	.076261	
	.001512	.077661	
	.003900	.078248	
	.015795	.080911	
	.001404	.081161	
	.001350	.081747	
	.001880	.082161	
	.003132	.082728	
	.006608	.089761	
	.001424	.090248	
	.001680	.094553	
	.003816	.094898	
	.001352	.098397	
	.002251	.103750	
	.001953	.138610	
	Gammas & X-rays:		
	.212950	.012000	
	.005500	.062900	
	.003200	.073830	
	.001500	.082900	
	.010156	.083230	
	.016815	.086100	
	.002900	.087380	
	.001600	.094900	
	.007660	.097500	
	.006500	.099550	
	.017000	.099800	
	.002800	.108400	
	.003200	.111500	
	.001900	.123800	
	.002000	.138200	
	.001300	.145000	
	.007100	.150090	
	.001900	.154000	
	.003100	.157250	
	.004600	.188000	
	.001400	.195690	
	.001000	.253500	
	.001100	.452400	
	.009257	.165160	
Fr-221[c]	Half-life: 4.8 minutes		
	Alphas:		
	.001300	5.938000	
	.001000	5.965000	
	.004900	5.979000	
	.001300	6.075000	
	.151000	6.125500	
	.013500	6.241800	
	.834000	6.339800	
	.001150	5.833200	
	Electrons:		
	.006400	.003770	
	.027697	.008520	
	.002160	.022470	
	.001100	.054270	
	.000788	.061200	
	.006880	.082007	
	.002400	.095183	
	.017500	.121870	
	.021750	.200110	
	.005750	.213280	
	.001962	.216560	
	Gammas & X-rays:		
	.022661	.011400	
	.007706	.078950	
	.012865	.081520	
	.005801	.092300	
	.001600	.099500	
	.125000	.217600	
	.001000	.412000	
	.003300	.210980	
At-217[c]	Half-life: .0323 seconds		
	Alphas:		
	.999340	7.066000	
	.000660	6.622300	
	Gammas & X-rays:		
	.000400	.594500	
Bi-213[c]	Half-life: 45.65 minutes		
	Alphas:		
	.001598	5.549000	
	.020002	5.870000	

[a] RSIC computer data file (DLC-80) contains x ray and photon data not in Kocher 1981. They are included in this table.

[b] Maximum energy for betas and positrons.

[c] Branching to radioactive daughter(s) shown in Table 8.13.

(continued)

Table 8.14 Energy and Probability by Radiation Type for Selected Radionuclides of Interest to Health Physicists (Continued)

Nuclide	Probability per Decay	Energy[b] (MeV)	Average Energy (MeV)
	Betas:		
	.010600	.319820	.090000
	.320000	.979580	.319000
	.007000	1.127200	.376000
	.640000	1.420000	.491000
	Electrons:		
	.024264	.008330	
	.001327	.059700	
	.003395	.199760	
	.040831	.347310	
	.007187	.423480	
	.002263	.436270	
	Gammas & X-rays:		
	.001327	.323810	
	.018304	.011100	
	.012519	.076862	
	.020970	.079290	
	.009410	.089800	
	.007397	.292860	
	.279670	.440420	
	.001479	.659810	
	.004438	.807360	
	.004790	1.100100	
Tl-209[c]	Half-life: 2.2 minutes		
	Betas:		
	1.000000	1.824800	.659000
	Electrons:		
	.125450	.007970	
	.183000	.029207	
	.006686	.056700	
	.035400	.101350	
	.008310	.113360	
	.002660	.116320	
	.023600	.377060	
	.007990	.449200	
	.002630	.461210	
	.002340	1.478900	
	Gammas & X-rays:		
	.087179	.010600	
	.058804	.072804	
	.099331	.074969	
	.044120	.084900	
	.770000	.117210	
	.965800	.465070	
	.996890	1.567000	
Pb-209	Half-life: 3.253 hours		
	Betas:		
	1.000000	.644600	.197600
Po-213[c]	Half-life: 4.2e-6 seconds		
	Alphas:		
	.999960	8.377000	
	.000040	7.612000	
	Gammas & X-rays:		
	.000039	.779000	
Ra-226	Half-life: 1600 years		
	Alphas:		
	.055500	4.601900	
	.945500	4.784500	
	.000078	4.314600	
	Electrons:		
	.009047	.008710	
	.000177	.062700	
	.006330	.087807	
	.012005	.168160	
	.003195	.181730	
	.001112	.185110	
	Gammas & X-rays:		
	.008023	.011700	
	.001802	.081070	
	.002994	.083780	
	.001357	.094900	
	.032800	.186210	
	.000067	.309700	
Rn-222[c]	Half-life: 3.8235 days		
	Alphas:		
	.999200	5.489700	
	.000785	4.986000	
	Gammas & X-rays:		
	.000760	.512000	
Po-218[c]	Half-life: 3.05 minutes		
	Alphas:		
	.999790	6.002500	
	.000011	5.181000	
Pb-214[c]	Half-life: 26.8 minutes		
	Betas:		
	.025500	.184940	.050000
	.008300	.490460	.145000
	.480000	.672080	.207000
	.425000	.728800	.227000
	.063000	1.024000	.337000
	Electrons:		
	.186500	.008150	
	.106790	.036839	
	.025093	.049227	
	.008446	.052288	
	.006827	.058200	
	.052889	.151460	
	.001879	.168260	
	.074676	.204690	
	.009214	.225590	
	.002899	.237980	
	.090792	.261400	
	.013357	.278830	
	.003156	.291210	
	.001051	.294270	
	.016000	.335530	
	.003758	.347920	
	.001250	.350980	
	Gammas & X-rays:		
	.135050	.010800	
	.011054	.053226	
	.062130	.074815	
	.104600	.077108	
	.046683	.087300	
	.074913	.241980	
	.005527	.258790	
	.003257	.274530	
	.192470	.295210	
	.372100	.351920	
	.001678	.462100	
	.003395	.480420	
	.004412	.487080	
	.001905	.533690	
	.003652	.580150	
	.010956	.785910	
	.005892	.839020	
	.003267	.280680	
Bi-214[c]	Half-life: 19.9 minutes		
	Betas:		
	.004100	.541410	.162000
	.002110	.550760	.165000
	.001180	.575300	.173000
	.001100	.761800	.239000
	.002050	.764390	.240000
	.010700	.787570	.248000
	.028100	.822270	.261000
	.005600	.976680	.318000
	.001400	1.003300	.328000
	.003360	1.061400	.350000
	.056100	1.065700	.352000
	.008900	1.077400	.357000
	.004300	1.122200	.374000
	.044300	1.151400	.385000
	.001440	1.181500	.397000
	.025000	1.252700	.425000
	.015000	1.259200	.427000
	.011900	1.275400	.434000
	.015900	1.379700	.475000
	.083400	1.422600	.492000
	.177000	1.505500	.525000
	.002560	1.527000	.534000
	.179000	1.540400	.539000
	.008800	1.608800	.567000
	.033800	1.726600	.615000
	.010100	1.854500	.668000

[a] RSIC computer data file (DLC-80) contains x ray and photon data not in Kocher 1981. They are included in this table.

[b] Maximum energy for betas and positrons.

[c] Branching to radioactive daughter(s) shown in Table 8.13.

Table 8.14 Energy and Probability by Radiation Type for Selected Radionuclides of Interest to Health Physicists (Continued)

	Probability per Decay	Energy[b] (MeV)	Average Energy (MeV)
	.078600	1.892300	.684000
	.002200	1.995200	.726000
	.006000	2.660700	1.007000
	.172000	3.270000	1.269000
	.003616	.526000	.158590
	Electrons:		
	.006911	.008330	
	.000382	.059700	
	.006942	.516210	
	.001948	.592370	
	.001924	1.027200	
	.003854	1.322700	
	Gammas & X-rays:		
	.005213	.011100	
	.003600	.076862	
	.006031	.079290	
	.002706	.089800	
	.001776	.273700	
	.003651	.387000	
	.004144	.389100	
	.001678	.405740	
	.001086	.426500	
	.003197	.454770	
	.001332	.469690	
	.001184	.474380	
	.462810	.609310	
	.015690	.665450	
	.004737	.703110	
	.004046	.719860	
	.001332	.752840	
	.050425	.768360	
	.003158	.786100	
	.012335	.806170	
	.001510	.821180	
	.001056	.904250	
	.032071	.934060	
	.003848	.964080	
	.003168	1.052000	
	.002862	1.070000	
	.151470	1.120300	
	.002556	1.133700	
	.016973	1.155200	
	.004618	1.207700	
	.059405	1.238100	
	.014802	1.281000	
	.001214	1.303800	
	.041051	1.377700	
	.007796	1.385300	
	.013914	1.401500	
	.024867	1.408000	
	.022203	1.509200	
	.004144	1.538500	
	.003553	1.543300	
	.007204	1.583200	
	.002664	1.594700	
	.003355	1.599300	
	.011545	1.661300	
	.002368	1.684000	
	.029702	1.729600	
	.158380	1.764500	
	.003848	1.838400	
	.020920	1.847400	
	.002270	1.873200	
	.001776	1.896300	
	.011743	2.118600	
	.049833	2.204200	
	.003256	2.293400	
	.015591	2.447900	
	.035073	1.158000	
Po-214[c]	Half-life: 6.37e-5 seconds		
	Alphas:		
	.999890	7.687100	
	.000106	6.892400	
	Gammas & X-rays:		
	.000105	.797300	
Ra-228[c]	Half-life: 5.75 years		
	Betas:		
	1.000000	.038930	.009900
	Electrons:		
	1.000000	.001668	
	Gammas & X-rays:		
	.000001	.006670	
Ac-228[c]	Half-life: 6.13 hours		
	Betas:		
	.001970	.126800	.033300
	.002900	.192540	.051700
	.001600	.237110	.064600
	.002150	.244270	.066700
	.002160	.377000	.107200
	.003700	.393300	.112300
	.001580	.401400	.114900
	.015900	.412900	.118500
	.024200	.448700	.130000
	.015400	.453950	.131700
	.049000	.491060	.143800
	.007800	.494390	.144900
	.013000	.499000	.146400
	.002600	.598200	.179600
	.080000	.605630	.182100
	.002200	.686780	.210000
	.001400	.792600	.247000
	.008200	.910390	.290000
	.001900	.962310	.309000
	.033000	.968710	.311000
	.070000	.983480	.317000
	.066000	1.014400	.328000
	.002400	1.046000	.340000
	.034000	1.114600	.366000
	.004600	1.121000	.368000
	.002100	1.157700	.382000
	.320000	1.168100	.386000
	.001500	1.193200	.396000
	.001100	1.617800	.538000
	.120000	1.740900	.611000
	.080000	2.079200	.748000
	.001030	.283000	.078844
	Electrons:		
	.361000	.009480	
	.007451	.019429	
	.571560	.037308	
	.001309	.044549	
	.155930	.052598	
	.057156	.056451	
	.001778	.069200	
	.048475	.074849	
	.040099	.078978	
	.009660	.094268	
	.003554	.098120	
	.003001	.099629	
	.071466	.108610	
	.019584	.123900	
	.007285	.127750	
	.001365	.160580	
	.009695	.164030	
	.001932	.169350	
	.003005	.179320	
	.002623	.228670	
	.001163	.231450	
	.001401	.353350	
	.001480	.685050	
	.002518	.801120	
	.001353	.859460	
	Gammas & X-rays:		
	.391080	.013000	
	.005014	.057780	
	.021326	.089953	
	.034846	.093350	
	.013019	.099450	
	.016121	.105000	
	.027700	.129080	
	.002105	.146100	
	.009418	.154200	
	.001163	.191200	
	.003324	.199700	
	.001634	.204400	
	.044320	.209280	

[a] RSIC computer data file (DLC-80) contains x ray and photon data not in Kocher 1981. They are included in this table.
[b] Maximum energy for betas and positrons.
[c] Branching to radioactive daughter(s) shown in Table 8.13.

(continued)

Table 8.14 Energy and Probability by Radiation Type for Selected Radionuclides of Interest to Health Physicists (Continued)

	Probability per Decay	Energy[b] (MeV)	Average Energy (MeV)
	.002161	.210000	
	.036010	.270230	
	.002216	.279000	
	.002410	.321700	
	.032132	.327640	
	.004432	.332360	
	.113570	.338320	
	.004155	.341100	
	.021329	.409510	
	.001385	.440300	
	.044320	.463000	
	.002299	.478200	
	.002050	.503600	
	.004709	.509600	
	.001163	.523000	
	.002105	.546300	
	.009418	.562300	
	.001773	.570700	
	.001551	.572100	
	.001440	.583200	
	.001136	.623800	
	.001884	.701500	
	.001496	.707100	
	.007756	.727000	
	.010526	.755180	
	.015512	.772170	
	.005263	.782000	
	.046259	.794700	
	.005900	.830500	
	.017451	.835500	
	.009418	.840000	
	.008310	.904500	
	.277000	.911070	
	.001025	.944100	
	.001163	.948000	
	.003019	.958500	
	.052076	.964600	
	.166200	.969110	
	.001828	.987800	
	.002161	1.033200	
	.001413	1.065100	
	.001274	1.095700	
	.003324	1.110400	
	.001523	1.153600	
	.005402	1.246400	
	.001136	1.287500	
	.009972	1.459300	
	.009972	1.495800	
	.005540	1.501500	
	.001939	1.556900	
	.006925	1.580200	
	.035456	1.588000	
	.003047	1.624700	
	.018614	1.630400	
	.005263	1.638000	
	.001994	1.666300	
	.001053	1.887000	
	.041168	.947770	
Th-228[c]	Half-life: 1.9132 years		
	Alphas:		
	.001800	5.175000	
	.003600	5.212000	
	.267000	5.340500	
	.727000	5.423300	
	.000500	5.138700	
	Electrons:		
	.095590	.009090	
	.191180	.065134	
	.051909	.079549	
	.018755	.083163	
	Gammas & X-rays:		
	.095590	.012300	
	.01210	.08426	
	.00128	.13150	
	.0082	.16643	
	.00277	.21575	
Ac-227[c]	Half-life: 21.773 years		
	Alphas:		
	.004968	4.938100	
	.006762	4.950500	
	.001875	4.836800	
	Betas:		
	.100000	.019201	.004800
	.350000	.034401	.008700
	.540000	.043701	.011100
	Electrons:		
	.005005	.008048	
	.022160	.004028	
	.414200	.004118	
	.010637	.009480	
	.068758	.010018	
	.007337	.019318	
	Gammas & X-rays:		
	.000982	.115350	
	.011523	.013000	
	.000362	.017357	
Fr-223[c]	Half-life: 21.8 minutes		
	Betas:		
	.001240	.221220	.060100
	.004900	.321790	.090200
	.001080	.344060	.097100
	.013500	.778070	.243000
	.001510	.813270	.255700
	.103000	.912660	.291900
	.170000	1.017400	.330900
	.127000	1.067900	.349900
	.570000	1.097500	.361100
	.003896	.670700	.208240
	Electrons:		
	.043667	.001063	
	.055408	.001478	
	.336810	.009090	
	.019681	.010363	
	.199380	.010673	
	.040161	.012393	
	.015139	.015478	
	.006257	.024778	
	.069783	.025088	
	.013757	.026808	
	.004108	.030663	
	.169270	.030863	
	.018157	.042263	
	.001004	.045078	
	.041208	.045278	
	.013915	.048892	
	.050590	.049463	
	.004919	.056678	
	.001762	.060292	
	.011716	.060563	
	.012895	.063878	
	.001336	.065900	
	.004603	.067492	
	.001902	.069478	
	.003796	.074978	
	.066281	.081163	
	.018068	.095578	
	.006523	.099192	
	.017890	.101080	
	.031597	.130980	
	.003438	.185760	
	.001121	.200180	
	.006065	.215660	
	.001972	.230080	
	Gammas & X-rays:		
	.001205	.006300	
	.336810	.012300	
	.007607	.020300	
	.007607	.049900	
	.316980	.050100	
	.003804	.068700	
	.076075	.079800	
	.014713	.085430	
	.024239	.088470	
	.011101	.100000	
	.009509	.100400	
	.005072	.134600	

[a] RSIC computer data file (DLC-80) contains x ray and photon data not in Kocher 1981. They are included in this table.

[b] Maximum energy for betas and positrons.

[c] Branching to radioactive daughter(s) shown in Table 8.13.

Table 8.14 Energy and Probability by Radiation Type for Selected Radionuclides of Interest to Health Physicists (Continued)

Nuclide	Probability per Decay	Energy[b] (MeV)	Average Energy (MeV)
	.001268	.173400	
	.002853	.184800	
	.010777	.205000	
	.028211	.234900	
	.002282	.289500	
	.005135	.319400	
	.001014	.369400	
	.003899	.775300	
	.012278	.482030	
Th-227[c]	Half-life: 18.718 days		
	Alphas:		
	.001760	5.585900	
	.001700	5.600600	
	.002160	5.613300	
	.020600	5.668000	
	.015000	5.693000	
	.036300	5.700800	
	.082000	5.709000	
	.048900	5.713200	
	.203000	5.757100	
	.002280	5.762300	
	.003110	5.795500	
	.012700	5.807500	
	.024200	5.866600	
	.001740	5.909900	
	.007800	5.916000	
	.030000	5.959700	
	.234000	5.977900	
	.029000	6.008800	
	.245000	6.038200	
	.001961	5.562500	
	Electrons:		
	.011480	.001063	
	.004600	.001478	
	.030800	.003478	
	.418000	.009090	
	.001523	.009178	
	.005322	.010363	
	.418000	.010673	
	.144800	.012393	
	.003980	.015478	
	.001769	.024463	
	.001692	.024778	
	.006860	.024863	
	.016900	.025063	
	.146000	.025088	
	.049600	.026808	
	.021000	.028963	
	.001080	.030663	
	.044856	.030863	
	.016000	.031463	
	.001192	.034963	
	.002930	.037313	
	.002380	.039278	
	.005850	.039478	
	.064440	.042263	
	.007500	.043378	
	.001134	.043463	
	.010920	.045278	
	.004320	.045878	
	.003688	.048892	
	.004389	.049463	
	.001600	.049492	
	.001030	.051728	
	.001520	.053663	
	.003600	.054463	
	.017460	.056678	
	.006255	.060292	
	.003080	.060563	
	.001518	.063878	
	.001278	.065900	
	.001300	.068878	
	.001396	.074763	
	.001073	.075963	
	.005576	.081163	
	.006817	.093863	
	.002072	.095578	
	.002822	.101080	
	.002516	.108280	
	.005152	.130980	
	.005669	.132080	
	.002695	.146180	
	.006552	.152280	
	.009840	.182180	
	.002436	.192680	
	.006426	.200480	
	.002206	.208680	
	.001068	.216760	
	.003818	.230280	
	.007182	.236960	
	.002602	.251380	
	.001920	.266860	
	.001304	.285160	
	Gammas & X-rays:		
	.001400	.008300	
	.418000	.012300	
	.002000	.020300	
	.001000	.029910	
	.002300	.043700	
	.002000	.049900	
	.084000	.050100	
	.002400	.062200	
	.020000	.079800	
	.014069	.085430	
	.023178	.088470	
	.014000	.094000	
	.010615	.100000	
	.001700	.113100	
	.005400	.113100	
	.001800	.117200	
	.001400	.141200	
	.002300	.204300	
	.001700	.205000	
	.002600	.206000	
	.012600	.210600	
	.004600	.234900	
	.115000	.236000	
	.004900	.250100	
	.001100	.252500	
	.009100	.254700	
	.063000	.256200	
	.001000	.262900	
	.004900	.273000	
	.001700	.281300	
	.016000	.286100	
	.004200	.296600	
	.018400	.299800	
	.002800	.300300	
	.013500	.304400	
	.004300	.312600	
	.004200	.314800	
	.029000	.329700	
	.011500	.334200	
	.003400	.342400	
	.001180	.350500	
	.017273	.184970	
Th-229[c]	Half-life: 7340 years		
	Alphas:		
	.001500	4.688000	
	.006300	4.761000	
	.012700	4.797800	
	.002200	4.809000	
	.093000	4.814600	
	.002900	4.833000	
	.048000	4.837000	
	.562000	4.845300	
	.001800	4.861000	
	.102000	4.901000	
	.001100	4.929000	
	.059700	4.967500	
	.031700	4.978500	
	.002400	5.033000	
	.052000	5.050000	
	.016000	5.052000	
	.002670	4.765500	

[a] RSIC computer data file (DLC-80) contains x ray and photon data not in Kocher 1981. They are included in this table.

[b] Maximum energy for betas and positrons.

[c] Branching to radioactive daughter(s) shown in Table 8.13.

(continued)

Table 8.14 Energy and Probability by Radiation Type for Selected Radionuclides of Interest to Health Physicists (Continued)

	Probability per Decay	Energy[b] (MeV)	Average Energy (MeV)
	Electrons:		
	.091168	.003248	
	.489090	.006153	
	.810550	.009090	
	.075888	.012063	
	.244490	.012538	
	.172430	.020568	
	.086904	.020578	
	.043268	.020778	
	.101020	.023523	
	.025174	.026478	
	.019584	.028048	
	.088128	.033108	
	.042758	.037363	
	.034435	.037938	
	.020520	.039028	
	.002039	.044378	
	.010812	.048943	
	.046563	.049663	
	.025525	.050478	
	.010216	.051778	
	.041626	.052558	
	.003623	.055392	
	.142010	.055963	
	.003652	.063358	
	.012566	.064078	
	.014961	.065900	
	.027286	.067063	
	.115970	.067203	
	.004522	.067692	
	.006261	.068978	
	.038547	.070378	
	.013837	.073992	
	.003237	.080078	
	.007095	.081478	
	.027754	.081618	
	.002551	.085092	
	.009914	.085232	
	.017063	.087933	
	.093177	.089708	
	.004073	.102350	
	.016157	.105260	
	.008078	.105460	
	.001464	.105960	
	.051898	.107050	
	.003656	.112730	
	.002071	.114180	
	.016483	.117790	
	.003880	.119680	
	.002619	.119880	
	.001383	.123290	
	.003813	.123710	
	.001185	.127150	
	.003917	.132210	
	.004734	.135160	
	.001400	.135820	
	.007719	.137240	
	.001238	.138130	
	.001538	.149580	
	.002502	.151660	
	.001162	.153660	
	.002550	.160560	
	.001037	.164760	
	.017258	.174390	
	.004126	.188810	
	.009661	.191730	
	.001460	.192420	
	.003117	.206150	
	Gammas & X-rays:		
	.810550	.012300	
	.001734	.017360	
	.040800	.031300	
	.001632	.042760	
	.003264	.056600	
	.001020	.068180	
	.001122	.068900	
	.005202	.075200	
	.164740	.085430	
	.003774	.086300	
	.030600	.086440	
	.271400	.088470	
	.124300	.100000	
	.008364	.107170	
	.012240	.124500	
	.006120	.124700	
	.003264	.131970	
	.016320	.137030	
	.004284	.142950	
	.013872	.148300	
	.006630	.154400	
	.011220	.156480	
	.002244	.172900	
	.005100	.179800	
	.002346	.184000	
	.045900	.193630	
	.032640	.210970	
	.001428	.218100	
	.000714	.130800	
Th-230[c]	Half-life: 77000 years		
	Alphas:		
	.001200	4.476000	
	.234000	4.621000	
	.763000	4.687500	
	.003100	4.367800	
	Electrons:		
	.084298	.009090	
	.168600	.048435	
	.045506	.062850	
	.016412	.066464	
	Gammas & X-rays:		
	.084298	.012300	
	.003730	.067672	
	.000689	.168090	
Th-232[c]	Half-life: 14050000000 years		
	Alphas:		
	.002000	3.830000	
	.230000	3.953000	
	.770000	4.010000	
	Electrons:		
	.083904	.009090	
	.166750	.039763	
	.045080	.054178	
	.016192	.057792	
	.001058	.105760	
	Gammas & X-rays:		
	.083904	.012300	
	.001900	.059000	
	.000420	.125000	
Th-234[c]	Half-life: 24.1 days		
	Betas:		
	.020000	.075770	.019500
	.068000	.095780	.024800
	.185000	.096200	.024900
	.725000	.188580	.050600
	Electrons:		
	.043625	.008385	
	.081484	.009680	
	.016744	.014653	
	.015779	.024123	
	.003465	.041755	
	.011778	.042185	
	.001202	.057493	
	.002889	.057923	
	.001006	.061903	
	.115260	.071275	
	.003011	.071695	
	.027793	.087013	
	.010245	.090993	
	Gammas & X-rays:		
	.095655	.013300	
	.038116	.063290	
	.027248	.092380	
	.026884	.092800	

[a] RSIC computer data file (DLC-80) contains x ray and photon data not in Kocher 1981. They are included in this table.
[b] Maximum energy for betas and positrons.
[c] Branching to radioactive daughter(s) shown in Table 8.13.

Table 8.14 Energy and Probability by Radiation Type for Selected Radionuclides of Interest to Health Physicists (Continued)

	Probability per Decay	Energy[b] (MeV)	Average Energy (MeV)
	.002418	.112810	
	.001284	.076765	
U-234[c]	Half-life: 244500 years		
	Alphas:		
	.002400	4.604700	
	.274000	4.723700	
	.724000	4.775800	
	.000001	4.216200	
	Electrons:		
	.096954	.009480	
	.200600	.032728	
	.054634	.048018	
	.020178	.051870	
	.001388	.100430	
	Gammas & X-rays:		
	.105030	.013000	
	.001180	.053200	
	.000401	.121430	
Pa-234[c]	Half-life: 6.7 hours		
	Betas:		
	.004700	.547740	.016300
	.012000	.563950	.091000
	.009800	.577090	.112700
	.040000	.583390	.121900
	.021000	.617390	.128600
	.023000	.680690	.136300
	.240000	.688690	.141000
	.110000	.692640	.141200
	.042000	.694390	.150800
	.160000	.710690	.198100
	.038000	.711240	.217600
	.009600	.767630	.296600
	.077000	.810390	.364300
	.023000	.833390	.372900
	.100000	1.183000	.390000
	.062000	1.237800	.410700
	.017000	1.244400	.413300
	.008000	1.259200	.418900
	Electrons:		
	.003121	.009794	
	.001031	.009890	
	.001359	.012543	
	.004068	.015594	
	.006711	.018764	
	.001434	.021723	
	.001836	.023433	
	.001856	.024694	
	.001519	.028394	
	.001387	.028752	
	.001281	.036443	
	.001297	.037094	
	.001091	.037932	
	.001958	.039642	
	.000000	.041243	
	.024674	.045343	
	.003123	.052652	
	.020859	.055094	
	.001158	.056759	
	.003460	.057452	
	.035129	.057933	
	.004080	.058994	
	.006740	.061552	
	.002491	.065659	
	.065484	.070394	
	.011919	.072600	
	.009719	.074142	
	.017564	.077994	
	.486170	.078103	
	.003635	.078249	
	.009996	.080794	
	.010331	.081653	
	.012876	.084094	
	.001750	.085374	
	.010771	.087394	
	.134640	.094312	
	.002864	.097862	
	.050918	.098419	
	.001080	.101970	
	.035394	.103640	
	.004100	.104190	
	.009568	.109440	
	.054583	.110790	
	.102660	.111590	
	.003384	.112610	
	.016616	.118540	
	.009833	.119850	
	.005712	.122240	
	.003692	.123960	
	.003162	.125650	
	.003142	.128440	
	.001120	.128820	
	.013586	.129590	
	.097726	.130940	
	.001357	.133290	
	.004443	.134750	
	.002035	.138450	
	.001652	.138860	
	.027063	.147150	
	.004080	.148940	
	.010114	.151260	
	.001573	.152840	
	.011322	.156490	
	.001591	.159890	
	.012811	.164240	
	.001346	.165150	
	.003433	.171840	
	.001928	.174640	
	.002516	.177940	
	.017861	.178090	
	.004847	.179220	
	.003101	.180450	
	.005361	.181240	
	.001126	.184560	
	.001132	.188050	
	.001829	.195430	
	.001255	.196890	
	.001934	.197450	
	.018475	.204640	
	.020028	.205440	
	.002203	.214990	
	.004736	.220850	
	.004841	.221650	
	.002653	.223440	
	.001739	.224960	
	.001762	.225760	
	.002203	.250340	
	.014169	.254190	
	.005052	.256790	
	.005132	.271940	
	.001778	.288150	
	.001851	.343190	
	.002733	.348040	
	.001053	.350640	
	.001459	.398090	
	.001120	.412390	
	.001571	.450290	
	.004590	.453090	
	.016262	.453890	
	.001012	.495890	
	1.136300	.013600	
	.001224	.043480	
	.032640	.063000	
	.002346	.069900	
	.001224	.079690	
	.156970	.094665	
	.254420	.098439	
	.048960	.099860	
	.001224	.103410	
	.118480	.111000	
	.010200	.125400	
	.204000	.131200	
	.002142	.134370	
	.001530	.137700	
	Gammas & X-rays:		
	1.136300	.013600	

[a] RSIC computer data file (DLC-80) contains x ray and photon data not in Kocher 1981. They are included in this table.
[b] Maximum energy for betas and positrons.
[c] Branching to radioactive daughter(s) shown in Table 8.13.

(continued)

Table 8.14 Energy and Probability by Radiation Type for Selected Radionuclides of Interest to Health Physicists (Continued)

Probability per Decay	Energy[b] (MeV)	Average Energy (MeV)	Probability per Decay	Energy[b] (MeV)	Average Energy (MeV)	Probability per Decay	Energy[b] (MeV)	Average Energy (MeV)
.001224	.043480		.002448	.472100		.002040	.777900	
.032640	.063000		.001836	.473500		.011220	.780700	
.002346	.069900		.003060	.478700		.005100	.783100	
.001224	.079690		.004080	.480400		.014280	.786270	
.156970	.094665		.003060	.482500		.015300	.793600	
.254420	.098439		.001020	.498900		.038760	.796300	
.048960	.099860		.016320	.506800		.004080	.804300	
.001224	.103410		.013260	.513700		.033660	.805600	
.118480	.111000		.006120	.520200		.005100	.812500	
.010200	.125400		.009180	.521000		.026520	.819600	
.204000	.131200		.006120	.528000		.040800	.826300	
.002142	.134370		.002040	.533200		.056100	.831600	
.001530	.137700		.001632	.537100		.001428	.841900	
.009180	.140300		.002652	.557000		.005100	.844000	
.003570	.144000		.014280	.565900		.001224	.851700	
.002040	.150200		.030600	.568700		.001224	.872900	
.068340	.152700		.109140	.569500		.040800	.876400	
.007140	.159100		.020400	.574000		.010200	.880500	
.005100	.170700		.001530	.585800		.122400	.880510	
.002040	.174600		.005100	.596600		.122400	.883240	
.020400	.186000		.009180	.602800		.041820	.899000	
.006120	.193600		.008160	.611500		.005100	.904370	
.004896	.199700		.002040	.616200		.004080	.920000	
.011220	.200980		.008160	.623600		.029580	.925000	
.012240	.203000		.008160	.627500		.112200	.926000	
.002040	.219800		.004080	.630600		.091800	.926720	
.060180	.226400		.003060	.634500		.122400	.946000	
.056100	.227200		.002040	.639700		.081600	.949000	
.009180	.245200		.002040	.643200		.001020	.960000	
.028560	.248900		.003060	.646000		.006120	.966000	
.001734	.267100		.009180	.653700		.014280	.978800	
.010200	.272100		.006120	.655000		.030600	.980500	
.002652	.275500		.009180	.658000		.020400	.980500	
.001428	.286100		.003060	.660600		.019380	.984000	
.001122	.289600		.013260	.664800		.006120	1.022600	
.039780	.293700		.016320	.666700		.008160	1.028300	
.001020	.309600		.014280	.669900		.005100	1.044900	
.003060	.312500		.002448	.683300		.002550	1.074600	
.001224	.316300		.002856	.687000		.007650	1.083200	
.001224	.320700		.015300	.692700		.003060	1.108500	
.003060	.328000		.046920	.699000		.005100	1.122300	
.006120	.330600		.031620	.706100		.008160	1.126000	
.006120	.351900		.002040	.711200		.003060	1.153100	
.029580	.369800		.001632	.713800		.002448	1.171300	
.013260	.372400		.087720	.733000		.003060	1.208000	
.004080	.409800		.010200	.738000		.003774	1.217500	
.001020	.416300		.024480	.742810		.003060	1.229000	
.006120	.426800		.001326	.746500		.005100	1.240500	
.001224	.446500		.014280	.755600		.003060	1.251000	
.015300	.458800		.001632	.760000		.002040	1.277400	
.001632	.461800		.003060	.766360		.006120	1.292700	
.004080	.467500		.005712	.768700		.017340	1.353300	

[a] RSIC computer data file (DLC-80) contains x ray and photon data not in Kocher 1981. They are included in this table.
[b] Maximum energy for betas and positrons.
[c] Branching to radioactive daughter(s) shown in Table 8.13.

Table 8.14 Energy and Probability by Radiation Type for Selected Radionuclides of Interest to Health Physicists (Continued)

	Probability per Decay	Energy[b] (MeV)	Average Energy (MeV)
	.001224	1.358500	
	.030600	1.394100	
	.002346	1.399700	
	.002040	1.427500	
	.004080	1.446000	
	.010200	1.452700	
	.003060	1.460000	
	.002040	1.493700	
	.004080	1.516000	
	.001020	1.549400	
	.001734	1.579700	
	.002550	1.585400	
	.006120	1.593800	
	.001530	1.627900	
	.004080	1.638000	
	.001530	1.656000	
	.012240	1.668500	
	.005100	1.686200	
	.012240	1.694600	
	.001530	1.699800	
	.001020	1.737600	
	.001020	1.741700	
	.002550	1.756000	
	.001020	1.772300	
	.003060	1.797300	
	.001938	1.890100	
	.001530	1.897100	
	.002856	1.905000	
	.005100	1.926000	
	.010099	.955590	
Pa-231[c]	Half-life: 32760 years		
	Alphas:		
	.001000	4.631000	
	.001000	4.642000	
	.015000	4.680000	
	.010000	4.712000	
	.084000	4.736000	
	.014000	4.851000	
	.030000	4.933000	
	.228000	4.950000	
	.004000	4.974000	
	.014000	4.984000	
	.254000	5.011000	
	.200000	5.028000	
	.025000	5.030500	
	.110000	5.057300	
	.000698	4.706200	
	Electrons:		
	.007550	.003760	
	.006680	.004860	
	.136800	.005700	
	.251100	.007520	
	.415150	.009280	
	.202400	.010110	
	.416640	.013898	
	.079566	.018360	
	.002410	.018598	
	.002140	.019698	
	.043560	.020538	
	.084537	.022358	
	.018000	.024320	
	.069276	.024948	
	.001402	.026530	
	.015045	.032900	
	.025926	.033198	
	.006600	.037260	
	.042900	.037350	
	.005742	.039158	
	.032800	.043830	
	.003621	.047738	
	.001309	.051471	
	.002530	.052098	
	.011700	.052188	
	.007900	.054340	
	.004212	.055921	
	.003937	.057520	
	.008950	.058668	
	.003230	.062401	
	.000540	.067500	
	.002925	.069178	
	.007867	.077040	
	.002362	.081080	
	.003023	.082660	
	.002930	.091878	
	.015065	.193330	
	.006552	.223320	
	.002806	.280240	
	.001219	.310230	
	Gammas & X-rays:		
	.093	.027396	
	.0159	.283673	
	.0238	.300070	
	.046	.302671	
	.0132	.330066	
	.006203	.087670	
	.010186	.090884	
	.004687	.102000	
	.001010	.255800	
	.001730	.260220	
	.016000	.283670	
	.023000	.300080	
	.023000	.302670	
	.013000	.330070	
	.001650	.340810	
	.001730	.357160	
	.014489	.165520	
Pa-233[c]	Half-life: 27 days		
	Betas:		
	.243000	.156510	.041500
	.157000	.173770	.046300
	.280000	.231800	.063000
	:330000	.260360	.071400
	Electrons:		
	.170920	.006783	
	.384370	.009890	
	.019489	.011712	
	.092640	.018593	
	.057668	.022992	
	.034740	.034802	
	.001223	.036143	
	.106580	.053523	
	.106490	.064833	
	.025922	.069732	
	.008230	.072600	
	.009413	.073839	
	.025912	.081042	
	.027421	.082103	
	.009457	.085149	
	.006744	.098312	
	.002446	.102420	
	.056101	.184510	
	.293750	.196370	
	.022581	.224890	
	.010888	.278360	
	.057128	.290220	
	.003592	.294570	
	.001670	.300150	
	.013742	.306430	
	.005018	.310540	
	.004742	.318740	
	.001581	.334950	
	Gammas & X-rays:		
	.489200	.013600	
	.012584	.075280	
	.018914	.086590	
	.108390	.094665	
	.175670	.098439	
	.007411	.103860	
	.081809	.111000	
	.003049	.271480	
	.066392	.300120	
	.386000	.311980	
	.045162	.340500	
	.006176	.375450	
	.012738	.398620	
	.016212	.415760	

[a] RSIC computer data file (DLC-80) contains x ray and photon data not in Kocher 1981. They are included in this table.
[b] Maximum energy for betas and positrons.
[c] Branching to radioactive daughter(s) shown in Table 8.13.

(continued)

Table 8.14 Energy and Probability by Radiation Type for Selected Radionuclides of Interest to Health Physicists (Continued)

	Probability per Decay	Energy[b] (MeV)	Average Energy (MeV)
	.002067	.120490	
U-233[c]	Half-life: 159200 years		
	Alphas:		
	.016100	4.729000	
	.001630	4.754000	
	.132000	4.783500	
	.002800	4.796000	
	.844000	4.824200	
	.002797	4.673600	
	Electrons:		
	.002034	.004798	
	.007322	.008678	
	.036209	.009480	
	.057600	.022008	
	.002346	.023968	
	.005416	.034268	
	.020736	.037298	
	.001935	.049558	
	.001015	.051368	
	.002046	.076668	
	Gammas & X-rays:		
	.039226	.013000	
	.001818	.114510	
U-232[c]	Half-life: 72 years		
	Alphas:		
	.002800	5.139000	
	.312000	5.263500	
	.686000	5.320300	
	.000034	4.983100	
	Electrons:		
	.110910	.009480	
	.229330	.037308	
	.062563	.052598	
	.022933	.056451	
	.001737	.108610	
	Gammas & X-rays:		
	.120160	.013000	
	.002012	.057780	
	.000729	.141980	
U-235[c]	Half-life: 703800000 years		
	Alphas:		
	.009000	4.150000	
	.057000	4.217000	
	.009000	4.219000	
	.004000	4.271000	
	.046000	4.325000	
	.015000	4.344000	
	.110000	4.364000	
	.060000	4.370000	
	.550000	4.396000	
	.021000	4.414000	
	.007000	4.435000	
	.017000	4.502000	
	.042000	4.556000	
	.050000	4.598000	
	Electrons:		
	.285350	.009480	
	.176000	.011078	
	.680000	.014408	
	.012000	.020928	
	.195570	.021488	
	.065600	.026368	
	.040400	.030828	
	.017376	.033628	
	.017220	.034109	
	.003840	.036218	
	.066780	.036778	
	.001976	.041289	
	.011040	.046118	
	.004464	.048918	
	.004080	.049971	
	.041470	.052228	
	.001632	.052770	
	.005687	.053699	
	.011330	.067518	
	.002275	.069200	
	.004191	.071370	
	.006000	.073049	
	.049572	.074064	
	.008686	.075618	
	.001069	.088668	
	.003259	.090908	
	.011000	.092469	
	.003328	.095660	
	.005211	.099528	
	.001962	.114820	
	.003664	.123290	
	.001197	.138580	
	.001180	.142880	
	.002180	.162230	
	.010044	.163240	
	.003278	.178530	
	.003810	.181650	
	.001330	.196940	
	Gammas & X-rays:		
	.309130	.013000	
	.001100	.072700	
	.027289	.089953	
	.044590	.093350	
	.020629	.105000	
	.015000	.109140	
	.001500	.120000	
	.002200	.140770	
	.105000	.143760	
	.047000	.163350	
	.004000	.182700	
	.540000	.185715	
	.005900	.194940	
	.010000	.202120	
	.047000	.205310	
	.001000	.221380	
	.009194	.190350	
Th-231[c]	Half-life: 25.52 hours		
	Betas:		
	.027000	.141670	.037400
		.170770	
	.003200		.045500
	.150000	.205510	.055400
	.012500	.214830	.058100
	.090000	.286740	.079300
	.410000	.287610	.079600
	.350000	.304790	.084800
	.004100	.311320	.086800
	.001153	.122100	.033364
	Electrons:		
	.004950	.003833	
	.486450	.004535	
	.007524	.004883	
	.602900	.009680	
	.453120	.011833	
	.197410	.012703	
	.167030	.020273	
	.001733	.022975	
	.005019	.023079	
	.001141	.033339	
	.546480	.037465	
	.005920	.042755	
	.003070	.047395	
	.005985	.050519	
	.150640	.053203	
	.055598	.057183	
	.002049	.058493	
	.079299	.060135	
	.023681	.061005	
	.145430	.063105	
	.001157	.063133	
	.001135	.068845	
	.000279	.070800	
	.020265	.075873	
	.005742	.076743	
	.022410	.078783	
	.006262	.095947	
	.002615	.097043	
	.002409	.100320	
	.002275	.862630	
	.001541	.906720	

[a] RSIC computer data file (DLC-80) contains x ray and photon data not in Kocher 1981. They are included in this table.
[b] Maximum energy for betas and positrons.
[c] Branching to radioactive daughter(s) shown in Table 8.13.

Table 8.14 Energy and Probability by Radiation Type for Selected Radionuclides of Interest to Health Physicists (Continued)

Nuclide	Probability per Decay	Energy[b] (MeV)	Average Energy (MeV)
	Gammas & X-rays:		
	.373890	.014300	
	.001023	.044080	
	.001112	.099550	
	.002094	.101880	
	.001788	.103760	
	.000841	.117000	
	.001023	.561150	
	.007592	.882630	
	.005141	.918690	
	.024752	.923980	
	.003308	.936610	
	.004546	.941380	
	.006093	.962770	
	.238000	.984450	
	.082110	1.025900	
	.173740	1.028500	
	.005445	.503940	
Pu-238[c]	Half-life: 87.75 years		
	Alphas:		
	.001000	5.357700	
	.283000	5.456500	
	.716000	5.499200	
	.000031	5.187500	
	Electrons:		
	.090948	.009890	
	.206700	.021723	
	.075660	.037932	
	Gammas & X-rays:		
	.115750	.013600	
	.000473	.055303	
Np-239[c]	Half life: 2.355 days		
	Betas:		
	.019600	.209570	.056500
	.350000	.329810	.092100
	.071000	.391290	.111200
	.520000	.435950	.125300
	.040000	.713540	.217800
	.000341	.219400	.059819
	Electrons:		
	.620400	.001927	
	.001194	.002598	
	.411920	.010300	
	.073320	.012467	
	.064070	.021566	
	.095105	.026315	
	.247430	.034176	
	.001015	.034203	
	.003442	.038383	
	.021748	.038730	
	.034037	.043479	
	.065604	.044744	
	.068948	.051340	
	.001160	.055547	
	.026251	.055714	
	.004489	.059897	
	.018319	.061908	
	.006966	.066282	
	.010101	.076000	
	.049942	.083033	
	.004171	.083403	
	.088534	.087932	
	.013621	.100200	
	.001616	.100570	
	.005821	.104570	
	.004994	.104570	
	.230390	.106370	
	.001572	.132590	
	.001016	.151020	
	.172020	.155790	
	.017772	.186650	
	.001391	.203290	
	.004313	.203820	
	.046186	.205090	
	.001608	.208190	
	.011252	.222250	
	.004190	.226630	
	.034686	.254510	
	.008474	.271670	
	.003158	.276050	
	Gammas & X-rays:		
	.617880	.014300	
	.001001	.049412	
	.001509	.057273	
	.009588	.061480	
	.147130	.099550	
	.236540	.103760	
	.227010	.106130	
	.111270	.117000	
	.001114	.181720	
	.032430	.209750	
	.003384	.226380	
	.107160	.228180	
	.001001	.254410	
	.141000	.277600	
	.007755	.285410	
	.015933	.315880	
	.020304	.334300	
	.003933	.151510	
Pu-239[c]	Half-life: 24131 years		
	Alphas:		
	.115000	5.104600	
	.151000	5.142900	
	.733000	5.155400	
	.001094	5.007500	
	Electrons:		
	.190000	.007392	
	.001785	.008333	
	.034683	.009890	
	.028128	.016933	
	.001071	.024463	
	.047840	.029863	
	.009962	.033142	
	.013208	.046072	
	.004930	.050179	
	Gammas & X-rays:		
	.044141	.013600	
	.000476	.112910	
Pu-240[c]	Half-life: 6569 years		
	Alphas:		
	.263900	5.123400	
	.735000	5.168300	
	.000730	5.017000	
	Electrons:		
	.086526	.009890	
	.196650	.023485	
	.072000	.039694	
	Gammas & X-rays:		
	.110120	.013600	
	.000525	.054327	
Pu-241	Half-life: 14.4 years		
	Betas:		
	.999980	.020811	.005230
Am-241	Half-life: 432.2 years		
	Alphas:		
	.014000	5.388000	
	.128000	5.443000	
	.852000	5.485700	
	.002000	5.512000	
	.003400	5.544300	
	.000339	5.308200	
	Electrons:		
	.160800	.003918	
	.309210	.010100	
	.148400	.010778	
	.016170	.020303	
	.055200	.020622	
	.090520	.020996	
	.049714	.027482	
	.008869	.033133	
	.005885	.037007	
	.308740	.037110	
	.031901	.037700	
	.003258	.049837	

[a] RSIC computer data file (DLC-80) contains x ray and photon data not in Kocher 1981. They are included in this table.
[b] Maximum energy for betas and positrons.
[c] Branching to radioactive daughter(s) shown in Table 8.13.

(continued)

Table 8.14 Energy and Probability by Radiation Type for Selected Radionuclides of Interest to Health Physicists (Continued)

	Probability per Decay	Energy[b] (MeV)	Average Energy (MeV)
	.076467	.053814	
	.026925	.058036	
	.002712	.076543	
	.001039	.093247	
	Gammas & X-rays:		
	.427000	.013900	
	.024000	.026345	
	.001060	.033205	
	.359000	.059537	
	.001793	.069231	
Pu-242[c]	Half-life: 375800 years		
	Alphas:		
	.224000	4.856300	
	.780000	4.900600	
	.000983	4.752500	
	Electrons:		
	.071755	.009890	
	.163080	.023158	
	.059760	.039367	
	Gammas & X-rays:		
	.091325	.013600	
	.000443	.056454	
Pu-244[c]	Half-life: 82600000 years		
	Alphas:		
	.197360	4.546000	
	.804990	4.589000	
	Electrons:		
	.062320	.009890	
	.141640	.022243	
	.051927	.038452	
	Gammas & X-rays:		
	.079317	.013600	
	.000283	.044000	
U-240[c]	Half-life: 14.1 hours		
	Betas:		
	1.000000	.436000	.125000
	Electrons:		
	.312060	.010100	
	.743000	.021673	
	.240000	.038377	
	Gammas & X-rays:		
	.430940	.013900	
	.016500	.044100	
Np-240[c]	Half-life: 65 minutes		
	Betas:		
	1.000000	.781380	.241000
	Electrons:		
	.729580	.010300	
	.729850	.019727	
	.055620	.025382	
	.016686	.030382	
	.270310	.036891	
	.121810	.070882	
	.624970	.075763	
	.005851	.076000	
	.175290	.092927	
	.066994	.097301	
	.024195	.124100	
	.143500	.129100	
	.006396	.141270	
	.002364	.145640	
	.039963	.146270	
	.058401	.148980	
	.015268	.150640	
	.043986	.169600	
	.006878	.173180	
	.001048	.185180	
	.011504	.186770	
	.004324	.191140	
	.017520	.247700	
	.004422	.264870	
	.001669	.269240	
	.001363	.271900	
	.001272	.283900	
	.002403	.326380	
	.026883	.444580	
	.001672	.479280	
	.006183	.543300	
	.002151	.560470	
	.001159	.865940	
	Gammas & X-rays:		
	1.094400	.014300	
	.001112	.042824	
	.050985	.098860	
	.085229	.099550	
	.137020	.103760	
	.064454	.117000	
	.003708	.134600	
	.013905	.147200	
	.083430	.152200	
	.060255	.175000	
	.009270	.182600	
	.067671	.192700	
	.083430	.270800	
	.003708	.280200	
	.006489	.295000	
	.013905	.307000	
	.166860	.448200	
	.013905	.462200	
	.020394	.467400	
	.018540	.507200	
	.268830	.566400	
	.203940	.601100	
	.015759	.606100	
	.046350	.847000	
	.083430	.867400	
	.037080	.884900	
	.011124	.888800	
	.129780	.896500	
	.013905	.915980	
	.023175	.959100	
	.213210	.973900	
	.046350	.987760	
	.009270	1.074400	
	.004635	1.088500	
	.006489	1.131300	
	.006489	1.163000	
	.046350	1.167600	
	.006489	1.180300	
	.004635	1.223200	
	.002002	.422690	
Am-242[c]	Half-life: 16.02 hours		
	Betas:		
	.420000	.619000	.184800
	.410000	.661200	.199000
	Electrons:		
	.084410	.010300	
	.077057	.021448	
	.028434	.038612	
	.002515	.076000	
	.110540	.010700	
	.307050	.017668	
	.114300	.035864	
	Gammas & X-rays:		
	.126620	.014300	
	.036628	.099550	
	.058888	.103760	
	.027700	.117000	
	.000138	.044545	
	.196510	.015000	
	.000364	.042200	
Cm-242[c]	Half-life: 163.2 days		
	Alphas:		
	.259000	6.069600	
	.741000	6.112900	
	.000399	5.948500	
	Electrons:		
	.076956	.010300	
	.192390	.020983	
	.071280	.038147	
	Gammas & X-rays:		
	.115430	.014300	
	.000386	.059249	

[a] RSIC computer data file (DLC-80) contains x ray and photon data not in Kocher 1981. They are included in this table.
[b] Maximum energy for betas and positrons.
[c] Branching to radioactive daughter(s) shown in Table 8.13.

Table 8.14 Energy and Probability by Radiation Type for Selected Radionuclides of Interest to Health Physicists (Continued)

Nuclide	Probability per Decay	Energy[b] (MeV)	Average Energy (MeV)
Am-242m[c]	Half-life: 152 years		
	Alphas:		
	.004236	5.205000	
	.000548	5.227500	
	Electrons:		
	.183420	.010500	
	.482690	.024824	
	.512550	.042505	
	.002787	.010100	
	.001220	.026943	
	.003046	.045473	
	.002369	.064273	
	Gammas & X-rays:		
	.299270	.014600	
	.000001	.048630	
	.003848	.013900	
	.001952	.049370	
	.001649	.108310	
Am-243[c]	Half-life: 7380 years		
	Alphas:		
	.011000	5.181000	
	.106000	5.233500	
	.879000	5.275400	
	.001200	5.321000	
	.001600	5.350000	
	.000155	5.032000	
	Electrons:		
	.399300	.008673	
	.282770	.010100	
	.077616	.020673	
	.048233	.021107	
	.145200	.025377	
	.008456	.032973	
	.027350	.037377	
	.016078	.037811	
	.003171	.049677	
	.138600	.052243	
	.034188	.068947	
	.012078	.073169	
	.001063	.076073	
	Gammas & X-rays:		
	.390500	.013900	
	.055440	.043534	
	.660000	.074670	
	.003366	.086720	
	.005544	.117660	
	.001254	.142180	
	.001644	.048438	
Cm-243[c]	Half-life: 28.5 years		
	Alphas:		
	.001397	5.639000	
	.001995	5.682000	
	.015962	5.686000	
	.114720	5.741600	
	.733240	5.784500	
	.005986	5.876000	
	.055866	5.993000	
	.009976	6.010000	
	.046887	6.057000	
	.014964	6.067000	
	.003411	5.700100	
	Electrons:		
	.678370	.001927	
	.405390	.010300	
	.069832	.012467	
	.084996	.021566	
	.094772	.026315	
	.229050	.034176	
	.017957	.034203	
	.028851	.038730	
	.033918	.043479	
	.099860	.044744	
	.063826	.051340	
	.005188	.051367	
	.024302	.055714	
	.001995	.055741	
	.027933	.061908	
	.010587	.066282	
	.009808	.076000	
	.001476	.083403	
	.089874	.087932	
	.227350	.106370	
	.001723	.132590	
	.001046	.151020	
	.170390	.155790	
	.018041	.186650	
	.004378	.203820	
	.045576	.205090	
	.001633	.208190	
	.011103	.222250	
	.004135	.226630	
	.034357	.254510	
	.008394	.271670	
	.003129	.276050	
	Gammas & X-rays:		
	.608090	.014300	
	.001197	.044663	
	.001397	.057273	
	.001397	.067841	
	.142860	.099550	
	.229680	.103760	
	.002594	.106130	
	.108040	.117000	
	.032921	.209750	
	.105750	.228180	
	.001097	.254410	
	.139660	.277600	
	.007282	.285410	
	.003342	.166970	
Cm-244[c]	Half-life: 18.11 years		
	Alphas:		
	.236000	5.762800	
	.764000	5.805000	
	.000260	5.633000	
	Electrons:		
	.068710	.010300	
	.171780	.019727	
	.063488	.036891	
	Gammas & X-rays:		
	.103070	.014300	
	.000284	.056867	
Cm-245[c]	Half-life: 8500 years		
	Alphas:		
	.003200	5.234600	
	.049700	5.303800	
	.931800	5.362000	
	.008300	5.488700	
	.005800	5.529200	
	.001190	5.318900	
	Electrons:		
	.424090	.010300	
	.313600	.011182	
	.467840	.018903	
	.170880	.036067	
	.153600	.052182	
	.009344	.076000	
	.163070	.109900	
	.042650	.127070	
	.016307	.131440	
	.060224	.150900	
	.015744	.168070	
	.005952	.172440	
	Gammas & X-rays:		
	.636130	.014300	
	.001152	.042000	
	.136110	.099550	
	.218820	.103760	
	.102930	.117000	
	.062720	.133000	
	.064000	.174000	
Cm-246[c]	Half-life: 4750 years		
	Alphas:		
	.209950	5.343000	
	.789790	5.386000	

[a] RSIC computer data file (DLC-80) contains x ray and photon data not in Kocher 1981. They are included in this table.
[b] Maximum energy for betas and positrons.
[c] Branching to radioactive daughter(s) shown in Table 8.13.

(continued)

Table 8.14 Energy and Probability by Radiation Type for Selected Radionuclides of Interest to Health Physicists (Continued)

	Probability per Decay	Energy[b] (MeV)	Average Energy (MeV)
	Electrons:		
	.061220	.010300	
	.153050	.021448	
	.056475	.038612	
	Gammas & X-rays:		
	.091830	.014300	
	.000276	.044545	
Cm-247[c]	Half-life: 15600000 years		
	Alphas:		
	.047000	4.818000	
	.710000	4.868000	
	.016000	4.941000	
	.02000	4.983000	
	.012000	5.145000	
	.057000	5.210000	
	.138000	5.265000	
	Electrons:		
	.039516	.010300	
	.058320	.034803	
	.015957	.051967	
	.006075	.056341	
	.000825	.076000	
	.003640	.153280	
	.001323	.156180	
	.022000	.165580	
	.001394	.211180	
	.001040	.252000	
	.004400	.264300	
	.012888	.280780	
	.001400	.281470	
	.002448	.379500	
	Gammas & X-rays:		
	.059275	.014300	
	.012016	.099550	
	.019318	.103760	
	.009087	.117000	
	.005200	.275100	
	.034000	.278000	
	.020000	.287400	
	.003400	.333000	
	.013000	.346000	
	.720000	.402600	
	.001060	.116110	
Pu-243[c]	Half-life: 4.956 hours		
	Betas:		
	.012300	.116280	.030300
	.002500	.472700	.136900
	.044000	.485600	.141000
	.290000	.498000	.145100
	.060000	.539790	.158700
	.590000	.582000	.172700
	.000239	.054000	.013880
	Electrons:		
	.021735	.010194	
	.072835	.010500	
	.007666	.017994	
	.090321	.018394	
	.008027	.027875	
	.029900	.030194	
	.002581	.035675	
	.031423	.036075	
	.008510	.047875	
	.003220	.052384	
	.037490	.060194	
	.002070	.072594	
	.000063	.077800	
	.009269	.077875	
	.003335	.082384	
	.003152	.256700	
	Gammas & X-rays:		
	.118840	.014600	
	.007590	.041800	
	.002300	.067000	
	.230000	.084000	
	.000919	.102050	
	.001473	.106490	
	.001610	.109300	
	.000696	.120000	
	.001311	.356400	
	.005520	.381700	
	.001792	.137170	
Cm-248[c]	Half-life: 339000 years		
	Alphas:		
	.165410	5.035100	
	.751350	5.078600	
	.000697	4.931100	
	Electrons:		
	.048447	.010300	
	.121120	.021103	
	.044858	.038267	
	Gammas & X-rays:		
	.072670	.014300	
	.000262	.056242	
Cf-252[c]	Half-life: 2.639 years		
	Alphas:		
	.002326	5.976600	
	.152150	6.075700	
	.815970	6.118300	
	.000020	5.820200	
	Electrons:		
	.040952	.010700	
	.112170	.018868	
	.041757	.037064	
	.001584	.076068	
	Gammas & X-rays:		
	.072804	.015000	
	.000268	.068180	

[a] RSIC computer data file (DLC-80) contains x ray and photon data not in Kocher 1981. They are included in this table.

[b] Maximum energy for betas and positrons.

[c] Branching to radioactive daughter(s) shown in Table 8.13.

References

Browne, E., Firestone, R.B. *Table of radioactive isotopes.* Shirley, V.S. Ed.; John Wiley & Sons, Inc.; New York; 1986.

Cember, H. *Introduction to Health Physics,* 2nd Edition; Pergamon Press; 1983.

Department of Energy. *Health Physics Manual of Good Practices for Uranium Facilities.* Idaho National Engineering Laboratory DE88-013620; EGG-2530; UC-41; 1988.

Department of Energy Environmental Measurements Laboratory. *Procedures Manual.* HASL-300; November 1990.

Eckerman, K. Personal Communication. Oak Ridge National Laboratory; Oak Ridge, TN; 1991.

International Commission on Radiological Protection. *Radionuclide Transformations Energy and Intensity of Emissions,* Publication 38; Pergamon Press; Oxford; 1983.

Kocher, D.C. ''Radioactive Decay Data Tables.'' DOE-TIC-11026; U.S. Department of Energy; Washington, DC; 1981. Obtained from RSIC computer data file (DLC-80 data library) and corrected as per ''RadDecay Version 4.0'' Grove Engineering, Inc.; Rockville, MD; 1991.

Peterson, H. Personal Communication. U.S. Department of Energy; Wheaton, MD; 1991.

Slaback, L. Personal Communication. Brookhaven Gamma Database; 1991.

Slaback, L. Personal Communication. National Institute of Standards and Technology; Gaithersburg, MD; 1991.

Siegbahn, K. *Alpha, Beta, and Gamma Ray Spectroscopy.* North-Holland Publishing Co.; Amsterdam; 1965.

Wapstra, A.H., Nijgh, G.J., Lieshout, R. *Nuclear Spectroscopy Tables.* North-Holland Publishing Co.; Amsterdam; 1959.

CHAPTER 9

RADIATION MEASUREMENT INSTRUMENTS

The requirements and characteristics of radiation measurement instruments vary according to the circumstances under which they are used (field, area, laboratory conditions) and according to their purpose (radiation survey, personal monitoring, use in emergencies, or alpha, beta or gamma counting). In fact, radiation measurement instruments are so varied that only an overview has been presented here. Groups of instruments for these and other conditions or uses are presented in tabular form together with their operational characteristics and requirements.

While examples of calibrations, efficiencies and variability of all the listed instruments are not given in this chapter, these parameters are illustrated for the most important types of gamma and beta survey instruments, in some cases with a specific instrument used as an example.

Some of the important parameters that need to be considered for laboratory counting of alpha and beta particles are presented. Charts for determination of optimum sample and background counting times, errors and statistics are given. (See Chapter 3, pages 55–56 and 64–65 for useful equations relevant to counting and counting statistics). Gamma spectral analysis is only slightly touched upon.

Mention of specific instruments does not infer any warranty or liability regarding their suitability for specific applications.

TABLE OF CONTENTS

Table 9.1 Main Applications of Radiation Detectors

Detector	Radiation	Energy Range	Overall Efficiency
Ionization Chamber	Alpha	All energies for counting and spectroscopy	High
	Beta	All energies	Moderate
	Gamma	All energies	<0.1%
	Neutrons	Thermal with BF_3 gas or boron lining, or fissionable material, fast proton recoil from hydrogenous material	Moderate
	X-rays	Common energies in radiological safety	Window thickness dependent at low energies
Proportional Counters	Alpha	All energies—spectroscopy	Window thickness dependent, high
	Beta and Electrons	Detects all energies: spectroscopy with low energy <200 keV	Moderate
	Gammas	All energies	<1%
	Neutrons	Thermal with BF_3 gas or boron lining	Moderate
	X-rays	Energy discrimination, spectra, radiological safety and diffraction studies	
GM Counters	Alpha	Insensitive to energy	Moderate
	Beta and Electrons	Insensitive to energy <3 MeV	Moderate
	Gamma	All energies through a secondary process	<1%
	Neutrons	Can use proton recoil or (n, α) reaction	Not too common
	X-rays	Common survey equipment	Window thickness dependent
Scintillation		Can do spectroscopic work with all scintillators with moderate resolutions.	
(a) Inorganic	Alpha	All energies—ZnS. No energy discrimination.	High
	Beta	Low energies—CsI(T1)	Moderate
	Gamma	All energies—NaI(T1), CsI(T1)	Moderate
	Neutrons	Thermal-LiI(Eu)	Moderate
	X-rays	Thin (1–3 mm) NaI(T1)—ultra thin beryllium window	High
Scintillation (b) Organic	Alpha	All energies—anthracene	Moderate
	Betas and Electrons	All energies—anthracene, stilbene, plastics	Moderate
	Gamma	All energies—plastics	Poor
	Neutrons	Plastic, liquids	Low
Semi-conductors		Can do spectroscopic work with resolutions that are at least a factor of 10 better than scintillators	
	Alpha	All energies with good resolution—Surface barrier, diffused junction	Low <0.1%
	Beta and Electrons	All energies under 2 MeV with good resolution—Surface barrier, diffused junction, lithium drifted silicon	Low <0.1%
	Gamma and X-rays	All energies—good resolution—with surface barrier and diffused junction—with lithium drifted germanium	Moderate for Gamma High for X-ray

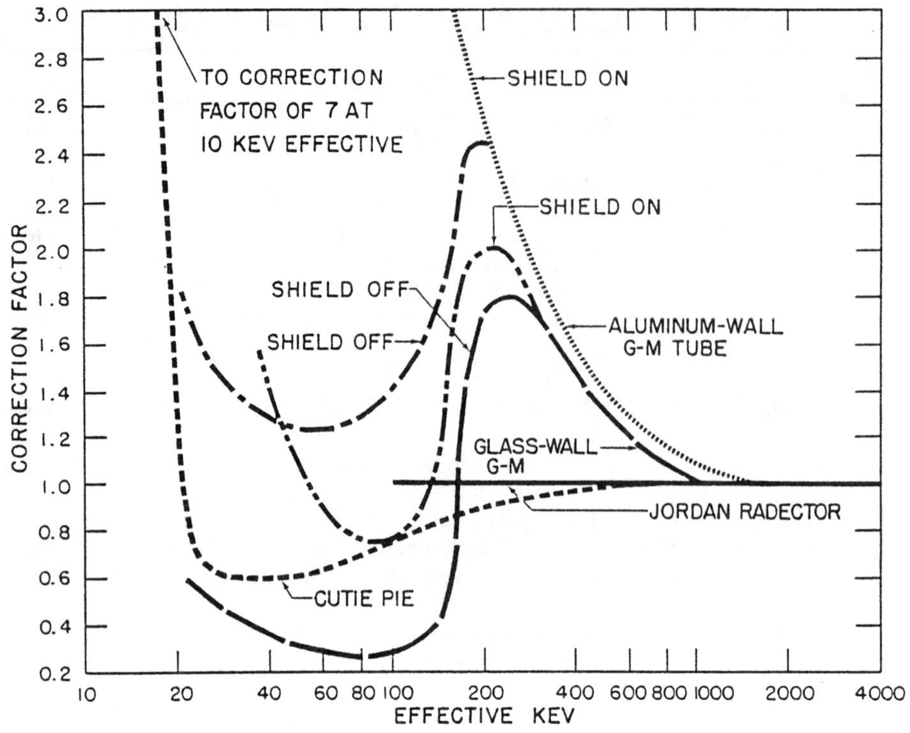

Figure 9.1 Typical Energy Dependence Correction Factors for Some Monitoring Instruments

Table 9.2 Personnel Monitoring Devices[a]

Instrument	Radiation Detected	Range (Nominal)	Application	Remarks
Film meter (badge).	γ, β, n_f, n_{th}	0.1–10,000 rad	Permanent record of dose of each type of mixed radiation. Au and In foils activated by criticality accident if incorporated in badge.	Film—density dependence on photon energy circumvented by filters. Orientation of film during exposure a problem. Expert examination of film can give added quantitative information.
Pocket chamber (indirect reading).	γ	To 100 + 5 mR To 200 ± 10 mR	Measurement of day-to-day gamma exposure.	Relatively energy independent for γ. Read by suitable meter.
Pocket chamber (direct reading).	γ, n_{th} (when coated with boron)	To 200 mR; available with higher ranges to 600 R.	Visual check on gamma and, when modified, thermal neutron exposure.	Position of electrometer fiber read through magnifying lens.
Personal radiation monitor. (''Chirpers'', electronic dosimeters)	γ, x	2 to 60 ''chirp''/min in a 1 mR/hr field, selectable on some instruments.	Audible warning of radiation field. Available different radiation ranges. Data can be transmitted for remote readout.	Signal frequency proportional to radiation intensity. Continuous tone above about 10 R/hr. to excess of 1500 R/hr.
Chemical dosimeter	γ	5 to 2 × 10^8 rad.	Measure gamma component of a mixed radiation field.	Read by titration, measurement of conductivity change, measurement of pH colorimetrically or electrometrically.
Glass dosimeter	γ	5 to several thousand rad.	Dose measurement of gamma exposure over a wide range.	Loosely bound electrons freed by radiation from photoluminescent centers with silver; centers excited by ultraviolet light emit photons (~6400 Å). Should not be read for 1 hr after exposure unless specifically calibrated.
''Bubble'' dosimeter	n	<1 mrem to?	Neutron dosimetry. Specific dosimeters have a limited dynamic range.	Can be made both energy independent for dosimeters and energy dependent for spectroscopy. Period of usage is limited, days to a few weeks.

[a] Characteristics for thermoluminescent dosimeters (TLDs) listed in Table 9.3.

Table 9.3 Characteristics of Thermoluminescent Dosimeters

Property/Type	LiF[d] (TLD-100)[c]	$Li_2B_4O_7$:Mn[d] (TLD-800)[c]	Al_2O_3:C (TLD-500)[c]	CaF_2:Mn[a] (TLD-400)[c]	CaF_2 (TLD-200)[ac]	$CaSO_4$:Mn[a]	$CaSO_4$:Dy[a] (TLD-900)[c]
Density (gm/cc) (Powder ½ of solid)	2.64	2.4	2.7	3.18	3.18	2.61	2.61
Effective atomic no. (Z) for photoelectric absorption	8.2	7.4	10.2	16.3	16.3	15.3	15.3
TL emission spectra	3500–6000 Å (4000 max)	5300–6300 Å (6050 max)	4200 Å	4400–6000 Å (5000 max)	Peaks at 4835 Å at 5765 Å	4500–6000 Å (5000 max)	4800 Å; 5700 Å
Temperature of main TL glow peak	195°C	200°C	185°C	260°C	180°C	110°C	220°C
Efficiency at ^{60}Co relative to LiF	1.0	0.15	30	10	30	70	20
Energy response 30 keV/^{60}Co	1.25	0.9	~2.9	~13	12.5	~10	~12.5
Useful range	mR–3×10^5 R	50 mR–10^6 R	50 μR–100 R	100 μR–3×10^5 R	10 μR–10^6 R	μR–10^4 R	100 μR–10^5 R
Fading	Negligible[b] 5%/yr. at 20°C	<5% in 3 months	3% per year	10% in first 24 hours; 15% total in 2 weeks	10% in first 24 hours[b]; 16% total in 2 weeks	50% in first 24 hours	8% in 6 months
Physical forms	Powder Ribbons Rods Bulbs Cards Cleaved Crystals	Powder Chips Bulbs Cards	Disk	Powder Chips Rods Bulbs	Powder Crystals Bulbs Cards	Powder	Powder

[a] The high sensitivity materials such as CaF_2 and $CaSO_4$ are extremely light (UV) sensitive, and fading is enhanced considerably. All of the high sensitivity materials should be handled, used and stored in opaque containers to prevent fading from light exposure.

[b] Post-irradiation, pre-evaluation anneal for 10 minutes with LiF and 20 minutes with CaF_2 (TLD-200 at 100°C normalizes these materials and eliminates fading).

[c] Harshaw Corporation designation for these TLD materials.

[d] Also available using ^6Li and ^7Li enriched material to enhance, or to reduce, the response to thermal neutrons, respectively. Other TLD materials include BeO:Mn, $CaSO_4$ (rare earth), Al_2O_3(Mn), $CaSO_4$(Tm), and Mg_2SiO_4(Tb).

Table 9.4 Characteristics of Selected Survey and Area Monitoring Instruments[a]

Instrument	Radiation Detected	Typical Ranges	Remarks
GM Counters	β, γ	Low range: 0.2–20 mR/hr 800–80,000 cpm High range: to 10,000 rem/h	Detection β >150 keV >20 keV for x-rays Rugged Strong energy dependence (can be flattened with filters) Possible paralysis of response at high count rates or exposure rates in old instruments Sensitive to microwave fields May be affected by ultra violet light
Ionization Chambers			
Pressurized	β, γ and x	0–0.5 to 0–5000 mR/h	10 μrem/h sensitivity
Unsealed	β, γ, and x	0–5 to 0–50 rem/hr, to 500 rem/h on some	Should be warmed up Typically have beta windows but beta correction factor required
Pocket Ion Chamber	x, γ	0–200 mR most common, up to 100 R available	No warm-up >50 keV Relatively inexpensive Gives estimate of integrated dose Small size Subject to accidental discharge Leakage discharge minimal on FEMA plastic PICs
Proportional Counters			
Air	α	100–100,000 cpm 500–500,000 cpm	~50% efficiency 2 geometry
Gas Flow	α, low energy β	—	~50% efficiency ~35% efficiency
Windowless Gas	α, low energy β	—	^{3}H surface contamination
Scintillation Counters			
Alpha	α	0–2000 k cpm 0–2,000,000 cpm	ZnS(Ag) Lin-Log scale
Low Energy Gamma	γ and x-rays	—	Thin NaI (Tl) 10–70 keV for ^{239}Pu, ^{241}Am, ^{125}I and x-rays
Thermal Neutron	n_{th}	60 cpm per n $cm^{-2}s^{-1}$	ZnS(Ag) n-alpha reaction
Fast Neutron	n_f	15 cpm per n $cm^{-2}s^{-1}$	ZnS(Ag) proton

[a] The electronic characteristics govern operational properties like ruggedness, warmup requirements, isotropism, and the impact of environmental factors (temperature, rate of temperature change, humidity, pressure, vibration).

(continued)

Table 9.4 Characteristics of Selected Survey and Area Monitoring Instruments[a] (Continued)

Instrument	Radiation Detected	Typical Ranges	Remarks
Neutron REM meters			
Bonner Sphere	n_{th}–n_f	5–5000 mrem/hr	Cd loaded polyethylene sphere plus BF_3 tube
Anderson-Braun	n_{th}–n_f	2–2000 mrem/hr	BF_3 proportional counter Gamma insensitive to 500 R/hr
Continuous beta-gamma air monitor (particulate)	β, γ	Includes DAC level	Features can include count ratemeter, strip chart, digital data storage, dynamic background subtration. GM based system does not distinguish between β and γ. Proportional based systems have α–β separation.
Continuous alpha-particulate air monitor	α, β		Alarm may be based on rate of increase of activity, rate of sample decay, change of normally constant—α–β ratio due to radon decay. Radon is a problem.
Continuous gaseous air monitor	Tritium	About $^1/_{100}$ to 10^3 × DAC for tritium	Ion chamber based system also responds to other radioactive gases. Proportional counting based system capable of limited selectivity.
Fast neutron dosimeter	n_f	From $^1/_{10}$ permissible exposure	Can be checked with internal source. Tissue-equivalent chamber.
Threshold detector unit	n_{th}, n_f	High intensity neutron flux	Should supplement, but never be substituted for, alarm-type instruments which warn of dose rate, but which do not measure dose.

[a] The electronic characteristics govern operational properties like ruggedness, warmup requirements, isotropism, and the impact of environmental factors (temperature, rate of temperature change, humidity, pressure, vibration).

Table 9.4 Characteristics of Selected Survey and Area Monitoring Instruments[a] (Continued)

Instrument	Radiation Detected	Range	Application	Remarks
Hand and foot monitor	β, γ	Low level	Simultaneous detection of β and γ contamination of hands and shoes. Will not detect α.	Most models have auxiliary probe for monitoring clothing. Typically GM based but some use proportional detectors.
Portal monitors	β, γ	Low level	Monitoring exits from areas of suspected contamination.	Slow passage through narrow portal (or a fixed count time) required for maximum instrument response. GM and proportional based systems have beta sensitivity. Plastic scintillator based systems are typically gamma only and are effective for screening certain internally deposited nuclides.
Whole body contamination monitors	α, β,	Low level	Monitor total body surface.	Typically counts half the body at a time. Typically can detect a few nCi with a 5–10 sec count. Radon can cause interference.
Water effluent monitor	γ, β		Monitoring water wastes or coolants. May be connected to rate meter, recorder, and alarm systems, or to the check and diversion valves for control of water flow.	Thin films of water (or other material) will absorb α. Monitoring for any radiation may be complicated by silt, algae, radioactive contamination of the detector, variability in water flow rate and surface levels.
''Stack'' monitors for gaseous effluents	Depends upon detectors chosen.		Rough estimate of the radioactivity of the effluent from a multiuse stack.	May require complicated and expensive sampling, collecting, detecting, counting, and data interpreting equipment.

[a] The electronic characteristics govern operational properties like ruggedness, warmup requirements, isotropism, and the impact of environmental factors (temperature, rate of temperature change, humidity, pressure, vibration).

Table 9.5 Health Physics Instrumentation Performance Criteria Comparison—Calibration Techniques (From Gillings et al., 1984)

Criteria	BNWL 1991[a]	ANSI N323[b]
Photon calibration sources	Use radionuclides, filtered x-rays, and K-fluorescent x-rays	Use radionuclides, filtered x-rays and K-fluorescent x-rays with a wide energy range
β particle calibration sources	Use accelerator or radioactive sources such as ^{90}Sr or natural uranium with a surface dose rate = 225 mrad/h	Use ^{90}Sr or U_3O_8 being sufficiently strong so it can be detected far enough away to make end window small when compared to distance of source
α particle calibration sources	Most are calibrated using radionuclide sources, plutonium, uranium, polonium or other α emitters, not point sources	Use radionuclide ^{148}Gd, ^{230}Th, ^{239}Pu, ^{210}Po, ^{241}Am, ^{238}Pu, ^{244}Cm, or ^{252}Cf
Neutron calibration sources	Calibrations may be accomplished with both isotopic neutron sources or neutron generating equipment; frequent sources include radium-beryllium, polonium-beryllium, americium-beryllium, antimony-beryllium and plutonium fluoride	Neutrons can be generated by (α, n), (γ, n), spontaneous fission, or by interaction with accelerated charged particle; sources for (α, n) or (γ, n) reactions generally consist of an α or γ emitter with beryllium
Temperature, pressure, and humidity	If temperature varies by more than 30°C from calibrated, the instrument should be calibrated over the expected temperature range; instrument shall be calibrated over the expected pressure and humidity during operation	If temperature varies by more than 30°C from calibrated, the instrument should be calibrated over the expected temperature range; instrument shall be calibrated over the expected pressure and humidity during operation
Directional dependence	Correction factors should be developed for different orientation relative to source	Correction factors should be developed for different orientation relative to source
Recalibration	After maintenance on or adjustment of instrument	After maintenance on or adjustment of instrument plus when instrument is subject to hand usage or corrosive environments
Performance field checks	Use check sources to test instrument and if reference reading differs $> \pm 20\%$ discrepancy should be corrected	Use check sources to test instrument and if reference reading differs $> \pm 20\%$ discrepancy should be corrected
Electronic calibrations	Electronically simulate radiation calibrations by 1) establishing a reference point with an appropriate radiation source, 2) match reference point with a nuclear pulse generator or current source, 3) vary pulse rate or current value to provide calibration check points	

[a] BNWL 1991 (Bramson et al., 1976), *Evaluation Testing and Calibration Methodology for Emergency Radiological Instrumentation.*
[b] ANSI N323, 1978, *Radiation Protection Instrumentation Test and Calibration.*

Table 9.5 Health Physics Instrumentation Performance Criteria Comparison—Calibration Techniques (Continued (From Gillings et al., 1984)

Criteria	BNWL 1991[a]	ANSI N323[b]
Primary photon calibration standard	Allowable error shall depend on state of the art	
Primary β, α and neutron calibration standard	Allowable error shall meet the state of the art	
Secondary photon standard	Allowable error of $\pm 2\%$ for exposure	
Secondary beta standard	Allowable error of $\pm 5\%$ for dose	
Secondary neutron standard accuracy	Allowable error of $\pm 5\%$ for dose	
Laboratory photon standard accuracy	Allowable error of $\pm 5\%$ for dose	
Laboratory beta standard accuracy	Allowable error of $\pm 10\%$ for dose	
Laboratory neutron standard accuracy	Allowable error of $\pm 10\%$ for dose	
Field photon standard accuracy	Allowable error of $\pm 20\%$ for exposure	
Field beta standard accuracy	Allowable error of $\pm 25\%$ for dose	
Field neutron standard accuracy	Allowable error of $\pm 25\%$ for dose	
Emergency photon standard accuracy	Allowable error of $\pm 40\%$ for dose	
Emergency beta standard accuracy	Allowable error of $\pm 40\%$ for dose	
Emergency neutron standard accuracy	Allowable error of $\pm 40\%$ for dose	
Precision	Shall be determined prior to calibration within $\pm 10\%$ of mean	Determined prior to calibration and be within $\pm 10\%$ of the mean
Linear readout instruments	Calibration shall be checked near ends of each scale 20% and 80% of full scale	Be checked near ends of each scale at 20% and 80% of full scale
Logarithmic readout instruments	Minimum calibration of one point near midpoint of each decade	Minimum calibration of one point near midpoint of each decade
Digital readout instruments	Calibrated at 20% and 80% of each scale	At 20% and 80% of each scale for scale switching readouts and at midpoint of each decade for nonswitching
Radiation energy	Calibrations shall be made at several energies over the energy range	At expected energies, or at several energies over range; an energy versus sensitivity curve will be plotted for energy dependence
Performance check frequency	Prior to intermittent use or several times a day during continuous use	Prior to intermittent use or several times a day during continuous use
Discrimination against unwanted radiation		Effects of radiation should be determined for all unwanted radiation

[a] BNWL 1991 (Bramson et al., 1976), *Evaluation Testing and Calibration Methodology for Emergency Radiological Instrumentation.*
[b] ANSI N323, 1978, *Radiation Protection Instrumentation Test and Calibration.*

Table 9.6 Requirements for Portable X or Gamma Radiation Exposure Rate Meters and Monitors

Test Characteristics	ANSI N42.17A, 1989
Alarm threshold	Alarm threshold shall be given as % of scale or decade of adjustment
Stability	±6% of reference for: 3 hrs: battery 24 hrs: AC power
Geotropism	Within ±6% of reference
Accuracy	±15%
Photon energy dependence	±20% from 80 keV to 1.25 MeV
Photon radiation overload	Instrument shall continue to operate and be offscale
Extracameral response	Not greater than 5%
Interfering ionizing radiation response	Not greater than stated by manufacturer
Temperature dependence	Reference 22°C: ±15%: 0 to 40°C ±20%: −10 to 50°C
Vibration	±15% following harmonic loading of 2 g/15 min w/freq. 10–33 Hz
Ambient pressure	±15%; 70–106 kPa reference 101 kPa
Mechanical shock	±15% following 50 g 18 msec sinusoid shock on 3 axes

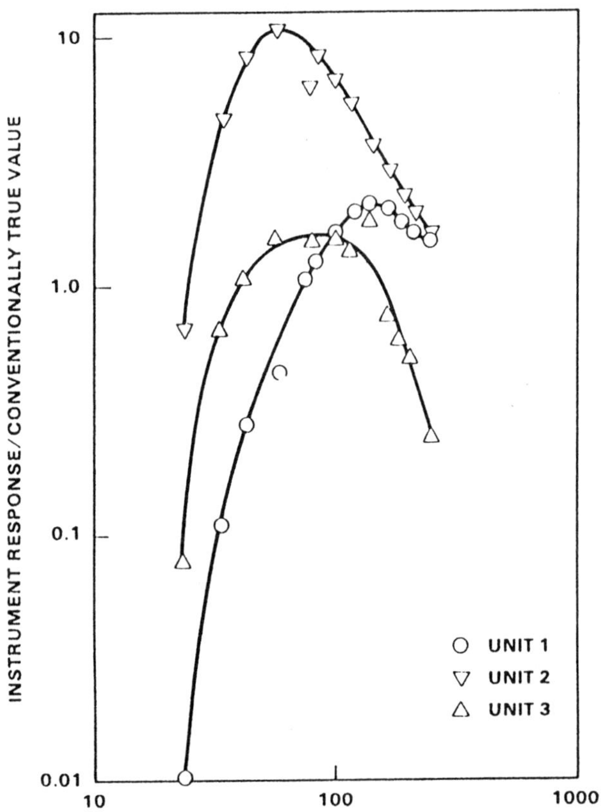

Figure 9.2 Energy Response of Three GM Detectors (From Swinth and Kenoyer, 1985)

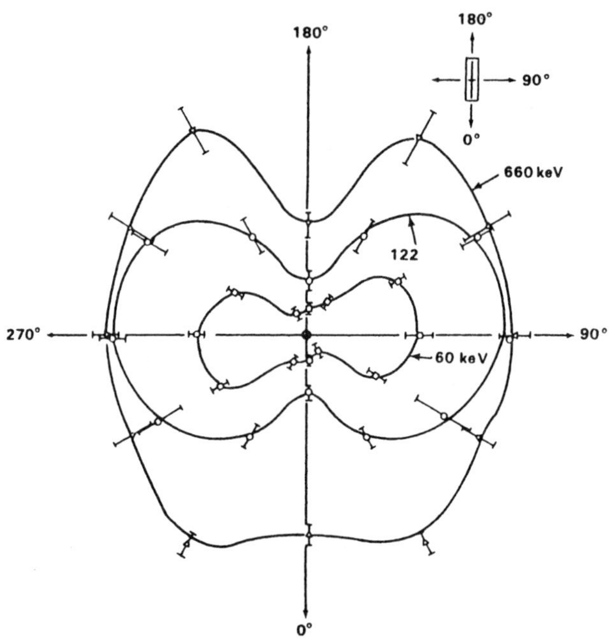

Figure 9.3 Angular Response of a GM Probe at Three Different Energies (From Swinth and Kenoyer, 1985)

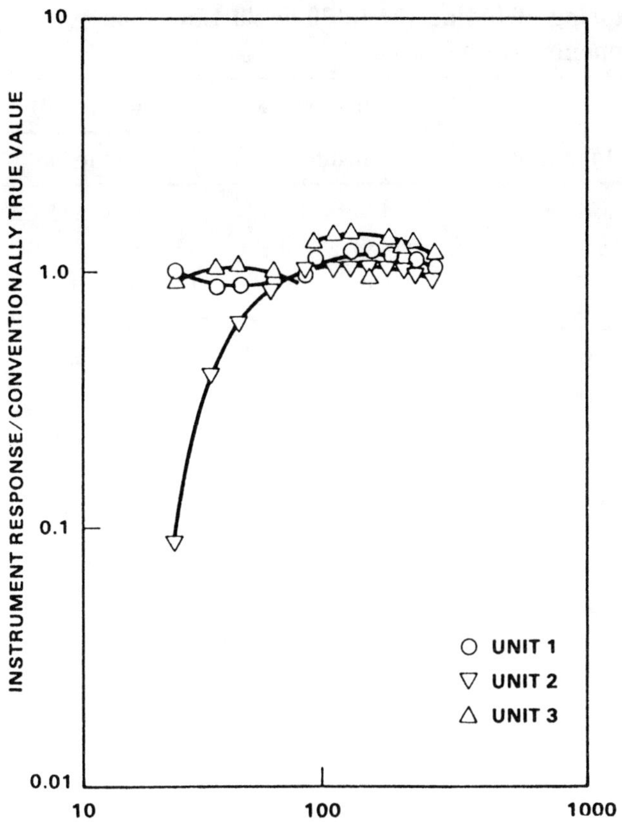

Figure 9.4 Energy Response of Three Ion Chamber Type Instruments (From Swinth and Kenoyer, 1985)

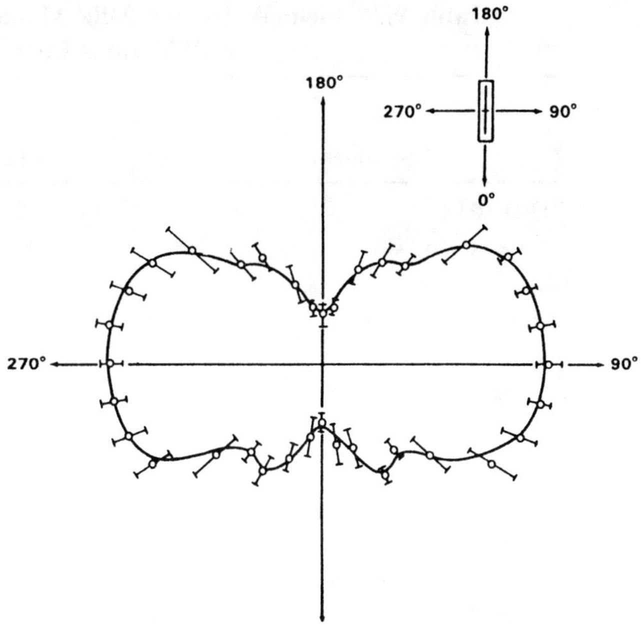

Figure 9.5 Angular Response of a GM Probe at 10° Increments with a 122 keV Test Source (From Swinth and Kenoyer, 1985)

Table 9.7 Field Water and Milk Monitoring of Iodine-131 in 20 or 40 Liter Can with Various Instruments (From Shleien, 1983)

Instrument[a]	Bkgd (cpm)	Net Count Rate (cpm per μCi/l)	
		Inside	Outside
OCD-D-103 (2)[b]	15[c] ± 8.5%[d]	134 ± 1.5%	55.9 ± 5.4%
Victoreen 6306 (4)[b]	54.4 ± 5%	1453 ± 1.4%	657 ± 2.0%
TGM-NP358 (2)[b]	19.1 ± 7%	685 ± 2%	310 ± 3.9%
Ludlum 44-3 (1)[b]	153 ± 2.6%	—	8052 ± 0.6%
CDV-700[b]	19	140	—
CDV-700[b]	50	134	56
CDV-700M[b]	20	1450	650
Al-walled GM tube[b]	50	1100	350
Mica-window GM[e]	50	700	250
3 mm thick bioplastic scintillator sprayed with ZnS. Effective area 6.4 cm^2 [e]	100	6,000	3300
Transportable single channel analyzer[e]	30	12,000	—

[a] Number in parentheses designates number of detectors used.
[b] 20 liter can.
[c] Mean of measurements.
[d] 1 standard deviation counting error.
[e] 40 liter can.

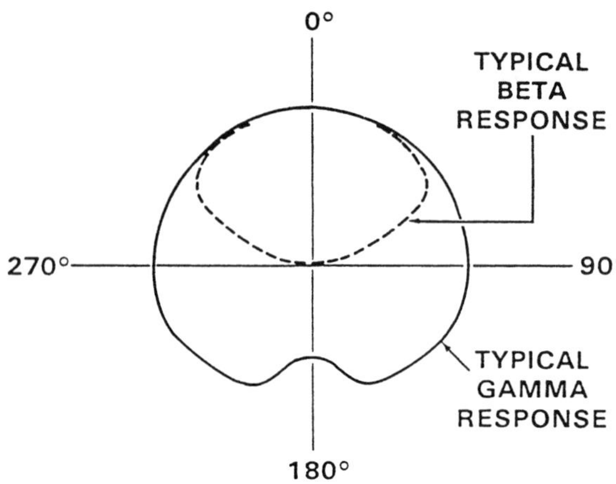

Figure 9.6 Typical Angular Dependence of "Cutie Pie" Response for Beta and Gamma Fields
(From Selby et al., 1978)

Table 9.8 Beta Dose Rate Correction Factor for an Ion Chamber Type Instrument at 30 cm from the Source (From Thompson, 1978)

Isotope	Maximum Energy (MeV)	Correction Factor
$^{90}Sr/^{90}Y$	0.546, 2.274	1.04
^{204}Tl	0.763	2.17
^{147}Pm	0.225	9.9

Table 9.9 Examples of Correction Factors Used When Measuring $^{90}Sr/^{90}Y$ Disk Source with a "Cutie Pie" Ion Chamber Survey Instrument[a] (From Hooker et al., 1980)

Source Diameter	Source to Window Distance			
	Contact	½ in.	1 in.	6 in.
½ in.	90	9	1.9	1
1 in.	35	5	2.0	1
6 in.	4.5	2.6	2.2	1
1 ft	4.5	2.5	2.3	1.3
6 ft	4.5	2.5	2.5	2.3

[a] In order to obtain the beta exposure/dose rate at the detector window, multiply the meter reading by the applicable correction factor. Note that this does not apply to point sources, e.g., "hot particles".

Table 9.10 Examples of Correction Factors For a Rectangular Volume Survey Meter "JUNO" Exposed to $^{90}Sr/^{90}Y$ Disk Sources[a] (From Hooker et al., 1980)

Source Diameter	Source to Window Distance			
	Contact	½ in.	1 in.	6 in.
½ in.	86	7	2.1	1
1 in.	31	5	2.0	1
6 in.	2	1.6	1.5	1
1 ft	2	1.8	1.7	1.3
6 ft	2	1.9	1.8	1.7

[a] In order to obtain the beta exposure/dose rate at the detector window, multiply the meter reading by the applicable correction factor. Note that this does not apply to point sources, e.g., "hot particles".

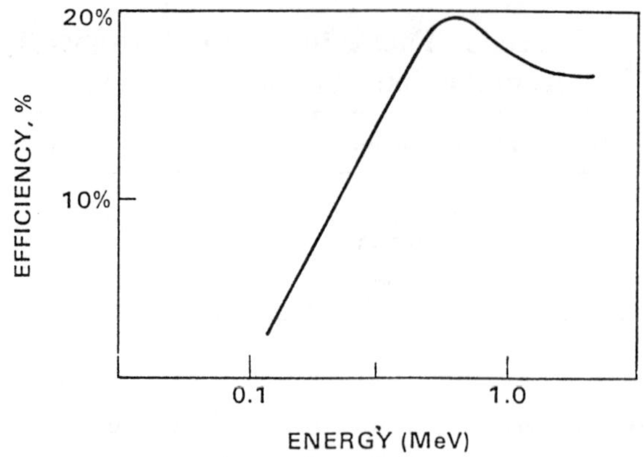

Figure 9.7 Beta Energy Response Curve for a Typical Pancake Geiger-Mueller (G.M.) Probe (From Selby et al., 1987)

Table 9.11 Beta Energy Dependence of Instruments (From Burgess and Iles, 1979 and 1981; Burgess, 1982a, 1982b)

Instrument	Response mR/h per mrad/h		
	$^{90}Sr/^{90}Y$	^{204}Tl	^{147}Pm
Eberline RO-1	0.76	0.38	0.25
Eberline RO-2	1.0	0.45	0.12
Victoreen 440RF	1.2	0.5	
Victoreen 470A	1.10	0.79	0.10
Victoreen 471RF	0.80	0.33	0.02
DCA 3795[a]	0.38	0.16	0.03
Keithley 36100[a]	0.80	0.16	0.01
Nuclear Enterprises PDR3	0.002		

[a] mrad in tissue; others mrad in air.

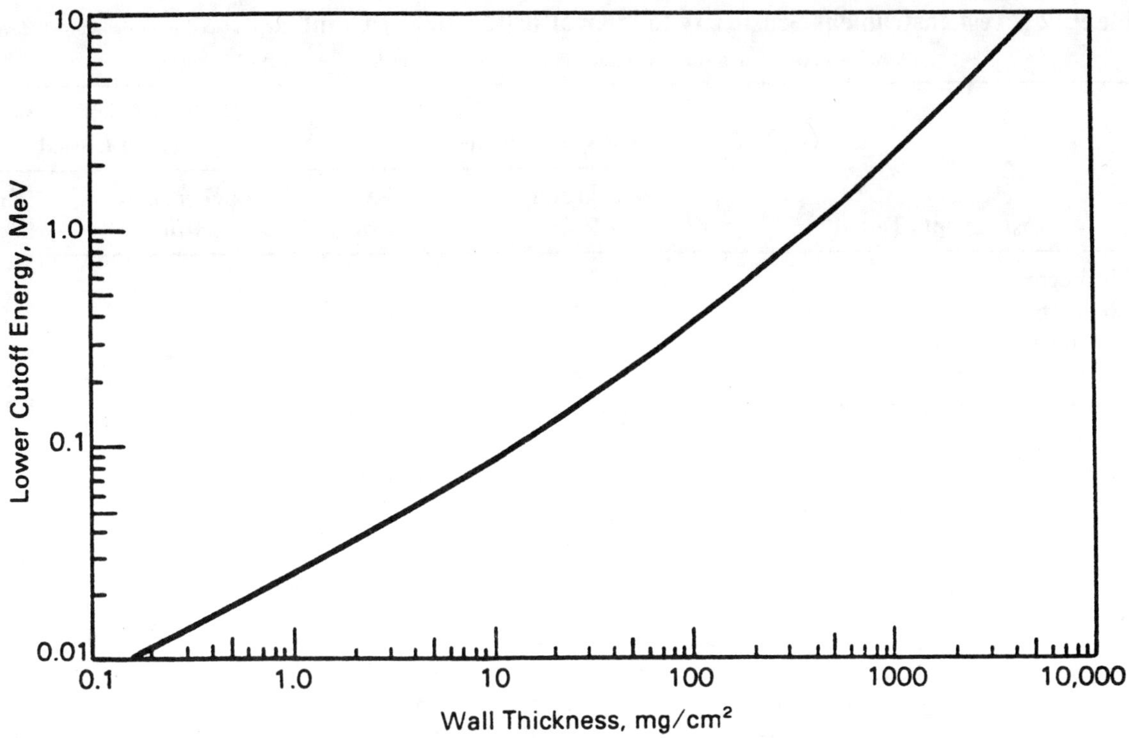

Figure 9.8 Lower Level Beta Cutoff Energy as a Function of Detector Wall Thickness (After The Health Physics and Radiological Health Handbook, 1984)

Table 9.12 Test Instrument Sensitivity to ^{85}Kr at 6.7 × 10^{-6} μCi/ml (Reproduced from the journal *Health Physics* with permission from the Health Physics Society from Jester et al., 1982)

	Beta Shield Open		No Beta Shield or Beta Shield Closed	
Instruments Tested	**Background μR/hr**	**^{85}Kr μR/hr**	**Background μR/hr**	**^{85}Kr μR/hr**
Ion Chambers				
Reuter Stokes, RSS-111 (Pressurized Ion Chamber)	NA	NA	7–10	8–10
Learsigler, 131500-1 (Suitcase-type)	NA	NA	8–13	10–15
Eberline RO-2 (Portable Survey Meter)	100–500	300–700	100–500	100–500
Scintillation Detectors				
Kimmel, MAB604 (Plastic Scintillator)	3–6	13–16	3–6	5–7
Elliott Process Rate Meter, 1597A	NA	NA	5–8	6–8
	cpm	**cpm**	**cpm**	**cpm**
GM Detectors[a]				
Eberline RM 14 ratemeter with Eberline HP 210 (Pancake Probe)	20–60	2000–2500	NA	NA
Ludlum-2A rate meter with Eberline-2A rate meter with Eberline HP 210 and HP 260 (Pancake Probes)	20–80	2000–2200	20–60	100–140
Eberline MS2 with following probes:				
HP 210 (Pancake Probe)	20–60	1700–2500	20–60	140–200
HP 260 (Pancake Probe)	20–60	2300–2700	30–60	150–160
HP 270 (Energy Compensated)	20–30	40–100	20–30	20–30
Gas Flow Proportional Counter				
Eberline PAC-4G rate meter with Eberline AC21B Beta Probe	150–200	30000–320000	100–200	300–400

NA = Not applicable.

[a] Beta shield for GM detectors was a 0.3 cm aluminum absorber.

Table 9.13 Continuous Air Monitor Specifications vs Selection Criteria (From Hickey et al., 1991)

Air Monitor Descriptions	Radiation Type	Ranges	Temperature Range	Alarm Capabilities	Background Compensation	Flow Rate		Weight (Lbs)	Dimensions	Filter	Detector	Efficiency (4 g)	Comments
						Ranges	Description						
Eberline Alpha 5A	Alpha	1–10 k cpm (Log Scale)	−7 to 54°C (System gain <5%)	Visual, audible; 0 to FS[a]; failure light	Electronic	10–100 lpm (60)[b]	Rotameter	19.7	36 cm H × 31 cm D × 40 cm L	47 mm membrane	Sillicon diffused junction diode, 490 mm^2	10% ^{239}Pu (4π)	
Eberline Alpha 6A	Alpha	N/A	0 to 40°C	Visual, audible; failure light, flowrate	Algorithm (Radon)	0.5–2 cfm (1)	Rotameter	15.0	36 cm H × 31 cm D × 40 cm L	47 mm membrane with 1″ effective diameter area	Silicone diffused junction diode, 490 mm^2	20% ^{239}Pu (4π)	Multichannel Analyzer
SAIC 452	Alpha	N/A		Audible; max. sensitivity; high level; flowrate	Algorithm (Radon)		Mass flow			47 mm membrane on a 2.5 × 3.5″ card	700 mm^2 ruggedized ion implant type standard		Multichannel Analyzer
Victoreen 758	Alpha	N/A		Audible	Algorithm (Radon)	0–140 lpm	Mass flow	20.0		47 mm membrane	1700 mm^2 solid state silicone		Multichannel Analyzer
Kurz 8300	Alpha	N/A		Aubible—low flow (optional)	Particle Size Discrimination (Radon)		Mass flow		8″ H × 4.5″	None (Deposit on detector)	490 mm^2 passivated diffused junction silicon diode	25% (4π)	To be used with separate electronics
NE America CAM 1A	Alpha		5 to 35°C	Visual, audible	Particle Size Discrimination (Radon)	30–50 lpm	Differential Thermistor			25 mm	314 mm^2 silicon	25% (4π)	
Eberline AMS-3	Beta-Photon	10–100 k cpm	−7 to 49°C (<20% change in calib.)	Visual, audible; failure light	Electronic (Photon)	10–100 lpm (60)	Rotameter	160	39.4 cm H × 39.4 cm D × 63.4 cm L	47 mm paper	Two pancake GM tubes (4.4 cm diameter)	13% ^{99}Tc 23% ^{90}Sr-T	
Ludlum 323-2	Beta-Photon	10–100 k cpm		Visual, audible	Electron (Photon)	10–100 lpm	Rotameter			47 mm paper	Two pancake GM tubes		
Johnston Triton (1C353)	Tritium	0–50 k $\mu Ci/m^3$		Audible	Gamma up to 5 mR/h	2 lpm	Fixed Flow Rate	24	11.5″ W × 10.5″ H × 11.5″ D	2″ diam. 0.5 micron fiberglass (Collect dirt, etc)	Flow through ion chamber (1.2 liters)		Can also be used for ^{14}C, ^{43}Ar, ^{85}Kr, and ^{133}Xe monitoring
Nuclear Research Corporation	Tritium	0–10 $\mu Ci/m^3$	0–50°C	Aubible 9–100% FS	Gamma 5 $\mu Ci/m^3$ or 5 mR/h)		Fixed Flow Rate	26	12.5″ W × 11.5″ H × 7.75″ D	N/A	Flow through ion chamber (2.6 liters)		Can also be used for ^{14}C, ^{43}Ar, ^{85}Kr, and ^{133}Xe monitoring
Nuclear Measurements Corporation	Particulate (P) Iodine (I) Noble Gas (NG)			Visual, audible	Lead shielding	0–4 cfm		1250	Cart: 44″ W × 44″ H × 22″ D	Charcoal, Ag Zn (1)	Beta Scintillator (P) NaI(T1) (I) Beta Scintillator 450 cc volume (NG)		

[a] FS = Full Scale [b] Usual

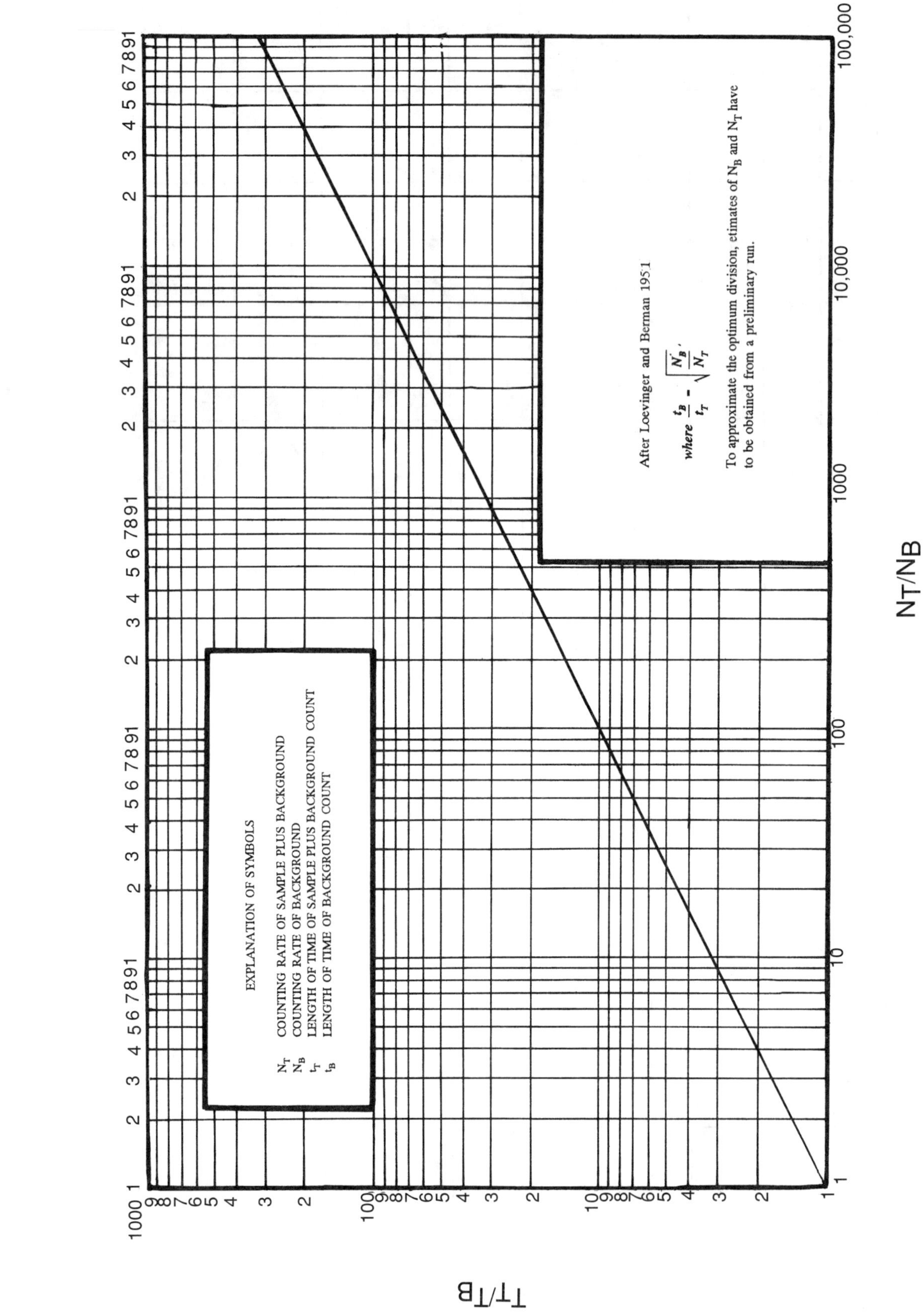

Figure 9.9 Graph Showing the Most Efficient Distribution of Counting Time Between Sample and Background

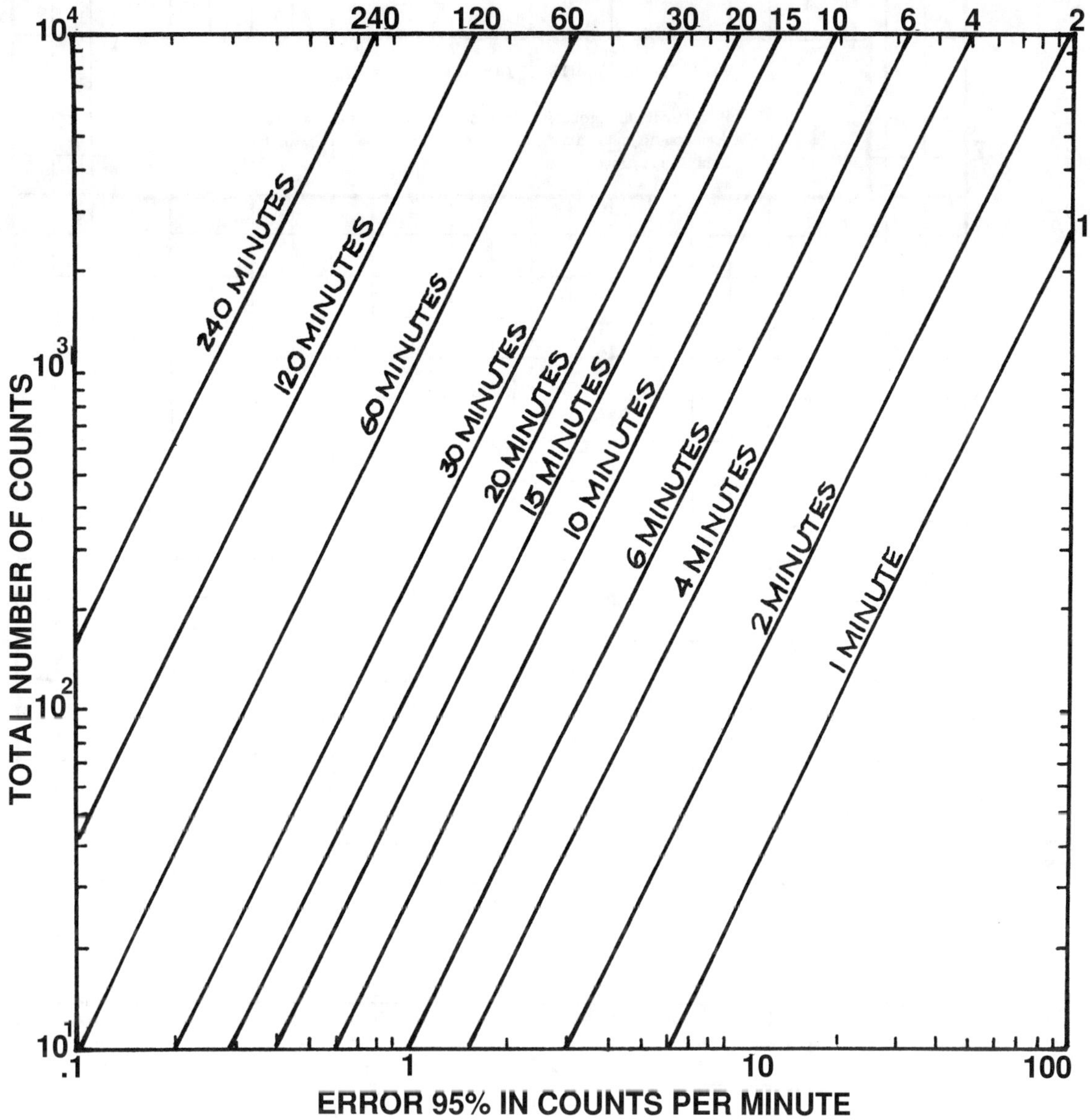

Figure 9.10 Error in Counts per Minute as a Function of Total Count and Length of Count (95% confidence level) (From Radiological Health Handbook, 1970)

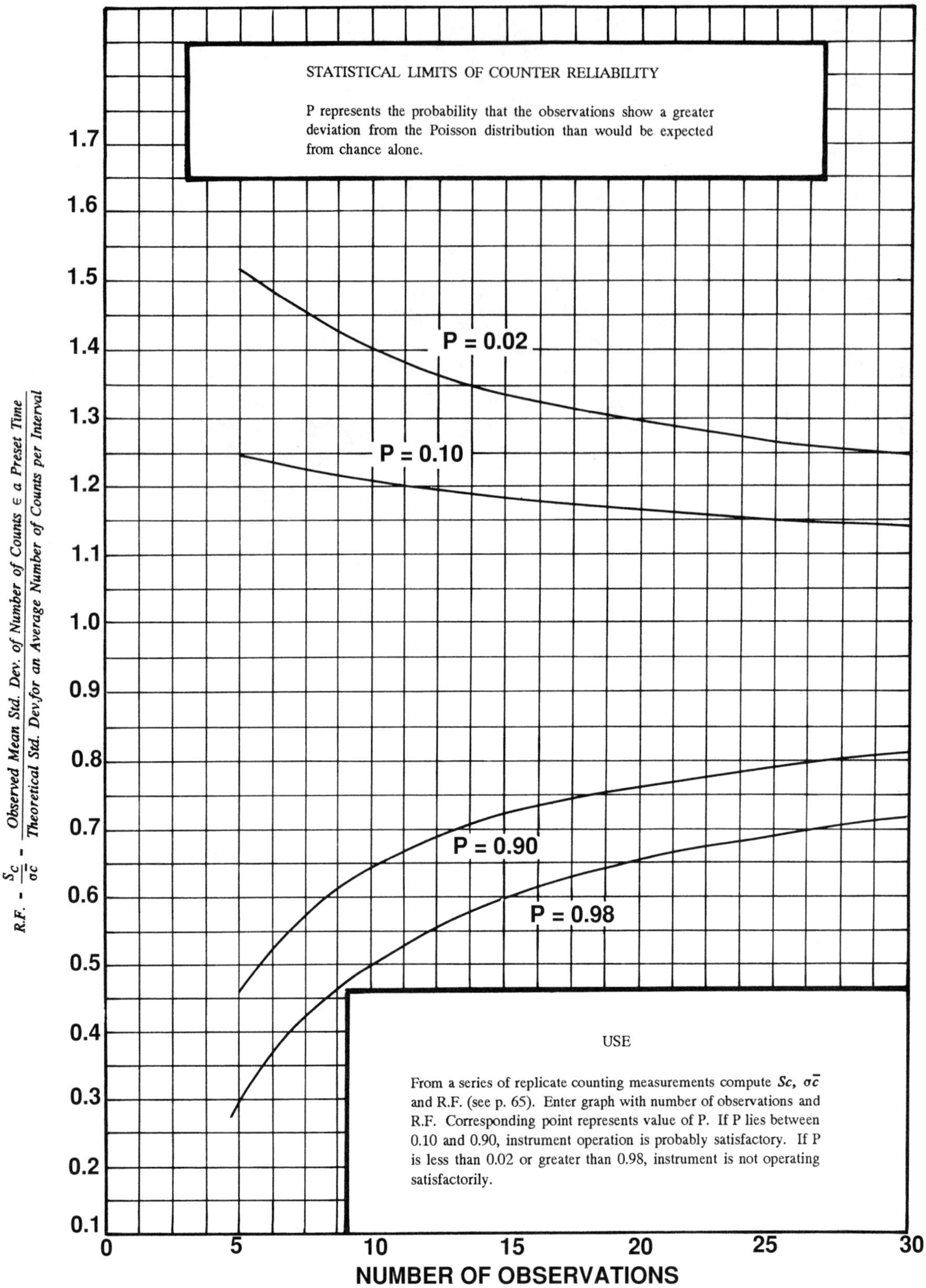

Figure 9.11 Statistical Limits of Counter Reliability (After Radiological Health Handbook, 1970)

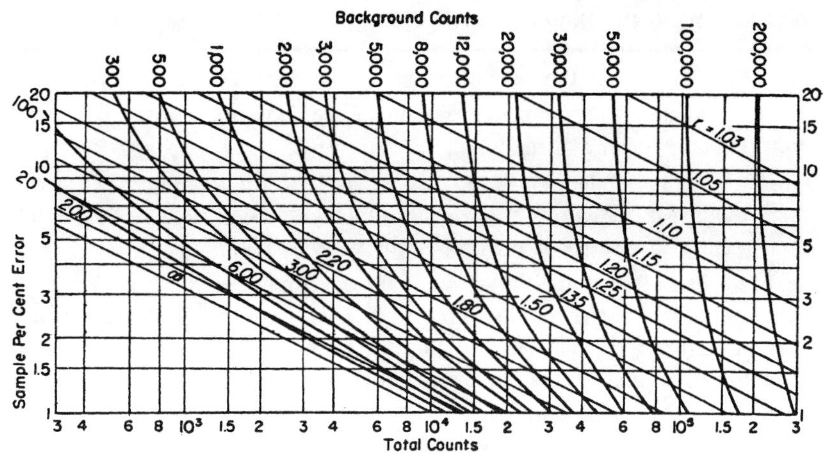

Figure 9.12 Optimum Number of Counts for Minimizing Combined Counting Time When Percent Error is Assigned and Total-to-Background Ratio is Known (After Loevinger and Berman, 1951)

The pertinent equations for Figure 9.12 are:

$$N_t = \left(\frac{100}{V_s}\right)^2 \frac{\sqrt{r}+1}{(r-1)^2} r^{3/2}$$

$$N_b = \frac{N_t}{r^{3/2}}$$

$$T_b = \frac{T_t}{\sqrt{r}}$$

$$T = T_t + T_b = \left(\frac{100}{V_s}\right)^2 \frac{1}{R_b(\sqrt{r}-1)^2}$$

where

N_t = total counts
N_b = background counts
V_s = sample percent error
R_b = background counting rate
T = combined time = $T_t + T_b$
R_T = total counting rate
r = ratio of R_T/R_b
and T_t = T_s (sample counting time) since sample can be counted only in the presence of background
T_b = background counting time

The use of Figure 9.12 may be somewhat clarified by a numerical example. Suppose it is desired to determine the sample counting rate to an error of 3%. Suppose also that $r = 1.5$. Then, from the graph, the horizontal 3% line crosses the $r = 1.5$ curve at the vertical line for 18,000 total counts. This point of intersection also lies about halfway between the background counts curves for 8,000 and 12,000. Hence, by interpolation, the total background count is about 10,000. For a counter with an ordinary background of 50 to 100 cpm these counts will run to many hours, so that the use of the optimum-time graph will be well worthwhile (Figure 9.9). A practical procedure would be to count background and sample for about 300 counts, or 5 min, each, and then estimate R_b and r as a basis for assigning the number of counts to be taken. It would be appropriate, in a case such as this, to take half the background counts before, and half after the sample count.

Table 9.14 Beta Particle Counting with End Window Geiger Counters

The counting rate should be corrected for the following factors for the individual isotope concerned:

Geometry. The solid angle subtended by the counter and the source is usually not equal to the physical solid angle because of the unknown sensitive volume of the tube.

Source size. The geometry for an extended source is smaller than for a point source because of the smaller solid angle subtended by the activity at the edge of the source. For this reason and because of the difficulty of producing a uniform coating on the plate, a large error is possible in the measurement.

Backscatter. A fraction of the particles leaving the source in the opposite direction from the counter will be scattered into the counter by the plate on which the source is mounted. This may be measured by placing a source on thin (0.2 to 0.5 mg/cm^2) film and measuring with and without the backing. This factor is reasonably constant for the same backing material with isotopes of maximum energy above about 0.6 MeV.

Absorption in window. Because of the continuous spectrum of particles emitted from a beta source, a fraction of the particles will be absorbed in the window of a mica-window counter and in the air between the counter and the source. As the first part of the absorption curve for a beta emitter is approximately linear on a semilogarithmic plot, this effect can be measured by counting the source with several thin absorbers and extrapolating through the thickness of the window and air to zero absorber. The slope of this line can be expressed as m in the equation $N/N_0 = e^{-mx}$ for use when the isotope is known. (N is the measured counting rate, N_0 is the extrapolated counting rate and x is the combined effective thickness of the window and air.)

Self-absorption. When the sample contains a large enough quantity of material, a fraction of the particles will be absorbed in the sample itself. This can be measured by preparing a series of plates with varying amounts of stable material and the same amount of an active isotope. This curve can then be used for correcting analytical results.

An approximation of the self-absorption factor can be made by use of the equation:

$$\frac{N}{N_0} = \frac{1}{mx}(1 - e^{-mx}),$$

where N is the measured counting rate, N_0 is the true counting rate, m is the absorption coefficient as measured above and x is the thickness of the sample.

Coincidence losses. With high counting rates some loss will occur because of a second particle arriving while the counter is inoperative from a previous discharge. A correction factor for coincidence losses can be obtained by counting several low activity sources individually and together.

Table 9.15 Determining Counting Efficiency for Internal Proportional Counters

Since internal proportional counters do not detect all beta rays emitted by a sample, it is necessary to divide the net counting rate by an appropriate efficiency correction decimal to determine the total beta emission. This efficiency (E), is the product of three factors—geometry (G), backscatter (B), and self absorption, generally expressed in terms of a transmission factor (T): $E = G \times B \times T$.

Geometry Factor (G)—Not all radiation from a sample is emitted in the direction of the detector. The geometry factor accounts for the fraction emitted in the proper direction. For internal proportional counters with hemispherical chambers, this factor is 0.50.

Backscatter Factor (B)—The backscattering of beta rays is a function of their energy and the atomic number (Z) of the counting dish. The following curves may be conveniently used for estimating this factor. To illustrate their use, consider a ^{32}P sample in a copper counting dish (Z = 29). From the appropriate value on the abscissa, draw a vertical line until it intersects the curve for ^{32}P. A horizontal line projected from the point of intersection to the ordinate reveals the resultant factor to be about 1.43 The *backscatter factor* is the ratio of the count with backscatter to that without backscatter.

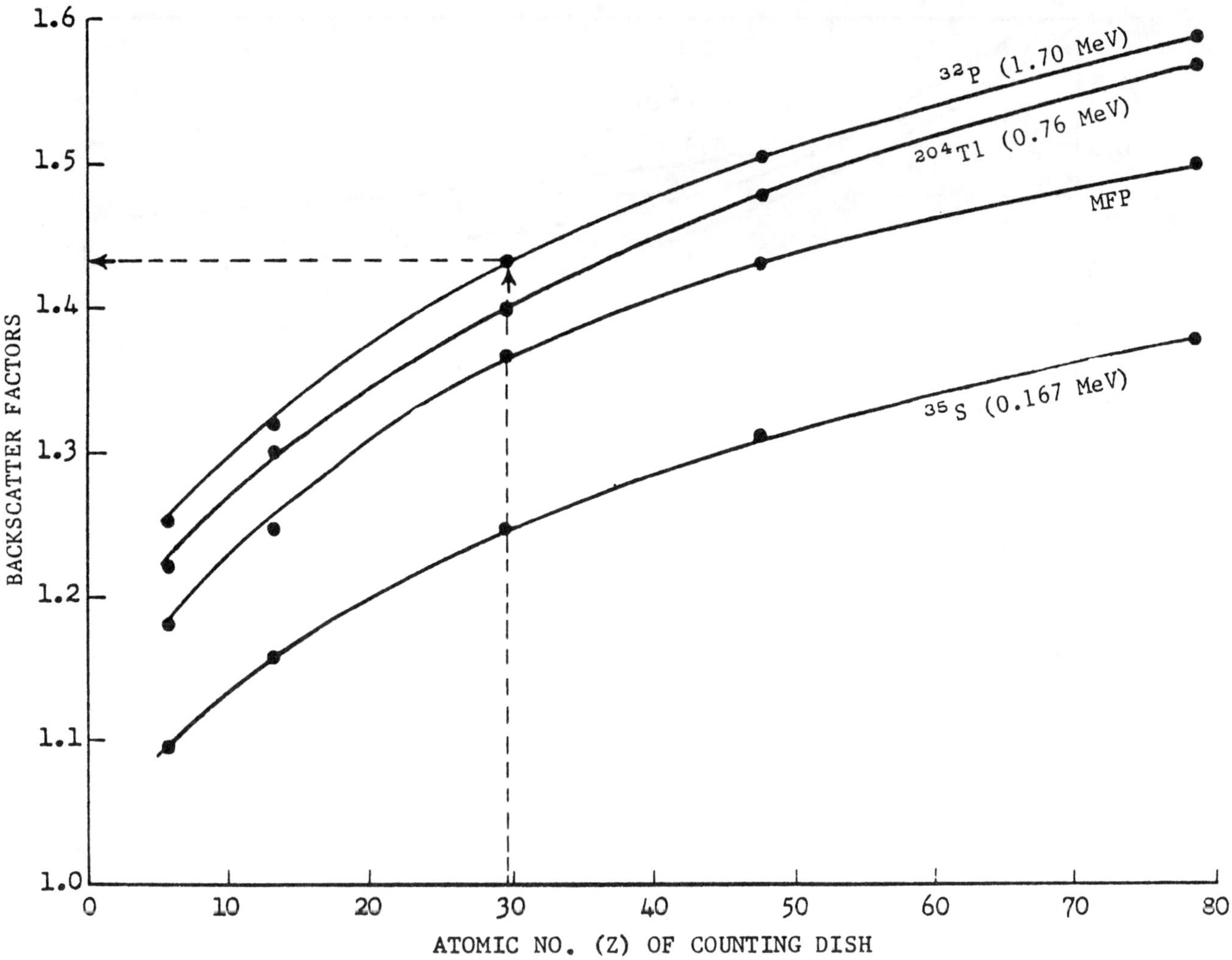

Figure 9.13 Backscatter Factors—Counting Efficiency (From Nader et al., 1954)

Self-Absorption or Transmission Factor (T)—A fraction of the beta particles emitted by a sample may be absorbed within the sample itself. This loss, which increases with sample thickness, is known as self-absorption. For counting purposes, it may be conveniently expressed in terms of a transmission factor, the fraction of the emitted beta particles not absorbed within a sample.

The transmission factor (T) may be estimated using the curves given below. If, for example, a sample containing ^{32}P weighs 200 milligrams and is evenly distributed on a 2 inch diameter dish, then the average sample thickness can be calculated to be 10 mg/cm^2. To estimate the factor, draw a vertical line from the appropriate value on the abscissa until it intersects the curve for ^{32}P. A horizontal line projected from the point of intersection to the ordinate reveals the resultant factor to be about 0.73.

Overall Counting Efficiency (E)—The efficiency correction decimal fraction for the previous example, in which a sample containing ^{32}P was counted, would be: $E = 0.50 \times 1.43 \times 0.73 = 0.52$.

If the net sample counting rate was 1,000 counts per minute, the disintegration rate could be calculated to be: dpm = net cpm/E = 1,000 cpm/0.52 = 1,920 dpm.

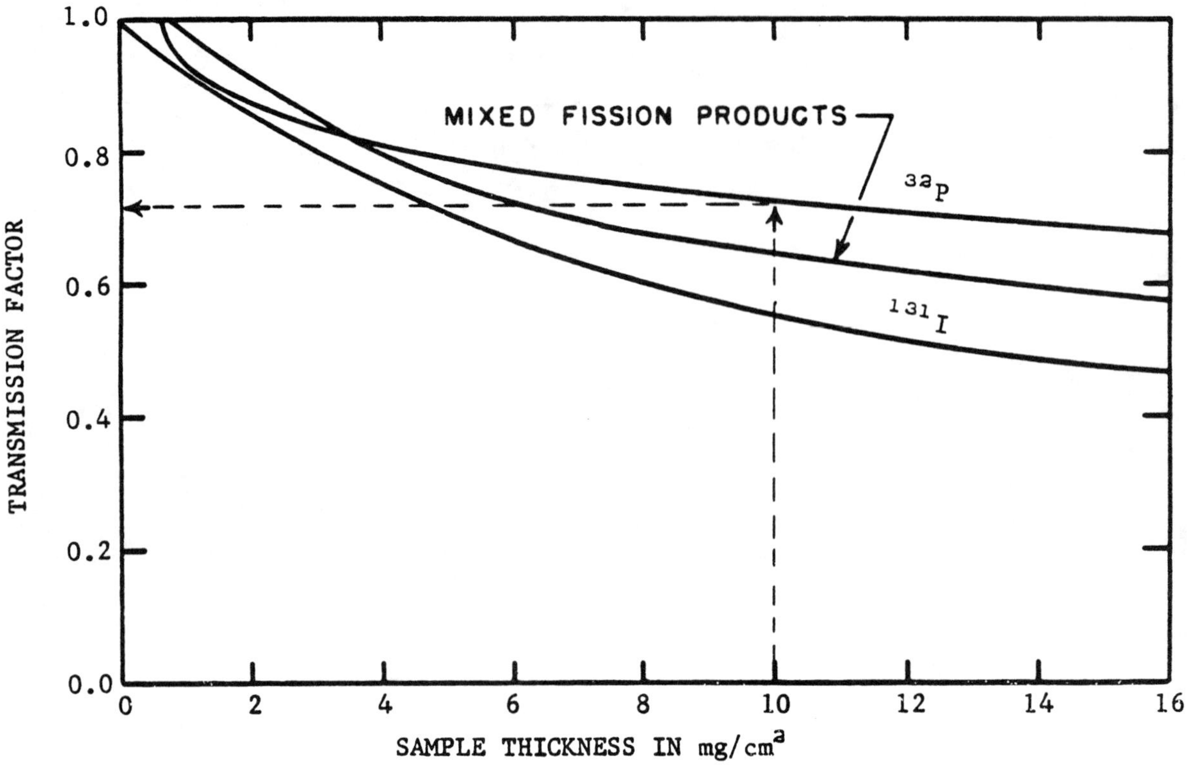

Figure 9.14 Transmission Factor—Counting Efficienc (From Setter et al., 1954)

Table 9.16 Backscatter of Normally Incident, Monoenergetic Electrons from Selected Materials[a]

(From Tabata, Ito and Okabe, 1971)

$$\text{Backscattering Factor} = a_1/(1 + a_2^{a_3})$$

where:

$$= \frac{\text{number of backscattered electrons}}{\text{number of incident electrons}}$$

$$= T/mc^2 \text{ (T = electron energy)}$$

$$a_1 = b_1 \exp(-b_2 Z^{-b_3})$$

$$a_2 = b_4 + b_5 Z^{-b_6}$$

$$a_3 = b_7 - b_8/Z$$

b_1	1.15 ± 0.06
b_2	8.35 ± 0.25
b_3	0.525 ± 0.020
b_4	0.0185 ± 0.0019
b_5	15.7 ± 3.1
b_6	1.59 ± 0.07
b_7	1.56 ± 0.02
b_8	4.42 ± 0.18

Note: The lower energy bound used in the data fit is 50 keV for Z 32, to 200 keV for Z 73. The relative rms deviation of the fit to the data is 2 to 8%, except that for carbon was 23%.

Note: These data are for a saturation thickness, i.e., typically 50% of the electron range for the material selected. Fig. 9.13 addresses isotropic backscatter from a surface into a detector.

[a] Figure 9.15 shows this function for several materials.

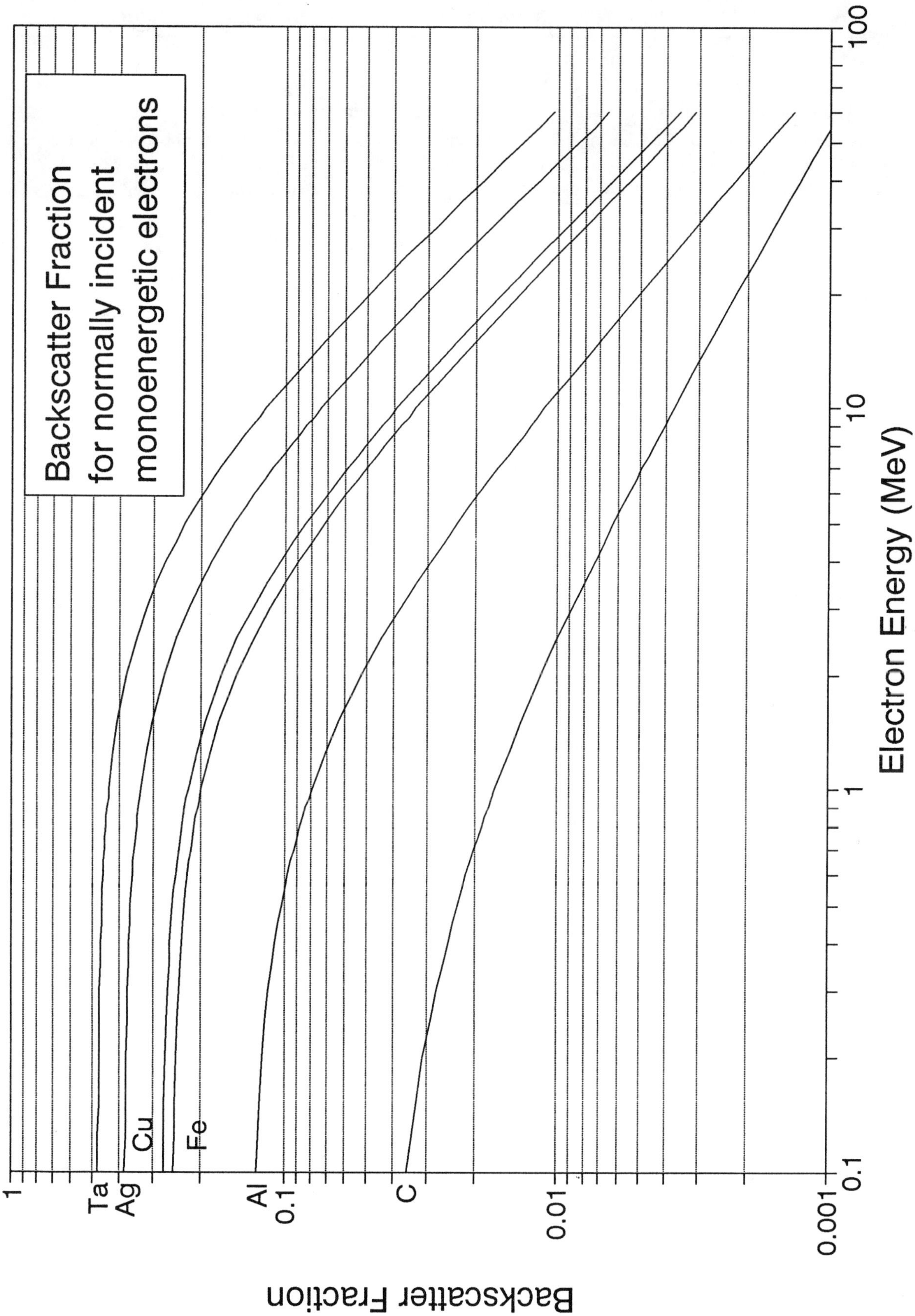

Figure 9.15 Backscatter of Normally Incident Electrons on Selected Materials

Table 9.17 Alpha Particle Counting with Pulse and Proportional Counters

Characteristics of the measurement which may introduce inaccuracies are:

Self-absorption. Because of the short range of the alpha particle, the self-absorption is usually very important. Generally, a chemical separation is advisable if the sample contains much inert substance.

Response across the chamber. Many chambers have a loss in sensitivity at the edge. The chamber should be checked with a point source to indicate the magnitude of this loss with the sample size used.

Coincidence losses. Those pulse counters which have long resolution times will have high resolution losses. This can be estimated by counting a number of low activity sources individually and then together.

Air samples collected on filter paper or with an electrostatic precipitator can be counted directly on pulse or proportional counters if correction is made for self-absorption and for the alpha emitting daughters of radon and thoron.

Table 9.18 Alpha Particle Counters—Typical Parameters for Current Systems (From Boecker et al., 1990)

Type of Detector	Minimum Detectable (mBq)[a,b]	Counting Time (min)	Background (c/m)	Efficiency (%)	Isotopic Selectivity[c]
Liquid scintillation	11.1	1000	10	80	poor
Gas flow proportional counter	7.4	1000	1	40	fair
Scintillation (ZnS)	0.4	1000	0.001	40	none
Surface barrier (Si)	0.7	1000	0.001	20	excellent

[a] Values given refer to measurement detectability and do not include consideration of chemical yield or sample size.
[b] 0.037 Bq = 1 pCi.
[c] Alpha particle energy resolution.

Table 9.19 Beta Particle Counters—Typical Parameters for Current Systems (From Boecker et al., 1990)

Type of Detector	Minimum Detectable (mBq)[a,b]	Counting Time (min)	Background (c/m)	Efficiency (%)	Isotopic Selectivity[c]
Gas flow GM and proportional counters	74	100	10	40	none
Liquid scintillation counter	37	100	10	80	poor
Anticoincidence, gas flow, GM, and proportional counters	3.7	1000	0.4	40	none
Plastic phosphor scintillation counter	7.4	1000	1	40	poor

[a] Values given refer to measurement detectability and do not include consideration of chemical yield or sample size.
[b] 37 mBq = 1 pCi.
[c] Beta particle energy resolution.

Table 9.20 Photon Counters—Typical Parameters for Current Systems (From Boecker et al., 1990)

Type of Detector	Minimum Detectable (mBq)[a,b]	Counting Time (min)	Background (c/m)	Efficiency (%)	Isotopic Selectivity[c]
Sodium iodide crystal NaI(Tl)	111	100	100	70	poor
High purity Ge and Ge(Li)	74	100	0.1	4	excellent
Si(Li)	5.6×10^3	100	0.5	0.1	excellent
Phoswich NaI/CsI	370	100	25	9	good

[a] 37 mBq = 1 pCi.
[b] Photon energy resolution.
[c] Resolution.

Table 9.21 Detection Capabilities[d]

Isotope	Mode of Detection	Typical Background (cpm)	System Detection Efficiency (%)	Estimated Lower Limit of Detection (pCi g^{-1})	Counting Time (min)	Sample Mass (g)	Minimum Detectable Concentration for Urinalysis[e] (pCi ml^{-1})
Gross	α	0.1	5–30	0.1–10	100–120	0.1–10	
Gross	β	1.2–2	19–51	0.3–10	100–120	0.1–10	
Gross	γ	5.0	variable	5[a]	500	500	
^{3}H	β	4.5–18	20–30	0.2–300	20–200	0.1–50	10
^{14}C	β	8–21	65–75	0.2–37	25–200	0.1–50	10
^{22}Na	γ	1	0.3	0.04–0.3	100	100–500	
^{36}Cl	β	22[b]	35[b]	0.5–10	100	50	
^{40}K	γ	1	0.3–35	0.35–3	100–120	100–500	
^{51}Cr	γ	1	1.2	0.2–2	100–120	100–500	
^{54}Mn	γ	1	0.5	0.2–0.3	100–500	100–500	
^{55}Fe	[c]	2.5–20	20–35	1–30	20–100	1–50	
^{58}Co	γ	1	0.5–30	0.007–0.3	120–500	100–750	
^{59}Fe	γ	1	0.4–30	0.05–0.5	100–500	100–500	
^{60}Co	γ	1	0.9–30	0.07–0.3	100–500	100–500	0.05
^{63}Ni	β	20	30–50	1–100	20–50	0.1–50	
^{65}Zn	γ	1	0.4–30	0.09–0.6	100–500	100–500	
^{89}Sr	β	0.05–1	45–58	0.5–1	100	1–25	0.02
^{90}Sr	β	0.5–1	20–58	0.03–5	100	1–25	0.02
^{90}Y	β	0.05–2	20–58	0.03–5	100	1–25	
^{99}Tc	β	2–30	20–33	0.3–15	50–100	1–10	
^{106}Ru	γ	1	0.7–30	0.2–1	100–500	100–500	
^{106}Rh	γ	1	0.7–30	0.35	100	1–500	

[a] Referenced to ^{137}Cs.
[b] Gamma data.
[c] Erroneous entry in reference. Probably x-ray.
[d] Results of a survey of 8 commercial labs and two DoE labs.
[e] After ANSI N13.30, 1996. Performance Criteria for Radiobioassay, Table C.2.

(continued)

Table 9.21 Detection Capabilities (Continued)[d]

Isotope	Mode of Detection	Typical Background (cpm)	System Detection Efficiency (%)	Estimated Lower Limit of Detection (pCi g^{-1})	Counting Time (min)	Sample Mass (g)	Minimum Detectable Concentration for Urinalysis[e] (pCi ml^{-1})
^{110m}Ag	γ	1	0.6–30	0.04	100–500	500	
^{125}Sb	γ	1	1–30	0.11	100–500	500	
^{129}I	β/γ	0.35–2	0.3–22	0.4–2	50–100	500	
^{133}Ba	γ	1	1.1–30	0.05–0.4	100–500	500	
^{134}Cs	γ	0.2–1	0.12–30	0.02–0.4	100–500	100–500	
^{137}Cs	γ	0.2–1	0.6–30	0.007–0.3	100–500	100–750	0.06
^{144}Ce	γ	1	2.2	0.23	100–500	500	
^{147}Pm	β	2–2.5	20–40	0.5–5	100	1–50	0.01
^{151}Sm	β	2.5	40	0.5	100	50	
^{154}Eu	γ	0.03–1	0.34–30	0.02–0.3	100–500	100–500	
^{204}Tl	β	0.5	40	1.0	100	50	
^{208}Tl	γ	1	0.7	0.14	100–500	500	
^{210}Pb	β/γ	2	20–36	0.5–5	100–200	1–10	0.005
^{210}Po	α	0.01	14–20	0.1–2	240–400	1–50	$1\ 10^{-4}$
^{210}Bi	β	2	20–35	0.1–5	100	1–50	
^{212}Pb	γ	1	1.6–30	0.08	100–500	500	
^{212}Bi	β	2,1	30,0.6	0.5–0.56	100	50–500	
^{212}Po	α	0.01	14–35	0.1	240–400	1–50	
^{214}Pb	γ	1	1.1	0.09	100–500	500	
^{214}Bi	γ	1	0.7	0.09	100–500	500	
^{224}Ra	β/γ	0.1–1	30/1.6	0.6/0.3–0.76	100–400	100–500	
^{226}Ra	γ	0.17–1	0.7–30	0.02–0.7	100–400	100–750	$1\ 10^{-4}$
^{228}Ra	γ	0.21–1	0.35–30	0.1–2	100–400	100–750	0.005
^{228}Th	γ	0.03	14–25	0.05–0.4	400–600	1–100	$1\ 10^{-4}$
^{230}Th	γ	0.01	14–25	0.05–0.5	400–700	1–10	$1\ 10^{-4}$
^{231}Th	β/γ	1	1.7	0.41	100–600	10–480	
^{232}Th	γ	0.01	25/–	0.05–2	400–700	1–10	$1\ 10^{-4}$
^{234}Th	β	0.4–1	0.23–30	0.1–5	100–600	1–500	
^{234}U	α	0.01	14–25	0.05–0.2	400–600	1–10	$1\ 10^{-4}$
^{235}U	α	0.004–0.01	14–25	0.02–0.3	400–1000	1–10	$1\ 10^{-4}$
^{236}U	α	0.01	14–25	0.05–0.2	400–600	1–10	
^{238}U	α	0.01	14–25	0.02–0.1	400–1000	1–10	$1\ 10^{-4}$
^{238}Pu	α	0.004–0.01	14–35	0.02–0.4	400–1000	1–10	$6\ 10^{-5}$
^{239}Pu	α	0.004–0.01	14–35	0.02–0.4	400–1000	1–10	$6\ 10^{-5}$
^{240}Pu	α	0.01	14–35	0.05–0.4	400–1000	1–10	$6\ 10^{-5}$
^{241}Pu	β	2–10	15–20	0.02–20	100–600	1–10	0.005
^{241}Am	α	0.008–0.01	14–35	0.05–0.5	400–700	1–10	$6\ 10^{-5}$
^{242}Cm	α	0.01	14–35	0.05–0.1	400–700	1–10	$6\ 10^{-5}$
^{244}Cm	α	0.005–0.01	14–35	0.05–0.1	400–700	1–10	$6\ 10^{-5}$
^{252}Cf	α	0	14	0.05	600	10	

[a] Referenced to ^{137}Cs.
[b] Gamma data.
[c] Erroneous entry in reference. Probably x-ray.
[d] Results of a survey of 8 commercial labs and two DoE labs.
[e] After ANSI N13.30, 1996. Performance Criteria for Radiobioassay, Table C.2.

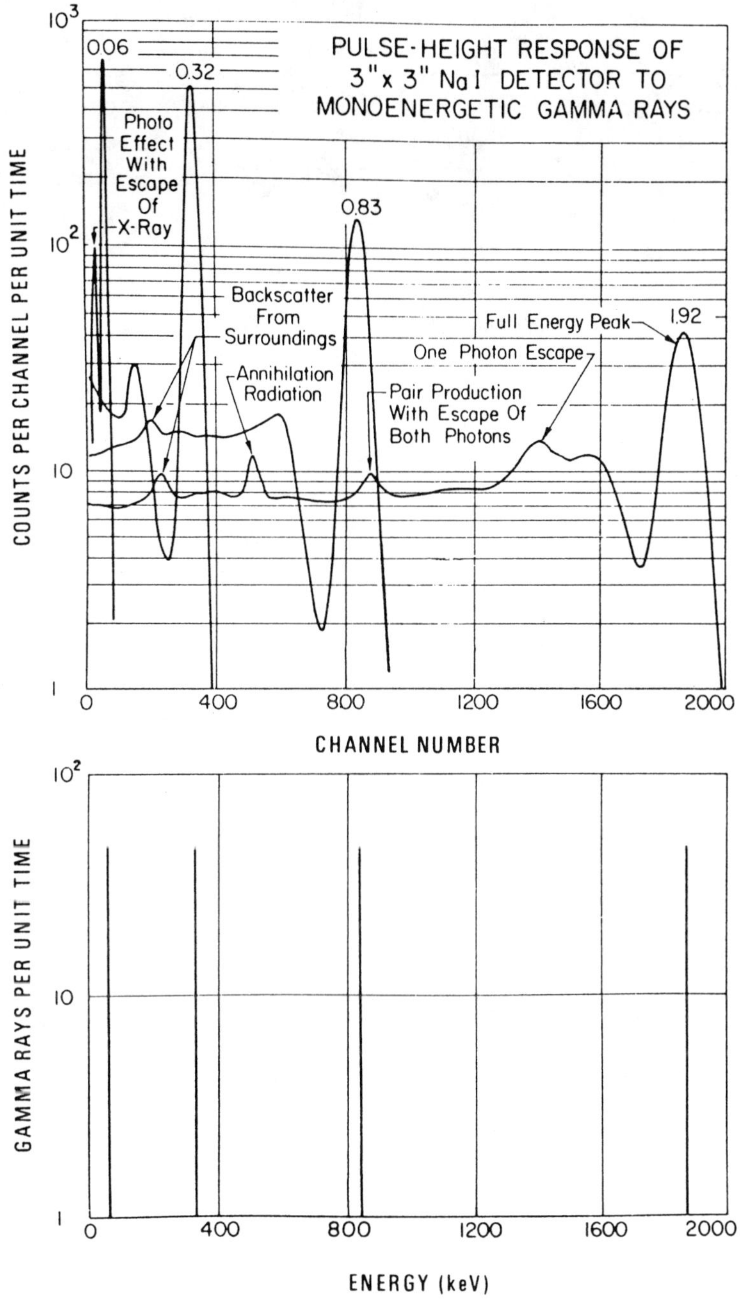

Figure 9.16 Pulse Height Distributions Obtained with a 3″ × 3″ NaI(Tl) Detector from monoenergetic gamma ray sources of 0.06, 0.32, 0.83, and 1.92 MeV normalized to equal emission rates. Pertinent features of these spectra are noted, including the decrease in detector efficiency with increasing energy. (Courtesy NCRP from Report No. 58, 1978, after Heath, 1964)

Table 9.22 Gamma-Ray Peaks in Residual Background of ImGe Detector[a] (Lindstrom, 1990)

Energy (keV)	Nuclide (source)	Origin	Count Rate (c/s)	Energy (keV)	Nuclide (source)	Origin	Count rate (c/s)
53.4	^{73m}Ge	cosmic	0.0004	511.0	β^{+} annih.	cosmic	0.029
66.7	^{73m}Ge	cosmic	0.003	569.5	^{207*}Pb	cosmic	0.0008
72.8	Pb $K_{\alpha 2}$	cosmic	0.009	583.1	^{208}Tl	thorium	0.0003
75.0	Pb $K_{\alpha 1}$	cosmic	0.015	596.1	^{74}Ge(n,n^{1})	cosmic	0.010
84.8	Pb $K_{\beta 1}$	cosmic	0.011	609.3	^{214}Bi	radon	0.001
87.3	Pb $K_{\beta 2}$	cosmic	0.003	693.4	^{72}Ge (n,n)	cosmic	0.007
109.9	^{19*}F[b]	cosmic	0.002				
122.1	^{57*}Fe	cosmic	0.0003	803.3	^{206*}Pb	cosmic	0.001
139.7	^{75m}Ge	cosmic	0.002	846.8	^{56*}Fe	cosmic	0.0006
159.7	^{77m}Ge	cosmic	0.001	911.2	^{228}Ac	thorium	0.0003
174.9	^{71*}Ge	cosmic	0.0003	1063.6	^{207*}Pb	cosmic	0.0003
197	^{71*}Ge + ^{19*}F[b]	cosmic	0.006	1120.3	^{214}Bi	radon	0.0003
				1173.2	^{60}Co	contamination	0.0006
238.6	^{212}Pb	thorium	0.0005	1332.5	^{60}Co	contamination	0.0006
295.2	^{214}Pb	radon	0.0004	1460.8	^{40}K	environmental	0.0003
352.0	^{214}Pb	radon	0.001				

[a] Using a 45% InGe detector surrounded by 15 cm of lead.
[b] The '*' indicates an excited nuclear state. The fluorine is in an inside teflon liner.

References

American National Standards Institute. *Radiation Protection Instrumentation Test and Calibration.* ANSI N323; 1978.

American National Standards Institute. *Performance Specifications for Health Physics Instrumentation.* ANSI N42.17A; 1989.

American National Standards Institute. *Performance Criteria for Radiobioassay.* ANSI N13.30; 1996.

Boecker, B., Hall, R., Inn, K., Lawrence, J., Ziemer, P., Eisele, G., Wacholz, B., Burr, W., Jr. ''Current status of bioassay procedures to detect and quantify previous exposures to radioactive materials,'' *Health Physics* **60:**(1):45–100; 1991.

Bramson et al. *Evaluation Testing and Calibration Methodology for Emergency Radiological Instrumentation.* BNWL; 1991.

Burgess, P.H. *Instrument Evaluation No. 27, Victoreen 471RF Radiation Survey Meter.* NRPB-IE27, National Radiological Protection Board Report. Chilton; 1982a.

Burgess, P.H. *Instrument Evaluation No. 28, Keithley Model 36100 Survey Meter.* NRPB-IE28, National Radiological Protection Board Report. Chilton 1982b.

Burgess, P.H.; Iles, W.J. *Instrument Evaluation No. 15, A Summary of the Performance of Exposure Rate and Dose Rate Instruments Contained in Instrument Evaluation Reports NRPB-IE1 to NRPB-IE13.* NRPB-IE15, National Radiological Protection Board Report; Chilton; 1979.

Burgess, P.H.; Iles, W.J. *Instrument Evaluation No. 22, Dosimeter Corporation of America Portable Survey Meter Type 3795 ''True Blue.''* NRPB-IE22, National Radiological Protection Board Report; Chilton; 1981.

Cox, F.M.; Guenther, C.F. ''An Industry Survey of Current Lower Limits of Detection for Various Radionuclides,'' *Health Physics* **69**(1):121–129; 1995.

Department of Health, Education and Welfare. *Radiological Health Handbook.* Public Health Service; Rockville, MD; 1970.

Gillings, J.C. et al. *Characterization of Emergency Preparedness at DOE Contractor Facilities.* PNL-4198; Battelle; 1984.

Heath, R.L. *Scintillation Spectrometry, Gamma-Ray Spectrum Catalogue, 2nd ed.* USAEC Report IDO-16880-1, U.S. Atomic Energy Commission; Idaho Falls, Idaho; 1964.

Hickey, E.E., Stoetzel, G.A., Olsen, P.C., McGuire, S.A. *Air Sampling in the Workplace.* U.S. Nuclear Regulatory Commission Report. NUREG-1400; 1991.

Hooker, C.D., Hadlock, D.E., Harrington, W.N., Gilchrist, R.L. *Interim Calibration and Field Use Guidance for Beta Portable Survey Instruments.* PNL-4378; Pacific Northwest Laboratory; Richland, WA; 1983.

Jester, W.A., Baratta, A.J., Granlund, R.W., Eidam, G.R. ''Evaluation of radiation monitor effectiveness for the detection of Kr,'' *Health Physics* **42:**827–832; 1982.

Kearney, C.H. *Trans-Pacific Fallout and Protective Countermeasures.* Oak Ridge National Laboratory Report ORNL-4900; Oak Ridge, TN; 1973.

Loevinger, R., Berman, M. ''Efficiency criteria in radioactivity counting,'' *Nucleonics* **9**(1):26; 1951.

Lindstrom, R., Lindstrom, D., Slaback, L., Langland, J. ''A low-background gamma-ray assay laboratory for activation analysis,'' *Nuc Inst and Methods in Physics Research* **A299**:425–429; 1990.

Nader, J.S., Hagee, G.R., Setter, L.R. ''Evaluating the performance of the internal counter,'' *Nucleonics* **12**(6): 1954.

National Council on Radiation Protection and Measurements. *A Handbook of Radioactivity Measurement Procedure.* NCRP Report No. 58; Bethesda, MD; 1978.

Selby, J.M., Swinth, K.L., Hooker, C.D., Kenoyer, J.L. *Field Measurement and Interpretation of Beta Dose and Dose Rates.* Proceedings of the International Beta Symposium. PNL-SA-15004; Battelle; 1987.

Setter, L.R., Goldin, A.S., Nader, J.S. ''Radioactivity assay of water and industrial wastes with internal proportional counter,'' *Analytical Chemistry* **26:**1305; American Chemical Society; 1954.

Shleien, B., Ed. *The Health Physics and Radiological Health Handbook.* Scinta, Inc.; Silver Spring, MD; 1984.

Shleien, B. *Preparedness and Response in Radiation Accidents.* National Center of Devices and Radiological Health, U.S. Dept. HHS; Rockville, MD; 1983.

Shlein, B., Schmidt, C.D., Chiacchierinni, R.P. *Background Document on Proposed Recommendations on Human Foods and Animal Feeds.* Food and Drug Administration; Rockville, MD; 1983.

Swinth, K.L., Kenoyer, J.L. ''Evaluation of health physics instrument performance,'' *IEEE Transactions on Nuclear Science* **NS-32**(1); 1985.

Tabata, T., Ito, R., Okabe, S. ''An empirical equation for the backscattering coefficient of electrons,'' *Nuclear Instruments and Methods* **94:**509–513; 1971.

Thompson, I.M.G. *International Standard Reference Radiations and Their Applications to the Type Testing of Dosimetric Apparatus. National and International Standardization of Radiation Dosimetry,* IAEA; Vienna; 1978.

U.S. Atomic Energy Commission, Report HW-70935; December 1962.

CHAPTER 10

PATIENT DOSES IN THE HEALING ARTS

Determinations of radiation doses to patients from x-ray procedures and radiopharmaceuticals are detailed in this chapter.

Instructions (after NCRP Report No. 102 adapted by J. Krohmer) are given for estimating doses from x-ray procedures. For selected pediatric procedures, the methodology developed by the Food and Drug Administration is presented. The effect of testicular and ovarian shielding is illustrated in tabular form.

Estimates of the Genetically Significant Dose (GSD) and mean annual bone marrow dose from diagnostic x-ray examinations are presented for the U.S. populations (1990).

This chapter also provides tables of patient doses from selected nuclear medicine procedures and estimates of fetal doses from ^{131}I.

TABLE OF CONTENTS

Table 10.1 Prospective Determination of Patient Doses for Various Diagnostic X-Ray Procedures (Adapted from NCRP 102, 1989 by Jack S. Krohmer)

The absorbed doses to selected organs during various diagnostic x-ray procedures included in ICRP Publication 34 are stated for an entrance kerma of 1 Gy (100 rad). The entrance kerma for any procedure is most accurately obtained or calculated from measurements made on the x-ray equipment which is used for the study. It may also be obtained from the data in Table 10.1.1 applying the actual kVp and mAs used for the diagnostic procedure in question. However, the entrance kerma can be determined *prospectively* as the product of the diagnostic receptor sensitivity (S) and the absorption factor (AF). The *receptor sensitivity* (S) is stated in tables 10.1.2, 10.1.3, 10.1.4 and 10.1.5 as air kerma to the front surface of the receptor in cGy or cGy/s while producing a good image. The *absorption factor* (AF) is the ratio of Entry to Exit dose in the patient; it is a function of the thickness of the patient part being studied and beam quality factors such as half-value-layer (See Table 10.1.4) or kVp and added filter, but it is nearly independent of the distance from the x-ray source to the entrance skin of the patient (SSD). Absorption factors are listed in Tables 10.1.6, 10.1.7 and 10.1.8.

Receptor sensitivities (S) are listed for the following x-ray receptors:

Radiographic screen-film systems used at 70 kVp and above	Table 10.1.2
Mammographic screen-film systems and other systems used below 70 kVp	Table 10.1.3
Xeromammographic systems	Table 10.1.4
Image intensifier fluoroscopic systems and associated static imaging systems	Table 10.1.5

Absorption factors (AF) are listed for the following x-ray procedures:

General radiography and fluoroscopy including associated static imaging	Table 10.1.6
Screen-film mammography	Table 10.1.7
Xeromammography	Table 10.1.8

Sample calculations using these data are as follows:

1. Radiographic study on patient part 20 cm thick using 120 kVp single phase xrays (HVL = 4.0 Al) and medium speed rare earth screens (2) with medium speed film.
   $S = 0.5 \times 10^{-3}$ cGy (From Table 10.1.2)
   $AF = 17.3$ (From Table 10.1.6)
   Entrance air kerma $= S \times AF = 8.65 \times 10^{-3}$ cGy
   Note that the choice of screen produces a spatial resolution of 6 line pairs per millimeter (lp/mm).
2. One minute (60 s) of fluoroscopy on patient part 15 cm thick using 100 kVp three phase x rays (HVL = 3.0 Al) with TV or video viewing.
   $S = 0.1 \times 10^{-3}$ cGy/s (From Table 10.1.5)
   $AF = 10.2$ (From Table 10.1.6)
   Entrance air kerma rate $= S \times AF = 1.02 \times 10^{-3}$ cGy/s
   Entrance air kerma $= (1.02 \times 10^{-3}) \times 60 = 6.12 \times 10^{-2}$ cGy
   Note that Video produces spatial resolution of about 2 lp/mm.
3. Screen-film mammogram on 6 cm thick breast with single slow rare earth screen and medium speed film and at 28 kVp with no filter using a molybdenum target tube (HVL = 0.31 mm Al).
   $S = 15 \times 10^{-3}$ cGy (From Table 10.1.3 A)
   $AF = 101$ (From Table 10.1.7)
   Entrance air kerma $= S \times AF = 1.515$ cGy
   Note that using the data in Table 10.1.9 the critical average glandular dose (AGD) is:
   AGD $=$ Entrance air kerma $\times 0.13 = 0.197$ cGy
   Note that spatial resolution for slow screen choice is 17 lp/mm.

The dose to structures below the entrance surface can be estimated by multiplying the percent depth dose (%DD) obtained from Table 10.1.1 by the kerma at the entrance surface. The %DD must be determined for the appropriate HVL, depth and field size.

The methods described here can be used, as stated, to prospectively estimate entrance air kerma for various diagnostic x-ray studies. They can also be used to prospectively compare various imaging techniques prior to patient exposure.[a]

[a] For an alternative method for estimation of diagnostic x-ray procedure doses see Rosenstein FDA 89–8031 1988.

Table 10.1.1 Average Air Kerma Rates Produced by Diagnostic X-Ray Equipment (Courtesy NCRP from Report 102, 1989)

Distance from Source to Point of Measurement	Tube Potential (kVp)											
	40	50	60	70	80	90	100	110	120	130	140	150
Centimeters	**Centigray per 100 milliampere-seconds**[a]											
30	1.8	3.3	5.1	6.9 (4.1)	8.9 (5.2)	11.3 (6.6)	12.8 (7.5)	14.7 (8.6)	17.8 (10.5)	21.1 (12.4)	22.9 (13.5)	25.6 (15.1)
45	0.79 (0.46)	1.5 (0.88)	2.3 (1.4)	3.1 (1.8)	3.9 (2.3)	5.0 (2.9)	5.7 (3.4)	6.5 (3.8)	7.9 (4.6)	9.4 (5.5)	10.2 (6.0)	11.4 (6.7)
60	0.44 (0.26)	0.83 (0.49)	1.3 (0.76)	1.7 (1.0)	2.2 (1.3)	2.8 (1.6)	3.2 (1.9)	3.7 (2.2)	4.4 (2.6)	5.3 (3.1)	5.7 (3.4)	6.4 (3.8)
100	0.16 (0.09)	0.30 (0.18)	0.46 (0.27)	0.62 (0.36)	0.80 (0.47)	1.0 (0.59)	1.1 (0.65)	1.3 (0.76)	1.6 (0.94)	1.9 (1.1)	2.1 (1.2)	2.3 (1.4)
137	0.09 (0.05)	0.16 (0.09)	0.24 (0.14)	0.33 (0.19)	0.42 (0.25)	0.54 (0.32)	0.61 (0.36)	0.70 (0.41)	0.85 (0.50)	1.0 (0.59)	1.1 (0.65)	1.2 (0.71)
183	0.05 (0.03)	0.09 (0.05)	0.14 (0.08)	0.18 (0.11)	0.24 (0.14)	0.30 (0.18)	0.34 (0.20)	0.39 (0.23)	0.48 (0.28)	0.57 (0.34)	0.62 (0.36)	0.69 (0.41)

[a] Calculated from Figure 3, Zamenhof et al., 1987. Values not in parentheses are for three phase generators. Values in parentheses are for single phase generators. All air kerma values are for total filtration equivalent to 2.5 mm aluminum. For total filtration above 2.5 mm aluminum, read value from Figure 10.1 Air Kerma for 3 Phase X-Ray Units.

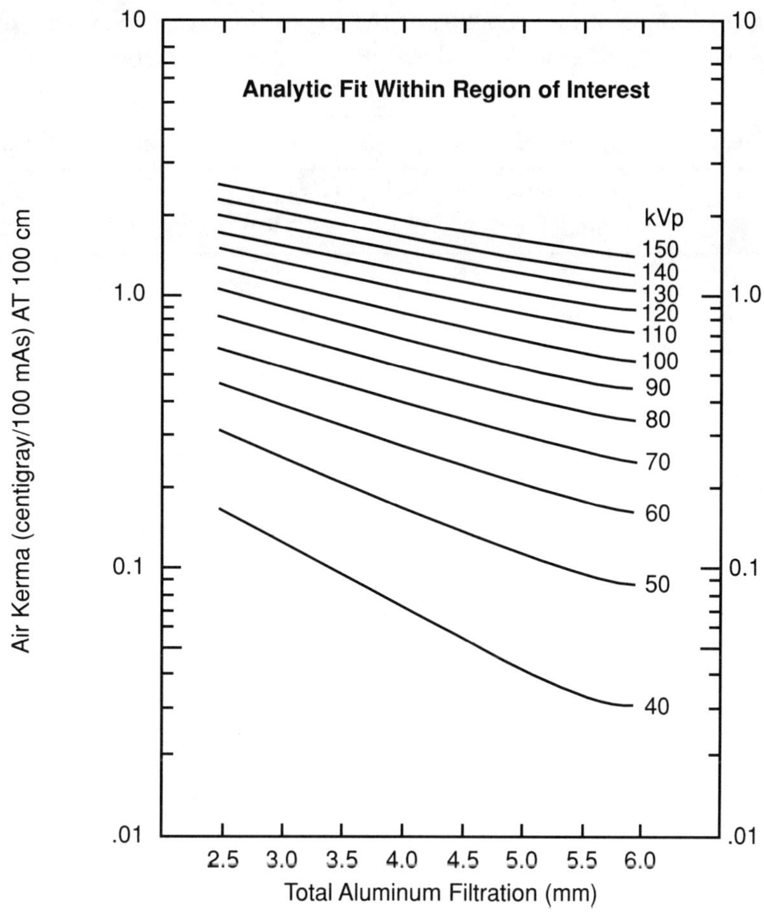

Figure 10.1 Air Kerma for 3 Phase X-Ray Units[a] (Courtesy NCRP from Report 102, 1989)

[a] To obtain air kerma for single phase units divide reading obtained from Figure by 1.7.

Table 10.1.2 Typical Values of Air Kerma[a] at the Front Surface of Screen-Film Systems Used at 70 kVp and above[b] with Resolution Values (Courtesy NCRP from Report 102, 1989 after Rao, Johns Hopkins University, personal communication)

A. $CaWO_4$ Screens (two) Used with Blue Sensitive Film (Double Emulsion)

Screen[b]	Slow Film[c] (0.5×)	Medium Film[c] (1×)	Fast Film[c] (2×)
Slow (0.5×) 7 lp/mm	4.0×10^{-3} cGy	2.0×10^{-3} cGy	1.0×10^{-3} cGy
Medium (1×) 5 lp/mm	2.0×10^{-3} cGy	1.0×10^{-3} cGy[d]	0.5×10^{-3} cGy
Fast (2×) 3.5 lp/mm	1.0×10^{-3} cGy	0.5×10^{-3} cGy	$.025 \times 10^{-3}$ cGy

B. Rare Earth Screens (two) Used with Green Sensitive Film (Double Emulsion)

Screen[b]	Slow Film[c] (0.5×)	Medium Film[c] (1×)	Fast Film[c] (2×)
Slow (1×) 8.5 lp/mm	2.0×10^{-3} cGy	1.0×10^{-3} cGy	0.5×10^{-3} cGy
Medium (2×) 6 lp/mm	1.0×10^{-3} cGy	0.5×10^{-3} cGy[e]	0.25×10^{-3} cGy
Fast (4×) 4.3 lp/mm	0.5×10^{-3} cGy	0.25×10^{-3} cGy	0.125×10^{-3} cGy
Extrafast (6×) 3.5 lp/mm	0.33×10^{-3} cGy	0.17×10^{-3} cGy	0.08×10^{-3} cGy

[a] When the air kerma is 1 cGy the exposure is approximately 1R.
[b] Screen speeds relative to Dupont Par speed $CaWO_4$ screens (2 screens).
[c] Film speeds relative to Dupont Cronex 4 film (double emulsion).
[d] Dupont Par speed screens with Cronex 4 film.
[e] 3M Trimax 4 screens with XD film.

Table 10.1.3 Typical Values of Air Kerma[a] at the Front Surface of Screen-Film Systems Used Between 50 and 70 kVp with Resolution Values (Courtesy NCRP from Report 102, 1989 after Rao, Johns Hopkins University, personal communication)

A. $CaWO_4$ Screens (two) Used with Blue Sensitive Film (Single Screen Emulsion)			
Screen[b]	**Slow Film[c] (0.25×)**	**Medium Film[c] (0.5×)**	**Fast Film[c] (1×)**
Slow (0.1×) 14 lp/mm	40×10^{-3} cGy	20×10^{-3} cGy	10×10^{-3} cGy
Medium (0.2×) 10 lp/mm	20×10^{-3} cGy	10×10^{-3} cGy	5×10^{-3} cGy
Fast (0.4×) 7 lp/mm	10×10^{-3} cGy	5×10^{-3} cGy	2.5×10^{-3} cGy
B. Rare Earth Screen Used with Green Sensitive Film (Single Screen Emulsion)			
Screen[b]	**Slow Film[c] (0.16×)**	**Medium Film[c] (0.33×)**	**Fast Film[c] (0.66×)**
Slow (0.2×) 17 lp/mm	30×10^{-3} cGy	15×10^{-3} cGy	7.5×10^{-3} cGy
Medium (0.4×) 12 lp/mm	15×10^{-3} cGy	15×10^{-3} cGy[e]	3.8×10^{-3} cGy
Fast (0.8×) 8.5 lp/mm	7.5×10^{-3} cGy	3.8×10^{-3} cGy	1.9×10^{-3} cGy

[a] When the air kerma is 1 cGy the exposure is approximately 1R.
[b] Screen speeds relative to Dupont Par speed $CaWO_4$ screens (2 screens). The resolution of a screen-film system is established by the screen and not the film.
[c] Film speeds relative to Dupont Cronex 4 film (double emulsion).

Table 10.1.4 Typical Values of Air Kerma at the Front Surface of Xerox Detectors to Produce Acceptable Images and Typical Values of the Resolution for High Contrast Objects (Courtesy NCRP from Report 102, 1989)

System	Air Kerma[a,b] (cGy)	Approximate Resolution Limit[c] (lp/mm)
Xerox 125 (neg. mode)	120×10^{-3}	10
Xerox 175 (neg. mode)	65×10^{-3}	10
(pos. mode)	80×10^{-3}	10

[a] When the air kerma is 1 cGy the exposure is approximately 1R.
[b] Speiser et al., 1986.

Table 10.1.5 Typical Values of Air Kerma[a] or Air Kerma Rate at the Front Surface of Image Intensifier Systems with Resolution Values (Courtesy NCRP from Report 102, 1989)

A. Air Kerma Rate Values to Produce Acceptable Fluoroscopy Images

System	$cGy\ s^{-1}$	lp/mm
1) Mirror[b]	0.05×10^{-3} to 0.15×10^{-3}	4
2) Video[b]	0.05×10^{-3} to 0.15×10^{-3}	1.4–2.6

B. Air Kerma to Produce Static Images Equivalent to that Produced by a Par Speed Screen-Film System

Recorder	Intensifier Input Field Diameter	cGy	lp/mm
1) SF Camera[c]	10 cm	0.5×10^{-3}	4
	15 cm	0.23×10^{-3}	4
	23 cm	0.10×10^{-3}	4
2) 35 mm cine[c]	23 cm	0.002×10^{-3}	4
3) Video-Digital[d]	23 cm	2.0×10^{-3}	1.4–2.6

[a] When the air kerma is 1 cGy the exposure is approximately 1 R.

[b] Private Communication from Picker X-ray Corp.

[c] P. Sprawls, 1977.

[d] Private communication from Technicare.

Table 10.1.6 General Radiography Absorption Factor (Ratio of Entry to Exit Dose) (Tungsten Target, Inherent Filter, 60 cm SSD, 35 × 35 cm Field Size) (Courtesy NCRP from Report 102, 1989 after Harrison, 1981)

Thickness of Overlying Tissue to Exit Surface (centimeters)	Absorption Factor (AF)[a]					
	Half-Value-Layer (mm Al)					
	1.0	1.5	2.0	3.0	4.0	5.0
0	1.00	1.00	1.00	1.00	1.00	1.00
1	1.39	1.25	1.18	1.07	1.02	1.01
2	2.04	1.64	1.47	1.28	1.15	1.06
3	3.29	2.10	1.81	1.54	1.35	1.17
4	3.79	2.75	2.20	1.78	1.55	1.35
5	5.13	3.45	2.62	2.11	1.82	1.56
6	6.67	4.35	3.13	2.50	2.12	1.80
7	8.33	5.26	3.73	2.94	2.48	2.09
8	10.5	6.41	4.42	3.42	2.90	2.40
9	13.3	7.69	5.13	3.98	3.34	2.76
10	17.2	9.35	5.99	4.61	3.82	3.20
11	21.8	11.5	7.10	5.43	4.50	3.75
12	26.3	13.7	8.20	6.25	5.18	4.30
13	33.2	16.9	9.70	7.40	6.11	4.90
14	40.0	20.0	11.2	8.55	7.04	5.70
15	53.3	24.3	13.3	10.2	8.28	6.60
16	66.7	28.6	15.4	11.8	9.52	7.00
20	168	63.0	29.5	22.0	17.3	13.7
25	550	165	65.5	49.0	36.5	27.8
30	1800	440	146	108	78.0	57.0
35		1150	330	240	166	118

[a] These Absorption Factors are for Source-Skin-Distance (SSD) of 60 cm; they are correct to within ±10% for all SSD's from 45 to 90 cm.

Table 10.1.7 Screen Film Mammography Absorption Factor[a] (Ratio of Entry to Exit Dose) (Molybdenum Target, 0.03 mm Molybdenum Filter, 55 cm SSD) (Courtesy NCRP from Report 102, 1989)

Thickness of Overlying Tissue to Exit Surface	Absorption Factor (AF)						
	kVp/mm Al Added Filter						
	24/0	25/0	26/0	28/0	30/0	32/0	35/0
	Half-value-layer (mm Al)						
Centimeters	0.305	0.31	0.32	0.335	0.35	0.365	0.39
0	1.00	1.00	1.00	1.00	1.00	1.00	1.00
1	3.16	3.07	2.98	2.82	2.72	2.66	2.36
2	7.81	7.45	7.09	6.49	6.10	5.81	5.32
3	18.0	16.8	15.6	13.9	12.7	11.8	10.8
4	39.1	36.0	32.8	28.4	25.2	23.0	20.1
5	82.6	74.4	66.2	55.2	47.8	42.6	35.3
6	169	148	127	101	84.7	73.0	59.5
7	294	257	220	173	143	120	93.5

[a] Adapted from Table A-2, Report No. 85 (NCRP, 1986).

Table 10.1.8 Xeromammography Absorption Factor[a] (Ratio of Entry to Exit Dose) (Tungsten Target, 72 cm SSD) (Courtesy NCRP from Report 102, 1989)

Thickness of Overlying Tissue to Exit Surface	Absorption Factor (AF)	
	kVp/mm Al Added Filter	
	45/1.6	50/2.1
	Half-value-layer (mm Al)	
Centimeters	0.94	1.33
0	1.00	1.00
1	1.58	1.39
2	2.34	1.93
3	3.36	2.58
4	4.67	3.38
5	6.37	4.41
6	8.33	5.59
7	10.9	7.14
8	14.4	9.17

[a] Adapted from Table A-2, Report No. 85 (NCRP, 1986).

Table 10.1.9 Average Glandular Dose in Mammography per Unit Entrance Air Kerma (cGy)[a]

(Courtesy NCRP from Report 102, 1989)

Thickness of Overlying Tissue to Exit Surface (cm)	Molybdenum Target HVL (mm Al)	Tungsten Target HVL (mm Al)					
	0.31	0.30	0.8	1.0	1.2	1.4	1.6
3.0	0.25	0.25	0.54	0.61	0.68	0.74	0.82
3.5	0.22	0.23	0.49	0.56	0.63	0.70	0.76
4.0	0.20	0.21	0.45	0.52	0.59	0.66	0.72
4.5	0.18	0.20	0.42	0.49	0.55	0.62	0.68
5.0	0.16	0.17	0.39	0.45	0.52	0.59	0.65
5.5	0.14	0.16	0.36	0.43	0.49	0.56	0.62
6.0	0.13	0.14	0.34	0.40	0.46	0.53	0.59
6.5	0.12	0.13	0.32	0.38	0.44	0.50	0.56
7.0	0.11	0.11	0.30	0.36	0.41	0.48	0.54
7.5	—	—	0.28	0.33	0.39	0.45	0.51
8.0	—	—	0.26	0.32	0.37	0.43	0.49

[a] Adapted from Table 3.3, Report No. 85 (NCRP 1986)

Table 10.1.10 Average Percentage Depth Doses for Diagnostic X-Ray Beams[a] (Courtesy NCRP from Report 102, 1989 after Harrison 1981)

	Half-Value Layer in Millimeters of Aluminum														
	1.0			1.5			2.0			3.0			4.0		
	Field Size in Centimeters														
	0	15 × 15	35 × 35	0	15 × 15	35 × 35	0	15 × 15	35 × 35	0	15 × 15	35 × 35	0	15 × 15	35 × 35
	Backscatter Factor (BSF)														
	1.00	1.22	1.25	1.00	1.26	1.28	1.00	1.27	1.32	1.00	1.37	1.39	1.00	1.40	1.42
Depth (cm)															
0	100	100	100	100	100	100	100	100	100	100	100	100	100	100	100
1	54.0	70.9	71.9	64.0	78.3	80.3	68.0	84.0	85.0	73.5	91.8	93.7	76.0	94.2	97.7
2	34.0	46.5	49.1	41.0	59.0	60.9	45.5	66.4	68.1	52.0	76.0	78.0	55.0	81.3	87.2
3	20.3	33.5	30.4	26.5	44.9	47.7	31.5	52.8	55.4	37.0	62.7	65.0	40.5	69.5	74.1
4	13.5	25.0	26.4	18.3	34.7	36.3	22.0	42.9	45.5	27.5	52.2	56.2	30.5	58.4	64.6
5	8.8	18.6	19.5	12.6	26.9	29.0	16.0	34.8	39.2	20.5	43.0	47.3	23.0	48.9	55.0
6	6.0	13.9	15.0	9.0	20.9	23.0	11.4	28.2	31.9	15.2	35.6	40.0	17.0	41.0	47.2
7	4.1	10.9	12.0	6.4	16.6	19.0	8.5	23.0	26.8	11.3	29.4	34.0	13.0	34.1	40.3
8	2.9	8.6	9.5	4.7	13.2	15.6	6.3	18.8	22.6	8.7	24.3	29.2	10.1	28.4	34.5
9	2.1	6.7	7.5	3.4	10.5	13.0	4.7	15.5	19.5	6.7	20.1	25.1	7.7	23.7	29.9
10	1.5	5.3	5.8	2.5	8.4	10.7	3.5	12.7	16.7	5.0	16.7	21.7	5.7	19.8	26.2
12	0.8	3.2	3.8	1.4	5.3	7.3	2.0	8.6	12.2	3.1	11.6	16.0	3.5	13.9	19.3
14	0.4	2.0	2.5	0.8	3.4	5.0	1.2	5.8	8.9	1.9	8.0	11.7	2.2	9.7	14.2
16	0.2	1.3	1.5	0.5	2.2	3.5	0.8	3.9	6.5	1.2	5.5	8.5	1.4	6.8	10.5
20	0.1	0.5	0.6	0.2	1.0	1.6	0.4	2.0	3.4	0.6	2.9	4.5	0.8	3.8	5.8
25	—	0.2	0.2	0.1	0.4	0.6	0.2	0.9	1.5	0.3	1.3	2.0	0.4	1.7	2.7
30	—	0.1	0.1	—	0.1	0.2	0.1	0.4	0.7	0.1	0.6	0.9	0.2	0.8	1.3
35	—	—	—	—	—	0.1	—	0.2	0.3	—	0.3	0.4	0.1	0.4	0.6

[a] Percentage depth doses are for Source to Skin-Distance (SSD) of 60 cm; they are correct to within 10% for all SSDs from 45 to 90 cm.

Table 10.2.1 Effect of Testicular Shielding on Absorbed Dose to the Testes (From Rosenstein FDA 89-8031, 1988)

AP View Field Size at Film 14″ × 17″ (35.6 cm × 43.2 cm)	SID = 40″ (102 cm)
Testes Center and X-ray Field Edge Separation[a] (cm)	**Relative Absorbed Dose to the Testes after Shielding**
−15	0.17
−10	0.15
−5	0.13
−4	0.12
−3	0.11
−2	0.10
−1	0.10
0	0.13
1	0.14
2	0.21
3	0.26
4	0.33
5	0.36
10	0.80
15	0.90

[a] This separation is measured between the testes center and the nearest edge of the entrance x-ray field on the patient surface.
For −15 cm: testes are centered in field. For −2 to 2 cm: testes are partially in field.
For −3 to −15 cm: testes are completely in field. For 3 to 15 cm: testes are out of field.

Table 10.2.2 Effect of Ovarian or Uterine Shielding on Absorbed Dose to the Ovaries or Uterus[a] (From Rosenstein FDA 89-8031, 1988)

AP or PA View Field Size at Film 14″ × 17″ (35.6 cm × 43.2 cm)	SID = 40″ (102 cm)
Separation (cm) Between the Ovaries or Uterus and the X-ray Field[b]	**Relative Absorbed Dose to the Ovaries or Uterus after Shielding**
Completely or partially in the field, or separated by less than 3 cm from field edge	0.65
Separated by 3 cm to 6 cm from field edge	0.80
Separated by more than 6 cm from field edge	1.00

[a] The relative absorbed doses were computed directly for shielding of the ovaries in the AP view. It is assumed that the same values would apply nominally for shielding of the ovaries in the PA view and the uterus in the AP and PA views.
[b] This separation is taken as the estimated vertical separation between the nearest point of the ovaries or uterus and the nearest edge of the entrance x-ray field on the patient surface.

Table 10.3.1 Estimating Organ Doses from Diagnostic X-Ray Examinations to Children (From Rosenstein et al. FDA 79-8079, 1979).

1. Assignment of organ doses to individual pediatric patients using the data in Tables 10.3.7.1 through 10.3.9 is not recommended unless the physical characteristics of the patient closely correlate with one of the three reference pediatric patients given in Table 10.3.4.
2. Select the radiographic projection (e.g., PA Abdomen). The field centers used in locating each of the radiographic projections are given in Table 10.3.5. The anatomical limits of the x-ray field sizes denoted as collimated to the body part are described in Table 10.3.6.
3. Determine the actual beam quality (HVL, mm Al) and entrance exposure free-in-air (R) at the facility. If not determined by direct measurement, beam quality and radiation output can be estimated from Tables 10.3.21 and 10.3.3 when the kVp, total filtration and waveform of the x-ray machine are known.
4. Look up the organ dose (mrad) for 1 R entrance exposure in Table 10.3.7.1 to 10.3.9. Since the listed HVLs are nominal and have not been fitted by a smooth function, selection of the closest table entry to the beam quality of interest is recommended. Source-to-image receptor distances (SID) within 10 inches (25 cm) of the listed SID will not result in variation in dose larger than 10%.
5. Multiply the organ dose (mrad) obtained in instruction 4 by the actual entrance exposure free-in-air (R) to obtain the organ dose for the projection. The dose represents the value for the reference pediatric patients described in HEW Publication (FDA) 79-8079.

Table 10.3.2 Diagnostic X-Ray Spectra Used to Determine Tissue Doses[a] (From Rosenstein FDA 89-8031, 1988)

Number of X ray Spectra	Range of kVp	Range of HVL (mm Al)
9	45 to 70	1.0 to 3.6
9	80 to 90	1.7 to 5.5
9	98 to 120	3.1 to 6.0

[a] The author has additional tabulations for each of the three separate ranges of kilovoltages, should the reader require these more detailed data. The number of tables prohibits inclusion of all the data in the Handbook, but the author can make all or part of the expanded tabulations available, upon request.

Table 10.3.2.1 Average Beam Qualities, Entrance Exposures and Number of Films Used for Various Examinations (Radiographic-Adults)[a]

Projection	Projection[b]	Beam Quality (HVL, mm Al)	Entrance Exposure (C/kg × 10^{-4})[c]	Average Number of Films per Examination	
				Projection	Total
Chest	AP	2.44	0.13	0.10	1.5
	PA	2.51	0.07	0.92	
	LAT	2.80	0.21	0.50	
	OBL	2.49	0.31	0.02	
Skull	AP	2.45	1.24	1.24	4.1
	PA	2.45	1.14	1.09	
	LAT	2.26	0.73	1.67	
	OBL	2.41	0.57	0.09	
Cervical Spine	AP	2.23	0.67	1.45	3.7
	PA	2.43	0.39	0.04	
	LAT	2.35	0.44	1.27	
	OBL	2.35	0.51	0.89	
Ribs	AP	2.24	0.92	0.87	3.0
	PA	2.44	0.75	0.80	
	LAT	2.98	0.48	0.08	
	OBL	2.38	1.62	1.20	
Shoulder (one)	AP	2.15	0.50	1.45	1.8
	PA	2.10	0.38	0.04	
	LAT	2.53	2.51	0.15	
	OBL	2.30	0.79	0.13	
Thoracic Spine	AP	2.37	1.71	1.07	2.1
	PA	2.50	1.33	0.00	
	LAT	2.42	3.76	0.93	
	OBL	2.42	1.95	0.12	
Cholecystogram	AP	2.46	1.40	0.48	3.2
	PA	2.41	1.41	1.41	
	LAT	2.51	1.94	0.13	
	OBL	2.52	1.92	1.21	
Lumbar Spine	AP	2.37	2.28	1.03	2.9
	PA	2.48	1.40	0.03	
	LAT	2.58	8.25	1.33	
	OBL	2.51	2.86	0.46	
Upper Gastrointestinal	AP	2.80	1.65	0.73	4.3
	PA	2.86	1.41	1.15	
	LAT	3.01	2.96	.051	
	OBL	2.94	2.00	1.93	

[a] From Laws and Rosenstein (1978), with exception of mammography.
[b] AP, Anterior-Posterior; PA, Posterior-Anterior; LAT, lateral; OBL, oblique (fluoroscopy not included).
[c] 2.58 × 10^{-4} C/kg - 1R.

(continued)

Table 10.3.2.1 Average Beam Qualities, Entrance Exposures and Number of Films Used for Various Examinations (Radiographic-Adults)[a] (Continued)

Projection	Projection[b]	Beam Quality (HVL, mm Al)	Entrance Exposure (C/kg × 10^{-4})[c]	Average Number of Films per Examination	
				Projection	Total
Abdomen (kidneys, ureters, bladder)	AP	2.54	1.71	1.28	1.7
	PA	2.45	1.08	0.23	
	LAT	2.51	5.41	0.07	
	OBL	2.44	3.15	0.11	
Barium Enema	AP	2.95	1.96	1.52	4.0
	PA	2.92	1.99	0.93	
	LAT	3.12	10.35	0.49	
	OBL	3.05	3.48	1.02	
Lumbosacral Spine	AP	2.40	2.35	1.21	3.4
	PA	2.35	5.04	0.08	
	LAT	2.65	8.98	1.43	
	OBL	2.54	4.14	0.70	
Intravenous Pyelogram	AP	2.47	1.54	4.51	5.5
	PA	2.53	1.14	0.20	
	LAT	2.59	1.36	0.04	
	OBL	2.59	2.36	0.70	
Pelvis	AP	2.39	1.41	1.04	1.3
	PA	2.40	0.79	0.02	
	LAT	2.64	3.46	0.13	
	OBL	2.61	3.72	0.14	
Hip	AP	2.36	1.16	1.21	2.0
	PA	1.80	1.11	0.01	
	LAT	2.44	2.34	0.76	
	OBL	2.30	2.39	0.07	
Full Spine (chiropractic)	AP	3.50	0.72	1.0	1.0
Mammography[d]	craniocaudal	[e]	2.5	1.0	2.0
	mediolateral		2.5	1.0	

[a] From Laws and Rosenstein (1978), with exception of mammography.
[b] AP, Anterior-Posterior; PA, Posterior-Anterior; LAT, lateral; OBL, oblique (fluoroscopy not included).
[c] 2.58 × 10^{-4} C/kg - 1R.
[d] The U.S. population x-ray survey (FDA, 1973) did not adequately represent current usage of mammography as a diagnostic modality. The HVLs and entrance exposures in current mammography vary according to technique. These conditions were chosen as representative for the purposes of this NCRP Report.
[e] Not specified.

Table 10.3.3 Half-Value Layers as a Function of Filtration and Tube Potential for Diagnostic Units (Courtesy NCRP from Report 102, 1989)

Total Filtration mm Al	Peak Tube Potential (kVp)									
	30	40	50	60	70	80	90	100	110	120
	Typical Half-Value Layers in Millimeters of Aluminum									
	Single Phase, Full wave[a]									
0.5	0.4	0.5	0.6	0.7	0.8	0.8	0.9	1.0	1.1	1.2
1.0	0.6	0.8	1.0	1.1	1.2	1.3	1.5	1.6	1.7	1.8
1.5	0.8	1.0	1.3	1.4	1.6	1.8	1.9	2.1	2.3	2.4
2.0	0.9	1.2	1.5	1.7	1.9	2.1	2.3	2.5	2.7	2.9
2.5	1.0	1.4	1.7	2.0	2.2	2.4	2.6	2.8	3.1	3.3
3.0	—	1.5	1.9	2.2	2.4	2.6	2.9	3.1	3.4	3.7
3.5	—	1.6	2.0	2.3	2.6	2.9	3.1	3.4	3.7	4.0
	Three Phase									
2.5[b]				2.2	2.4	2.7	3.1	3.3	3.6	4.0
3.0[b]				2.3	2.6	3.0	3.3	3.6	4.0	4.3
3.5[b]				2.6	2.9	3.2	3.6	3.9	4.3	4.6

[a] Derived from Hale (1966) by interpolation and extrapolation
[b] Estimated from Kelley and Trout (1971)

Table 10.3.4 Anthropomorphic Characteristics of Reference Pediatric Phantoms

	Newborn	1-Year Old	5-Year Old
Height	52 cm	76 cm	112 cm
Weight	3.96 kg	10.4 kg	20.0 kg
Distance from vertex to:			
External acoustic meatus (EAM)	7.7 cm	12.0 cm	12.6 cm
Thyroid (center)	11.5 cm	15.8 cm	17.2 cm
Sternal notch	13.3 cm	18.2 cm	20.2 cm
Nipples	17.7 cm	25.5 cm	29.7 cm

PO Bladder		
5-year	Umbilicus to 9.3 cm below symphysis pubis	5.6 cm to either side of bladder center
1-year	Umbilicus to 0.7 cm below symphysis pubis	4.4 cm to either side of bladder center
AP Pelvis		
5-year	2.5 cm above umbilicus to 11.1 cm below hip joint	1 cm beyond width of trunk
1-year	2.5 cm above umbilicus to 8.9 cm below hip joint	1 cm beyond width of trunk
Newborn	2.5 cm above umbilicus to 6.1 cm below hip joint	1 cm beyond width of trunk
AP, PO, Hip		
5-year	Iliac crest to 8.6 cm below hip joint	to width of upper leg
1-year	Iliac crest to 6.4 cm below hip joint	to width of upper leg

Table 10.3.5 Field Centers for X-Ray Projections

Projection	Distance from Phantom Vertex (cm)	Distance from Nearest Anatomical Landmark: Landmark	Distance from Nearest Anatomical Landmark: (cm)	Distance from Phantom Midline (cm)
		Newborn		
AP, LAT Skull	3.7	ext. acoustic meatus	4 above	0
AP, LAT Chest	15.2	nipples	2.5 above	0
AP Pelvis	31.3	symphysis pubis	0.4 above	0
		One-Year-Old		
AP, LAT Skull	8.0	ext. acoustic meatus	4 above	0
AP, LAT Chest	22.8	nipples	2.7 above	0
AP Pelvis, PO Hip	46.4	symphysis pubis	0.5 above	0
		Five-Year Old		
AP, LAT Skull	10.1	ext. acoustic meatus	2.5 above	0
AP, LAT Chest	26.4	nipples	3.3 above	0
AP Pelvis	57.0	symphysis pubis	0.7 above	0

Table 10.3.6 Description of X-Ray Fields Collimated to the Body Part

Projection	Vertical Limits of Field in Phantom Midplane	Horizontal Limits of Field in Phantom Midplane
AP, LAT Chest		
All ages	EAM[a] to bottom of 12th rib	1 cm beyond chest walls[b]
AP Pelvis		
5-year	2.5 cm above umbilicus to 11.1 cm below hip joint	1 cm beyond width of trunk
1-year	2.5 cm above umbilicus to 8.9 cm below hip joint	1 cm beyond width of trunk
Newborn	2.5 cm above umbilicus to 6.1 cm below hip joint	1 cm beyond width of trunk

[a] External acoustic meatus.

[b] Abdominal and chest walls defined as the width of the ribcage plus two layers of skin.

Table 10.3.7.1 AP Skull Pediatric—Organ Dose (mrad) for 1R Entrance Exposure (free-in-air)

Reference Patient	SID and Field Size (centimeters [inches]) Newborn		1-Year Old		5-Year Old	
Source-to-image receptor distance (SID)	102 [40]		102 [40]		91 [36]	
Field size at image receptor						
Collimated to film size #1	20 × 25 [8 × 10]		20 × 25 [8 × 10]			
Collimated to film size #2			25 × 20 [10 × 12]		25 × 30 [10 × 12]	
			Organ Dose (mrad/R)[a]			
Beam Quality (HVL mm Al)	**2.0**		**2.5**		**3.0**	
Collimation	**Film #1**	**Film #2**	**Film #1**	**Film #2**	**Film #1**	**Film #2**
Thyroid						
Newborn	682		802		857	
1-year	509	509	540	540	585	585
5-year		467		530		636
Active Bone Marrow						
Newborn	45		58		62	
1-year	26	38	35	51	36	54
5-year		26		34		37

[a] Only organ doses with a coefficient of variation less than 10% listed. For others trend in mrad/R as a function of HVL could not be resolved.

Table 10.3.7.2 LAT Skull Pediatric—Organ Dose (mrad) for 1R Entrance Exposure (free-in-air)

Reference Patient	SID and Field Size (centimeters [inches]) Newborn		1-Year Old		5-Year Old	
Source-to-image receptor distance (SID)	102 [40]		102 [40]		91 [36]	
Field size at image receptor						
Collimated to film size #1	25 × 20 [10 × 8]		25 × 20 [10 × 8]			
Collimated to film size #2			30 × 25 [12 × 10]		30 × 25 [12 × 10]	
	Organ Dose (mrad/R)					
Beam Quality (HVL mm Al)	**2.0**		**2.5**		**3.0**	
Collimation	**Film #1**	**Film #2**	**Film #1**	**Film #2**	**Film #1**	**Film #2**
Active Bone Marrow						
Newborn	35		46		48	
1-year	28	34	38	47	39	51
5-year		26		35		38

Table 10.3.8.1 AP Chest Pediatric—Organ Dose (mrad) for 1R Entrance Exposure (free-in-air)

Reference Patient	SID and Field Size (centimeters [inches]) Newborn	1-Year Old	5-Year Old
Source-to-image receptor distance (SID)	102 [40]	102 [40]	183 [72]
Field size at image receptor			
Collimated to body part[a]	13 × 16 [5.1 × 6.3]	17 × 23 [6.7 × 9.1]	21 × 30 [8.3 × 11.8]
Collimated to film size	20 × 25 [8 × 10]	25 × 30 [10 × 12]	28 × 36 [11 × 14]

Organ Dose (mrad/R)

Beam Quality (HVL mm Al) Collimation	2.0		2.5		3.0		3.5	
	Body Part	Film Size	Body Part	Film Size	Body Part	Film Size	Body Part	Film Size
Thyroid								
Newborn	682	682	802	802	857	857		
1-year	509	509	540	540	585	585		
5-year			650	650	770	770	880	880
Active Bone Marrow								
Newborn	81	129	111	169	116	188		
1-year	69	84	92	113	101	122		
5-year			88	103	121	140	127	153

Table 10.3.8.2 LAT Chest Pediatric—Organ Dose (mrad) for 1R Entrance Exposure (free-in-air)

Reference Patient	SID and Field Size (centimeters [inches]) Newborn	1-Year Old	5-Year Old
Source-to-image receptor distance (SID)	102 [40]	102 [40]	183 [72]
Field size at image receptor			
Collimated to body part[a]	13 × 16 [5.1 × 6.3]	16 × 14 [6.3 × 5.5]	21 × 30 [8.3 × 11.8]
Collimated to film size	20 × 25 [8 × 10]	25 × 30 [10 × 12]	28 × 36 [11 × 14]

Organ Dose (mrad/R)

Beam Quality (HVL mm Al) Collimation	2.0		2.5		3.0		3.5	
	Body Part	Film Size	Body Part	Film Size	Body Part	Film Size	Body Part	Film Size
Active Bone Marrow								
Newborn	102	160	146	225	173	281		
1-year	83	101	120	147	150	182		
5-year			93	111	132	153	138	162

[a] See description of x-ray fields collimated to the body part, Table 10.3.6 Body part collimation in subsequent tables have same reference table.

Table 10.3.9 AP Pelvis Pediatric—Organ Dose (mrad) for 1R Entrance Exposure (free-in-air)

Reference Patient	Newborn	1-Year Old	5-Year Old
	SID and Field Size (centimeters [inches])		
Source-to-image receptor distance (SID)	102 [40]	102 [40]	102 [40]
Field size at image receptor			
Collimated to body part	15 × 15 [5.9 × 5.9]	21 × 21 [8.3 × 8.3]	28 × 25 [11.0 × 9.8]
Collimated to film size	25 × 20 [10 × 8]	30 × 25 [12 × 10]	36 × 28 [14 × 11]

Organ Dose (mrad/R)

Beam Quality (HVL mm Al) Collimation	2.0		2.5		3.0	
	Body Part	Film Size	Body Part	Film Size	Body Part	Film Size
Testes						
Newborn	910	910	1000	1000	1120	1120
Ovaries						
Newborn	390	390	560	560	580	580
1-year	270	270	370	370	400	400
5-year	270	270	370	370	400	400
Active Bone Marrow						
Newborn	97	117	132	155	138	164
1-year	67	76	96	106	104	119
5-year	48	50	72	73	76	80

Table 10.4 Estimate of Dose to Embryo-Fetus from X-Ray Examinations (Courtesy NCRP from Report 54, 1977)

1. Use uterine doses listed below to determine the estimated number of millirads to the uterus of a ''standard woman'' per roentgen exposure at the skin. For this data, the center of the uterus (and hence the fetus) is assumed to be located 8 cm below the anterior surface of the abdomen. This method works reasonably well for average-sized women in early pregnancy.
2. If the patient is considerably larger or smaller than average, and/or if the patient is in the latter stages of pregnancy, a somewhat better method is to use appropriate tissue-air-ratio (TAR) tables in Schulz, R.J. and Gignac, C., Radiology, 120, 687 (1976) for large fields at the depth (corresponding to the center of the uterus) below the skin where the beam enters the patient.

Embryo (uterine) Doses for Selected X-Ray Projections (mrad/R)[a,b]

Projection	View	SID (in.)	Image Receptor Size (in.)[c]	Beam Quality (HVL, mm Al) 1.5	2.0	2.5	3.0	3.5	4.0
Pelvis, lumbopelvic	AP	40	17″ × 14″	142	212	283	353	421	486
	LAT	40	14″ × 17″	13	25	39	56	75	97
Abdominal[d]	AP	40	14″ × 17″	133	199	265	330	392	451
	PA	40	14″ × 17″	56	90	130	174	222	273
	LAT	40	14″ × 17″	13	23	37	53	71	91
Lumbar Spine	AP	40	14″ × 17″	128	189	250	309	366	419
	LAT	40	14″ × 17″	9	17	27	39	53	68
Hip	AP (one)	40	10″ × 12″	105	153	200	244	285	324
	AP (both)	40	17″ × 14″	136	203	269	333	395	454
Full Spine (Chiropractic)	AP	40	14″ × 36″	154	231	308	384	457	527
Urethrogram Cystography	AP	40	10″ × 12″	135	200	265	327	386	441
Upper G.I.	AP	40	14″ × 17″	9.5	16	25	34	45	56
Femur (one side)	AP	40	7″ × 17″	1.6	3.0	4.8	6.9	9.4	12
Cholecystography	PA	40	10″ × 12″	0.7	1.5	2.6	4.1	6.0	8.3
Chest	AP	72	14″ × 17″	0.3	0.7	1.3	2.0	3.1	4.3
	PA	72	14″ × 17″	0.3	0.6	1.2	2.0	3.0	4.5
	LAT	72	14″ × 17″	0.1	0.3	0.5	0.8	1.2	1.8
Ribs, Barium, Swallow	AP	40	14″ × 17″	0.1	0.3	0.5	0.9	1.4	2.0
	PA	40	14″ × 17″	0.1	0.3	0.5	0.9	1.5	2.2
	LAT	40	14″ × 17″	0.03	0.08	0.2	0.3	0.4	0.6
Thoracic Spine	AP	40	14″ × 17″	0.2	0.4	0.8	1.4	4.1	3.0
	LAT	40	14″ × 17″	0.04	0.1	0.2	0.4	0.5	0.8
Skull, Cervical Spine, Scapula, Shoulder, Humerus	—	40	—	<.01	<.01	<.01	<.01	<.01	

[a] Average dose to the uterus (mrad) for 1R entrance skin exposure (free-in-air).
[b] From Rosenstein, M. Organ Doses in Diagnostic Radiology, DHEW Publication (FDS) 76-8030, 1976.
[c] Field size is collimated to the image receptor size.
[d] Includes: Retrograde Pyelogram, KUB, Barium Enema, Lumbosacral Spine, IVP, Renal Arteriogram.

Table 10.5 Factors Included in Calculation of Genetically Significant Dose (GSD) for 1980 by Sex and Examination Type[a] (Courtesy NCRP from Report 100, 1989)

Sex	Exam Type	Mean Gonadal Dose μGy (mrad)	Relative Frequency (10^{-3})	Relative Child Expectancy	GSD for Exam Type μGy (mrad)
Male	Head & neck	—	40	0.57	—
	Chest	10 (1)	298	0.31	0.9 (0.09)
	Cervical spine	—	23	0.47	—
	Lumbar spine	2,180 (218)	59	0.15	19.3 (1.93)
	Hips/pelvis	6,000 (600)	18	0.38	41.0 (4.10)
	Upper extremities	—	106	0.65	—
	Lower extremities	150 (15)	119	0.70	12.5 (1.25)
	Abdomen (kidneys, ureters, bladder)	970 (97)	35	0.31	10.5 (1.05)
	Upper gastrointestinal & small bowel	10 (1)	28	0.22	0.1 (0.01)
	Barium enema	1,750 (175)	17	0.17	5.1 (0.51)
	Gall bladder	—	11	0.20	—
	Intravenous pyelogram	2,070 (207)	18	0.24	8.9 (0.89)
	Head CT	—	11	0.13	—
	Body CT	—	3	0.21	—
				Male Total	98 (9.8)
Female	Head & neck	—	32	0.41	
	Chest	10 (1)	270	0.21	0.6 (0.06)
	Cervical spine	—	22	0.30	—
	Lumbar spine	7,210 (721)	56	0.21	84.8 (8.48)
	Hips/pelvis	2,100 (210)	25	0.21	11.0 (1.10)
	Upper extremities	—	72	0.15	—
	Lower extremities	—	103	0.41	—
	Abdomen (kidneys, ureters, bladder)	2,210 (221)	35	0.38	29.4 (2.94)
	Upper gastrointestinal and small bowel	1,710 (171)	39	0.26	17.3 (1.73)
	Barium enema	9,030 (903)	26	0.17	39.9 (3.99)
	Gall bladder	780 (78)	19	0.14	2.1 (0.21)
	Intravenous pyelogram	5,880 (588)	20	0.20	23.5 (2.35)
	Head CT	—	13	0.33	—
	Body CT	—	3	0.21	—
				Female Total	209 (20.9)

(—) indicates less than 0.01 μGy.

[a] There are a number of examination types which are usually included in the category of ''others'' which have not been included in this table. Inclusion of these may increase the GSD by 10 to 20%.

Table 10.6 Mean Annual Bone Marrow Dose to Adults for All U.S. Radiographic Procedures: 1980 (After NCRP from Report 100, 1989)

Examination	Active Marrow Dose (mGy)[a] Per Examination		Annual per Capita Exam Rate	Adult per Capita Mean Active Marrow Dose (mGy)[a]	
	Shleien[b] et al. (1978)	Rosenstein[c] (1976)		Shleien[b] et al. (1978)	Rosenstein[c] (1976)
Skull	0.780	0.730	0.022	0.017	0.016
Head CT	2.200	2.200[d]	0.015	0.033	0.033
Body CT	3.500	3.500[e]	0.003	0.011	0.011
Chest	0.100	0.060	0.335	0.034	0.020
Abdomen (kidneys, ureters, bladder)	1.470	0.850	0.043	0.063	0.037
Biliary	1.680	1.260	0.019	0.032	0.024
Thoracic Spine	2.470	1.210	0.010	0.025	0.012
Lumbar/Lumbosacral Spine	4.000	2.400	0.072	0.288	0.173
Full Spine	0.640	0.350[f]	0.008	0.005	0.003
Upper Gastrointestinal	5.350	3.640	0.042	0.225	0.153
Barium Enema	8.750	5.690	0.027	0.236	0.154
Intravenous Pyelogram	4.200	2.350	0.023	0.097	0.054
Pelvis, hip	0.830	0.390	0.026	0.022	0.010
Cervical Spine & Other Head and Neck	0.520	0.270	0.044	0.009	0.012
Dental	0.090	0.080	0.430	0.040	0.034
Total Diagnostic Radiology				1.14	0.75

[a] 1 Gy = 100 rad
[b] Shleien et al (1978)
[c] Rosenstein (1976)
[d] Huda (1984)
[e] Huda (1984) and Ewen et al (1983)
[f] Kereiakes and Rosenstein (1980)

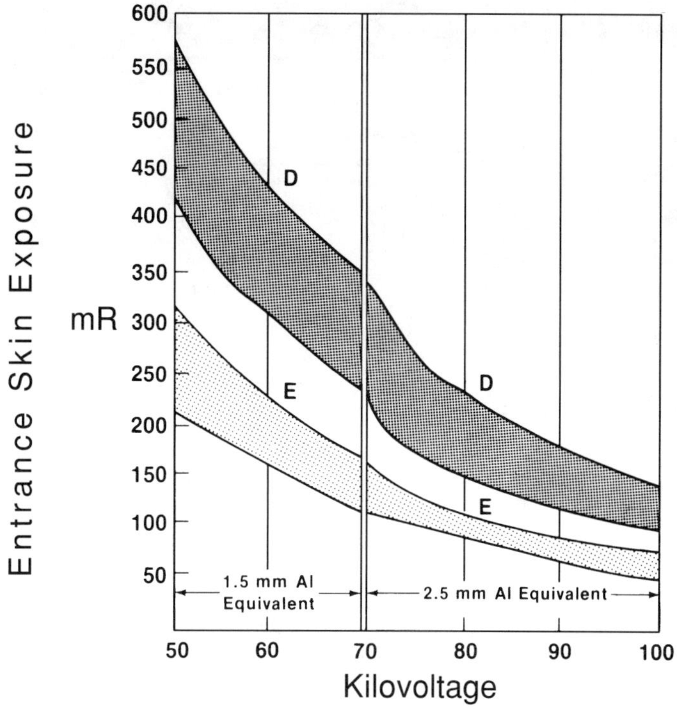

Figure 10.2 Acceptable X-Ray Exposure (mR) Ranges Speed Group "D" and "E" Film (From FDA 85-8245, 1985)

Table 10.7 Radiation Doses to Patients from Cardiac Radiological Procedures Summary of Dose Results (mGy)

Dosemeters	Adult Cardiac Catheterization			Paediatric Cardiac Catheterization			PTCA[a]		
	Mean	Standard Deviation	Range	Mean	Standard Deviation	Range	Mean	Standard Deviation	Range
Total of four trunk dosemeters	59.2	40.8	21.1–127.1	66.3	57.9	5.2–145.7	151.9	76.0	50.6–298.1
Xiphisternum	5.9	4.6	2.8–15.3	4.2	4.9	0.3–13.7	10.5	7.0	2.8–26.7
Right mid-auxillary line	20.3	23.8	1.4–98.8	20.8	24.2	0.1–119.7	75.7	85.6	0.6–280.7
Left mid-auxillary line	13.8	9.3	2.8–25.7	4.4	5.0	0.2–12.2	4.7	4.4	0.6–18.1
Spinous process T9	19.4	32.8	3.6–75.9	37.0	45.5	4.6–73.5	55.1	64.6	3.3–200.7
Thyroid	1.7	0.8	0.8–2.7	1.2	1.3	0.2–3.7	2.0	0.9	0.8–4.1
Iliac crest	0.4	0.3	0.1–0.9	0.7	0.7	0.0–1.8	1.2	1.1	0.0–3.2
Thigh	0.1	0.1	0.1–0.2	—	—	—	0.3	0.2	0.0–0.8
Diamentor reading (Rcm^2)	4800	3010	180–12500	490	360	150–570	3270	1440	2320–5780
Energy imparted (mJ)	473.0	296.8	17.7–1232.6	42.9	31.5	13.1–49.9	322.5	142.0	228.8–570.0

[a] Percutaneous transluminal coronary angioplasty.
(From Faulkner, K. et al Br. J. Radiol. 59:359–363; 1986)

Table 10.8 Mean Tissue Doses From CT Examinations[a]

	Mean Dose Per Examination (mGy)		
Organ or Tissue	**Head[b]**	**Chest[c]**	**Upper Abdomen**
Ovary	0.003	0.105	0.614
Testis	0.002	0.053	0.103
Breast	0.107	15.90	0.778
Red bone marrow	1.454	5.69	2.16
Lung	0.080	19.60	1.678
Thyroid	0.548	1.855	0.171
Bone surface	8.95	8.34	2.37
Other			
Stomach	0.020	9.19	26.9
Liver	0.021	8.96	27.77
Lg Intest.	0.004	0.145	0.995
Rectum	0.003	0.115	0.424
Bladder	0.003	0.091	0.421
Effective dose male	0.489	6.85	3.67
Equivalent (mSv) female	0.489	6.86	3.78
Eye Dose (mGy)	22.40	—	—
Surface dose (mGy)			
max	39.8	26.4	35.9
ave.	32.1	22.7	28.6

[a] Japanese Population
[b] Tube Voltage (kVp) 120
Mas/scan 3 (mAs) 533–520,400
[c] Tube Voltage (kVp) 120–125
Mas/Scan (mAs) 200–533
(Adapted from Nishizawa, K. et al. Determination of Organ Doses and Effective Dose Equivalent from Computed Tomographic Examinations, B.J. Radiol 64, 20–28, 1991.)

Table 10.9 Estimated Tissue Dose For Entire Fluoroscopic and Cineangiographic Examination of the Coronary Arteries[a]

Tissue	Tissue Dose (rad)
Entrance Skin in primary field	84
Brain	0.005
Thyroid	0.14
Thymus	1.8
Active Bone Marrow	3.5
Esophagus	10.1
Lung	16.5
Heart	19
Adrenal	15.5
Spleen	2.6
Pancreas	3.5
Stomach	1.6
Liver	3.0
Kidney	1.8
Colon	0.082
Small Intestine	0.105
Urinary Bladder	0.005
Testis	<0.001

[a] Mean of two methods of calculation described in FDA 95-8288 to an adult male.

Table 10.10 Absorbed Dose (mGy) and Effective Dose (mSv) per unit Administered Activity (MBq) in Normal Adults (With Permission ICRP from Summary of Current ICRP Report of Committee 3 "Principles for Protection of Patient in Nuclear Medicine," 1993)

Function or Organ Examined	Radionuclide	Pharmaceutical	Most Highly Irradiated Organs: Organ 1 (mGy/MBq)	Organ 2 (mGy/MBq)	Organ 3 (mGy/MBq)	Conceptus (mGY/MBq)	Effective dose (mSv/MBq)
Bone	^{99m}Tc	phosphate/ phosphonate	6.3×10^{-2} (bone surface)	5.0×10^{-2} (bladder)	9.6×10^{-3} (red marrow)	6.1×10^{-3}	5.8×10^{-3}
Renal (normal renal function)	^{51}Cr	EDTA	2.3×10^{-2} (bladder)	2.8×10^{-3} (uterus)	1.8×10^{-3} (kidneys)	2.8×10^{-3}	2.1×10^{-3}
	^{123}I	hippurate	2.0×10^{-1} (bladder)	1.7×10^{-2} (uterus)	7.3×10^{-3} (lower large intestine)	1.7×10^{-2}	1.2×10^{-2}
	^{131}I	hippurate	9.6×10^{-1} (bladder)	3.5×10^{-2} (uterus)	3.0×10^{-2} (kidneys)	3.5×10^{-2}	5.3×10^{-2}
	^{99m}Tc	DTPA	6.5×10^{-2} (bladder)	7.9×10^{-3} (uterus)	4.4×10^{-3} (kidneys)	7.9×10^{-3}	5.2×10^{-3}
	^{99m}Tc	DMSA	1.7×10^{-1} (kidneys)	1.9×10^{-2} (bladder)	1.3×10^{-2} (adrenals, spleen)	4.6×10^{-3}	8.7×10^{-3}
	^{99m}Tc	MAG_3	1.1×10^{-1} (bladder)	1.2×10^{-2} (uterus)	5.7×10^{-3} (lower large intestine)	1.2×10^{-2}	7.3×10^{-3}
Thyroid	^{99m}Tc	pertechnetate (no blocking)	6.2×10^{-2} (upper large intestine)	2.9×10^{-2} (stomach)	2.3×10^{-2} (thyroid)	8.1×10^{-3}	1.2×10^{-2}
	^{131}I	iodide (35% uptake)	5.0×10^{2} (thyroid)	4.6×10^{-1} (stomach)	4.0×10^{-1} (bladder)	5.0×10^{-2}	24
	^{123}I	iodide (35% uptake)	4.5 (thyroid)	6.8×10^{-2} (stomach)	6.0×10^{-2} (bladder)	1.4×10^{-2}	2.2×10^{-1}
Liver (+gall bladder)	^{99m}Tc	colloid (large)	7.7×10^{-2} (spleen)	7.4×10^{-2} (liver)	1.2×10^{-2} (pancreas)	1.9×10^{-3}	9.2×10^{-3}
	^{99m}Tc	colloid (small)	7.7×10^{-2} (spleen)	7.4×10^{-2} (liver)	1.5×10^{-2} (red marrow)	1.8×10^{-3}	9.7×10^{-3}
	^{99m}Tc	HIDA	1.1×10^{-1} (gall bladder)	9.2×10^{-2} (upper large intestine)	6.2×10^{-2} (lower large intestine)	1.3×10^{-2}	1.5×10^{-2}
	^{57}Co	B_{12} (no carrier)	5.1×10 (liver)	5.4 (adrenals, pancreas)	5.0 (kidneys)	1.8	4.4
Brain	^{99m}Tc	pertechnetate (blocked thyroid)	3.2×10^{-2} (bladder)	6.6×10^{-3} (uterus)	4.7×10^{-3} (kidneys, ovaries)	6.6×10^{-3}	4.7×10^{-3}
	^{99m}Tc	gluconate/ lucoheptonate	5.6×10^{-2} (bladder)	4.9×10^{-2} (kidneys)	7.7×10^{-3} (uterus)	7.7×10^{-3}	5.4×10^{-3}
	^{99m}Tc	HMPAO	3.4×10^{-2} (kidneys)	2.6×10^{-2} (thyroid)	2.3×10^{-2} (bladder)	6.6×10^{-3}	9.3×10^{-3}
	^{18}F	FDG	1.7×10^{-1} (bladder)	6.5×10^{-2} (heart)	2.6×10^{-2} (brain)	2.0×10^{-2}	2.0×10^{-2}

Table 10.10 Absorbed Dose (mGy) and Effective Dose (mSv) per unit Administered Activity (MBq) in Normal Adults (With Permission ICRP from Summary of Current ICRP Report of Committee 3 "Principles for Protection of Patient in Nuclear Medicine," 1993)

Function or Organ Examined	Radionuclide	Pharmaceutical	Most Highly Irradiated Organs: Organ 1 (mGy/MBq)	Organ 2 (mGy/MBq)	Organ 3 (mGy/MBq)	Conceptus (mGy/MBq)	Effective dose (mSv/MBq)
Lung	^{99m}Tc	MAA	6.7×10^{-2} (lungs)	1.6×10^{-2} (liver)	1.0×10^{-2} (bladder)	2.4×10^{-3}	1.1×10^{-2}
	^{99m}Tc	aerosol (fast clearance)	4.7×10^{-2} (bladder)	1.7×10^{-2} (lungs)	5.9×10^{-3} (uterus)	5.9×10^{-3}	6.1×10^{-3}
	^{99m}Tc	aerosol (slow clearance)	9.3×10^{-2} (lungs)	1.3×10^{-2} (bladder)	6.4×10^{-3} (breasts)	1.7×10^{-3}	1.4×10^{-2}
	^{133}Xe	gas, 5 min (re-breathing)	1.1×10^{-3} (lungs)	8.4×10^{-4} (red marrow)	8.3×10^{-4} (breasts)	7.4×10^{-4}	7.3×10^{-4}
	^{133}Xe	gas, 30 s 1 breath	7.7×10^{-4} (lungs)	1.2×10^{-4} (bone surfaces, red marrow, breasts)	1.1×10^{-4} (small and large intestines, liver, pancreas, spleen, uterus)	1.1×10^{-4}	1.8×10^{-4}
	^{81m}Kr	gas	2.1×10^{-4} (lungs)	4.6×10^{-6} (breasts)	3.5×10^{-6} (pancreas)	1.3×10^{-7}	9.5×10^{-4}
Heart	^{201}Tl	thallous ion	5.6×10^{-1} (testes)	5.4×10^{-1} (kidneys)	3.6×10^{-1} (lower large intestine)	5.0×10^{-2}	2.3×10^{-1}
	^{99m}Tc	RBC	2.3×10^{-2} (heart)	1.5×10^{-2} (sleen)	1.4×10^{-2} (lungs)	4.7×10^{-3}	6.6×10^{-3}
Abscess	^{111}In	white cells	5.5 (spleen)	7.1×10^{-1} (liver)	6.9×10^{-1} (red marrow)	1.2×10^{-1}	3.6×10^{-1}
	^{67}Ga	citrate	5.9×10^{-1} (bone surfaces)	2.0×10^{-1} (lower large intestine)	1.9×10^{-1} (red marrow)	7.9×10^{-2}	1.1×10^{-1}
Thrombi	^{125}I	fibrinogen (thyroid totally blocked)	3.2×10^{-1} (heart)	2.4×10^{-1} (spleen)	2.3×10^{-1} (lungs)	5.5×10^{-2}	8.0×10^{-2}
	^{111}In	platelets	7.5 (spleen)	7.3×10^{-1} (liver)	6.6×10^{-1} (pancreas)	9.5×10^{-2}	3.9×10^{-1}
	^{51}Cr	platelets	2.6 (spleen)	3.0×10^{-1} (liver)	1.9×10^{-1} (red marrow)	2.8×10^{-2}	1.4×10^{-1}
Pancreas	^{75}Se	methionine	6.2 (liver)	5.3 (kidneys)	3.9 (spleen)	2.6	2.5
Adrenals	^{75}Se	methyl cholesterol	5.1 (adrenals)	2.0 (liver)	1.8 (small intestine, pancreas, uterus, red marrow)	1.8	1.5
	^{131}I	MIBG	8.3×10^{-1} (liver)	5.9×10^{-1} (bladder)	4.9×10^{-1} (spleen)	8.0×10^{-2}	1.4×10^{-1}
Spleen	^{51}Cr	RBC denatured	5.6 (spleen)	3.0×10^{-1} (pancreas)	1.7×10^{-1} (liver)	1.3×10^{-2}	1.8×10^{-1}
GIT	^{99m}Tc	pertechnetate (oral, no blocking agent)	7.4×10^{-2} (upper large intestine)	5.0×10^{-2} (stomach)	3.0×10^{-2} (small intestine)	8.7×10^{-3}	1.4×10^{-2}

Table 10.11 Radiation Absorbed Dose for Various PET Studies (Adapted from Kearfott, 1982a; 1982b; Courtesy NCRP from Report 124, 1996)

Radio-pharmaceutical	Activity Administered (MBq)	Organ of Interest	Organ Absorbed Dose (μGy MBq^{-1})	Absorbed Dose to Patient (μGy MBq^{-1})
^{11}CO	740	Spleen, lungs, intestine	14 to 23	5.0
$C^{15}O$	1,850	Spleen, lungs, intestine	4, 3, 4	0.4
$CO^{15}O$	1,850	Lungs	1.3	0.4
$H_2{}^{15}O$	1,850	Blood, kidneys, liver, lungs	3	0.4
^{18}F-FDG	370	Bladder	120	10.5
^{82}Rb	1,850	Heart, kidneys	3.5 to 5	0.4

References

Aboul-Khair, S.A., Buchanan, T.J., Crooks, J., Turnbill, A.C. ''Structural and functional development of the human foetal thyroid,'' *Clin Sci* **31:**415–424; 1966.

Department of Health Education and Welfare. *Evaluation of Radiation Exposure from Diagnostic Radiology Examinations—Technique/Exposure Guide for the Dental Bite Wing Projection.* FDA 85-8245; 1985.

Dyer, N.C., Brill, A.B. ''Maternal-fetal transport of iron and iodine in human subjects,'' *Advances in Experimental Medicine and Biology, Vol 27: Drugs and Fetal Development.* M.A. Klingberg, A. Abramovici, J. Chemke, eds.; Plenum Press; New York; 1972.

Hale, J. ''The homogeneity factor for pulsating potential x-ray beams in the diagnostic energy region,'' *Radiology* **86:** 147–148; 1966.

Harrison, R.M. ''Central axis depth-dose data for diagnostic radiology,'' *Phys Med Biol* **26:**657–670; 1981.

Huda, W. ''Is energy imparted a good measure of the radiation risk associated with CT examinations?'' *Phys Med Biol* **19:** 1137; 1984.

Huda, W., Ewen, V.K., Lackner, K., Fisher, P. ''Das Somatische Strahlenmiskobei Herzuntersuchungen mit der digitalenageographic und der computertomographic,'' *Fortschr Rontgerstr* **139:**440; 1984.

Johnson, J.R. ''A review of age dependent radioiodine dosimetry,'' *Age-Related Factors in Radionuclide Metabolism and Dosimetry.* G.B. Gerber, H. Metivier, H. Smith, eds.; Martinus Nijhoff Publishers; Dordrecht; 249–259; 1987.

Kelley, J.P., Trout, E.D. ''Physical characteristics of the radiations from 2-pulse, 12-pulse, and 1,000-pulse x-ray equipment,'' *Radiology* **100:**653–661; 1971.

Kereiakes, J.G., Rosenstein, M. *Handbook of Radiation Doses in Nuclear Medicine and Diagnostic X-ray.* CRC Press; Boca Raton, FL; 1980.

National Council on Radiation Protection and Measurements. *Medical Radiation Exposure of Pregnant and Potentially Pregnant Women.* NCRP Report 54; Bethesda, MD; 1977.

National Council on Radiation Protection and Measurements. *Mammography: A User's Guide.* NCRP Report 85; Bethesda, MD; 1986.

National Council on Radiation Protection and Measurements. *Exposure of the U.S. Population from Diagnostic Medical Radiation.* NCRP Report 100; Bethesda, MD; May 1, 1989.

National Council on Radiation Protection and Measurements. *Medical X-Ray, Electron Beam and Gamma Ray Protection for Energies up to 50 MeV (Equipment Design, Performance, and Use).* NCRP Report 102; Bethesda, MD; 1989.

National Council on Radiation Protection and Measurements. *Sources and Magnitude of Occupational and Public Exposure from Nuclear Medicine Procedures.* NCRP Report 124; Bethesda, MD; 1996.

Nishizakawa, K., et al. ''Determination of organ doses and effective dose equivalent from computed tomographic examinations,'' *British Journal of Radiology* **64:**20–28; 1991.

Roedler, H.D. ''Assessment of fetal activity concentration and fetal dose for selected radionuclides based on animal and human data,'' *Age-related Factors in Radionuclide Metabolism and Dosimetry*, G.B. Gerber, H. Metivier, and H. Smith, eds.; Martinus Nijhoff Publishers; Dordrecht; 327–337; 1987.

Rosenstein, M. *Organ Doses in Diagnostic Radiology*, Department of Health Education and Welfare Publication FDA 76–8030; 1976.

Rosenstein, M.; Beck, T.J.; and Warner, O.C. *Handbook of Selected Organ Doses for Projections Common in Pediatric Radiology*, Department of Health Education and Welfare FDA 79–8079; 1979.

Rosenstein, M. *Handbook of Selected Tissue Doses for Projections Common in Diagnostic Radiology*, Department of Health Education and Welfare Publication FDA 89–8031; 1988.

Shleien, B., Tucker, T.T. and Johnson, D.W. ''The mean active bone marrow dose to the adult population of the United States from diagnostic radiology,'' *Health Physics*, **34:**587; 1978.

Speiser, R.C., Zanrosso, E.M., Jeromin, L.S. and Carlson, R.A. ''Dose comparisons for mammographic systems,'' *Med. Phys.* **13:**667–673; 1986.

Sprawls, P. *The Physical Principles of Diagnostic Radiology*, University Park, Baltimore, Maryland; 1977.

Watson, E.E. ''Radiation Dose Estimates to the Fetal Thyroid at Various Stages of Development,'' Presentation; Oak Ridge Associated Universities; Oak Ridge, TN; 1989.

Watson, E.E. ''Radiation absorbed dose to the human fetal thyroid,'' *Proceedings of the Fifth International Radiopharmaceutical Dosimetry Symposium Held in Oak Ridge, TN, May 7–10, 1991*; 1991.

Zamenhof, R.G., Shahabi, S. and Morgan, H.T. ''An improved method for estimating the entrance exposure in diagnostic x-ray systems,'' *Amer. J. Roentgenol.* **149:**637; 1987.

CHAPTER 11

OPERATIONAL HEALTH PHYSICS

This Chapter emphasizes the practical everyday good work practices[a] in various aspects of health physics. The breadth of operational health physics is such that the Chapter is organized into sections on:

SECTION 1. LABORATORY OPERATION AND GOOD WORK PRACTICES
SECTION 2. NUCLEAR POWER PLANTS
SECTION 3. ATMOSPHERIC DISPERSION AND ENVIRONMENTAL MONITORING
SECTION 4. MEDICAL/ACCELERATOR/X-RAY DIFFRACTION
SECTION 5. EMERGENCIES

Included are pertinent data related to reactor source terms, atmospheric dispersion, radiation surveys, contamination guidance and release levels and surface decontamination techniques.

[a] Good work practice guides reflect the ''common sense'' basis for the indicated activities. Specific regulatory, license, organizational procedural, or operational requirements may override any of these guides. These guides reflect what experienced workers consider common sense.

SECTION 1 LABORATORY OPERATION AND GOOD WORK PRACTICES

Section 1 is concerned with laboratory operation and good work practices. Hence, it contains information on the classification of laboratories, levels of radioisotopes used in various processes, decontamination guides, use of respirators, radiation survey information, and good work practices guides for use under different conditions. The good work practice guides are intended as an abridged summary to supplement specific training. They are not detailed proscriptive procedures.

TABLE OF CONTENTS

Table 11.1.1 Classification of Workplaces (From International Labor Office *Guidelines for the Radiation Protection of Workers in Industry (Ionizing Radiations)* Occupational Safety and Health Series 62 ©International Labour Organization, 1989)

Introduction

1. In view of the extreme diversity of processes carried out with unsealed radioactive sources and the great variety of potential risks, working areas and workshops should be classified according to the relative radiotoxicity of the radionuclides taking into account the nature of the operations and the total amount used.
2. Specialized installations should be divided into three types of workplaces depending, to the extent practicable, on the factors referred to in paragraph 1 and in accordance with Table 11.1.1.1 for radiotoxicity classification. The types of workplace are commonly referred to as:
   (a) type I workplace or type C workplace;
   (b) type II workplace or type B workplace;
   (c) type III workplace or type A workplace.
3. The activity limits for use of radionuclides in the various types of workplace are given in Table 11.1.1.2.
4. Workplaces of all three types should be:
   (a) reserved exclusively for work with radioactive substances and isolated from other workplaces as far as is practicable;
   (b) subject to classification according to the potential risks involved: normally areas where radioactive substances are used will be classified as controlled areas; however, areas where workers are not likely to receive more than three tenths of the dose limits may be either included in a controlled area or defined as supervised areas, if this is duly justified and considered more convenient.
5. A changing area should be provided at the entrances of areas where radioactive substances are prepared or used, in order to prevent contamination from being transported by persons to outside areas. The changing area should contain a foot barrier. Places for clean clothes should be left outside the barrier and protective clothing, equipment and containers for discarded contaminated clothing should be provided on the active side of the barrier.
6. Washing facilities should be set up appropriate to the level of radioactivity present in the workplace. The wash basins should be elbow, knee or foot operated.
7. Changing areas should contain monitoring and control equipment, appropriate to the levels of radioactive materials present, to monitor the hands, feet, shoes and clothes of workers leaving controlled or supervised areas. Additional check points should be established within controlled areas when necessary, depending on the type of work being carried out.
8. Separate rooms should be assigned to different types of work when such work involves widely varying levels of activity, and in accordance with the classification of workplaces as given in this chapter. Counting apparatus should normally be placed in a separate room. The design should take into account, as far as practicable, the transfer of radioactive materials from one workplace to another, where necessary, without passing through the surrounding area.

Type I Workplace

1. The design, construction and equipment of a type I (type C) workplace should be similar to those of a good quality modern chemical laboratory.
2. Normal ventilation is usually sufficient, and could be complemented with continuous movement of air into a fume hood.

Type II Workplace

1. A type II (type B) workplace should be specifically designed, constructed and equipped for work with radioisotopes.
2. The levels of airborne activity should be kept as low as reasonably achievable by the use of totally or partially ventilated fume hoods or glove boxes.

Table 11.1.1 Classification of Workplaces (Continued)

3. The workplace should have reduced air pressure relative to the surrounding areas. The ventilation exhaust should be via a fume hood. There should be a space for an absolute filter to be put between the fume hood and the ventilation duct allowing for easy change of the filter and for monitoring the negative pressure gradient. Special attention should be given to avoiding the recirculation of air and the dispersion of contamination to other occupied areas.
4. The surfaces of the fume hood and the ventilation duct should be smooth and made of non-absorbent material that can withstand the chemicals normally used in the hood.
5. The speed of the air flow should be regular, without eddies, and should be such that there can be no escape of air from the fume hood into the workplace under typical operating conditions, including the opening of windows and doors and the suction of other fume hoods. This should be checked using smoke tests. The gas, water and electrical outputs should be operated from outside the hood.
6. Fume hoods and glove boxes where ''active'' work is carried out should be properly marked with the radiation symbol and the appropriate explanatory text.
7. A waste bin with a foot-operated lid should be available for the collection of low activity waste. The bin should bear the radiation warning sign. A plastic bottle which could withstand the effects of the various solvents and the effects of radiation should be provided for the temporary retention of liquid waste.
8. Facilities for washing hands should be foot or elbow operated.
9. A special room should be provided for storing radioactive substances.

Type III Workplace

1. A type III (type A) workplace should be specifically designed, constructed and equipped for handling large quantities of radioactive material in accordance with the specifications and requirements laid down by the competent authority.
2. Processes involving risks of air contamination should be carried out in completely enclosed glove boxes or hot cells under negative pressure and provided with filters and transfer boxes.
3. Radioactive substances should be stored only in a special room equipped with suitable shielding and ventilation, and in accordance with the provisions as regards waste storage.

Table 11.1.1.1 Toxicity Classification of Radionuclides[a] (From International Labor Office *Guidelines for the Radiation of Workers in Industry (Ionizing Radiations)* Occupational Safety and Health Series 62 ©International Labour Organization, 1989)

Very High Radiotoxicity (Group 1)

^{210}Pb	^{228}Ra	^{229}Th	^{232}U	^{236}Pu	^{241}Pu	^{243}Am	^{244}Cm	^{248}Cm	^{251}Cf
^{210}Po	^{227}Ac	^{230}Th	^{233}U	^{238}Pu	^{242}Pu	^{240}Cm	^{245}Cm	^{248}Cf	^{252}Cf
^{223}Ra	^{227}Th	^{231}Pa	^{234}U	^{239}Pu	^{241}Am	^{242}Cm	^{246}Cm	^{249}Cf	^{254}Cf
^{225}Ra	^{228}Th	^{230}U	^{237}Np	^{240}Pu	^{242m}Am	^{243}Cm	^{247}Cm	^{250}Cf	^{254}Es
^{226}Ra									

High Radiotoxicity (Group 2)

^{22}Na	^{90}Sr	^{110m}Ag	^{124}I	^{140}Ba	^{170}Tm	^{212}Pb	^{228}Ac	^{244}Pu	^{253}Cf
^{36}Cl	^{91}Y	^{115m}Cd	^{125}I	^{144}Ce	^{181}Hf	^{207}Bi	^{232}Th	^{242}Am	^{253}Es
^{45}Ca	^{93}Zr	^{114m}In	^{126}I	^{152}Eu	^{182}Ta	^{210}Bi	Th Nat[b]	^{241}Cm	^{254m}Es
^{46}Sc	^{94}Nb	^{124}Sb	^{131}I	^{154}Eu	^{192}Ir	^{211}At	^{230}Pa	^{249}Bk	^{255}Fm
^{60}Co	^{106}Ru	^{125}Sb	^{134}Cs	^{160}Tb	^{204}Tl	^{224}Ra	^{236}U	^{246}Cf	^{256}Fm

Moderate Radiotoxicity (Group 3)

^{7}Be	^{52}Fe	^{82}Br	^{97}Zr	^{105}Ag	^{134}Te	^{143}Ce	^{171}Tm	^{198}Au	^{237}U
^{14}C	^{55}Fe	^{74}Kr	^{90}Nb	^{111}Ag	^{120}I	^{142}Pr	^{175}Yb	^{199}Au	^{240}U
^{18}F	^{59}Fe	^{77}Kr	^{93m}Nb	^{109}Cd	^{123}I	^{143}Pr	^{177}Lu	^{197}Hg	^{239}Np
^{24}Na	^{55}Co	^{87}Kr	^{95}Nb	^{115}Cd	^{130}I	^{147}Nd	^{181}W	^{197m}Hg	^{240}Np
^{31}Si	^{56}Co	^{88}Kr	^{96}Nb	^{115m}In	^{132m}I	^{149}Nd	^{185}W	^{203}Hg	^{234}Pu
^{32}P	^{57}Co	^{86}Rb	^{90}Mo	^{113}Sn	^{133}I	^{147}Pm	^{187}W	^{200}Tl	^{237}Pu
^{33}P	^{58}Co	^{83}Sr	^{93}Mo	^{125}Sn	^{135}I	^{149}Pm	^{183}Re	^{201}Tl	^{245}Pu
^{35}S	^{63}Ni	^{85}Sr	^{99}Mo	^{122}Sb	^{135}Xe	^{151}Sm	^{186}Re	^{202}Tl	^{238}Am
^{38}Cl	^{65}Ni	^{89}Sr	^{96}Tc	^{121}Te	^{132}Cs	^{153}Sm	^{188}Re	^{203}Pb	^{240}Am
^{41}Ar	^{64}Cu	^{91}Sr	^{97m}Tc	^{121m}Te	^{136}Cs	^{152m}Eu	^{185}Os	^{206}Bi	^{244m}Am
^{42}K	^{65}Zn	^{92}Sr	^{97}Tc	^{123m}Te	^{137}Cs	^{155}Eu	^{191}Os	^{212}Bi	^{244}Am
^{43}K	^{69m}Zn	^{90}Y	^{99}Tc	^{125m}Te	^{131}Ba	^{153}Gd	^{193}Os	^{220}Rn	^{238}Cm
^{47}Ca	^{72}Ga	^{92}Y	^{97}Ru	^{127m}Te	^{140}La	^{159}Gd	^{190}Ir	^{222}Rn	^{250}Bk
^{47}Sc	^{73}As	^{93}Y	^{103}Ru	^{129m}Te	^{134}Ce	^{165}Dy	^{194}Ir	^{226}Th	^{244}Cf
^{48}Sc	^{74}As	^{86}Zr	^{105}Ru	^{131}Te	^{135}Ce	^{166}Dy	^{191}Pt	^{231}Th	^{254}Fm
^{48}V	^{76}As	^{88}Zr	^{105}Rh	^{131m}Te	^{137m}Ce	^{166}Ho	^{193}Pt	^{234}Th	
^{51}Cr	^{77}As	^{89}Zr	^{103}Pd	^{132}Te	^{139}Ce	^{169}Er	^{197}Pt	^{233}Pa	
^{52}Mn	^{75}Se	^{95}Zr	^{109}Pd	^{133m}Te	^{141}Ce	^{171}Er	^{196}Au	^{231}U	
^{54}Mn									

Low Radiotoxicity (Group 4)

^{3}H	^{60m}Co	^{81}Kr	^{91m}Y	^{99m}Tc	^{120m}I	^{127}Cs	^{138}Cs	^{207}Po	^{243}Pu
^{15}O	^{61}Co	^{83m}Kr	^{88}Nb	^{103m}Rh	^{121}I	^{129}Cs	^{137}Ce	^{227}Ra	^{237}Am
^{37}Ar	^{62m}Co	^{85m}Kr	^{89}Nb	^{113m}In	^{128}I	^{130}Cs	^{191m}Os	^{235}U	^{239}Am
^{51}Mn	^{59}Ni	^{85}Kr	^{97}Nb	^{116}Te	^{129}I	^{131}Cs	^{193m}Pt	^{238}U	^{245}Am
^{52m}Mn	^{69}Zn	^{80}Sr	^{98}Nb	^{123}Te	^{134}I	^{134m}Cs	^{197m}Pt	^{239}U	^{246m}Am
^{53}Mn	^{71}Ge	^{81}Sr	^{93m}Mo	^{127}Te	^{131m}Xe	^{135}Cs	^{203}Po	U Nat	^{246}Am
^{56}Mn	^{76}Kr	^{85m}Sr	^{101}Mo	^{129}Te	^{133}Xe	^{135m}Cs	^{205}Po	^{235}Pu	^{249}Cm
^{58m}Co	^{79}Kr	^{87m}Sr	^{96m}Tc	^{133}Te	^{125}Cs				

[a] Based on the classification published in the *Official Journal of the European Communities,* No. L246, Vol. 23; Luxembourg; 17 Sep. 1980.
[b] One becquerel of natural thorium corresponds to 1 alpha disintegration per second (dps) (0.5 dps of ^{232}Th and 0.5 dps of ^{228}Th). One curie of natural thorium corresponds to 3.7×10^{10} alpha disintegrations per second (1.85×10^{10} dps of ^{232}Th and 1.85×10^{10} dps of ^{228}Th).

Table 11.1.1.2 Activity Limits for Use of Radionuclides in Various Types of Workplace[a] (From International Labor Office *Guidelines for the Radiation Protection of Workers in Industry (Ionizing Radiation)* Occupational Safety and Health Series 62 ©International Labour Organization, 1989)

Radionuclide Group	Type of Workplace		
	Type I	Type II	Type III
1. Very high	500 KBq or less	500 KBq–500 MBq	500 MBq or more
2. High	5 MBq or less	5 MBq–5 G Bq	5 GBq or more
3. Moderate	50 MBq or less	50 MBq–50 G Bq	50 GBq or more
4. Low	500 MBq or less	500 MBq–500 G Bq	500 GBq or more

[a] The above table provides, as precisely as the complexity of the subject will allow, a basis for assessing the type of workplace required for normal operations. According to the nature of the operations, the following modifying factors should be applied:

Operation	Modifying Factor
Storage (stock solutions)	×100
Very simple wet operations	×10
Normal operations	×1
Complex wet operations with risk of spills and simple dry operations	×0.1
Dry and dusty operations	×0.01

Table 11.1.1.3 Hazard Index (HI) (Hickey, 1991)

The HI may be used to assess workplace air monitoring requirements and the potential intake of workers. Using this formula an HI of 100 represents a potential intake of 1 ALI.

$$HI = \frac{Q \times 10^{-6} \times R \times F}{ALI \times C} \times 100$$

where:

Q = average annual activity used
ALI = annual limit of intake
C = confinement factor (see table below)
R = Release Fraction factor (see table below)

F = other modifying factors (For instance: added dispersibility due to added energy, e.g., chemistry, grinding; adjustments due to less than annual work duration) ['F' is not in final 1993 report.]

Table 11.1.1.4 Release Fractions

Condition	Factor[b]
Gases or volatile material	1
Nonvolatile powders, β- γ	0.01
Nonvolatile powders, α[a]	0.001
Solid, e.g., metals	0.00001 (.001)
Liquid	0.001 (0.01)
Surface contamination, β- γ[a]	0.001
Surface contamination, α[a]	0.0001
Encapsulated material	0

[a] From the 1991 draft report. Not in the 1993 final report.
[b] The second value is from the 1993 final report.

Table 11.1.1.5 Containment Factors

Condition	Factor[b]
Glovebox	10 (100)
Hood (well ventilated)	1 (10)
Open bench, normal ventilation	0.1 (1)
Non-routine or special jobs where the ventilation is unknown	0.01[a]

[a] From the 1991 draft report. Not in the 1993 final report.
[b] The second value is from the 1993 final report.

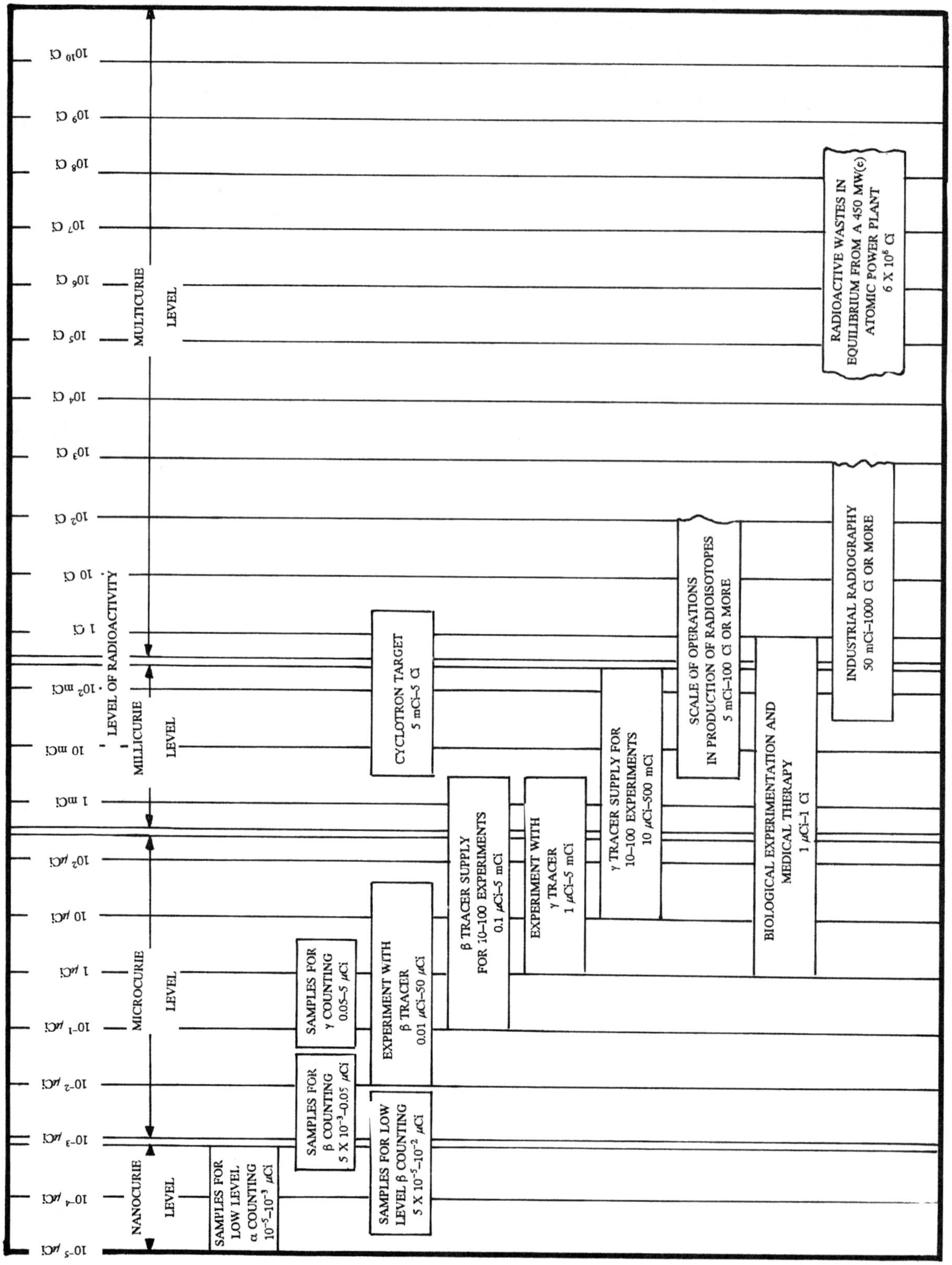

Figure 11.1 Source Strengths of Radioactive Material Typically Encountered

Table 11.1.2 Typical Uses of Radionuclides in Industry (From NUREG/CR-3332, 1983. Adapted from EPA-520/4-73-002, 1974)

Application	Radionuclides	Typical Source Strengths
Encapsulated Sources		
Industrial radiography	^{192}Ir, ^{137}Cs, ^{170}Tm, ^{60}Co	10–100 Ci (0.4–4 TBq)
Borehold logging	^{137}Cs, ^{60}Co	10 mCi–2 Ci (~0.4–70 GBq)
	Pu-Be, Am-Be	50 mCi–20 Ci (~1.9–700 GBq)
	^{252}Cf	100 μCi (~4 MBq)
Radiation gauges, automatic weighing equipment	^{90}Sr, ^{147}Pm, ^{144}Ce, ^{137}Cs, ^{60}Co	5–200 mCi (~0.2–7 GBq)
Smoke detectors	^{241}Am	5 μCi (~200 kBq)
Luminous signs	^{3}H	0.5 Ci (~20 GBq)
Mössbauer analysis	^{57}Fe, ^{57}Co	2–50 μCi (~0.4 MBq)
Tracer Applications		
Hydrological tracers	^{3}H	1–100 Ci (~4 TBq)
	^{82}Br	10–100 mCi (~4 GBq)
Reservoir engineering	^{85}Kr	200 mCi (~7 GBq)

Table 11.1.3 Typical Radiation Sources for Industrial Radiography (From IAEA Safety Series No. 102, 1990)

X-Rays	Up to 8 MV	140–300 kVp	60–140 kVp
Gamma ray sources	Co-60	Ir-192	Tm 170
Typical	100 GBq	few tens of GBq to 1 TBq	
Up to:	100 TBq	10 TBq	1 TBq
Materials		**Optimum Working Thickness:**	
Steel	50–150 mm	10–60 mm	2.5–12.5 mm
Light alloy	150–450 mm	40–190	7.5–37 mm
Others	40–120 g cm $^{-2}$	10–50 g cm $^{-2}$	2–10 g cm $^{-2}$

Table 11.1.4 Derived Values for Exemption of Sealed Sources from Inventory[a] (From Kerr and Eckerman, 1990a)

Unlimited source activities						
^{87}Rb	^{113}Cd	^{115}In	^{123}Te	^{152}Gd	^{180}Ta	^{187}Re

Less than 1000 μCi (4×10^7 Bq)						
^{3}H	^{7}Be	^{14}C	^{35}S	^{41}Ca	^{45}Ca	^{49}V
^{53}Mn	^{55}Fe	^{59}Ni	^{63}Ni	^{73}As	^{79}Se	^{99}Tc
^{107}Pd	^{135}Cs	^{141}Ce	^{181}W	^{185}W	^{188}W	^{204}Tl

Less than 100 μCi (4×10^6 Bq)						
^{36}Cl	^{40}K	^{59}Fe	^{57}Co	^{58}Co	^{75}Se	^{84}Rb
^{85}Sr	^{89}Sr	^{91}Y	^{95}Zr	^{93m}Nb	^{95}Nb	^{97m}Tc
^{103}Ru	^{105}Ag	^{114m}In	^{113}Sn	^{119m}Sn	^{121m}Sn	^{123}Sn
^{123m}Te	^{125m}Te	^{127m}Te	^{129m}Te	^{125}I	^{137}La	^{139}Ce
^{143}Pm	^{145}Pm	^{147}Pm	^{145}Sm[b]	^{151}Sm	^{149}Eu	^{155}Eu
^{151}Gd	^{153}Gd	^{157}Tb	^{159}Dy	^{170}Tm	^{171}Tm	^{169}Yb
^{173}Lu	^{174}Lu	^{174m}Lu	^{175}Hf	^{181}Hf	^{179}Ta	^{184}Re
^{186m}Re	^{192}Ir	^{193}Pt	^{195}Au	^{203}Hg	^{205}Pb	^{235}Np
^{237}Pu						

Less than 10 μCi (4×10^5 Bq)						
^{10}Be	^{22}Na	^{26}Al	^{32}Si	^{46}Sc	^{44}Ti	^{54}Mn
^{60}Fe	^{56}Co	^{60}Co	^{65}Zn	^{68}Ge	^{83}Rb	^{90}Sr
^{88}Y	^{88}Zr	^{93}Zr	^{94}Nb	^{93}Mo	^{95m}Tc	^{97}Tc
^{98}Tc	^{106}Ru	^{101}Rh	^{102}Rh	^{102m}Rh	^{108m}Ag	^{110m}Ag
^{109}Cd	^{126}Sn	^{124}Sb	^{125}Sb	^{121m}Te	^{129}I	^{134}Cs
^{137}Cs	^{133}Ba	^{138}La	^{144}Ce	^{144}Pm	^{146}Pm	^{148m}Pm
^{148}Eu	^{150}Eu	^{152}Eu	^{154}Eu	^{146}Gd	^{158}Tb	^{160}Tb
^{166m}Ho	^{176}Lu	^{177m}Lu	^{172}Hf	^{182}Ta	^{184m}Re	^{195}Os
^{194}Os	^{192m}Ir	^{194m}Ir	^{194}Hg	^{202}Pb	^{207}Bi	^{241}Cm

Less than 1 μCi (4×10^4 Bq)						
^{113m}Cd	^{178m}Hf	^{182}Hf	^{210m}Bi	^{210}Po	^{226}Ra	^{228}Ra
^{249}Bk						

Less than 0.1 μCi (4×10^3 Bq)						
^{146}Sm	^{147}Sm	^{210}Pb	^{233}U	^{234}U	^{235}U	^{236}U
^{238}U	^{241}Pu	^{242}Cm	^{248}Cf	^{254}Es	^{257}Fm	^{258}Md

Less than 0.01 μCi (4×10^2 Bq)						
^{148}Gd	^{228}Th	^{230}Th	^{232}U	^{236}Np	^{237}Np	^{236}Pu
^{238}Pu	^{239}Pu	^{240}Pu	^{242}Pu	^{244}Pu	^{241}Am	^{242m}Am
^{243}Am	^{243}Cm	^{244}Cm	^{245}Cm	^{246}Cm	^{247}Cm	^{247}Bk
^{249}Cf	^{250}Cf	^{251}Cf	^{252}Cf	^{254}Cf		

Less than 0.001 μCi (4×10^1 Bq)						
^{227}Ac	^{229}Th	^{232}Th	^{231}Pa	^{248}Cm	^{250}Cm	

[a] The criteria for exemption are: (1) the annual occupational dose from external radiation at 1 m from the source is approximately 100 μSv (10 mrem) or less; and (b) the source activity is approximately equal to the annual limit on intake by inhalation or less than 4×10^7 Bq (1000 μCi). These criteria were selected to correspond to an annual occupational dose of approximately 50 to 500 μSv (5 to 50 mrem) and a small potential annual risk of approximately 1×10^{-6} to 1×10^{-5} fatal cancers or less.

Table 11.1.5 NRC Guidelines for Decontamination of Facilities and Equipment Prior to Release for Unrestricted Use or Termination of Licenses for Byproduct, Source, or Special Nuclear Material (From NRC Div. of Industrial and Medical Nuclear Safety, 1987)

	Acceptable Surface Contamination Levels		
Nuclides[a]	Average[b,c,f]	Maximum[b,d,f]	Removable[b,e,f]
U-nat, ^{235}U, ^{238}U, and associated decay products	5,000 dpm α/100 cm^2	15,000 dpm α/100 cm^2	1,000 dpm α/100 cm^2
Transuranics, ^{226}Ra, ^{228}Ra, ^{230}Th, ^{228}Th, ^{231}Pa, ^{227}Ac, ^{125}I, ^{129}I	100 dpm/100 cm^2	300 dpm/100 cm^2	20 dpm/100 cm^2
Th-nat, ^{232}Th, ^{90}Sr, ^{223}Ra, ^{224}Ra, ^{232}U, ^{126}I, ^{131}I, ^{133}I	1,000 dpm/100 cm^2	3,000 dpm/100 cm^2	200 dpm/100 cm^2
Beta-gamma emitters (nuclides with decay modes other than alpha emission or spontaneous fission) except ^{90}Sr and others noted above.	5,000 dpm $\beta\gamma$/100 cm^2	15,000 dpm $\beta\gamma$/100 cm^2	1,000 dpm $\beta\gamma$/100 cm^2

[a] Where surface contamination by both alpha and beta-gamma emitting nuclides exists, the limits established for alpha and beta-gamma emitting nuclides should apply independently.

[b] As used in this table, dpm (disintegrations per minute) means the rate of emission by radioactive material as determined by correcting the counts per minute observed by an appropriate detector for background, efficiency, and geometric factors associated with the instrumentation.

[c] Measurements of average contaminant should not be averaged over more than 1 square meter. For objects of less surface area, the average should be derived for each such object.

[d] The maximum contamination level applies to an area of not more than 100 cm^2.

[e] The amount of removable radioactive material per 100 cm^2 of surface area should be determined by wiping that area with dry filter or soft absorbent paper, applying moderate pressure, and assessing the amount of radioactive material on the wipe with an appropriate instrument of known efficiency. When removable contamination on objects of less surface area is determined, the pertinent levels should be reduced proportionally and the entire surface should be wiped.

[f] The average and maximum radiation levels associated with surface contamination resulting from beta-gamma emitters should not exceed 0.2 mrad/hr at 1 cm and 1.0 mrad/hr at 1 cm, respectively, measured through not more than 7 milligrams per square centimeter of total absorber.

Table 11.1.6 Guidelines for Radioactive Surface Contamination (From Health Physics Society Draft standard ANSI N13.12, 1987)

Group No.	Group Description	Activity Guide (dpm/100 cm^2) Removable	Total[a]
(1)	All alpha emitters (except those in Group II) plus $^{210}Pb(^{210}Po)$ and $^{228}Ra(^{228}Th)$	20	100
(4)	Uranium (natural, depleted, enriched [<100 %]), Thorium (natural)	200	1,000
(2)	^{90}Sr, ^{125}I, ^{126}I, ^{129}I, ^{131}I	200	5,000
(3)	All β, γ-emitters not in Groups I, II, or III except β-emitters with $E_{max} \leq 0.15$ MeV[b]	1,000	5,000

[a] "Total" includes removable and fixed contamination.

[b] Pure beta-emitting radionuclides with maximum beta energies less than 0.15 MeV must be handled on a case-by-case basis because they are not detectable by conventional monitoring instruments.

Note: for recommended action levels for removable surface contamination in medical institutions see Table 11.4.8.

Table 11.1.7 Contamination Level Guides for Respiratory Protection Equipment Used by Nuclear Facilities

Equipment	Removable $\beta-\gamma$	Fixed $\beta-\gamma$
Respiratory Protection		
Inside Facepieces, Outside Facepieces, and Filter (Outside Canister)	1000 dpm/100 cm^2	1.5 mR/hr[a]

[a] The average over the entire facepiece should not exceed 0.2 mR/hr.

Table 11.1.8 Guideline for Protective Clothing Used by Nuclear Facilities[a]

Garment	Radiation Level $\beta-\gamma$[b]
Coveralls, Lab Coats and Hats or Hoods	2.5 mR/hr[c]
Gloves and Shoe Covers	10 mR/hr

[a] Clothing normally laundered after each use. May be re-worn when previously worn in areas less than 10,000 dpm/100 cm^2 removable contamination.

[b] If guideline exceeded, the clothing should be stored for use in the contaminated area.

[c] This is an average value over the garment as long as any one spot does not exceed 10 mR/hr.

Table 11.1.9 Acceptable Frequencies for Surveys (From NRC Reg. Guide 8.21, 1979)

Radionuclide Group		External Radiation Surveys (nuclides with asterisks only)[a]		Amounts (Curies) in Process at Any One Time or Placed into Process in Any 3 Mo. Period Within Any Room Requiring Surveys					
				Air Sampling[b]			Surface Contamination		
		Weekly	Monthly	Weekly	Monthly	Quarterly	Weekly	Monthly	Quarterly
I:	^{3}H, ^{14}C, ^{18}F,* ^{42}K,* ^{64}Cu,* ^{99m}Tc,* ^{113m}In*	If point source of activity could exceed 50 mrad/h at 1 meter	If point source of activity could exceed 0.5 mrad/h at 1 meter	≥ 10	≥ 1 < 10	< 1	≥ 100	≥ 10 < 100	< 10
II:	^{82}Br, ^{51}Cr,* ^{55}Fe, ^{123}I,* ^{197}Hg*			≥ 1	≥ 0.1 < 1	< 0.1	≥ 10	≥ 1 < 10	< 1
III:	^{35}S, ^{198}Au, ^{47}Ca, ^{132}I, ^{141}Ce, Mixed fission products,* ^{85}Sr, ^{140}La, ^{95}Nb, ^{65}Zn, ^{58}Co,* ^{59}Fe,* ^{24}Na,* ^{57}Co,* ^{75}Se,* ^{99}Mo*			≥ 0.1	≥ 0.001 < 0.1	< 0.01	≥ 1	≥ 0.1 < 1	< 0.1
IV:	^{181}Hf, ^{147}Pm, ^{32}P,* ^{140}Ba,* ^{234}Th, ^{85}Kr, ^{192}Ir,* ^{36}Cl, ^{91}Y, ^{192}Ta, ^{45}Ca, ^{89}Sr, ^{137}Cs, ^{60}Co,* ^{144}Ce,* ^{126}I, ^{154}Eu, ^{131}I,* ^{125}I,* ^{170}Tm, ^{22}Na,* ^{54}Mn,* ^{110m}Ag,* ^{203}Hg,* ^{222}Rn,* ^{113}Sn*			≥ 0.01	≥ 0.001 < 0.01	< 0.001	≥ 0.1	≥ 0.01 < 0.1	< 0.01
V:	^{99}Tc, ^{129}I, ^{106}Ru			≥ 0.001	$\geq 10^{-4}$ < 0.001	$< 10^{-4}$	≥ 0.01	≥ 0.001 < 0.01	< 0.001
VI:	^{223}Ra, ^{210}Po, ^{227}Th, ^{90}Sr, ^{210}Pb, ^{242}Cm, ^{233}U*			$\geq 10^{-4}$	$\geq 10^{-5}$ $< 10^{-4}$	$< 10^{-5}$	≥ 0.001	$\geq 10^{-4}$ < 0.001	$< 10^{-4}$
VII:	^{147}Sm, ^{144}Nd, ^{226}Ra,* ^{244}Cm, ^{228}Ra, ^{241}Pu			$\geq 10^{-5}$	$\geq 10^{-6}$ $< 10^{-5}$	$< 10^{-6}$	$\geq 10^{-4}$	$\geq 10^{-5}$ $< 10^{-4}$	$< 10^{-5}$
VIII:	^{243}Am, ^{241}Am,* ^{237}Np, ^{227}Ac, ^{230}Th, ^{242}Pu, ^{238}Pu, ^{240}Pu, ^{239}Pu, ^{228}Th, ^{252}Cf			$\geq 10^{-6}$	$\geq 10^{-7}$ $< 10^{-6}$	$< 10^{-8}$	$\geq 10^{-5}$	$\geq 10^{-6}$ $< 10^{-5}$	$< 10^{-6}$

[a] Nuclides with Asterisks are those more likely to require external radiation surveys. Editorial note: Reg Guide 8.21 is for manufacturing facilities. Other facilities may consider external radiation surveys for gamma emitting nuclides not so marked.

[b] Assuming continuous sampling is unnecessary.

Table 11.1.10 Good Work Practice Guide for Performing a Laboratory Survey (Personal communication Slaback, 1991)

(NOTE: For a particular survey, it is good practice to select several items for emphasized review.)

Getting Started:

- Check previous survey results for any special problems.
- Check usage of area, e.g., user names, nuclides used, processes, amounts.
- Initiate survey form, where applicable.

General Audit:

- How is waste being collected, identified, stored, and disposed?
- Is any radioactive material being disposed via the lab sink?
- Is the room posted ''CAUTION, RADIOACTIVE MATERIAL''?
- Are all sources and source containers labeled with a ''CAUTION RAM'' label and identified as to nuclide, amount, and assay date?
- Is radioisotope hood labeled with a current flow check? Is the hood functioning?
- Is there an instrument available for contamination checks, if required?

Observe General Conditions:

- Food or drink present? In refrigerator with nuclides?
- Smoking restrictions being followed?
- Waste container full?
- Spill containment available for liquid radionuclides?
- Proper pipetting techniques being used? i.e., no mouth pipetting.
- Work area neat?
- Are users wearing required dosimetry?

Contamination Surveys Technique:

- Smear general access areas first, then do source storage and usage areas. That is, work from areas expected to be low to those that might be high. If the actual results show aberrant results considered the possibility of cross-contamination of smears. Do not smear posted contaminated areas except as a separate special survey.
- Prime survey points include: floor at entrance, door handle at entrance, floor in front of work area or hood, apron on hood, lab sink, ventilation exhaust grill or duct, and drawer and cabinet handles near the work area.
- Low energy beta emitters (^{3}H, ^{14}C) and pure photon emitters require special counting consideration.

Radiation Survey Technique:

- Check all occupiable areas for radiation levels >2.5 mR/h. Under ALARA objectives extended occupancy areas should be less than 0.5 mR/h.
- Check adjacent rooms located behind source storage areas, particularly if lead shielding is being used. Also check above and below storage areas.
- For fixed contamination checks include all surfaces near the work area, including the ceiling and difficult to smear items like lab coats.

When Finished:

- Record all results.
- Notify user of survey results.

Table 11.1.11 Sample Checklist for Radiation Surveyor (After NRC Regulatory Guide 8.23 Rev. 1, 1982)[a]

Initiate Contamination Survey Report for Each Lab:

- Check card for previous survey results, e.g., successive red circles (problems?), nobody in.
- Fill in name of Authorized User, Department, Building and Room Number, and Survey Date.
- Sketch floor plan.

Ask Lab Personnel (and record answers on report form):

- What isotopes are being used? (Compare with what User is cleared for.)
- Where in the lab are they used?
- Where are isotopes stored?
- What was last order? (Compare with card record.)
- Is Authorized User available if needed? If not, give reason, e.g., on leave, out of country, terminated employment.
- In what other labs are isotopes used? (Compare with card record.)
- Where is waste stored and disposed of?
- Who is currently handling—primary solutions? diluted solutions? Are these persons on bioassay programs?

Check Labeling:

- Lab Door—''Caution, Radioactive Material''
- Liquid Waste Container—''Contaminated Liquid Waste.'' Is container log posted? Is it being used?
- Radioactive Hood—''Caution, Radioactive Material'' (Survey card should indicate radioactive hood—RH). ''Air Flow Check'' white label wth date no older than 4 months required.
- Refrigerator and other storage areas—''CRM,'' including those in corridors.
- Radioactive waste containers—''CRM'' or ''Contaminated Waste'' should be lined with yellow plastic bag.
- Any area with external radiation over 2.5 mR/h should be labeled with ''Caution, Radiation Area'' and should be noted on survey form.
- 10 CFR Part 19 signs.

Observe General Laboratory Conditions:

- Food and drink preparation and use in radioactive material areas?
- Waste container overfilled?
- Dosimeters being worn?
- Mouth pipetting?
- Secondary containment in liquid RAM user area.

Conduct Laboratory Survey Using Portable Survey Meter:

- Record external dose rate from accessible storage
- Record exposure rate from contaminated surfaces

Conduct Smear Survey:

- Take first smear near or in lab entrance.
- Take several smears from floor and benches and equipment as indicated by answers to earlier questions.
- Do smears in suspected contaminated areas.
- Sample frost in refrigerator for contamination.

Table 11.1.11 Sample Checklist for Radiation Survey (Continued)

Discuss 10 CFR Part 19 (Instructions to Workers) Requirements.

Complete Results:

- Count smears and list results on survey form.
- Notify lab personnel of contamination, and note on form who was called and date of notification.
- Identify all abnormal radiation safety conditions on survey form.
- Complete survey card, replace in file, and mail survey form copy to User.
- If lab has contamination (significant), isolate lab if necessary, call User, request cleanup, and resmear.
- Resmear when notified or call User if no resmear was called for.
- File carbon copy of results form.

Table 11.1.12 Good Work Practice Guide for Using Radiation Survey Instruments (Personal communications Slaback, 1991)

Choosing an Instrument:

- Choose an instrument with the appropriate energy response and range for your needs. If you do not know anything about the field to be surveyed you cannot select an instrument! Consult a supervisory health physicist.
- NaI crystals are good low level detectors but are not for dose rate measurements; pancake GMs are good contamination detectors but also are not for dose rate measurements; energy compensated GMs are not for low energy photon measurements; open window instruments calibrated with photons are not calibrated for betas unless so indicated.

Before You Turn the Instrument On:

- **Do Not Use** an instrument you have never used before; that is one for which you have no prior experience on the way it behaves. Always ''learn'' an instrument in a non-operational situation and become comfortable with is peculiarities.
- **Do Not Use** an instrument for which you have not read the manual. You simply cannot guess with surety at special features or limitations that might be incorporated into a new instrument.
- **Do Not Use** an instrument with an out-of-date calibration sticker. If it is even one day out of calibration it is not usable, and must be removed from service.

Turn Instrument On:

- Do a battery check. On some instruments there is more than one battery check to be done.
- Do a High Voltage check, if present.
- Observe the behavior of the instrument after the range switch is turned to the desired setting. Look for any peculiarities based on your previous experience with this instrument. Do not use the instrument if there is any doubt as to its operational condition.
- Do a performance check, if available. This might be done with a built-in check source, with a nearby operational check source, or by performing an internal electronic check.

Using the Instrument:

- Select the proper window for the type of radiation to be monitored.
- Observe the instrument as you enter a radiation field. If the trend from the readings do not make sense, leave the area. Then think about it.
- Use the instrument in the manner for which it is calibrated. Usually this requires uniform chamber irradiation with photons. Field gradients close to point sources, small beams, beta fields all require special calibrations.
- For a long survey, regularly check the condition of the batteries.
- Notify area users of survey results, with emphasis on changed or extraordinary conditions.
- Record all results. If nothing is on paper the survey was never done! Include date, time, instrument model and serial number, and your name.

When Finished, TURN OFF. Recheck the battery and performance when finished to verify that the instrument is still working properly.

Table 11.1.13.1 Good Work Practice Guide for the Use of Laboratory Hoods (Personal Communication Slaback, 1991)

Fume hoods may be of many different designs (also see 11.1.13.2). This guide is restricted to five sided, front sash type laboratory hoods. Even with proper usage a laboratory hood provides only a limited measure of protection, typically in the range of a factor of 5 to 50 exposure reduction. Hence the exposure potential of the materials being used and the work being done should be carefully reviewed, and strong consideration should be given to a glove box for very hazardous operations.

Design Features:

- **Base:** For flammables this should meet NFPA 30 and 20CFR1910.106 (double wall, unvented). For corrosives the construction should be acid resistant and be vented front and back.
- **Hood Liner:** For radionuclides this should be a seamless stainless steel surface. The working surface should be dished with a front lip.
- **Baffle:** This is a panel at the back to control the exhausted air. Typically there are three horizontal slots (bottom, middle top) to provide an even air flow pattern in the hood.
- **Jamb:** This is the flange around the front face of the hood. This makes the hood opening smaller than the internal cross section which serves to minimize eddies.
- **Sill:** Typically this is an airfoil which reduces eddies by shaping the air flow both above and below the sill. Without this, careless hand movements would spill high concentrations from those eddies to the room.
- **Location:** Away from air supplies, doors, people pathways. Competing air movements by these can seriously compromise the hood effectiveness.

Usage Guide:

- Consider additional protective measures: gloves, mask, apron, labcoat . . .
- Use secondary containment for liquid sources.
- Verify that an adequate air flow is present before starting work.
- Keep the sash as low as possible. Equipment in the hood can induce a rollover pattern which carries fumes back towards your face.
- When the hood is unattended completely close the sash. This is particularly important for chemical hoods where the exhaust fan is turned off since there is a potential for backflow into the lab from the exhaust system.
- Keep all operations at least 8″ from the front edge of the hood. Keep all equipment at least 12″ from the front hood edge. In general keep sources as far back in the hood as possible and towards the sides of the hood. Air ''spillage'' from the center and front of the hood is greater than the sides and back.
- **Do not block** the baffle slots or the opening under the sill with equipment or absorbent paper. Blocked baffles or airfoils greatly decrease the hood protection factor.
- Keep material and equipment in the hood to a minimum. If the equipment does not have legs place it on 3″ blocks to allow air flow underneath.
- Adjust baffles so that the lower slot is wide open and the top slot is open ½″ to 1″. For most operations this will minimize rollover.
- Keep hand movements slow and deliberate. Normal hand movements create eddies that extract contaminants from the hood atmosphere to the room.
- Do not allow foot traffic in front of a hood in use. Eddies created by the passage of a person will extract air from a working hood.
- Perform regular inspections and maintenance.

Table 11.1.13.2 Exhaust and Laminar-Flow Hoods

Two types of hoods are used in radioisotope laboratories: conventional exhaust hoods and laminar-flow exhaust hoods. An exhaust hood, normally used in chemical laboratories, is an enclosure from which the toxic and/or radioactive fumes of a chemical reaction are removed by means of an exhaust fan. An exhaust hood should be equipped with a filter in the exhaust line if radioactive material is expected in the exhaust. These hoods may also be equipped with lead shielding and remote handling devices if necessitated by the level of radioactivity and the time spent on the procedure. A properly placed mirror makes it possible to follow the operations without direct exposure to the head. Exhaust hoods with remotely-controlled manipulators and adequate construction to support the heavy weight of lead shielding are available commercially.

In nuclear medicine, the worker is interested in protecting an open container of radioactive material, usually a solution, from bacterial contamination while also protecting personnel from contamination by radioactivity from the material. To accomplish this, a laminar-flow exhaust hood is required. This containment-type cabinet not only provides a workspace that is protected from the ambient working environment, it also provides an ambient working environment that is protected from the experiment done in the work space. A diagram of this type of hood showing the design, HEPA filtering system, air-flow patterns is given in Figure 11.2. This type of hood is sold primarily as a biological hazard hood. With some structural modification, the work area can handle the heavy load of a lead brick shield that may be required for some procedures.

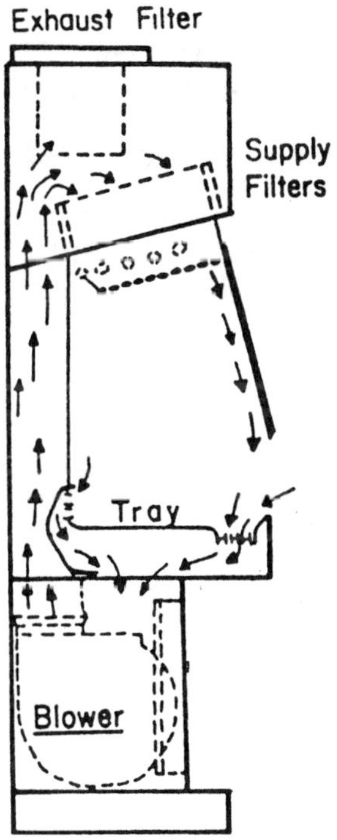

Figure 11.2 Laminar-Flow Exhaust Hood

Table 11.1.14 Good Work Practice Guide for the Use of Sealed Sources[a] (Personal Communication Slaback, 1991)

1. Ensure that all personnel using the source(s) are trained in the hazards, safety precautions, and proper use of the radioactive material.
2. Store sources in shielded locations or locations remote from day-to-day occupancy. Do not store sources in the vicinity of dosimeter storage locations. Maintain security for all sources.
3. Be aware of external and surface dose rates. Use time-distance-shielding techniques whenever possible. Use remote handling devices where appropriate. This should be considered for even small check sources to reduce finger exposures.
4. Whenever handling or removing a source from its container, look for abnormalities. If in doubt about the condition of a source, return it to storage and contact Health Physics immediately to perform a leak test.
5. Do not leave an exposed source that produces more than 5 mrem/h at 12 inches unattended unless specific arrangements are made with Health Physics.
6. Wear[b] a radiation dosimeter when using sources that can produce whole body dose rates in excess of 2 mrem/h or is otherwise required.
7. Have a radiation survey instrument immediately available when radiation levels in excess of 2 mrem/hr are being produced.
8. Protect personnel in adjoining areas.
9. Maintain a use log for those sources that can produce significant personnel exposures. This log should contain sufficient detail so that any operation with the source can be reconstructed.
10. Be aware of and follow the usage restrictions specified on the source usage approval form.

[a] Radioactive Material encased in a capsule or having a bonded cover to prevent leakage or the escape of the radioactive material under conditions of use for which it is designed.

[b] If a dosimeter is assigned, wear it for all work. Frequency of usage and other work can affect this criteria. The underlying fundamental criteria is total annual exposure. Consult your radiation safety office for a specific assessment.

Table 11.1.15 Good Work Practice Guide for the Use of Unsealed Sources (Including Uranium and Thorium) (Personal Communication Slaback, 1991)

1. Ensure that all involved persons are trained in the hazards, safety precautions, and proper use of the material.
2. Wear gloves to prevent hand contamination. Additional protective clothing such as lab coats, aprons, face shields, and caps may be advisable, depending on the level of activity, the hazard of the nuclide, and the type of work planned. Contamination prevention is far less costly than decontamination.
3. Monitor hands, clothing and work areas for contamination after each procedure. Wash hands immediately following work completion.
4. Never pipette by mouth.
5. Control aerosols resulting from the use of blenders, opening recently centrifuged test tubes, the use of ultrasonic devices, heating, or other similar procedures.
6. Minimize hood air flow disturbances by keeping the work space uncluttered, by reducing the front opening as far as possible, and by careful and deliberate hand movements. (See Table 11.1.13.2)
7. Be aware of external and container surface dose rates. Use remote handling devices where appropriate.
8. Use shielding whenever possible and if appropriate. Pipette from shielded containers, put containers behind or into shields when not actually in use. Transport sources in shielded containers.
9. Use secondary spill containment whenever possible. That is, work in a tray and/or on diaper paper. Store the source in a secondary container in case of leakage, transport the source in the unbreakable container, e.g., a plastic bag, in case of droppage.
10. Visually inspect source containers for damage or leakage before putting them into use.
11. Label all containers of radioactive material. This includes vials, test tubes, flasks, beakers, etc., in addition to the primary and diluted source solutions.
12. Collect all waste for transfer to Health Physics. Collect all liquid waste separately.
13. Wear radiation dosimetry as required by Health Physics.
14. Do not eat, drink, smoke, or apply cosmetics in any area where radioactive material is stored or in use. Do not store food or drink with radioactive material.
15. Be aware of the chemical properties of the radionuclide you are working with to avoid uncontrolled releases of activity. Tritium, radioiodines, polonium, ruthenium, plutonium and many others form chemically mobile (i.e., volatile) compounds. Others such as ^{226}Ra give rise to volatile daughter products.

(continued)

Table 11.1.15 Good Work Practice Guide for the Use of Unsealed Sources (Including Uranium and Thorium) (Continued)

Uranium and Thorium Users' Addendum

Characteristics

Material	Specific Activity (μCi/g)	Gamma Dose Rate[b] at 10 cm from 1 g (μR/h)	Committed Internal Dose for Intake of 1 mg (rem/mg)	Normal Daily Intake (μg)	Radiations Emitted
Natural Thorium	0.22[e]	44	9.0[c]	3	α, β, γ
Natural Uranium	0.71[f]	9	0.3[d]	1.9	α, β, γ
Depleted Uranium[a]	0.33[g]	5	0.3[d]	—	α, β, γ

[a] Many chemicals are in fact made from depleted uranium, i.e., depleted in ^{235}U. Also be aware that the chemical toxicity of uranium is equally or more important than the radiological toxicity.

[b] Assuming equilibrium with short-lived daughters. Natural background is 6–10 μR/h.

[c] For inhalation of ^{232}Th only, dose to bone surfaces.

[d] For inhalation of insoluble ^{238}U, dose to lungs.

[e] ^{232}Th + first daughter.

[f] ^{238}U + other natural occurring uranium isotopes.

[g] ^{238}U only.

Addendum

Accounting: Each person using uranium or thorium compounds must be prepared to account for all material acquired. A normal research notebook is adequate for this purpose. Amounts in excess of 10 g shall be registered with Health Physics.

Disposal: All wastes containing uranium or thorium compounds shall be collected and transferred to Health Physics for disposal.

Dosimetry: External radiation dosimeters are not needed or required. Bioassays (urinalysis, fecal analysis) may be required for complex procedures which could lead to airborne materials. 10CFR20 (e) limits soluble uranium intake to 10 mg/week.

Contamination Monitoring: This is normally required only for dry operations or for significant quantities.

Table 11.1.16 Good Work Practice Guide for Radioluminous Materials (Personal Communication Slaback, 1991)

Radioactive materials are frequently used to produce devices that emit light, e.g., wrist watches, laboratory light sources, etc. The main advantage of such devices is not needing electrical power to produce the light and constancy of the light produced, at least over a short period of time. But these sources are radioactive so you should be aware of some basic safety precautions.

Radionuclides Used:

The majority of the radioluminous devices use low energy beta emitters as the energizing material. The two most common radionuclides are tritium (^{3}H), the only radioactive isotope of hydrogen, and promethium-147 (^{147}Pm). Some charactetristics are

	^{3}H	^{147}Pm
Half-life	12.28 y	2.62 y
Beta Energy maximum:	18.6 keV	224.7 keV
average:	5.7 keV	62.0 keV
Other Radiations	none[a]	none[a]
Range of Average Beta	0.02 mg/cm^2	5 mm in air

Hazards and Precautions:

There is in essence no external exposure risk from these sources. The range of the primary emissions is such that the betas do not escape the encapsulation or containment. If there is sufficient radioactive material, i.e., enough activity, the very low rate of bremsstrahlung (photon) production may result in measurable external dose rates. For tritium even this is very unlikely to be a concern because this low energy spectrum cannot penetrate the body. For ^{147}Pm and other radionuclides this is also unlikely to be significant but a measurement should be made.

The primary risk of concern is internal exposure. This can only occur if the source containment is broken in some way. If a source is suspected to be broken **do not handle or disturb it in any way.** ***Contact Health Physics*** immediately.

All radioluminous sources must be labeled as radioactive material so that anyone who encounters the source will be aware of its nature. Such labels are available from Health Physics.

The manufacturer of the source is required by the Nuclear Regulatory Commission to provide safety instructions and hazardous material data. Keep these instructions available and make certain that all users of the sources are familiar with this information.

[a] Excluding beta produced bremsstrahlung.

Table 11.1.17 Protection Factors for Respirators[a] (Appendix A to 20.1001–20.2401) (Reproduced from 10CFR 20, 1991)

Description[b]	Modes[c]	Protection Factors[d]: Particulates Only	Protection Factors[d]: Particulates, Gases, & Vapors[c]	Tested & Certified Equipment: National Institute for Occupational Safety and Health/Mine Safety and Health Administration Tests for Permissibility
I. Air Purifying Respirators:[f]				
Facepiece, half mask[g]	NP	10		30 CFR Part 11, Subpart K
Facepiece, full	NP	50		
Facepiece, half mask full, 000or hood	PP	1000		
II. Atmosphere Supplying Respirators:				
1. Air line respirator:				
Facepiece, half mask	CF		1,000	30 CFR Part 11, Subpart J
Facepiece, half mask	D		5	
Facepiece, full	CF		2,000	
Facepiece, full	D		5	
Facepiece, full	PD		2,000	
Hood	CF		[h]	
Suit	CF		[i]	[j]
2. Self contained breathing apparatus (SCBA):				
Facepiece, full	D		50	30 CFR Part 11, Subpart H
Facepiece, full	PD		10,000[k]	
Facepiece, full	RD		50	
Facepiece, full	RP		5,000[l]	
III. Combination Respirators				
Any combination of air purifying and atmosphere supplying respirators	Protection factor for type and mode of operation as listed above.			30 CFR Part 11, § 11.63(b)

[a] For use in the selection of respiratory protective devices to be used only where the contaminants have been identified and the concentrations (or possible concentrations) are known.

[b] Only the shaven faces and where nothing interferes with the seal of tight-fitting facepieces against the skin. (Hoods and suits are excepted.)

[c] The mode symbols are defined as follows:

CF = continuous flow
D = demand
NP = negative pressure (i.e., negative phase during inhalation)
PD = pressure demand (i.e., always positive pressure)
PP = positive pressure
RD = demand, recirculating (closed circuit)
RP = pressure demand, recirculating (closed circuit)

[d] 1. The protection factor is a measure of the degree of protection afforded by a respirator, defined as the ratio of the concentration of airborne radioactive material outside the respiratory protective equipment to that inside the equipment (usually inside the facepiece) under conditions of use. It is applied to the ambient airborne concentration to estimate the concentrations inhaled by the wearer according to the following formula:

$$\text{concentration inhaled} = \frac{\text{Ambient airborne concentration}}{\text{Protection factor}}$$

2. The protection factors apply:

(a) Only for individuals trained in using respirators and wearing properly fitted respirators that re used and maintained under supervision in a well planned respiratory protective program.

(b) For air purifying respirators only when high efficiency particulate filters (above 99.97% removal efficiency by thermally generated 0.3 μ dioctyl phthalate (DPO) test or equivalent) are used in atmospheres not deficient in oxygen and not containing radioactive gas or vapor respiratory hazards.

(c) No adjustment is to be made for the use of sorbents against radioactive material in the form of gases or vapors.

(d) For atmosphere-supplying respirators only when supplied with adequate respirable air. Respirable air shall be provided of the quality and quantity required in accordance with NIOSH/MSHA certification (described in 30 CFR part 11). Oxygen and air shall not be used in the same apparatus.

[e] Excluding radioactive contaminants that present an absorption or submersion hazard. For tritium oxide, approximately one-third of the intake occurs by absorption through the skin so that an overall protection factor of less than 2 is appropriate when atmosphere-supplying respirators are used to protect against tritium oxide. If the protection factor for a device is 5 the effective protection factor for tritium is about 1.4; for devices with protection factors of 10 the effective factor for tritium oxide is about 1.7, and for devices with protection factors of 100 or more the effective factor for tritium oxide is about 1.9. Air-purifying respirators are not suitable for protection against tritium oxide. See also footnote i concerning supplied-air suits.

[f] Canisters and cartridges shall not be used beyond service-life limitations.

[g] Under-chin type only. This type of respirator is not satisfactory for use where it might be possible (e.g., if an accident or emergency were to occur) for the ambient airborne concentrations to reach instantaneous values greater than 10 times the pertinent values in table 1, column 3 of appendix B to §§20.1001–20.2401 of this part. This type of respirator is not suitable for protection against plutonium or other high-toxicity materials. The mask is to be tested for fit prior to use, each time it is donned.

[h] 1. Equipment shall be operated in a manner that ensures that proper air flow-rates are maintained. A protection factor of no more than 1,000 may be utilized for tested-and-certified supplied-air hoods when a minimum air flow of 6 cubic feet (0.17 cubic meters) per minute is maintained and calibrated air-line pressure gauges or flow measuring devices are used. A protection factor of up to 2,000 may be used for tested and certified hoods only when the air flow is maintained at the manufacturer's recommended maximum rate for the equipment, this rate is greater than 6 cubic feet (0.17 cubic meters) per minute, and calibrated air-line pressure gauges or flow measuring devices are used.

2. The design of the supplied-air hood or helmet (with a minimum flow of 6 cfm (0.17 m^3 per minute) of air) may determine its overall efficiency and the protection it provides. For example, some hoods aspirate contaminated air into the breathing zone when the wearer works with hands-overhead. This aspiration may be overcome if a short cape-like extension to the hood is worn under a coat or overalls. Other limitations specified by the approval agency shall be considered before using a hood in certain types of atmospheres (see footnote i)

[i] Appropriate protection factors shall be determined, taking into account the design of the suit and its permeability to the contaminant under conditions of use. There shall be a standby rescue person equipped with a respirator or other apparatus appropriate for the potential hazards and communications equipment whenever supplied-air suits are used.

[j] No approval schedules are currently available for this equipment. Equipment is to be evaluated by testing or on the basis of reliable test information.

[k] This type of respirator may provide greater protection and be used as an emergency device in unknown concentrations for protection against inhalation hazards. External radiation hazards and other limitations to permitted exposure, such as skin absorption, must be taken into account in such circumstances.

[l] Quantitative fit testing shall be performed on each individual and no more than 0.02% leakage is allowed with this type of apparatus. Perceptible outward leakage of gas from this or any positive pressure self-contained breathing apparatus is inacceptable because service life will be reduced substantially. Special training in the use of this type of apparatus shall be provided to the wearer.

Note 1: Protection factors for respirators as may be approved by the U.S. Bureau of Mines/National Institute for Occupational Safety and health (NIOSH), according to applicable approvals for respirators for type and mode of use to protect against airborne radionuclides, may be used to the extent that they do not exceed the protection factors listed in this table. The protection factors listed in this table may not be appropriate to circumstances where chemical or other respiratory hazards exist in addition to radioactive hazards. The selection and use of respirators for such circumstances should take into account applicable approvals of the U.S. Bureau of Mines/NIOSH.

SECTION 2 NUCLEAR REACTORS/FUEL CYCLE

Locations of operating power reactors throughout the United States and schematics for boiling and pressurized water power reactors begin this section. Data in this section pertain to reactor source term characteristics and variables. Data on research reactors are at the end of the section.

TABLE OF CONTENTS

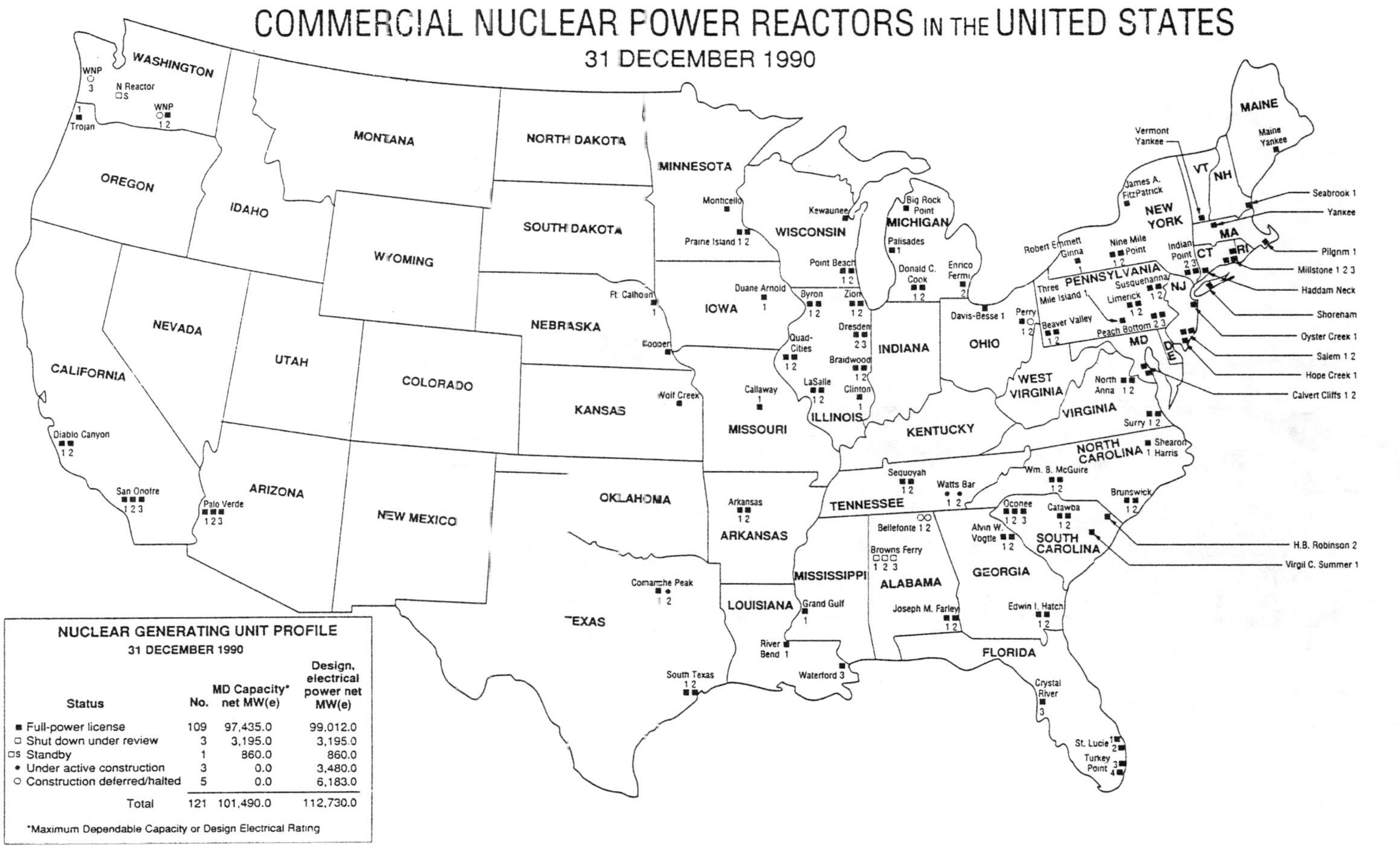

NUCLEAR GENERATING UNIT PROFILE
31 DECEMBER 1990

Status	No.	MD Capacity* net MW(e)	Design, electrical power net MW(e)
■ Full-power license	109	97,435.0	99,012.0
□ Shut down under review	3	3,195.0	3,195.0
□S Standby	1	860.0	860.0
• Under active construction	3	0.0	3,480.0
○ Construction deferred/halted	5	0.0	6,183.0
Total	121	101,490.0	112,730.0

*Maximum Dependable Capacity or Design Electrical Rating

Figure 11.2.1 Locations of Existing and Planned Commercial Reactors as of December 31, 1990 (From DOE/OSTI-8200-R53, 1991)

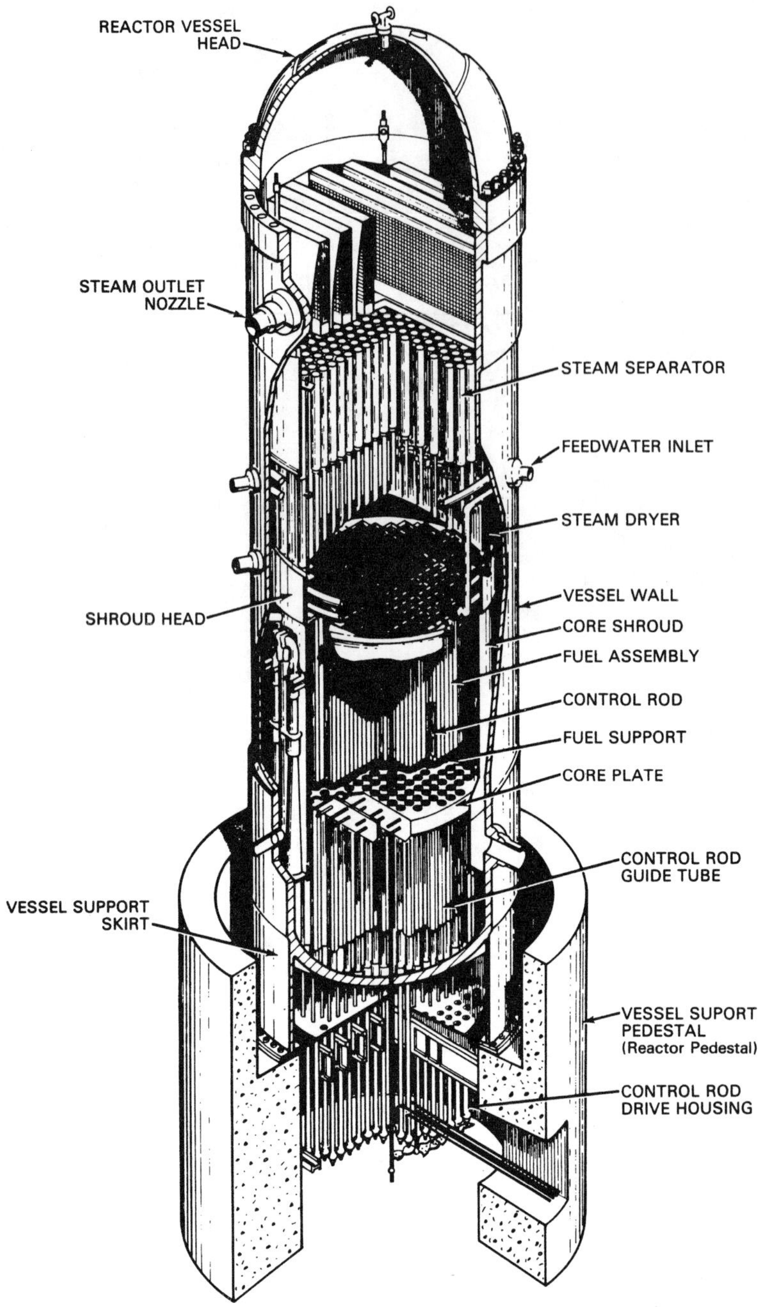

Figure 11.2.2 Schematic of BWR Reactor Vessel Internal Structure (From NUREG-0956, 1986)

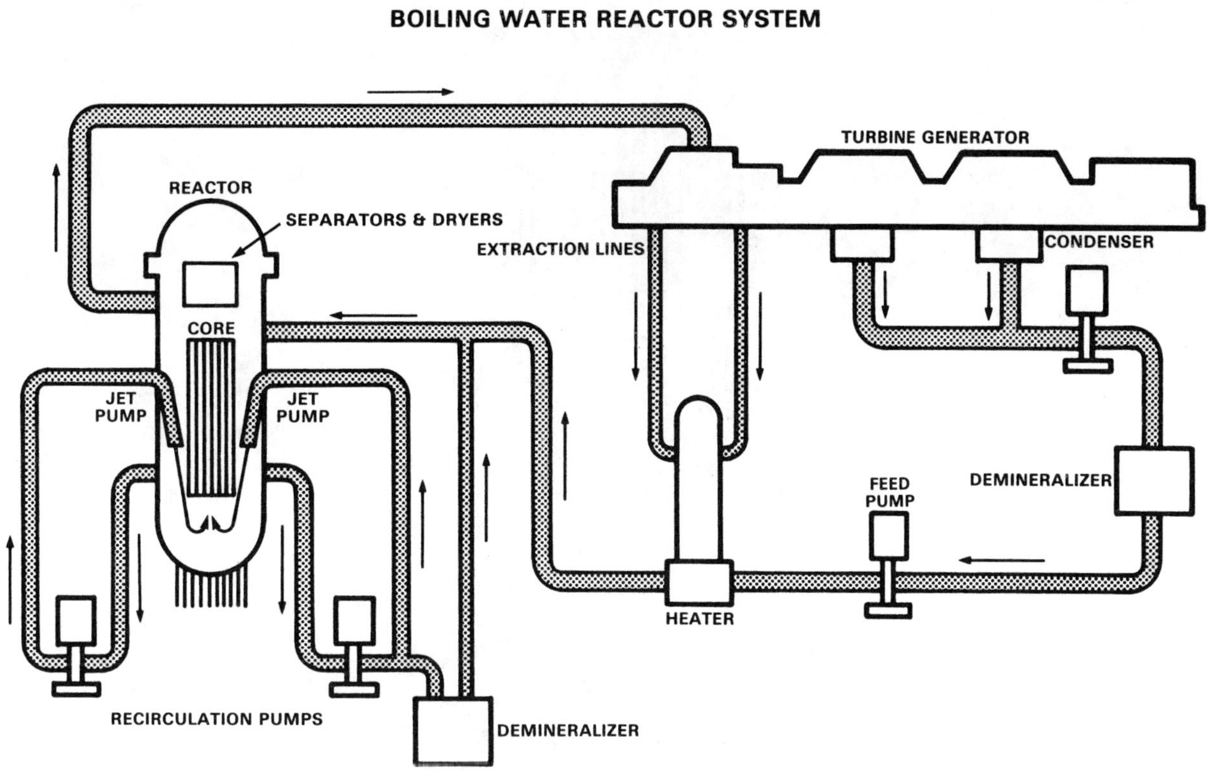

Figure 11.2.3 Schematic of BWR Plant Design (From NUREG-0956, 1986)

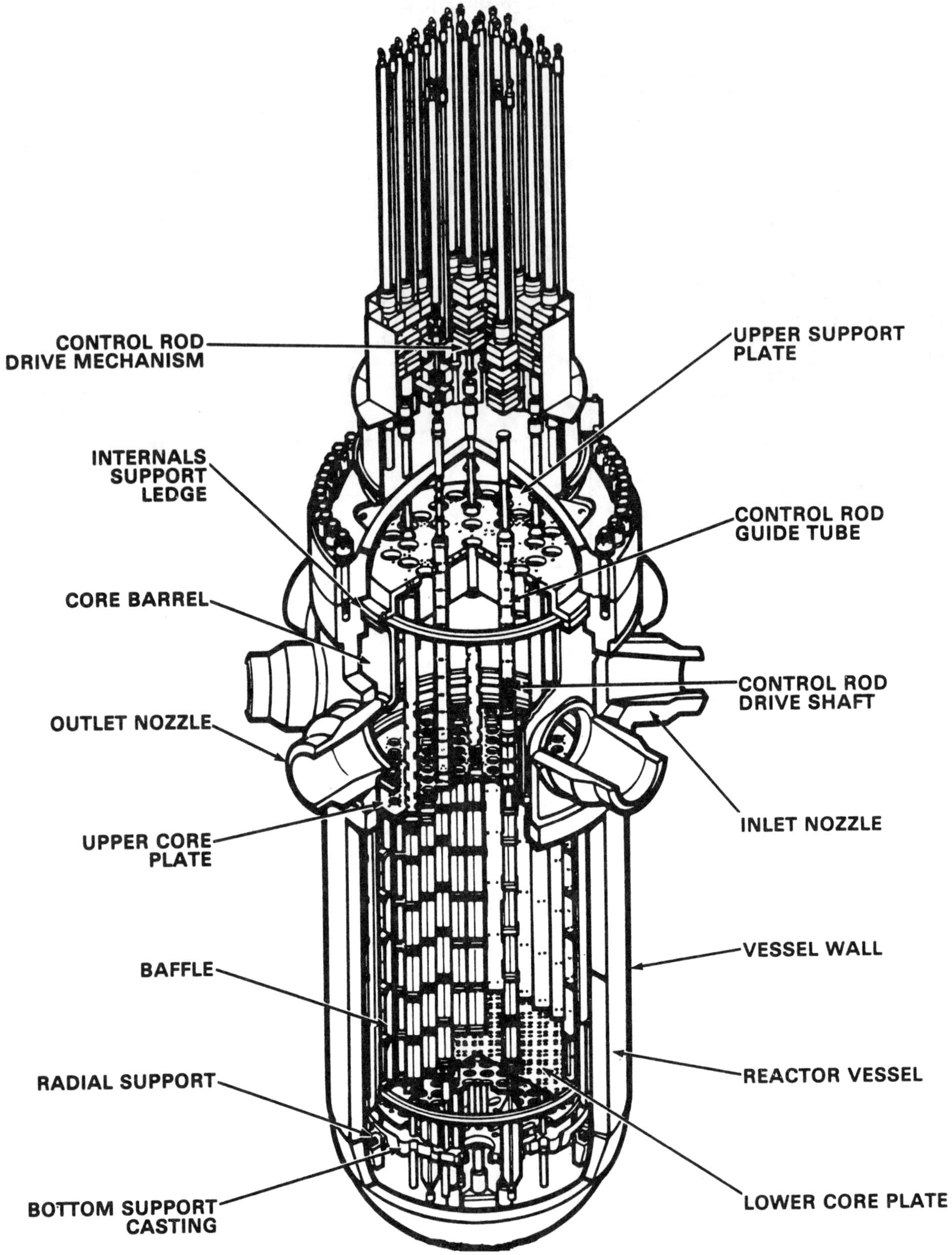

Figure 11.2.4 Schematic of PWR Reactor Vessel Internal Structure (From NUREG-0956, 1986)

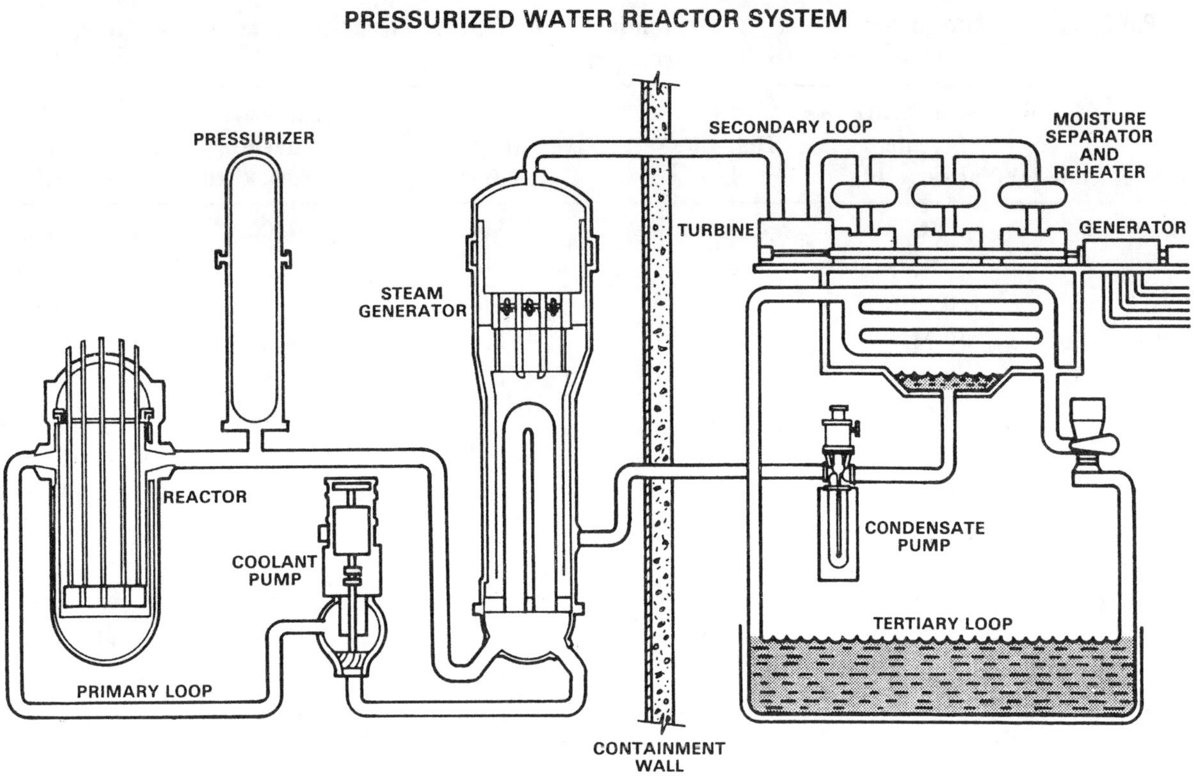

Figure 11.2.5 Schematic of PWR Plant Design (From NUREG-0956, 1986)

Table 11.2.1 Initial Activity of Radionuclides in the Nuclear Reactor Core at the Time of a Hypothetical Accident (From NUREG-0956, 1986)[a]

Radionuclide	Radioactive Inventory (curies × 10^{-8})	Half-Life[b] (days)	Radionuclide	Radioactive Inventory (curies × 10^{-8})	Half-Life[b] (days)
^{58}Co	0.0078	70.8	^{127}Sb	0.061	3.85
^{60}Co	0.0029	1924	^{129}Sb	0.33	0.183
^{85}Kr	0.0056	3913	^{131}I	0.85	8.04
^{85m}Kr	0.24	0.187	^{132}I	1.2	0.0958
^{87}Kr	0.47	0.0530	^{133}I	1.7	0.867
^{88}Kr	0.68	0.118	^{134}I	1.9	0.0365
^{86}Rb	0.00026	18.7	^{135}I	1.5	0.275
^{89}Sr	0.94	50.5	^{133}Xe	1.7	5.245
^{90}Sr	0.037	10629	^{135}Xe	0.34	0.379
^{91}Sr	1.1	0.396	^{134}Cs	0.075	753
^{90}Y	0.039	2.67	^{136}Cs	0.030	13.1
^{91}Y	1.2	58.5	^{137}Cs	0.047	11,012
^{95}Zr	1.5	64.0	^{140}Ba	1.6	12.74
^{97}Zr	1.5	0.704	^{140}La	1.6	1.678
^{95}Nb	1.5	35.15	^{141}Ce	1.5	32.5
^{99}Mo	1.6	2.75	^{143}Ce	1.3	1.38
^{99m}Tc	1.4	0.251	^{144}Ce	0.85	284
^{103}Ru	1.1	39.28	^{143}Pr	1.3	13.56
^{105}Ru	0.72	0.185	^{147}Nd	0.60	10.98
^{106}Ru	0.25	368.2	^{239}Np	16.4	2.355
^{105}Rh	0.49	1.535	^{238}Pu	0.00057	32,025
^{127}Te	0.059	0.390	^{239}Pu	0.00021	8.78×10^{6}
^{127m}Te	0.011	109	^{240}Pu	0.00021	2.39×10^{6}
^{129}Te	0.31	0.048	^{241}Pu	0.034	5,260
^{129m}Te	0.053	33.6	^{241}Am	0.000017	1.58×10^{5}
^{131m}Te	0.13	1.25	^{242}Cm	0.0050	163
^{132}Te	1.2	3.258	^{244}Cm	0.00023	6,610

[a] From the *Reactor Safety Study*, Appendix VI to WASH-1400, October 1975, Table VI 3-1.
[b] The half-life entries are from the Radiological Health Handbook.

Table 11.2.2 Radioactive Effluent Source Terms for Steam Generator Replacements Compared with Typical 1986 Effluent Data for Boiling Water Reactors (BWRs) and Pressurized Water Reactors (PWRs)

Type of Radioactive Effluent	Surry[a] Measurement (Ci)		Turkey Point[a] Measurement (Ci)		Point Beach[b] Estimate (Ci/unit)	H.B. Robinson[c] Estimate (Ci/unit)	Typical 1986 Effluent Data	
	Unit 1	Unit 2	Unit 3	Unit 4			BWRs[d,e] (Ci)	PWRs[e] (Ci)
Gaseous								
Noble gases	510	101	—	875	Negligible	140	53%, 1000	57%, 1000
Iodines	3.3×10^{-3}	6.9×10^{-1}	—	0.039	7×10^{-6}	4×10^{-5}	63%, 0.01	26%, 0.01
Particulates	2.7×10^{-3}	1.3×10^{-3}	2.1×10^{-4}	1.2×10^{-3}	1.5×10^{-4}	9×10^{-5}	63%, 0.01	26%, 0.01
Tritium	4.2	—	—	0.027	Negligible	7×10^{-1}	—	—
Liquid								
Mixed fission & activation products (excluding tritium)	0.52	0.26	0.12	0.078	0.23	1.3×10^{-3}	50%, 0.1	30%, 1.0
Tritium	8.5[f]	—	—	47	125	14	26%, 10	85%, 100

[a] NUREG/CR-3540
[b] NUREG-10011
[c] NUREG-1003
[d] Adapted from NUREG/CR-2907
[e] Read as: 53% of the BWR nuclear power reactor sites released annually at least 1000 Ci of noble gases per reactor unit in 1986.
[f] Estimated value NUREG-0692

Table 11.2.3 Average Fission Energy[a] for a PWR Reactor (Personal Communication, Heeb and Little, 1992)

A	B	C	D
Isotope	MeV/fis	30 GWd/metric ton[b] micro sig × N	B × C[c]
U-234	200	0.18	36.00
U-235	202	7.96	1607.92
U-236	200	3.81	762.00
U-238	208	94.80	19718.40
Pu-239	211	5.37	1133.07
Pu-240	212	2.10	445.20
Pu-241	213	1.15	244.95
	Sums	115.37	23947.54
	AVERAGE MEV/FIS		207.57

[a] Point average, not cumulative average.
[b] Note that the entry in Column C is the microscopic cross section times the nuclei density = macroscopic cross section in units of reciprocal cm, i.e., barns × nuclei per barn-cm.
[c] Specific Reaction Rate at a given flux.

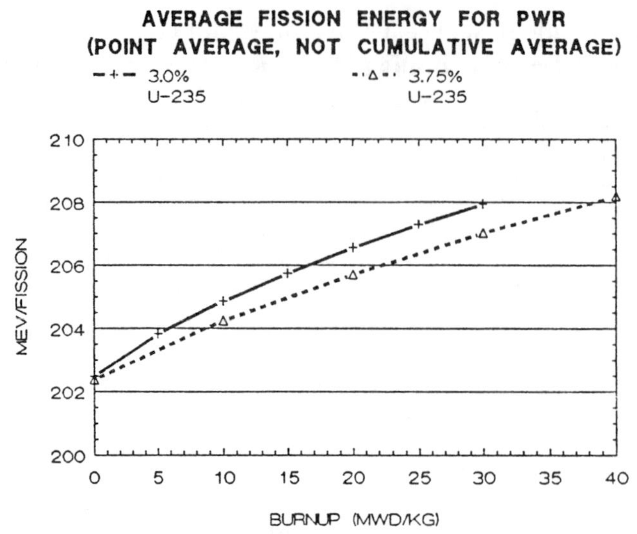

Figure 11.2.6 Average Fission Energy for PWR Reactor (Personal Communication, Heeb and Little, 1992)

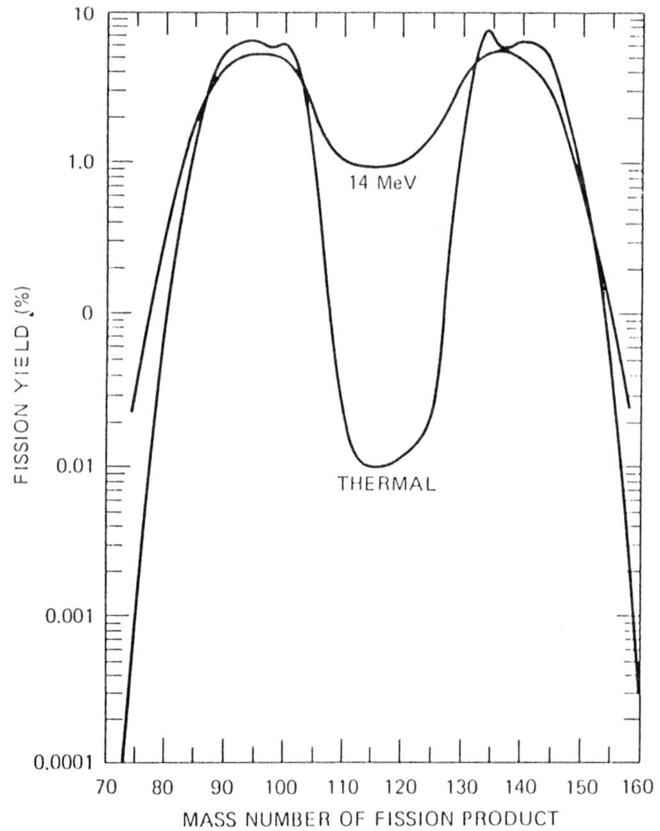

Figure 11.2.7 Fission Product Yield for the Thermal Fissioning of Uranium-235 (From NUREG 0956, 1986)

Table 11.2.4 Predicted Reactor Coolant Inventory of Fission Products and Corrosion Products [1000 MW(e) PWR at 578°F][a] From NUREG/CR-3332, 1983, source Eicholz, 1977)

Noble Gas Fishion Products

Isotope	μCi/ml
^{85}Ke	1.11
^{85m}Kr	1.46
^{87}Kr	0.87
^{88}Kr	2.58
^{133}Xe	1.74×10^{2}
^{133m}Xe	1.97
^{135m}Xe	0.14
^{138}Xe	0.36
Total Noble Gases	187.3[b]

Corrosion Products

Isotope	μCi/ml
^{54}Mn	4.2×10^{-3}
^{56}Mn	2.2×10^{-2}
^{58}Co	8.1×10^{-3}
^{59}Fe	1.8×10^{-3}
^{60}Co	1.4×10^{-3}
Total Corrosion Products	3.7×10^{-2}
^{84}Br	3.0×10^{-2}

Fission Products

Isotope	μCi/ml
^{88}Rb	2.56
^{89}Rb	6.7×10^{-2}
^{89}Sr	2.52×10^{-3}
^{90}Sr	4.42×10^{-3}
^{90}Y	5.37×10^{-5}
^{91}Y	4.77×10^{-4}
^{92}Sr	5.63×10^{-4}
^{92}Y	5.54×10^{-4}
^{95}Zr	5.04×10^{-4}
^{95}Nb	4.70×10^{-4}
^{99}Mo	2.11
^{131}I	1.55
^{132}Te	0.17
^{132}I	0.62
^{133}I	2.55
^{134}Te	2.2×10^{-2}
^{134}I	0.39
^{134}Cs	7.0×10^{-2}
^{135}I	1.4
^{136}Cs	0.33
^{137}Cs	0.43
^{138}Cs	0.48
^{144}Ce	2.3×10^{-4}
^{144}Pr	2.3×10^{-4}
Total Fission Products	12.8[b]

[a] Contamination concentration corresponding to 1% failed fuel near end of fuel life.
[b] 187.3 μCi/ml = 6.9 GBq/l; 12.8 μCi/ml = 0.47 GBq/l.

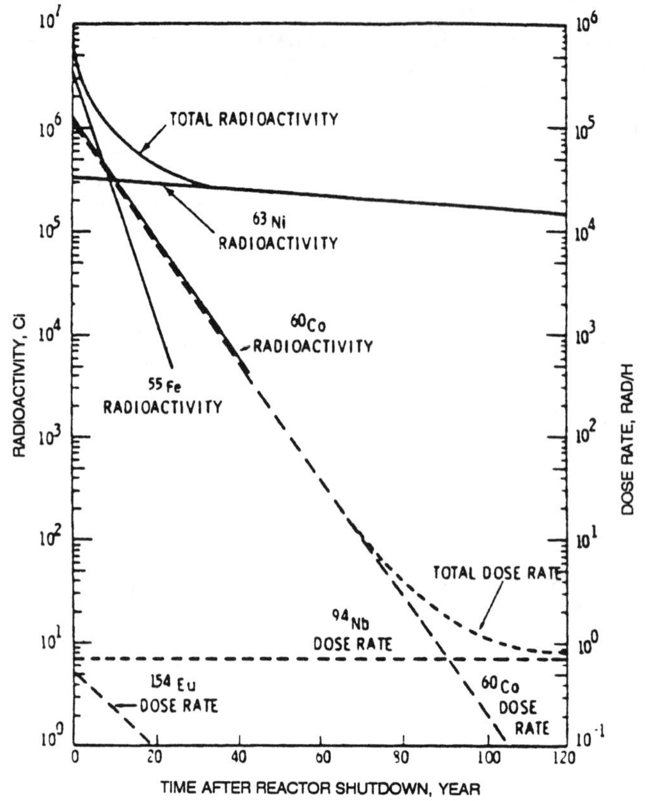

Figure 11.2.8 Time Dependence of Radioactivity and Dose Rate in a Boiling Water Reactor Core Shroud After 40 Years of Operation (From NUREG 1437, 1991)

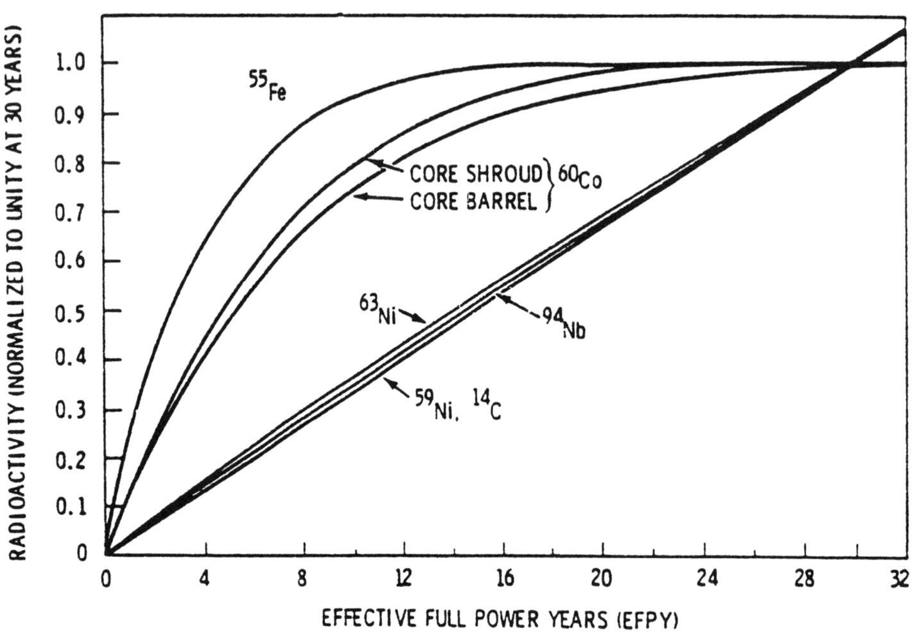

Figure 11.2.9 Buildup of Activation Products in Pressurized Water Reactor Internal Components as a Function of Effective Full Power Years (From NUREG 1437, 1991)

Table 11.2.5 Arrhenius-Type Constants Used in Calculation of Release Rate Coefficients in M-Version of CORSOR (From NUREG 0656, 1986)

Species	k_o (min^{-2})	Q (kcal/mol)
Cs, I, Kr, Xe, Te	2.0×10^5	63.8
Ag	7.9×10^3	61.4
Sb	[a]	[a]
Ba	2.95×10^5	100.2
Sn (clad)	5.95×10^3	70.8
Ru	1.62×10^6	152.8
UO_2	1.46×10^7	143.1
Zr (clad)	8.55×10^4	139.5
Zr	2.67×10^8	188.2
Fe	2.94×10^4	87.0
Mo	[b]	[b]
Sr	4.40×10^5	117.0
Cr	4.62×10^4	84.5
Ni	5.36×10^4	92.2
Mn	5.04×10^3	56.8
La group	0	[c]

[a] Omitted from consideration due to potential chemical reaction with in-core surfaces and lack of radiological significance.

[b] Omitted from consideration due to very low pressure and lack of radiological significance.

[c] La_2O_3 exhibits no significant vapor pressure prior to conversion to LaO, which is not believed to occur in vessel.

Table 11.2.6 Melting Point and Boiling Point of Materials of Interest (From NUREG 0956, 1986)

Material	Melting Point (°C)	Boiling Point (°C)
Volatile Fission Products		
I_2	114	185
HI	−51	−35
CsI	626	1280
CsOH	315	990
Te	450	988
Refractory Fission Products		
BaO	1923	2808
Ru	2250	4150
SrO	2430	3249
La_2O_3	2315	>4000
Control Rods		
Ag	961	2163
In	157	2073
Cd	321	767
B_4C	2470	>3500
Hf	2222	4450
Zircaloy		
Zr	1852	4409
Sn	232	2603
Stainless Steel		
Fe	1535	2862
Cr	1890	2672
Ni	1453	2914
Mn	1244	2062
Fuel		
UO_2	2840[a]	3293

[a] Oxidized Zr will form a liquified two-phase mixture with UO_2 at about 1,900°C.

Table 11.2.7 Actinide and Fission-Product Activities of Research Reactor Cores (After Kahook, 1995)

Radio-nuclide	Half-Life	Activity (Ci)		Radio-nuclide	Half-Life	Activity (Ci)	
		MURR	RHF			MURR	RHF
^{3}H	12.346 y	$1.66\ 10^{1}$	$3.41\ 10^{1}$	^{144}Ce	284.3 d	$2.13\ 10^{4}$	$4.78\ 10^{4}$
^{85}Kr	10.72 y	$4.61\ 10^{2}$	$9.48\ 10^{2}$	^{144}Pr	17.28 m	$2.13\ 10^{4}$	$4.78\ 10^{4}$
^{89}Sr	50.5 d	$1.57\ 10^{1}$	$4.92\ 10^{1}$	^{144m}Pr	7.2 m	$2.56\ 10^{2}$	$5.73\ 10^{2}$
^{90}Sr	28.6 y	$3.91\ 10^{3}$	$8.08\ 10^{3}$	^{147}Pm	2.623 y	$8.52\ 10^{3}$	$1.88\ 10^{4}$
^{90}Y	2.67 d	$3.92\ 10^{3}$	$8.08\ 10^{3}$	^{148m}Pm	41.3 d	$1.19\ 10^{-2}$	—
^{91}Y	58.5 d	$7.15\ 10^{1}$	$2.13\ 10^{2}$	^{151}Sm	90. y	$2.49\ 10^{1}$	$1.97\ 10^{1}$
^{95}Zr	64.0 d	$1.57\ 10^{2}$	$4.54\ 10^{2}$	^{154}Eu	8.8 y	$5.20\ 10^{1}$	$1.58\ 10^{2}$
^{95}Nb	35.15 d	$3.48\ 10^{2}$	$1.01\ 10^{3}$	^{155}Eu	4.96 y	$6.18\ 10^{1}$	$9.34\ 10^{1}$
^{95m}Nb	86.6 h	1.16	3.37	^{231}Th	25.52 h	$9.90\ 10^{-3}$	$1.14\ 10^{-2}$
^{99}Tc	$2.13\ 10^{5}$ y	$5.90\ 10^{-1}$	—	^{234}Th	24.1 d	$1.54\ 10^{-4}$	$2.16\ 10^{-4}$
^{103}Ru	39.28 d	$6.42\ 10^{-1}$	2.17	^{233}Pa	27. d	$4.81\ 10^{-3}$	$2.71\ 10^{-3}$
^{103m}Rh	56.1 m	$5.78\ 10^{-1}$	1.96	^{234m}Pa	1.17 m	$1.54\ 10^{-4}$	$2.16\ 10^{-4}$
^{106}Ru	368.2 d	$1.97\ 10^{3}$	$4.13\ 10^{3}$	^{234}U	$2.445\ 10^{5}$ y	$4.28\ 10^{-4}$	$1.50\ 10^{-4}$
^{106}Rh	29.9 s	$1.97\ 10^{3}$	$4.13\ 10^{3}$	^{235}U	$7.038\ 10^{8}$ y	$9.90\ 10^{-3}$	$1.14\ 10^{-2}$
^{110m}Ag	249.8 d	$8.25\ 10^{-1}$	—	^{236}U	$2.242\ 10^{7}$ y	$1.96\ 10^{-2}$	$3.28\ 10^{-2}$
^{119m}Sn	293 d	$8.66\ 10^{-2}$	1.42	^{237}U	6.75 d	$6.52\ 10^{-5}$	$4.40\ 10^{-5}$
^{123}Sn	129.2 d	4.93	$1.01\ 10^{1}$	^{238}U	$4.468\ 10^{9}$ y	$1.54\ 10^{-4}$	$2.16\ 10^{-4}$
^{125}Sb	2.77 y	$1.76\ 10^{2}$	$3.03\ 10^{2}$	^{237}Np	$2.14\ 10^{6}$ y	$4.81\ 10^{-3}$	$2.71\ 10^{-3}$
^{125m}Te	58. d	$4.29\ 10^{1}$	$7.39\ 10^{1}$	^{236}Pu	2.85 y	$8.32\ 10^{-4}$	$3.63\ 10^{-3}$
^{127}Te	9.35 h	$1.06\ 10^{1}$	$2.38\ 10^{1}$	^{238}Pu	87.75 y	5.29	1.56
^{127m}Te	109 d	$1.09\ 10^{1}$	$2.43\ 10^{2}$	^{239}Pu	24131 y	$9.75\ 10^{-2}$	$8.53\ 10^{-2}$
^{129}Te	69.6 m	$1.60\ 10^{-3}$	—	^{240}Pu	6569 y	$4.58\ 10^{-2}$	$4.32\ 10^{-2}$
^{129m}Te	33.6 d	$2.46\ 10^{-3}$	—	^{241}Pu	14.4 y	2.66	1.79
^{134}Cs	2.062 y	$9.41\ 10^{2}$	$1.43\ 10^{3}$	^{241}Am	432.2 y	$9.28\ 10^{-3}$	$6.10\ 10^{-3}$
^{137}Cs	30.17 y	$4.07\ 10^{3}$	$8.34\ 10^{3}$	^{242}Cm	163.2 d	$1.09\ 10^{-3}$	$3.22\ 10^{-4}$
^{137m}Ba	2.55 m	$3.85\ 10^{3}$	$7.89\ 10^{3}$	^{244}Cm	18.11 y	$1.74\ 10^{-4}$	$4.32\ 10^{-5}$
^{141}Ce	32.5 d	$8.61\ 10^{-2}$	—				

[a] MURR is the University of Missouri reactor. MURR uses an 8 element, HEU core. These values are for a uniform irradiation (as opposed to a cycled operation), 120 d at 11 MW (1320 MWd), with a 2 yr cooling period. Total activity is $7.35\ 10^{4}$ Ci. A cycled operation produced $6.45\ 10^{4}$ Ci.

[b] RHF is the Reactor á Haut Flux, France. The RHF core consists of two fuel tubes with a total of 280 plates with D_2O moderation. These data are for natural uranium fuel exposed for 50 d at 62.7 MW (3135 MWd), with a 2 yr cooling period. Total activity is $1.6\ 10^{5}$ Ci, for either the natural or the enriched uranium fuel.

Table 11.2.8 Types of Research Reactors[a]

Type	Number
Pool	89 (84)
Tank	40 (37)
Argonaut[b]	15 (12)
Homogeneous(S)	19 (18)
TRIGA[c]	51 (50)
Heavy Water	16 (15)
Slowpoke MNSR[d]	13 (13)
Homogeneous(L)	9 (5)
Critical Assembly	22 (30)
Others[e]	47 (32)

Table 11.2.9 Number of Research Reactors[a]

Year	Number	Total Thermal Power (MW)
1955	38	166
1960	178	1339
1965	319	2415
1970	362	3204
1975	373	3992
1980	362	4591
1985	339	3977
1990	323	4037
(1995)	(297)	(3392)

Table 11.2.10 Research Reactor Power Levels[a]

Thermal Power (kW)	Number
0	45 (30)
0.001–0.5	33 (34)
1–10	34 (30)
18–50	21 (24)
60–700	51 (46)
1,000–4,000	54 (50)
5,000–20,000	51 (49)
23,000–45,000	14 (14)
50,000–70,000	7 (8)
100,000–563,000[f]	12 (11)

[a] After IAEA, 1991. In parentheses, after IAEA, 1994.

[b] Argonaut reactors are simply a specific design utilizing MTR-type fuel. These were popular at universities at one time, but there are only two currently operational in the U.S. (University of Florida and Iowa State University).

[c] A pool type reactor designed and sold by General Atomics with reactor powers up to 15 MW.

[d] A tank type reactor originally designed by Canada with reactor powers typically of 20 kW.

[e] Pressurized Water Reactors, Zero Power, Sodium Fast, Sodium Cooled.

[f] The 563 MW reactor is a sodium-cooled fast breeder reactor in France.

SECTION 3 ATMOSPHERIC DISPERSION

(Contributed by Harold T. Peterson Personal Communication, 1991)

This section discusses atmospheric dispersion of radioactive materials and the resulting gamma and beta radiation exposure rates. It continues with guidance on sampling sites, collection frequency and analysis frequency for various types of facilities.

TABLE OF CONTENTS

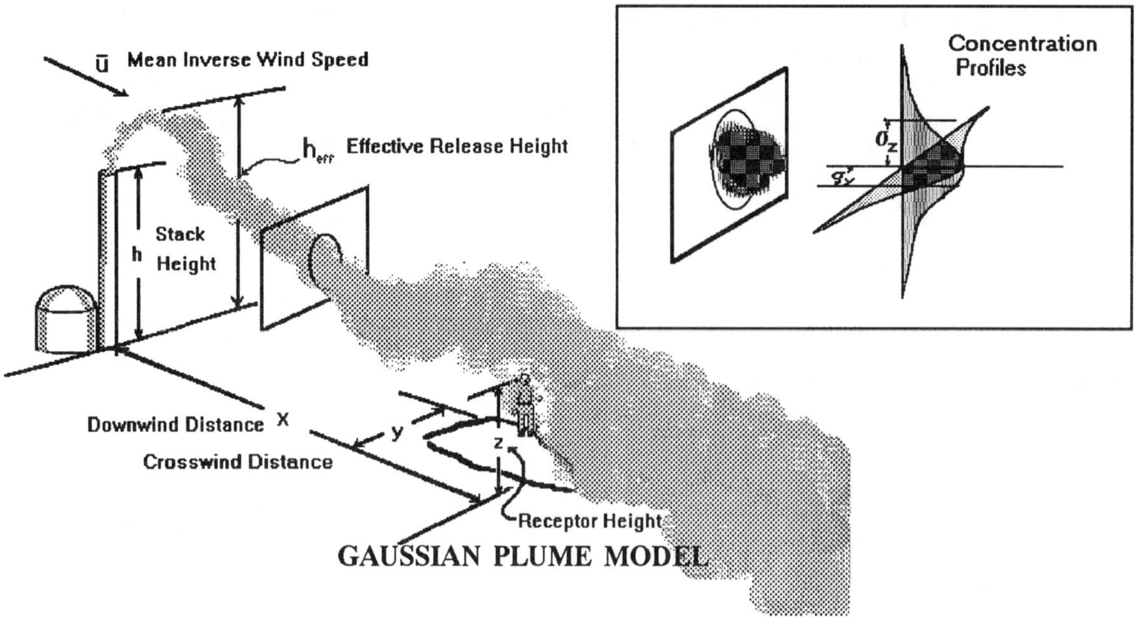

Figure 11.3.1 Atmospheric Dispersion

Table 11.3.1.1 Continuous Point Sources

A. Elevated Source, Elevated Receptor

(source height = $h(h_{eff})$; receptor height = z)

$$\chi(x,y,z) = \frac{\dot{Q}}{2\pi\sigma_y\sigma_z\bar{u}}\left[\exp\left\{-\frac{(h+z)^2}{2\sigma_z^2}\right\} + \exp\left\{-\frac{(h-z)^2}{2\sigma_z^2}\right\}\right]\left[\exp\left\{-\frac{y^2}{2\sigma_y^2}\right\}\right]$$

$\chi(x,y,z)$ = air concentration (Bq m^{-3} or Ci m^{-3}) at downwind distance x, crosswind distance y, and height z;

$\dot{Q}$ = Activity release rate (Bq sec^{-1} or Ci sec^{-1})

σ_y = horizontal dispersion parameter (m)

σ_z = vertical dispersion parameter (m)

$\bar{u}$ = mean inverse wind speed (m sec^{-1})

$$\left(\frac{1}{\bar{u}}\right) = \frac{1}{N}\sum_{i-1}^{N}\frac{1}{u_i}$$

B. Elevated Source, Elevated Receptor, Centerline

(source height = $h(h_{eff})$; receptor height = z; y = 0)

$$\chi(x,0,z) = \frac{\dot{Q}}{2\pi\sigma_y\sigma_z\bar{u}}\left[\exp\left\{-\frac{(h+z)^2}{2\sigma_z^2}\right\} + \exp\left\{-\frac{(h-z)^2}{2\sigma_z^2}\right\}\right]$$

C. Elevated Source, Ground-Level Receptor

(source height = $h(h_{eff})$; receptor height, z = 0)

$$\chi(x,y,0) = \frac{\dot{Q}}{\pi\sigma_y\sigma_z\bar{u}}\left[\exp\left\{-\frac{h^2}{2\sigma_z^2}\right\}\right]\left[\exp\left\{-\frac{y^2}{2\sigma_y^2}\right\}\right]$$

D. Elevated Source, Ground-Level Receptor, Centerline

(source height = h(h_{eff}); receptor height, z = 0; y = 0)

$$\chi(x,0,0) = \frac{\dot{Q}}{\pi\sigma_y\sigma_z\bar{u}}\left[\exp\left\{-\frac{h^2}{2\sigma_z^2}\right\}\right]$$

Approximate Maximum Concentration:

$$\chi_{\max} \sim \frac{2\dot{Q}}{\pi e\bar{u}h^2}\left(\frac{\sigma_z}{\sigma_y}\right)$$

where e is the base of natural logarithms (e = 2.71 + . . .). This maximum occurs when $\sigma_z = h/\sqrt{2}$. The distance that the maximum occurs can be read off the graphs for σ_z versus distance.

E. Ground-Level Source, Ground-Level Receptor

(source height, h = 0; receptor height, z = 0)

$$\chi(x,y,0) = \frac{\dot{Q}}{\pi\sigma_y\sigma_z\bar{u}}\left[\exp\left\{-\frac{y^2}{2\sigma_y^2}\right\}\right]$$

F. Ground-Level Source, Ground-Level Receptor, Centerline

(Release height, h = 0; receptor height, z = 0; y = 0)

$$\chi(x,0,0) = \frac{\dot{Q}}{\pi\sigma_y\sigma_z\bar{u}}$$

G. Crosswind Integrated Concentration

$$\chi_{CWI} = \frac{\dot{Q}}{\pi\sigma_z\bar{u}}\left[\exp -\left(\frac{h^2}{2\sigma_z^2}\right)\right]\frac{1}{\sigma_y}\int_{-\infty}^{\infty}\exp -\left(\frac{y^2}{2\sigma_y^2}\right)dy$$

$$= \left(\frac{2}{\pi}\right)^{1/2}\frac{\dot{Q}}{\sigma_z\bar{u}}\left[\exp -\left(\frac{h^2}{2\sigma_z^2}\right)\right]$$

H. Sector-Averaged Long-Term Concentration

$$\chi_{sector\text{-}averaged} = \frac{\dot{Q}}{\pi\sigma_z\bar{u}}\left[\exp -\left(\frac{h^2}{2\sigma_z^2}\right)\right]\frac{1}{\sigma_y}\int_{-\infty}^{\infty}\exp -\left(\frac{y^2}{2\sigma_y^2}\right)dy$$

$$= \left(\frac{2}{\pi}\right)^{1/2}\frac{\dot{Q}}{\sigma_z\bar{u}}\left[\exp -\left(\frac{h^2}{2\sigma_z^2}\right)\right]\times\frac{0.01\,f}{2\pi(x/n)}$$

The sector-averaged equation uses the crosswind-integrated model but distributes the y-concentration evenly over a sector. The width of a sector is equal to the circumference (= 2πx) at distance x from the source divided by the number of sectors, n (typically n = 16 so that there are 16 22½° sectors in a full circle of 360°). The concentration in each sector is weighted by the fraction of the time that the wind blows into the sector of interest (0.01 × the percentage of the time, f, that wind is blowing into the sector of interest). Sector-averaging is an artifice for representing long-term meandering of the plume.

Table 11.3.1.2 Instantaneous Point Sources

A. Elevated Source, Elevated Receptor

(source height = h (h_{eff}); receptor height = z)

$$\chi(x,y,z,t) = \frac{Q}{(2\pi)^{3/2}\sigma_{xI}\sigma_{yI}\sigma_{zI}\bar{u}}\left[\exp\left\{-\frac{(h+z)^2}{2\sigma_{zI}^2}\right\} + \exp\left\{-\frac{(h-z)^2}{2\sigma_{zI}^2}\right\}\right]\cdot\left[\exp\left\{-\frac{y^2}{2\sigma_{yI}^2}\right\}\right]\left[\exp -\left\{\frac{(x-\bar{u}t)^2}{2\sigma_{xI}^2}\right\}\right]$$

where σ_{xI}, σ_{yI}, and σ_{zI} are instantaneous dispersion parameters in the x, y, and z directions rather than the 15–20 minute average parameters normally used, and Q is the total activity released rather than the activity release rate.

B. Elevated Source, Ground-Level Receptor

$$\chi(x,y,0,t) = \frac{Q}{2^{1/2}\pi^{3/2}\sigma_{xI}\sigma_{yI}\sigma_{zI}\bar{u}}\left[\exp\left\{-\frac{h^2}{2\sigma_{zI}^2}\right\}\right]\left[\exp\left\{-\frac{y^2}{2\sigma_{yI}^2}\right\}\right]\left[\exp -\left\{\frac{(x-\bar{u}t)^2}{2\sigma_{xI}^2}\right\}\right.$$

C. Ground-Level Source, Ground-Level Receptor

$$\chi(x,y,0,t) = \frac{Q}{2^{1/2}\pi^{3/2}\sigma_{xI}\sigma_{yI}\sigma_{zI}\bar{u}}\left[\exp\left\{-\frac{y^2}{2\sigma_{yI}^2}\right\}\right]\left[\exp -\left\{\frac{(x-\bar{u}t)^2}{2\sigma_{xI}^2}\right\}\right]$$

D. Ground-Level Source, Ground-Level Receptor, Centerline

$$\chi(x,0,0,t) = \frac{Q}{2^{1/2}\pi^{3/2}\sigma_{xI}\sigma_{yI}\sigma_{zI}\bar{u}}\left[\exp -\left\{\frac{(x-\bar{u}t)^2}{2\sigma_{xI}^2}\right\}\right]$$

Table 11.3.2 Specialized Equations

A. Fumigation (Trapping) Inversion at Height H (H > h)

$$\chi_F(x,y,0) = \frac{\dot{Q}}{(2\pi)^{1/2} H\sigma_y\bar{u}}\left[\exp\left\{-\frac{y^2}{2\sigma_y{}^2}\right\}\right]$$

This equation is used for uniform vertical mixing between an inversion lid at height H and the ground. Very high airborne concentrations of a pollutant may be attained.

B. Gamma Dose Rate from a Radioactive Plume

$$\dot{D}(x,y,z,t) = 0.0404\mu_a\bar{E}_\gamma \times \int_0^\infty \int_0^\pi \frac{(1 + k\mu r)\exp(-\mu r)}{r^2}\chi(x,y,z,t) \times 2\pi r^2 \sin\phi\, d\phi\, dr$$

where $r^2 = x^2 + y^2 + z^2$, μ_a is the mass energy absorption coefficient for average gamma energy E_γ, and k is $(\mu - \mu_a)/\mu_a$. The integration is usually done numerically or graphically. Use of the ground-level radionuclide concentration for estimating the gamma dose rate from an elevated source (h > 0) can seriously underestimate the dose for the condition close to the release point before the plume reaches the ground. And use of a semi-infinite cloud approximation where the plume is in close proximity to the ground may significantly overestimate the dose for high energy gamma emitters.

C. Radioactive Cloud (Beta and Gamma Exposure)

(From USNRC Reg Guide 1.4, June, 1979)

(1) *Beta Exposure*

For an infinite uniform cloud containing χ curies of beta radioactivity per cubic meter, the beta dose in air at the cloud center is:

$$D(\beta)_\infty = 0.457\bar{E}_\beta\chi$$

The dose rate to the body surface (skin) from beta emitters in the infinite cloud can be approximated as being one-half this amount; i.e.,

$$D(\beta)_{\infty,s} = 0.23\bar{E}_\beta\chi$$

(2) *Gamma Exposure*

For gamma emitting material, the dose rate in air at the spherical cloud center is:

$$D(\gamma)_\infty = 0.507\bar{E}_\gamma\chi$$

From a semispherical-infinite cloud, the gamma dose rate in air is:

$$D(\gamma)_{\infty/2} = 0.25\bar{E}_\gamma\chi$$

where χ = concentration of beta or gamma emitting isotope in the cloud (curie/m^3)
$D(\beta)_\infty$ = beta dose rate from an infinite cloud (rad/sec)
$D(\beta)_{\infty,s}$ = beta dose rate to skin from an infinite cloud (rad/sec)
$D(\gamma)_\infty$ = gamma dose rate from an infinite cloud (rad/sec)
$D(\gamma)_{\infty/2}$ = gamma dose rate from a semi-infinite cloud (rad/sec)
$\bar{E}_\beta$ = average beta energy per disintegration (MeV/dis)
$\bar{E}_\gamma$ = average gamma energy per disintegration (MeV/dis)

$$\bar{E}_\gamma = \sum f_i E_i$$

The ith gamma of energy E_i, f_i is the fractional abundance of the ith gamma per disintegration.

For a finite semispherical cloud the dose rate, as a fraction of that for a semispherical infinite cloud, is shown in Figure 11.3.2. For ‘small clouds’, e.g., room-sized volumes, ICRP multiplies this by 2 since a person standing in a room more closely approximates exposure at the center of a cloud.

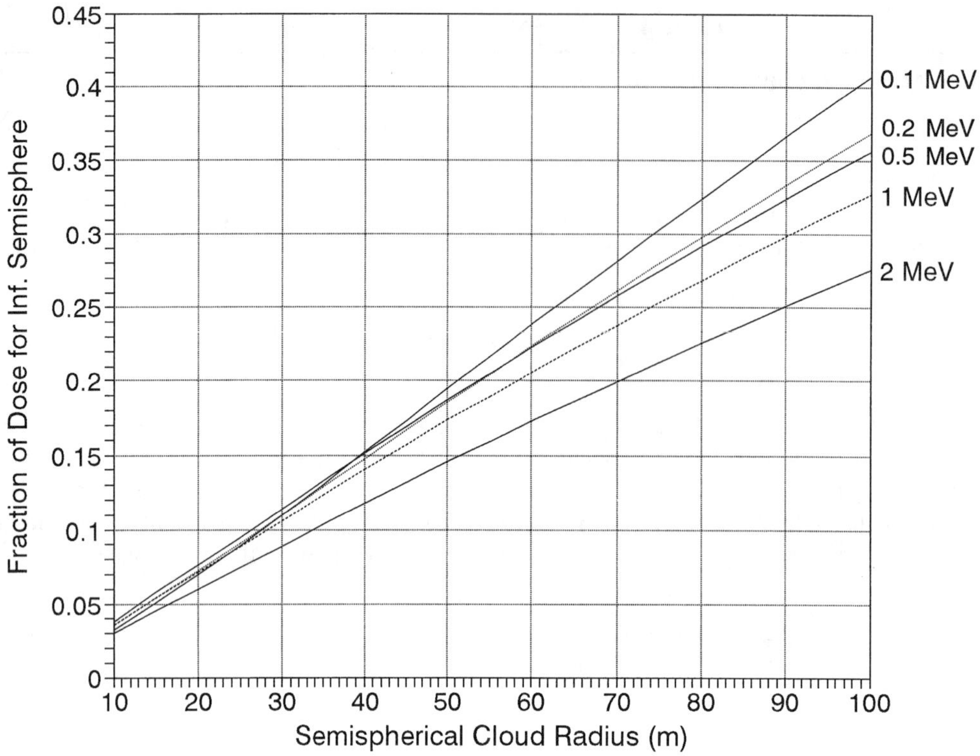

Figure 11.3.2 Fraction of Dose Rate of an Infinite Radius Semisphere

Table 11.3.3 Determination of Atmospheric Stability Conditions [Based on Table A.1 in Appendix A of *Meteorology and Atomic Energy,* USAEC, 1968)

	STABILITY CLASS				
				Nighttime Conditions	
Surface Wind Speed ($m\ s^{-1}$)	Daytime Solar Insolation*			Thin Overcast or ≥ 50% Cloud Cover	≤ 40% Cloud Cover
	Strong	Moderate	Light		
<2	A	A–B	B	—	—
2	A–B	B	C	E	F
4	B	B–C	C	D	E
6	C	C–D	D	D	D
>6	C	D	D	D	D

PASQUILL-GIFFORD STABILITY CLASSES

Stability Class	
A	***Extremely Unstable*** (good vertical & horizontal mixing—most common on bright sunny days—peak downwind concentration near release point)
B	***Moderately Unstable*** (common on sunny days with higher winds or with some cloudiness)
C	***Slightly Unstable*** (common on cloudy days with low wind speeds)
D	***Neutral Stability*** (most common condition with heavy overcast, day or night)
E	***Slightly stable*** (at night with low winds)
F	***Moderately stable*** (very low wind speeds at night or just before dawn—peak concentration furthest from the release point).
G	***Very Stable*** (USNRC origin, not Pasquill-Gifford, use parameters $\sigma_{yG} \sim 2/3\ \sigma_{yF}$; $\sigma_{zG} \sim 2/3\ \sigma_{zF}$; use at night with very low windspeeds).

* Intensity of sunlight.

Table 11.3.4 Parameters for Instantaneous Releases [Based on Table A.2 in Appendix A of *Meteorology and Atomic Energy—1968,* USAEC Report TID-24190 (July, 1968)]

Parameter	Power Function Approximation	Atmospheric Stability	Values at 0.1 km	Values at 4 km
σ_{yI} (m)	$0.14\ x^{0.92}$	Unstable	10.0	300
	$0.06\ x^{0.92}$	Neutral	4.0	120
	$0.02\ x^{0.89}$	Very Stable	1.3	35
σ_{zI} (m)	$0.53\ x^{0.73}$	Unstable	15.0	220
	$0.15\ x^{0.70}$	Neutral	3.8	50
	$0.05\ x^{0.61}$	Very Stable	0.75	7

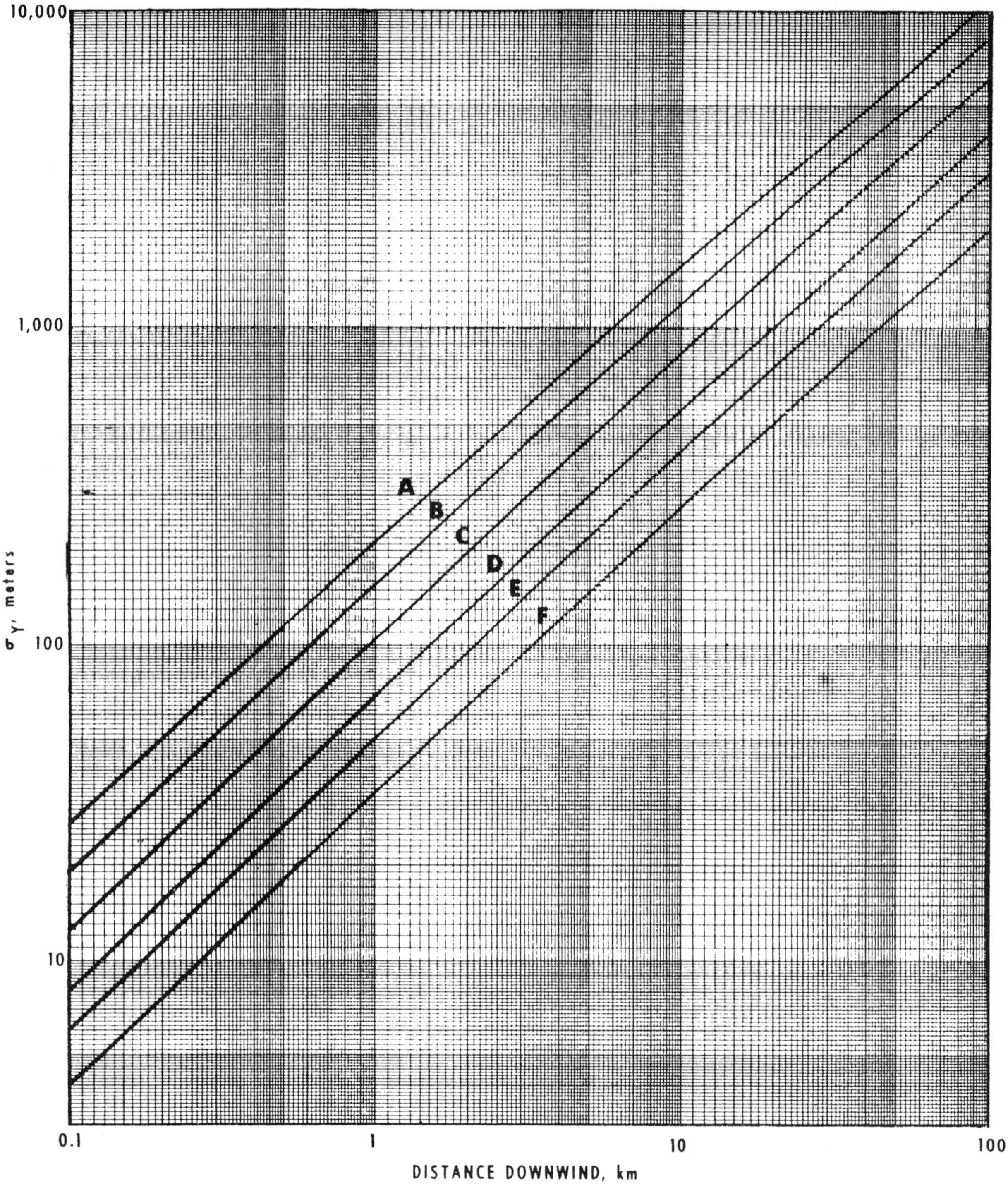

Figure 11.3.3 Horizontal Dispersion parameter (σ_y) as a Function of Downwind Distance from the Source (From USAEC TID 24190, 1968)

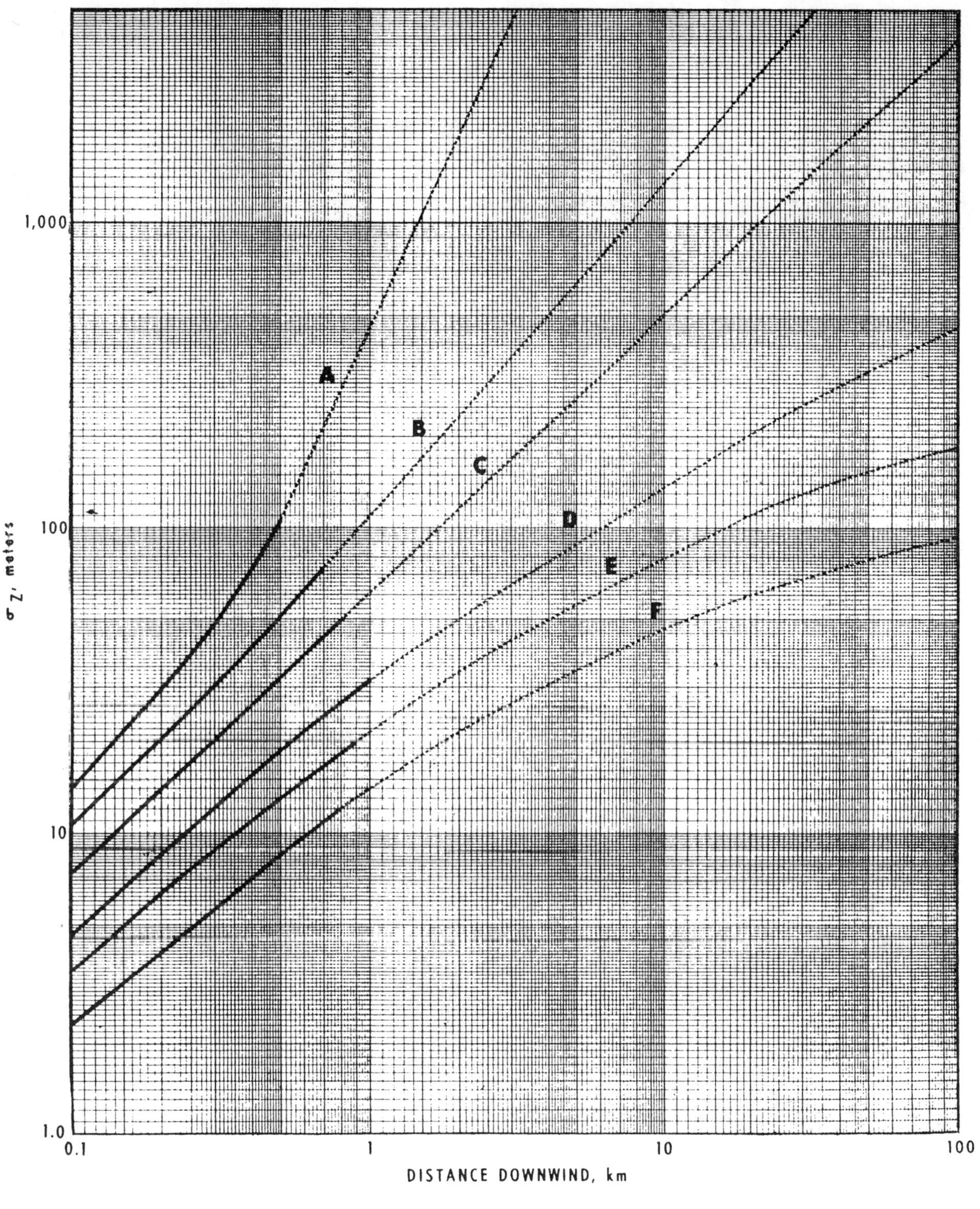

Figure 11.3.4 Vertical Dispersion Parameter (σ_z) as a Function of Downwind Distance from the Source (From USAEC TID-24190, 1968)

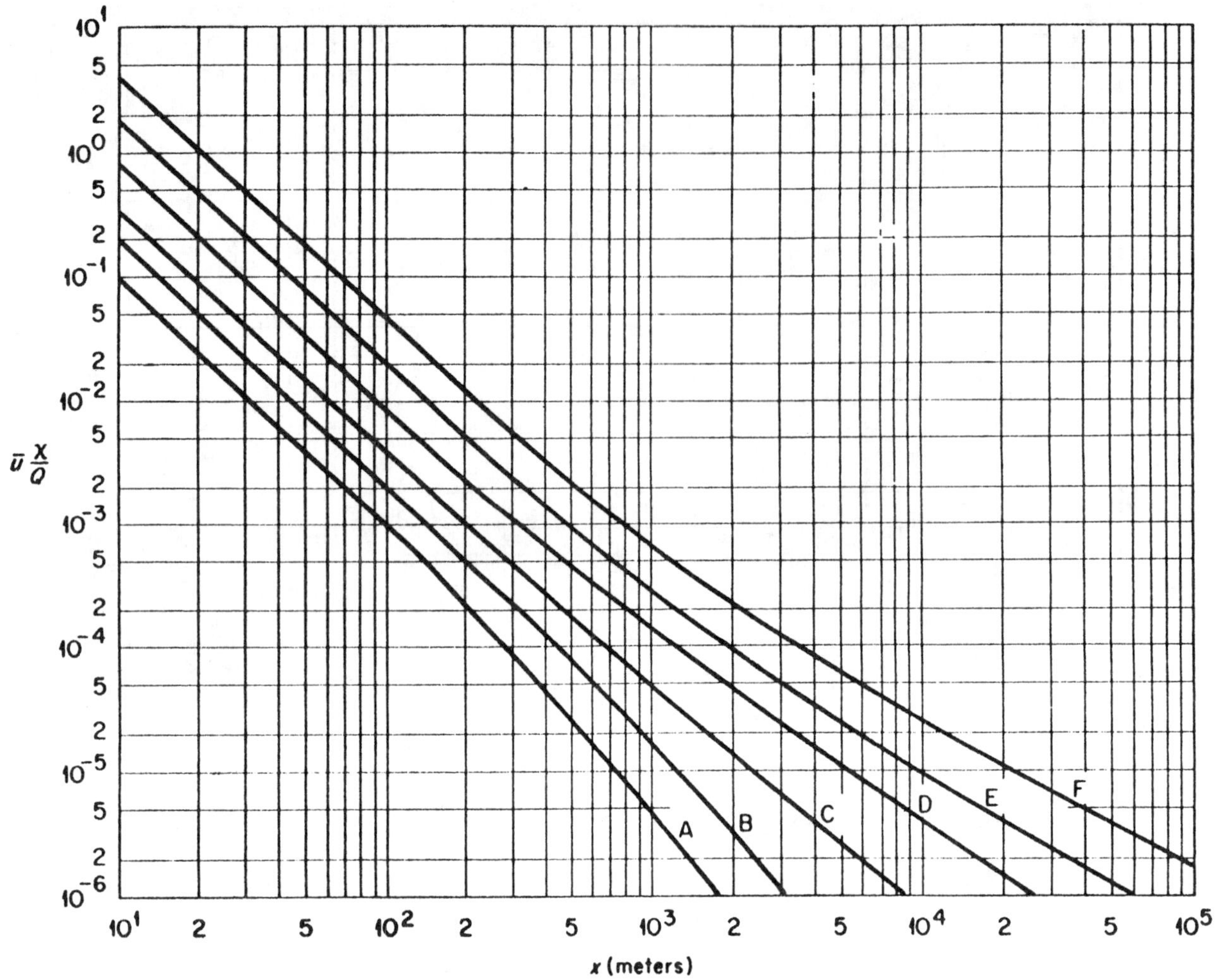

Figure 11.3.5 Values of the Normalized Dispersion Function ($\bar{u}\chi/Q$) as a Function of Downwind Distance, x, for a Release Height, h, of 0 m (From Hilsmeier et al., 1962)

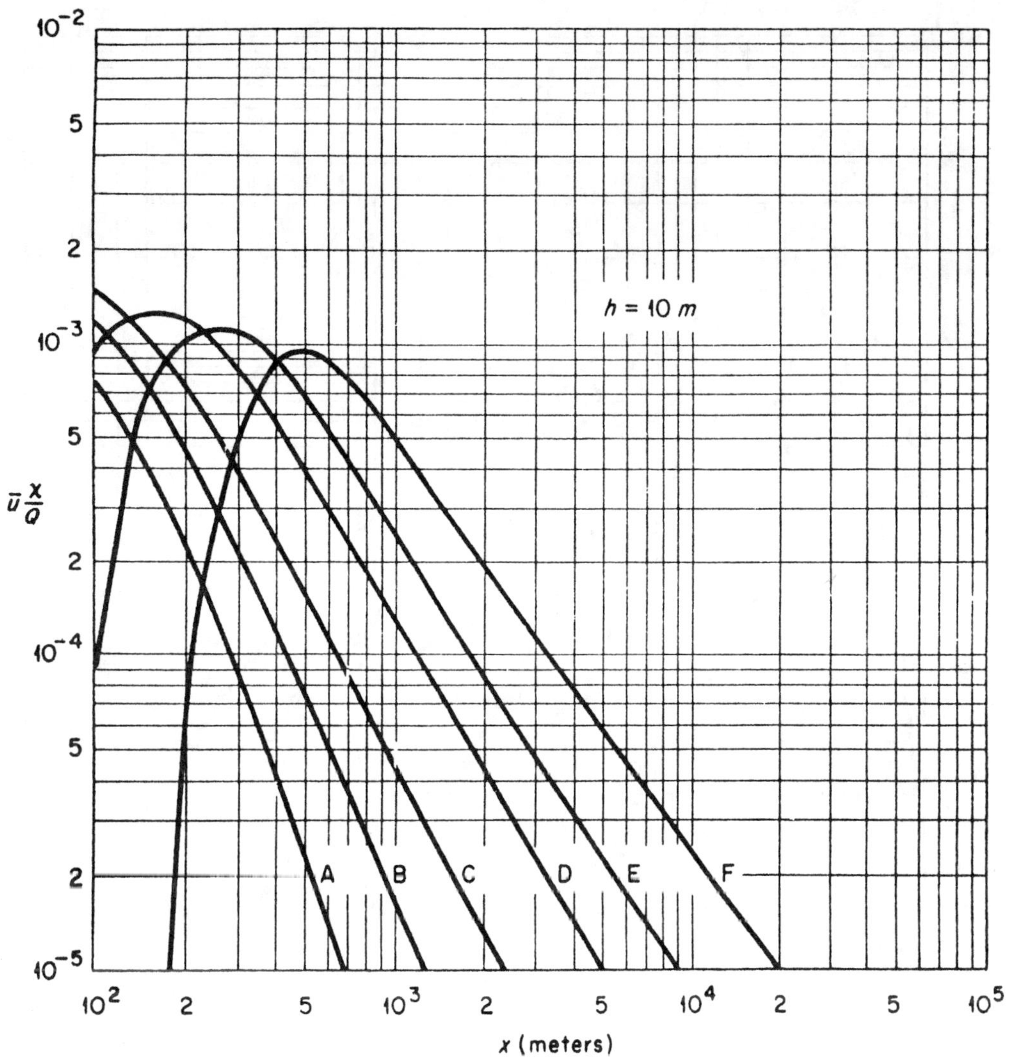

Figure 11.3.6 Values of the Normalized Dispersion Function ($\bar{u}\chi/Q$) as a Function of Downwind Distance, x, for a Release Height, h, of 10 m (From Hilsmeier et al., 1962)

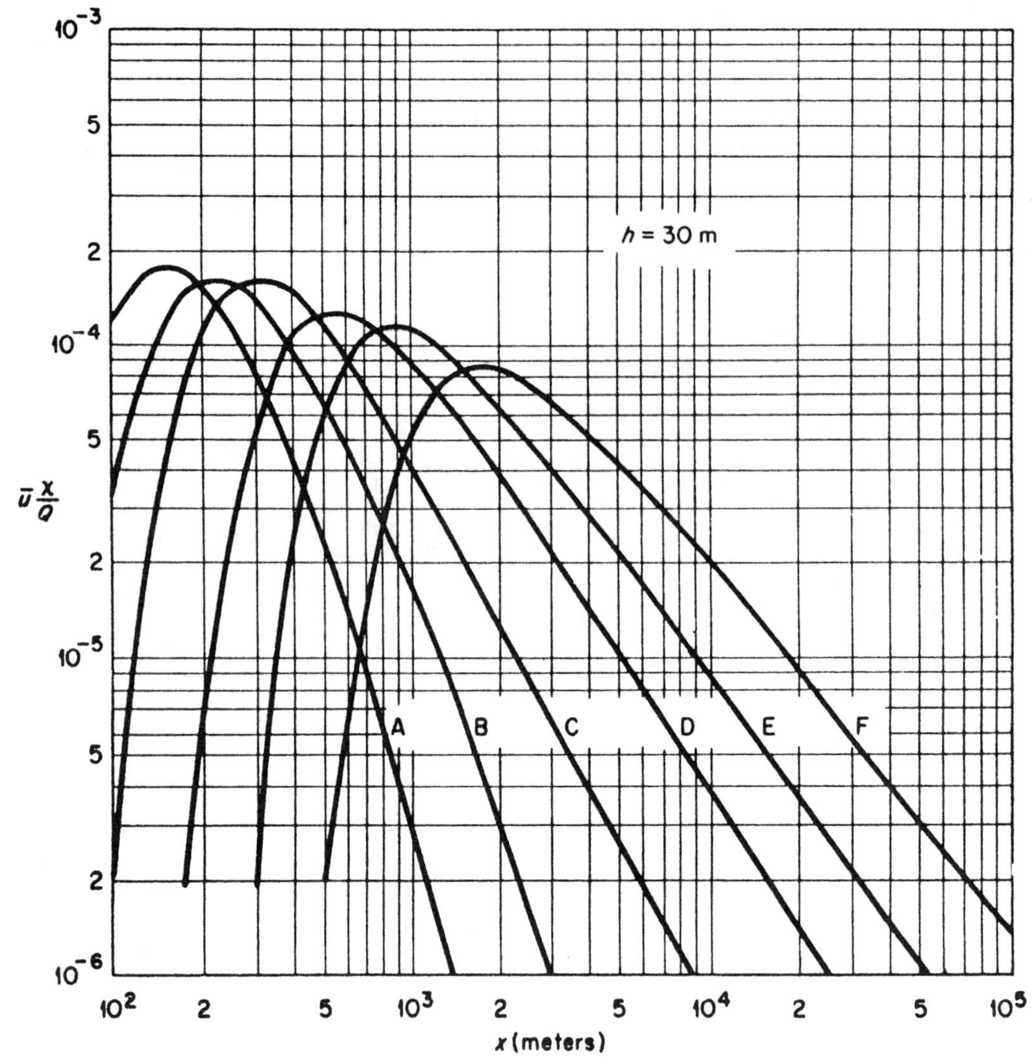

Figure 11.3.7 Values of the Normalized Dispersion Function ($\bar{u}\chi/Q$) as a Function of Downwind Distance, x, for a Release Height, h, of 30 m (From Hilsmeier et al., 1962)

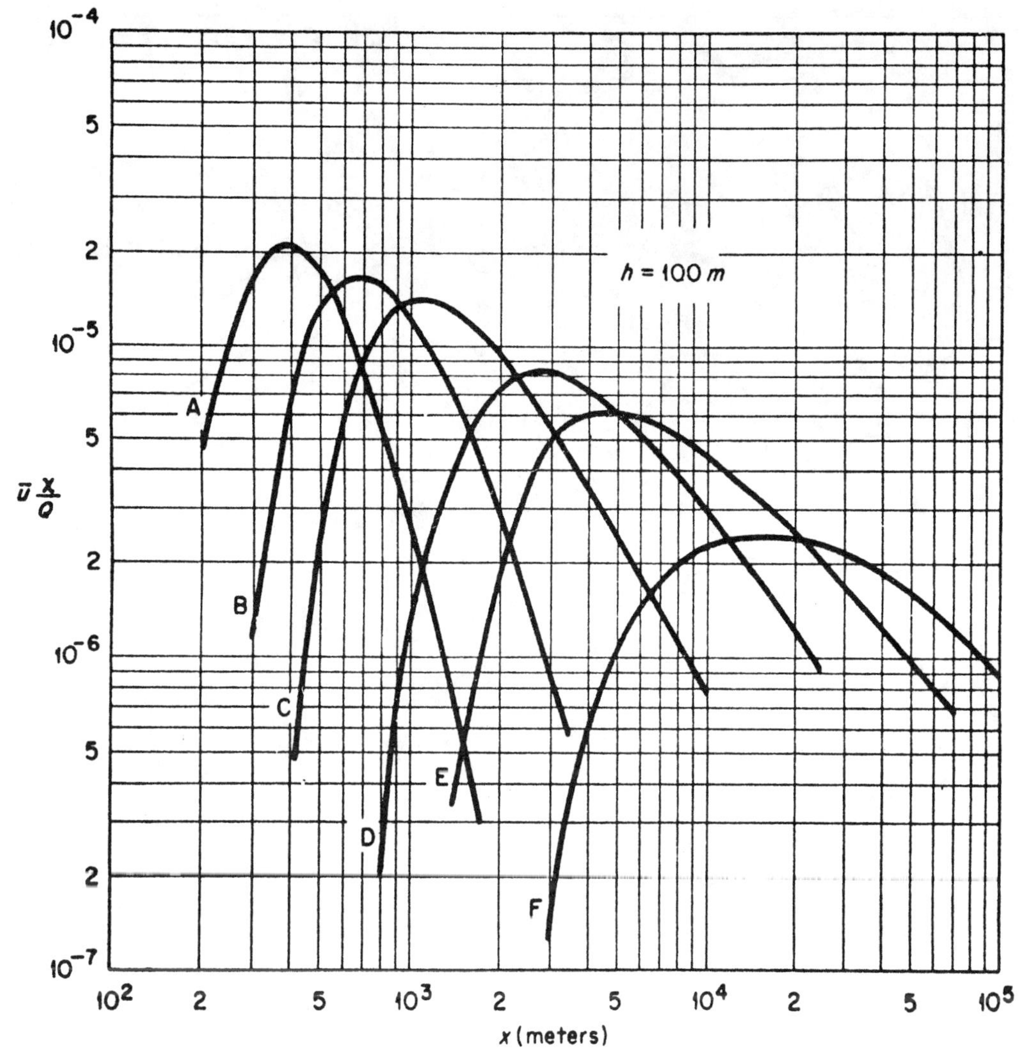

Figure 11.3.8 Values of the Normalized Dispersion Function ($\bar{u}\chi/Q$) as a Function of Downwind Distance, x, for a Release Height, h, of 100 m (From Hilsmeier et al., 1962)

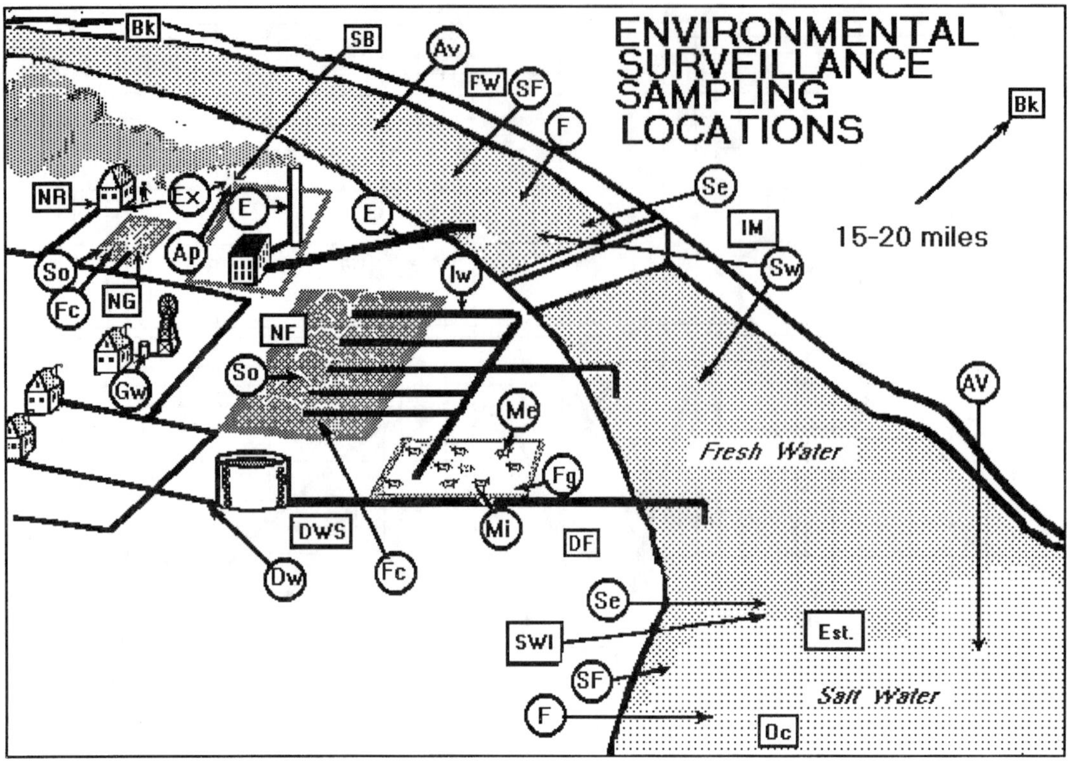

KEY

Locations		Types of Samples	
Bk	Background Location	AP	Airborne Particulates
DF	Dairy Farm	AV	Aquatic Vegetation
DWS	Drinking Water Supply	DW	Drinking Water
Est	Estuary	E	Effluents
FW	Freshwater	Ex	External Dose
IM	Impoundment	F	Fish
NF	Nearest Farms	FC	Food Crops
NG	Nearest Garden		
NR	Nearest Residences	Fg	Forage & Feed
OC	Ocean		
SB	Site Boundary	GW	Groundwater
SWI	SaltWater [\Freshwater] Interface	IW	Irrigation Water
		M	Meat
		Mi	Milk
		Se	Sediment
		SF	Shellfish
		So	Soil

Figure 11.3.9 Locations and Types of Environmental Monitoring Samples

Table 11.3.5 Nuclear Power Reactor-1

Sample Type	Sampling Sites	Collection Frequency	Analysis Frequency
External Radiation Thermoluminescent Dosimeters (TLDs)	20+ Sites [SB] (each sector), [NR]+, [Bk], [Ntown] [NSchool]	Monthly	Monthly readout
Noble Gases Ionization Chamber	1 Site: [E]	Continuously	Continuous readout
Airborne Particulates Low-velocity Air Sampler	4+ Sites: [E, SB+, NR+, Bk]	Weekly	Continuous monitor on effluent; γ-spectrometry: weekly
Airborne Radio-iodines Charcoal canister	6+ Sites: [E, Bk, SB+, NR+, NF, DF]	Weekly	Continuous monitor on effluent; γ-spectrometry: Weekly
Liquid Effluent	Effluent [E]	Continuous on effluent line; batch samples from waste tanks prior to release	Continuous monitoring, γ-spectrometry on each batch sample, ^{90}Sr, ^{3}H on monthly composites
Surface Water	Surface waters upstream [Bk] and freshwater [FW] and [IM], estuary [Est] and ocean [OC]	Monthly	γ-spectrometry on each batch sample, ^{90}Sr, ^{3}H on quarterly composites
Groundwater	Nearest wells in direction of groundwater flow [GW]	Quarterly	γ-spectrometry on each batch sample, ^{90}Sr, ^{3}H, ^{226}Ra on annual composites

Table 11.3.6 Nuclear Power Reactor-2

Sample Type	Sampling Sites	Collection Frequency	Analysis Frequency
Drinking Water	Nearest downstream public water supply [DWS]	Semicontinuous composite (collected by water supply operator every 3–6 hours)	γ-spectrometry, ^{90}Sr, ^{3}H on monthly composites
Milk	Nearest dairy farms [DF] + Dairy	Weekly or biweekly at farms, monthly at dairy	γ-spectrometry weekly; ^{90}Sr, ^{3}H on monthly composites
Food Crops	Nearest garden [NG] and nearby farms [NF]	At harvest (either annually or semi-annually)	γ-spectrometry; ^{90}Sr if other nuclides are detected
Fish	Water source receiving effluent [FW], [IMP], [Oc] & [Bk]	During fishing season or semi-annually	γ-spectrometry; ^{90}Sr if other nuclides are detected
Shellfish	Water source receiving effluent [FW], [IMP], [Oc] & [Bk]	Semi-annually	γ-spectrometry; ^{90}Sr if other nuclides are detected
Sediments	Water source receiving effluent [FW], [IMP], [Oc] & [Bk]	Semi-annually	γ-spectrometry

Table 11.3.7 Research Reactors [Power $\geq$ 1 megawatt (thermal)]

Sample Type	Sampling Sites	Collection Frequency	Analysis Frequency
External Radiation Thermoluminescent dosimeters (TLDs)	3 Sites: [SB, NR, Bk]. More for significant releases	Quarterly	Quarterly readout
Airborne Particulates Low-velocity air sampler (e.g., moving tape sampler)	1 Site: [E]	Continuously	As needed
Noble Gases Ionization chamber	1 Site: Effluent [E]	Continuously	Continuous readout
Liquid Effluent	1 Site: Effluent [E]	Batch or continuously	Each release or continuous; γ-spectrometry on monthly composite
Drinking Water	Pathway to nearest downstream public water supply [DWS]	Semi-continuous or periodic composite samples depending on the nature and level of the released nuclides	γ-spectrometry (^{3}H for D_2O reactors) on quarterly composites

Table 11.3.8 Uranium Mill or Fuel Cycle Facility

Sample Type	Sampling Sites	Collection Frequency	Analysis Frequency
External Radiation Thermoluminescent dosimeters (TLDs)	3 Sites: [SB, NR, Bk]	Quarterly	Quarterly readout
Airborne Particulates Low-velocity air sampler	4+ Sites: [E, SB+, NR+, Bk]	Continuous monitor on primary vents; weekly on environmental samples	Quarterly composites for U (mills and fuel cycle), and ^{226}Ra, ^{230}Th, and ^{210}Po at mills
Radon Gas [at Mill] Charcoal filter	4+ Sites: [E, SB+, NR+, Bk]	At least one week per month at each location	Monthly
Liquid Effluent	Effluent [E]	Continuous on effluent line; batch samples from waste tanks prior to release	Monthly composite of batch samples for U (mills and fuel cycle), and ^{226}Ra, ^{230}Th, and ^{210}Po at mills
Surface Water	Surface waters upstream [Bk] and downstream	Monthly	Quarterly composites for U (mills and fuel cycle), and ^{226}Ra, ^{230}Th, and ^{210}Po at mills

Table 11.3.9 Uranium Mill or Fuel Cycle Facility-2

Sample Type	Sampling Sites	Collection Frequency	Analysis Frequency
Drinking Water	Nearest downstream public water supply [DWS]	Semicontinuous composite (collected by water supply operator every 3–6 hours)	Quarterly composites for U (mills and fuel cycle), and ^{226}Ra, ^{230}Th, and ^{210}Po at mills
Groundwater At mills and other U recovery facilities (e.g., *in situ*)	Nearest wells in direction of groundwater flow [GW]	Quarterly	Total U, ^{226}Ra, ^{230}Th, and ^{210}Po
Food Crops	Nearest garden [NG] and nearby farms [NF]	At harvest (either annually or semi-annually)	U (mills and fuel cycle), and ^{226}Ra, ^{230}Th, and ^{210}Po at mills
Soil	4+ Sites: [E, SB+, NR+, Bk]	Annually	U (mills and fuel cycle), and ^{226}Ra at mills

Table 11.3.10 Low-Level Waste Disposal Site

Sample Type	Sampling Sites	Collection Frequency	Analysis Frequency
External Radiation Thermoluminescent dosimeters (TLDs)	3 Sites: [SB, NR, Bk]	Quarterly	Quarterly readout
Airborne Particulates Low-velocity air sampler [while disposal operations are in progress]	3+ Sites: [SB+, NR+, Bk]	Weekly	γ-spectrometry: weekly
Airborne Tritium (water bubbler or condensation collector)	3+ Sites: [SB+, NR+, Bk]	Weekly	^{3}H on quarterly composites
Surface Water	Surface waters upstream [Bk] and freshwater [FW] and [IM], downstream of site	Monthly	γ-spectrometry on each batch sample, ^{90}Sr, ^{3}H on quarterly composites
Groundwater	Nearest wells (public private and monitoring wells) [GW] in all directions	Quarterly Monthly in direction of groundwater flow	γ-spectrometry on each batch sample, ^{90}Sr, ^{3}H, ^{226}Ra on quarterly composites for each site
Drinking Water	Nearest downstream public water supply [DWS]	Semicontinuous composite (collected by water supply operator every 3–6 hours)	γ-spectrometry, ^{90}Sr, ^{3}H on monthly composites

Table 11.3.11 Medical Facilities and Research Laboratories

Sample Type	Sampling Sites	Collection Frequency	Analysis Frequency
External Radiation Thermoluminescent dosimeters (TLDs)	3 Sites: [SB, NR, Bk]	Quarterly	Quarterly readout
Airborne particulates Low-velocity air sampler (e.g., moving tape sampler)	1 Site: [E]	Continuously	Continuous readout, γ-spectrometry on monthly composite
Airborne Radioiodines [Hospitals doing ^{131}I therapy] Charcoal canister	2+ Sites: [Em SB]	Weekly	Continuous monitor on effluent; γ-spectrometry on weekly canisters
Liquid Effluent	1 Site: Effluent [E]	Continuously on discharge line, monthly sample on holdup tank (if used)	Continuous readout; γ-spectrometry on monthly composite; ^{3}H and ^{90}Sr [if used] on quarterly composite; more frequent analysis if ^{32}P or other short-lived nuclides used

Table 11.3.12 Suggestions for Improving Accuracy of Dose Assessments

Media Specific

Individual calibration and use of duplicate TLDs at each monitoring site can improve reliability of **external dose** measurements

Air particulate samples should be collected more frequently if dust loading is high.

Use of particle sizing samplers (e.g., cascade impactors) can improve dose estimates where **airborne particulates** are principal contributors to dose (e.g., uranium fuel fabrication plants).

Edible **fish and shellfish** should be cleaned and prepared as for consumption or cooking. (The fish skin and viscera often have higher radionuclide concentrations than the muscle).

Food crops should be cleaned and only the edible portions prepared for analysis. (This will result in more representative estimates of actual radionuclide intakes.)

Facility Specific

Fuel fabrication facilities handling high enriched (i.e., >4%) and low enriched uranium should perform isotopic uranium analyses for ^{234}U, ^{235}U, and ^{238}U on representative air and water samples.

Power reactors should place external dosimeters at site boundary locations that are likely to receive direct external doses from turbines (^{16}N ''turbine shine'') or outside radioactive waste storage tanks (e.g., PWR demineralized coolant water storage tank).

Low-level Waste Sites should consider sampling atmospheric methane and similar hydrocarbons which are formed by decomposition of organic materials and could contain ^{3}H or ^{14}C.

Table 11.3.13 Concentration Factors for Marine and Freshwater Organisms

$$\text{Concentration Factor (L/kg)} = \frac{\text{Equilibrium Concentration in Aquatic Organism [activity/fresh weight(kg)]}}{\text{Equilibrium Concentration in Water (activity/liter)}}$$

	Concentration Factor[a] (Liters/Kilogram)			
	Freshwater		Seawater	
Element	Fish	Molluscs & Crustaceans	Fish	Molluscs & Crustaceans
H (tritium)	9.0E − 01	9.0E − 01	9.0E − 01	9.0E − 01
Carbon	4.6E + 03	9.1E + 03	1.8E + 03	1.4E + 03
Sodium	1.0E + 02	2.0E + 02	6.7E − 02	1.9E − 01
Phosphorus	1.0E + 05	2.0E + 04	2.9E + 04	3.0E + 04
Chromium	2.0E + 02	2.0E + 03	4.0E + 02	2.0E + 03
Manganese	4.0E + 02	9.0E + 04	5.5E + 02	4.0E + 02
Iron	1.0E + 02	3.2E + 03	3.0E + 03	2.0E + 04
Cobalt	5.0E + 01	2.0E + 02	1.0E + 02	1.0E + 03
Nickel	1.0E + 02	1.0E + 02	1.0E + 02	2.5E + 02
Copper	5.0E + 01	4.0E + 02	6.7E + 02	1.7E + 03
Zinc	2.0E + 03	1.0E + 04	2.0E + 03	5.0E + 04
Bromine	4.2E + 02	3.3E + 02	1.5E − 02	3.1E + 00
Rubidium	2.0E + 03	1.0E + 03	8.3E + 00	1.7E + 01
Strontium	3.0E + 01	1.0E + 02	2.0E + 00	2.0E + 01
Yttrium	2.5E + 01	1.0E + 03	2.5E + 01	1.0E + 03
Zirconium	3.3E + 00	6.7E + 00	2.0E + 02	8.0E + 01
Niobium	3.0E + 04	1.0E + 02	3.0E + 04	1.0E + 02
Molybdenum	1.0E + 01	1.0E + 01	1.0E + 01	1.0E + 01
Technetium[b]	1.5E + 01	5.0E + 00	1.0E + 01	5.0E + 01
Ruthenium	1.0E + 01	3.0E + 02	3.0E + 00	1.0E + 03
Rhodium	1.0E + 01	3.0E + 02	1.0E + 01	2.0E + 03
Tellurium	4.0E + 02	6.1E + 03	1.0E + 01	1.0E + 02
Iodine	1.5E + 01	5.0E + 00	1.0E + 01	5.0E + 01
Cesium	2.0E + 03	1.0E + 03	4.0E + 01	2.5E + 01
Barium	4.0E + 00	2.0E + 02	1.0E + 01	1.0E + 02
Rare Earths (La)	2.5E + 01	1.0E + 03	2.5E + 01	1.0E + 03
Radium[b]	5.2E + 02	1.3E + 03	1.1E + 02	1.3E + 03
Uranium[b]	7.5E + 00	1.0E + 03	2.1E + 01	—
Neptunium	1.0E + 01	4.0E + 02	1.0E + 01	1.0E + 01
Plutonium[c]	4.0E + 00	1.0E + 02	1.0E + 00	1.0E + 03
Americium[c]	3.0E + 01	1.0E + 03	1.0E + 01	2.0E + 03

[a] From NRC Regulatory Guide 1.109 (NRC, 1977).
[b] Values from Peterson, 1983.
[c] Values from IAEA, 1982.

SECTION 4 MEDICAL/ACCELERATOR/X-RAY DIFFRACTION

This section gives guidance on surveys and contamination levels, and good work practices for uses of medical x-rays and radiopharmaceuticals, accelerators and x-ray diffraction equipment. Guidance pertinent to laboratories using radioactive materials (section 1 of this chapter) also apply to uses of radiopharmaceuticals.

TABLE OF CONTENTS

Table 11.4.1 Data on Dose Equivalent Rates from Adult Patients (Courtesy NCRP from Report 105, 1989 after Syed et al., 1982; Castronovo et al., 1982; Jankowski, 1984)

Study	Radiopharmaceutical	Administered Amount MBq	(mCi)	Time After Administration	Distance (cm)	Dose Equivalent Rate μSv/h	(mrem/h)
Bone	^{99m}Tc MDP	740	(20)	0	100	9	(0.9)
				1 h	100	6.3	(0.63)
				2 h	100	4.7	(0.47)
				3 h	100	3.5	(0.35)
Liver	^{99m}Tc S colloid	150	(4)	0	100	2	(0.2)
Blood pool	^{99m}Tc RBC	740	(20)	0	100	14	(1.4)
Tumor	^{67}Ga citrate	110	(3)	0	100	3.5	(0.35)
CSF	^{111}In DTPA	19	(0.5)	0	100	0.8	(0.08)
Heart	^{201}Tl chloride	740	(20)	0	[a]	20	(2)
Heart	^{99m}Tc HSA	190	(5)	0	[a]	15	(1.5)
Bone	^{99m}Tc MDP	740	(20)	0	[a]	25	(2.5)
Heart	^{99m}Tc RBC	1000	(27)	20 min	100	18	(1.8)

[a] Side of stretcher

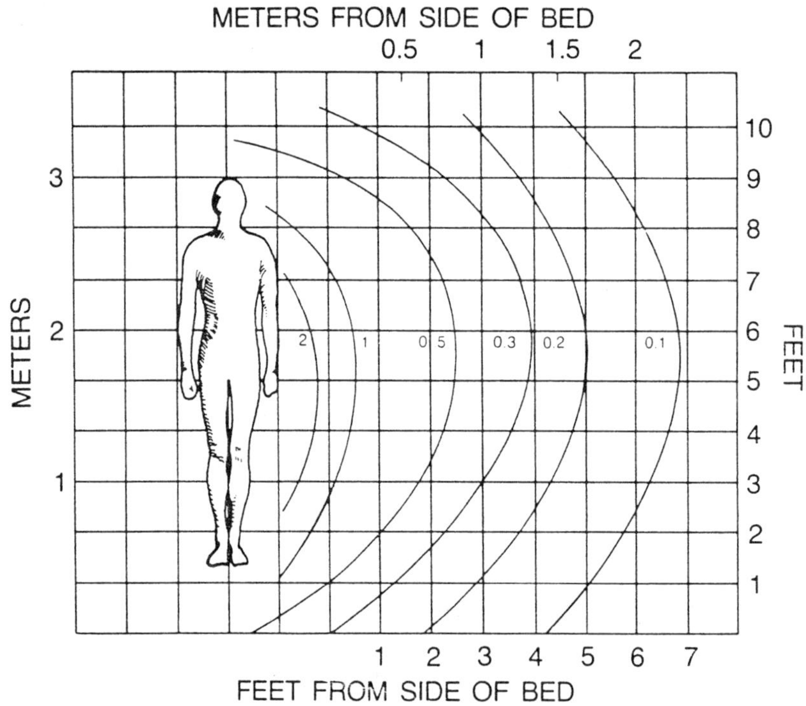

Figure 11.4.1 Approximate Dose Equivalent Rates from a Patient Containing Cs-137 or I-131 in mSv h^{-1} (mrem h^{-1} × 100) in regions around the bed of a patient containing 3700 MBq (100 mCi) cesium-137 or 5550 MBq (150 mCi) of iodine-131. Note that although only one side is shown, the exposure pattern completely surrounds the body. (Courtesy NCRP from Report 105, 1989)

Table 11.4.2 Estimated Radiation Dose Rates at Various Times and Distances after the Administration of 3.7 GBq (100 mCi) of ^{131}I for Thyroid Metastases[a] (μSv h^{-1}) (From Castronovo et al., 1986, with permission)

Distance From Patient (cm)	Time Post Administration (h)							
	0	6	12	18	24	36	48	72
10	16000[b]	7311	5087	4950	4612	3450	2855	750
30.5	1891	1511	1051	1023	953	713	590	155
100	216	173	120	117	109	81.4	67.4	17.7

[a] Skeletal, residual thyroid bed or lung metastasis.
[b] Average measurement for 5 patients directly over stomach immediately after the oral administration of ^{131}I (NaI).

Table 11.4.3 Radiation Doses (μSv) Accumulated for Various Contact Times with Therapy Patients Administered 3.7 GBq (100 mCi) ^{131}I (From Castronovo et al., 1986, with permission)

Contact Time (min)	Distance (cm)	Position	Time Post Administration (h)			
			0	24	48	72
1	10	Hands	267.0[b]	77.1	47.7	12.5
	30.5	WB[a]	31.5	15.9	9.8	2.6
	100	WB[a]	3.6	1.8	1.1	0.3
5	10	Hands	333	385.5	238.5	62.5
	30.5	WB	158	79.6	49.3	12.9
	100	WB	18	9.1	5.6	1.5
15	10	Hands	4000	1157	716	188
	30.5	WB	473	238	148	38.6
	100	WB	54	27.2	16.8	4.4
30	10	Hands	8000	2313	1432	375
	30.5	WB	945	945	295	77.2
	100	WB	108	54.4	33.6	8.8

[a] WB = Whole body.
[b] Average measurement for 5 patients directly over stomach immediately after the oral administration of ^{131}I (NaI).

Table 11.4.4 Dose Received By Nuclear Medicine Technologist From Selected Routine Procedures (From NCRP 105, 1989)

Procedure	Agent[b]	Activity Administered (MBq)	Dose from Single Routine Procedure (μGy)			
			Prep[c]	Administration	Imaging	Total
Bone	TcDiphos	555	0.2	0.1	5.4	5.7
Brain	TcO_4	740	0.4	0.2	2.2	2.8
CBF[a]	TcO_4	740	0.4	0.2	0.3	0.9
Infarct	TcPyro	555	0.1	0.1	0.2	0.4
Liver	TcSC	148	0.1	0.2	0.3	0.6
Thyroid	TcO_4	74	0.2	0.1	0.4	0.7

[a] Cerebral blood flow.
[b] Using ^{99m}Tc.
[c] Dosage preparation and assay.

Table 11.4.5 Projected Personnel Radiation Doses at 30.5 cm for Various Patient Care Times per 3.7 GBq (100 mCi) of ^{131}I Patient Dose at Administration (From Castronovo et al., 1986, with permission)

Classification	Task	Time (min)	Whole Body Dose (μSv)
Moderate care (1–3 times per shift)	Greeting, shift rounds	2	62.8
	Complete visit	5	157
	Give medicine	2–5	62.8–157
	Straighten linen	2–5	62.8–157
	Give back rub	2	62.8
Moderate to intense care	Patient assessment	5	157
	Ambulate to and from bathroom	5	157
	IV mainline (total care)	15	471
	Set IV dose and resetting mainline	5	157
	Central venous pressure or subclavian dressing change (includes total parenteral nutrition)	20–45	628–1413
	Assess for and administer cardiac medicines	2–5	62.8–157
	Chest physiotherapy	20	628
	Endotracheal or track suctioning	10	314
	Troubleshoot problems (IV site)	5–10	157–314
	Set 12-lead ECG	10	314

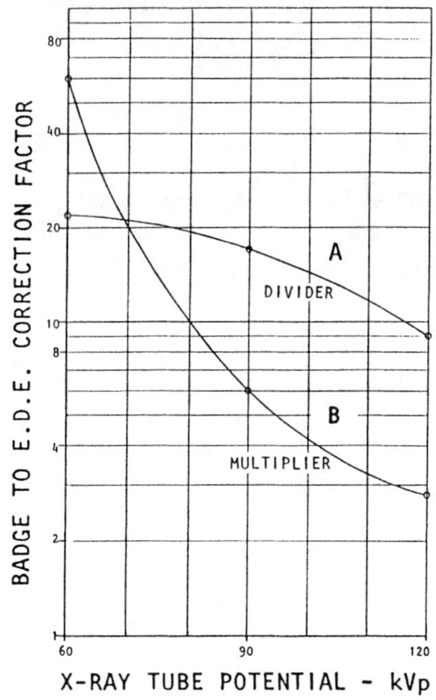

Figure 11.4.2 Correction Factors for Deriving Effective Dose Equivalent from Film Badge Dose Equivalents for medical personnel wearing lead aprons with 0.5 mm lead equivalents exposed to scattered x-rays generated at 60, 90 and 120 kVp. *Curve A*: Division factors for neck badge above apron. *Curve B*: Multiplication factors for waist badge under apron. (From Webster, 1989, with permission)

Table 11.4.6 Healing Arts X-Ray Survey Measurement Criteria (From CRCPD NBSGCR 79-174, 1979)

		Measurement		
Application	Regulatory Criteria	Range Expected	Accuracy Requirements	Instrument Considerations
Unrestricted area	States regs only. 2 mrem in one hour. 100 mrem in 7 consecutive days.	Few mR/hr	Screening ±50% Verification ±20%	Survey meter, ion chambers. 20–120 kV capability. <1 sec. response time. Long-term integrate mode. Temperature insensitive.
Occupational exposure	1250 mrem/calendar qtr. 5 rem/yr whole body. 75 rem/yr extremities. 30 rem/yr skin of whole body	Personnel monitoring: background to several rem per year	Screening ±50% low end of exposure	Pocket dosimeters, TLD, film badge. Survey meter, up to 150 kV range. (250 kV for therapy)
		Radiation area Monitoring: Few mR/hr to R/hr	Verification ±10% above 25% of regulatory criteria	TLDs of known energy response. Portable survey meter: integrating, rate and direction independent, wide exposure range.
Overexposures	State regulations. Defined as anything over 1.25 rem/qtr.	Several rem to thousands of rem	±20% over 5 rem	Use same instrumentation as for occupational exposure. Stop watch to reproduce time involved. Film badge readout is critical. TLD not a permanent record [can't tell if fixed or moving relative to sources].
Fluoroscopic output (useful beam)	State regulations. Old equipment, <10 R/min. New equipment with image intensifier, <5 R/min. BRH performance standard. Manual <5 R/min. Hi Level Control <10 R/min.	<1 R/min to 100 R/min.	±10%	Ionization chamber. Measured at skin entrance. Energy independent at 50 kV to 150 kV.

Table 11.4.6 Healing Arts X-Ray Survey Measurement Criteria (Continued)

<table>
<tr><th rowspan="2">Application</th><th rowspan="2">Regulatory Criteria</th><th colspan="2">Measurement</th><th rowspan="2">Instrument Considerations</th></tr>
<tr><th>Range Expected</th><th>Accuracy Requirements</th></tr>
<tr><td>Half-value layer</td><td>State Regulations for old equipment. BRH performance standard for new equip. (HVL shall not be less than values shown below.)</td><td>HVL range: 0.2–6 mm aluminum (type 1100)</td><td>+40% to −0%</td><td>Small ion chambers (must be completely covered by beam). Exposure rate independent. 20–120 kV</td></tr>
<tr><td></td><td>
<table>
<tr><th>Design Operating Range (Kilovolt Peak)</th><th>Measured Potential (Kilovolts Peak)</th><th>Half-Value Layer (Millimeters of aluminum)</th></tr>
<tr><td>Below 50</td><td>30</td><td>0.3</td></tr>
<tr><td></td><td>40</td><td>0.4</td></tr>
<tr><td></td><td>49</td><td>0.5</td></tr>
<tr><td>50 to 70</td><td>50</td><td>1.2</td></tr>
<tr><td></td><td>60</td><td>1.3</td></tr>
<tr><td></td><td>70</td><td>1.5</td></tr>
<tr><td>Above 70</td><td>71</td><td>2.1</td></tr>
<tr><td></td><td>80</td><td>2.3</td></tr>
<tr><td></td><td>90</td><td>2.5</td></tr>
<tr><td></td><td>100</td><td>2.7</td></tr>
<tr><td></td><td>110</td><td>3.0</td></tr>
<tr><td></td><td>120</td><td>3.2</td></tr>
<tr><td></td><td>130</td><td>3.5</td></tr>
<tr><td></td><td>140</td><td>3.8</td></tr>
<tr><td></td><td>150</td><td>4.1</td></tr>
</table>
</td><td>Radiation range: 10 mR to 0.5 R integrated.
Rates 1 R/sec to several R/sec.</td><td>±20%</td><td></td></tr>
<tr><td>Leakage</td><td>BRH performance standard. 100 mR in an hour at 1 meter from tubehead; 2 mR in an hour at 5 cm from rest of unit.</td><td>Few mR/hr to R/hr</td><td>Screening ±50%
Verification ±20%</td><td>Survey meter, ion chamber 20 kV–120 kV, <1 sec. response time; rate and/or integrate mode. Temperature insensitive. Ionization chamber with 100 cm^2 surface. No detector linear dimension greater than 20 cm.</td></tr>
<tr><td>Diagnostic beam output (useful beam)</td><td>State and BRH regs. Reproducibility, linearity. Federal guidance—NEXT, DENT and BENT programs.</td><td>Integrate 10 mR to several R
Rates 1 R/sec to several R/sec</td><td>±10%</td><td>Ion chamber capable 20 kV to 150 kV, energy and rate independent. Tape measure (cm).</td></tr>
<tr><td>Therapy beam output (useful beam)</td><td>Range of exposures for accepted medical practice. Reproducibility.</td><td>Up to 100 R/min (at skin entrance)</td><td>±10%
Reproducibility and linearity ±1%</td><td>TLD. Ion chamber. Dose rate and energy independent. Integrating up to 100 R. Rate, 100 R/sec. 0–250 kV.</td></tr>
</table>

Table 11.4.7 Survey Frequencies at Medical Institutions (From NRC Regulatory Guide 8.23 Rev. 1, 1981)

1. All elution, preparation, and injection areas should be surveyed daily with a survey meter and decontaminated if necessary.
2. Laboratory areas where only small quantities of radioactive material (less than 200 μCi at any one time) are used should be surveyed monthly.
3. All other laboratory areas should be surveyed weekly.
4. The weekly and monthly surveys should consist of the following:
   a. A measurement of radiation levels with a survey meter sufficiently sensitive to detect 0.1 mR/h.
   b. A series of smear tests to measure contamination levels. The method for performing smear tests should be sufficiently sensitive to detect the limits in Table 11.4.8 to one significant digit.
   c. Any air sample measurements necessary to determine compliance with §20.103 of 10 CFR Part 20 in cases where calculations alone are not sufficient.

Table 11.4.8 Recommended Action Levels for Removable Surface Contamination in Medical Institutions[a] (From NRC Regulatory Guide 23 Rev. 1, 1981)

	Type of Radioactive Material[b]					
	Alpha Emitters		Beta or X-Ray Emitters		Low-Risk Beta or X-Ray Emitters	
Type of Surface	(μCi/cm^2)	(dpm/100 cm^2)	(μCi/cm^2)	(dpm/100 cm^2)	(μCi/cm^2)	(dpm/100 cm^2)
1. Unrestricted areas	10^{-7}	22	10^{-6}	220	10^{-5}	2,200
2. Restricted areas	10^{-6}	220	10^{-5}	2,200	10^{-4}	22,000
3. Personal clothing worn outside restricted areas	10^{-7}	22	10^{-6}	220	10^{-5}	2,200
4. Protective clothing worn only in restricted areas	10^{-6}	220	10^{-5}	2,200	10^{-4}	22,000
5. Skin	10^{-6}	220	10^{-6}	220	10^{-5}	2,200

[a] Averaging is acceptable over nonliving areas of up to 300 cm or, for floors, walls, and ceiling, 100 cm. Averaging is also acceptable over 100 cm^2 for skin or, for the hands, over the whole area of the hand, nominally 300 cm^2.

[b] Beta or x-ray emitter values are applicable for all beta or x-ray emitters other than those considered low risk. Low risk nuclides include C-14, H-3, S-35, Tc-99m, and others whose beta energies are less than 0.2 MeV maximum, whose gamma or x-ray emission is less than 0.1 R/h at 1 meter per curie, and whose permissible concentration in air (see 10 CFR Part 20, Appendix B, Table 1) is greater than 10^{-6} μCi/ml.

Table 11.4.9 Types of Particle Accelerators (Modified from, courtesy NCRP from Report 51, 1977, by R. Thomas)

Direct (Potential-drop) accelerators
(Single-stage for acceleration of either ions or electrons)
(Two-stage [tandem] for acceleration of ions)

1. Electrostatic high-voltage generators:
   a. belt-charging system (e.g., Van de Graaff, Pelletron)
   b. rotating-cylinder charging system
2. High-voltage transformers:
   a. transformer-rectifier set
   b. voltage-multiplying system (e.g., Cockcroft-Walton, Dynamitron)
   c. cascaded transformer system (e.g., Insulating-Core transformer)

Indirect (Radio-frequency, plasma) accelerators

1. Linear beam trajectory:
   a. radiofrequency quadruple accelerator,
   b. ion linear accelerator.
   c. electron linear accelerator.
2. Circular or spiral beam trajectory:
   a. cyclotron (ions only)
   b. synchrotron (ions or electrons)
   c. betatron (electrons only)
   d. microtron (electrons only)
3. Combined/complex accelerators
   a. race track microtron (electrons only),
   b. colliding beam, storage ring

Table 11.4.10 Applications of Particle Accelerators (Augmented and adapted from, courtesy NCRP from Report 51, 1977, by R. Thomas)

	Electron	X-Ray	Ion	Neutron
Diagnostic radiology		*		
Radiotherapy	*	*	*	*
Industrial radiography		*		
Analysis of materials, e.g.				
activation analysis			*	*
microscopy, electron or ion	*		*	
x-ray fluorescence analysis	*	*	*	
geological well-logging	*	*		*
neutron scattering			*	*
synchrotron light sources	*	*		
ion separation			*	
Ion implantation, polishing			*	*
Surface conditioning, roughening	*	*		
Radioisotope production			*	*
Radiation processing	*	*		
Radiation sterilization	*	*		
Research and training, e.g.,	*	*	*	*
nuclear-structure physics				
neutron physics				
atomic and solid-state physics				
biology, chemistry				
radiation effects on materials.				

Table 11.4.11 Radiation of Possible Concern in Occupiable Areas of Particle Accelerator Facilities

Accelerator	Particles Accelerated	Beam Energy (MeV)	Purpose of Operation	Radiation of Possible Concern in Occupiable Areas[a]
Potential-drop	Protons Deuterons Alpha Particles	1–10 1–10 2–20	Research Neutron Production Neutron Radiography Activation Analysis	Fast Neutrons Thermal Neutrons Gamma Rays
	Electrons	1–10	Processing Radiography	X-rays
Electron Linear	Electrons	1–10	Processing Radiography Therapy	X-rays
	Electrons	>10	Research Neutron Production Neutron Radiography Activation Analysis	Electrons X-rays Fast Neutrons Thermal Neutrons Gamma Rays
Cyclotron	Protons Deuterons Alpha Particles	15–50 7.5–24 15–50	Research Isotope Production Neutron Production Neutron Radiography Activation Analysis	Fast Neutrons Thermal Neutrons Gamma Rays
Betatron	Electrons	1–50	Radiography Therapy	X-rays

[a] Excluding occupancy of primary beam areas where the accelerated beam is the primary issue.

Table 11.4.12 Propensity for Inducing Radioactivity of Accelerated Particles (From NBS Handbook 107, 1970)

Particle	Energy Range	Induced Radioactivity in Target	Induced Radioactivity in Vicinity
Electrons	below 1.67[a] MeV	none	none
Electrons	1.67[a] to 10 MeV	limited	very slight
Electrons	above 10 MeV	probable	suspect
Protons, Helium ions	below 1 MeV	limited	none
Protons, Helium ions	1 to 10 MeV	limited	suspect
Deuterons, tritons	any energy	limited	suspect
All ions of light atomic weight	above 10 MeV	probable	suspect

[a] if ^{3}H and Be are excluded as possible target materials this value is 7 MeV.

Table 11.4.13 Summary of Radionuclides Commonly Identified in Materials Irradiated in Accelerator Radiation Environments (With permission of publisher from Patterson et al. 1973, with additions)

Target Material	Radionuclides	Half-Life
Plastics and oils	^{7}Be	53.6 days
	^{11}C	20.4 minutes
Duralumin	As above, plus	
	^{18}F	110 minutes
	^{22}Na	2.60 years
	^{24}Na	15.0 hours
Steel	As above, plus	
	^{42}K	12.47 hours
	^{43}K	22.4 hours
	^{44}Sc	3.92 hours
	^{44m}Sc	2.44 days
	^{46}Sc	84 days
	^{47}Sc	3.43 days
	^{48}Sc	1.83 days
	^{48}V	16.0 days
	^{51}Cr	27.8 days
	^{52}Mn	5.55 days
	^{52m}Mn	21.3 minutes
	^{54}Mn	300 days
	^{56}Co	77 days
	^{57}Co	270 days
	^{58}Co	72 days
	^{55}Fe	2.94 years
	^{59}Fe	45.1 days
Stainless steel	As above, plus	
	^{60}Co	5.27 years
	^{57}Ni	37 hours
	^{60}Cu	24 minutes
Copper	As above, plus	
	^{65}Ni	2.56 hours
	^{61}Cu	3.33 hours
	^{62}Cu	9.80 minutes
	^{64}Cu	12.82 hours
	^{63}Zn	38.3 minutes
	^{65}Zn	245 days
Concrete	^{152}Eu	13.4 years
	^{154}Eu	8.5 years

Table 11.4.14 Production of Ozone by External Electron Beams (Courtesy NCRP from Report No. 51, 1977)

Assumptions:

No disassociation of ozone (O_3) during period of irradiation;
No ventilation of the room in which the external electron beam is contained;
O_3 is distributed uniformly throughout the volume of the room during irradiation.

The ozone concentration in air, C_{O_3}, after an irradiation period t, is given by

$$C_{O_3} = \left[\frac{C_{O_2} G \epsilon}{N}\right]\left[\frac{S_{col}\, I \times t}{v}\right] \times 10^6$$

$$= 3.25 \times 10^6 \left[\frac{S_{col}\, I \times t}{v}\right] ppm$$

where C_{O_2} = the fractional concentration of oxygen in air (0.232);
G = the G-value for O_3 production by electron irradiation of oxygen (~6 molecules per 100 electron volts)[a] See also Table 11.4.16.
ϵ = the number of electronic charges per milliampere-second of electron-beam current (6.28×10^{15} mA^{-1} s^{-1});
N = Avogadro's Number (6.02×10^{23} molecules per 22.4 liters of gas at NTP);
S_{col} = the collision stopping power of electrons in air at NTP (keV cm^{-1})[b]
I = the external electron beam current (mA);
x = the distance in air traversed by the external electron beam (cm);
t = the irradiation period (s);
and v = the volume of the room containing the external electron beam (l).

As an example of ozone production, a 1 mA external beam of 10 MeV electrons, traversing a 300 cm distance in a room 4 m × 4 m × 3 m (about $5 \times 10^4 l$), can produce an ozone concentration of about 15 ppm after a 5 minute irradiation period. Reference is made to Table 11.4.15 for threshold limit values for ozone.

[a] Frequently reported G-values are between 3 and 9. For the purpose of this report, a value of 6 is used (Brynjolfsson and Martin 1967).
[b] Typical values for S_{col}:

0.5 MeV 2.3 keV cm^{-1}
1.0 MeV 2.2 keV cm^{-1}
10 MeV 2.5 keV cm^{-1}
50 MeV 3.0 keV cm^{-1}

Table 11.4.15 Threshold Limit Values for Ozone and Certain Oxides of Nitrogen in Workroom Air[a] (Courtesy NCRP from Report No. 51, 1977)

Substance	Threshold Limit Values (TLV)[a] (ppm)
Ozone	0.1
Nitric oxide	25
Nitrogen dioxide	5

According to ACGIH (American Conference of Governmental Industrial Hygienists Documentation of the Threshold Limit Values for Substances in Workroom Air, 3rd ed., 1971), ozone is a highly injurious and lethal gas at relatively low concentrations (a few ppm) and at short exposure periods (a few hours). Ozone is apparently radiomimetic, i.e., it mimics, in its effects on health, those of ionizing radiation. The TLV of 0.1 ppm for ozone represents a limit which, although it results in no ostensible or manifest injury, may result in premature aging in a manner similar to that from continued exposure to ionizing radiation, if exposure is sufficiently prolonged.

If electron beam exposures to the air are prolonged (as for electron beam processing), it may be necessary to provide for very high ventilation for the ozone contaminated volume of air. Facilities for electron beam generators *should* be designed so that the path of the electron beam in air is short. A high capacity air exhaust system *should* preferably be close to the beam output.

After machine shutoff, the concentration of ozone in the affected volume of air is given by[b]:

$$C'_{O_3} = C_{O_3} e^{-ft'/v}$$

where C'_{O_3} = ozone concentration (ppm) at time t',
C_{O_3} = ozone concentration at shutoff,
f = pump exhaust rate (liters s^{-1}),
t' = time after shutoff (s),
v = volume of the room (liters).

[a] ACGIH (American Conference of Governmental Industrial Hygienists, Threshold Limit Values of Airborne Contaminants and Physical Agents with Intended Changes Adopted by ACGIH for 1971).

[b] Note that equation does not allow for breakup of ozone.

Table 11.4.16 Toxic Gases Produced by Radiation at Electron LINAC Installations (Courtesy IAEA from Publication No. 188, 1979)

Gas		TLV[a] (ppm)	G (air)[b] (molecules per 100 eV)		Decomposition Time Assumed[c] (min)
			Low $\dot{D}$	High $\dot{D}$	
Ozone	O_3	0.1	7.4	10.3	50
Nitric oxide	NO	25			
Nitrogen dioxide	NO_2	5[d]	(4.8)	(<0.15)	
Nitrogen trioxide	NO_3				
Nitrogen tetroxide	N_2O_4	5[d]			
Nitric anhydride	N_2O_5				
Nitrous oxide	N_2O				

[a] Threshold limit value. Maximum concentration averaged over any 8 hour work shift, assuming 40 hour work week.
[b] Values from Willis et al., 1970. High dose rate means instantaneous dose rate (during beam pulse) greater than about 5×10^8 Gy s^{-1} (5×10^{10} rad s^{-1}) ($\approx 3 \times 10^{24}$ eV g^{-1} s^{-1}) to air. Theoretical values are in parentheses.
[c] Decomposition time for ozone may depend strongly on size of room and nature of materials present.
[d] Value also represents ceiling value: maximum concentration allowed at any time.

Table 11.4.17 Radionuclides Identified in the Air Around Several Accelerators (With permission of Publisher from Patterson and Thomas, 1973)

Laboratory	Accelerator	Radionuclides Identified	Comments
RPI	50 MeV electron linac	^{15}O, ^{13}N	
Saclay	330 to 560 MeV, 100 kW beam power	^{13}N, ^{15}O, ^{11}C, ^{41}Ar, ^{38}Cl, ^{7}Be	
CERN	600 MeV proton synchrotron	^{11}C, ^{13}N, ^{41}Ar	
PPA	3 GeV proton synchrotron, 10^{11} p/sec	^{14}O, ^{15}O, ^{13}N, ^{11}C	^{13}N, ^{11}C, levels negligible ^{14}O, ^{15}O same order of magnitude as $(MPC)_a$
RHEL	7 GeV proton synchrotron	^{16}N, ^{15}O, ^{13}N, ^{11}C	Maximum concentrations $\approx 2 \times 10^{-6}$ μCi/cm^3 close to target
CERN	25 GeV proton synchrotron	^{13}N, ^{11}C, ^{41}Ar	
BNL	30 GeV proton synchrotron	^{13}N, ^{11}C, ^{41}Ar	

Table 11.4.18 Radiation Safety Program for Particle Accelerators (Personal Communication Thomas, 1992)

The requirements for an Operational Radiation Safety Program at an accelerator facility include the basic elements set out in NCRP Report 59 titled, ''Operational Radiation Safety Program'' [NCRP, 1978]. These basic elements are:

- Organization
- Facility Design
- Warning and Personnel Security Systems
- Monitoring and Control Programs
- Personnel Protective Equipment
- Orientation and Training
- Emergency Planning
- Occupational Medicine

At particle accelerator facilities the specific operational requirements do not, in general, differ from these basic elements listed above but there are, in some instances, special considerations which apply to accelerator facilities.

A convenient checklist for use in determining whether the principal components of an accelerator radiation safety program are in place is appended to this section.

Organization and Administration

An extensive discussion of the organization of an accelerator radiation safety program is given by Thomas and Stevenson (Chapter 5, IAEA Tech. Rept. 283, 1988).

The one essential element of the radiological safety organization for an accelerator facility is personnel with both a sound educational basis in radiological protection and appropriate experience in accelerator health physics. An outline of the experience required may be found in Patterson and Thomas 1973 or Thomas and Stevenson (IAEA Tech. Rept. 283, 1988).

The range of radiological problems to be found at particle accelerators varies widely with accelerator characteristics, particles accelerated, and beam energy and intensity. It is therefore essential that appropriately qualified personnel have overall responsibility for the radiological safety program. Otherwise, the general organization required for the radiological safety program at an accelerator facility is, in most respects, similar to that discussed in NCRP Report 59.

Facility Design

The most important parameter that influences the design of an accelerator facility is the characteristics of the primary radiation sources. These in turn are influenced by the particles being accelerated, the beam energy and its intensity.

Specific issues which must be addressed during facility design are:

- *Access or Egress*—must balance the conflicting demands of rapid evacuation during emergencies with the need to limit radiation leakage through access ways.
- *Ventilation*—at high intensities/energies accelerators may produce radioactive and toxic gases. Toxic gases are also often used in experimental apparatuses in conjunction with accelerators. Optimum ventilation rates are required to provide adequate cooling, to minimize the release of toxic or radioactive gases to the environment, and to limit the influence of corrosive gases on accelerator components.
  It may be necessary to obtain appropriate permits for the release of radioactive gas to the environment and local jurisdictions should be consulted on this matter.
- *Multiplicity of Hazards*—major accelerator facilities are extremely complex. The combination of accelerators with experimental apparatuses or experimental equipment gives rise to a wide range of hazards. In addition to ionizing radiations it is not uncommon to find hazards due to, for example: UV; infrared light; lasers; RF; high voltages, magnetic fields; high pressures as well as the usual toxicological and industrial safety hazards found in most large industrial facilities. The facility design must take account of such hazards.

Personnel Security

- Access to many areas associated with particle accelerators must be strictly controlled because of a variety of hazards (see *Facility Design*). In some instances access to areas for maintenance or, for example, to adjust equipment is required during accelerator operation. Access Control is a particularly serious problem at larger accelerator facilities where access points may be remote from the central control facilities. The design of complex interlock systems and appropriate administrative controls to prevent improper entry to hazardous areas is imperative. An excellent discussion of these issues is given in NCRP Report 88 1986.

Control of Radioactive Materials and Contamination

The prompt accelerator radiation environment may induce radioactivity in accelerator components and surrounding materials. Movement of material from the accelerator area must therefore be strictly controlled to prevent both the release of radioactive materials to the environment and the spread of radioactive contamination about the accelerator.

Control of Radioactive Materials

The control of radioactive material is achieved by:

- Setting a lower limit of what constitutes ''radioactivity''. Many facilities consider material whose radioactivity is more than twice the background level to be radioactive.
- Labeling radioactive materials—indicating, for example, external dose rate, specific activity.
- Providing well designed radioactive storage facilities.
- Providing particular attention to ensuring that materials surrounding the accelerator facility that may have become activated are monitored and controlled. Examples would be: shielding materials around beams (lead, iron, concrete, earth); air in accelerator vaults; accelerator components such as magnets, vacuum chambers, beam pipes, etc.
- Ensuring appropriate procedures for the transportation of radioactive materials to and from the accelerator facility are prepared and implemented.

Contamination Control

Many accelerator produced nuclides have emission characteristics which are different from those of the radionuclides routinely monitored in the nuclear industry (see, for example, Patterson and Thomas, 1973, and Thomas and Stevenson IAEA, 1988).

In certain cases care must be taken to ensure that the accelerator-produced materials are detected. Examples of accelerator produced radionuclides (which do not emit β particles) are ^{7}Be, ^{54}Mn and ^{51}Cr. Monitoring programs designed to identify activation products using simple beta particle detectors might overlook such radionuclides. In some circumstances these radionuclides might present problems; for example, in water purification systems, even after considerable radioactive decay, in resin beds where ^{7}Be is collected; in stainless steels rich in cobalt and nickel; or on the surfaces of equipment which have become contaminated by the deposition of Be aerosols formed in the air (the latter example has been observed at LAMPF).

Contamination Standards

The surface contamination limits recommended for β particle emitting radionuclides are appropriate for accelerator facilities but there are special considerations which apply to the ''unusual'' accelerator-produced radionuclides.

Training

In general the radiation safety training for accelerator users and operators is described in NCRP Report 59, 1978. However, accelerator facilities can be extremely complex and—particularly at large accelerators—the multiplicity of operators and users coupled with the potential for dangerous radiation exposures—mandates essential and comprehensive training. Patterson and Thomas, 1973 is a textbook which summarizes a training program developed for the USAEC (DOE) in the 1960s. Much of this material is of value to the present day. Busick and Warren, 1979 have stressed the importance of including discussions of recent relevant accidents in the program of training.

Occupational Medicine-Accident Dosimetry

One area of interest to occupational health physicists at accelerator facilities might be the estimate of dose to workers after an accident. Miller and Patterson, 1972 first discussed the estimation of dose strategy after an exposure to a high energy accelerator beam by determining the production of ^{11}C (20 min.) in the victim's trunk. Tatcher et al., 1987 have recently discussed this technique in conjunction with radiotherapy facilities.

Accelerator Radiation Safety Checklist (Courtesy IAEA from Technical Report 283, 1988 after Patterson and Thomas, 1973)

The Lawrence Berkeley Laboratory has used the following checklist as an aid in assessing accelerator radiation safety programs. It is reproduced here in slightly modified form for the convenience of the reader.

The list, though not applicable to all accelerators, should prove useful in many circumstances. The reader may wish to add items or put greater emphasis on some, but probably nothing should be omitted.

I. Shielding

A. *Design and calculations.* Are the calculations available on which shielding design is based? What is the source of the input data for the calculations?

B. *Measurements.* Have measurements been made to check the accuracy of the calculations and the efficacy of the shield?

II. Radiation Damage Estimates for Sensitive Components

Are sensitive components of the radiation monitoring system or the interlock system so located that their function cannot be impaired by exposure to very high radiation doses?

III. Accelerator Controls

Is access to the accelerator controls restricted to those persons who are authorized to operate the accelerator or can the accelerator controls be locked to prevent unauthorized use?

IV. Interlocks

A. *Manual reset.* Can tripped interlocks be reset only manually at the location of the interlock, rather than remotely from the control console?

B. *Run-safe switches.* Are there switches in the radiation and high radiation areas that make it impossible for the accelerator to operate or beam to be admitted to the area when the switch is in the 'safe' position or is each person entering the zone forced to take a key or other token with him that cuts accelerator operation until all keys (tokens) are returned to their distribution point?

C. *Regular tests.* Is the function of the entire interlock system tested at regular intervals and are the results recorded?

D. *Up to date circuit diagrams.* Are up to date circuit diagrams maintained?

V. Exclusion Areas and High Radiation Areas

A. Have all areas that must be cleared of personnel before the accelerator can be allowed to operate been properly marked and interlocked? Have the responsibilities of the persons who will effect the search and secure procedure been set down in writing? Has special attention been paid to the possibilities of holes in the enclosures of exclusion areas?

B. Can all areas where high radiation levels could occur be locked, or has a visible and audible alarm system been provided to warn of the presence of radiation? Have staff working in such areas been instructed concerning the correct course of action should alarms occur?

C. Is an audible warning or other suitable indication given to alert personnel that the accelerator is about to be turned on, or that beam is about to be admitted to a specific area?

D. Are suitable radiation monitors available to indicate the presence of radiation in areas where personnel may have access?

1. Are functioning of the monitors calibrated at regular intervals?
2. Is the functioning of the monitors and any associated alarms checked regularly?
3. Is the readout from these monitors and alarms conveniently available to the operators?
4. Are suitable records maintained concerning calibration, testing and radiation levels?

5. Is there a need to carry a portable instrument to monitor for unsuspected radiation upon entry to a shutdown accelerator (induced radioactivity or x-rays from high voltage equipment) or into a shutdown beam area (beam in an adjacent area)?

VI. Procedures

A. *Widespread understanding.* Are procedures posted, read, and familiar to operators and support personnel and to visitors?

B. *Validity.* Are procedures reviewed and updated at suitable intervals?

C. *Inclusiveness.* Do procedures include:

1. A clear statement of responsibilities of management, accelerator operators, and radiation safety officers?
2. Standard operating procedures and procedures for emergency situations?
3. Access rules and regulations and search procedures to be used before turning on the accelerator?
4. Instructions for the proper handling of radioactivity and disposal of radioactive waste?
5. Descriptions of the facility and the accelerator giving enough information so that people unfamiliar with it can make some estimate of the relative hazard that prevails? Are any special problems described?

VII. Personnel Monitoring

A. *Requirement.* Is suitable personnel monitoring required?

B. *Calibration.* Is the calibration correct for the circumstances under which the monitors are used?

C. *Interpretation.* Is there adequate justification for the interpretation of results and assumptions made in deriving dose equivalent?

D. *Records.* Are adequate monitoring records maintained and are they available to the supervisor and employees?

VIII. Area Monitoring and Surveys

A. *Instruments*

1. *Calibration.* Is their calibration correct for the circumstances under which monitoring or survey instruments are used?
2. *Interpretation.* Is there adequate justification for the interpretation of results and assumptions made in deriving dose equivalent?

B. *Repetition.* Are area radiation surveys performed at regular intervals?

C. *Records.* Do the records of radiation surveys include:

1. Date and time and person doing?
2. Particle, energy, and current?
3. Target?
4. Collimator and magnets?
5. Purpose and detector used?
6. Location?
7. Results and recommendations?

D. *Induced activity*

1. *Accelerator.* Have suitable measurements been made of the radioactivity induced in the accelerator itself, in targets, and in shielding? Are suitable methods used to reduce personnel exposures from this source?
2. *Atmosphere.* Have suitable measurements or estimates been made of radioactivity induced in air? If this is a problem, is ventilation adequate, and where does the exhausted air go?
3. *Water.* Have measurements been taken to ensure pipes carrying radioactive water do not pass through occupied areas, or are adequately shielded? Have suitable measures been taken for the storage and regeneration or disposal of deionizing resins? Is a program for monitoring the release of radioactivity in water necessary?

4. *Workers.* Are bioassay and whole body counting procedures used occasionally to check for ingested or inhaled radioactivity?

IX. Education and Training of Operators, Support Personnel, and Others

Is there a regular program of education training available? Does it include at least the following topics?

A. *Radiation safety*
   1. Interaction of radiation with matter
   2. Units of dose and radioactivity
   3. Biological hazards
   4. Methods of control of exposure
   5. Procedures

B. *Radiation detection*
   1. Use of instruments and personnel monitors
   2. Survey and measurement techniques

C. *Equipment*
   1. Accelerator
   2. Remote handling devices
   3. Interlocks

X. Relations Between Health Physics, Accelerator Operators, and Experiments

Are the technical and personal relations between health physics, accelerator operators, experiments, and management good? Are there frequent interchanges of views and positions? Is there a radiation safety committee? If not, what takes its place?

Table 11.4.19 Good Work Practice for X-Ray Diffraction and X-Ray Fluorescence Units

(Personal Communication Slaback, 1991)

This guide reflects various standards and regulations but is not intended in itself as a ''regulation''.

Applicable portions of this guide may be used for other x-ray producing machines that can produce exposures to the eyes or a significant portion of the body in excess of 2 mR in one hour.

Enclosed/Open Systems: Definition

An *enclosed system* is one that meets the definition of NBS Handbook 111, 1972. This includes the requirement that all areas with exposure rates greater than 0.25 mR/hr are enclosed within an interlocked barrier to prevent personnel exposures. An interlock on the barrier is not required when its removal inherently prevents exposure to the x-rays, such as when the chamber and x-ray tube have a common vacuum system.

All other systems are considered *open systems*. *Open systems* are further subdivided based on their potential for exposures greater than or less than 2 mR/hr during normal use (i.e., excluding failure of engineered protective devices).

Protection Program

The protection program for these x-ray units consists of the following elements. These elements are implemented to differing degrees depending upon the system type and exposure potential.

- Designated Responsible Operator
- User Training
- Operating Procedures/Instructions
- Engineered Protection Systems
- Surveillance Programs

Enclosed X-Ray Systems

1. The head of the organizational unit to which the x-ray unit is assigned shall ensure that only those individuals who are qualified as specified below use the x-ray unit and that the unit is maintained in a manner that is in compliance with the safety requirements below.
2. Users authorized to operate this unit shall be trained in the following topics:
    - Hazards of exposure to x-rays.
    - General methods to minimize radiation exposure.
    - Protective devices incorporated into the x-ray unit to minimize or prevent radiation exposures.
    - Proper operating procedure for the x-ray unit.
    - How to recognize failures of protection systems or other unusual conditions which could lead to radiation exposures.
3. Operating procedures beyond those provided by the manufacturer are not required except that supplementary procedures shall be provided to describe any changes to the manufacturer's procedures necessitated by modifications to the system or if the manufacturer's procedures do not address the following points:
    - Proper operating sequence.
    - Description of personnel protective mechanisms and warning devices.
    - Prohibition of altering or bypassing interlocks on the system.

A copy of these procedures shall be readily available to the users of the x-ray unit.

4. The engineered protection system shall include:
   - Failsafe interlocks on all protective barriers of the unit needed to meet the 0.25 mR/hr limitation. Interlocks shall be tested at least annually.
   - Shielding adequate to reduce the exposure rate at 5 cm from any accessible surface to less than 0.25 mR/hr for normal operations.
   - A console ''power-ON'' indicator should be present.
   - A warning light of size and brightness adequate to warn anyone present in the room that x-rays are being produced shall be present. This light shall be labeled as to its meaning. (Note that commercial devices in the form of illuminated signs are available.)
   - The system shall bear a label ''Caution: This equipment produces x-rays when energized—to be operated only by qualified personnel,'' or the equivalent.
5. Personal radiation monitoring devices are not required for Enclosed X-ray Systems.

Limited Open X-Ray Systems (<2 mR/hr)

Those x-ray systems in this category are those that would otherwise meet the requirements for an enclosed system except that:

- Accessible areas have exposure rates not exceeding 2 mR/hr. For small beams, e.g., less than 1 cm^2, this is approximately equivalent to a limit of 4000 photons/sec. An accessible area is any area outside a barrier, shield, or curtain or one routinely occupied by personnel.
- Protective barriers are not fail safe. That is, some protective coverings, e.g., port covers, are only mechanically secured—bolted on, not interlocked; or the interlocked barrier can be defeated without activating the interlock; e.g., ducking under an interlocked curtain.

These are generally systems that use a variety of enclosed or fluorescence beam lines that require periodic plumbing changes and hence present the possibility of operating with a port or other protective cover removed. Also included are older systems that do not have all the protective features but are safely operable by qualified and aware personnel.

The requirements for enclosed systems shall apply with the following additional requirements:

- A log book of major changes to the system shielding, enclosures, and configuration shall be maintained.
- A list of authorized operators shall be maintained in the system's log book.
- Key control on the unit's operability shall be maintained. Alternatively room access controls may be established.
- In the absence of *personal* knowledge or documentation that the system is unchanged from previous operations the operator will perform a radiation survey of potential leakage points at the start of his operations. In particular, a survey will be performed of any modifications or alterations to the system shielding and enclosures and around any covers that have been removed since the last operation. Results of these surveys shall be recorded in the logbook for the system.

Open X-Ray Systems

1. A Designated Responsible Operator shall be clearly identified. This individual shall have the responsibility and authority to control the use of the system and to ensure its continued compliance with the safety requirements.
2. Users authorized to operate this unit shall be trained in the following topics. Receipt of this training shall be documented in the system log book. A list of authorized operators shall be maintained in the front of the system logbook. Users shall be trained in the following topics:
   - Hazards of Exposure to x-rays.
   - Exposure potential of this x-ray system with emphasis on in-beam exposure rates.
   - General methods to minimize radiation exposure.
   - Specific protective procedures for this system and any protective devices incorporated into the system.
   - Proper operating sequence for the system.
   - How to recognize failures of protection systems or other conditions which could lead to radiation exposures.
   - Proper survey procedures and limitations of available survey instruments.
   - Proper use of radiation dosimetry (if required).

3. Specific operating procedures that prescribe the precautions to minimize or avoid radiation exposure for the manner in which this system is used as required. These, together with any provided by the manufacturer, shall prescribe or describe the:

    - Proper operating sequence.
    - Specific procedural precautions to avoid or minimize radiation exposures.
    - Limitations on operating parameters and use of the system.
    - System shielding requirements.
    - Radiation survey requirements.
    - Dosimetry requirements for operators.
    - Training requirements for system operators.

For systems dedicated for permanent use by one or two individuals this information is documented in the Health Physics Survey Report for the system and a separate document is not required. The operating procedures shall be readily available to the users of the x-ray system.

4. The engineered protection system shall include:

    - Failsafe interlocks on all removable protective barriers[a].
    - Protective barriers which reduce exposure rates to accessible areas to less than 2 mR/hr at 5 cm from any surface[a].
    - Key control on the production of x-rays[a].
    - A console ''power on'' indicator.
    - A warning light or illuminated sign of a size and brightness adequate to warn anyone present in the room the x-rays are being produced. A simple light must have an explanatory sign near it.
    - The system shall bear a label ''Caution: This equipment produces x-rays when energized—to be operated by authorized personnel,'' or an equivalent label.
    - The entrance to the room shall bear a sign ''Caution: X-ray device in this area,'' or an equivalent sign.

5. Dosimetry requirements will be established by Health Physics upon a review of each facility. In general if partial body exposures could be in excess of 0.5 rem/hr a whole body dosimeter shall be required. If hand exposures could exceed 5 rem/yr extremity monitoring shall be required.

Health Physics Support

Health Physics will perform periodic facility reviews to ensure compliance with this guidance. Radiation surveys and specific facility evaluations may be requested by x-ray users. These will be appropriately scheduled.

Routine surveys such as those following instrument realignments shall be performed by users. Instruments used for such surveys shall be on the Health Physics Instrument Calibration and Quality Assurance Program.

NOTE: Local/State regulations may have specific requirements more stringent than the above, particularly in regard to open sysems.

---

[a] Variance to these requirements may be obtained from Health Physics. Such a variance is intended primarily for older systems for which an additional investment is not economically justified or the protective features simply are not available and for systems using highly variable geometries. In such instances even greater emphasis will be placed on operator qualifications and training and on survey procedures.

SECTION 5 EMERGENCIES

Practical steps to guide health physicists and medical personnel responding to a radiation accident have been formulated, some many years ago. They have passed the test of time and are summarized in this Chapter. Governmental regulations and guides for radiation accidents are found in Chapter 4, Section 1, Part D of this text.

TABLE OF CONTENTS

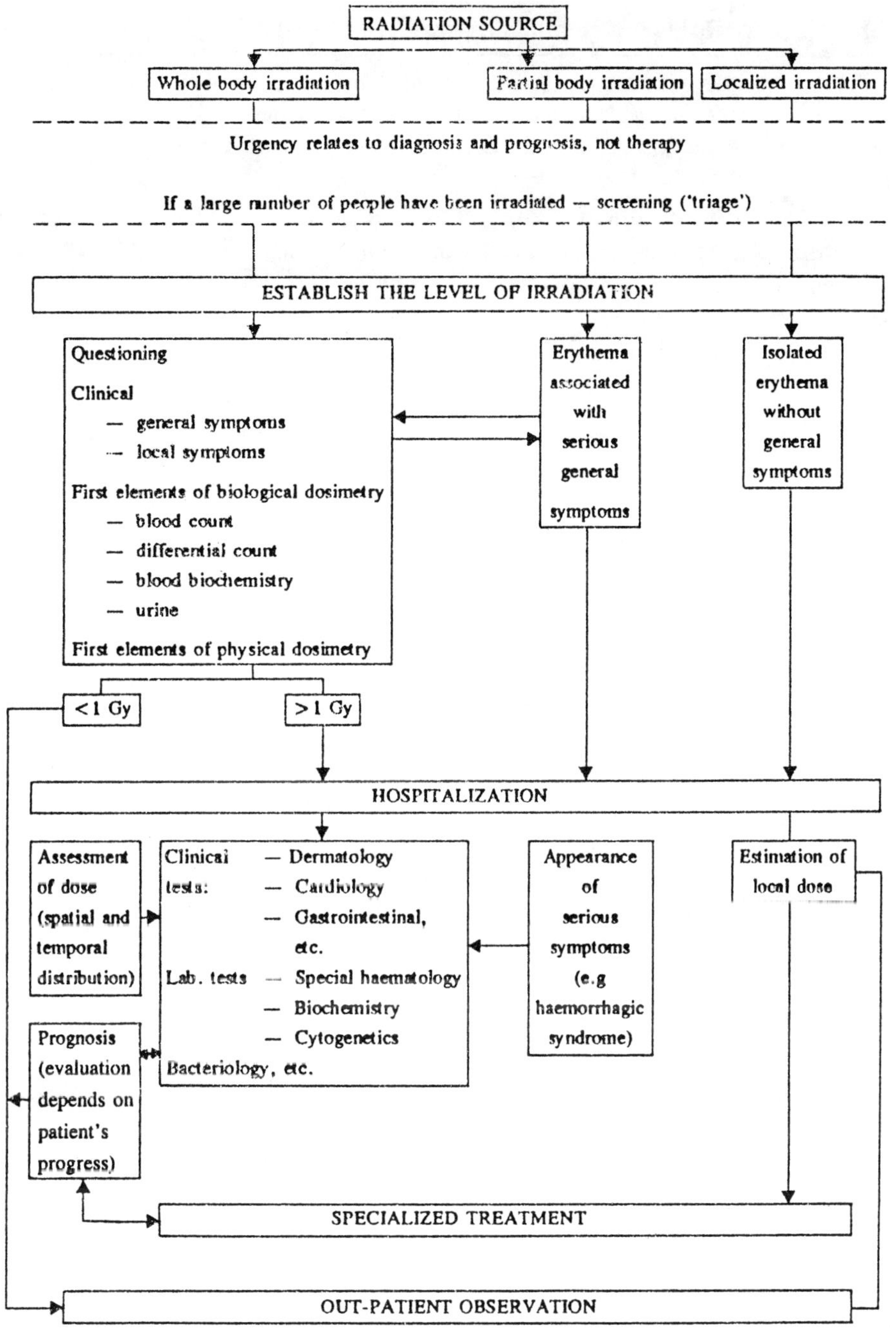

Figure 11.5.1 Main Steps to be Taken in Response to Accidental Overexposure to a Source External to the Body (Courtesy IAEA from Safety Series 88, 1988)

Table 11.5.1 General Rules for Health Physicists in a Radiation Accident (After Saenger, 1963)

Rule 1	When and if accident is suspected, evacuate personnel and segregate them. Determine the medical status of involved personnel (see rule 4). Remove all personnel dosimeters and/or film badges immediately from exposed personnel. Read dosimeters and record the reading. Send dosimeters and films immediately to a safe area.
Rule 2	Notify Radiological Safety Officer or Emergency Director who will then activate emergency plan.
Rule 3	Close off radiation area. Shut off ventilation. Seal area if contamination is likely. This step is unnecessary if the radiation source is some type of x-ray generator or sealed source, where no radionuclides are produced or released.
Rule 4	Evaluate situation and personnel in regard to: (a) Personnel medical status (b) Current environs status (primary event controlled, source removed, etc.) (c) Extent of contamination (d) Nature and level of the radiation exposure (external, internal, gamma/neutron, etc.) (e) Contamination of environs
Rule 5	Save all samples of clothing, blood, urine, stool, vomitus. Label with name, date, time. Send film badges for emergency processing by standard technique.
Rule 6	Do not release patients to hospitals before preliminary decontamination, if medical condition permits. Do not delay life-saving (i.e., any significant) medical treatment. Notify hospitals before patients are sent there. Send a health physicist to the hospital to advise on the patient's radiological status.
Rule 7	It is often difficult to determine that a criticality accident has occurred. The search for neutron induced radioactivity of small metal objects at the accident site is valuable. Such objects may require preliminary decontamination.
Rule 8	Portable battery operated tape recorders will be very useful in collecting and storing information and for obtaining a complete history of the accident. It is often difficult to record all of the events, opinions, and statements available in an emergency situation. The taped records can be typed later, thus providing a more complete history of the accident.
Rule 9	A video camera will provide an excellent method of showing exactly what happened. If a video camera is not available, suitable still photographs will be useful.
Rule 10	In a major accident, management should obtain the aid of 50–100 health physicists on an emergency standby basis. These individuals can be found in neighboring installations and will be essential for the proper handling of the accident during the first week, particularly if it is necessary to work a 24-hour day. Experts in public communication will also be needed since the impact on public health can be significant, even in the absence of released radiation.

Table 11.5.2 Medical Information Check List (Courtesy NCRP from Report 65, 1980)

NOTE: These questions can be used by the attending physician at the hospital for obtaining historical information to assist in the early management of radioactively contaminated persons. The best information in industrial cases can probably be obtained from plant personnel, such as the health physicist or occupational physician familiar with the plant and accident details.

- When did the accident occur? What are the circumstances and what are the most likely pathways for exposure? How much radioactive material is involved potentially?
- What injuries have occurred? What potential medical problems may be present besides the radionuclide contamination?
- Are toxic or corrosive chemicals involved in addition to the radionuclides? Have any treatments been given for these?
- What radionuclides now contaminate the patient? Where? What are the radiation measurements at the surface?
- What information is available about the chemistry of the compounds containing the radionuclides? Soluble or insoluble? Any information about the probable particle size?
- What radioactivity measurements have been made at the site of the accident, i.e., air monitors, smears, fixed radiation monitors, nasal smear counts, and skin contamination levels?
- What decontamination efforts, if any, have already been attempted? What success?
- Have any therapeutic measures such as blocking agents or isotopic dilution been given?
- Was the victim also exposed to penetrating radiation? If so, what has been learned from processing personal dosimeters, e.g., film badge, TLD, or pocket ionization chamber? If not yet known, when is the information expected?
- Has clothing removed at the site of accident been saved in case the contamination still present on it is needed for radiation energy spectrum analysis and particle size studies?
- What excreta have been collected? Who has the samples? What analyses are planned? When will they be done?

Table 11.5.3 Hospital Decontamination Procedures for Protection of Personnel and Facilities

(Courtesy NCRP from Report 65, 1980)

- Personnel should wear surgical scrub suits, surgical caps and gowns, and rubber gloves (surgical, household, or industrial depending upon duties).
- The team leader should be trained to recognize the rare instance where there may be a need for masks, respirators, or supplied airpacks due to the presence of high levels of alpha or beta radionuclides.
- Rubber or plastic shoe covers are desirable. Those performing the actual decontamination with water should wear plastic or rubber laboratory aprons. Good temporary shoe covers for dry areas can be improvised with brown paper bags held on with adhesive or masking tape.
- Air conditioning and forced air heating systems should be turned off so radioactive particulates are not carried into ducts or to other rooms unless a special filter system has been designed for use under these conditions.
- The floors should be protected with a disposable covering to reduce ''tracking'' by keeping cleaner surfaces and to aid the clean up tasks. The covering should be changed when significant contamination is present. Brown paper rolls (36 inches wide, 60 pound weight) are ideal where water is not used. Plastic sheets are useful where spillage of liquids is a problem, although ribbed or non-skid types should be used to reduce the change of slips and falls.
- All contaminated clothing should be placed carefully into plastic or paper bags to reduce secondary contamination of area.
- Splashing of solutions used in decontamination should be avoided.
- Patients and other potentially contaminated personnel may move to clean areas only after surveys show satisfactory decontamination.
- All passage of persons and property between contaminated and clean areas must be surveyed and regulated by monitoring teams.
- Supplies are passed through monitoring stations from clean areas to contaminated areas. Reverse flow must not occur unless supplies are monitored and found clean.
- All individuals on the decontamination team shall be trained in radiological monitoring and decontamination techniques. Persons not working on the team should be excluded from the work area.
- Fiberboard or steel drums with tight fitting tops should be obtained for contaminated materials. Labels describing the contents should be affixed so that proper disposal can be carried out without reopening them. They may be sealed with masking tape or some other type of sealing tape.
- Personal dosimeters (pocket chambers, film badge or TLD dosimeters) should be supplied to all personnel working in the decontamination area. Personnel should be rotated after a dose of 5 rems (or less if possible) is received.
- The entry of all non-essential personnel including family, visitors, and administrative persons should be restricted.

Table 11.5.4 Personnel Decontamination

To properly decontaminate personnel, it is necessary to first define the areas of contamination by means of proper monitoring techniques. Special emphasis should be placed on the location of any hot spots on the individual. The mildest methods of cleansing should be attempted first, progressing to more harsh methods when necessary. Cleansing methods in order of harshness are as follows:

1. Lifting off with sticky tape[a]
2. Flushing with water
3. Soap and warm water, commercial skin cleaner
4. Mild abrasive soap, soft brush, and water
5. Skin cleaner with a mild abrasive, e.g., cornmeal
6. Complexing solution[b]
7. Mild organic acid (citric acid)[b]

After removal of contamination, individuals should take a thorough shower with special attention to washing the hair, hands, and fingernails.

In all personnel decontamination procedures every effort should be made to prevent the spread of contamination.

All cleaning action should be from periphery of contaminated area towards the center to avoid spreading contamination.

Be aware of personal and ethnic privacy issues when initiating any body surveys or decontamination procedures.

[a] Some individuals are allergic to certain adhesives. Strong adhesives can disturb the skin barrier enabling internal uptake of the contamination.

[b] Any agents not designed and approved for use on the human skin should have medical approval before use.

Table 11.5.5 Techniques for Reducing Internal Contamination (Wald, 1991)

There are several elements for which dose reduction techniques have some effect. All require medical supervision for administration. These are:

Method	Radioisotope	Agent
Dilution	H-3	Water
	P-32	Phosphorous (Neutrophos)
Blocking	Cs-137	Ferric ferrocyanide (Prussian blue)
	I-131, Tc-99m	KI (Lugol's solution)
	Sr-89, Sr-85	Al-phosphate, Al-hydroxide
Mobilization	Rb-86	Chlorthalidone (Hygroton)
Chelatin	Cf-252, Cm-242, Am-241, Pu-239, Ce-144, Pm-143, La-140, Y-90, Zn-65, Sc-46, rare earths	DTPA
	Pb-210	EDTA, penicillamine
	Hg-203, Co-60	Penicillamine

Table 11.5.6 Recommended Surface Contamination Screening Levels for Emergency Screening of Persons and Other Surfaces at Screening or Monitoring Stations in High Background Radiation Areas (0.1 mR/h to 5 mR/h Gamma Exposure)[a] (From EPA 5201 1-75-001-A, 1990)

Condition	Geiger Counter Shielded Window Reading	Recommended Action
Before decontamination	$<2 \times$ bkgd and <0.5 mR/h above background	Unconditional release
	$>2 \times$ bkgd or >0.5 mR/h above background	Decontaminate. Equipment may be stored or disposed of as appropriate.
After decontamination	$<2 \times$ bkgd and <0.5 mR/h above background	Unconditional release
	$>2 \times$ bkgd or >0.5 mR/h above background	Continue to decontaminate or refer to low background monitoring and d-con station. Equipment may also be stored for decay or disposed of as appropriate.

[a] Monitoring stations in these high exposure rate areas are for use only during the early phase of an incident involving major atmospheric releases of particulates. Otherwise use Table 11.5.7.

Table 11.5.7 Recommended Surface Contamination Screening Levels for Persons and Other Surfaces at Monitoring Stations in Low Background Radiation Areas (<0.1 mR/h Gamma Exposure Rate) (After EPA 5201 1-75-001-A, 1990)

Condition	Geiger Counter Thin Window[a] Reading	Recommended Action
Before decontamination	$<2 \times$ bkgd	Unconditional release
	$>2 \times$ bkgd	Decontaminate
After simple[b] decontamination	$<2 \times$ bkgd	Unconditional release
	$>2 \times$ bkgd	Full decontamination[c]
After full[c] decontamination effort	$<2 \times$ bkgd	Unconditional release
	$>2 \times$ bkgd	Continue to d-con persons
	<0.5 mR/h[d]	Release animals and equipment
After additional full decontamination effort	$<2 \times$ bkgd	Unconditional release
	$>2 \times$ bkgd	Send persons for special evaluation
	<0.5 mR/h[d]	Release animals and equipment
	>0.5 mR/h[d]	Refer, or use informed judgment on further control of animals and equipment

[a] Window thickness of approximately 30 mg/cm^2 is acceptable for most commonly encountered radionuclides. Other detectors or techniques may be required for certain radionuclides, e.g., low energy beta emitters. Recommended limits for open window readings are expressed as twice the existing background (including background) in the area where measurements are being made. Corresponding levels, expressed in units related to instrument designations, may be adopted for convenience. Levels higher than twice background (not to exceed the meter reading corresponding to 0.1 mR/h) may be used to speed the monitoring of evacuees in very low background areas.

[b] Flushing with water and wiping is an example of a simple decontamination effort.

[c] Washing or scrubbing with soap or solvent followed by flushing is an example of a full decontamination effort.

[d] Closed shield reading including background.

Table 11.5.8 Procedure for Dealing with Minor Spills and Personnel Contamination (After Saenger, 1963)

Most spills in the laboratory will likely involve less than millicurie quantities, frequently of short half-life radioactive materials. The following procedure can be used for dealing with this type of spill:

1. Wash hands first if they are contaminated as a result of the accident. Put on rubber gloves to prevent contamination of the hands.
2. Cover liquid spill with absorbent material to limit spread of contamination. It is highly unlikely that a dry spill will occur in a nuclear medicine laboratory; but if encountered, it should be dampened to avoid spreading due to air currents, but carefully so as not to spread it unnecessarily.
3. If fans, ventilators, or air conditioners that circulate air to other areas are operating, they should be shut off; preferably, this should be done by someone not involved in the contaminated area. Direct exhaust ventilation should be left on.
4. Mark off contaminated area with chalk, marker, rope, etc., and restrict traffic to that area.
5. Do not allow anyone to leave contaminated area without first being monitored to be sure he/she is not contaminated.
6. Notify the radiation protection officer of the accident.
7. Start decontamination procedures as soon as possible. Cleaning agents normally used in the laboratory should be adequate. Start at the periphery of the contaminated area and work inward, reducing systematically the contaminated area.
8. Put all contaminated, disposable materials into plastic bags for disposal. Contaminated cleaning equipment, such as brushes or mops, should be stored in plastic bags until the radioactivity has sufficiently decayed before it is used.
9. A survey meter or wipe tests should be used to monitor effectiveness of the decontamination procedure.
10. Area should be cleaned if the contamination level exceeds 200 dpm/100 cm^2.

It is advisable to have a specific tray or cart prepared and set aside that is equipped with plastic bags and cleaning materials such as disposable towels, detergents, cotton swabs, and so forth, that can be used in case of a spill.

Personnel Contamination

When radioactive materials are prepared in a well ventilated hood, most contamination occurs on the outer surfaces of personnel. When body surfaces or clothing become contaminated, it is important that the contamination be removed as soon as possible to prevent its spread to other surfaces and to eliminate it as a source of internal contamination by way of ingestion, absorption, inhalation, and wound contamination. See Table 11.5.4 for detailed decontamination procedures. Personnel suspected of being contaminated should be monitored with a survey meter to identify problem areas. Clothing that is significantly contaminated should be removed and stored in plastic bags until the activity has decayed to an acceptable level of activity (approximately 200 dpm per 100 cm^2).

Table 11.5.9 Summary of Surface Decontamination Methods (From FDA 83-8211, 1983)

Method	Surfaces	Action	Technique	Advantages	Disadvantages
Vacuum Cleaning	Dry contaminated surfaces.	Removal of contaminated dust by suction.	Use conventional vacuum technique with efficient filter.	Good on dry porous surfaces. Avoids water reactions.	All dust must be filtered out of exhaust. Machine is contaminated.
Water	All nonporous surfaces (metal, paint, plastic, etc.). ***Not suitable for porous materials***, such as wood, concrete, canvas, etc.	Solution and erosion.	Use gross decontamination employing water shot from high pressure hoses. Work from top to bottom to avoid recontamination; from upwind to avoid spray; 15 to 20 feet from the surface is the optimum operating distance. Vertical surface should be hosed at an incident angle of 30 to 45 degrees. Determine cleaning rate experimentally if possible. Otherwise, use a rate of 4 square feet per minute.	All water equipment may be utilized. Allows operation to be carried out from a distance. Contamination may be reduced by 50%. Water solutions of other decontaminating agents may utilize water equipment.	Draininage must be controlled. Porous materials will absorb contaminants. Oiled surfaces cannot be decontaminated. Not applicable on dry contaminated surfaces (use vacuum). Spray will be contaminated.
Steam	Nonporous surfaces (especially painted or oiled surfaces.	Solution and erosion.	Work from top to bottom and from upwind. Clean surface at a rate of 4 square feet per minute. The cleaning efficiency of steam may be greatly increased by using detergents.	Steam reduces contamination by approximately 90% on painted surfaces.	Steam subject to same limitations as water. Spray hazard makes the wearing of waterproof outfits necessary.
Detergents	Nonporous surfaces (especially industrial film).	Emulsifying agent. Wetting agent.	Rub surface for 1 minute and wipe with dry rag. Use clean surface of the rag for each application. A powered rotary brush (with pressure feed) is more efficient. Moist application is all that is desired. Solution should not be allowed to drip onto other surfaces. Solution may be applied from a distance with a pressure proportioner.	Dissolves industrial film which holds contamination. Contamination may be reduced by 90%.	May require contact with surface. Mild method not efficient on long-standing contamination.
Complexing Agents Oxalates Carbonates Citrates	Nonporous surfaces (especially unweathered surfaces; i.e., no rust or calcareous growth).	Forms soluble complexes with contaminated material.	Solution should contain 3% (by weight) of agent. Spray surface with solution. Keep surface moist for 30 minutes by spraying with solution periodically. After allotted time, flush material off with water. Agents may be used on vertical and overhead surfaces by employing mechanical foam.	Holds contamination in solution. Contamination (unweathered surfaces) reduced 75% in 4 minutes. Easily stored. Carbonates and citrates are non-toxic, non-corrosive.	Requires application from 5 to 30 minutes. Little penetrating power; of small value on weathered surfaces.

Table 11.5.9 Summary of Surface Decontamination Methods (Continued)

Method	Surfaces	Action	Technique	Advantages	Disadvantages
Organic Solvents	Nonporous surfaces (greasy or waxed surfaces, paint or plastic finishes, etc.).	Solution of organic materials (oil, paint, etc.)	Entire unit may be immersed in solvent. Also may be applied by standard wiping procedures. (See Detergents.)	Quick dissolving action. Recovery of solvent possible by distillation.	Requires good ventilation and fire precautions. Toxic to personnel. Material bulky.
Inorganic Acids	Metal surfaces, especially those with porous deposits (i.e., rust or calcareous growth). Circulatory pipe systems.	Strong dissolving power on metals and porous deposits.	Dip-bath technique is advisable for movable items. Acid should be kept at a concentration of from 1 to 2 Normal (9 to 18% hydrochloric, 3 to 6% sulfuric acid). Reaction time on weathered surfaces should be 1 hour. Pipe systems, 2 to 4 hours. Afterwards, surface should be neutralized and rinsed.	Corrosive action on metal and porous deposits. Corrosive action may be moderated by addition of corrosion inhibitors to solution	Good ventilation required because of toxicity and explosive gases. Acid mixtures should not be heated. Possibility of excessive corrosion if used without inhibitors. Sulfuric acid not effective on calcareous deposits.
Acid Mixtures Hydrochloric Sulfuric Acetic Acid Citric Acid Acetates Citrates	Nonporous surfaces (especially those having porous deposits). Circulatory pipe systems.	Dissolving action.	Applied in same manner as inorganic acids. Mixture consists of 0.1 gal. hydrochloric, 0.2 lb. sodium acetate, 1.0 gal of water	Dissolving action may reduce contamination 90% in 1 hour (unweathered surfaces).	Weathered surfaces may require prolonged treatment.
Caustics Lye (sodium hydroxide) Calcium Hydroxide Potassium Hydroxide	Painted surfaces (horizontal).	Dissolving power softens paint (harsh method).	Lye paint-removal mixture: 10 gal. water, 4 lb lye, 5 lb. boiler compound, 0.75 lb cornstarch. Allow lye paint remover solution to remain on surface until paint is softened to the point there it may be washed off with water. Remove remaining paint with long handled scrapers.	Minimum contact with contaminated surfaces. Easily stored.	Personnel danger (painful burns). Reaction slow: thus, it is not efficient on vertical surfaces or overheads. Should not be used on aluminum or magnesium. Method is difficult on vertical or overhead surfaces.
Tri Sodium Phosphate	Painted surfaces (vertical, overhead).	Dissolving power (mild method).	Hot 10% solution applied by standard wiping technique. (See Detergents.) One minute rub	Reduces activity to tolerance in one or two applications.	Destructive effect on paint. Not to be used on aluminum or magnesium.
Abrasion	Nonporous surfaces.	Surface removal.	Use conventional procedures, but keep surface damp to avoid dust hazard.	Activity may be reduced to as low a level as may be desired.	Impracticable for porous surfaces because of surface penetration by moisture. Contamination spread over area must be recovered.
Wet Sandblasting	Nonporous surfaces.		Wet sandblasting is most practical on large surface areas. Collect used abrasive.		
Vacuum Blasting	Porous and nonporous surfaces.	Abrasion with controlled removal by vacuum suction.	Hold tool flush to surface to prevent escape of contamination.	Controlled disposal.	Contamination of equipment.

References

Atomic Energy Commission. *Meteorology and Atomic Energy,* USAEC Report TID-24190; July, 1968.

Baes, C.F., III, Sharp, R.D., Sjoreen, A.L., Shor, R.W. *A Review and Analysis of Parameters for Assessing Transport of Environmentally Released Radionuclides through Agriculture.* Oak Ridge National Laboratory Report ORNL-5786; 1984.

Blaylock, B.G., "Radionuclide data bases available for bioaccumulation factors for freshwater biota" *Nuclear Safety* **23**(4): 427–438; 1982.

Brynjolfsson, A., Martin, T.G., III. "*Radiation Protection Problems Associated With Electron Accelerators.*" Radiation Protection Symposium. U.S. Army, Edgewood Arsenal, Maryland; 1967.

Busick, D.D., Warren, G.J. *A Unique Safety Manual for Experimental Personnel.* SLAC-PUB-2384. Presented at 13th Topical Health Physics Symposium; Hawaii; December 13–16, 1978; August 1979.

Department of Commerce. *Ionizing Radiation Measurement Criteria for Regulatory Purposes Conference of Radiation Control Program Directors, Inc.* NBSGCR 79-174; National Bureau of Standards; November 1979.

Castronovo, F.P., Jr., Beh, R.A., Veilleux, N.M. "Iodine 131 therapy patients: Dose to staff" *Rad Prot Dosimetry* **15**(1): 45–49; Nuclear Technology Printing; 1986.

Coughtrey, P.C. et al. *Radionuclide Distribution and Transport in Terrestrial and Aquatic Ecosystems, 2 Vols.* A.A. Balkema; Netherlands; 1983.

Department of Energy. *Nuclear Reactors Built, Being Built, or Planned.* DOE/OSTI-8200-R53; Washington, DC; 1991.

Environmental Protection Agency (EPA). *Manual of Protective Actions for Nuclear Incidents.* EPA 520/1-75-001-A; Washington, DC; 1990.

Food and Drug Administration. *Preparedness and Response in Radiation Accidents.* FDA 93-8211 R; Rockville, MD; 1983.

Health Physics Society. *Surface Radioactivity Guides for Materials, Equipment, and Facilities to be Released for Uncontrolled Use.* American National Standards Institute, ANSI N13.12, Table 1, page 4; November 1987.

Heeb, C.M., Little, W.W. Personal Communication; 1992.

Hickey, E.E.; Stoetzel, G.A.; Olsen, P.C., McGuire, S.A.. *Air Sampling in the Workplace.* NUREG/CR-1400; Washington, DC; 1991.

Hilsmeier, W.F. et al. *Graphs for Estimating Atmospheric Dispersion.* Oak Ridge National Laboratory Report ORO-545; July 1962.

International Atomic Energy Agency. *Radiological Safety Aspects of the Operation of Electron Linear Accelerators.* IAEA Technical Report Series No. 188; Vienna; 1979.

International Atomic Energy Agency. *Generic Models and Parameters for Assessing the Environmental Transfer of Radionuclides from Routine Releases—Exposures of Critical Groups.* IAEA Safety Series No. 57, IAEA; Vienna; 1982.

International Atomic Energy Agency. *Medical Handling of Accidentally Exposed Individuals.* IAEA Safety Series No. 88; IAEA; Vienna; 1988.

International Atomic Energy Agency. *Nuclear Research Reactors In the World.* Reference Data Series No 3, May 1991; 1994.

International Labour Office (ILO). *Guidelines for the Protection of Workers in Industry (Ionizing Radiation).* Occupational Safety and Health Series 62; Geneva; 1989.

International Organization of Legal Metrology. *Vocabulary of Legal Metrology: Fundamental Terms.* Paris; 1976.

Miller, A.J, Patterson, H.W. "Measurement of induced radioactivity to estimate personnel radiation exposures received from accelerator beams," *Health Physics* **23:**671; 1972.

National Bureau of Standards (NBS). *Radiological Safety in the Design and Operation of Particle Accelerators.* NBS Handbook 107; Washington, DC; 1970.

National Council on Radiation Protection and Measurements. *Radiation Alarms and Access Control Systems.* NCRP Report 88; Bethesda, MD; 1986.

National Council on Radiation Protection and Measurements. *Management of Persons Accidentally Contaminated with Radionuclides.* NCRP Report No. 65; Bethesda, MD; 1980.

National Council on Radiation Protection and Measurements. *Operational Radiation Safety Program.* NCRP Report 59; Bethesda, MD; 1978.

National Council on Radiation Protection and Measurements. *Radiation Protection Design Guidelines for 0.1–100 MeV Particle Accelerator Facilities.* NCRP Report No. 51; Bethesda, MD; 1977.

National Council on Radiation Protection and Measurements. *Radiation Protection for Medical and Allied Health Personnel.* NCRP Report 105; Bethesda, MD; 1989.

National Council on Radiation Protection and Measurements. *Screening Models for Releases of Radionuclides to Atmosphere, Surface Water, and Ground.* NCRP Report No. 123 I; Bethesda, MD; 1996.

Ng, Y.C., Colsher, C.S., Thompson, S.E. *Soil-to-Plant Concentration Factors for Radiological Assessments.* Nuclear Regulatory Commission NUREG/CR-2975; Washington, DC; 1982.

Nuclear Regulatory Commission. *Health Physics Surveys for Byproduct Material at NRC Licensed Processing and Manufacturing Plants.* NRC Regulatory Guide 8.21; Washington, DC; 1979.

Nuclear Regulatory Commission. *Calculation of Annual Doses to Man from Routine Releases of Reactor Effluents for the Purpose of Evaluating Compliance with 10 CFR Part 50, Appendix I.* NRC Regulatory Guide 1.109; Washington, DC: 1977.

Nuclear Regulatory Commission. *Radiation Surveys at Medical Institutions.* NRC Regulatory Guide 8.23, Rev. 1; Washington, DC; 1981.

Nuclear Regulatory Commission. *Reassessment of the Technical Base for Estimating Source Terms.* NUREG-0956; Washington, DC; 1986

Nuclear Regulatory Commission. *Standards for Protection Against Radiation: Final Rule.* 10CFR20 et al. Part VI; *Federal Register 56*(98); Government Printing Office; Washington, DC; May 21, 1991.

Nuclear Regulatory Commission. *Generic Environmental Impact Statement for License Renewal of Nuclear Plants—Draft Report for Comment.* NUREG-1437; Washington, DC; 1991.

Nuclear Regulatory Commission. *Guidelines for Decontamination of Facilities and Equipment Prior to Release for Unrestricted Use or Termination of Licenses for Byproduct, Source, or Special Nuclear Material.* NRC Division of Industrial and Medical Nuclear Safety; Washington, DC; August 1987.

Patterson, H.W., Thomas, R.H. *Accelerator Health Physics.* Academic Press; New York, NY; 1973.

Peterson, H. Personal Communication; 1991.

Peterson, H. ''Terrestrial and Aquatic Food Chain Pathways,'' Chapter 5 in *Radiological Assessment—A Textbook on Environmental Dose Analysis.* Till, J.E., Meyer, H.R., eds., Nuclear Regulatory Commission NUREG/CR-3332; Washington, DC; 1983.

Randerson, D., ed. *Atmospheric Science and Power Production.* U.S. Department of Energy Report DOE/TIC-27601; 1984.

Saenger, E.L. *Medical Aspects of Radiation Accidents.* U.S. Atomic Energy Commission; Washington, DC; 1963.

Slaback, L. Personal Communication; 1991.

Smith, M., ed. *Recommended Guide for the Prediction of the Dispersion of Airborne Effluents.* American Society of Mechanical Engineers; New York, NY; 1968.

Tatcher, M., Rosenberg, I., Couch, J.G. ''Dose to radiotherapy technologists from activation of patients at a fast neutron therapy facility,'' *Health Physics* **53:**311–312; 1987.

Thomas, R.H. Personal Communication; 1991.

Thomas, R.H., Stevenson, G.R. *Radiological Safety Aspects of the Operation of Proton Accelerators.* International Atomic Energy Agency Technical Report 283; Vienna; 1988.

Thompson, S.E., Burton, C.A., Quinn, D.J., Ng, Y.C. *Concentration Factors of Chemical Elements in Edible Aquatic Organisms.* Lawrence Livermore National Laboratory Report UCRL-50564 Rev. 1; October 10, 1972.

Till, J.E., Meyer, H.R., eds. *Radiological Assessment—A Textbook on Environmental Dose Analysis.* Nuclear Regulatory Commission NUREG/CR-3332; Washington, DC; 1983.

U.S. Atomic Energy Commission. *Meteorology and Atomic Energy—1968.* USAEC Report TID-24190; July 1968.

Webster, E.W. ''EDE for exposure with protective aprons,'' *Health Physics* **56**(4):568; 1989.

Wald, N. ''Acute radiation injuries and their medical management,'' *The Biological Basis of Radiation Protection Practice.* Proceedings of the 1991 HPS Summer School, Williams and Wilkins.

Willis, C., Boyd, A.W., Young, M.J. ''Radiolysis of air and nitrogen-oxygen mixtures with intense pulses: Determinations of a mechanism by comparison of measured and computed yields,'' *Can J Chem* **48:**1515; 1970.

CHAPTER 12

BIOASSAY AND RADIOBIOLOGICAL DATA

This chapter reviews the recommendations for bioassay of the International Commission on Radiological Protection (Publication 54 1987) together with bioassay modeling information from other sources.

Also included in this chapter are specifications for reference man from the International Commission on Radiological Protection (Publication 23 1974), data on dietary and fluid intake, activity levels and body organ weights.

TABLE OF CONTENTS

Table 12.1 A Discussion of Bioassay

The following outline was derived mainly from an excellent paper by Boecker et al., 1991.

I. *INTRODUCTION*

A) Bioassay-definition

The determination of the kind, quantity or concentration, and, in some cases, location of radioactive material in the human body by direct measurement (*in vivo* counting) or by analysis and evaluation of materials excreted or removed from the human body.

B) Purpose—in protection program

1. Assess the adequacy of control over intake of radionuclide.
2. Detects accumulation of body burden.
3. Provide basis for calculating radiation dose from internal radioactivity.

C) Evaluation of Internal Radiation Exposure

The Individual:

a. Intake
b. Excretion and Exhalation = Indirect Assay
c. Direct Assay (*in vivo*)

Categories b and c comprise ''bioassay'' as the term is used in health physics, although it is usually reserved for b while ''whole-body counting'' is used for c.

D) Internal Radioactivity and Dose

1. Measurement yields radionuclide content.
2. Content yields dose rate.
3. Content vs. Time yields the retention function needed to calculate the committed dose.

II. *IN VIVO ANALYSIS (DIRECT BIOASSAY)*

A) Definition: Measurement of radioactivity in the body by means of detectors located external to the body.

Advantages:

1. Provides a direct measurement of internally deposited radionuclides.
2. More accurate than excreta analysis when sufficient quantities are present.
3. It can measure retained insoluble compounds that are not readily excreted.
4. Analysis is simple and short in duration.
5. Organ or body contents are immediately and directly determined without the use of metabolic models.
6. Multiple radionuclides can be analyzed simultaneously.

Disadvantagcs:

1. Detection sensitivity is less than excreta analysis.
2. Discrimination between externally and internally deposited radionuclides is difficult. Avoid contamination of the subject or the counter itself.
3. Expense: dedicated facility, massive shielding, detectors, and computers.

B) *In Vivo* Analysis—Applications

1. Radiation Protection Program—Internal radioactivity
2. Human and animal tracer studies—An administered tracer is used to measure biological turnover in specific organs and the whole body.
3. Body Composition—K-40 activity can be used to determine lean muscle mass since elemental tissue composition and abundance are known.

C) Types of radiation detected: Gamma emissions and bremsstrahlung from beta emitters. Bremsstrahlung from beta emitters like Y-90 and P-32 can be adequately detected. Photon emissions in excess of 200 keV can be readily detected by most whole-body counters in common use.

D) Body Regions Counted:

1. Total body
2. Partial body; e.g., trunk, lung, liver, thyroid, skull.

E) Detectors:
1. GM or ion chamber: used for the first measurements of radionuclides *in vivo* on radium dial painters around 1925. Low sensitivity and non-specificity led to development of better systems used today.
2. Thallium-activated sodium iodide [NaI(T1)] detectors developed in the 1940s and 1950s. These are the most popular detectors in use today. Crystals can be up to 30 cm (12 in.) in diameter yielding a higher gamma detection efficiency than the smaller germanium detectors. In situations where fine energy resolution is not necessary or the highest sensitivity is needed, NaI(T1) is the detector of choice.
3. Germanium (Ge) semiconductor detectors. These detectors came into use in the late 1970s and early 1980s. The hyperpure, or intrinsic Ge detectors are now more commonly used than lithium drifted, or Ge(Li) types. The big advantage here is in energy resolution, i.e., radionuclide selectivity.
4. The ''phoswich'' (phosphor sandwich) consists of a NaI(T1) crystal optically coupled to a CsI(T1) crystal. This detector functions as an anticoincidence shield. Signals are separated on the basis of different scintillation decay times. It is used for low-energy photon detection (e.g., ^{239}Pu and ^{241}Am). These detectors are commonly supplemented with Ge detectors which are more sensitive for Pu.
5. Organic scintillators: Liquid (toluence based), or plastic.
Advantage: sensitivity is good (>20%) compared to Ge (as low as 2%), but less than NaI(T1) at close to 99%. The subject can be surrounded by the detector yielding 4π geometry. Energy resolution is very poor, therefore this detector should be used by labs analyzing known and well-separated radionuclides.

F) Shielding: Low background Pb, iron or steel. Pb walls are 3–4 inches thick; steel walls are 5 to 6 inches thick. Pre-World War II naval armor plate is preferred because global fallout contaminants and Co-60 used in manufacturing are not present. Levels of radiation are typically reduced to 1–2% of outside levels. Cosmic-ray background is reduced with facility depth underground. Rn can be eliminated with air purifiers.

G) Detector orientations: The subject may be supine or seated in a tilting chair with fixed or movable detectors provided as single units or arrays. Measurement times are from a few minutes to an hour with multiple counting sessions sometimes required.

H) Calibration: Known amounts of the radionuclide of interest are placed in an anthropomorphic phantom or phantom organ (some have cavities or tanks which may be filled with tagged solutions) and counted in the same reproducible geometry to be used with humans.

I) Sensitivity: The minimum detectable amount (MDA) is that amount of radionuclide in the body that will be detected 95 times out of 100 in a subject containing that amount, and will be reported as being exceeded only 5 times out of 100 in an individual whose true content is 0. One of the many factors determining the MDA is the background counting rate. That rate can be subdivided into ''detector'', ''room'' and ''subject'' backgrounds. In sensitive counters the subject background due to K-40 greatly exceeds the other two.

III. *IN VITRO ANALYSIS (INDIRECT BIOASSAY)*

A) Definition: The identification and quantification of radionuclides in the body by analysis of material excreted or removed from the body.
Advantages:
1. Avoids attenuation by the body encountered in whole-body counting. Sample self-absorption must still be considered. Detection sensitivity is enhanced.
2. Internal and external contamination are easily discriminated.
3. Expense: Common detection equipment may be used. A standard laboratory with no additional shielding is adequate.

Disadvantages:
1. The measurement of internally deposited radionuclides is indirect.
2. Delineation of deposition sites is not possible.
3. Compounds that are not readily excreted may not be detected.
4. Excreted samples are subject to possible cross-contamination during the collection process.
5. Repetitive sampling is necessary, and sample-to-sample variability is unavoidable.
6. Chemical processing and preparation of the analyte for counting may be complex and lengthy.

7. Contamination by multiple radionuclides in different forms may require separate chemical procedures so that the available sample for any particular sample is reduced.
8. Quantification requires back-calculation using metabolic models. Since the human metabolism of most radionuclides is not well known, the models described in ICRP Publication No. 30 are frequently used. They were designed to derive standards for occupational exposures. The assumptions contained therein lead to conservative estimates, i.e. not necessarily an accurate estimate of the body burden.

B) Compartment Model: Mathematical models are based on empirical data and simplifying assumptions about radionuclide deposition and retention in the body. The body has been divided into compartments with entrance and exit rates specific to each radionuclide. Clearance from the body is by one or more of the excretion pathways combined with radioactive decay. The respiratory and gastrointestinal tracts are further compartmentalized. Biokinetic assumptions include instantaneous uptake to compartments followed by fractional losses with no recycling of material between compartments. These oversimplifications do not introduce much error, however alternative models for specific elements that are based on better experimental data should be used when available. The previous ICRP respiratory tract model contains anatomical compartments where deposition is based on differences in impaction and diffusion between aerosols according to Activity Median Aerodynamic Diameter (AMAD) and solubility. Those compartments are the nasopharyngeal region (N-P), tracheobronchial region (T-B), and pulmonary region (P). This model has now been revised as a much more complex treatment. The gastrointestinal tract is divided into the stomach, small intestine, upper large intestine, and lower large intestine. Transfer and uptake rates are specified, and the mucosal layer of cells lining the tract is considered to be target of concern along its length. Excretion data are also useful for calculation of doses to endosteal bone cells and red bone marrow from deposited bone-seekers.

C) Sampling: Common samples collected for analysis include urine, feces, and exhaled air. Other samples may include saliva, blood, sweat, hair, tissue (biopsy), fingernails, and teeth.

1. Urine samples: the most frequently used *in vitro* sample especially for radionuclides in a soluble form. The usual procedure is to analyze periodic 24-hour collections of urinary excretion. This type of sampling provides verification of the intake, and information about the excretion rate.
2. Fecal samples: daily sampling is less common and less desirable for aesthetic reasons. A fecal sample taken soon after a known ingestion indicates the amount of the radionuclide that was not absorbed during passage through the GI tract. Of that fraction that is absorbed, a portion is returned to the GI tract via bile from the liver, and is eliminated in the feces. Inhaled radionuclides may also be detected in fecal samples. Some fraction of the soluble portion will be excreted from the liver as described above. Some portion is also removed from the respiratory tract by the mucociliary escalator and swallowed into the GI tract. Fecal analysis is also useful in studying relatively insoluble radionuclides that pass through the GI tract with little or no absorption, but irradiate tissue in transit.
3. Tissue samples: useful for postmortem analysis or for living subjects when biopsy samples are available from medical procedures. Direct evidence of radionuclide deposition is provided as well as direct measurement of specific tissue concentrations. Time of intake and retention half-life in the organ can not be determined from removed tissue specimens.
4. Others: used in special circumstances, e.g., breath samples for gaseous forms such as $^{14}CO_2$ and ^{222}Rn.
5. Variability: in addition to the variability (often considerable) between individual metabolisms leading to estimation errors based on standard man models, there will be biological variation in day-to-day biological turnover, and sampling technique variability which will all affect the committed dose equivalent estimate.

D) Radiochemical Analysis: The in vitro bioassay sample must be chemically processed to a purity and form amenable to quantification via an appropriate counting system. Sample size will be about 1.0 liter for urine and the entire voiding for feces. The sample matrix must be removed from the relatively minute amount of analyte before counting. This often involves heating the sample in acid solutions, or ashing at high temperatures with subsequent dissolution in acid. During the preparation a yield monitor (radioactive or non-radioactive) should be added and brought into equilibrium with the analyte before chemical manipulations lead to losses. The percent loss of the monitor will then indicate the analyte loss. Multiple purification steps are often necessary to separate the analyte from other chemicals and radionuclides. The purified sample will be prepared for counting as a liquid or solid dried in a planchet or electroplated onto a disc.

E) Detectors: Considerations in the choice of detection system include radiation types, energies, precision requirements, isotopic specificity, sensitivity, and time constraints.
   1. Alpha emitters: Detectors include gas-flow proportional counters, ZnS phosphor systems, liquid scintillation spectrometers, and surface-barrier semiconductor detectors. Low-level samples requiring selectivity and sensitivity should be counted using the surface-barrier detector.
   2. Beta emitters: Detectors include shielded anti-coincidence and nonshielded gas-flow GM and proportional counters, liquid scintillation (especially for routine surveys on tritium users), and solid scintillation.
   3. Photon emitters: Detectors include NaI(Tl), Ge(Li) or intrinsic Ge semiconductors. NaI(Tl) is best used for radionuclides well-separated in energies, or when high counting efficiency is needed. Ge semiconductors are useful when fine energy resolution is required, or for counting low-energy photons. For bulky (self-attenuating) samples phoswich (NaI/CsI) detectors are preferred especially for ^{238}Pu, ^{239}Pu, and ^{241}Am.

F) MDA: Factors that should be optimized to increase sensitivity include counting time, sample size, yield, and background variability. An advantage afforded by increased sensitivity is that the time window for analysis for each radionuclide is increased, especially those with the long effective half-lives.

G) Recent Developments:
   1. Fission track analysis (FTA): Useful for ^{239}Pu analysis. The sample is irradiated with neutrons and the resulting fission tracks are proportional to the amount of ^{239}Pu present. The fission tracks are formed on a quartz slide which is subsequently etched with hydrofluoric acid prior to optical counting with a microscope. Facilities must be cleaned to remove ^{235}U contamination since indistinguishable tracks would result.
   2. Mass spectrometry: Isotopic content is analyzed by ionizing the sample in a vacuum, followed by separation of the ions by momentum and energy so that selected ions can be counted.

IV. *AN ALTERNATIVE METHOD* (summarized from Piechowski and Menoux, 1996)

The interpretation of bioassay in exposed workers is a complex subject undergoing constant evolution. This evolution essentially concerns the quality and detection limit of the measurements and the representation of metabolic and dosimetric models. On the other hand, the approach to the interpretation of individual monitoring data is not often questioned. The present idea is to try to determine the intake as well as possible by using the metabolic models that describe the overall kinetics of the radionuclide from the time it enters the organism until its excretion. It is precisely this question that deserves to be reconsidered, and a different approach may yield new information. The approach employed here is to use the smallest possible number of useful parameters, i.e., minimal modeling. In practice, this leads to less uncertainty regarding the estimates of the activities that have entered the organism. From an anatomo-physiological point of view, two main regions can be distinguished: (a) the routes of entry: respiratory tract, gastrointestinal tract, skin and outer mucous membranes; and (b) the systemic part of the organism, which is involved once the radioactive product has entered the blood. In most cases, the essential problem, in terms of the dose and health hazards, is systemic contamination. However, for relatively insoluble products, the dose to the routes of entry may not be negligible. The authors approach the interpretation of measurement data by separating these two main regions of the organism and concentrate on the systemic region. The aim is to estimate the activity transferred from the routes of entry to the blood on the basis of systemic retention and excretion measurements. The point of capital importance in this approach is to treat the systemic and route of entry burdens separately. This means that in the calculations, one can avoid the use of transfer parameters whose nature is often difficult to analyze and whose value cannot always be proved.

The activity absorbed comprises a variously large fraction of the activity incorporated. This fraction, which is related to transferability, depends on the nature of the product and on the route of entry. Consequently, the activity absorbed is not directly comparable to the Annual Limit on Intake (ALI). The amount of radionuclide transferred daily from the routes of entry to the blood contributes to systemic retention and excretion measurements made subsequently. Retention and excretion can be considered to be the sum of elementary activities resulting from successive systemic transfers of the radionuclide: $A(\tau)$ represents activity absorbed on day τ, and $q_s(t - \tau + 1)$ represents systemic retention or excretion resulting, at time $t \geq \tau$, from a unit absorption on day τ. Then, the Q(t) values for the systemic amounts measured on day t are given by the general equation: $Q(t) = \Sigma$ (from $\tau = 1$ to t) $q_s(t - \tau + 1)A(\tau)\ t \geq \tau$. The $A(\tau)$ values are easy to determine from the above system of equations since each equation includes one unknown quantity. Mathematically speaking, this is a discrete deconvolution. The amount of radionuclide absorbed between the two dates τ_1 and τ_2 is equal to the sum of daily absorptions during the period between them: A (from τ_1 to τ_2) $= \Sigma A(\tau)$.

The interpretation of measurement data, as currently recommended by the ICRP, requires the design of complete metabolic models, starting from intake up to retention and excretion (ICRP 1979; ICRP 1988). Difficulties arise, in particular, when the kinetics of entry towards the systemic compartment have to be defined. The more the model takes into account the latest information acquired about the mechanisms of clearance of entry route tissue, the more complicated the modeling becomes. The difficulty is that, for lack of sufficient information, most of the values attributed to the different parameters are not personalized or adapted to the individual cases encountered. The variations in the parameters are related to the nature of the contaminating products and to the particular physiological characteristics of each individual. In addition, a model cannot include absolutely everything down to the smallest details without paralyzing the interpretation procedure by taking account of too many factors. Lastly, it is clearly not possible to create a model for all potentially conceivable routes of entry, with specific modalities of contamination for each case. The time course of contamination also plays a very important role, and apart from recognized incidents, it is seldom possible to know exactly how the intake occurred. The approach proposed here makes it possible to become independent of many of these problem factors. In theory, it is sufficient to master the q_s function describing systemic retention or excretion after absorption of a single unit of activity. The refinement of this function is an objective that one may justifiably hope to achieve with far more limited theoretical or experimental means than those required for a model that starts with intake. The important point is to have chemical forms of product available that are representative of the form in which the radionuclide enters the extra-cellular fluids, especially as regards redox conditions, valences, and the ions or associated complexing molecules.

The real difficulty that remains is connected with the number of Q(t) measurements available. To apply the proposed system of equations correctly, the number of measurements must be as large as possible. However, for practical reasons, this is rarely the case. In certain situations, there could perhaps be more measurements if all those concerned in the monitoring protocol were convinced of the soundness and advantages of the method. Nevertheless, excessively strict constraints would produce undesirable results. The procedure used for interpretation must therefore be adapted to a limited number of measurements and use them to the best advantage. The solution chosen here consists of considering the value measured as the Q(t) value and keeping it unchanged until the next measurement, and so on. In other words, the measurement made at a given time is the reference measurement throughout the entire period of time elapsing until the next one. The result of this procedure is that the $A(\tau)$ values found for absorption are more like mathematical increments than real values. Thus, if the calculations made over a certain period overestimate absorption, there will be a series of negative $A(\tau)$ values during the following period. The main thing is to calculate the sum of the $A(\tau)$ values over fairly long periods, especially if measurements are infrequent. This summing of increments, which are sometimes positive and sometimes negative, makes it possible, in the end, to counterbalance an under or an overestimation. Lastly, algebraic addition of the $A(\tau)$ values allows an absorption value to be reached that is fairly representative of reality. The procedure proposed comprises a gradual process of self-correction, sometimes reflecting reality by overstatement and sometimes by understatement. This amounts to taking account of the different measurements in a way that resembles the calculation of an average.

In practice, the new approach emerges as a more reliable way of determining the radioactivity entering the blood. It could be applied as a complement to current practice and even replace it in the future, once a solution has been found for the problems concerning the frequency of monitoring and the determination of the radioactivity present in the routes of entry. Already now, dosimetry can be applied to the activity, absorbed, using the appropriate dose factors (Sv Bq^{-1} absorbed). On the other hand, its application to the radioactivity in the routes of entry requires further development of the method.

V. *PHYSIOLOGICALLY BASED BIOKINETIC MODELS*

The ICRP and NCRP are increasingly promoting complex physiologically-based biokinetic models that extend the ability to model persons who do not conform to standard man and deal with chemically similar radionuclides. The drawback is that such models are unwieldy and can not be implemented without a computer. Indeed, a program (LUDEP) has already been written to handle the new ICRP lung model. That model's complexity is illustrated by Tables 12.5–12.8 generated by Huston (1995) after ICRP figures. In an examination of uncertainty in lung dose from plutonium oxide aerosols using the ICRP model, Huston characterized over sixty input parameters for that model. It is evident that the operational health physicist sometimes needing to make rapid assessments and decisions would tend to rely on the older, simpler model. For a more in-depth discussion see Health Phys. 70(5):656–664; 1996 (Khursheed, et al.).

Table 12.1.1 Recommendations of the International Commission on Radiological Protection Relevant to Bioassay (Courtesy ICRP from Publication 54, 1987)

1. The dose equivalent limits relate to the sum of the dose equivalent from external exposure during one year and the committed dose equivalent from that year's intake of radionuclides. For internal exposures, the Commission has confirmed that its policy is to limit the risk ''committed'' by each year of operation and that this is achieved by the use of annual limits on intake calculated from the committed dose equivalent, with a 50 year integrating period (ICRP, 1984). In practice, use may be made of secondary limits; for intakes of radionuclides, the ALI is the appropriate limit. The procedure under which both internal and external exposures are expressed as fractions of the relevant limits, and the sum compared with unity may be unnecessarily restrictive; in this case, doses should be calculated and compared with the Commission's dose equivalent limits. This report is concerned with procedures for evaluating the dose related to the internal exposure.
2. In ICRP Publication 35 (ICRP 1982), it is suggested that the need for individual monitoring may be based on independent evaluations of the likely magnitude of external and internal exposure. Thus, classification of a working environment as Working Condition A on the basis of external exposure would not indicate the need for individual monitoring for internal exposure unless intakes of radionuclides might exceed three-tenths of the annual limit. For example, a working environment in which workers handle sealed sources or unsealed sources in good containment may be classified as Working Condition A on the basis of external exposure, but individual monitoring for intakes of radionuclides would not be required unless monitoring of the working environment, by measurement of surface contamination or airborne activity, suggested that a failure of containment had occurred. Conversely, workers handling tritium or ^{125}I may require monitoring for intakes of these radionuclides, but not for external irradiation. This classification should also apply when annual dose equivalents both from external irradiation and from intakes of radionuclides might exceed three-tenths of relevant annual limits (for example, in some parts of the nuclear fuel cycle).
3. In the case of intakes of mixtures of radionuclides, the total intake should not give rise to a dose equivalent in excess of the dose equivalent limit and reference levels should be adjusted accordingly. It may not be practicable or, indeed, necessary to undertake individual monitoring for every radionuclide in the mixture.

Table 12.2 ICRP Bioassay Levels (Courtesy ICRP from Publication 54, 1987)

1. **Reference Levels**
   Reference levels are described in *ICRP Publication 26* (ICRP, 1977). ''Reference levels may be established for any of the quantities determined in the course of radiation protection programs, whether or not there are limits for these quantities. A reference level is not a limit and is used to determine a course of action when the value of a quantity exceeds or is predicted to exceed the reference level. The action to be initiated may range from simply recording the information, through investigations into causes and consequences, up to intervention measures. It is important to define the general scope of this action when defining the reference level. The most common forms of reference level are recording levels, investigation levels and intervention levels.''
2. **Investigation Level**
   The investigation level is a value of committed dose equivalent or intake above which the result is regarded as sufficiently important to justify further investigation. In this report, investigation levels are calculated separately for each radionuclide. For routine monitoring, the investigation level is set in relation to the monitoring interval to which the measurement result refers and is taken as three-tenths of that fraction of the annual limit corresponding to the monitoring interval. Thus, for N monitoring intervals per year, the investigation level for intake, IL_R, of any radionuclide is:

$$IL_R = \frac{3}{10}\frac{ALI}{N}$$

where ALI is the annual limit on intake for that radionuclide. For other types of monitoring programs, the investigation level will depend upon the objectives of the program and the type of investigation to be carried out. In this report, the investigation level for special (and operational) monitoring is taken as one-tenth of the limit since it is unlikely that more than a few unusual events involving the same individual will occur in a year. Thus, for intakes of radionuclides:

$$IL_S = \frac{1}{10} ALI.$$

3. **Recording Level**
The Commission recommends the use of the concept of a recording level. The recording level is a formally defined value of committed dose equivalent or intake above which a result from a monitoring program is of sufficient interest to be worth keeping and interpreting. In this report, recording levels are calculated separately for each radionuclide. For routine monitoring, the Commission has recommended that the recording level for individual monitoring should be based on one-tenth of that fraction of the annual limit corresponding to the monitoring period to which the measurement refers [paragraph 181 of *ICRP Publication 26* (ICRP, 1977)]. Thus, for N monitoring intervals per year, the recording level for intake is:

$$RL_R = \frac{1}{30} \frac{ALI}{N}.$$

In this report, the recording level for special (or operational) monitoring is taken as one-thirtieth of the annual limit, i.e.,

$$RL_S = \frac{1}{30} \frac{ALI}{N}.$$

Although the Commission has recommended the values of recording level given above, it is necessary to consider any subsidiary purposes of the monitoring program and to ensure that the results recorded are appropriate for these purposes. Such subsidiary objectives could be related to the need to keep records for the assessment of collective dose and optimization purposes or, for individuals, the need to keep adequate records for use in the event of compensation claims. The Commission recognizes that such considerations may justify the use of recording levels lower than those generally recommended.

4. **Derived Reference Levels**
The quantities normally measured in individual monitoring programs for intakes of radionuclides are body or organ content or activity excreted per unit time and it is convenient to compare the measurement results directly with derived reference levels, i.e., derived investigation level (DIL) and derived recording level (DRL). Calculations of derived reference levels require assumptions about the time and pattern of intake and the use of models of intake, deposition, metabolism and retention. Derived investigation and recording levels are calculated separately for each radionuclide. These calculations form the main subject of this report and derived reference levels for a number of radionuclides of importance in occupational exposure are given in the Appendix of ICRP 54, 1987.

A measured value in excess of the derived recording level should be interpreted in terms of intake or committed dose equivalent and recorded in the formal dose record. A measured value below the derived recording level need not be interpreted in terms of committed dose equivalent or intake.

Table 12.2.1 Confirmatory Monitoring (Courtesy ICRP from Publication 54, 1987)

One method of confirmation that working conditions are satisfactory is to carry out occasional individual monitoring. Such measurements can be interpreted only qualitatively, but unexpected findings give grounds for further investigations and may suggest the need for a monitoring program designed to assess individual doses or intakes. Confirmatory monitoring of this type is only useful for those radionuclides that can be easily detected in the body or in excreta at low levels, such as many fission and activation products.

Table 12.2.2 Use of Derived Reference Levels in Routine Bioassay Monitoring[a] (Courtesy ICRP from Publication 54, 1987)

1. The models outlined in Figures 12.1 and 12.2 can be described by systems of equations which may be solved to give values of body or organ content or excretion rate as a function of time following unit intake. These functions give the predicted values per unit intake of the various quantities that can be measured; i.e., activity in the body or an organ, or activity excreted per unit time, at time, t after a unit intake. They are denoted in the text by the generic function m(t). The corresponding measured values following an unknown intake are denoted by M. As defined in Table 12.2, the investigation level for routine monitoring is:

$$IL_R = \frac{3}{10}\frac{ALI}{N}$$

or

$$IL_R = \frac{3}{10} ALI \frac{T}{365}$$

for N monitoring periods each of T days. Similarly the recording level for routine monitoring is:

$$RL_R = \frac{1}{10} ALI \frac{T}{365}$$

The derived investigation level for routine monitoring is then:

$$DIL_R = IL_R\, m(T/2)$$

since intake is assumed to occur at the mid-point of the monitoring interval. Similarly, the derived recording level is:

$$DIL_R = RL_R\, m\,(T/2)$$

2. As an additional, long-term check it may be useful to compare the individual monitoring results with the values that would result from a continuing intake at the rate of ALI/365 per day. Results regularly approaching these values would indicate the need to re-examine the monitoring programs and the control procedures in the workplace.

[a] The DILs for routine and special monitoring for some radionuclides can be found in the Appendix of ICRP Publication 54, 1987. ALI values are published in ICRP Publication 61, 1990.

Table 12.2.3 Bioassay—Special and Operational Monitoring[a] (Courtesy ICRP Publication 54, 1987)

1. Special monitoring refers to monitoring carried out in actual or suspected abnormal conditions. Operational monitoring is monitoring carried out to provide information about a particular operation. Since both special and operational monitoring relate to distinct events, either real or suspected, many of the problems encountered in interpretation of routine monitoring results do not apply. In particular, the time of possible intake is likely to be known and there is likely to be more information about the physical and chemical form of the contaminant.
2. In the case of special and operational monitoring, the time of intake is known and measurements are likely to be made in the few days following intake.
3. The values of m(t) are also used to calculate derived reference levels for 1 to 7 days after intake. As defined in table 12.2, the investigation level for special or operational monitoring is:

$$IL_S = \frac{1}{10} ALI$$

and the recording level is:

$$RL_S = \frac{1}{30} ALI$$

The corresponding derived investigation and recording levels are:

$$DIL_S = IL_S\, m(t)$$

and

$$DRL_S = RL_S\, m(t)$$

Values of DIL_S are given in the Appendix of ICRP Publication 54. These values have been calculated for inhalation of a 1 μm AMAD aerosol by Reference Man (ICRP, 1975). Values for the appropriate inhalation class should be used. If the AMAD is known to be different from 1 μm, appropriate values of m(t) and DIL_S may be calculated.

[a] The DILs for routine and special monitoring for some radionuclides can be found in the Appendix of ICRP Publication 54, 1987. ALI values are published in ICRP Publication 61, 1990.

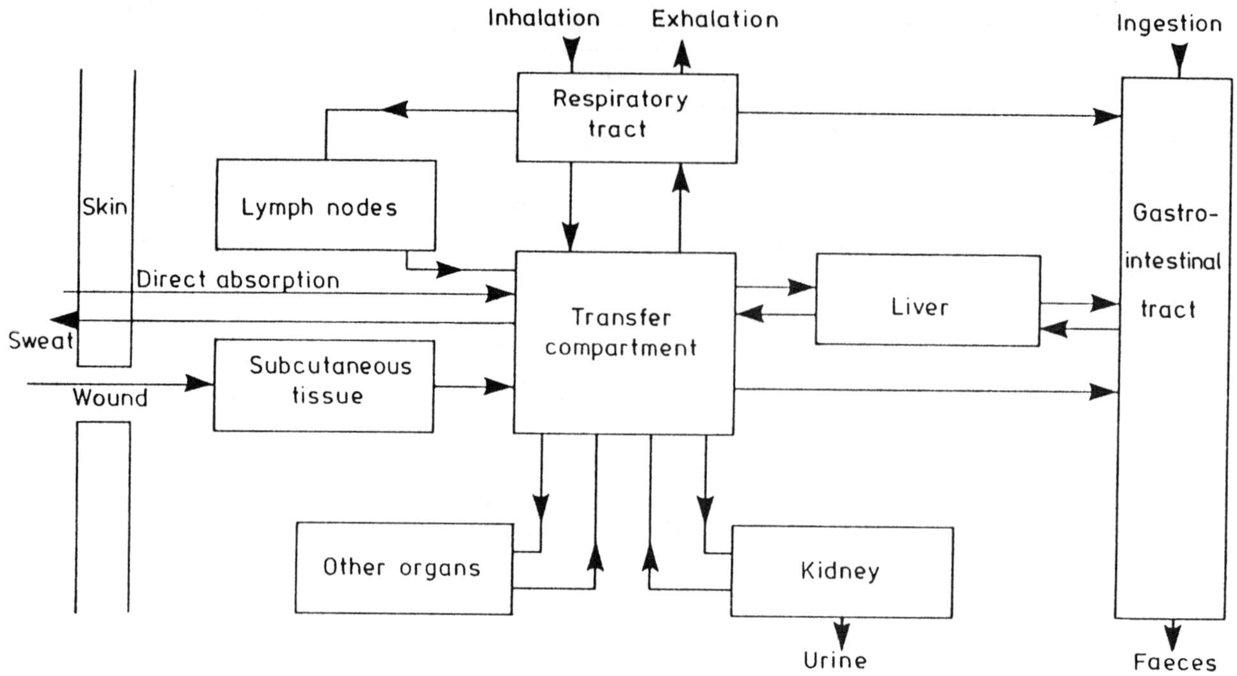

Figure 12.1 Routes of Intake, Transfers and Excretion (Courtesy ICRP from Publication 54, 1987)

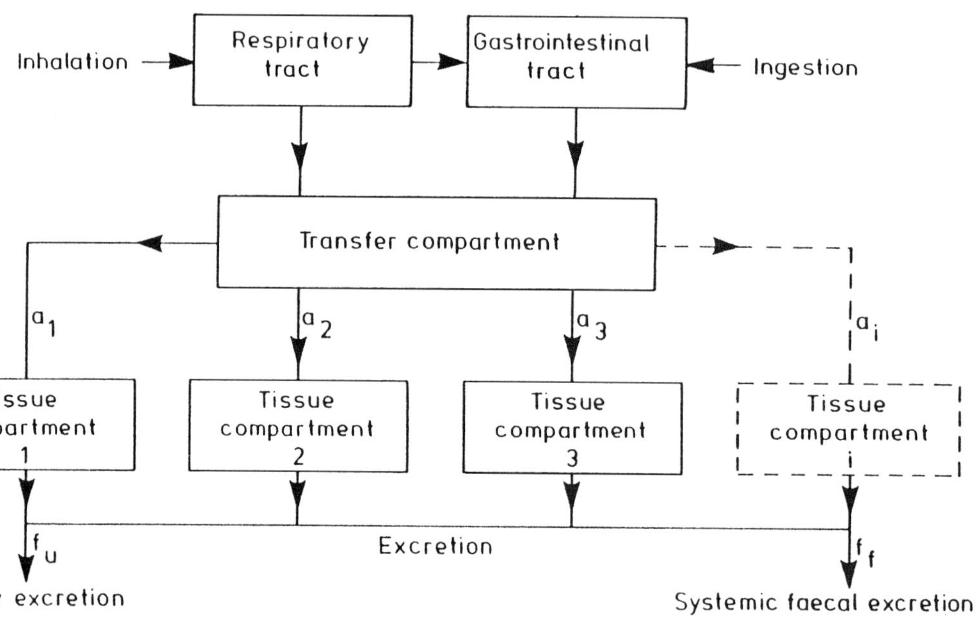

Figure 12.2 General Model Used to Represent the Kinetics of Radionuclides in Body Compartments (Courtesy ICRP from Publication 54, 1987)

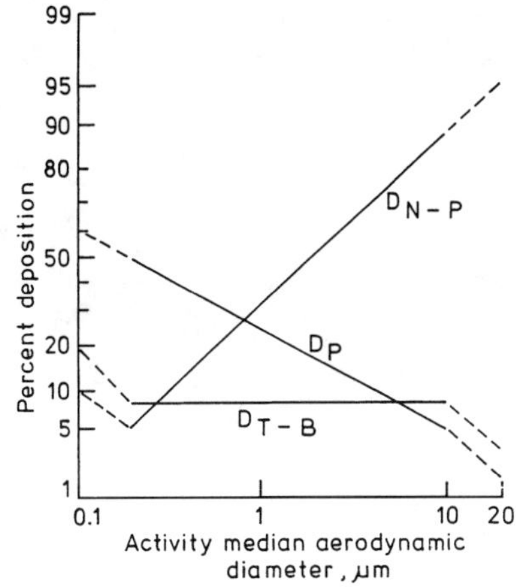

Figure 12.3 Deposition of Dust in the Respiratory System. The percentage of activity or mass of an aerosol which is deposited in the N-P, T-B and P regions is given in relation to the Activity Median Aerodynamic Diameter (AMAD) of the aerosol distribution. The model is intended for use with aerosol distributions with AMADs between 0.2 and 10 μm and with geometric standard deviations of less than 4.5. Provisional estimates of deposition further extending the size range are given by the dashed lines. For an unusual distribution with an AMAD of greater than 20 μm, complete deposition in N-P can be assumed. The model does not apply to aerosols with AMADs of less than 0.1 μm. (Courtesy ICRP from Publication 54, 1987)

		Class					
		D		W		Y	
Region	**Compartment**	**T (day)**	**F**	**T (day)**	**F**	**T (day)**	**F**
N-P	a	0.01	0.5	0.01	0.1	0.01	0.01
(D_{N-P} = 0.30)	b	0.01	0.5	0.40	0.9	0.40	0.99
T-B	c	0.01	0.95	0.01	0.5	0.01	0.01
(D_{T-B} = 0.08)	d	0.2	0.05	0.2	0.5	0.2	0.99
	e	0.5	0.8	50	0.15	500	0.05
P	f	n.a.	n.a.	1.0	0.4	1.0	0.4
(D_p = 0.25)	g	n.a.	n.a.	50	0.4	500	0.4
	h	0.5	0.2	50	0.05	500	0.15
L	i	0.5	1.0	50	1.0	1000	0.9
	j	n.a.	n.a.	n.a.	n.a.	∞	0.1

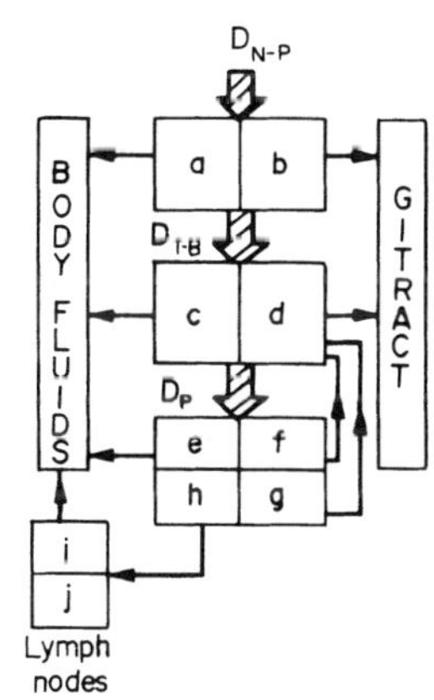

Figure 12.4 Mathematical Model Used to Describe Clearance From the Respiratory System. The values for the clearances T_{a-j} and compartmental fractions, F_{a-j} are given in the tabular portion of the figure for each of the three classes of retained materials. The values given for D_{N-P}, D_{T-B}, and D_P (left column) are the regional depositions for an aerosol with an AMAD of 1 μm. The schematic drawing identifies the various clearance pathways from compartments a-j in the four respiratory regions, N-P, T-B, P and L. n.a. = not applicable. (Courtesy ICRP from Publication 54, 1987)

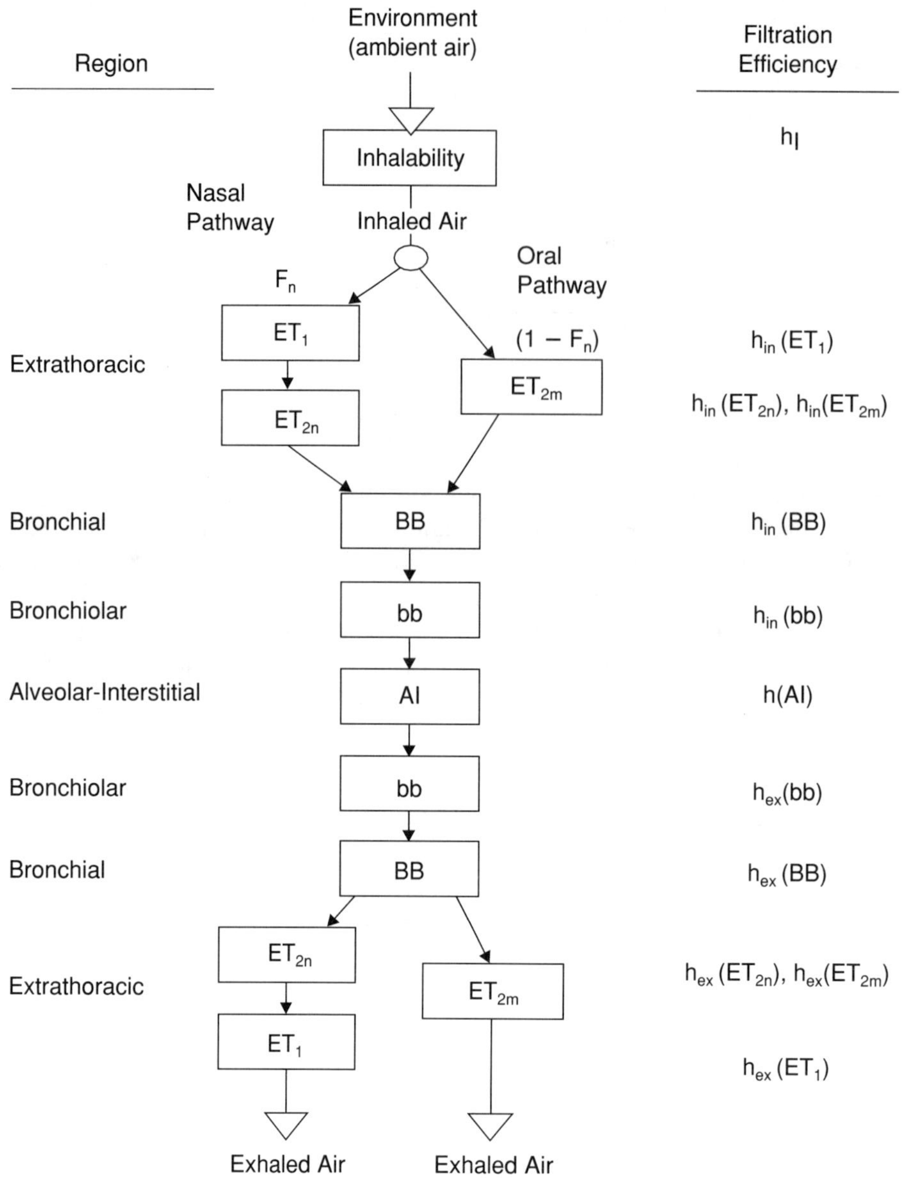

Representation of the deposition component of the revised ICRP respiratory tract model. The respiratory tract is modeled as a series of filters with characteristic volumes and deposition efficiencies. After (Figure 8 in ICRP,1994).

Figure 12.5 Deposition Component of the Revised ICRP Respiratory Tract Model (Courtesy of Huston, 1995)

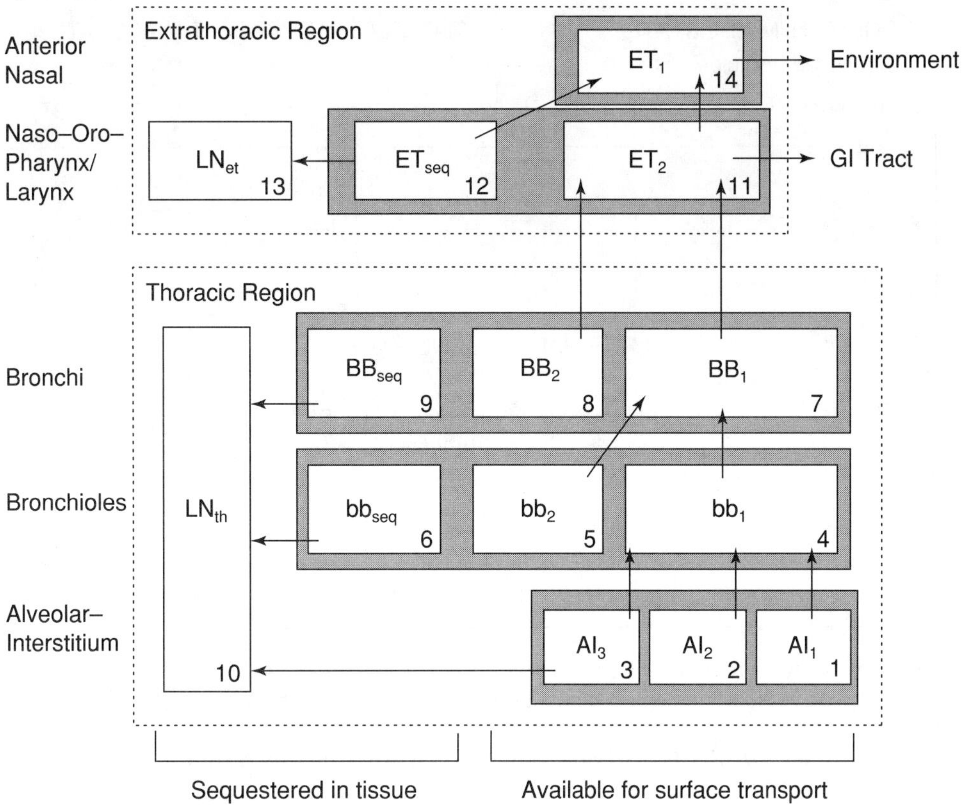

Representation of particle transport model recommended by the ICRP (1994) for mucociliary and macrophage transport mechanisms to the gastrointestinal tract and lymph nodes (no absorption pathways shown).

Figure 12.6 ICRP Model for Mechanical Clearance from the Respiratory Tract (Courtesy of Huston, 1995)

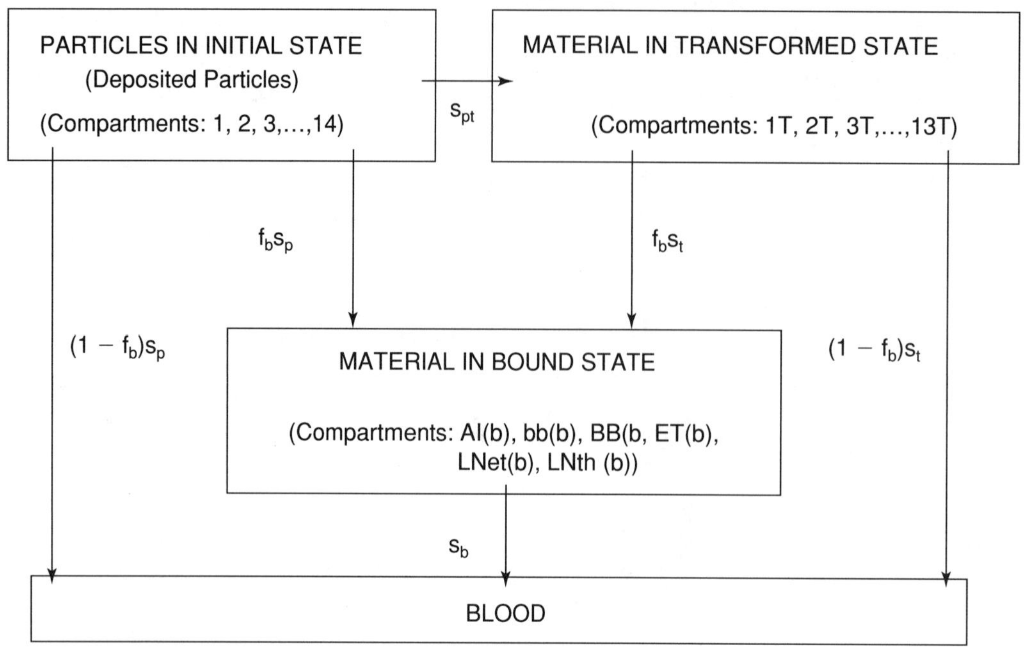

Compartment model recommended by ICRP (1994) to represent dissolution and absorption to blood and lung tissues for materials deposited in the respiratory tract.

Figure 12.7 ICRP Model for Dissolution and Absorption to Blood (Courtesy of Huston, 1995)

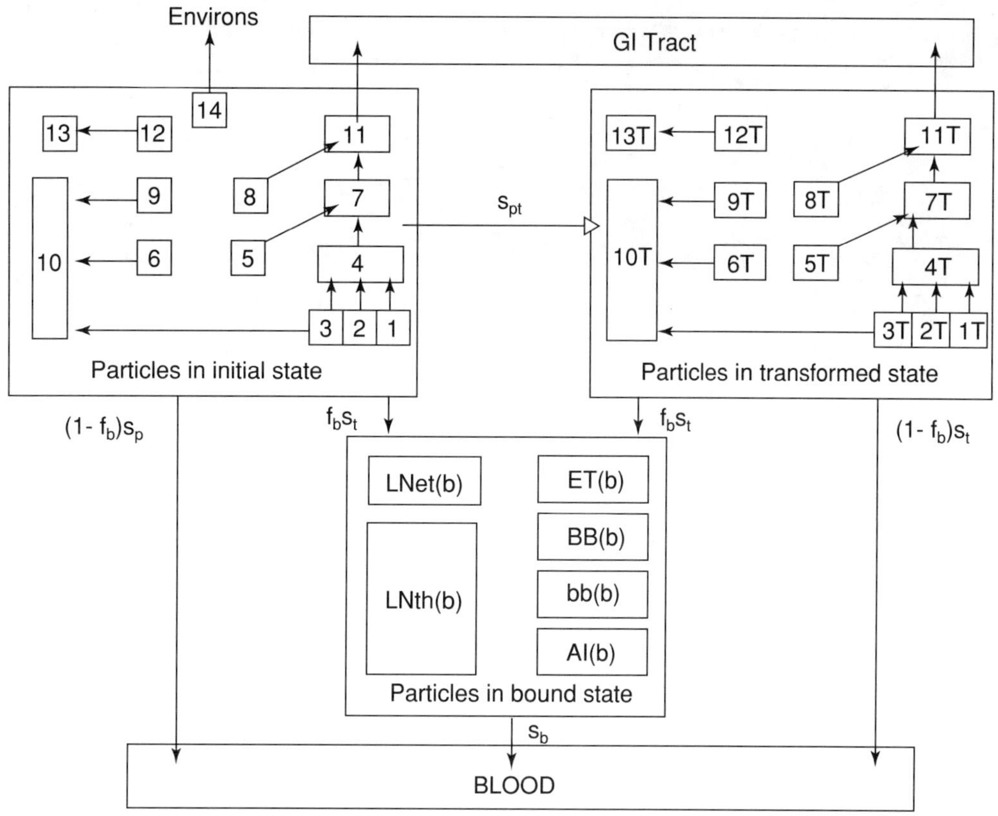

Schematic of the overall compartment model to represent clearance of material from the respiratory tract by mechanical and absorptive processes.

Figure 12.8 Overall ICRP Model for Respiratory Tract Clearance (Courtesy of Huston, 1995)

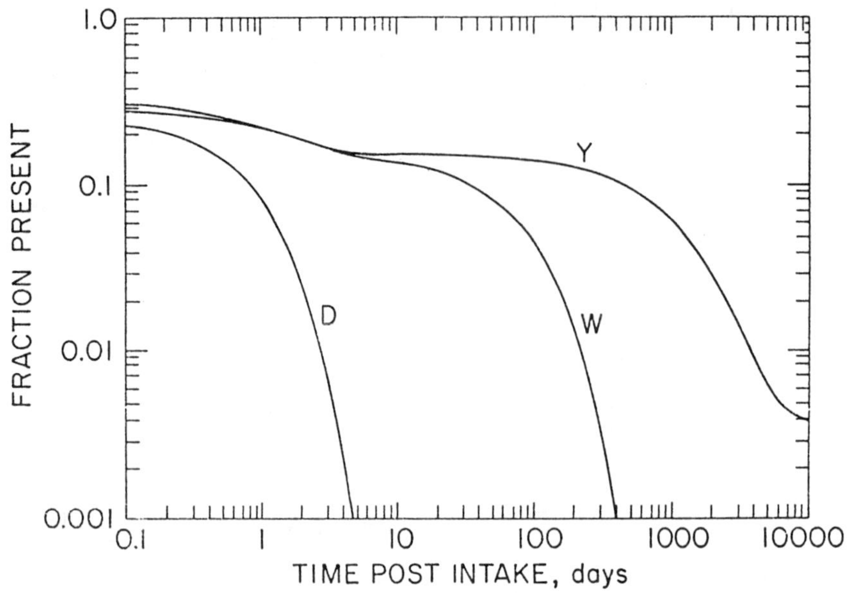

Figure 12.9 Inhalation Intake Retention Functions for Lungs for 1 Micron AMAD Aerosols of Stable Class D, W, or Y Compounds (From NRC NUREG/CR-4884, 1987)

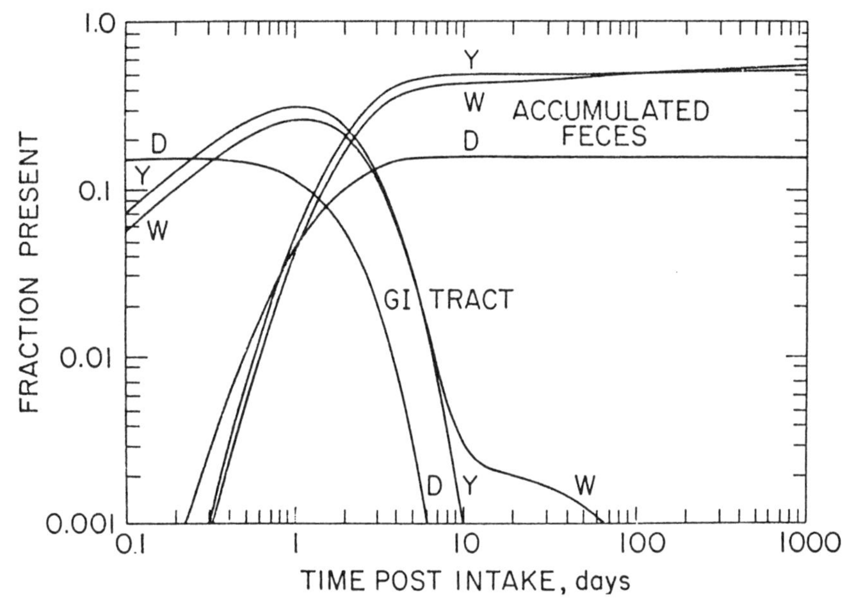

Figure 12.10 Inhalation Intake Retention Functions for GI Tract and Accumulated Feces for 1 Micron AMAD Aerosols of Stable Class D, W, or Y Compounds for Which f_1 and f_f = Zero (From NRC NUREG/CR-4884, 1987)

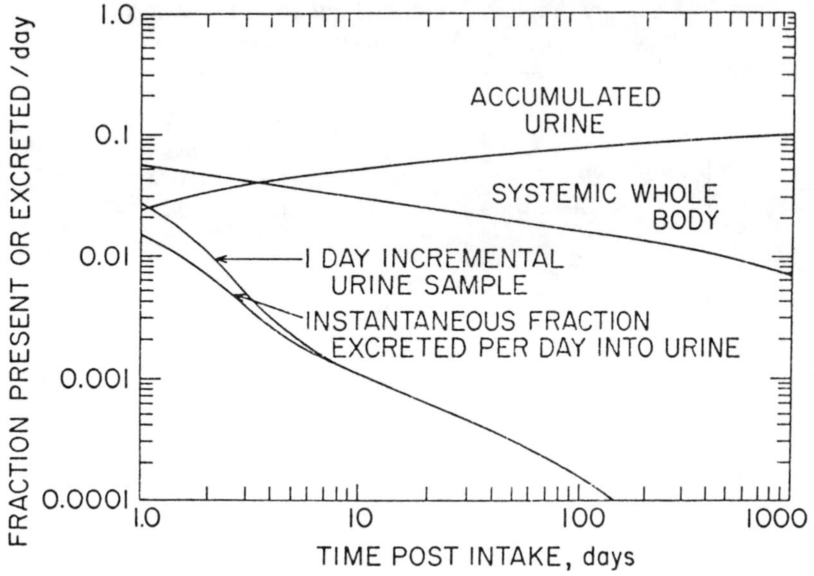

Figure 12.11 Systemic Retention and Urinary Excretion Post Single Inhalation Intake of 1 Micron AMAD Aerosols of Stable Class W Cobalt for Which f_1 = 0.05 and f_u = 0.8 (From NRC NUREG/CR-4884, 1987)

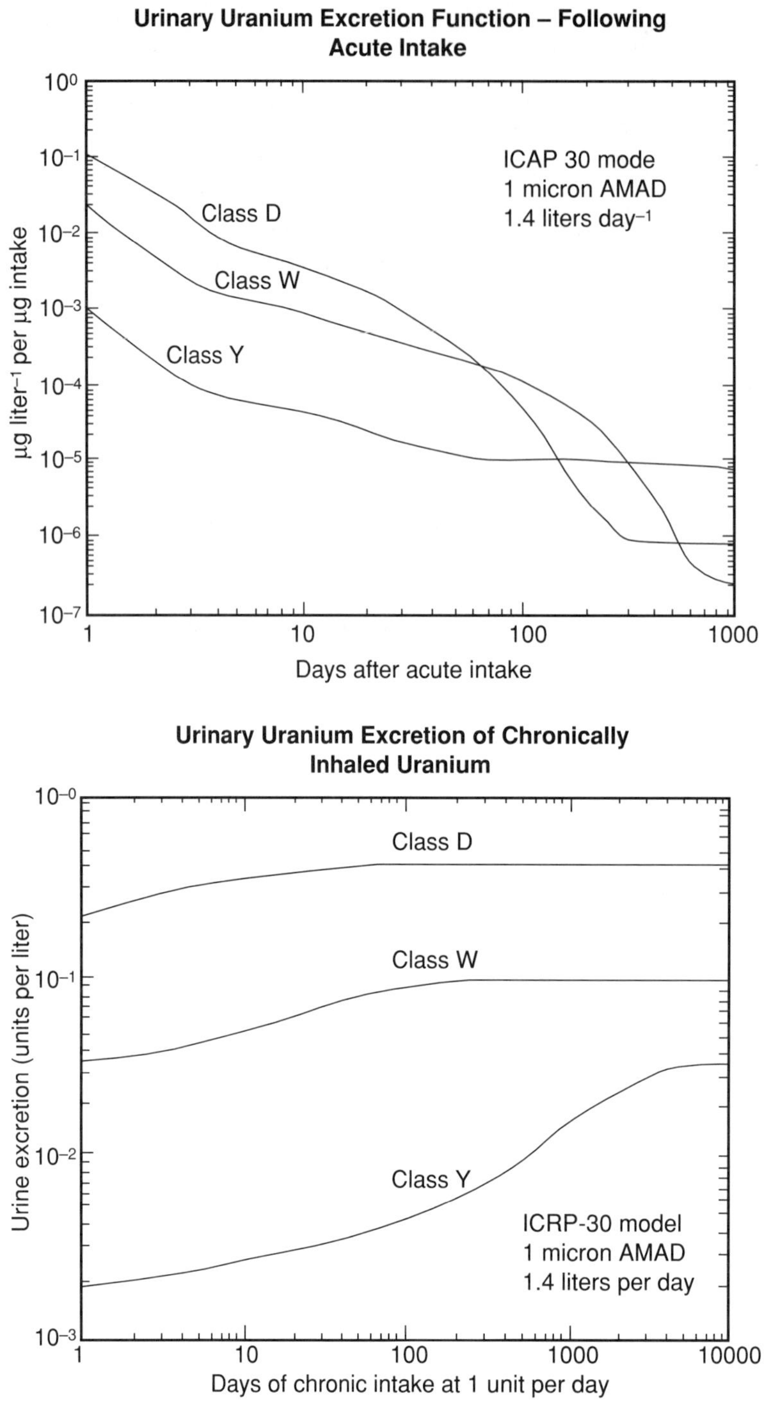

Figure 12.12 Urinary Uranium Excretion (Courtesy Health Physics Society N13.22, 1995)

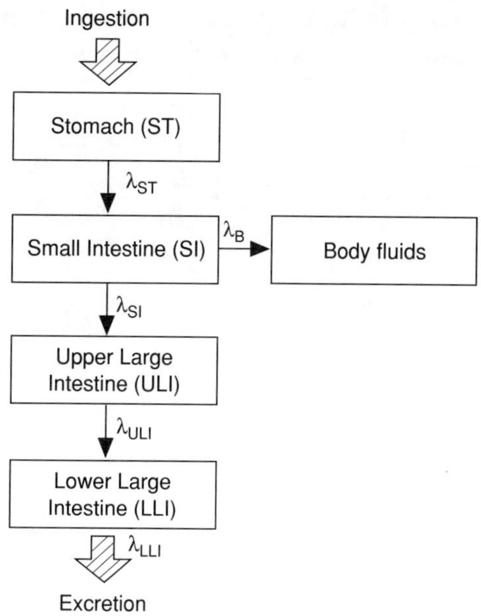

Figure 12.13 Schematic of the GI Tract Model (Courtesy ICRP from Publication 30, 1978)

Table 12.3 Mathematical Model Used to Describe the Kinetics of Radionuclides in the Gastrointestinal Tract (After ICRP Publications 23, 1975; 30, 1978; and 54, 1987)

Section of GI Tract	Mass of Walls (g)	Mass of Contents (g)	Mean Residence Time (day)	γ (day^{-1})
Stomach (ST)	150	250	1/24	24
Small Intestine (SI)	640	400	4/24	6
Upper Large Intestine (ULI)	210	220	13/24	1.8
Lower Large Intestine (LLI)	160	135	24/24	1

Table 12.4 Explanation of Bioassay Terms

(Courtesy ICRP from Publication 54, 1987)

1. ***Intake*** is the quantity of material entering the body, the principal routes being inhalation, ingestion or through intact or wounded skin.
2. ***Uptake*** is the quantity transferred from the site of intake to body organs or tissues.
3. ***Retained quantity*** in a specific organ or tissue is the quantity of deposited material in that organ or tissue at a given time after intake, deposition or uptake. Material taken up by body fluids is known as systemic material. The quantity in the whole body is the sum of systemic material and material retained within the respiratory and the gastrointestinal tracts.
4. Removal of material from the body occurs by urinary and fecal excretion, by perspiration and sometimes by exhalation. ***Urinary excretion*** is the removal in urine of material from the extracellular fluid. ***Fecal excretion*** has two components: system fecal excretion which represents removal of systemic material via the gastrointestinal tract; and direct fecal excretion of the material passing unabsorbed through the gastrointestinal tract.
5. Retention and excretion are expressed as functions of time. These functions take into account both the biological transfers and the radioactive decay of the radionuclide and can be normalized to unit intake or uptake, if required.
6. It is convenient to distinguish between (i) models representing routes of entry, such as the models for the respiratory tract and the gastrointestinal tract, for which parameters are defined by the physical and chemical properties of materials, and (ii) models that describe the processes of retention and excretion following uptake.

Table 12.5 Reference Organ Masses for Individuals of Various Ages (Courtesy ICRP from Publication 56, 1989)

	Mass of Organ (g)					
Organ	Newborn 3.4 kg	Age 1 Year 9.8 kg	Age 5 Year 19 kg	Age 10 Year 32 kg	Age 15 Year 55 kg	ICRP Reference Man[a] 70 kg
Adrenals	5.83	3.52	5.27	7.22	10.5	14.0
Brain	325	884	1260	1360	1410	1400
Breasts	0.107	0.732	1.51	2.60	360	360
Gall bladder wall	0.408	0.910	3.73	7.28	9.27	10.0
GI tract						
LLI[b] wall	7.96	20.6	41.4	70.0	127	160
SI[b] wall	32.6	84.9	169	286	516	640
Stomach wall	6.41	21.8	49.1	85.1	118	150
ULI[b] wall	10.5	27.8	55.2	93.4	168	210
Heart wall	25.4	50.6	92.8	151	241	330
Kidneys	22.9	62.9	116	173	248	310
Liver	121	292	584	884	1400	1800
Lungs	50.6	143	290	453	651	1000
Ovaries	0.328	0.714	1.73	3.13	11.0	11.0
Pancreas	2.80	10.3	23.6	30.0	64.9	100
Skeleton						
Active marrow	47	150	320	610	1050	1500
Endosteal tissue	15.0	26.0	37.0	68.0	120	120
Skin	118	271	538	888	2150	2600
Spleen	9.11	25.5	48.3	77.4	123	180
Testes	0.843	1.21	1.63	1.89	15.5	35.0
Thymus	11.3	22.9	29.6	31.4	28.4	20.0
Thyroid	1.29	1.78	3.45	7.93	12.4	20.0
Urinary bladder wall	2.88	7.70	14.5	23.2	35.9	45.0
Uterus	3.85	1.45	2.70	4.16	80.0	80.0

[a] Acc. to *ICRP Publication 23*.

[b] LLI = lower large intestine, ULI = upper large intestine, and SI = small intestine.

Table 12.5.1 Organ Masses for Japanese Children (After ICRU Report No. 48, 1992)

Organ Masses for Male (M) and Female (F) Japanese Children[a,b]

Organs	Newborn/Infant (0 to 1 month) M	Newborn/Infant (0 to 1 month) F	Child (1 to 2 yr) M	Child (1 to 2 yr) F	Child (5 to 6 yr) M	Child (5 to 6 yr) F	Child (9 to 10 yr) M	Child (9 to 10 yr) F	Child (15 to 16 yr) M	Child (15 to 16 yr) F
	Mass (g)									
Total Body Mass[c]	3200	3200	11100	10500	19000	18600	32500	32800	57500	51800
Adrenals (2)	4	4	5	4	6	6	8	8	11	11
Brain	475	467	1185	1099	1406	1321	1438	1306	1486	1355
Heart	28	27	62	61	103	121	167	170	309	250
Kidneys (2)	30	29	75	72	122	119	177	154	260	247
Liver	169	173	450	416	712	670	920	853	1454	1265
Lungs (2)	90	90	211	205	339	305	503	446	972	666
Pancreas	6	7	27	25	45	49	67	62	106	99
Spleen	13	13	45	39	66	63	88	81	121	114
Testes (2)	2	—	3	—	3	—	4	—	34	—
Thyroid	2	2	3	3	5	6	8	8	16	16

[a] Tanaka et al., 1989.
[b] Tabulated data are mean values as presented by authors.
[c] From Table A.2.3 (ASIATIC)

Table 12.5.2 Organ Masses for European and European Ancestry Children (After ICRU Report No. 48, 1992)

Organs	Newborn (1 yr) M	Newborn (1 yr) F	Child (1 yr) M	Child (1 yr) F	Child (2 yr) M	Child (2 yr) F	Child (5 yr) M	Child (5 yr) F	Child (10 yr) M	Child (10 yr) F	Child (15 yr) M	Child (15 yr) F
	Mass (g)											
Total Body Mass	3500	3400	10200	9700	12700	12200	18500	18200	31300	31200	53900	51700
Adrenals (2)	5	5	6	6	—	—	—	—	—	—	—	—
Brain	403	347	925	894	1064	1012	1237	1206	1290	1226	1356	1318
Heart	23	21	50	49	60	58	94	88	150	145	224	222
Kidneys (2)	27	—	71	—	98	—	129	—	187	—	—	—
Liver	155	—	288	—	394	—	596	—	852	—	—	—
Lungs (2)	55	—	121	—	164	—	211	—	343	—	—	—
Pancreas	6	5	14	15	—	—	—	—		—		
Spleen	10	—	26	—	33	—	47	—	85	—	—	—
Testes (2)	0.4	—	1.4	—	1.8	—	1.8	—	1.6	—	13.6	—
Thyroid	2	—	—	—	—	—	—	—	—	—	—	—

[a] Altman and Dittmer, 1962; Potter and Craig, 1975; Ludwig, 1979.
[b] Tabulated data are mean values as presented by authors.

Table 12.6 Specifications for Reference Man (Courtesy ICRP after Publication 23, 1974)

	Adult Man	Adult Woman	Child 10 Years	Infant 1 Year	Newborn
Weight (kg)	70	58	—	—	3.5 (M) 3.4 (F)
Length (cm)	170	160	—	—	50.8 (M) 50.0 (F)
Surface Area (cm^2)	18000	16000	—	—	2200
Specific Gravity	1.07	1.04	—	—	1.026 (M) 1.022 (F)
Total Body Water (ml/kgW)	600	500	—	—	757
Extracellular Water	260	200	—	—	—
Intracellular	340	300	—	—	—
Total Blood Volume (ml)	5200	3900	—	—	—
Red Cell Volume (ml)	2200	1350	—	—	—
Plasma Volume (ml)	3000	2500	—	—	—
Total Body Weight (g)	5500	4100	—	—	—
Red Cell Weight (g)	2400	1500	—	—	—
Plasma Weight (g)	3100	2600	—	—	—
Total Adipose Tissue (kg)	15	19	—	—	—
Subcutaneous	7.5	13	—	—	—
Separable	5.0	4	—	—	—
Yellow Marrow	1.5	1.3	—	—	—
Interstitial	1.0	0.7	—	—	—
Total Connective Tissue (g)	5050	4100	—	—	
Cartilage	2500	2000	—	—	—
Tendons and Fascia	850	700	—	—	—
Other	1700	1400	—	—	—
Total Fat (kg)	13.5	16	—	—	—
Nonessential	12	15	—	—	—
Essential	1.5	1.2	—	—	—
Total bone marrow (g)	3000	2600	—	—	—
Red bone marrow (g)	1500	1300	—	—	—
Yellow bone marrow (g)	1500	1300	—	—	—
Total Skin (g)	2600	1790	—	—	200
Epidermis	100	90	—	—	—
Dermis	2500	1700	—	—	—
Hypodermis	7500	13000	—	—	480
Energy expenditure (Kcal/d)	3000	2100	2000	—	—
Resting Metabolic Rate (cal/min-kg)	17	16	25	35	—
Oxygen Inhaled (g/day)	920	640	600	—	—
Carbon Dioxide Exhaled (g/day)	1000	700	660	—	—
Total Lung Capacity (liters)	5.6	4.4	—	—	—
Functional Residual	2.2	1.8	—	—	—
Vital	4.3	3.3	—	—	—
Dead Space	0.16	0.13	—	—	—

Table 12.6 Specifications for Reference Man (Continued)

	Adult Man	Adult Woman	Child 10 Years	Infant 1 Year	Newborn
Minute Volume (liters/min)					
Resting	7.5	6.0	4.8	1.5	0.5
Light Activity	20	19	13	4.2	1.5
Total Air Breathed (liters)	23000	21000	15000	3800	800
8 hr working (light)	9600	9100	6240	2500 (10 hr)[a]	90 (1 hr)[a]
8 hr nonoccupational	9600	9100	6240	—	—
8 hr resting	3600	2900	2300	1300	690
Dietary Intake (g)					
Protein	95	66	63	—	—
Carbohydrate	390	270	260	—	—
Fat	120	85	81	—	—
Water in Diet	1000	700	—	—	—
Water in Fluid	1700	1200	—	—	—
Water in Oxidation	300	200	—	—	—
Elements (g/day)					
Carbon	300	210	200	—	—
Hydrogen	350	245	230	—	—
Nitrogen	15	10	10	—	—
Oxygen	2600	1800	1700	—	—
Sulfur	1	0.7	0.7	—	—
Milk Consumption (ml/day)	300	200	470	700	700[b]
Fecal Components (g/day)					
Weight	135	110	85	24	—
Water	105	90	70	19	—
Solids	30	20	19	5	—
Ash	17	15	6	1	—
Fats	5	4.5	4	3	—
Nitrogen	1.5	1.3	1	0.3	—
Other Substances	6.5	5.0	8	0.7	—
Elements					
Carbon	7	6	4.2	1.2	—
Hydrogen	13	11	8.6	2.5	—
Nitrogen	1.5	1.3	1.0	0.3	—
Oxygen	100	90	62	17	—

(continued)

Table 12.6 Specifications for Reference Man (Continued)

	Adult Man	Adult Woman	Child 10 Years	Infant 1 Year	Newborn
Urine					
Volume (ml/day)	1400	1000	1000	450	—
Specific Gravity	1.02	—	—	1.01	—
pH	6.2	—	—	—	—
Solids (g/day)	60	50	47	19	19
Urea (g/day)	22	—	—	—	—
''Sugars'' (g/day)	1	—	—	—	—
Bicarbonates (g/day)	0.14	0.12	—	—	—
Elements (g/day)					
Nitrogen	15	13	11	5	—
Hydrogen	160	130	110	50	—
Oxygen	1300	1100	970	420	—
Carbon	5	4	3	0.5	—
Water Balance (ml/day)					
Total Gains	3000	2100	2000	—	—
Fluid Intake	1950	1400	1400	—	—
Milk	300	200	450	—	—
Tap Water	150	100	200	—	—
Others	1500	1100	750	—	—
In Food	700	450	400	—	—
By Oxidation in Food	350	250	200	—	—
Total Losses (ml/day)	3000	2100	2000	—	—
Urine	1400	1000	1000	—	—
Feces	100	80	70	—	—
Insensible Loss	850	600	580	—	—
Sweat	650	420	350	—	—

[a] Period sustained if different from 8 hours

[b] From HHS Publication, FDA 82-8196 1982

Table 12.7 Reference Man: Summary of Weights of Organs and Tissues

(Courtesy ICRP from Publication 23, 1974)

	Weight (g)		Weight (g)
Adipose tissue	15,000	Lenses (2)	0.40
Subcutaneous	7,500	Liver	1,800
Separable	5,000	Lung tissue (plus arterial and venous blood)	1,000
Yellow marrow	1,500	Lymphocytes	1500
Interstitial	1,000	Lymphatic tissue ("fixed")	700
Adrenal glands (2)	14	Muscles (skeletal)	28,000
Blood (total)	5,500	Palatine tonsils (2)	4
Red blood cells	2,400	Pancreas	100
Plasma	3,100	Parathyroid glands (4)	0.12
Body (total)	70,000	Periarticular tissue (total)	1,500
Bone marrow (total)	3,000	Pineal gland	0.18
Red bone marrow	1,500	Pituitary gland	0.60
Yellow bone marrow	1,500	Prostate gland	16
Brain	1,400	Pulmonary blood	530
Breasts (2)	26	Salivary glands (3 prs.)	85
Bronchial tree	30	Parotid (2)	50
Cartilage (skeletal)	1,100	Submaxillary (2)	25
Connective tissue	5,050	Sublingual (2)	10
Cartilage	2,500	Skeleton	10,000
Tendons and fascia	850	Bone	5,000
Other	1,700	Marrow	3,000
Esophagus	40	Other tissue	2,000
Eyes (2)	15	Skin (total)	2,600
Fat (total)	13,500	Epidermis	100
Nonessential	12,000	Dermis	2,500
Essential	1,500	Spinal Cord	30
Fingernails and toenails	3	Spleen	180
Gallbladder	10	Stomach	150
GI tract (without contents)	1,200	Superficial fascia	500
Esophagus	40	Teeth	46
Stomach	150	Tendons and deep fascia	850
Small intestine	640	Testes (2)	35
Large intestine	370	Thymus	20
GI tract contents	1,005	Thyroid	20
Stomach	250	Tongue	70
Small intestine	400	Tonsils (2 palatine)	4
Upper large intestine	220	Trachea	10
Lower large intestine	135	Ureters (2)	16
Hair	20	Urethra	10
Heart (without blood)	330	Urinary bladder	45
Heart (at end of diastole)	570		
Heart (at end of systole)	425		
Hypodermis	7,500		
Kidneys (2)	310		
Larynx	28		

Table 12.7.1 A Comparison of ICRP Reference Persons and Japanese Reference Persons (Courtesy ICRU after Publication 48, 1992)

Organs	Mass (g)			
	ICRP[a]		Japanese[b]	
	M	F	M	F
Total body mass	70000	58000	60000	51000
Adipose Tissue[c]	12500	17000	11000	—
Adrenals (2)	14	14	14	13
Aorta	100	—	87	—
Blood Vessels	200	—	170	—
Blood (whole)	5500	4100	4800	—
Brain	1400	1200	1500	1300
Breasts (2)	26	360	—	—
Connective tissue (separable)	1600	—	1400	—
Eyes (2)	15	15	15	—
Gallbladder	10	8	8	—
Gallbladder-bile	62	—	40	—
Gastrointestinal tract	1200	1100	1100	—
Gastrointestinal tract (contents)	1005	—	900	—
Heart	330	240	360	280
Kidneys (2)	310	275	320	280
Larynx	28	19	24	—
Liver	1800	1400	1600	1400
Lungs (2)	1000	800	1100	900
Lymphatic tissue	700	580	600	—
Muscle (skeletal)	28000	17000	24000	—
Ovaries (2)	—	11	—	—
Pancreas	100	85	130	100
Prostate	16	—	14	—
Salivary glands (6)	85	70	72	—
Skeleton-cartilage	1100	900	1000	—
Skeleton-osseous tissue	5000	2600	4500	—
Skeleton-periarticular tissue	900	700	800	—
Skeleton-red marrow	1500	1300	1000	—
Skeleton-yellow marrow	1500	1300	1200	—
Skin	2600	1790	2200	—
Spleen	180	150	140	120
Testes (2)	35	—	37	—
Thyroid	20	17	19	17
Urinary bladder	45	45	38	—
Urinary bladder (contents)	102	102	70	—

[a] ICRP, 1975.
[b] Tanaka, 1988 (Female data from Tanaka et al., 1979a)
[c] Excludes yellow marrow and interstitial adipose tissue.

Table 12.8 Reference Man: Other Anatomical Values (Courtesy ICRP from Publication 23, 1974)

Alveoli (surface area)	75 m^2
Blood (distribution of in total body)	
Arterial system	1000 ml
Venous system	3200 ml
Pulmonary system	500 ml
Heart cavity (av. value)	500 ml
Blood volume (total)	5200 ml
Volume of red blood cells	2200 ml
Volume of plasma	3000 ml
Body (length)	170 cm
Body water (total)	600 ml/kgW
Extracellular water	260 ml/kgW
Intracellular water	340 ml/kgW
Bronchial tree, mean wall thickness	75 μm
Bronchial tree, surface area	3950 cm^2
Cerebrospinal fluid, volume	120 ml
Hypodermis (thickness)	3750 μm
Intestinal tract (length)	660 cm
Small intestine	500 cm
Large intestine	160 cm
Lens (depth and size)	
Anterior aspect of lens to anterior pole of cornea	0.3–0.4 cm
Anterior aspect of lens to anterior aspect of closed lid	0.8 cm
Equator of lens to anterior of corneal border	0.3 cm
Equatorial diameter of lens	0.9 cm
Axial thickness of lens	0.4 cm
Nose (specifications)	
Surface area of both vestibules	21 cm^2
Surface area of turbinates and nasal passages	160 cm^2
Thickness of mucus	0.5 mm
Thickness of epithelium	0.1 mm
Thickness of entire mucosa	2 mm
Weight of mucosa	32 g
Skin (total thickness)	1300 μm
Epidermis	50 μm
Dermis	1250 μm
Specific gravity of total body	1.07
Surface area of body	18,000 cm^2
Urinary bladder capacity	
Capacity (distress)	500 ml
Physiological capability	200 ml

Table 12.9 Rule of Nines for Estimating Surface Area of Regions of the Total Body (Courtesy ICRP from Publication 23, 1974)

Region	Percent
Head and Neck	9%
Upper Limbs (each 9%)	18%
Lower Limbs (each 18%)	36%
Front of Trunk	18%
Back of Trunk	18%
Perineum	1%
Outstretched Palms and Fingers	1%

Table 12.10 Skin Thickness (μm) (Courtesy ICRP from Publication 23, 1974)

	Thickness (μm)	
	Male	**Female**
Total Skin Thickness	1300	1300
Epidermis	50	50
Dermis	1250	1250
Hypodermis	3750	6600

Table 12.11 Distribution of Total Body Water in Adult Male (Courtesy ICRP from Publication 23, 1974)

	Volume[a] (ml/kg)	% Total Body Water
Plasma	41	7
Interstitial Lymph	121	20
Dense Connective Tissue and Cartilage	41	7
Inaccessible Bone	41	7
Transcellular	15	2.5
Intraluminal GI	8.4	1.4
Total extracellular Water	260	43
Total intracellular Water	340	57
Total Body Water	600	100

[a] Volume = (ml/kg).

Table 12.12 Lean Body Mass (Courtesy ICRP from Publication 23, 1974)

Total Body Water	724 ml/kg	± 100
Extracellular Fluid	334 ml/kg	± 57
Blood Volume (Male)	84 ml/kg	± 14.5
Red Cell Volume (Male)	34 ml/kg	± 7.4
Red Cell Volume (Female)	29 ml/kg	± 2.6
Plasma Volume	50.7 ml/kg	± 7.8

Table 12.13 Distribution of Intracellular Water (Courtesy ICRP from Publication 23, 1974)

	ml/kg W[a]
Muscle Cell Water	235
Bone Cell Water	20
Connective Tissue Cell Water	20
Erythrocytes	30
Other Tissues	35
Total	340

[a] W is weight in kg.

Table 12.14 Elemental Composition of Body Components
(Used in calculation of concentrations of these elements in tissue) (Courtesy ICRP from Publication 23, 1974)

Component	Carbon (%)	Hydrogen (%)	Nitrogen (%)	Oxygen (%)
Water		11		89
Fat	77	12		11
Protein	52	7	16	23
Carbohydrate	42	6		52
Bone Ash				40

Table 12.15 Elemental Content of Body Fat and Body Water (Courtesy ICRP from Publication 23, 1974)

		Elemental Content (g)		
Component	**Mass (g)**	**Carbon**	**Hydrogen**	**Oxygen**
Body Fat	113,500	1.0×10^4	1.6×10^3	1.5×10^3
Essential	1,500	1.2×10^3	1.8×10^2	1.7×10^2
Nonessential	12,000	9.2×10^2	1.4×10^3	1.3×10^3
Body Water	42,000		4.6×10^3	3.7×10^4
Extracellular	18,000		2.0×10^3	1.6×10^4
Intracellular	24,000		2.6×10^3	2.1×10^4

Table 12.16 Assumed Physical Characteristics of the Human Embryo/Fetus
(From NRC NUREG/CR-5631, 1990)

Stage of Gestation (days)	Length (cm)	Mass (g)	Major Axis (cm)	Minor Axis (cm)
30	0.4	0.0335	0.2	0.2
60	3.34	5.24	1.7	0.85
90	10.6	28.1	5.3	1.1
120	18.9	146	9.5	1.9
150	26.8	421	13	2.7
180	33.7	859	17	3.4
210	39.8	1432	20	4.1
240	45.1	2103	23	4.6
270	49.6	2836	25	5.1

Table 12.17 Mean and Standard Error for the Daily Intake of Food Class and Subclass by Regions (in grams)[a] (From EPA 52011-84-015, 1984)

Food Class/Subclass	U.S. Population	Region			
		Northeast	North Central	South	West
Daily Products	308.6 ± 5.3	318.6 ± 10.4	336.1 ± 10.0	253.6 ± 8.4	348.1 ± 12.3
Fresh cow's milk	253.5 ± 4.9	256.1 ± 9.7	279.7 ± 9.4	211.0 ± 7.8	283.5 ± 11.5
Other	55.1 ± 1.2	62.5 ± 2.3	56.5 ± 2.2	42.6 ± 1.9	64.6 ± 2.7
Eggs	26.9 ± .5	23.8 ± 1.0	23.5 ± .9	31.0 ± .8	29.1 ± 1.2
Meats	172.2 ± 1.6	169.9 ± 5.3	176.9 ± 3.1	171.9 ± 2.6	168.6 ± 3.9
Beef & veal	87.6 ± 1.1	82.3 ± 2.3	92.9 ± 2.2	84.0 ± 1.8	92.9 ± 2.7
Pork	28.2 ± .6	28.8 ± 1.1	29.6 ± 1.1	30.1 ± .9	22.1 ± 1.3
Poultry	31.3 ± .8	31.7 ± 1.5	26.6 ± 1.4	36.5 ± 1.2	28.9 ± 1.8
Other	25.1 ± .4	27.1 ± .9	27.8 ± .8	21.3 ± .7	24.7 ± 1.0
Fish	17.5 ± .5	20.5 ± 1.1	14.7 ± 1.0	17.0 ± .8	18.5 ± 1.2
Fin fish	14.7 ± .4	16.7 ± .9	13.1 ± .8	14.2 ± .7	15.2 ± 1.0
Shellfish	2.6 ± .2	3.6 ± .5	1.5 ± .4	2.6 ± .4	2.8 ± .5
Produce	282.6 ± 3.5	270.6 ± 6.9	282.4 ± 6.7	280.7 ± 5.6	303.1 ± 8.2
Leafy	39.2 ± .8	38.1 ± 1.5	37.1 ± 1.5	38.4 ± 1.2	45.3 ± 1.8
Exposed	86.0 ± 1.5	88.5 ± 3.0	87.8 ± 2.9	76.9 ± 2.4	95.5 ± 3.6
Protected	150.4 ± 2.3	137.2 ± 4.5	150.1 ± 4.3	160.1 ± 3.6	152.5 ± 5.3
Other	7.0 ± .3	6.9 ± .6	7.3 ± .5	5.4 ± .4	9.8 ± .7
Grain	200.0 ± 3.0	203.5 ± 5.8	192.8 ± 5.6	202.2 ± 4.7	202.6 ± 6.9
Breads	147.3 ± 1.4	153.1 ± 2.8	150.9 ± 2.7	143.9 ± 2.3	139.5 ± 3.3
Cereals	29.9 ± 1.3	24.6 ± 2.5	28.7 ± 2.4	34.6 ± 2.0	30.9 ± 3.0
Other	22.9 ± 1.7	25.9 ± 3.3	13.3 ± 3.2	23.7 ± 2.7	32.1 ± 4.0
Beverages	1434. ± 13.7	1288. ± 27.0	1448 ± 26.0	1513 ± 21.8	1480 ± 32.1
Tap water	662.5 ± 9.9	520.9 ± 19.5	659.8 ± 18.8	748.5 ± 15.7	714.4 ± 23.1
Water based	457.1 ± 6.7	418.5 ± 13.3	476.0 ± 12.8	470.5 ± 10.7	458.2 ± 15.8
Soups	45.9 ± 1.2	52.2 ± 2.4	48.9 ± 2.3	36.8 ± 1.9	48.1 ± 2.9
Other	269.9 ± 4.7	297.2 ± 9.4	264.5 ± 9.0	258.1 ± 7.5	260.6 ± 11.1
Miscellaneous	34.6 ± .7	31.4 ± 1.4	37.0 ± 1.3	32.3 ± 1.1	39.2 ± 1.6

[a] Data based on 1977–1978 USDA National Food Consumption Survey.

Table 12.18 Average Daily Fluid Consumption Rate by Age Group (With permission of the Journal of the American Dietetic Association from Pennington, 1983)

	Total Average Daily Consumption Rate l/day	
Age Group	**Total Fluids[a]**	**Water and Water-Based Foods[b]**
6–11 months	0.689	0.201
2 years	0.930	0.499
14–16 years	1.470	0.746
25–30 years	1.750	1.066
60–65 years	1.645	1.295

[a] Includes milk/formula/milk-based soup, carbonated soda, alcoholic beverages, canned juices, water, coffee, tea, reconstituted juices, and reconstituted soups. From the Total Diet Study.

[b] Includes water, coffee, tea, reconstituted juices, and reconstituted soups.

Table 12.19 Mean and Standard Error for the Daily Intake of Beverages[a] and Tap Water by Age (From USEPA EPA-520/1-84-021, 1984)

Age	Beverage Intake (ml)	Tap Water Intake (ml)
All ages	1434 ± 13.7	662.5 ± 9.9
Under 1	307 ± 89.2	170.7 ± 64.5
1 to 4	743 ± 43.5	434.6 ± 31.4
5 to 9	861 ± 36.5	521.0 ± 26.4
10 to 14	1025 ± 34.2	620.2 ± 24.7
15 to 19	1241 ± 35.9	664.7 ± 26.0
20 to 24	1484 ± 46.9	656.4 ± 33.9
25 to 29	1531 ± 48.0	619.8 ± 34.6
30 to 39	1642 ± 37.7	636.5 ± 27.2
40 to 59	1732 ± 29.3	735.3 ± 21.1
60 and over	1547 ± 32.8	762.5 ± 23.7

[a] Includes tap water; water-based drinks such as coffee, tea, soups, and other drinks such as soft drinks, fruitades, alcoholic drinks.

Table 12.20 Measured Fluid Intakes (ml/day) (Courtesy ICRP from Publication 23, 1974)

Subject	Total Fluids (Range)	Milk	Tap Water	Water-Based Drinks[a]
Adults (''normal'' conditions)	1000–2400	120–450	45–730	320–1450
Adults (high environmental temperature to 32°C)	2840–3410 3256 ± (SD = 900)			
Adults (moderately active)	3700			
Children				
5 yr	1100–1200	330–500	ca. 200	ca. 380
14 yr	1310–1670	540–650		540–790

[a] Includes tea, coffee, soft drinks, beer, cider, wine, etc.

Table 12.21 Estimated Minute Ventilation Associated with Activity Level for Average Male Adult (Adapted from USEPA EPA/600/8-85-009, 1985)

Level of Work	l/min	Representative Activities
Light	13	Level walking at 2 mph; washing clothes
Light	19	Level walking at 3 mph; bowling; scrubbing floors
Light	25	Dancing; pushing wheelbarrow with 15 kg load; simple construction; stacking firewood
Moderate	30	Easy cycling; pushing wheelbarrow with 75 kg load; using a sledgehammer
Moderate	35	Climbing stairs; playing tennis; digging with spade
Moderate	40	Cycling at 13 mph; walking on snow, digging trenches
Heavy	55	Cross-country skiing; rock climbing; stair climbing with load; playing squash or handball; chopping with axe
Heavy	63	
Very heavy	72	
Very heavy	85	Level running at 10 mph; competitive cycling
Severe	100+	Competitive long distance running; cross-country skiing

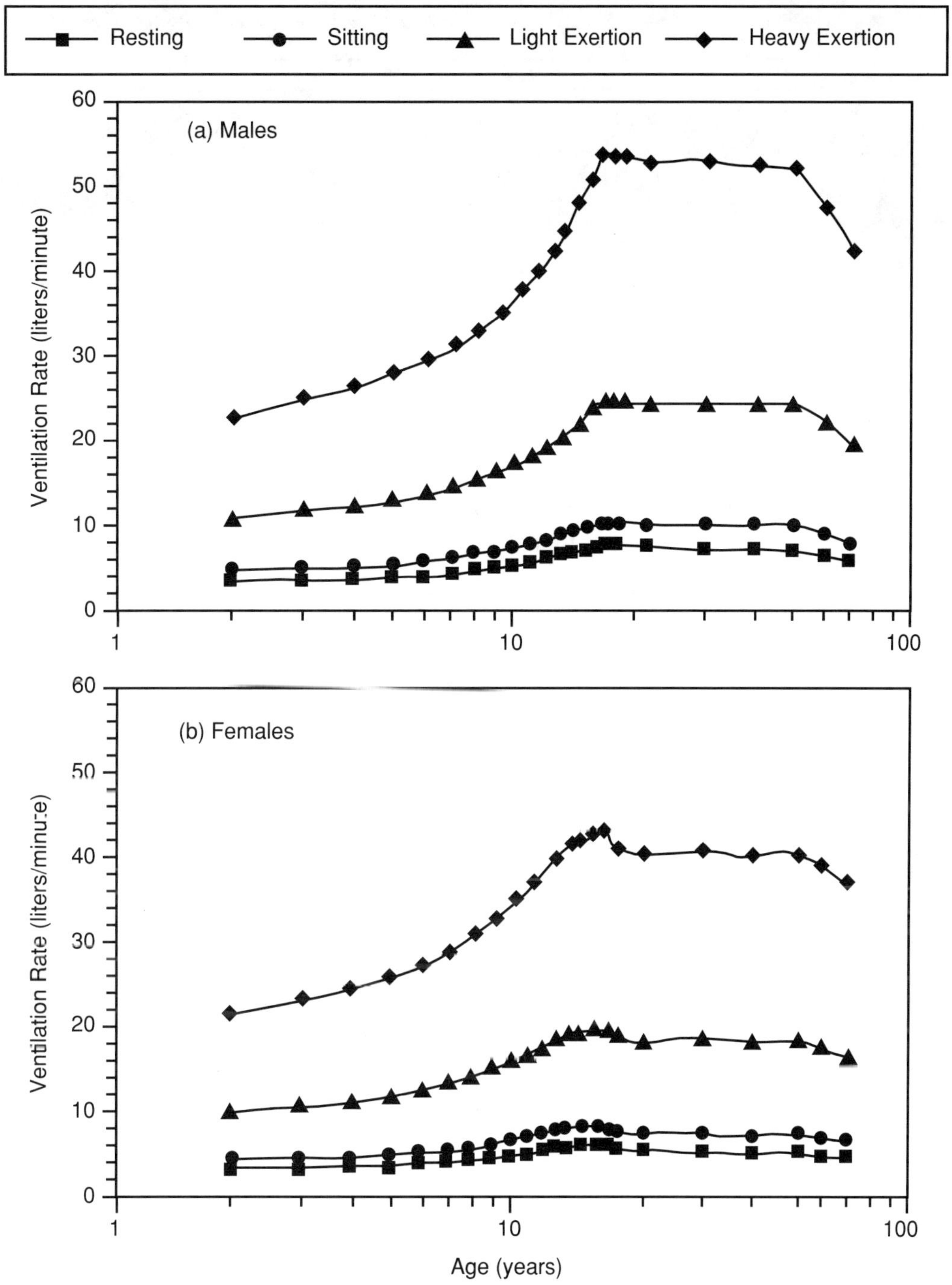

Figure 12.14 Ventilation Rate versus Age for Various Exertion Levels. Predicted average values for ventilation rate as a function of age for (a) males and (b) females. Each data point is based on 1000 trials using Latin hypercube sampling techniques. (Courtesy of Huston, 1995)

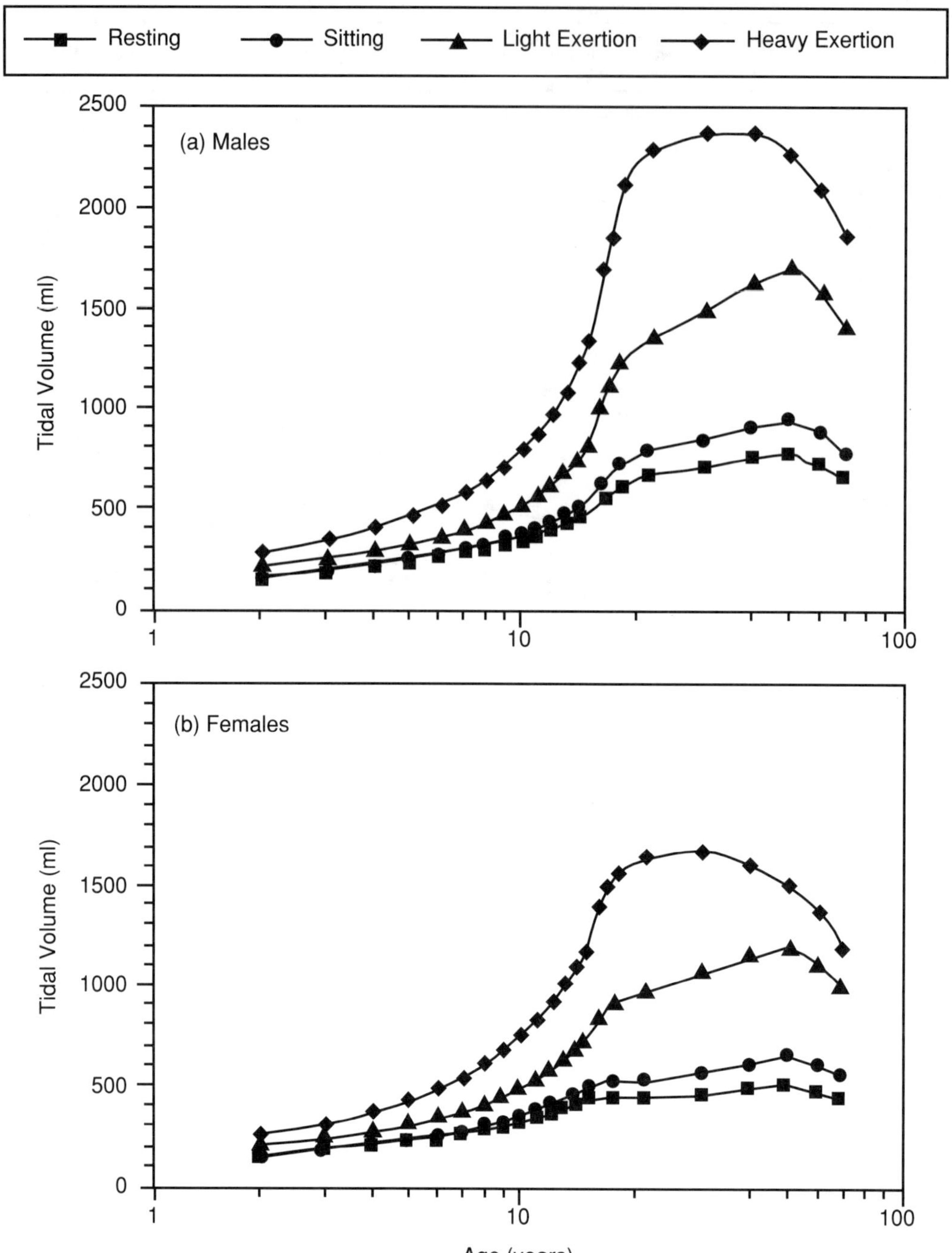

Tidal volume at various physical exertion levels for (a) males and (b) females at different ages. Based on 1000 realizations using Latin hypercube sampling techniques.

Figure 12.15 Tidal Volume Versus Age for Various Exertion Levels (Courtesy of Huston, 1995)

Table 12.22 Surface Area by Body Part for Adults (m^2) (Adapted from USEPA EPA/600/8-85-010, 1985)

Body Part	Men Mean (s.d.)[a]	Men Min	Men Max.[b]	Men n	Women Mean (s.d.)[a]	Women Min.	Women Max[b]	Women n
Head	0.118 (0.0160)[c]	0.090	0.161	29	0.110 (0.00625)[c]	0.0953	0.127	54
Trunk	0.569 (0.0140)	0.306	0.893	29	0.542 (0.0712)	0.437	0.867	54
Upper extremities	0.319 (0.0461)	0.169	0.429	48	0.276 (0.0241)	0.215	0.333	57
Arms	0.228 (0.0374)	0.109	0.292	32	0.210 (0.0129)	0.193	0.235	13
Upper arms	0.143 (0.0143)	0.122	0.156	6	—		—	—
Forearms	0.114 (0.0127)	0.0945	0.136	6	—		—	—
Hands	0.084 (0.0127)	0.0596	0.113	32	0.0746 (0.00510)	0.0639	0.0824	12
Lower extremities	0.636 (0.0994)	0.283	0.858	48	0.626 (0.0675)	0.492	0.809	57
Legs	0.505 (0.0885)	0.221	0.656	32	0.488 (0.0515)	0.423	0.585	13
Thighs	0.198 (0.1470)	0.128	0.403	32	0.258 (0.0333)	0.258	0.360	13
Lower legs	0.207 (0.0379)	0.093	0.296	32	0.194 (0.0240)	0.165	0.229	13
Feet	0.112 (0.0177)	0.0811	0.156	32	0.0975 (0.00903)	0.0834	0.115	13
Total	1.94 (0.00374)[a]	1.66	2.28[b]	48	1.69 (0.00374)[a]	1.45	2.09[b]	58

[a] s.d. = standard deviation
[b] percentiles (5th–95th)
[c] median (standard error)
n = number of observations

Table 12.23 Intakes of Uranium of Various Enrichments To Produce 25-rem Effective Dose Equivalent (From NUREG–1391)

Uranium Enrichment (% U-235)	Specific Activity (μCi g^{-1})[a]	Effective Dose Equivalent per gram U (rem)	Intake to Produce 25-rem Effective Dose Equivalent (milligrams)
0.71	0.67	1.7	14,700
4	1.97	5.0	5,000
20	9.36	23.7	1,060
50	27.90	70.7	353
93	65.2	165.0	151

[a] Specific activity is controlled by the U-234 content that is assumed for each enrichment level, e.g., see Table 12.25.

Table 12.24 Uranium Activity Versus Isotopic Enrichments (After HPS N13.22, with permission from the Health Physics Society, 1995)

Percent U-235	Bq Total Uranium Activity for 7.4 Bq of U-235 (HPS 1987)[a]
3	180
5	163
7	158
10	156
15	159
20	161
30	170
40	180
50	192
60	203
70	214
80	226
93	240

Percent of U-235	Percent of U-238	Bq Total Uranium Activity for 110 Bq U-238 (HPS 1987)[a]
0.0	100.0	110
0.2	99.8	143
0.7	99.3	228
1.0	99.0	279

[a] The values of 7.4 Bq (0.2 nCi) U-235 and 110 Bq (3 nCi) U-238 were estimated to be reasonably attainable MDAs for in-vivo counting (Health Physics Society, 1987). Recent determinations of specific activity at the Portsmouth Gaseous Diffusion Plant have shown that variations of about a factor of two from the specific activity formulae in 10 CFR Part 20 can be obtained, but these variations are limited to variations of about 30% for enrichments used in commercial fuel (Manninen, 1994). Variations are due mainly to variations in the U-234 to U-238 ratio for different gaseous diffusion processes.

Table 12.25 Specific Activities of Each Uranium Isotope as a Function of Weight Percent U-235 and Average Alpha Energies for Each Isotope (From HPS N13.22-1995, with permission from the Health Physics Society, 1995)

	dpm mg^{-1} of Total Uranium[a]				
Percent U-235	**U-234**	**U-235**	**U-236**	**U-238**	**Total**
Normal	.745	.033	.001	.745	1.524
2%	1.514	.095	.002	.725	2.336
4%	3.854	.190	.004	.710	4.758
93%	144.52	4.427	.294	.041	149.28
Average Alpha Energy	4.76	4.26	4.48	4.18	

[a] Note that exact proportions of these isotopes can vary for different enrichment processes (Manninen, 1994).

References

Boecker, et al. ''Current status of bioassay procedures to detect and quantify previous exposures to radioactive materials,'' *Health Physics* **60(1)**:45–100; 1991.

Environmental Protection Agency. *Development of Statistical Distributions or Ranges of Standard Factors Used in Exposure Assessment.* Office of Health and Environmental Assessment, Exposure Assessment Group, USEPA. EPA-600/8–85–010; Washington, DC; 1985.

Environmental Protection Agency. *An Estimation of the Daily Food Intake Based on Data from the 1977–1978 USDA Nationwide Food Consumption Survey.* Office of Radiation Prog., USEPA. EPA-520/1–84–015; Washington, DC; 1984.

Environmental Protection Agency. *An Estimation of the Daily Average Food Intake by Age and Sex for Use in Assessing the Radionuclide Intake of Individuals in the General Population.* Office of Radiation Prog., USEPA. EPA-520/1–84–021; Washington, DC; 1984.

Health Physics Society. *An American National Standard-Bioassay Programs for Uranium.* HPS N13.22–1995; McLean, VA; 1995.

Huston, T.E. *Quantifying Uncertainties in Lung Dosimetry With Application to Plutonium Oxide Aerosols.* Doctoral Dissertation; University of Florida, Gainesville, FL; 1995.

International Commission on Radiation Units and Measurements. *Phantoms and Computational Models in Therapy, Diagnosis and Protection.* ICRU Report 48; Bethesda, MD; 1992.

International Commission on Radiological Protection. *Human Respiratory Tract Model for Radiological Protection.* ICRP Publication 66; Annals of the ICRP.24 (1–3); 1994.

International Commission on Radiological Protection. *Age-dependent Doses to Members of the Public from Intake of Radionuclides.* ICRP Publication 56; Pergamon Press; Oxford; 1989.

International Commission on Radiological Protection. *Individual Monitoring for Intakes of Radionuclides by Workers: Design and Interpretation.* ICRP Publication 54; Pergamon Press; Oxford; 1987.

International Commission on Radiological Protection. *General Principles of Monitoring for Radiation Protection of Workers.* ICRP Publication 35; Pergamon Press; Oxford; 1982.

International Commission on Radiological Protection. *Limits for Intakes of Radionuclides by Workers.* ICRP Publication 30, Part 1; Pergamon Press; Oxford; 1978.

International Commission on Radiological Protection. *Recommendations of the Oxford International Commission on Radiological Protection.* ICRP Publication 26; Pergamon Press; Oxford; 1977.

International Commission on Radiological Protection. *Report of the Task Group on Reference Man.* ICRP Publication 23; Pergamon Press; Oxford; 1974.

Nuclear Regulatory Commission. *Contribution of Material Radionuclide Burdens to Prenatal Radiation Doses-Interim Recommendations.* NUREG/CR-5631; 1990.

Nuclear Regulatory Commission. *Interpretation of Bioassay Measurements.* NUREG/CR-4884; Brookhaven National Laboratory; Upton, NY; 1987.

Nuclear Regulation Commission. NUREG-1391.

Pennington, J.A.T. ''Revision of the total diet study food list and diets,'' *J Am Dietetic Assoc* **82:**166–173; 1983.

Piechowski, J., Menoux, B. ''Assessment of radioactive systemic uptakes by deconvolution of individual monitoring results,'' *Health Physics* **70(4)**:537–545; 1996.

Shleren, B., Schmidt, G.D., Chiacchierini, R.P. *Background for Protection Action Recommendation: Accidental Radioactive Contamination of Food and Animal Feeds.* Food and Drug Administration. HHS Publication. FDA 82-8196; Rockville, MD; 1982.

CHAPTER 13

RADIATION DOSIMETRY

This chapter presents information on photon, alpha, radon, beta, neutron and proton dosimetry. It begins with a brief discussion of dosimetric quantities and units, and factors influencing the calculation of radiation dose, then continues its discussion with data on external radiation dosimetry from varying geometric configurations and sources; these include radionuclides deposited on the ground, in a radioactive cloud or in an aqueous environment.

A short discussion of alpha particle dosimetry with particular emphasis on radon is included. Beta dosimetry from point sources and beta emitters uniformly deposited on the skin is presented in several figures and tables.

This chapter also provides reference material on shallow and deep dose equivalents on the International Commission on Radiation Units and Measurement (ICRU) sphere from various incident beam geometries for an anthropomorphic phantom.

Selected organ doses from external sources of photons and neutrons supplement extensive tables of dose factors for internally deposited radionuclides which enter the body through ingestion and inhalation.

TABLE OF CONTENTS

Table 13.1 Quantities and Units Used in 10CFR20 (After NUREG-1437, 1991 and 10CFR20, 1991)

Quantities and Units

The unit *rad* is usually used for the quantity *radiation absorbed dose* whenever early biological effects are the concern. When latent effects (e.g., cancer and genetic effects) are being considered, the unit *rem* is used for the *dose equivalent* (DE) quantity. The absorbed dose in rads is multiplied by an overall efficiency factor Q to obtain the dose equivalent in rem. Each type of radiation has its own value of Q which, in a very rough way, makes absorbed doses from different radiations additive for latent effects.

These values of Q reflect the overall efficiency of a given type of radiation in causing latent effects and are not used for early effects such as acute radiation syndrome. In the old Part 20, these Q values are also applied to protection of the eye lens from cataracts and protection of the skin from cosmetic effects. The values were derived in consideration of the ability of the various radiations to ionize atoms in water as well as the Relative Biological Effectiveness factors (RBEs) observed for specific effects. Most of the dose limits given in the old Part 20 are DE, and the rem unit is used.

Table 13.1.1 presents Q for all types of radiation except neutrons and the relationship between absorbed dose and dose equivalent. Quality Factors and fluence per unit dose equivalent as a function of neutron energy from the 10CFR20 regulations are presented in Table 13.1.2.

Table 13.1.1 Quality Factors and Absorbed Dose Equivalencies

Type of Radiation	Quality Factor (Q)[a]	Absorbed Dose Equal to a Unit Dose Equivalent[b]
X, gamma, or beta radiation	1	1
Alpha particles, multiple-charged particles, fission fragments and heavy particles of unknown charge	20	0.05
Neutrons of unknown energy	10	0.1
High-energy protons	10	0.1

[a] See Table 4.2.3.2 for ICRP *Radiation Weighting Factors.*

[b] Absorbed dose in rad equal to 1 rem or the absorbed dose in gray equal to 1 sievert.

Table 13.1.2 Mean Quality Factors, Q, and Fluence per Unit Dose Equivalent for Monoenergetic Neutrons[a]

	Neutron Energy (MeV)	Quality Factor[b] (Q)	Fluence per Unit Dose Equivalent[c] (Neutrons cm^{-2} rem^{-1})
(thermal)	2.5×10^{-8}	2	980×10^6
	1×10^{-7}	2	980×10^6
	1×10^{-6}	2	810×10^6
	1×10^{-5}	2	810×10^6
	1×10^{-4}	2	840×10^6
	1×10^{-3}	2	980×10^6
	1×10^{-2}	2.5	1010×10^6
	1×10^{-1}	7.5	170×10^6
	5×10^{-1}	11	39×10^6
	1	11	27×10^6
	2.5	9	29×10^6
	5	8	23×10^6
	7	7	24×10^6
	10	6.5	24×10^6
	14	7.5	17×10^6
	20	8	16×10^6
	40	7	14×10^6
	60	5.5	16×10^6
	1×10^2	4	20×10^6
	2×10^2	3.5	19×10^6
	3×10^2	3.5	16×10^6
	4×10^2	3.5	14×10^6

[a] See Figure 4.2.3.1 for ICRP *Radiation Weighting Factors* for neutrons.

[b] Value of quality factor (Q) at the point where the dose equivalent is maximum in a 30 cm diameter cylinder tissue equivalent phantom.

[c] Monoenergetic neutrons incident normally on a 30 cm diameter cylinder tissue-equivalent phantom.

Collective Dose

The collective dose equivalent (person-rem) is used extensively by the NRC in risk analyses and in its decision-making processes. The collective dose equivalent may be obtained as the sum of all individual doses or as the product of the average individual dose and the number of people exposed.

Penetrating and Shallow DE

Part 20 requires measurement of the penetrating DE at a tissue depth of 1 cm (1000 mg/cm^2) or less. It is recognized, of course, that this DE is not representative of the DE to the internal organs—particularly those located at considerable depth. However, measurement at 1 cm or less is comparatively simple and inexpensive; and this depth is adequate for regulatory control. The shallow DE is used only in the protection of the skin and must be measured at a depth of 0.007 cm or less. The basal cell layer is assumed to be located at this depth, and the DE limits are based on the risk to these cells, which renew the skin. The *penetrating dose equivalent* is now called the *deep dose equivalent.*

In addition to the above quantities and units, 10CFR20 employs concepts introduced by the International Commission on Radiation Protection such as Annual Limit of Intake, Dose Equivalent (or ICRP's Equivalent Dose), Effective Dose Equivalent (or ICRP's Effective Dose), Committed Effective Dose Equivalent, Annual Limit of Intake and Derived Air Concentrations. These are reviewed in Chapter 4 (Tables 4.2.3–4.2.7) ***The NRC tissue weighting factors differ from those of the ICRP 60 (Table 4.2.3.3) and are presented below.***

Table 13.1.3 Organ Dose Weighting Factors (W_T Defined by the NRC for Calculating the Effective Dose Equivalent)[a]

Organ or Tissue	W_T
Gonads	0.25
Breast	0.15
Red bone marrow	0.12
Lung	0.12
Thyroid	0.03
Bone surfaces	0.03
Remainder	0.30[b]
Whole Body	1.00[c]

[a] For ICRP *Tissue Weighting Factors* see Table 4.2.3.3.
[b] 0.30 results from 0.06 for each of 5 ''remainder'' organs (excluding the skin and the lens of the eye) that receive the highest doses.
[c] For the purpose of weighting the external whole body dose (for adding it to the internal dose) single weighting factor, $W_T = 1.0$, has been specified. The use of other weighting factors for external exposure will be approved on a case-by-case basis at such time as specific guidance is issued.

Table 13.2 Summary of Estimated RBE_M Values for Fission Neutrons Versus Gamma Rays

(Courtesy NCRP from Report No. 104, 1990)

End Point	Range of Values[a]
Cytogenetic studies, human lymphocytes in culture	34–53
Transformation	3–80[b]
Genetic endpoints in mammalian systems	5–70[c]
Genetic endpoints in plant systems	2–100
Life shortening, mouse	10–46
Tumor induction	16–59

[a] Values taken from larger tables or data given in earlier sections of NCRP Report No. 104, 1990.
[b] This value of 80 was derived from one set of experiments only.
[c] The value of 70; derived from data on specific locus mutations in mice, is not necessarily an RBE_M.

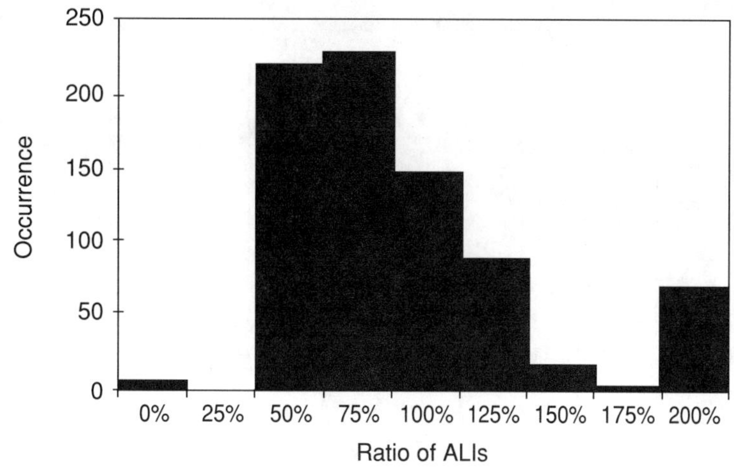

Histogram of ratio of ALIs for ingestion intakes from 10 CFR Part 20 (U.S. NRC, 1991) to ICRP Publication 61 (ICRP, 1990), following an adjustment for differing dose limits.

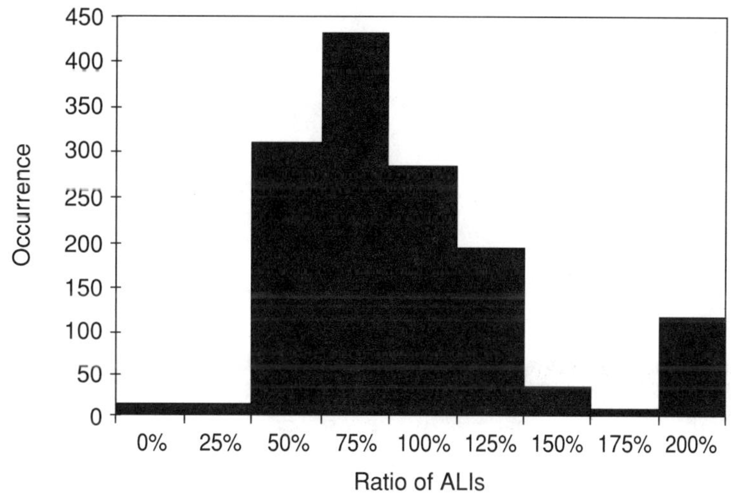

Histogram of ratio of ALIs for inhalation intakes from 10 CFR Part 20 (U.S. NRC, 1991) to ICRP Publication 61 (ICRP, 1990), following an adjustment for differing dose limits.

Figure 13.1 A Comparison of 10CFR20 and ICRP 61 ALIs. These illustrations point out the differences between 10CFR20 and ICRP61 Annual Limits on Intake (ingestion and inhalation) even when differing dose limits are considered. It is evident that care should be taken in choosing an ALI and in interpretation of information based on them. (From Kearfott and Zhu, 1996)

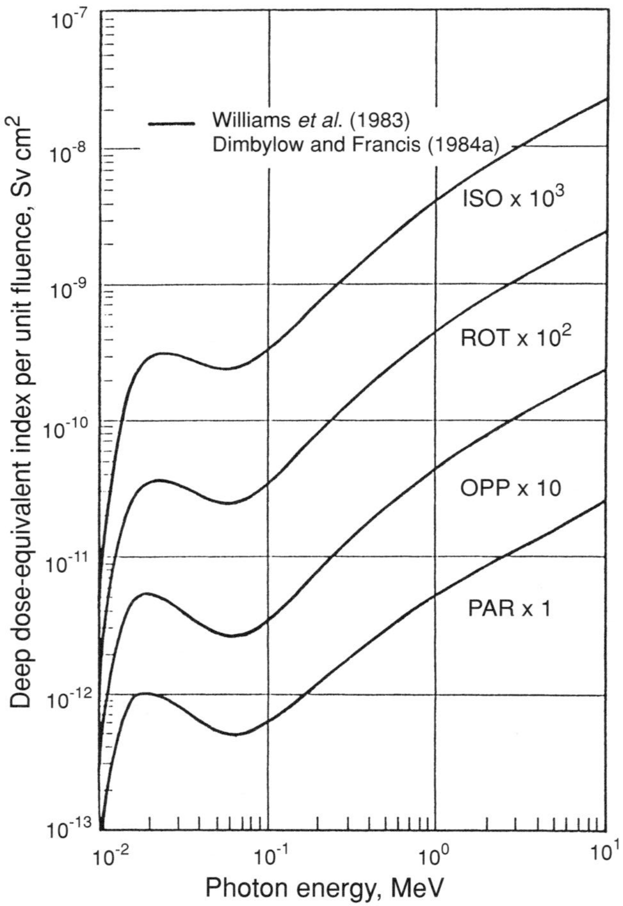

Figure 13.2 Deep Dose-Equivalent Index, $H_{I,d'}$ per unit fluence for photons incident in various geometries on the ICRU sphere. See notes to figures 13.2, 13.3 and 13.4 which follow figure 13.4 for further information. (Courtesy ICRP from Publication 51, 1987)

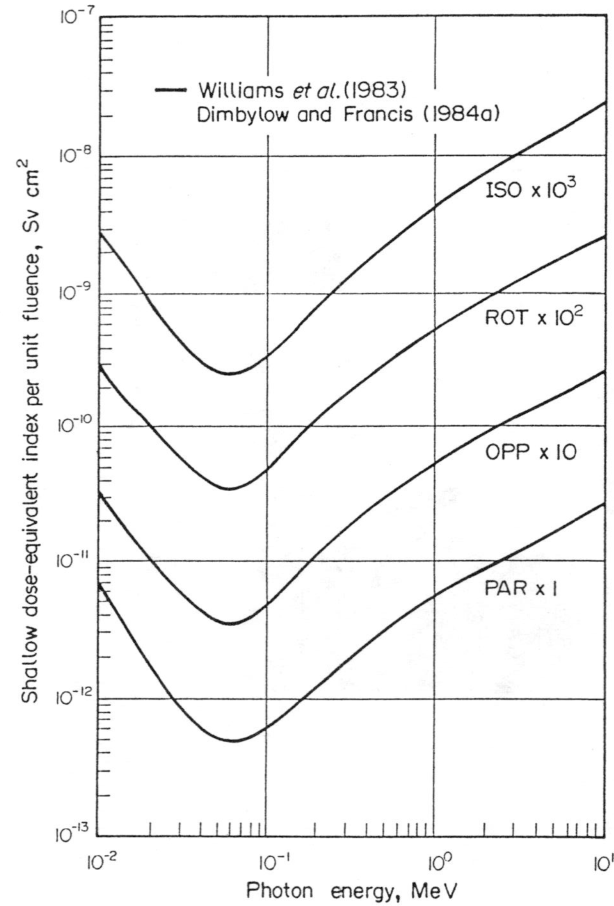

Figure 13.3 Shallow Dose-Equivalent Index $H_{I,s'}$ per unit fluence for photons incident in various geometries on the ICRU sphere. See notes to figures 13.2 13.3, and 13.4 which follow figure 13.4 for further information. (Courtesy ICRP from Publication 51, 1987)

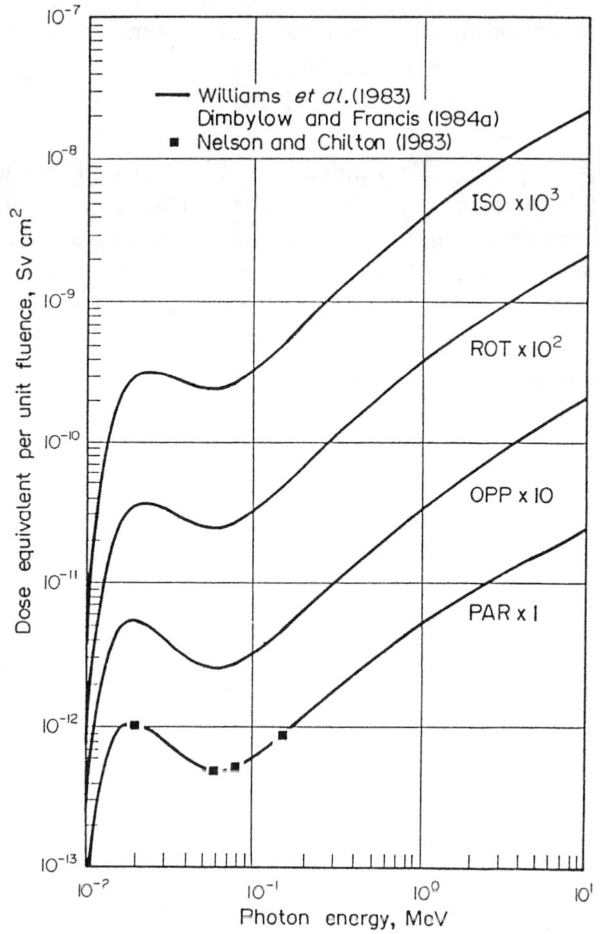

Figure 13.4 Dose Equivalent per Unit Fluence on the Principal Axis at a depth of 10 mm for photons incident in various geometries on the ICRU sphere. See notes to figures 13.2, 13.3, and 13.4 which follow for further information. (Courtesy ICRP from Publication 51, 1987)

Notes to Figures 13.2, 13.3, and 13.4

The anteroposterior (AP) geometry refers to irradiation from the front of the body to the back with the beam at right angles to the long axis of the body. Conversely, the posteroanterior (PA) geometry refers to irradiation from the back to the front. The LAT geometry refers to lateral irradiation from either side. These geometries are intended to represent irradiation of a person whose orientation is fixed relative to the location of the source.

There are two ways of defining the rotational geometry, which is labelled ROT. It is created by rotating the body about its long axis at a uniform rate in a broad unidirectional beam at right angles to the axis of rotation. The same effect is created by rotating such a field at a uniform rate around the long axis of the fixed body. This geometry may be seen as an approximation to the irradiation pattern of a person moving around unsystematically relative to the location of a source.

Isotropic irradiation occurs with a radiation field in which the flux of particles per unit solid angle is independent of direction. Such geometry would be approximated by a body suspended in a cloud of radioactive gas virtually infinite in extent, although the radiation would not be monoenergetic. Other applications of the results for isotropic irradiation are discussed in ICRP Publication 51, 1987.

For the ICRU sphere, four idealized geometries are sometimes discussed, three involving, broad beams—single plane parallel beam, two opposed plane parallel beams, rotating plane parallel beam—with the fourth being an isotropic field. They are identified as PAR, OPP, ROT, and ISO respectively.

Conversion coefficients are presented in figures 13.2, 13.3 and 13.4 for monoenergetic photons with energies from 10 keV to MeV incident on the ICRU sphere. The data refer to the relationship between fluence and various quantities comprising the restricted dose-equivalent indices, $H_{I,d'}$ and $H_{I,s'}$ and the dose equivalents on the principal axis at a depth of 10 mm; the principal axis is the axis of symmetry for a parallel beam. Irradiation geometries are a plane parallel beam, two opposed plane parallel beams, and a 360° rotating plane parallel beam. Data for an isotropic field are also given. The values for the single plane parallel beam at a depth of 10 mm are numerically the same as for the ambient dose equivalent at the recommended depth (ICRU, 1986a).

Table 13.3 Conversion Factors for Monenergetic Photons for Computing Dose Equivalent from Exposure in Free Air (1 rem $= 10^{-2}$ Sv; 1 R $= 2.58 \times 10^{-4}$ C kg^{-1}) (With permission of publisher Ehrlich, 1981)

Photon Energy (keV)	Conversion Factor (rem R^{-1}) to Dose Equivalent in the ICRU Sphere at a Depth of 1.0 cm ("deep")	0.3 cm	0.007 cm ("shallow")
15	0.28	0.67	0.90
20	0.58	0.79	0.94
30	1.00	1.07	1.11
40	1.28	1.29	1.34
50	1.46	1.46	1.50
60	1.47	1.47	1.52
70	1.45	1.45	1.50
80	1.43	1.43	1.48
90	1.41	1.41	1.45
100	1.39	1.39	1.43
110	1.37	1.37	1.40
120	1.35	1.35	1.36
130	1.33	1.33	1.34
140	1.32	1.32	1.32
150	1.30	1.30	1.30
662	1.03	1.01	1.03

Table 13.4 Comparison of Average Conversion Factors for Computing Dose Equivalent from Exposure in Free Air (1 rem = 10^{-2} Sv; 1 R = 2.58×10^{-4} C kg^{-1}) With permission of publisher Ehrlich, 1981)

	Bremsstrahlun Technique[a]				Conversion Factor ($rem\ R^{-1}$) to [b]		
Constant Potential (kV_cP)	Added Filter (Al mm)	Added Filter (Cu mm)	Half Value Layer (Al mm)	Homogeneity Coefficient (1st Al HVL / 2nd Al HVL)	Average Energy (keV)	Deep Dose Equivalent	Shallow Dose Equivalent
30	0.5	—	0.36	0.64	20	0.40 (0.45)	0.92 (1.08)
50	1.0	—	1.02	0.66	29	0.72 (0.81)	1.03 (1.13)
75	1.5	—	1.86	0.63	39	0.95 (1.00)	1.14 (1.21)
100	3.50	—	5.03	0.73	51	1.20 (1.25)	1.30 (1.25)
150	3.49	0.25	10.25	0.89	70	1.38 (1.47)	1.43 (1.41)
^{137}Cs gamma radiation						1.03 (1.03)	1.03 (—)

[a] The inherent filtration for the bremsstrahlung spectra produced at constant potentials of 30 to 75 keV is 1.0 mm Be, that for the higher energies is 1.5 mm Al.

[b] Shown are both the factors specified in the standard for the bremsstrahlung spectra to be used in the testing program and those measured by Yoder et al (in parentheses).

Table 13.5 Conversion Coefficients Relating Air Kerma in Free Air, K_a, Fluence, ϕ, and Exposure, X, for Monoenergetic Photons The quantity g is the fraction of kerma lost to bremsstrahlung (ICRU 47, 1992)

Photon Energy (keV)	K_a/ϕ (pGy cm^2)	X/ϕ nR (nR cm^2)	K_a/X (mGy R^{-1})	1-g
10	7.43	0.848	8.76	1.00
15	3.12	0.357	8.76	1.00
20	1.68	0.192	8.76	1.00
30	0.721	0.0823	8.76	1.00
40	0.429	0.0489	8.76	1.00
50	0.323	0.0369	8.76	1.00
60	0.289	0.0330	8.76	1.00
80	0.307	0.0350	8.76	1.00
100	0.371	0.0424	8.76	1.00
150	0.599	0.069	8.76	1.00
200	0.856	0.098	8.76	1.00
300	1.38	0.157	8.76	1.00
400	1.89	0.216	8.76	1.00
500	2.38	0.271	8.76	1.00
600	2.84	0.324	8.76	1.00
800	3.69	0.422	8.76	1.00
1000	4.47	0.509	8.76	1.00
1500	6.14	0.699	8.76	0.996
2000	7.54	0.857	8.83	0.995
3000	9.96	1.127	8.85	0.991
4000	12.1	[a]	[a]	0.988
5000	14.1			0.984
6000	16.1			0.980
8000	20.1			0.972
10000	24.0			0.964

[a] The exposure, X, is not accurately determined at energies above 3 MeV since there is significant departure from electronic equilibrium.

Table 13.6 Conversion Coefficients for Monoenergetic Photons, Relating Ambient Dose Equivalent, H*(10), Fluence, ϕ, Air Kerma, K_a, and Exposure, X, and Relating Directional Dose Equivalent, H′(0.07), to Fluence and Air Kerma. Values of $H^*(10)/K_a$ and $H'(0.07)/K_a$, are derived from the empirical functions of Wagner et al. (1985) (with the exception of values of $H^*(10)/K_a$, at energies less than 20 keV) and other quantities are calculated from these and the values of Table 13.5.

(After ICRU 47, 1992)

Photon Energy (keV)	$H^*(10)/\phi$ (pSv cm^2)	$H^*(10)/K_a$ (Sv Gy^{-1})	$H^*(10)/X$ (cSv R^{-1})	$H'(0.07)/\phi$ (pSv cm^2)	$H'(0.07)/K_a$ (Sv Gy^{-1})
10	0.077	0.0103	0.0091	7.1	0.95
15	0.85	0.271	0.237	3.10	0.99
20	1.00	0.60	0.521	1.76	1.05
30	0.79	1.10	0.96	0.88	1.22
40	0.63	1.47	1.29	0.60	1.41
50	0.54	1.67	1.46	0.50	1.53
60	0.50	1.74	1.52		
80	0.53	1.72	1.51		
100	0.61	1.65	1.44		
150	0.89	1.49	1.31		
200	1.20	1.40	1.22		
300	1.80	1.31	1.14		
400	2.38	1.26	1.10		
500	2.93	1.23	1.08		
600	3.44	1.21	1.06		
800	4.38	1.19	1.04		
1000	5.2	1.17	1.03		
1500	7.0	1.15	1.01		
2000	8.6	1.14	1.00		
3000	11.2	1.13	0.99		
4000	13.6	1.12	[a]		
5000	15.7	1.11			
6000	17.9	1.11			
8000	22.3	1.11			
10000	26.4	1.10			

[a] Exposure is not accurately determined at energies above 3 MeV since there is significant departure from electronic equilibrium.

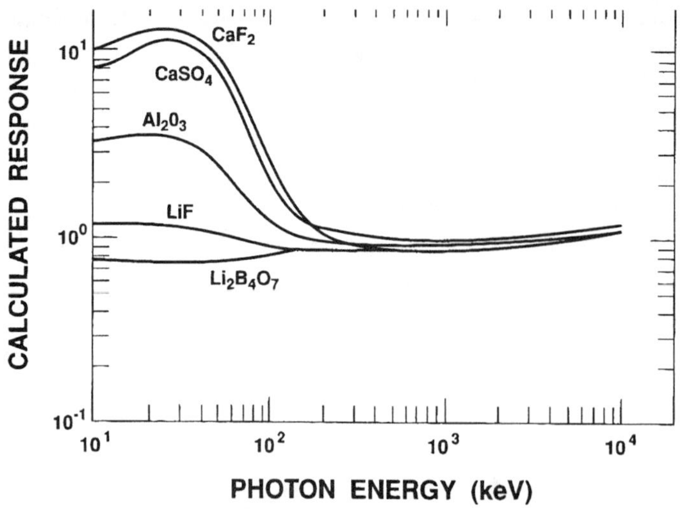

Relative variation of the calculated kerma in thermoluminescent materials, as a function of photon energy. These curves give an approximation to the relative energy response, per unit exposure, for several unshielded TLD materials. Below 100 keV the relative responses of dosimeters will differ significantly from these curves because of the dependence of light output on LET and because of attenuation in the cover.

Figure 13.5 Relative response of TLD materials as a function of photon energy. (From ICRU 47, 1992)

Table 13.7.1 Selected Organ Dose Equivalent per Unit Fluence for Photons Incident in Various Geometries on a Male Anthropomorphic Phantom (Courtesy ICRP from Publication 51, 1987)

Photon Energy (MeV)	AP	PA	LAT	ROT	ISO
		Testes, 10^{-12} Sv cm^2			
$1.0\ 10^{-2}$	0.043	0.000	0.000	0.009	0.043
$1.5\ 10^{-2}$	0.448	0.000	0.000	0.140	0.140
$2.5\ 10^{-2}$	0.662	0.025	0.005	0.218	0.245
$5.0\ 10^{-2}$	0.569	0.104	0.069	0.207	0.209
$6.0\ 10^{-2}$	0.561	0.124	0.084	0.216	0.213
$7.0\ 10^{-2}$	0.592	0.152	0.103	0.248	0.229
$8.0\ 10^{-2}$	0.586	0.166	0.113	0.270	0.243
$1.0\ 10^{-1}$	0.670	0.204	0.137	0.341	0.288
$1.5\ 10^{-1}$	0.984	0.329	0.211	0.507	0.464
$2.0\ 10^{-1}$	1.31	0.510	0.311	0.688	0.632
$3.0\ 10^{-1}$	1.93	0.918	0.571	1.08	0.997
$5.0\ 10^{-1}$	3.00	1.77	1.17	1.91	1.69
$1.0\ 10^{0}$	5.18	3.74	2.85	3.73	3.35
$3.0\ 10^{0}$	11.4	9.43	8.90	8.77	8.44
$6.0\ 10^{0}$	18.4	16.0	15.0	14.7	14.3
$1.0\ 10^{1}$	27.4	23.7	23.1	22.4	24.2
		Red Bone Marrow, 10^{-12} Sv cm^2			
$1.0\ 10^{-2}$	0.000	0.000	0.000	0.000	0.000
$1.5\ 10^{-2}$	0.029	0.004	0.011	0.011	0.004
$2.5\ 10^{-2}$	0.032	0.100	0.031	0.054	0.042
$5.0\ 10^{-2}$	0.119	0.236	0.101	0.151	0.119
$6.0\ 10^{-2}$	0.149	0.297	0.128	0.194	0.147
$7.0\ 10^{-2}$	0.187	0.358	0.154	0.230	0.177
$8.0\ 10^{-2}$	0.213	0.388	0.181	0.255	0.202
$1.0\ 10^{-1}$	0.279	0.478	0.234	0.324	0.261
$1.5\ 10^{-1}$	0.453	0.728	0.374	0.510	0.415
$2.0\ 10^{-1}$	0.628	0.973	0.538	0.713	0.585
$3.0\ 10^{-1}$	0.989	1.44	0.843	1.11	0.911
$5.0\ 10^{-1}$	1.72	2.32	1.47	1.91	1.58
$1.0\ 10^{0}$	3.37	4.19	3.14	3.68	3.11
$3.0\ 10^{0}$	8.42	9.28	8.08	8.75	7.84
$6.0\ 10^{0}$	14.5	15.3	14.0	14.7	13.6
$1.0\ 10^{1}$	21.9	22.6	21.0	22.6	21.1

See notes to Figures 13.2, 13.3 and 13.4 for irradiation geometries.

Table 13.7.2 Selected Organ Dose Equivalent per Unit Fluence for Photons Incident in Various Geometries on a Female Anthropomorphic Phantom (Courtesy ICRP from Publication 51, 1987)

Photon Energy (MeV)	AP	PA	LAT	ROT	ISO
		Ovaries, 10^{-12} Sv cm^2			
$1.0\ 10^{-2}$	0.000	0.000	0.000	0.000	0.000
$1.5\ 10^{-2}$	0.000	0.000	0.000	0.000	0.000
$2.5\ 10^{-2}$	0.077	0.035	0.002	0.029	0.011
$5.0\ 10^{-2}$	0.284	0.217	0.072	0.174	0.125
$6.0\ 10^{-2}$	0.327	0.284	0.098	0.201	0.154
$7.0\ 10^{-2}$	0.378	0.337	0.126	0.240	0.198
$8.0\ 10^{-2}$	0.404	0.361	0.140	0.265	0.214
$1.0\ 10^{-1}$	0.500	0.443	0.175	0.335	0.253
$1.5\ 10^{-1}$	0.708	0.636	0.277	0.510	0.375
$2.0\ 10^{-1}$	0.920	0.858	0.392	0.694	0.520
$3.0\ 10^{-1}$	1.37	1.32	0.649	1.06	0.840
$5.0\ 10^{-1}$	2.26	2.21	1.19	1.81	1.51
$1.0\ 10^{0}$	4.15	4.17	2.49	3.52	3.11
$3.0\ 10^{0}$	9.43	9.66	6.85	8.67	8.19
$6.0\ 10^{0}$	15.7	16.1	12.8	14.7	14.6
$1.0\ 10^{1}$	23.5	24.3	20.1	22.4	22.0
		Breast, 10^{-12} Sv cm^2			
$1.0\ 10^{-2}$	0.376	0.000	0.128	0.179	0.111
$1.5\ 10^{-2}$	0.573	0.000	0.190	0.287	0.207
$2.5\ 10^{-2}$	0.599	0.025	0.237	0.309	0.315
$5.0\ 10^{-2}$	0.450	0.101	0.199	0.243	0.234
$6.0\ 10^{-2}$	0.441	0.111	0.197	0.245	0.235
$7.0\ 10^{-2}$	0.471	0.129	0.221	0.273	0.248
$8.0\ 10^{-2}$	0.481	0.144	0.233	0.284	0.265
$1.0\ 10^{-1}$	0.568	0.194	0.288	0.344	0.317
$1.5\ 10^{-1}$	0.848	0.332	0.461	0.524	0.494
$2.0\ 10^{-1}$	1.15	0.484	0.651	0.725	0.696
$3.0\ 10^{-1}$	1.75	0.831	1.06	1.14	1.11
$5.0\ 10^{-1}$	2.86	1.59	1.83	1.94	1.92
$1.0\ 10^{0}$	5.13	3.37	3.58	3.72	3.72
$3.0\ 10^{0}$	10.5	8.53	8.77	8.83	8.99
$6.0\ 10^{0}$	16.7	14.5	15.1	14.9	15.0
$1.0\ 10^{1}$	25.5	22.4	22.9	22.9	22.0

Table 13.7.2 Selected Organ Dose Equivalent per Unit Fluence for Photons Incident in Various Geometries on a Female Anthropomorphic Phantom (Continued)

Photon Energy (MeV)	AP	PA	LAT	ROT	ISO
			Red Bone Marrow, 10^{-12} Sv cm^2		
$1.0\ 10^{-2}$	0.000	0.000	0.000	0.000	0.000
$1.5\ 10^{-2}$	0.029	0.004	0.011	0.011	0.004
$2.5\ 10^{-2}$	0.032	0.100	0.032	0.154	0.042
$5.0\ 10^{-2}$	0.119	0.259	0.109	0.151	0.120
$6.0\ 10^{-2}$	0.157	0.308	0.136	0.194	0.152
$7.0\ 10^{-2}$	0.200	0.370	0.162	0.236	0.183
$8.0\ 10^{-2}$	0.224	0.402	0.186	0.265	0.214
$1.0\ 10^{-1}$	0.288	0.502	0.242	0.336	0.268
$1.5\ 10^{-1}$	0.467	0.760	0.390	0.528	0.423
$2.0\ 10^{-1}$	0.648	1.01	0.555	0.722	0.600
$3.0\ 10^{-1}$	1.02	1.51	0.881	1.12	0.938
$5.0\ 10^{-1}$	1.76	2.44	1.53	1.92	1.60
$1.0\ 10^{0}$	3.46	4.48	3.18	3.68	3.11
$3.0\ 10^{0}$	8.59	10.0	8.08	8.75	7.84
$6.0\ 10^{0}$	14.5	16.5	13.9	14.7	13.6
$1.0\ 10^{-1}$	21.9	21.5	21.0	22.6	21.1

See notes to figures 13.2, 13.3 and 13.4 for irradiation geometries.

Table 13.8 Alpha Particle Dosimetry (After National Academy of Science BEIR IV Report, 1988)

Alpha particles have a fairly sharply defined range (R), which is the average distance that they travel in coming to rest in a material. Figure 13.6 shows the ranges of alpha particles in soft tissue of unit density. For comparison, the average distances traveled by electrons, neglecting energy straggling, are also given. Because of their very much lower stopping powers, the electrons travel 2 or 3 orders of magnitude farther than alpha particles.

The stopping powers and ranges in tissue suffice for most applications to alpha particle dosimetry. Occasionally, however, it is necessary to consider alpha particle paths that lie partly in one material, partly in another (e.g., partly in soft tissue and partly in bone). Fortunately, the ranges of an alpha particle of a given energy in different materials are proportional to one another, independently of the energy, to within a few percent.

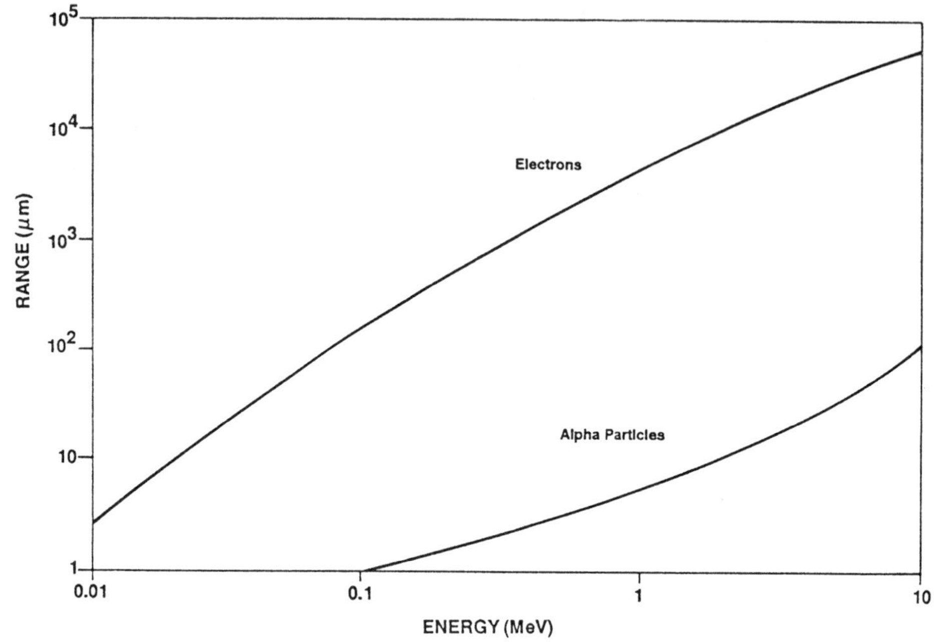

Figure 13.6 Ranges of Alpha Particles and Electrons in Soft Tissue of Unit Density (Reprinted with permission from *Health Risks of Radon and Other Internally Deposited Alpha-Emitters; BEIR IV*, c. 1988 by the National Academy of Sciences. Published by National Academy Press, Washington, DC.)

If one does not require much accuracy, for example, if one is making just a trial or illustrative calculation, the variation of the stopping power E/R Figure 13.7 shows the results of a calculation done in the $e(r) = E/R$ approximation to illustrate the doses from non-equilibrium distribution of alpha particle emitters. In this instance, C alpha particles per unit mass of energy E were emitted from spherical regions of radius a in uniform tissue in which the range of the particles is R. The doses are shown as functions of x, the distance from the center of the sphere. All distances are normalized to the alpha particle range R. Under charged particle equilibrium conditions, the density C would produce a uniform dose, CE; all the doses in Figure 13.7 are normalized to CE.

Figure 13.7 illustrates the conditions required to obtain charged particle equilibrium. For the two largest spheres, radii of 2 and 3 times the range, the dose equals the equilibrium dose CE in the central region of the sphere. There each point is surrounded by emitters out to a distance at least equal to the range of the alpha particles; emitters farther away have no influence on the dose because the particles cannot reach the point. This example illustrates the requirement discussed above that C must be uniform out to distances equal to the range beyond the edge of the region before charged particle equilibrium can exist within it.

Inside the largest spheres, at points less than the alpha particle range from the edge, the dose is less than CE because there are regions within the range that contain no emitters. At the edge of these spheres (that is, for $x = a$), the dose is roughly one half CE (the dose would be exactly one-half CE at a plane surface in an equilibrium region if all the emitters were removed from one side of the plane; small parts of the surfaces of large spheres are shaped much like planes). Outside a sphere of any size, at distances greater than the alpha particle range from the edge, the dose drops to zero because particles cannot penetrate that far.

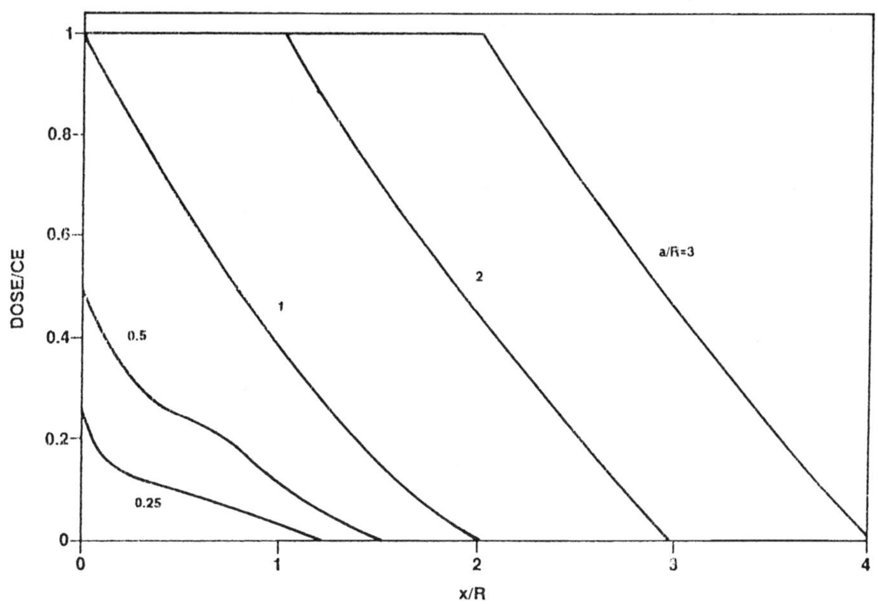

Figure 13.7 Absorbed Dose from Alpha Particles of Energy *E* and Range *R* as a Function of Distance *x* from the Centers of Spherical Regions of Radius *a* that Contain Uniform Concentrations *C* of the Emitter [in the e(r) = *E*/*R* Approximation]. (Reprinted with permission from *Health Risks of Radon and Other Internally Deposited Alpha-Emitters; BEIR IV*, c. 1988 by the National Academy of Sciences. Published by National Academy Press, Washington DC)

The figure also suggests that the average dose *(D)* discussed above in the sphere is a reasonable estimate of the dose throughout the sphere. Clearly, it is reasonable if the lower doses at the inner edge of the sphere are negligible in the average. Since the mass involved is proportional to the square of the distance from the center, the sphere must be quite large relative to the range of the alpha particles. For about 10% accuracy, the radius of the sphere must be roughly 30 times the range; this usually means that spheres with radii of 1 to 2 mm are needed to give meaningful averages.

When the radius of the sphere equals the range, the dose *CE* is attained only at the exact center. For smaller spheres, the dose *CE* is never attained. [In the e(r) = *E/R* approximation only, the relative dose at the center is *a/R*.] In general, for uniform distributions in *C*, the absorbed dose does not exceed *CE* anywhere. If the sphere (or any other small volume) is very small, then at distances several times its radius:

$$D = [CV\, e(x)]/(4\pi x^2),^{a}$$

where *V* is the volume of the sphere and, hence, *CV* is the number of alpha particles emitted.

[a] The average absorbed dose *(D)* = *(C)* where *(D)* is in gray (Gy), *(C)* in becquerels (Bq) times a time per unit mass and *E* is in million electron volts. To convert to conventional units use $D = k(C)E$ where $k = 2.13\ J\ kg^{-1}/\mu Ci\text{-}h\ MeV\ g^{-1}$. *D* in rads and *C* in microcurie-hours per gram.

Table 13.9 Some Physical Properties of ^{222}Rn and Its Short-Lived Decay Products (Reprinted with permission from *Health Risks of Radon and Other Internally Deposited Alpha-Emitters; BEIR IV*, c. 1988 by the National Academy of Sciences. Published by National Academy Press, Washington, DC)

Element	Historical Symbol	Principal Radiation(s)	Decay Energies (MeV)	Half-Life	No. of Atoms Per μCi	No. of Atoms Per Bq
^{222}Ra	Ra	α	4.8	1,620 yr	2.7×10^{15}	7.4×10^{10}
^{222}Rn	Rn	α	5.5	3.82 day	1.8×10^{10}	4.8×10^{5}
^{218}Po	RaA	α	6.0	3.05 min	9.77×10^{6}	2.6×10^{2}
^{214}Pb	RaB	β, γ	1.0 max	26.8 min	8.58×10^{7}	2.3×10^{3}
^{214}Bi	RaC	β, γ	3.3 max	19.7 min	6.31×10^{7}	1.7×10^{3}
^{214}Po	RaC′	α	7.7	164 μs	8.8	2.4×10^{-4}

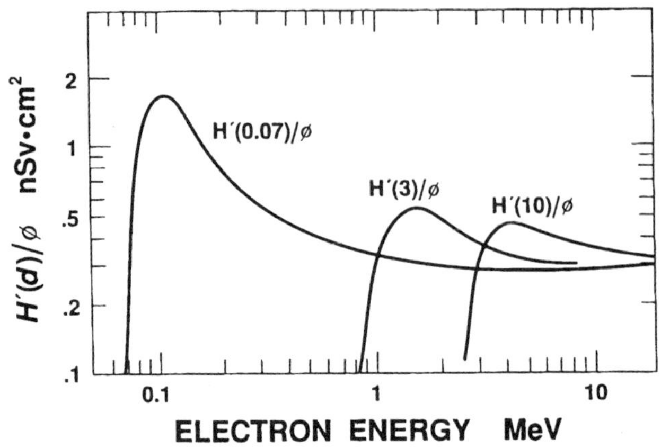

Conversion coefficients relating *H*′(0.07), *H*′(3) and *H*′(10) to the fluence of monoenergetic electrons incident on the ICRU sphere, normal to the surface (Cross *et al.*, 1991).

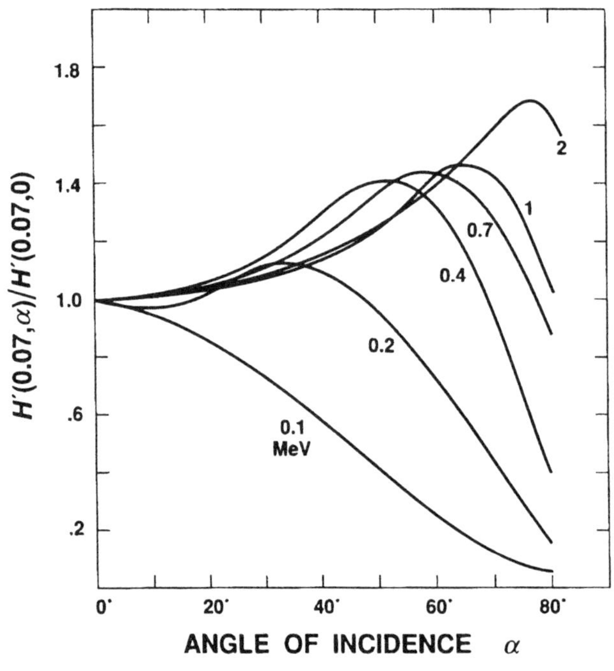

Relative variation of directional dose equivalent *H*′(0.07,α) with angle of incidence, α, for a given fluence of monoenergetic electrons. The numbers on the curves give the electron energies in MeV (Cross, 1988).

Figure 13.10 Variation in Absorbed Dose with Energy and Angle of Incidence for Monoenergetic Electrons. (From ICRU 47, 1992)

Table 13.12.1 Electron Dose Rate Factors in Skin from Selected Radionuclides Deposited on the Body Surface (Reproduced from the journal *Health Physics* with permission from the Health Physics Society from Kocher and Eckerman, 1987)

Nuclide	Dose Rate Factors (Sv/y per Bq/cm^2) Versus Depth in Tissue[a]			
	4 mg cm^{-2}	8 mg cm^{-2}	40 mg cm^{-2}	7 mg cm^{-2}
^{3}H	0.0	0.0	0.0	0.0
^{14}C	7.9×10^{-3}	2.1×10^{-3}	0.0	2.9×10^{-3}
^{32}P	2.4×10^{-2}	2.0×10^{-2}	1.1×10^{-2}	2.1×10^{-2}
^{51}Cr	0.0	0.0	0.0	0.0
^{54}Mn	0.0	0.0	0.0	0.0
^{55}Fe	0.0	0.0	0.0	0.0
^{58}Co	3.6×10^{-3}	2.6×10^{-3}	4.4×10^{-4}	2.8×10^{-3}
^{60}Co	1.6×10^{-2}	8.7×10^{-3}	2.5×10^{-4}	9.9×10^{-3}
^{86}Rb	2.3×10^{-2}	1.9×10^{-2}	1.0×10^{-2}	2.0×10^{-2}
^{89}Sr	2.3×10^{-3}	1.9×10^{-2}	9.8×10^{-3}	2.0×10^{-2}
^{90}Sr	2.1×10^{-2}	1.5×10^{-2}	3.4×10^{-3}	1.6×10^{-2}
^{90}Y	2.4×10^{-2}	2.0×10^{-2}	1.2×10^{-2}	2.1×10^{-2}
^{91}Y	2.3×10^{-2}	1.9×10^{-2}	9.9×10^{-3}	2.0×10^{-2}
^{95}Zr	1.7×10^{-2}	1.0×10^{-2}	7.4×10^{-4}	1.2×10^{-2}
^{95}Nb	6.4×10^{-3}	1.7×10^{-3}	1.8×10^{-5}	2.3×10^{-3}
^{99}Mo	2.3×10^{-2}	1.8×10^{-2}	7.1×10^{-3}	1.9×10^{-2}
^{99m}Tc	2.9×10^{-3}	1.8×10^{-3}	0.0	2.1×10^{-3}
^{103}Ru	1.1×10^{-2}	4.8×10^{-3}	2.1×10^{-4}	5.8×10^{-3}
^{106}Ru	0.0	0.0	0.0	0.0
^{105}Rh	1.8×10^{-2}	1.2×10^{-2}	2.1×10^{-3}	1.3×10^{-2}
^{127}Sb	2.2×10^{-2}	1.7×10^{-2}	5.9×10^{-3}	1.8×10^{-2}
^{127}Te	2.1×10^{-2}	1.5×10^{-2}	4.0×10^{-3}	1.6×10^{-2}
^{127m}Te	1.6×10^{-2}	2.5×10^{-3}	9.4×10^{-5}	4.7×10^{-3}
^{129}Te	2.3×10^{-2}	1.9×10^{-2}	9.1×10^{-3}	2.0×10^{-2}
^{129m}Te	2.3×10^{-2}	1.1×10^{-2}	3.5×10^{-3}	1.3×10^{-2}
^{131}Te	2.8×10^{-2}	2.2×10^{-2}	1.0×10^{-2}	2.3×10^{-2}
^{132}Te	1.3×10^{-2}	5.9×10^{-3}	4.7×10^{-5}	7.0×10^{-3}
^{131}I	2.1×10^{-2}	1.4×10^{-2}	3.0×10^{-3}	1.5×10^{-2}
^{132}I	2.3×10^{-2}	1.8×10^{-2}	8.2×10^{-3}	1.9×10^{-2}
^{135}I	2.2×10^{-2}	1.7×10^{-2}	6.5×10^{-3}	1.8×10^{-2}
^{134}Cs	1.6×10^{-2}	1.1×10^{-2}	2.7×10^{-3}	1.2×10^{-2}
^{136}Cs	2.0×10^{-2}	1.2×10^{-2}	5.9×10^{-4}	1.3×10^{-2}
^{137}Cs	2.0×10^{-2}	1.3×10^{-2}	2.3×10^{-3}	1.4×10^{-2}
^{137m}Ba	2.4×10^{-3}	2.0×10^{-3}	1.2×10^{-3}	2.1×10^{-3}
^{140}Ba	2.2×10^{-2}	1.6×10^{-2}	5.0×10^{-3}	1.7×10^{-2}
^{140}La	2.4×10^{-2}	1.9×10^{-2}	9.2×10^{-3}	2.0×10^{-2}
^{141}Ce	2.5×10^{-2}	1.5×10^{-2}	1.6×10^{-3}	1.7×10^{-2}
^{143}Ce	2.4×10^{-2}	1.8×10^{-2}	7.7×10^{-3}	1.9×10^{-2}

(continued)

Table 13.12.1 Electron Dose Rate Factors in Skin from Selected Radionuclides Deposited on the Body Surface (Continued)

Nuclide	Dose Rate Factors (Sv/y per Bq/cm^2) Versus Depth in Tissue[a]			
	4 mg cm^{-2}	8 mg cm^{-2}	40 mg cm^{-2}	7 mg cm^{-2}
^{144}Ce	1.5×10^{-2}	7.6×10^{-3}	1.7×10^{-4}	8.9×10^{-3}
^{143}Pr	2.2×10^{-2}	1.7×10^{-2}	6.2×10^{-3}	1.8×10^{-2}
^{147}Nd	2.3×10^{-2}	1.5×10^{-2}	4.2×10^{-3}	1.7×10^{-2}
^{239}Np	3.6×10^{-2}	2.0×10^{-2}	1.2×10^{-3}	2.3×10^{-2}
^{238}Pu	0.0	0.0	0.0	0.0
^{239}Pu	3.8×10^{-6}	0.0	0.0	0.0
^{241}Pu	0.0	0.0	0.0	0.0
^{241}Am	4.8×10^{-4}	1.1×10^{-5}	0.0	2.2×10^{-5}
^{242}Cm	0.0	0.0	0.0	0.0
^{244}Cm	0.0	0.0	0.0	0.0

[a] First three depths are values recommended by Whitton (1973) for various parts of body surface; last depth is average value over body surface recommended in ICRP Publication 26, 1977.

Table 13.12.2 Dose Conversion Factors for Selected Radionuclides on Skin (After Faw, 1992)

Radionuclides	Normalized Dose (Sv y^{-1} per Bq cm^{-2})					
	With Air Reflection Depth (mg cm^{-2})			Without Air Reflection Depth (mg cm^{-2})		
	3–5	5–10	30–50	3–5	5–10	30–50
^{11}C	0.0242	0.0198	0.0081	0.0163	0.0138	0.0066
^{14}C	0.0082	0.0028	0.0000	0.0070	0.0025	0.0000
^{18}F	0.0241	0.0186	0.0050	0.0167	0.0135	0.0043
^{22}Na	0.0215	0.0162	0.0035	0.0151	0.0120	0.0030
^{32}P	0.0241	0.0207	0.0113	0.0158	0.0139	0.0086
^{33}P	0.0141	0.0075	0.0000	0.0111	0.0063	0.0000
^{35}S	0.0081	0.0030	0.0000	0.0068	0.0027	0.0000
^{40}K	0.0213	0.0181	0.0093	0.0141	0.0122	0.0072
^{45}Ca	0.0140	0.0075	0.0001	0.0011	0.0063	0.0001
^{46}Sc	0.0179	0.0114	0.0007	0.0135	0.0091	0.0006
^{59}Fe	0.0173	0.0110	0.0011	0.0129	0.0087	0.0009
^{57}Co	0.0010	0.0007	0.0000	0.0007	0.0006	0.0000
^{58}Co	0.0037	0.0028	0.0005	0.0026	0.0021	0.0004
^{60}Co	0.0162	0.0098	0.0003	0.0124	0.0079	0.0003
^{65}Zn	0.0003	0.0002	0.0000	0.0002	0.0002	0.0000
^{67}Ga	0.0079	0.0025	0.0000	0.0067	0.0024	0.0000
^{68}Ga	0.0218	0.0190	0.0111	0.0142	0.0127	0.0083
^{75}Se	0.0017	0.0009	0.0000	0.0013	0.0007	0.0000

Table 13.12.2 Dose Conversion Factors for Selected Radionuclides on Skin (Continued)

	Normalized Dose (Sv y^{-1} per Bq cm^{-2})					
	With Air Reflection Depth (mg cm^{-2})			Without Air Reflection Depth (mg cm^{-2})		
Radionuclides	3–5	5–10	30–50	3–5	5–10	30–50
^{86}Rb	0.0237	0.0200	0.0104	0.0156	0.0136	0.0079
^{85}Sr	0.0002	0.0001	0.0001	0.0001	0.0001	0.0001
^{90}Sr	0.0213	0.0157	0.0035	0.0151	0.0117	0.0030
^{90}Y	0.0242	0.0210	0.0123	0.0159	0.0141	0.0091
^{95}Zr	0.0177	0.0114	0.0009	0.0133	0.0090	0.0008
^{95}Nb	0.0066	0.0022	0.0000	0.0056	0.0020	0.0000
^{95m}Nb	0.0191	0.0157	0.0023	0.0129	0.0114	0.0020
^{99}Mo	0.0230	0.0184	0.0074	0.0157	0.0129	0.0059
^{99}Tc	0.0174	0.0107	0.0003	0.0132	0.0086	0.0003
^{99m}Tc	0.0030	0.0021	0.0000	0.0023	0.0017	0.0000
^{103}Ru	0.0112	0.0055	0.0001	0.0090	0.0047	0.0001
^{109m}Ag	0.0186	0.0043	0.0000	0.0165	0.0041	0.0000
^{109}Cd	0.0186	0.0043	0.0000	0.0165	0.0041	0.0000
^{111}In	0.0043	0.0033	0.0002	0.0030	0.0026	0.0002
^{113m}In	0.0089	0.0076	0.0037	0.0058	0.0051	0.0032
^{123m}Te	0.0216	0.0076	0.0000	0.0182	0.0069	0.0000
^{123}I	0.0044	0.0031	0.0000	0.0033	0.0026	0.0000
^{129}I	0.0086	0.0030	0.0000	0.0073	0.0028	0.0000
^{131}I	0.0211	0.0152	0.0032	0.0151	0.0113	0.0028
^{132}I	0.0235	0.0192	0.0086	0.0158	0.0133	0.0067
^{133}I	0.0231	0.0187	0.0079	0.0156	0.0130	0.0062
^{134}Cs	0.0160	0.0117	0.0029	0.0113	0.0086	0.0025
^{137}Cs	0.0206	0.0149	0.0031	0.0147	0.0111	0.0027
^{137m}Ba	0.0025	0.0022	0.0013	0.0016	0.0014	0.0010
^{140}La	0.0241	0.0200	0.0096	0.0161	0.0137	0.0075
^{141}Ce	0.0252	0.0166	0.0018	0.0187	0.0131	0.0016
^{147}Pm	0.0110	0.0053	0.0000	0.0089	0.0045	0.0000
^{154}Eu	0.0310	0.0187	0.0038	0.0235	0.0145	0.0031
^{169}Yb	0.0144	0.0087	0.0001	0.0111	0.0072	0.0001
^{192}Ir	0.0235	0.0172	0.0038	0.0166	0.0128	0.0032
^{198}Au	0.0235	0.0186	0.0067	0.0161	0.0131	0.0055
^{203}Hg	0.0151	0.0086	0.0004	0.0117	0.0070	0.0004
^{201}Tl	0.0055	0.0022	0.0000	0.0046	0.0020	0.0000
^{208}Tl	0.0261	0.0218	0.0103	0.0174	0.0149	0.0080

Upper (i.e., with air reflection) and lower (i.e., without air reflection) bounds for normalized doses are given for three ranges of depth in skin. The upper bound corresponds to an inclusion for atmospheric reflection of electrons to the skin. The factors 422.1 and 197.8 convert units to rad h^{-1} per μCi cm^{-2} and MeV g^{-1} s^{-1} per Bq cm^{-2}, respectively. The dose factor reflects initial dose rate and does not account for radioactive decay. The dose factor is averaged over the indicated depth.

Table 13.13 Electron Dose Rate Factors for Skin for Immersion in Contaminated Air (Reproduced from the journal *Health Physics* with permission from the Health Physics Society from Kocher and Eckerman, 1981)

	Dose Rate Factor (Sv/y per Bq/cm^3)		
Nuclide	Half-Life	Value at 70 μm Depth	Value Averaged over Dermis
^{3}H	12.28 y	0.0	0.0
^{14}C	5.73E3 y	5.9E − 03	1.1E − 03
^{85}Kr	10.72 y	4.1E − 01	1.1E − 01
^{85m}Kr	4.48 h	4.2E − 01	1.2E − 01
^{88}Kr	2.84 h	6.6E − 01	3.7E − 01
^{88}Rb	17.8 m	4.6E 00	3.8E 00
^{90}Sr	28.6 y	2.9E − 01	6.2E − 02
^{90}Y	64.1 h	2.0E 00	1.3E 00
^{95}Zr	64.02 d	1.1E − 01	2.4E − 02
^{95}Nb	35.06 d	6.9E − 03	2.8E − 03
^{99}Tc	2.13E5 y	5.4E − 02	1.8E − 02
^{106}Ru	368.2 d	0.0	0.0
^{106}Rh	29.92 s	3.1E 00	2.3E 00
^{129}I	1.57E7 y	3.5E − 03	6.6E − 04
^{131}I	8.040 d	2.6E − 01	5.8E − 02
^{133}I	20.8 h	7.6E − 01	3.2E − 01
^{131m}Xe	11.84 d	1.1E − 01	1.5E − 02
^{133}Xe	5.245 d	8.2E − 02	2.6E − 02
^{133m}Xe	2.19 d	2.5E − 01	5.3E − 02
^{135}Xe	9.11 h	5.4E − 01	1.7E − 01
^{134}Cs	2.062 y	2.3E − 01	5.7E − 02
^{137}Cs	30.17 y	2.3E − 01	5.5E − 02
^{137m}Ba	2.552 m	1.3E − 01	5.6E − 02
^{154}Eu	8.8 y	3.7E − 01	1.5E − 01
^{210}Pb	22.26 y	0.0	0.0
^{214}Pb	26.8 m	4.2E − 01	1.0E − 01
^{210}Bi	5.013 d	7.1E − 01	2.8E − 01
^{214}Bi	19.9 m	1.3E 00	7.5E − 01
^{210}Po	138.378 d	0.0	0.0
^{222}Rn	3.8235 d	0.0	0.0
^{226}Ra	1600 y	3.2E − 03	4.9E − 04
^{230}Th	7.7E4 y	0.0	2.2E − 07
^{231}Th	25.52 h	4.6E − 02	1.6E − 02
^{234}Th	24.10 d	7.9E − 03	1.9E − 03
^{234m}Pa	1.17 m	1.7E 00	1.1E 00
^{234}U	2.445E5 y	3.4E − 05	2.6E − 06
^{235}U	7.038E8 y	5.0E − 03	1.0E − 03
^{236}U	2.3415E7 y	1.9E − 05	1.5E − 06
^{238}U	4.468E9 y	1.3E − 05	1.1E − 06
^{238}Pu	87.75 y	0.0	0.0
^{240}Pu	6537 y	0.0	0.0
^{241}Pu	14.4 y	0.0	0.0
^{241}Am	432.2 y	1.5E − 05	1.8E − 06

The coefficients are tabulated in SI units. To convert to conventional units (mrem/y per μCi/cm^3) multiply table entry by 3.7×10^9.

Table 13.14 Electron Dose Rate Factors for Skin for Immersion in Contaminated Water (From Kocher and Eckerman, 1981)

Nuclide	Half-Life	Value at 70 μm Depth	Value Averaged over Dermis
^{3}H	12.28 y	0.0	0.0
^{14}C	5.73E3 y	6.2E − 06	1.2E − 06
^{85}Kr	10.72 y	4.4E − 04	1.1E − 04
^{85m}Kr	4.48 h	4.5E − 04	1.3E − 04
^{88}Kr	2.84 h	7.0E − 04	4.0E − 04
^{88}Rb	17.8 m	5.0E − 03	4.1E − 03
^{90}Sr	28.6 y	3.1E − 04	6.6E − 05
^{90}Y	64.1 h	2.1E − 03	1.4E − 03
^{95}Zr	64.02 d	1.2E − 04	2.5E − 03
^{95}Nb	35.06 d	7.5E − 06	3.0E − 06
^{99}Tc	2.13E5 y	5.7E − 05	1.9E − 05
^{106}Ru	368.2 d	0.0	0.0
^{106}Rh	29.92 s	3.3E − 03	2.4E − 03
^{129}I	1.57E7 y	3.7E − 06	6.9E − 07
^{131}I	8.040 d	2.8E − 04	6.1E − 05
^{133}I	20.8 h	8.0E − 04	3.4E − 04
^{131m}Xe	11.84 d	1.4E − 04	1.8E − 05
^{133}Xe	5.245 d	8.7E − 05	2.8E − 05
^{133m}Xe	2.19 d	3.1E − 04	6.4E − 05
^{135}Xe	9.11 h	5.7E − 04	1.8E − 04
^{134}Cs	2.062 y	2.5E − 04	6.0E − 05
^{137}Cs	30.17 y	2.4E − 04	5.8E − 05
^{137m}Ba	2.552 m	1.5E − 04	6.8E − 05
^{154}Eu	8.8 y	4.0E − 04	1.6E − 04
^{210}Pb	22.26 y	0.0	0.0
^{214}Pb	26.8 m	4.6E − 04	1.1E − 04
^{210}Bi	5.013 d	7.6E − 04	3.0E − 04
^{214}Bi	19.9 m	1.4E − 03	8.0E − 04
^{210}Po	138.378 d	0.0	0.0
^{222}Rn	3.8235 d	0.0	0.0
^{226}Ra	1600 y	3.9E − 06	5.9E − 07
^{230}Th	7.7E4 y	0.0	2.7E − 10
^{231}Th	25.52 h	4.9E − 06	1.7E − 05
^{234}Th	24.10 d	8.4E − 06	2.0E − 06
^{234m}Pa	1.17 m	1.8E − 03	1.1E − 03
^{234}U	2.445E5 y	4.2E − 08	3.1E − 09
^{235}U	7.038E8 y	6.0E − 06	1.2E − 06
^{236}U	2.3415E7 y	2.3E − 08	1.9E − 09
^{238}U	4.468E9 y	1.5E − 08	1.3E − 09
^{238}Pu	87.75 y	0.0	0.0
^{240}Pu	6537 y	0.0	0.0
^{241}Pu	14.4 y	0.0	0.0
^{241}Am	432.2 y	1.8E − 08	2.2E − 09

The coefficients are tabulated in SI units. To convert to conventional units (mrem/y per μCi/cm^3 multiply table entry by 3.7×10^9. This table does not include dose related to absorption into the skin of the radionuclide.

Table 13.15 Electron Dose Rate Factors for Skin for Exposure 1 m Above a Contaminated Ground Surface (From Kocher and Eckerman, 1981)

		Dose Rate Factor ($Sv\ y^{-1}$ per $Bq\ cm^{-2}$)	
Nuclide	**Half-Life**	**Value at 70 μm Depth**	**Value Averaged over Dermis**
^{3}H	12.28 y	0.0	0.0
^{14}C	5.73E3 y	0.0	0.0
^{85}Kr	10.72 y	2.6E − 04	5.3E − 05
^{85m}Kr	4.48 h	3.6E − 04	9.5E − 05
^{88}Kr	2.84 h	7.7E − 04	5.3E − 04
^{88}Rb	17.8 m	5.1E − 03	4.0E − 03
^{90}Sr	28.6 y	4.4E − 05	1.3E − 05
^{90}Y	64.1 h	3.4E − 03	2.3E − 03
^{95}Zr	64.02 d	6.9E − 06	2.2E − 06
^{95}Nb	35.06 d	4.7E − 06	2.2E − 06
^{99}Tc	2.13E5 y	0.0	0.0
^{106}Ru	368.2 d	0.0	0.0
^{106}Rh	29.92 s	4.4E − 03	3.3E − 03
^{129}I	1.57E7 y	0.0	0.0
^{131}I	8.040 d	5.8E − 05	1.1E − 05
^{133}I	20.8 h	1.2E − 03	5.1E − 04
^{131m}Xe	11.84 d	0.0	0.0
^{133}Xe	5.245 d	0.0	0.0
^{133m}Xe	2.19 d	0.0	0.0
^{135}Xe	9.11 h	5.6E − 04	1.6E − 04
^{134}Cs	2.062 y	1.0E − 04	2.3E − 05
^{137}Cs	30.17 y	7.4E − 05	2.8E − 05

Table 13.15 Electron Dose Rate Factors for Skin for Exposure 1 m Above a Contaminated Ground Surface (Continued)

		Dose Rate Factor ($Sv\ y^{-1}$ per $Bq\ cm^{-2}$)	
Nuclide	Half-Life	Value at 70 μm Depth	Value Averaged over Dermis
^{137m}Ba	2.552 m	2.9E − 04	8.6E − 05
^{154}Eu	8.8 y	4.0E − 04	2.0E − 04
^{210}Pb	22.26 y	0.0	0.0
^{214}Pb	26.8 m	1.9E − 04	4.6E − 05
^{210}Bi	5.013 d	1.1E − 03	4.2E − 04
^{214}Bi	19.9 m	2.1E − 03	1.2E − 03
^{210}Po	138.378 d	0.0	0.0
^{222}Rn	3.8235 d	0.0	0.0
^{226}Ra	1600 y	0.0	0.0
^{230}Th	7.7E4 y	0.0	0.0
^{231}Th	25.52 h	0.0	0.0
^{234}Th	24.10 d	0.0	0.0
^{234m}Pa	1.17 m	3.0E − 03	1.9E − 03
^{234}U	2.445E5 y	0.0	0.0
^{235}U	7.038E8 y	0.0	0.0
^{236}U	2.3415E7 y	0.0	0.0
^{238}U	4.468E9 y	0.0	0.0
^{238}Pu	87.75 y	0.0	0.0
^{240}Pu	6537 y	0.0	0.0
^{241}Pu	14.4 y	0.0	0.0
^{241}Am	432.2 y	0.0	0.0

The coefficients are tabulated in SI units. To convert to conventional units (mrem/y per $\mu Ci/cm^{-2}$) multiply table entry by 3.7×10^9.

Table 13.16 Beta Ray Dose Rates for an Isotropic Source in Air of Density 1.205 mg/cm³ (From Cross et al., 1982)

For each nuclide the dose rates in mGy/h at R cm from a 1 MBq point source are given by dividing entries in the second column by R^2. The dose rates in rad/h at R cm from a 1 mCi source are 3.7 times larger.

The third column for each nuclide gives dose rates in mGy/h at R cm from a plane isotropic source of 1 MBq/cm² and of infinite area. Dose rates in rad/h at R cm from a plane source of 1 mCi/cm² are 3.7 times larger.

The number of significant figures given in the table does not reflect the accuracy of the values. In general, the uncertainty in dose rates is a few percent except near the end of the range.

Examples: At 12 cm in air from a 37 MBq point source of ^{32}P, the dose rate is 37/1 × 93.2/144 mGy/h = 23.9 mGy/h.

At 12 cm from a 1 mCi point source of ^{32}P, the dose rate is 1 × 3.7 × 93.2/144 rad/h = 2.39 rad/h.

At 12 cm in air from a large area plane source of 37 MBq/cm² of ^{32}P, the dose rate is 37 × 1786 mGy/h = 66.1 Gy/h. For a similar source of 1 mCi/cm² the dose rate is 3.7 × 1786 rad/h = 6.61 krad/h.

R (cm)	^3H $R^2J'(R)$	Plane Source	R (cm)	^{11}C $R^2J'(R)$	Plane Source	R (cm)	^{14}C $R^2J'(R)$	Plane Source
0.00	2245.2	*****	0.0	108.8	*****	0.0	518.8	*****
.02	1922.3	17291	3.0	114.9	2565	1.0	335.5	2962
.04	1534.0	10052	6.0	116.1	2082	2.0	270.7	1692
.06	1256.0	6546	9.0	116.7	1789	3.0	221.3	1074
.08	1035.7	4489	12.0	117.0	1579	4.0	181.1	713
.10	857.7	3167	15.0	117.1	1416	5.0	147.6	483
.12	710.8	2271	30.0	114.2	932	6.0	119.4	331
.14	587.1	1644	45.0	107.8	653	7.0	95.8	227
.16	483.8	1195	60.0	99.1	467	8.0	76.0	155
.18	396.1	870	75.0	89.1	336	9.0	59.5	105
.20	322.9	633	90.0	78.1	240	10.0	45.8	70
.22	261.3	458	105.0	66.9	170	11.0	34.6	46
.24	209.6	329	120.0	55.9	119	12.0	25.6	29
.26	166.5	235	135.0	45.5	81	13.0	18.4	18
.28	130.8	165	150.0	36.0	54	14.0	12.9	11
.30	101.4	115	165.0	27.6	35	15.0	8.7	6
.32	77.5	79	180.0	20.5	22	16.0	5.6	4
.34	58.2	53	195.0	14.6	13	17.0	3.4	2
.36	42.9	35	210.0	9.9	8	18.0	1.9	1
.38	30.9	22	225.0	6.3	4	19.0	1.0	
.40	21.6	14	240.0	3.8	2	20.0	.5	
.42	14.7	8	255.0	2.1	1	21.0	.2	
.44	9.6	5	270.0	1.0		22.0	.1	
.46	5.9	3	285.0	.4				
.48	3.5	1	300.0	.1				
.50	1.9	1						
.52	.9							
.54	.4							
.56	.1							

Table 13.16 Beta Ray Dose Rates for an Isotropic Source in Air of Density 1.205 mg/cm^3 (Continued)

R (cm)	^{18}F $R^2J'(R)$	Plane Source	R (cm)	^{22}Na $R^2J'(R)$	Plane Source	R (cm)	^{24}Na $R^2J'(R)$	Plane Source
0.0	128.5	*****	0.0	128.3	*****	0.0	101.9	*****
1.5	139.8	3115	1.5	142.5	2955	4.0	99.7	2383
3.0	141.6	2525	3.0	144.6	2354	8.0	99.8	1966
4.5	142.1	2169	4.5	144.9	1990	12.0	110.2	1714
6.0	141.9	1914	6.0	144.2	1731	16.0	100.5	1534
7.5	141.4	1716	7.5	143.0	1530	20.0	100.9	1394
15.0	135.6	1136	15.0	133.0	952	40.0	101.1	971
22.5	126.6	807	22.5	119.4	635	60.0	99.1	719
30.0	115.9	589	30.0	104.6	434	80.0	95.1	545
37.5	104.5	435	37.5	89.5	299	100.0	89.4	416
45.0	92.7	322	45.0	74.9	205	120.0	82.4	318
52.5	81.1	238	52.5	61.4	139	140.0	74.6	242
60.0	69.8	175	60.0	49.0	93	160.0	66.5	183
67.5	59.2	127	67.5	38.1	60	180.0	58.2	137
75.0	49.3	91	75.0	28.7	38	200.0	50.1	101
82.5	40.3	65	82.5	20.9	23	220.0	42.3	73
90.0	32.3	45	90.0	14.6	14	240.0	35.0	52
97.5	25.2	30	97.5	9.7	8	260.0	28.3	36
105.0	19.2	20	105.0	6.0	4	280.0	22.3	25
112.5	14.2	13	112.5	3.5	2	300.0	17.0	16
120.0	10.1	8	120.0	1.8	1	320.0	12.5	10
127.5	6.9	5	127.5	.9		340.0	8.8	4
135.0	4.5	3	135.0	.3		360.0	5.9	3
142.5	2.8	1	142.5	.1		380.0	3.7	2
150.0	1.6	1				400.0	2.2	1
157.5	.8					420.0	1.2	
165.0	.4					440.0	.6	
172.5	.2					460.0	.2	
180.0	.1					480.0	.1	

(continued)

Table 13.16 Beta Ray Dose Rates for an Isotropic Source in Air of Density 1.205 mg/cm^3 (Continued)

R (cm)	^{32}P $R^2J'(R)$	Plane Source	R (cm)	^{35}S $R^2J'(R)$	Plane Source	R (cm)	^{40}K $R^2J'(R)$	Plane Source
0.0	94.6	*****	0.0	581.6	*****			
6.0	92.8	2176	1.0	317.2	2821	0.0	91.4	*****
12.0	93.2	1786	2.0	251.9	1629	4.0	87.1	2122
18.0	93.8	1551	3.0	206.1	1054	8.0	86.6	1759
24.0	94.4	1382	4.0	170.1	716	12.0	86.6	1541
30.0	94.9	1250	5.0	140.7	499	16.0	86.6	1386
60.0	95.7	851	6.0	116.0	353	20.0	86.8	1265
90.0	93.4	614	7.0	95.3	251	40.0	87.0	901
120.0	88.4	450	8.0	77.7	178	60.0	86.1	683
150.0	81.5	332	9.0	62.9	126	80.0	84.0	530
180.0	73.4	243	10.0	50.3	89	100.0	80.7	415
210.0	64.7	176	11.0	39.8	62	120.0	76.2	326
240.0	55.8	126	12.0	31.0	42	140.0	71.0	255
270.0	46.9	88	13.0	23.8	29	160.0	65.1	198
300.0	38.3	60	14.0	17.9	19	180.0	58.9	152
330.0	30.2	39	15.0	13.1	12	200.0	52.5	115
360.0	22.9	25	16.0	9.4	8	220.0	45.9	86
390.0	16.5	15	17.0	6.5	5	240.0	39.4	62
420.0	11.3	8	18.0	4.4	3	260.0	32.9	44
450.0	7.2	4	19.0	2.8	2	280.0	26.7	30
480.0	4.2	2	20.0	1.7	1	300.0	20.9	20
510.0	2.2	1	21.0	1.0		320.0	15.6	12
540.0	1.0		22.0	.5		340.0	11.1	7
570.0	.4		23.0	.2		360.0	7.4	4
600.0	.1		24.0	.1		380.0	4.5	2
						400.0	2.5	1
						420.0	1.2	
						440.0	.5	
						460.0	.1	

Table 13.16 Beta Ray Dose Rates for an Isotropic Source in Air of Density 1.205 mg/cm^3 (Continued)

R (cm)	^{41}Ar $R^{2\prime}(R)$	Plane Source	R (cm)	^{42}K $R^2J'(R)$	Plane Source	R (cm)	^{45}Ca $R^2J'(R)$	Plane Source
0.0	111.5	*****	0.0	83.5	*****	0.0	414.4	*****
6.0	106.5	2065	12.0	83.1	2006	2.0	236.8	2207
12.0	106.0	1620	24.0	83.6	1657	4.0	193.4	1306
18.0	105.7	1354	36.0	84.2	1446	6.0	161.7	860
24.0	105.2	1164	48.0	84.6	1295	8.0	136.0	593
30.0	104.5	1018	60.0	85.0	1176	10.0	114.4	418
60.0	97.6	595	120.0	85.1	820	12.0	95.7	298
90.0	86.0	364	180.0	82.6	609	14.0	79.6	213
120.0	71.6	223	240.0	78.7	464	16.0	65.6	153
150.0	56.4	133	300.0	74.0	358	18.0	53.6	109
180.0	42.0	77	360.0	68.6	276	20.0	43.2	77
210.0	29.5	43	420.0	62.7	213	22.0	34.3	53
240.0	19.2	22	480.0	56.7	163	24.0	26.9	37
270.0	11.4	11	540.0	50.6	123	26.0	20.6	25
300.0	6.0	5	600.0	44.7	92	28.0	15.5	16
330.0	2.8	3	660.0	38.7	67	30.0	11.4	10
360.0	1.2	1	720.0	32.8	47	32.0	8.1	4
390.0	.6	1	780.0	26.9	32	34.0	5.6	4
420.0	.4	1	840.0	21.1	21	36.0	3.7	2
450.0	.3	1	900.0	15.8	13	38.0	2.3	1
480.0	.3		960.0	11.2	8	40.0	1.4	1
510.0	.3		1020.0	7.4	4	42.0	.8	
540.0	.2		1080.0	4.4	2	44.0	.4	
570.0	.2		1140.0	2.4	1	46.0	.2	
600.0	.1		1200.0	1.1		48.0	.1	
630.0	.1		1260.0	.4				
660.0	.1		1320.0	.1				
690.0	.1							

(continued)

Table 13.16 Beta Ray Dose Rates for an Isotropic Source in Air of Density 1.205 mg/cm³ (Continued)

R (cm)	^{47}Sc $R^2J'(R)$	Plane Source	R (cm)	^{49}Sc $R^2J'(R)$	Plane Source	R (cm)	^{56}Mn $R^2J'(R)$	Plane Source
0.0	232.4	*****	0.0	90.7	*****	0.0	106.3	*****
1.2	188.1	3268	6.0	88.9	2212	10.0	98.4	1829
2.4	167.7	2504	12.0	89.2	1839	20.0	96.1	1421
3.6	168.9	2070	18.0	89.6	1615	30.0	93.7	1183
4.8	162.6	1772	24.0	90.2	1453	40.0	91.1	1017
6.0	157.1	1549	30.0	90.7	1327	50.0	88.4	892
12.0	134.8	938	60.0	92.2	944	100.0	73.4	553
18.0	116.1	623	90.0	91.9	713	150.0	60.6	384
24.0	99.3	429	120.0	89.4	550	200.0	52.2	283
30.0	84.0	301	150.0	85.3	428	250.0	46.9	214
36.0	70.2	213	180.0	80.1	334	300.0	43.1	162
42.0	57.9	151	210.0	74.1	259	350.0	39.6	122
48.0	47.1	107	240.0	67.6	200	400.0	35.7	91
54.0	37.8	76	270.0	60.7	152	450.0	31.3	66
60.0	29.9	53	300.0	53.6	115	500.0	26.7	47
66.0	23.3	37	330.0	46.4	85	550.0	22.1	32
72.0	18.0	26	360.0	39.2	61	600.0	17.6	21
78.0	13.7	18	390.0	32.4	43	650.0	13.4	14
84.0	10.3	13	420.0	26.0	30	700.0	9.7	8
90.0	7.8	9	450.0	20.2	20	750.0	6.7	5
96.0	5.8	6	480.0	15.1	13	800.0	4.2	2
102.0	4.3	4	510.0	10.8	8	850.0	2.5	1
108.0	3.2	3	540.0	7.3	4	900.0	1.3	
114.0	2.3	2	570.0	4.7	2	950.0	.6	
120.0	1.7	1	600.0	2.8	1	1000.0	.2	
126.0	1.1	1	630.0	1.5	1	1050.0	.1	
132.0	.8		660.0	.7				
138.0	.5		690.0	.3				
144.0	.3		720.0	.1				
150.0	.2							

Table 13.16 Beta Ray Dose Rates for an Isotropic Source in Air of Density 1.205 mg/cm^3 (Continued)

R (cm)	^{58}Co $R^2J'(R)$	Plane Source	R (cm)	^{59}Fe $R^2J'(R)$	Plane Source	R (cm)	^{60}Co $R^2J'(R)$	Plane Source
0.0	20.4	*****	0.0	318.0	*****	0.00	358.5	*****
1.0	22.7	559	1.0	230.1	3359	0.60	262.4	4177
2.0	24.0	461	2.0	206.8	2444	1.20	239.6	3126
3.0	24.7	400	3.0	190.9	1944	1.80	224.4	2543
4.0	25.1	356	4.0	178.3	1613	2.40	212.5	2151
5.0	25.4	320	5.0	167.6	1371	3.00	202.4	1861
10.0	25.3	214	10.0	128.1	752	6.00	165.2	1091
15.0	23.9	153	15.0	100.4	465	9.00	137.8	710
20.0	22.0	111	20.0	79.0	304	12.00	115.5	483
25.0	19.9	82	25.0	62.3	205	15.00	96.4	335
30.0	17.6	61	30.0	49.1	142	18.00	79.9	234
35.0	15.4	45	35.0	38.9	99	21.00	65.6	164
40.0	13.2	33	40.0	31.0	70	24.00	53.2	114
45.0	11.1	24	45.0	24.8	49	27.00	42.6	79
50.0	9.2	17	50.0	19.9	34	30.00	33.5	54
55.0	7.5	12	55.0	15.8	24	33.00	25.9	36
60.0	6.1	8	60.0	12.3	16	36.00	19.5	24
65.0	4.7	6	65.0	9.4	11	39.00	14.4	15
70.0	3.6	4	70.0	6.9	7	42.00	10.3	9
75.0	2.6	2	75.0	5.0	4	45.00	7.1	6
80.0	1.9	1	80.0	3.5	3	48.00	4.7	3
85.0	1.3	1	85.0	2.3	1	51.00	2.9	2
90.0	.8		90.0	1.4	1	54.00	1.7	1
95.0	.5		95.0	.9		57.00	1.0	
100.0	.3		100.0	.5		60.00	.5	
105.0	.2		105.0	.2		63.00	.2	
110.0	.1		110.0	.1		66.00	.1	

(continued)

Table 13.16 Beta Ray Dose Rates for an Isotropic Source in Air of Density 1.205 mg/cm^3 (Continued)

R (cm)	^{63}Ni $R^2J'(R)$	Plane Source	R (cm)	^{64}Cu $R^2J'(R)$	Plane Source	R (cm)	^{65}Zn $R^2J'(R)$	Plane Source
0.00	1262.0	*****	0.0	98.7	*****	0.00	2.4	*****
0.20	631.3	5038	1.5	85.5	1697	0.50	2.7	70
0.40	464.6	2742	3.0	83.0	1345	1.00	2.8	59
0.60	360.5	1706	4.5	81.3	1138	1.50	2.9	52
0.80	285.5	1126	6.0	79.8	994	2.00	3.0	46
1.00	228.3	767	7.5	78.5	883	2.50	3.1	42
1.20	183.1	532	15.0	72.2	568	5.00	3.1	29
1.40	146.8	373	22.5	65.7	394	7.50	3.0	21
1.60	117.4	262	30.0	59.0	282	10.00	2.8	16
1.80	93.3	184	37.5	52.1	205	12.50	2.6	12
2.00	73.7	129	45.0	45.4	149	15.00	2.4	9
2.20	57.7	90	52.5	39.0	108	17.50	2.1	7
2.40	44.6	62	60.0	33.0	78	20.00	1.9	5
2.60	34.1	42	67.5	27.4	56	22.50	1.6	4
2.80	25.6	28	75.0	22.4	39	25.00	1.4	3
3.00	18.9	18	82.5	17.9	27	27.50	1.2	2
3.20	13.7	12	90.0	14.0	18	30.00	1.0	2
3.40	9.6	7	97.5	10.7	12	32.50	.8	1
3.60	6.6	4	105.0	7.9	8	35.00	.7	1
3.80	4.3	3	112.5	5.7	5	37.50	.5	1
4.00	2.8	1	120.0	4.0	3	40.00	.4	
4.20	1.7	1	127.5	2.6	2	42.50	.3	
4.40	.9		135.0	1.7	1	45.00	.3	
4.60	.5		142.5	1.0	1	47.50	.2	
4.80	.2		150.0	.6		50.00	.1	
5.00	.1		157.5	.3		52.50	.1	
			165.0	.3		55.00	.1	
			172.5	.1				

Table 13.16 Beta Ray Dose Rates for an Isotropic Source in Air of Density 1.205 mg/cm^3 (Continued)

R (cm)	^{68}Ga $R^2J'(R)$	Plane Source	R (cm)	^{74}As $R^2J'(R)$	Plane Source	R (cm)	^{82}Br $R^2J'(R)$	Plane Source
0.0	72.6	*****	0.0	74.4	*****	0.0	274.4	*****
6.0	75.6	1968	4.0	70.8	1441	1.0	209.6	3447
12.0	77.3	1648	8.0	70.7	1145	2.0	193.1	2604
18.0	78.8	1452	12.0	70.6	968	3.0	182.2	2132
24.0	80.0	1309	16.0	70.3	841	4.0	173.5	1813
30.0	81.1	1197	20.0	69.8	743	5.0	166.3	1576
60.0	84.3	850	40.0	65.4	460	10.0	138.7	937
90.0	84.6	638	60.0	58.7	304	15.0	117.7	614
120.0	82.3	488	80.0	50.8	206	20.0	99.8	419
150.0	78.3	376	100.0	42.6	141	25.0	84.0	291
180.0	73.1	290	120.0	34.8	97	30.0	69.9	203
210.0	67.2	222	140.0	27.7	66	35.0	57.5	142
240.0	60.7	168	160.0	21.7	46	40.0	46.7	98
270.0	53.8	126	180.0	16.8	31	45.0	37.2	67
300.0	46.8	93	200.0	12.9	22	50.0	29.1	45
330.0	39.7	67	220.0	9.8	15	55.0	22.3	30
360.0	32.9	47	240.0	7.4	10	60.0	16.6	19
390.0	26.4	32	260.0	5.6	7	65.0	12.0	12
420.0	20.5	21	280.0	4.2	5	70.0	8.4	7
450.0	15.3	13	300.0	3.1	3	75.0	5.6	4
480.0	10.9	8	320.0	2.3	2	80.0	3.5	2
510.0	7.4	5	340.0	1.6	1	85.0	2.1	1
540.0	4.7	2	360.0	1.1	1	90.0	1.2	1
570.0	2.7	1	380.0	.7		95.0	.6	
600.0	1.5	1	400.0	.4		100.0	.3	
630.0	.7		420.0	.3		105.0	.1	
660.0	.3		440.0	.1				
690.0	.1		460.0	.1				

(continued)

Table 13.16 Beta Ray Dose Rates for an Isotropic Source in Air of Density 1.205 mg/cm³ (Continued)

R (cm)	^{85}Kr $R^2J'(R)$	Plane Source	R (cm)	^{86}Rb $R^2J'(R)$	Plane Source	R (cm)	^{88}Kr-Rb[a] $R^2J'(R)$	Plane Source
0.0	179.4	*****	0.0	108.4	*****	0.0	250.4	*****
2.0	145.2	2742	6.0	98.7	2108	20.0	186.9	2670
4.0	137.4	2150	12.0	96.7	1699	40.0	152.6	1959
6.0	132.4	1811	18.0	95.4	1457	60.0	128.1	1606
8.0	128.6	1577	24.0	94.3	1287	80.0	112.4	1390
10.0	125.5	1399	30.0	93.3	1156	100.0	103.7	1239
20.0	113.9	898	60.0	88.1	776	200.0	95.1	823
30.0	104.0	624	90.0	82.3	562	300.0	91.2	589
40.0	94.1	446	120.0	76.2	420	400.0	85.6	430
50.0	84.1	322	150.0	70.1	318	500.0	78.2	316
60.0	74.0	231	180.0	64.1	241	600.0	69.7	231
70.0	63.8	165	210.0	58.1	182	700.0	61.0	168
80.0	53.9	116	240.0	52.0	136	800.0	52.4	121
90.0	44.3	79	270.0	45.7	100	900.0	44.3	85
100.0	35.3	53	300.0	39.2	72	1000.0	36.5	58
110.0	27.3	34	330.0	32.8	50	1100.0	29.1	39
120.0	20.2	21	360.0	26.6	34	1200.0	22.3	25
130.0	14.3	13	390.0	20.7	22	1300.0	16.4	15
140.0	9.6	7	420.0	15.3	13	1400.0	11.3	8
150.0	6.0	4	450.0	10.8	8	1500.0	7.3	4
160.0	3.4	2	480.0	7.0	4	1600.0	4.2	2
170.0	1.8	1	510.0	4.2	2	1700.0	2.1	1
180.0	.8		540.0	2.3	1	1800.0	.8	
190.0	.3		570.0	1.1		1900.0	.2	
200.0	.1		600.0	.4				
			630.0	.1				

Table 13.16 Beta Ray Dose Rates for an Isotropic Source in Air of Density 1.205 mg/cm^3 (Continued)

R (cm)	^{89}Sr $R^2J'(R)$	Plane Source	R (cm)	^{90}Sr $R^2J'(R)$	Plane Source	R (cm)	^{90}Y $R^2J'(R)$	Plane Source
0.0	111.4	*****	0.00	209.6	*****	0.0	93.0	*****
5.0	100.9	2198	.80	174.2	3676	8.0	88.7	2060
10.0	98.9	1779	1.60	164.7	2966	16.0	88.3	1689
15.0	97.8	1532	2.40	158.9	2559	24.0	88.1	1467
20.0	97.0	1357	3.20	154.6	2278	32.0	88.1	1309
25.0	96.3	1222	4.00	151.0	2064	40.0	88.0	1186
50.0	92.7	826	4.80	148.0	1894	80.0	87.0	819
75.0	88.5	599	5.60	145.4	1752	120.0	84.1	605
100.0	83.1	445	6.40	143.0	1631	160.0	79.8	457
125.0	76.7	333	7.20	140.8	1526	200.0	74.9	349
150.0	69.7	250	8.00	138.8	1434	240.0	69.6	267
175.0	62.4	186	16.00	122.9	886	280.0	63.8	202
200.0	55.0	137	24.00	109.4	594	320.0	57.6	152
225.0	47.5	99	32.00	96.4	409	360.0	50.9	112
250.0	40.1	70	40.00	83.5	283	400.0	44.0	80
275.0	32.9	48	48.00	70.9	195	440.0	37.0	56
300.0	26.2	32	56.00	58.8	133	480.0	30.0	38
325.0	20.0	20	64.00	47.5	88	520.0	23.3	24
350.0	14.5	12	72.00	37.1	57	560.0	17.2	15
375.0	9.9	7	80.00	27.9	35	600.0	11.9	8
400.0	6.2	4	88.00	20.0	21	640.0	7.7	4
425.0	3.6	2	96.00	13.6	12	680.0	4.5	2
450.0	1.9	1	104.00	8.7	6	720.0	2.4	1
475.0	.8		112.00	5.1	3	760.0	1.1	
500.0	.3		120.00	2.7	1	800.0	.4	
525.0	.1		128.00	1.3		840.0	.1	
			136.00	.5				
			144.00	.1				

(continued)

Table 13.16 Beta Ray Dose Rates for an Isotropic Source in Air of Density 1.205 mg/cm³ (Continued)

R (cm)	^{90}Sr-Y[a] $R^2J'(R)$	Plane Source	R (cm)	^{91}Y $R^2J'(R)$	Plane Source	R (cm)	^{95}Zr $R^2J'(R)$	Plane Source
0.0	282.3	*****	0.0	110.3	*****	0.0	292.3	*****
5.0	235.5	4165	5.0	100	2203	1.5	214.2	2859
10.0	222.3	3206	10.0	98.1	1788	3.0	190.6	2011
15.0	212.3	2660	15.0	97.0	1543	4.5	174.5	1553
20.0	203.5	2287	20.0	96.1	1370	6.0	161.5	1251
25.0	195.1	2008	25.0	95.4	1236	7.5	150.3	1033
30.0	186.9	1790	50.0	92.1	844	9.0	140.4	867
35.0	178.8	1613	75.0	88.2	617	10.5	131.4	736
40.0	170.7	1467	100.0	83.2	463	12.0	123.1	629
45.0	162.8	1344	125.0	77.3	351	13.5	115.3	541
50.0	155.0	1239	150.0	70.8	267	15.0	108.0	467
100.0	96.5	712	175.0	64.0	201	30.0	53.3	130
150.0	81.0	489	200.0	57.0	151	45.0	21.9	35
200.0	74.9	349	225.0	50.0	111	60.0	6.8	9
250.0	68.1	249	250.0	43.0	80	75.0	1.7	3
300.0	60.7	175	275.0	36.1	57	90.0	.7	2
350.0	52.6	121	300.0	29.4	39	105.0	.6	1
400.0	44.0	80	325.0	23.2	26	120.0	.5	1
450.0	35.2	51	350.0	17.5	16	135.0	.4	1
500.0	26.6	30	375.0	12.6	10	150.0	.3	
550.0	18.7	17	400.0	8.5	6	165.0	.2	
600.0	11.9	8	425.0	5.3	3	180.0	.1	
650.0	6.8	4	450.0	3.1	1	195.0	.1	
700.0	3.3	1	475.0	1.6	1	210.0	.1	
750.0	1.3		500.0	.7				
800.0	.4		525.0	.2				
850.0	.1		550.0	.1				

Table 13.16 Beta Ray Dose Rates for an Isotropic Source in Air of Density 1.205 mg/cm^3 (Continued)

R (cm)	^{95}Nb $R^2J'(R)$	Plane Source	R (cm)	^{99}Mo $R^2J'(R)$	Plane Source	R (cm)	^{103}Ru $R^2J'(R)$	Plane Source
0.0	654.4	*****	0.0	145.6	*****	0.0	443.2	*****
1.0	316.4	2569	4.0	120.8	2207	1.5	252.9	2311
2.0	238.0	1408	8.0	114.5	1714	3.0	197.5	1368
3.0	186.9	874	12.0	110.2	1431	4.5	161.0	918
4.0	148.9	572	16.0	106.6	1237	6.0	133.7	653
5.0	119.1	385	20.0	103.4	1090	7.5	112.1	481
6.0	95.2	263	40.0	90.3	684	15.0	47.7	147
7.0	75.7	180	60.0	79.7	471	22.5	19.3	63
8.0	59.8	123	80.0	70.9	336	30.0	8.6	38
9.0	46.8	84	100.0	63.0	242	37.5	5.9	27
10.0	36.1	57	120.0	55.3	175	45.0	5.2	21
11.0	27.4	38	140.0	47.6	125	52.5	4.7	16
12.0	20.5	25	160.0	40.0	88	60.0	4.2	13
13.0	14.9	16	180.0	33.0	61	67.5	3.7	10
14.0	10.6	10	200.0	26.5	42	75.0	3.2	7
15.0	7.3	6	220.0	20.7	27	82.5	2.8	6
16.0	4.9	3	240.0	15.6	18	90.0	2.4	4
17.0	3.1	2	260.0	11.4	11	97.5	2.0	3
18.0	1.9	1	280.0	7.9	6	105.0	1.6	2
19.0	1.0		300.0	5.2	3	112.5	1.3	2
20.0	.5		320.0	3.2	2	120.0	1.1	1
21.0	.3		340.0	1.8	1	127.5	.8	1
22.0	.1		360.0	.9		135.0	.6	1
			380.0	.4		142.5	.5	
			400.0	.1		150.0	.4	
						157.5	.2	
						165.0	.2	
						172.5	.1	
						180.0	.1	

(continued)

Table 13.16 Beta Ray Dose Rates for an Isotropic Source in Air of Density 1.205 mg/cm³ (Continued)

R (cm)	^{106}Ru $R^2J'(R)$	Plane Source	R (cm)	^{106}Rh $R^2J'(R)$	Plane Source	R (cm)	^{129}I $R^2J'(R)$	Plane Source
0.00	1799.0	*****	0.0	82.8	*****	0.0	801.0	*****
0.10	873.4	6221	12.0	81.8	1999	1.0	297.9	2118
0.20	605.9	3122	24.0	82.1	1656	2.0	202.6	1070
0.30	443.9	1803	36.0	82.6	1449	3.0	148.3	629
0.40	332.3	1106	48.0	83.1	1300	4.0	112.1	395
0.50	250.5	—	60.0	83.5	1184	5.0	86.0	257
0.60	188.8	449	120.0	84.5	832	6.0	66.4	170
0.70	141.6	289	180.0	83.5	621	7.0	51.2	113
0.80	105.3	185	240.0	81.1	473	8.0	39.3	75
0.90	77.3	118	300.0	77.4	362	9.0	29.9	49
1.00	55.8	74	360.0	72.6	277	10.0	22.4	32
1.10	29.5	45	420.0	66.7	209	11.0	16.5	20
1.20	27.3	27	480.0	59.9	156	12.0	11.9	13
1.30	18.3	16	540.0	52.6	115	13.0	8.3	8
1.40	11.8	9	600.0	45.0	83	14.0	5.6	4
1.50	7.3	5	660.0	37.4	58	15.0	3.6	2
1.60	4.2	2	720.0	30.2	39	16.0	2.2	1
1.70	2.3	1	780.0	23.5	26	17.0	1.3	1
1.80	1.1		840.0	17.6	16	18.0	.7	
1.90	.5		900.0	12.6	10	19.0	.3	
2.00	.2		960.0	8.5	6	20.0	.1	
2.10	.1		1020.0	5.4	3			
			1080.0	3.1	1			
			1140.0	1.6	1			
			1200.0	.7				
			1260.0	.3				
			1320.0	.1				

Table 13.16 Beta Ray Dose Rates for an Isotropic Source in Air of Density 1.205 mg/cm³ (Continued)

R (cm)	^{131}I $R^2J'(R)$	Plane Source	R (cm)	^{132}Te $R^2J'(R)$	Plane Source	R (cm)	^{132}I $R^2J'(R)$	Plane Source
0.0	222.7	*****	0.0	497.0	*****	0.0	121.8	*****
1.0	182.5	3402	1.5	261.6	2361	6.0	107.4	1965
2.0	170.1	2664	3.0	206.8	1380	12.0	103.7	1523
3.0	162.1	2246	4.5	169.7	907	18.0	101.2	1265
4.0	155.9	1961	6.0	141.3	628	24.0	99.0	1086
5.0	150.8	1746	7.5	118.2	447	30.0	96.8	949
6.0	146.2	1577	9.0	98.9	323	60.0	85.3	568
7.0	142.3	1437	10.5	82.7	235	90.0	73.0	369
8.0	138.6	1320	12.0	68.8	172	120.0	60.6	249
9.0	135.2	1219	13.5	56.9	125	150.0	49.5	172
10.0	132.0	1130	15.0	46.7	91	180.0	40.2	121
20.0	106.7	630	16.5	37.9	66	210.0	32.5	86
30.0	87.0	387	18.0	30.5	47	240.0	26.2	61
40.0	70.4	246	19.5	24.3	33	270.0	21.0	44
50.0	56.2	157	21.0	19.0	23	300.0	16.8	31
60.0	44.0	100	22.5	14.6	16	330.0	13.3	22
70.0	33.6	62	24.0	11.1	11	360.0	10.5	16
80.0	24.9	38	25.5	8.2	7	390.0	8.2	11
90.0	17.7	22	27.0	5.9	4	420.0	6.3	8
100.0	12.0	12	28.5	4.1	3	450.0	4.8	5
110.0	7.6	7	30.0	2.8	2	480.0	3.6	3
120.0	4.5	3	31.5	1.8	1	510.0	2.7	2
130.0	2.5	1	33.0	1.1	1	540.0	1.9	1
140.0	1.2	1	34.5	.7		570.0	1.4	1
150.0	.5		36.0	.4		600.0	.9	
160.0	.2		37.5	.2		630.0	.6	
170.0	.1		39.0	.1		660.0	.3	
						690.0	.2	
						720.0	.1	

(continued)

Table 13.16 Beta Ray Dose Rates for an Isotropic Source in Air of Density 1.205 mg/cm³ (Continued)

R (cm)	^{133}I $R^2J'(R)$	Plane Source	R (cm)	^{133}Xe $R^2J'(R)$	Plane Source	R (cm)	^{134}Cs $R^2J'(R)$	Plane Source
0.0	136.5	*****	0.00	353.8	*****	0.0	377.6	*****
4.0	117.0	2241	.40	270.8	4919	1.0	202.9	2861
8.0	112.0	1761	.80	249.2	3730	2.0	157.7	2106
12.0	108.9	1484	1.20	235.2	3121	3.0	133.4	1740
16.0	106.3	1290	1.60	224.4	2709	4.0	119.1	1514
20.0	104.1	1144	2.00	215.4	2402	5.0	110.5	1353
40.0	94.3	728	2.40	207.7	2160	6.0	105.3	1230
60.0	85.4	503	2.80	200.8	1963	7.0	101.9	1130
80.0	76.8	357	3.20	194.6	1797	8.0	99.6	1045
100.0	67.9	256	3.60	188.9	1656	9.0	97.7	972
120.0	59.1	183	4.00	183.6	1532	10.0	96.0	908
140.0	50.3	130	8.00	143.6	847	20.0	81.8	536
160.0	42.0	92	12.00	115.2	522	30.0	69.8	345
180.0	34.3	63	16.00	92.6	335	40.0	58.9	230
200.0	27.4	43	20.00	74.0	219	50.0	49.0	154
220.0	21.3	28	24.00	58.4	144	60.0	40.1	104
240.0	16.0	18	28.00	45.3	93	70.0	32.1	69
260.0	11.7	11	32.00	34.5	60	80.0	25.1	45
280.0	8.1	7	36.00	25.7	38	90.0	19.1	28
300.0	5.4	4	40.00	18.6	23	100.0	14.0	18
320.0	3.3	2	44.00	13.0	14	110.0	9.9	10
340.0	1.9	1	48.00	8.7	8	120.0	6.7	6
360.0	1.0		52.00	5.6	4	130.0	4.2	3
380.0	.5		56.00	3.4	2	140.0	2.5	2
400.0	.2		60.00	1.9	1	150.0	1.4	1
420.0	.1		64.00	.9		160.0	.7	
			68.00	.4		170.0	.3	
			72.00	.2		180.0	.1	

Table 13.16 Beta Ray Dose Rates for an Isotropic Source in Air of Density 1.205 mg/cm^3 (Continued)

R (cm)	^{135}I $R^2J'(R)$	Plane Source	R (cm)	^{137}Cs-Ba[a] $R^2J'(R)$	Plane Source	R (cm)	^{140}Ba-La[a] $R^2J'(R)$	Plane Source
0.0	145.7	*****	0.0	226.7	*****	0.0	285.9	*****
6.0	119.4	1863	2.0	176.4	2906	6.0	235.9	3815
12.0	111.2	1380	4.0	162.9	2195	12.0	220.8	2858
18.0	105.3	1108	6.0	153.7	1798	18.0	210.0	2316
24.0	100.3	923	8.0	146.7	1528	24.0	200.8	1948
30.0	95.7	786	10.0	140.7	1327	30.0	192.3	1673
60.0	76.6	425	12.0	135.4	1170	60.0	157.6	940
90.0	61.3	252	14.0	130.6	1041	90.0	130.4	579
120.0	48.0	154	16.0	126.0	934	120.0	106.5	366
150.0	36.6	95	18.0	121.7	842	150.0	84.3	233
180.0	27.1	59	20.0	117.6	763	180.0	64.6	148
210.0	19.5	36	40.0	81.3	346	210.0	48.0	93
240.0	13.8	22	60.0	52.0	179	240.0	34.7	59
270.0	9.5	14	80.0	31.7	104	270.0	24.6	37
300.0	6.4	8	100.0	21.4	67	300.0	17.2	23
330.0	4.3	5	120.0	18.9	44	330.0	11.8	14
360.0	2.8	3	140.0	18.9	25	360.0	8.0	9
390.0	1.8	2	160.0	15.0	11	390.0	5.3	5
420.0	1.2	1	180.0	7.1	3	410.0	3.5	3
450.0	.8	1	200.0	.8		450.0	2.3	2
480.0	.5	1	220.0	.2		480.0	1.6	1
510.0	.4		240.0	.1		510.0	1.0	1
540.0	.3		260.0	.1		540.0	.7	
570.0	.2					570.0	.4	
600.0	.2					600.0	.3	
630.0	.1					630.0	.2	
660.0	.1					660.0	.1	
						690.0	.1	

(continued)

Table 13.16 Beta Ray Dose Rates for an Isotropic Source in Air of Density 1.205 mg/cm³ (Continued)

R (cm)	^{141}Ce $R^2J'(R)$	Plane Source	R (cm)	^{144}Ce-Pr[a] $R^2J'(R)$	Plane Source	R (cm)	^{147}Pm $R^2J'(R)$	Plane Source
0.00	264.2	*****	0.0	401.8	*****	0.0	503.8	*****
0.80	209.5	3720	6.0	231.3	3161	1.5	262.3	2338
1.60	194.2	2875	12.0	176.3	2307	3.0	206.2	1357
2.40	183.9	2400	18.0	142.4	1907	4.5	168.4	886
3.20	176.0	2076	24.0	121.2	1670	6.0	139.4	610
4.00	169.4	1835	30.0	107.0	1511	7.5	116.0	431
4.80	163.6	1645	36.0	97.5	1394	9.0	96.7	310
5.60	158.4	1490	42.0	91.3	1303	10.5	80.4	224
6.40	153.6	1359	48.0	87.7	1228	12.0	66.5	613
7.20	149.3	1247	54.0	86.0	1164	13.5	54.7	118
8.00	145.2	1150	60.0	85.3	1107	15.0	44.6	85
16.00	112.9	609	120.0	84.9	750	16.5	36.0	61
24.00	88.3	356	180.0	82.5	540	18.0	28.8	43
32.00	68.2	216	240.0	78.6	395	19.5	22.7	30
40.00	51.6	132	300.0	73.3	289	21.0	17.6	21
48.00	38.2	81	360.0	66.7	209	22.5	13.5	14
56.00	27.5	49	420.0	58.9	149	24.0	10.1	9
64.00	19.2	30	480.0	50.4	103	25.5	7.4	6
72.00	13.1	18	540.0	41.5	69	27.0	5.2	4
80.00	8.7	10	600.0	32.8	44	28.5	3.6	2
88.00	5.7	6	660.0	24.6	27	30.0	2.4	1
96.00	3.7	3	720.0	17.4	16	31.5	1.5	1
104.00	2.4	2	780.0	11.4	8	33.0	.9	
112.00	1.5	1	840.0	6.9	4	34.5	.5	
120.00	.9	1	900.0	3.7	2	36.0	.3	
128.00	.5		960.0	1.7	1	37.5	.1	
136.00	.2		1020.0	.7		39.0	.1	
144.00	.1		1080.0	.2				

Table 13.16 Beta Ray Dose Rates for an Isotropic Source in Air of Density 1.205 mg/cm^3 (Continued)

R (cm)	^{192}Ir $R^2J'(R)$	Plane Source	R (cm)	^{198}Au $R^2J'(R)$	Plane Source	R (cm)	^{203}Hg $R^2J'(R)$	Plane Source
0.0	222.1	*****	0.0	158.6	*****	0.0	532.9	*****
1.5	170.3	2805	1.5	136.3	2991	1.5	265.1	2239
3.0	165.4	2121	3.0	130.7	2431	3.0	203.6	1258
4.5	147.2	1740	4.5	127.0	2108	4.5	162.7	798
6.0	139.9	1482	6.0	124.1	1882	6.0	131.8	533
7.5	133.8	1291	7.5	121.8	1711	7.5	107.3	366
15.0	111.2	778	9.0	119.8	1573	9.0	87.3	255
22.5	94.5	519	10.5	118.0	1458	10.5	70.7	179
30.0	80.7	362	12.0	116.4	1359	12.0	56.9	125
37.5	68.8	258	13.5	114.9	1274	13.5	45.4	87
45.0	58.3	185	15.0	113.5	1198	15.0	35.9	61
52.5	49.0	133	30.0	101.5	748	16.5	28.0	41
60.0	40.7	96	45.0	90.7	506	18.0	21.4	28
67.5	33.3	68	60.0	80.2	353	19.5	16.1	19
75.0	26.9	49	75.0	69.8	248	21.0	11.9	12
82.5	21.5	34	90.0	59.6	174	22.5	8.6	8
90.0	16.8	24	105.0	49.8	121	24.0	6.0	5
97.5	12.9	16	120.0	40.8	83	25.5	4.0	3
105.0	9.8	11	135.0	32.6	56	27.0	2.6	2
112.5	7.2	7	150.0	25.3	37	28.5	1.6	1
120.0	5.3	5	165.0	19.1	24	30.0	.9	
127.5	3.7	3	180.0	14.0	15	31.5	.5	
135.0	2.6	2	195.0	9.8	9	33.0	.2	
142.5	1.7	1	210.0	6.5	5	34.5	.1	
150.0	1.1	1	225.0	4.1	3			
157.5	.7		240.0	2.4	1			
165.0	.4		255.0	1.3	1			
172.5	.2		270.0	.6				
180.0	.1		285.0	.3				
			300.0	.1				

(continued)

Table 13.16 Beta Ray Dose Rates for an Isotropic Source in Air of Density 1.205 mg/cm^3 (Continued)

R (cm)	^{204}Tl $R^2J'(R)$	Plane Source	R (cm)	^{210}Pb $R^2J'(R)$	Plane Source	R (cm)	^{210}Bi $R^2J'(R)$	Plane Source
0.0	194.2	*****	0.00	2759.6	*****	0.0	167.3	*****
2.0	150.2	2609	0.20	213.4	1114	3.0	134.6	2367
4.0	138.9	2004	0.40	87.0	485	6.0	126.2	1821
6.0	131.5	1664	0.60	65.8	293	9.0	120.6	1511
8.0	125.8	1433	0.80	51.0	188	12.0	116.1	1298
10.0	121.0	1261	1.00	39.9	125	15.0	112.2	1139
20.0	103.8	790	1.20	31.3	84	30.0	96.9	701
30.0	90.9	545	1.40	24.5	57	45.0	84.1	473
40.0	80.1	392	1.60	19.1	39	60.0	72.8	333
50.0	70.5	287	1.80	14.8	26	75.0	62.5	238
60.0	61.6	211	2.00	11.3	18	90.0	53.2	172
70.0	53.5	155	2.20	8.6	12	105.0	44.8	125
80.0	45.9	114	2.40	6.4	8	120.0	37.3	90
90.0	38.8	83	2.60	4.7	5	135.0	30.7	65
100.0	32.3	59	2.80	3.3	3	150.0	25.0	47
110.0	26.4	41	3.00	2.3	2	165.0	20.1	33
120.0	21.1	28	3.20	1.6	1	180.0	16.0	23
130.0	16.4	19	3.40	1.0	1	195.0	12.5	16
140.0	12.4	12	3.60	.6		210.0	9.6	11
150.0	9.0	8	3.80	.4		225.0	7.3	7
160.0	6.3	5	4.00	.2		240.0	5.4	5
170.0	4.2	3	4.20	.1		255.0	3.9	3
180.0	2.6	1	4.40	.1		270.0	2.7	2
190.0	1.5	1				285.0	1.8	1
200.0	.8					300.0	1.2	1
210.0	.4					315.0	.7	
220.0	.2					330.0	.4	
						345.0	.2	
						360.0	.1	

Table 13.16 Beta Ray Dose Rates for an Isotropic Source in Air of Density 1.205 mg/cm³ (Continued)

R (cm)	^{212}Pb $R^2J'(R)$	Plane Source	R (cm)	^{234}mTh-Pa[a] $R^2J'(R)$	Plane Source
0.0	348.8	*****	0.0	562.4	*****
1.0	244.2	3289	8.0	155.8	2203
2.0	214.7	2327	16.0	105.7	1655
3.0	194.7	1813	24.0	91.9	1407
4.0	179.2	1477	32.0	89.8	1244
5.0	166.2	1236	40.0	89.5	1119
10.0	120.7	635	80.0	87.3	749
15.0	90.8	370	120.0	82.9	535
20.0	68.7	227	160.0	77.0	391
25.0	51.6	143	200.0	70.2	289
30.0	38.2	91	240.0	63.1	212
35.0	27.9	59	280.0	55.6	155
40.0	20.0	39	320.0	48.1	112
45.0	14.3	27	360.0	40.7	79
50.0	10.2	18	400.0	33.5	54
55.0	7.3	13	440.0	26.7	36
60.0	5.5	10	480.0	20.5	23
65.0	4.3	7	520.0	15.1	14
70.0	3.4	5	560.0	10.6	8
75.0	2.8	4	600.0	7.0	5
80.0	2.3	3	640.0	4.3	2
85.0	1.9	2	680.0	2.4	1
90.0	1.6	2	720.0	1.2	
95.0	1.2	1	760.0	.5	
100.0	1.0	1	800.0	.2	
105.0	.7	1			
110.0	.5				
115.0	.4				
120.0	.3				
125.0	.2				

[a] Parent-Daughter for 1 MBq of the parent in transient equilibrium with its daughter.

Table 13.17 Beta Dose Rate (nGy h^{-1}) at Various Depths in Water, on the Axis of a 1 Bq cm^{-2} Plane Isotopic Source Distributed Uniformly over a 1 cm^2 Circular Area on an Air-Water Boundary (After Cross et al., 1992b)*

	nGy h^{-1}				nGy h^{-1}		
Nuclide	**0.07 mm**	**3 mm**	**10 mm**	**Nuclide**	**0.07 mm**	**3 mm**	**10 mm**
^{14}C	290			^{113m}Cd	1341		
^{22}Na	1442			^{122}Sb	1617		
^{24}Na	1692	32.8		^{123}Sn	1030		
^{28}Al	1846	298	2	^{123}I	305		
^{31}Si	1715	48.3		^{124}Sb	1389	46.6	
^{32}P	1726	89.5		^{125}Sb	679		
^{35}S	310			^{126}I	697	1.8	
^{36}Cl	1577			^{129}I	149		
^{38}Cl	1856	270	27.7	^{131}I	1319		
^{42}K	1852	314	13.2	^{132}I	1576	43.2	
^{45}Ca	747			^{134}Cs	1000		
^{52m}Mn	1757	268	0.8	^{135}I	1508	14.2	
^{52}Fe	974			^{137}Cs	1432		
^{56}Mn	1701	163	1	^{140}Ba	1455	0.7	
^{56}Ni	25.5			^{140}La	1639	28.5	
^{57}Co	68.4			^{141}Ce	1538		
^{58}Co	245			^{143}Pr	1524	0.3	
^{59}Fe	1027			^{144}Ce	815		
^{60}Co	935			^{144}Pr	1815	285	3
^{64}Cu	813			^{147}Pm	535		
^{65}Zn	21.7			^{153}Sm	1425		
^{66}Cu	1819	243	0.5	^{154}Eu	1840	11.6	
^{74}As	1060	7.8		^{155}Eu	270		
^{82}Br	1181			^{182}Ta	1780		
^{85}Sr	8.9			^{192}Ir	1384		
^{88}Rb	1940	364	38.6	^{198}Au	1564	0.4	
^{89}Sr	1667	54.6		^{201}Tl	208		
^{90}Sr	1377			^{203}Hg	820		
^{90}Y	1756	200		^{204}Tl	1346		
^{95}Zr	1058			^{208}Tl	1737	54.9	
^{95}Nb	230			^{210}Bi	1471	2.4	
^{99}Mo	1537	9.6		^{212}Pb	1707		
^{99}Tc	922			^{212}Bi	1071	81.8	
^{99m}Tc	207			^{214}Pb	1499		
^{105}Rh	1168			^{214}Bi	1639	86.5	1.1
^{106}Rh	1845	326	10.3	^{228}Ac	1542	16.6	
^{109}Cd	491			^{231}Th	738		
^{110}Ag	1821	278	1.9	^{234}Th	348		
^{110m}Ag	407	57.9		^{234m}Pa	1724	152	

* This data for a 1 cm^2 source serves equally well for a point source, and underestimates a 100 cm^2 circular area of 1 Bq cm^{-2} by no more than 11%.

Table 13.18 Dose Rates for Beta Emitters[a] in an Infinite Water Medium (After Cross et al., 1992)

^{14}C			^{22}Na			^{24}Na			^{32}P		
R	$R^2J'(R)$	Plane Source	R	$R^2J'(R)$	Plane Source	R	$R^2J'(R)$	Plane Source	R	$R^2J'(R)$	Plane Source
0.000	611.5	inf.	0.0000	147.9	inf.	0.000	114.9	inf.	0.000	106.4	inf.
0.001	373.7	3429	0.0015	162.4	3421	0.004	112.4	2710	0.006	104.5	2473
0.002	304.3	2009	0.0030	164.7	2736	0.008	112.6	2239	0.012	105.0	2035
0.003	252.3	1310	0.0045	164.7	2322	0.012	112.9	1956	0.018	105.5	1770
0.004	209.9	895	0.0060	163.8	2027	0.016	113.1	1753	0.024	105.8	1581
0.005	174.7	626	0.0075	162.4	1800	0.020	113.1	1595	0.030	106.0	1433
0.006	144.7	444	0.0150	151.2	1143	0.040	112.0	1123	0.060	105.3	990
0.007	119.2	316	0.0225	136.9	781	0.060	108.9	846	0.090	102.5	729
0.008	97.5	226	0.0300	121.4	549	0.080	104.5	654	0.120	98.0	549
0.009	79.0	160	0.0375	105.9	391	0.100	99.1	512	0.150	92.0	417
0.010	63.4	113	0.0450	90.8	278	0.120	92.8	403	0.180	84.8	316
0.011	50.2	79	0.0525	76.5	197	0.140	85.9	316	0.210	76.6	238
0.012	39.2	55	0.0600	63.3	139	0.160	78.4	247	0.240	67.7	177
0.013	30.2	37	0.0675	51.4	96	0.180	70.6	192	0.270	58.7	130
0.014	22.8	25	0.0750	40.8	66	0.200	62.6	148	0.300	49.7	95
0.015	16.8	16	0.0825	31.7	44	0.220	54.7	113	0.330	41.2	67
0.016	12.2	11	0.0900	24.0	29	0.240	47.0	85	0.360	33.4	47
0.017	8.6	7	0.0975	17.7	18	0.260	39.7	64	0.390	26.3	32
0.018	5.9	4	0.1050	12.6	11	0.280	33.0	47	0.420	20.2	21
0.019	3.9	2	0.1125	8.7	7	0.300	26.9	34	0.450	15.0	14
0.020	2.5	1	0.1200	5.7	4	0.320	21.5	24	0.480	10.7	8
0.021	1.5		0.1275	3.6	2	0.340	16.9	16	0.510	7.3	5
0.022	0.9		0.1350	2.1	1	0.360	12.9	11	0.540	4.8	3
0.023	0.5		0.1425	1.2		0.380	9.6	7	0.570	3.0	1
0.024	0.3		0.1500	0.6		0.400	6.9	5	0.600	1.7	
0.025	0.1		0.1575	0.3		0.420	4.8	3	0.630	0.9	
0.026	0.0		0.1650	0.1		0.440	3.2	2	0.660	0.4	
						0.460	2.1	1	0.690	0.2	
						0.480	1.3				
						0.500	0.7				

(continued)

Table 13.18 Dose Rates for Beta Emitters[a] in an Infinite Water Medium (Continued)

^{35}S			^{45}Ca			^{59}Fe			^{60}Co		
R	R²J′(R)	Plane Source	R	R²J′(R)	Plane Source	R	R²J′(R)	Plane Source	R	R²J′(R)	Plane Source
0.000	685.9	inf.	0.000	476.2	inf.	0.000	366.3	inf.	0.0000	407.3	inf.
0.001	354.2	3266	0.002	265.0	2558	0.001	258.2	3839	0.0006	294.8	4757
0.002	283.8	1929	0.004	218.1	1546	0.002	232.2	2812	0.0012	268.1	3578
0.003	234.9	1278	0.006	184.2	1041	0.003	214.3	2251	0.0018	251.2	2926
0.004	196.7	890	0.008	157.0	734	0.004	200.6	1878	0.0024	238.4	2486
0.005	165.3	638	0.010	134.1	531	0.005	189.2	1606	0.0030	227.3	2161
0.006	139.0	464	0.012	114.2	389	0.010	146.5	903	0.0060	186.6	1294
0.007	116.6	340	0.014	96.9	287	0.015	116.7	572	0.0090	157.4	862
0.008	97.5	251	0.016	81.7	213	0.020	93.5	383	0.0120	133.6	601
0.009	81.1	185	0.018	68.5	157	0.025	75.2	266	0.0150	113.4	428
0.010	66.9	136	0.020	56.8	116	0.030	60.5	188	0.0180	95.8	309
0.011	54.8	99	0.022	46.8	85	0.035	48.8	135	0.0210	80.4	224
0.012	44.5	72	0.024	38.1	62	0.040	39.6	98	0.0240	66.9	162
0.013	35.7	52	0.026	30.6	44	0.045	32.3	72	0.0270	55.2	117
0.014	28.3	37	0.028	24.3	31	0.050	26.4	52	0.0300	45.0	84
0.015	22.2	26	0.030	19.0	22	0.055	21.5	38	0.0330	36.2	60
0.016	17.1	18	0.032	14.7	15	0.060	17.4	27	0.0360	28.7	42
0.017	13.0	12	0.034	11.1	10	0.065	14.0	19	0.0390	22.4	29
0.018	9.7	8	0.036	8.2	7	0.070	11.0	14	0.0420	17.2	20
0.019	7.1	5	0.038	6.0	4	0.075	8.6	9	0.0450	13.0	13
0.020	5.0	3	0.040	4.2	3	0.080	6.5	6	0.0480	9.6	9
0.021	3.5	2	0.042	2.9	2	0.085	4.8	4	0.0510	6.9	6
0.022	2.4	1	0.044	1.9	1	0.090	3.5	3	0.0540	4.8	3
0.023	1.6		0.046	1.2		0.095	2.5	2	0.0570	3.3	2
0.024	1.0		0.048	0.8		0.100	1.7	1	0.0600	2.1	1
0.025	0.6		0.050	0.5		0.105	1.1		0.0630	1.3	
0.026	0.3		0.052	0.3		0.110	0.7		0.0660	0.8	
0.027	0.2		0.054	0.1		0.115	0.4		0.0690	0.5	
0.028	0.1		0.056	0.1		0.120	0.2		9.0720	0.2	
0.029	0.0					0.125	0.1		0.0750	0.1	

Table 13.18 Dose Rates for Beta Emitters[a] in an Infinite Water Medium (Continued)

^{67}Ga			^{89}Sr			^{90}Sr			^{90}Y		
R	$R^2J'(R)$	Plane Source	R	$R^2J'(R)$	Plane Source	R	$R^2J'(R)$	Plane Source	R	$R^2J'(R)$	Plane Source
0.0000	69.9	inf.	0.000	125.8	inf.	0.0000	239.8	inf.	0.000	104.0	inf.
0.0015	83.3	1516	0.005	114.1	2507	0.0008	195.9	4186	0.008	99.6	2343
0.0030	109.3	1113	0.010	111.9	2034	0.0016	185.7	3386	0.016	99.2	1927
0.0045	150.3	786	0.015	110.5	1754	0.0024	179.0	2928	0.024	98.9	1678
0.0060	191.8	479	0.020	109.3	1557	0.0032	174.2	2611	0.032	98.6	1501
0.0075	178.3	221	0.025	108.2	1405	0.0040	170.3	2371	0.040	98.3	1363
0.0090	87.6	69	0.050	103.1	963	0.0048	166.8	2178	0.080	96.4	956
0.0105	18.9	18	0.075	97.8	710	0.0056	163.7	2018	0.120	93.5	717
0.0120	3.1	8	0.100	92.1	540	0.0064	161.0	1882	0.160	89.7	552
0.0135	1.2	7	0.125	86.1	416	0.0072	158.5	1764	0.200	85.1	430
0.0150	1.1	6	0.150	79.8	321	0.0080	156.1	1660	0.240	79.6	336
0.0165	1.2	5	0.175	73.1	247	0.0160	138.1	1044	0.280	73.6	262
0.0180	1.3	5	0.200	65.9	189	0.0240	123.3	716	0.320	67.1	203
0.0195	1.4	4	0.225	58.5	143	0.0320	109.6	506	0.360	60.4	156
0.0210	1.5	3	0.250	50.9	107	0.0400	96.5	363	0.400	53.5	119
0.0225	1.5	3	0.275	43.5	78	0.0480	83.7	260	0.440	46.6	89
0.0240	1.5	2	0.300	36.4	56	0.0560	71.4	185	0.480	39.7	65
0.0255	1.3	1	0.325	29.8	40	0.0640	59.6	130	0.520	33.2	47
0.0270	1.2		0.350	23.7	27	0.0720	48.7	90	0.560	27.0	33
0.0285	1.0		0.375	18.3	18	0.0800	38.9	61	0.600	21.3	22
0.0300	0.7		0.400	13.7	12	0.0880	30.1	40	0.640	16.3	15
0.0315	0.5		0.425	9.9	7	0.0960	22.7	26	0.680	12.0	9
0.0330	0.3		0.450	6.8	4	0.1040	16.4	16	0.720	8.5	6
0.0345	0.1		0.475	4.4	2	0.1120	11.4	9	0.760	5.7	3
0.0360	0.1		0.500	2.7	1	0.1200	7.6	5	0.800	3.6	2
0.0375	0.0		0.525	1.6		0.1280	4.8	3	0.840	2.2	1
			0.550	0.8		0.1360	2.8	1	0.880	1.2	
			0.575	0.4		0.1440	1.5		0.920	0.6	
			0.600	0.2		0.1520	0.8		0.960	0.2	
						0.1600	0.3				

(continued)

Table 13.18 Dose Rates for Beta Emitters[a] in an Infinite Water Medium (Continued)

^{91}Y			^{95}Zr			^{95}Nb			^{99m}Tc		
R	R²J′(R)	Plane Source	R	R²J′(R)	Plane Source	R	R²J′(R)	Plane Source	R	R²J′(R)	Plane Source
0.000	124.5	inf.	0.0000	333.2	inf.	0.000	777.4	inf.	0.000	18.1	inf.
0.005	113.0	2513	0.0015	240.7	3283	0.001	354.3	2987	0.001	18.9	508
0.010	110.9	2044	0.0030	214.7	2329	0.002	269.8	1680	0.002	20.2	427
0.015	109.5	1767	0.0045	197.1	1811	0.003	214.9	1071	0.003	21.8	374
0.020	108.3	1572	0.0060	182.2	1471	0.004	174.1	721	0.004	23.8	333
0.025	107.3	1421	0.0075	170.5	1225	0.005	142.1	501	0.005	26.3	298
0.050	102.4	982	0.0090	159.6	1036	0.006	116.2	353	0.006	29.3	266
0.075	97.5	731	0.0105	149.9	886	0.007	94.8	251	0.007	32.9	236
0.100	92.2	560	0.0120	141.1	765	0.008	77.0	179	0.008	37.0	207
0.125	86.7	436	0.0135	132.7	663	0.009	62.2	128	0.009	41.2	178
0.150	80.8	340	0.0150	124.9	578	0.010	49.8	91	0.010	45.2	149
0.175	74.5	265	0.0300	66.2	178	0.011	39.5	64	0.011	48.4	121
0.200	67.8	205	0.0450	31.0	56	0.012	31.0	45	0.012	49.8	95
0.225	60.8	158	0.0600	12.1	17	0.013	24.0	31	0.013	47.9	70
0.250	53.7	120	0.0750	3.9	6	0.014	18.3	21	0.014	43.1	49
0.275	46.6	90	0.0900	1.3	3	0.015	13.7	14	0.015	35.5	32
0.300	39.7	66	0.1050	0.7	2	0.016	10.1	9	0.016	26.2	19
0.325	33.1	48	0.1200	0.6	1	0.017	7.3	6	0.017	17.3	11
0.350	27.0	34	0.1350	0.5		0.018	5.1	4	0.018	10.4	6
0.375	21.5	24	0.1500	0.4		0.019	3.5	2	0.019	6.0	3
0.400	16.6	16	0.1650	0.3		0.020	2.3	1	0.020	3.4	2
0.425	12.5	10	0.1800	0.2		0.021	1.5		0.021	2.1	1
0.450	9.0	6	0.1950	0.2		0.022	0.9		0.022	1.2	
0.475	6.2	4	0.2100	0.1		0.023	0.5		0.023	0.7	
0.500	4.1	2	0.2250	0.1		0.024	0.3		0.024	0.3	
0.525	2.5	1	0.2400	0.1		0.025	0.2				
0.550	1.5		0.2550	0.0		0.026	0.1				
0.575	0.8		0.2700	0.0							
0.600	0.4		0.2850	0.0							
0.625	0.2		0.3000	0							

Table 13.18 Dose Rates for Beta Emitters[a] in an Infinite Water Medium (Continued)

^{106}Rh			^{123}I			^{125}I			^{131}I		
R	R²J′(R)	Plane Source	R	R²J′(R)	Plane Source	R	R²J′(R)	Plane Source	R	R²J′(R)	Plane Source
0.000	91.5	inf.	0.000	290.2	inf.	0.00000	59.4	inf.	0.000	267.3	inf.
0.012	91.0	2268	0.001	781.0	2339	0.00007	62.3	1880	0.001	225.0	4125
0.024	91.5	1886	0.002	38.4	623	0.00014	65.3	1613	0.002	226.3	3179
0.036	92.0	1656	0.003	29.4	538	0.00021	68.9	1444	0.003	201.8	2642
0.048	92.5	1490	0.004	31.7	483	0.00028	73.6	1316	0.004	177.6	2301
0.060	92.9	1360	0.005	34.4	437	0.00035	79.1	1209	0.005	171.7	2057
0.120	94.1	969	0.006	37.7	395	0.00042	85.3	1116	0.006	166.6	1864
0.180	93.5	733	0.007	41.5	357	0.00049	92.6	1030	0.007	162.1	1705
0.240	91.1	567	0.008	46.1	320	0.00056	101.1	948	0.008	157.9	1571
0.300	87.1	443	0.009	51.2	284	0.00063	110.5	870	0.009	154.3	1456
0.360	81.8	346	0.010	56.3	249	0.00070	121.2	794	0.010	150.8	1355
0.420	75.6	270	0.011	61.2	214	0.00077	133.0	718	0.020	123.2	781
0.480	68.8	210	0.012	65.5	179	0.00084	145.3	642	0.030	102.3	497
0.540	61.7	161	0.013	68.0	146	0.00091	155.6	566	0.040	85.2	329
0.600	54.4	123	0.014	67.1	114	0.00098	163.3	492	0.050	70.9	220
0.660	47.2	93	0.015	62.7	86	0.00105	168.4	420	0.060	58.2	146
0.720	40.2	69	0.016	55.3	62	0.00112	170.4	351	0.070	46.3	96
0.780	33.6	50	0.017	45.3	43	0.00119	166.3	287	0.080	35.3	62
0.840	27.6	36	0.018	34.1	29	0.00126	156.2	229	0.090	25.8	39
0.900	22.1	25	0.019	23.8	19	0.00133	141.7	179	0.100	18.7	24
0.960	17.3	17	0.020	15.7	13	0.00140	124.7	136	0.110	13.3	15
1.020	13.1	12	0.021	10.5	9	0.00147	105.9	100	0.120	9.1	9
1.080	9.7	7	0.022	7.4	6	0.00154	86.1	72	0.130	6.0	5
1.140	6.9	5	0.023	5.8	4	0.00161	66.9	51	0.140	3.7	3
1.200	4.7	3	0.024	4.5	3	0.00168	50.5	35	0.150	2.2	1
1.260	3.1	2	0.025	3.3	2	0.00175	37.1	24	0.160	1.2	
1.320	1.9	1	0.026	2.3	1	0.00182	26.9	16	0.170	0.6	
1.380	1.1		0.027	1.5		0.00189	19.4	11	0.180	0.3	
1.440	0.6		0.028	0.9		0.00196	13.7	7	0.190	0.1	
1.500	0.3		0.029	0.5		0.00203	9.2	4	0.200	0	

(continued)

Table 13.18 Dose Rates for Beta Emitters[a] in an Infinite Water Medium (Continued)

^{133}Xe			^{135}Xe			^{137}Cs-Ba			^{140}Ba		
R	R²J′(R)	Plane Source	R	R²J′(R)	Plane Source	R	R²J′(R)	Plane Source	R	R²J′(R)	Plane Source
0.000	596.3	inf.	0.000	186.5	inf.	0.000	257.8	inf.	0.000	225.0	inf.
0.003	487.7	2921	0.003	156.0	2945	0.002	200.9	3350	0.003	163.7	2737
0.006	237.1	1403	0.006	149.7	2305	0.004	185.1	2541	0.006	153.0	2074
0.009	158.5	906	0.009	145.8	1934	0.006	174.8	2089	0.009	146.4	1698
0.012	132.9	644	0.012	143.1	1674	0.008	166.6	1782	0.012	141.3	1439
0.015	114.3	472	0.015	141.0	1476	0.010	159.8	1555	0.015	134.5	1247
0.018	98.2	350	0.030	134.9	898	0.012	153.9	1375	0.030	106.2	743
0.021	84.2	262	0.045	107.5	594	0.014	148.4	1229	0.045	88.7	498
0.024	71.9	197	0.060	91.4	415	0.016	143.3	1107	0.060	74.6	351
0.027	60.9	148	0.075	79.6	296	0.018	138.6	1003	0.075	63.2	255
0.030	51.3	111	0.090	68.4	211	0.020	134.0	913	0.090	54.0	188
0.033	42.8	82	0.105	57.9	150	0.040	95.3	432	0.105	46.3	140
0.036	35.4	61	0.120	48.1	106	0.060	64.3	232	0.120	39.8	104
0.039	29.0	45	0.135	39.2	74	0.080	41.2	137	0.135	33.9	77
0.042	23.5	33	0.150	31.3	50	0.100	27.5	89	0.150	28.6	56
0.045	18.8	23	0.165	24.4	34	0.120	21.7	61	0.165	23.7	40
0.048	14.8	17	0.180	18.4	22	0.140	20.2	41	0.180	19.3	29
0.051	11.5	12	0.195	13.5	14	0.160	18.6	25	0.195	15.3	20
0.054	8.8	8	0.210	9.6	8	0.180	14.7	12	0.210	11.9	14
0.057	6.6	5	0.225	6.5	5	0.200	8.4	5	0.225	9.0	9
0.060	4.8	4	0.240	4.3	3	0.220	2.9	1	0.240	6.7	6
0.063	3.5	2	0.255	2.6	1	0.240	0.6		0.255	4.8	4
0.066	2.4	1	0.270	1.5		0.026	0.2		0.270	3.3	2
0.069	1.6		0.285	0.8		0.028	0.1		0.285	2.2	1
0.072	1.1		0.300	0.4		0.300	0.1		0.300	1.4	
0.075	0.7		0.315	0.2		0.320	0.0		0.315	0.8	
0.078	0.4		0.330	0.1		0.340	0.0		0.330	0.4	
0.081	0.2					0.360	0.0		0.345	0.2	
0.084	0.1					0.380	0.0		0.360	0.1	
0.087	0.1					0.400	0.0		0.375	0.0	

Table 13.18 Dose Rates for Beta Emitters[a] in an Infinite Water Medium (Continued)

^{140}La			^{141}Ce			^{144}Pr			^{147}Pm		
R	$R^2J'(R)$	Plane Source	R	$R^2J'(R)$	Plane Source	R	$R^2J'(R)$	Plane Source	R	$R^2J'(R)$	Plane Source
0.000	128.1	inf.	0.0000	340.7	inf.	0.000	95.6	inf.	0.0000	585.5	inf.
0.008	115.8	2135	0.0008	275.0	5241	0.006	93.9	2614	0.0015	294.4	2715
0.016	113.5	1654	0.0016	260.6	4119	0.012	93.8	2221	0.0030	233.3	1609
0.024	111.5	1372	0.0024	253.1	3474	0.018	93.9	1985	0.0045	192.8	1074
0.032	109.6	1173	0.0032	248.7	3023	0.024	94.0	1816	0.0060	161.5	756
0.040	107.6	1022	0.0040	246.9	2677	0.030	94.1	1685	0.0075	136.6	548
0.080	96.6	594	0.0048	246.7	2395	0.036	94.2	1578	0.0090	115.6	404
0.120	83.7	367	0.0056	248.7	2156	0.042	94.3	1486	0.0105	98.0	300
0.160	69.7	230	0.0064	252.0	1946	0.048	94.4	1407	0.0120	82.8	225
0.200	55.4	143	0.0072	256.3	1758	0.054	94.5	1337	0.0135	69.6	168
0.240	41.9	87	0.0080	260.0	1588	0.060	94.6	1275	0.0150	58.3	126
0.280	30.3	52	0.0160	139.6	751	0.120	94.5	879	0.0165	48.4	94
0.320	21.0	30	0.0240	103.2	446	0.180	92.5	644	0.0180	40.0	70
0.360	13.9	18	0.0320	81.1	280	0.240	88.7	481	0.0195	32.8	52
0.400	8.9	10	0.0400	63.3	179	0.300	83.0	361	0.0210	26.6	38
0.440	5.6	6	0.0480	48.7	115	0.360	76.1	271	0.0225	21.3	28
0.480	3.4	3	0.0560	36.7	74	0.420	68.3	201	0.0240	16.9	20
0.520	2.1	2	0.0640	27.1	48	0.480	59.9	147	0.0255	13.3	14
0.560	1.3	1	0.0720	19.6	30	0.540	51.4	106	0.0270	10.2	10
0.600	0.8		0.0800	14.0	19	0.600	42.9	75	0.0285	7.8	7
0.640	0.5		0.0880	9.8	12	0.660	34.9	52	0.0300	5.8	5
0.680	0.3		0.0960	6.8	8	0.720	27.5	35	0.0315	4.3	3
0.720	0.2		0.1040	4.6	5	0.780	20.9	22	0.0330	3.0	2
0.760	0.1		0.1120	3.2	3	0.840	15.3	14	0.0345	2.1	1
0.800	0.1		0.1200	2.1	2	0.900	10.7	8	0.0360	1.5	
0.840	0.0		0.1280	1.4	1	0.960	7.2	5	0.0375	1.0	
0.880	0.0		0.1360	0.9		1.020	4.5	2	0.0390	0.6	
			0.1440	0.6		1.080	2.6	1	0.0405	0.4	
			0.1520	0.3		1.140	1.4		0.0420	0.2	
			0.1600	0.2		1.200	0.7		0.0435	0.1	

(continued)

Table 13.18 Dose Rates for Beta Emitters[a] in an Infinite Water Medium (Continued)

^{170}Tm			^{198}Au			^{204}Tl			^{210}Pb		
R	$R^2J'(R)$	Plane Source	R	$R^2J'(R)$	Plane Source	R	$R^2J'(R)$	Plane Source	R	$R^2J'(R)$	Plane Source
0.000	210.9	inf.	0.000	184.3	inf.	0.000	221.6	inf.	0.0000	4271.9	inf.
0.003	208.4	3241	0.012	136.4	1658	0.002	169.5	2984	0.0002	381.0	4184
0.006	234.5	2314	0.024	125.0	1111	0.004	156.7	2301	0.0004	238.0	2887
0.009	144.9	1837	0.036	116.1	808	0.006	148.6	1918	0.0006	239.1	2288
0.012	132.0	1588	0.048	108.6	606	0.008	142.1	1657	0.0008	259.4	1840
0.015	129.0	1406	0.060	100.8	460	0.010	136.9	1462	0.0010	279.7	1464
0.030	115.9	893	0.072	90.9	350	0.020	117.4	929	0.0012	279.9	1144
0.045	104.0	617	0.084	79.1	268	0.030	103.1	652	0.0014	249.6	888
0.060	92.5	441	0.096	68.4	206	0.040	91.2	478	0.0016	214.6	694
0.075	81.5	319	0.108	59.5	159	0.050	80.9	358	0.0018	195.2	543
0.090	70.9	232	0.120	51.4	122	0.060	71.5	271	0.0020	190.9	415
0.105	60.9	168	0.132	44.3	94	0.070	63.0	206	0.0022	184.2	303
0.120	51.5	121	0.144	37.9	71	0.080	55.1	156	0.0024	165.6	207
0.135	42.8	86	0.156	32.1	54	0.090	47.8	118	0.0026	135.0	132
0.150	34.9	61	0.168	26.8	40	0.100	41.1	89	0.0028	100.1	77
0.165	27.8	42	0.180	22.1	29	0.110	34.9	66	0.0030	65.0	41
0.180	21.7	29	0.192	17.9	21	0.120	29.2	49	0.0032	38.2	20
0.195	16.5	19	0.204	14.2	15	0.130	24.1	35	0.0034	19.7	9
0.210	12.2	12	0.216	11.1	11	0.140	19.5	25	0.0036	9.4	4
0.225	8.8	8	0.228	8.5	7	0.150	15.5	18	0.0038	4.0	2
0.240	6.1	5	0.240	6.4	5	0.160	12.0	12	0.0040	1.7	1
0.255	4.1	3	0.252	4.7	3	0.170	9.1	8	0.0042	0.8	
0.270	2.6	1	0.264	3.3	2	0.180	6.7	5	0.0044	0.3	
0.285	1.6		0.276	2.3	1	0.190	4.8	3	0.0046	0.2	
0.300	0.9		0.288	1.5		0.200	3.3	2	0.0048	0.1	
0.315	0.5		0.300	1.0		0.210	2.2	1	0.0050	0.1	
0.330	0.2		0.312	0.6		0.220	1.4		0.0052	0.0	
0.345	0.1		0.324	0.3		0.230	0.8		0.0054	0.0	
0.360	0.0		0.336	0.2		0.240	0.4				
			0.348	0.1		0.250	0.2				

[a] J′(R) is the dose rate (nGy h^{-1}) at distance R (cm) from a 1-Bq point isotropic source. The third column for each nuclide gives the dose rate (nGy H^{-1}) at distance R (cm) from a uniform plane source of 1 Bq cm^{-2} and infinite lateral extent.

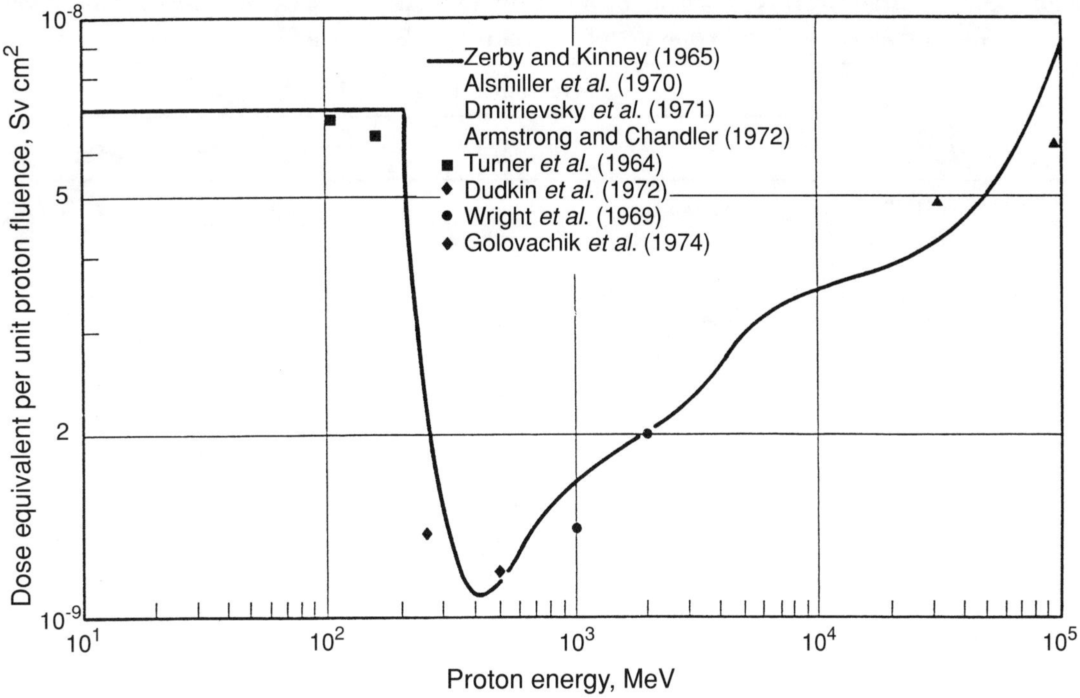

Figure 13.11 Maximum Dose Equivalent per Unit Fluence for Protons Incident in a Plane Parallel Beam on a 30 cm Thick Semi-Infinite Slab Phantom. (Courtesy ICRP from Publication 51, 1987)

Table 13.19 Statement on Neutron Quality Factor 1985 (Courtesy ICRP from Publication 45, 1985b)

The ICRP issued the following statement from its meeting in Paris during March 1985 on the value of the quality factor in the case of neutrons (ICRP, 1985b). "The information now available on the relative biological effectiveness (RBE) for neutrons for a variety of cellular effects *in vitro,* and for life shortening in the mouse, is being reviewed by the Commission. The implications of this information will be considered as part of a larger review of recommendations to be undertaken by the Commission over the next four years or so. Meanwhile, in the case of neutrons, the Commission recommends an increase in Q by a factor of 2. The permitted approximation for Q for fast neutrons thus changes from 10 to 20. These changes relate only to neutrons, and no other changes in Q are recommended at this time."

The available conversion coefficients for neutrons are based on the established L_∞-Q relationship for the secondary charged particles (ICRP, 1977), which is incorporated in the calculations. Until this relationship is redefined, it is not appropriate to recalculate the coefficients nor the contributions that the various charged particles make to the total dose equivalent. Neither is it relevant to make approximate adjustments for some of the contributions such as recoil protons and capture photons. All that should be done is simply to apply the factor of 2 as the Commission recommends. Since all the calculations referred to predate the statement or do not take it into account, the results relate to dose equivalent for neutrons as defined before 1985. When the results are multiplied by a factor of 2, they relate to the dose equivalent as redefined in 1985 for neutrons. A note to this effect is attached to all the data presented here.

Since the change in Q for neutrons may not be introduced into all national procedures at the same time, it seems appropriate for statements of the dose equivalent for neutrons to indicate whether the change has been applied.

Table 13.20 Effective Dose Equivalent per Unit Fluence for Neutrons Incident in Various Geometries on an Anthropomorphic Phantom (Courtesy ICRP from Publication 51, 1987)

Neutron Energy (MeV)	Conversion Coefficient, 10^{-12} Sv cm^2			
	AP	PA	LAT	ROT
2.5×10^{-8}	(4.00)	(2.60)	(1.30)	(2.30)
1.0×10^{-7}	(4.40)	(2.70)	(1.40)	(2.40)
1.0×10^{-6}	4.82	2.81	1.43	2.63
1.0×10^{-5}	4.46	2.78	1.33	2.48
1.0×10^{-4}	4.14	2.63	1.27	2.33
1.0×10^{-3}	3.83	2.49	1.19	2.18
1.0×10^{-2}	4.53	2.58	1.27	2.41
2.0×10^{-2}	5.87	2.79	1.46	2.89
5.0×10^{-2}	10.9	3.64	2.14	4.70
1.0×10^{-1}	19.8	5.69	3.57	8.15
2.0×10^{-1}	38.6	8.60	6.94	15.3
5.0×10^{-1}	87.0	30.8	18.7	38.8
1.0×10^{0}	143	53.5	33.3	65.7
1.5×10^{0}	183	85.8	52.1	93.7
2.0×10^{0}	214	120	71.8	120
3.0×10^{0}	264	174	105	162
4.0×10^{0}	300	215	131	195
5.0×10^{0}	327	244	151	219
6.0×10^{0}	347	265	167	237
7.0×10^{0}	365	283	181	253
8.0×10^{0}	380	296	194	266
1.0×10^{1}	410	321	218	292
1.4×10^{1}	(480)	(415)	(280)	(365)

See notes to Figures 13.2, 13.3 and 13.4 for irradiation geometries.
These values of the conversion coefficient relate to the dose equivalent for neutrons as defined before 1985. They should be multiplied by a factor of 2 to obtain the dose equivalent as redefined for neutrons in 1985 (ICRP, 1985b). See Table 13.19.
Values in parenthesis are extrapolated from original data.

Table 13.21 Dose-Equivalent Indices per Unit Fluence for Neutrons Incident in a Plane Parallel Beam on the ICRU Sphere (Courtesy ICRP from Publication 51, 1987)

Neutron Energy (MeV)	Conversion Coefficient, 10^{-12} Sv cm^2	
	$H_{I,d}$[a]	$H_{I,s}$[b]
2.5×10^{-8}	8.00	9.50
1.0×10^{-7}	10.1	11.1
1.0×10^{-6}	11.8	11.2
1.0×10^{-5}	11.6	9.20
1.0×10^{-4}	11.0	7.10
1.0×10^{-3}	9.50	6.20
1.0×10^{-2}	8.60	9.50
2.0×10^{-2}	14.5	19.9
5.0×10^{-2}	35.0	50.6
1.0×10^{-1}	69.0	96.0
2.0×10^{-1}	124	151
5.0×10^{-1}	258	279
1.0×10^{0}	339	364
1.5×10^{0}	363	375
2.0×10^{0}	358	369
3.0×10^{0}	388	418
4.0×10^{0}	418	439
5.0×10^{0}	396	402
6.0×10^{0}	402	415
7.0×10^{0}	416	444
8.0×10^{0}	435	464
1.0×10^{1}	464	481
1.4×10^{1}	520	520
1.7×10^{1}	610	640
2.0×10^{1}	650	660

These values of the conversion coefficient relate to the dose equivalent for neutrons as defined before 1985. They should be multiplied by a factor of 2 to obtain the dose equivalent as redefined for neutrons in 1985 (ICRP, 1985b). See table 13.19.

[a] Deep dose-equivalent index.

[b] Shallow dose-equivalent index.

Table 13.22 Dose-Equivalent Indices per Unit Fluence for Neutrons Incident Isotropically on the ICRU Sphere (Courtesy ICRP from Publication 51, 1987)

Neutron Energy (MeV)	Conversion Coefficient, 10^{-12} Sv cm^2	
	$H_{I,d}$[a]	$H_{I,s}$[b]
2.5×10^{-8}	2.10	3.00
1.0×10^{-7}	2.80	3.40
1.0×10^{-6}	3.40	3.30
1.0×10^{-5}	3.30	2.80
1.0×10^{-4}	3.10	2.40
1.0×10^{-3}	3.00	2.00
1.0×10^{-2}	3.10	4.30
2.0×10^{-2}	4.30	9.27
5.0×10^{-2}	9.76	25.0
1.0×10^{-1}	22.0	49.0
2.0×10^{-1}	42.7	91.6
5.0×10^{-1}	84.0	136
1.0×10^{0}	135	184
1.5×10^{0}	159	195
2.0×10^{0}	175	211
3.0×10^{0}	205	224
4.0×10^{0}	236	252
5.0×10^{0}	239	247
6.0×10^{0}	250	258
7.0×10^{0}	266	277
8.0×10^{0}	277	300
1.0×10^{1}	306	340
1.4×10^{1}	380	400
1.7×10^{1}	420	440
2.0×10^{1}	490	520

These values of the conversion coefficient relate to the dose equivalent for neutrons as defined before 1985. They should be multiplied by a factor of 2 to obtain the dose equivalent as redefined for neutrons in 1985 (ICRP, 1985b). See Table 13.19.

[a] Deep dose-equivalent index.

[b] Shallow dose-equivalent index.

Table 13.23 Dose-Equivalent per Unit Fluence at Depths of 0.07 mm, 3 mm and 10 mm on the Principal Axis for Neutrons Incident in a Plane Parallel Beam on the ICRU Sphere (Courtesy ICRP from Publication 51, 1987)

Neutron Energy (MeV)	Conversion Coefficient, 10^{-12} Sv cm^2		
	0.07 mm	3 mm	10 mm
2.5×10^{-8}	7.20	8.00	8.00
1.0×10^{-7}	5.50	8.50	10.4
1.0×10^{-6}	3.70	6.90	11.2
1.0×10^{-5}	2.80	5.30	9.20
1.0×10^{-4}	2.50	4.40	7.10
1.0×10^{-3}	2.80	3.90	6.20
1.0×10^{-2}	8.90	9.20	8.60
2.0×10^{-2}	18.2	18.3	14.6
5.0×10^{-2}	46.6	48.1	35.0
1.0×10^{-1}	95.0	95.0	69.0
2.0×10^{-1}	168	186	126
5.0×10^{-1}	219	266	258
1.0×10^{0}	292	332	340
1.5×10^{0}	292	344	362
2.0×10^{0}	283	335	352
3.0×10^{0}	305	358	380
4.0×10^{0}	329	387	409
5.0×10^{0}	301	358	378
6.0×10^{0}	302	364	383
7.0×10^{0}	312	384	403
8.0×10^{0}	341	407	417
1.0×10^{1}	368	446	446
1.4×10^{1}	359	520	520
1.7×10^{1}	421	610	610
2.0×10^{1}	516	670	650

These values of the conversion coefficient relate to the dose equivalent for neutrons as defined before 1985. They should be multiplied by a factor of 2 to obtain the dose equivalent as redefined for neutrons in 1985 (ICRP, 1985b). See Table 13.19.

Table 13.24 Dose-Equivalent per Unit Fluence at Depths of 0.07 mm, 3 mm and 10 mm for Neutrons Incident in an Isotropic Field on the ICRU Sphere (Courtesy ICRP from Publication 51, 1987)

Neutron Energy (MeV)	Conversion Coefficient, 10^{-12} Sv cm^2		
	0.07 mm	3 mm	10 mm
2.5×10^{-8}	2.70	2.70	2.10
1.0×10^{-7}	2.80	3.10	2.90
1.0×10^{-6}	2.30	2.80	3.30
1.0×10^{-5}	1.70	2.10	2.80
1.0×10^{-4}	1.40	1.80	2.40
1.0×10^{-3}	1.30	1.50	2.00
1.0×10^{-2}	4.30	4.20	3.10
2.0×10^{-2}	9.31	8.25	4.32
5.0×10^{-2}	25.0	20.7	9.76
1.0×10^{-1}	49.0	45.0	22.0
2.0×10^{-1}	90.5	79.3	43.2
5.0×10^{-1}	134	117	84.8
1.0×10^{0}	184	165	135
1.5×10^{0}	194	186	160
2.0×10^{0}	209	193	176
3.0×10^{0}	223	219	205
4.0×10^{0}	288	250	238
5.0×10^{0}	259	252	239
6.0×10^{0}	232	278	249
7.0×10^{0}	260	317	265
8.0×10^{0}	277	310	276
1.0×10^{1}	281	303	300
1.4×10^{1}	276	380	370
1.7×10^{1}	345	480	460
2.0×10^{1}	400	510	500

These values of the conversion coefficient relate to the dose equivalent for neutrons as defined before 1985. They should be multiplied by a factor of 2 to obtain the dose equivalent as redefined for neutrons in 1985 (ICRP, 1985b). See Table 13.19.

Table 13.25 Maximum Dose Equivalent per Unit Fluence and Dose Equivalent per Unit Fluence at a Depth of 10 mm for Neutrons Incident in a Plane Parallel Beam on a 30 cm Thick Semi-Infinite Slab Phantom (Courtesy ICRP from Publication 51, 1987)

Neuron Energy (MeV)	Conversion Coefficient, 10^{-12} Sv cm^2	
	Max.	10 mm
2	3.30	3.30
10	4.10	3.60
20	4.25	3.66
60	4.50	3.60
100	4.69	3.51
200	5.08	2.95
400	6.30	2.80
700	10.5	7.09
1,000	13.1	8.10
1,500	15.8	9.70
3,000	19.5	11.5
5,000	23.4	12.3
10,000	30.3	12.8
30,000	44.0	13.0
100,000	55.0	14.0

These values of the conversion coefficient relate to the dose equivalent for neutrons as defined before 1985. They should be multiplied by a factor of 2 to obtain the dose equivalent as redefined for neutrons in 1985 (ICRP, 1985b). See Table 13.19.

Table 13.26 Red Bone Marrow Dose Equivalent per Unit Fluence for Neutrons Incident in Various Geometries on an Anthropomorphic Phantom (Courtesy ICRP from Publication 51, 1987)

Neutron Energy (MeV)	Red Bone Marrow, 10^{-12} Sv cm^2			
	AP	PA	LAT	ROT
1.00×10^{-6}	3.17	4.33	2.00	2.87
1.00×10^{-5}	3.01	4.07	1.85	2.69
1.00×10^{-4}	2.87	3.78	1.69	2.51
1.00×10^{-3}	2.74	3.67	1.59	2.40
1.00×10^{-2}	2.91	3.93	1.85	2.64
2.30×10^{-2}	3.52	4.74	2.57	3.35
5.00×10^{-2}	5.31	7.24	4.42	5.35
1.00×10^{-1}	9.49	13.4	8.51	9.97
2.52×10^{-1}	24.5	26.0	21.6	23.4
5.00×10^{-1}	50.8	72.7	41.8	51.8
1.00×10^{0}	84.7	121	68.1	85.5
2.10×10^{0}	175	227	128	165
4.50×10^{0}	277	334	203	254
7.50×10^{0}	330	381	245	300
1.10×10^{1}	380	429	291	348
1.35×10^{1}	447	499	343	408

See notes to Figures 13.2, 13.3 and 13.4 for irradiation geometries. These values of the conversion coefficient relate to the dose equivalent for neutrons as defined before 1985. They should be multiplied by a factor of 2 to obtain the dose equivalent as redefined for neutrons in 1985 (ICRP, 1985b). See Table 13.19.

Table 13.27 Calculation of Internal Dose by Several Methods

(After Snyder et al. 1969, 1975, and ICRP Publication 30, 1977)

1. Medical Internal Radiation Dose (MIRD) Method

$$D(t \leftarrow s) = \tilde{A} \Sigma \Delta \phi (t \leftarrow s)$$

where $D(t \leftarrow s)$ = total dose (in rad) (source to target organ)
$\tilde{A}$ = cumulated activity (in microcurie–hours) the time integral of the activity
ϕ = specific absorbed fraction, fraction of energy absorbed in target compound to amount released in source (unique for each target, source pair and radionuclide)
Δ = average energy released per transformation divided by a constant.

For non-penetrating radiation (B^-, $B+$, ICE, and AE) target and source organs are the same.

$$A = 1.443\, T_{eff}\, A_0 \left(1 - e^{-0.693t/T_{eff}}\right).$$

For **t** very long

$$A = 1.443\, T_{eff}\, (in\ hours)\, A_0\, (in\ \mu Ci).$$

2. Equation with ''S'' Factor

$$D(t \leftarrow s) = \tilde{A}\ ``S",$$

where ''S'' $= \Delta \phi$.

''S'' gives the rads per μCi hrs of cumulated activity of a specifc radionuclide for a specific target, source organ pair.

3. ICRP Report No. 30 Dose Model

$$H_{50}(T \leftarrow S) = (1.6 \times 10^{-10}) U_s SEE(T \leftarrow S)$$

where H_{50} is the 50 year dose equivalent commitment in sieverts.

Where SEE is the *Specific Effective Energy* modified by a quality factor for radiation absorbed in the target organ (T) for each transformation in the source organ (S) expressed in MeV/g.

$$SEE = \sum \frac{Y \cdot E \cdot AF \cdot Q}{M_T}.$$

where:

Y = yield of radiations per transformation
E = average energy of the radiation
AF = absorbed faction of energy absorbed in the target organ (T) per emission of radiation in the source organ (S).
Q = quality factor
M_T = Mass of the target organ

and U_S is the number of nuclear transformations in the source organ (S) during the time interval for which the dose is to be calculated.

Table 13.28 Committed Dose Equivalent Per Unit Intake for Selected Radionuclides Used in Medicine and Industry and of Environmental Importance (After Eckerman et al., 1988)

The committed dose equivalent is the total dose delivered to a tissue of the body in the 50 year period following the intake. The committed effective dose equivalent is the weighted sum of the committed dose equivalent in the various tissues. That is:

$$H_E = \sum_T W_T H_T{}^a$$

Weighting Factors

Tissue/Organ	W_T
Gonads	0.25
Breast	0.15
R. Marrow	0.12
Lung	0.12
Thyroid	0.03
Endosteal	0.03
Remainder	0.30

The weighting factor for the *remainder* tissue group (0.30) is applied to the average dose among the five organs or tissues not given in the table which received the highest dose equivalent excluding skin. In the tabulations the committed dose equivalent for the remainder tissue group is tabulated in the column headed by H_{rem}. The last column in the tabulations, headed by H_{eff}, is the committed effective dose equivalent per unit intake.

The column headed f_1, in the case of inhalation intake , gives the lung clearance class (D, W, or Y) and the fractional uptake to blood from the gastrointestinal tract (f_1) for common chemical forms of the radionuclide. The aerosol is assumed to be characterized by an activity median aerodynamic diameter of one micron. Vapor forms are noted by *V* in the tabulations.

In the case of ingestion, the column headed by f_1 gives the fractional uptake to blood for chemical compounds of the radionuclide.

[a] W_T in this case is appropriate for use with 10CFR20 (see Table 13.1.3), but differs from those employed in the 1990 ICRP recommendations (see Table 4.2.1.3)

Table 13.29.1 Committed Dose Equivalent per Unit Intake via Ingestion (Sv/Bq)[a]

Nuclide	f1	Gonad	Breast	Lung	R Marrow	Endosteal	Thyroid	Hrem	Heff
^{3}H	1.00E + 00	1.73E − 11	1.73E − 11	1.73E − 11	1.73E − 11	1.73E − 11	1.73E − 11	1.73E − 11	1.73E − 11
^{10}Be	5.00E − 03	2.42E − 11	2.42E − 11	2.42E − 11	7.23E − 10	2.15E − 09	2.42E − 11	3.66E − 09	1.26E − 09
^{11}C	1.00	3.41E − 12	2.98E − 12	3.09E − 12	3.18E − 12	3.03E − 12	2.97E − 12	3.54E − 12	3.29E − 12
^{14}C	1.00	5.64E − 10	5.64E − 10	5.64E − 10	5.64E − 10	5.64E − 10	5.64E − 10	5.64E − 10	5.64E − 10
^{22}Na	1.00	2.81E − 09	2.58E − 09	2.51E − 09	4.29E − 09	5.54E − 09	2.50E − 09	3.18E − 09	3.10E − 09
^{24}Na	1.00	3.43E − 10	2.71E − 10	2.60E − 10	3.74E − 10	4.68E − 10	2.60E − 10	5.31E − 10	3.84E − 10
^{32}P	8.00E − 01	6.55E − 10	6.55E − 10	6.55E − 10	8.09E − 09	7.87E − 09	6.55E − 10	2.67E − 09	2.37E − 09
^{41}Ca	3.00E − 01	2.71E − 12	3.19E − 12	2.84E − 12	1.78E − 09	4.01E − 09	2.84E − 12	2.74E − 11	3.44E − 10
^{46}Sc	1.00E − 04	2.01E − 09	2.51E − 10	4.86E − 11	4.03E − 10	1.39E − 10	7.69E − 12	3.78E − 09	1.73E − 09
^{51}Cr	1.00E − 01	4.00E − 11	7.51E − 12	4.38E − 12	1.25E − 11	7.86E − 12	3.71E − 12	8.75E − 11	3.98E − 11
	1.00E − 02	3.96E − 11	4.49E − 12	9.47E − 13	8.52E − 12	3.19E − 12	4.26E − 13	9.17E − 11	3.93E − 11
^{54}Mn	1.00E − 01	9.48E − 10	2.77E − 10	2.29E − 10	4.89E − 10	5.71E − 10	1.33E − 10	1.21E − 09	7.48E − 10
^{56}Mn	1.00E − 01	8.53E − 11	1.76E − 11	8.80E − 12	2.43E − 11	1.06E − 11	2.40E − 12	7.84E − 10	2.64E − 10
^{55}Fe	1.00E − 01	1.07E − 10	1.04E − 10	1.02E − 10	1.05E − 10	1.05E − 10	1.10E − 10	3.00E − 10	1.64E − 10
^{59}Fe	1.00E − 01	1.66E − 09	7.37E − 10	6.35E − 10	8.45E − 10	6.61E − 10	6.03E − 10	3.56E − 09	1.81E − 09
^{57}Co	5.00E − 02	1.83E − 10	4.10E − 11	2.89E − 11	8.84E − 11	4.92E − 11	1.93E − 11	4.42E − 10	2.01E − 10
	3.00E − 01	2.94E − 10	1.58E − 10	1.63E − 10	2.67E − 10	2.12E − 10	1.15E − 10	5.39E − 10	3.20E − 10
^{60}Co	5.00E − 02	3.19E − 09	1.10E − 09	8.77E − 10	1.32E − 09	9.39E − 10	7.88E − 10	4.97E − 09	2.77E − 09
	3.00E − 01	7.23E − 09	5.08E − 09	4.96E − 09	5.49E − 09	4.18E − 09	4.68E − 09	1.06E − 08	7.28E − 09
^{59}Ni	5.00E − 02	3.83E − 11	3.58E − 11	3.50E − 11	3.66E − 11	3.62E − 11	3.90E − 11	1.03E − 10	5.67E − 11
^{63}Ni	5.00E − 02	8.50E − 11	8.50E − 11	8.50E − 11	8.50E − 11	8.50E − 11	8.50E − 11	3.20E − 10	1.56E − 10
^{65}Ni	5.00E − 02	2.43E − 11	5.63E − 12	2.75E − 12	7.26E − 12	2.89E − 12	6.79E − 13	5.32E − 10	1.68E − 10
^{64}Cu	5.00E − 01	4.78E − 11	1.59E − 11	1.28E − 11	1.94E − 11	1.39E − 11	1.13E − 11	3.57E − 10	1.26E − 10
^{65}Zn	5.00E − 01	3.56E − 09	3.28E − 09	3.08E − 09	4.50E − 09	4.50E − 09	3.21E − 09	4.59E − 09	3.90E − 09
^{69}Zn	5.00E − 01	4.17E − 13	4.17E − 13	4.17E − 13	5.36E − 13	5.18E − 13	4.17E − 13	7.91E − 11	2.40E − 11
^{79}Se	8.00E − 01	9.06E − 10	9.06E − 10	9.06E − 10	9.06E − 10	9.06E − 10	9.06E − 10	5.73E − 09	2.35E − 09
	5.00E − 02	5.66E − 11	5.66E − 11	5.66E − 11	5.66E − 11	5.66E − 11	5.66E − 11	1.04E − 09	3.51E − 10
^{82}Br	1.00E + 00	4.48E − 10	3.81E − 10	3.84E − 10	4.14E − 10	3.80E − 10	3.83E − 10	5.80E − 10	4.62E − 10
^{83}Br	1.00E + 00	7.35E − 12	7.34E − 12	7.35E − 12	7.35E − 12	7.33E − 12	7.33E − 12	6.54E − 11	2.47E − 11
^{84}Br	1.00E + 00	6.75E − 12	6.62E − 12	6.99E − 12	6.21E − 12	5.56E − 12	5.20E − 12	1.48E − 10	4.91E − 11
^{86}Rb	1.00E + 00	2.15E − 09	2.14E − 09	2.14E − 09	3.72E − 09	6.86E − 09	2.14E − 09	2.33E − 09	2.53E 09
^{87}Rb	1.00E + 00	1.14E − 09	1.14E − 09	1.14E − 09	2.02E − 09	3.80E − 09	1.14E − 09	1.17E − 09	1.33E − 09
^{88}Rb	1.00E + 00	2.78E − 12	2.82E − 12	2.91E − 12	2.76E − 12	2.75E − 12	2.43E − 12	1.50E − 10	4.71E − 11
^{89}Rb	1.00E + 00	3.32E − 12	3.38E − 12	3.68E − 12	3.53E − 12	4.19E − 12	2.21E − 12	8.04E − 11	2.65E − 11
^{89}Sr	3.00E − 01	2.40E − 10	2.40E − 10	2.40E − 10	3.23E − 09	4.81E − 09	2.40E − 10	6.11E − 09	2.50E − 09
	1.00E − 02	8.05E − 12	7.98E − 12	7.97E − 12	1.08E − 10	1.61E − 10	7.97E − 12	8.25E − 09	2.50E − 09
^{90}Sr	3.00E − 01	1.51E − 09	1.51E − 09	1.51E − 09	1.94E − 07	4.19E − 07	1.51E − 09	6.14E − 09	3.85E − 08
	1.00E − 02	5.04E − 11	5.04E − 11	5.04E − 11	6.45E − 09	1.39E − 08	5.04E − 11	6.70E − 09	3.23E − 09
^{91}Sr	3.00E − 01	2.10E − 10	4.98E − 11	3.05E − 11	1.08E − 10	7.90E − 11	2.41E − 11	1.98E − 09	6.74E − 10
	1.00E − 02	2.48E − 10	3.57E − 11	9.81E − 12	5.53E − 11	2.02E − 11	1.90E − 12	2.54E − 09	8.39E − 10
^{92}Sr	3.00E − 01	8.01E − 11	2.69E − 11	1.89E − 11	3.87E − 11	2.13E − 11	1.35E − 11	1.37E − 09	4.43E − 10
	1.00E − 02	8.18E − 11	1.70E − 11	7.22E − 12	2.29E − 11	8.49E − 12	1.30E − 12	1.72E − 09	5.43E − 10
^{90}Y	1.00E − 04	1.43E − 14	1.27E − 14	1.26E − 14	3.70E − 13	3.67E − 13	1.26E − 14	9.68E − 09	2.91E − 09
^{91}Y	1.00E − 04	3.54E − 12	5.54E − 13	2.02E − 13	6.59E − 12	6.13E − 12	1.29E − 13	8.57E − 09	2.57E − 09
^{91m}Y	1.00E − 04	6.94E − 12	1.84E − 12	1.28E − 12	2.24E − 12	8.71E − 13	1.17E − 13	2.92E − 11	1.12E − 11
^{92}Y	1.00E − 04	1.96E − 11	3.55E − 12	1.39E − 12	4.91E − 12	1.75E − 12	1.77E − 13	1.70E − 09	5.15E − 10
^{93}Y	1.00E − 04	2.20E − 11	3.13E − 12	8.67E − 13	4.93E − 12	1.73E − 12	1.26E − 13	4.09E − 09	1.23E − 09
^{93}Zr	2.00E − 03	9.23E − 14	1.97E − 13	1.15E − 13	7.42E − 10	9.14E − 09	7.31E − 14	2.83E − 10	4.48E − 10
^{95}Zr	2.00E − 03	8.16E − 10	1.05E − 10	2.34E − 11	2.14E − 10	4.86E − 10	8.27E − 12	2.53E − 09	1.02E − 09

(continued)

Table 13.29.1 Committed Dose Equivalent per Unit Intake via Ingestion (Sv/Bq)[a] (Continued)

Nuclide	f1	Gonad	Breast	Lung	R Marrow	Endosteal	Thyroid	Hrem	Heff
^{97}Zr	2.00E − 03	6.22E − 10	8.12E − 11	1.76E − 11	1.30E − 10	4.55E − 11	2.66E − 12	6.98E − 09	2.28E − 09
^{93m}Nb	1.00E − 02	3.34E − 11	2.57E − 12	2.45E − 12	2.32E − 11	5.98E − 11	2.44E − 12	4.25E − 10	1.41E − 10
^{95}Nb	1.00E − 42	8.05E − 10	1.07E − 10	2.74E − 11	1.99E − 10	2.94E − 10	1.18E − 11	1.47E − 09	6.95E − 10
^{97}Nb	1.00E − 02	1.45E − 11	3.30E − 12	1.98E − 12	4.20E − 12	1.60E − 12	2.11E − 13	1.94E − 10	6.30E − 11
^{93}Mo	8.00E − 01	1.27E − 10	9.96E − 11	1.06E − 10	2.82E − 10	1.15E − 09	9.42E − 11	7.79E − 10	3.64E − 10
	5.00E − 02	2.54E − 11	6.78E − 12	6.63E − 12	1.97E − 11	7.22E − 11	5.89E − 12	1.74E − 10	6.52E − 11
^{99}Mo	8.00E − 01	2.21E − 10	1.83E − 10	1.93E − 10	5.33E − 10	7.69E − 10	1.64E − 10	2.08E − 09	8.22E − 10
	5.00E − 02	2.18E − 10	3.43E − 11	1.51E − 11	8.32E − 11	6.32E − 11	1.03E − 11	4.28E − 09	1.36E − 09
^{99}Tc	8.00E − 01	6.04E − 11	6.04E − 11	6.04E − 11	6.04E − 11	6.04E − 11	1.62E − 09	1.02E − 09	3.95E − 10
^{99m}Tc	8.00E − 01	9.75E − 12	3.57E − 12	3.14E − 12	6.29E − 12	4.06E − 12	8.46E − 11	3.34E − 11	1.68E − 11
^{101}Tc	8.00E − 01	6.29E − 13	4.06E − 13	4.13E − 13	4.36E − 13	2.55E − 13	3.89E − 12	3.66E − 11	1.14E − 11
^{103}Ru	5.00E − 02	5.72E − 10	1.20E − 10	7.31E − 11	1.66E − 10	9.63E − 11	6.25E − 11	2.10E − 09	8.24E − 10
^{105}Ru	5.00E − 02	9.67E − 11	1.59E − 11	6.21E − 12	2.35E − 11	8.89E − 12	1.82E − 12	8.54E − 10	2.87E − 10
^{106}Ru	5.00E − 02	1.64E − 09	1.44E − 09	1.42E − 09	1.46E − 09	1.43E − 09	1.41E − 09	2.11E − 09	7.40E − 09
^{105}Rh	5.00E − 02	5.80E − 11	8.97E − 12	3.86E − 12	1.47E − 11	6.75E − 12	2.91E − 12	1.27E − 09	3.99E − 10
^{107}Pd	5.00E − 03	9.91E − 15	9.91E − 15	9.91E − 15	5.36E − 14	1.43E − 13	9.91E − 15	1.35E − 10	4.04E − 11
^{109}Pd	5.00E − 03	7.90E − 12	6.27E − 13	1.49E − 13	2.04E − 12	1.02E − 12	9.48E − 14	1.95E − 09	5.87E − 10
^{100m}Ag	5.00E − 02	2.99E − 09	7.51E − 10	8.30E − 10	9.42E − 10	4.93E − 10	1.81E − 10	6.08E − 09	2.92E − 09
^{111}Ag	5.00E − 02	3.58E − 11	1.09E − 11	8.84E − 12	1.38E − 11	9.67E − 12	7.48E − 12	4.51E − 09	1.37E − 09
^{113m}Cd	5.00E − 02	3.44E − 09	3.44E − 09	3.44E − 09	3.44E − 09	3.44E − 09	3.44E − 09	1.37E − 07	4.35E − 08
^{115m}Cd	5.00E − 02	1.84E − 10	1.66E − 10	1.64E − 10	1.68E − 10	1.64E − 10	1.61E − 10	1.42E − 08	4.37E − 09
^{123}Sn	2.00E − 02	3.80E − 11	3.22E − 11	3.15E − 11	2.41E − 10	6.62E − 10	3.13E − 11	7.35E − 09	2.27E − 09
^{125}Sn	2.00E − 02	2.88E − 10	4.41E − 11	1.60E − 11	2.08E − 10	2.38E − 10	9.78E − 12	1.07E − 08	3.33E − 09
^{126}Sn	2.00E − 02	2.41E − 09	7.96E − 10	5.99E − 10	2.72E − 09	5.06E − 09	5.51E − 10	1.33E − 08	5.27E − 09
^{124}Sb	1.00E − 01	1.74E − 09	3.21E − 10	1.65E − 10	6.16E − 10	7.99E − 10	1.18E − 10	6.81E − 09	2.65E − 09
	1.00E − 02	1.78E − 09	2.30E − 10	5.40E − 11	3.81E − 10	1.89E − 10	1.76E − 11	7.34E − 09	2.74E − 09
^{125}Sb	1.00E − 01	5.24E − 10	1.00E − 10	6.03E − 11	2.26E − 10	5.86E − 10	4.62E − 11	1.86E − 09	7.59E − 10
	1.00E − 02	5.27E − 10	6.22E − 11	1.36E − 11	1.21E − 10	9.05E − 11	5.58E − 12	1.99E − 09	7.57E − 10
^{126}Sb	1.00E − 01	2.73E − 09	4.17E − 10	1.66E − 10	7.23E − 10	5.17E − 10	1.05E − 10	6.29E − 09	2.76E − 09
	1.00E − 02	2.89E − 09	3.53E − 10	6.85E − 11	5.93E − 10	2.27E − 10	1.74E − 11	6.77E − 09	2.89E − 09
^{127}Sb	1.00E − 01	5.88E − 10	9.76E − 11	4.38E − 11	2.11E − 10	1.50E − 10	3.16E − 11	5.39E − 09	1.81E − 09
	1.00E − 02	6.14E − 10	7.60E − 11	1.57E − 11	1.33E − 10	5.24E − 11	4.64E − 12	5.87E − 09	1.95E − 09
^{125m}Te	2.00E − 01	1.27E − 10	4.64E − 11	4.36E − 11	1.21E − 09	1.27E − 08	3.93E − 11	1.40E − 09	9.92E − 10
^{127}Te	2.00E − 01	4.02E − 12	3.00E − 12	2.89E − 12	6.57E − 12	6.46E − 12	2.86E − 12	6.13E − 10	1.87E − 10
^{127m}Te	2.00E − 01	1.25E − 10	9.74E − 11	9.62E − 11	5.43E − 09	2.07E − 08	9.43E − 11	2.98E − 09	2.23E − 09
^{129}Te	2.00E − 01	1.59E − 12	6.05E − 13	4.91E − 13	7.64E − 13	5.40E − 13	3.36E − 13	1.79E − 10	5.45E − 11
^{129m}Te	2.00E − 01	2.41E − 10	1.66E − 10	1.59E − 10	3.50E − 09	7.99E − 09	1.57E − 10	7.08E − 09	2.89E − 09
^{131}Te	2.00E − 01	1.57E − 11	4.96E − 12	3.39E − 12	6.60E − 12	3.69E − 12	4.21E − 09	3.73E − 10	2.44E − 10
^{131m}Te	2.00E − 01	7.38E − 10	1.35E − 10	6.26E − 11	2.42E − 10	3.24E − 10	4.29E − 08	3.07E − 09	2.46E − 09
^{132}Te	2.00E − 01	5.41E − 10	3.50E − 10	3.30E − 10	4.44E − 10	8.30E − 10	5.95E − 08	1.49E − 09	2.54E − 09
^{133m}Te	2.00E − 01	3.68E − 11	1.14E − 11	8.33E − 12	1.31E − 11	6.61E − 12	4.17E − 09	2.89E − 10	2.26E − 10
^{134}Te	2.00E − 01	2.03E − 11	1.37E − 11	1.29E − 11	1.49E − 11	1.23E − 11	8.82E − 10	9.65E − 11	6.63E − 11
^{129}I	1.00	1.38E − 10	3.31E − 10	1.65E − 10	2.21E − 10	2.17E − 10	2.48E − 06	1.99E − 10	7.46E − 08
^{130}I	1.00	5.52E − 11	7.32E − 11	7.18E − 11	6.74E − 11	6.12E − 11	3.94E − 08	1.97E − 10	1.28E − 09
^{131}I	1.00	4.07E − 11	1.21E − 10	1.02E − 10	9.44E − 11	8.72E − 11	4.76E − 07	1.57E − 10	1.44E − 08
^{132}I	1.00	2.33E − 11	2.52E − 11	2.64E − 11	2.46E − 11	2.19E − 11	3.87E − 09	1.65E − 10	1.82E − 10
^{133}I	1.00	3.63E − 11	4.68E − 11	4.53E − 11	4.30E − 11	4.07E − 11	9.10E − 08	1.55E − 10	2.80E − 09
^{134}I	1.00	1.10E − 11	1.17E − 11	1.26E − 11	1.09E − 11	9.32E − 12	6.21E − 10	1.34E − 10	6.66E − 11
^{135}I	1.00	3.61E − 11	3.85E − 11	3.75E − 11	3.65E − 11	3.36E − 11	1.79E − 08	1.54E − 10	6.08E − 10

Table 13.29.1 Committed Dose Equivalent per Unit Intake via Ingestion (Sv/Bq)[a] (Continued)

Nuclide	f1	Gonad	Breast	Lung	R Marrow	Endosteal	Thyroid	Hrem	Heff
^{134}Cs	1.00	2.06E − 08	1.72E − 08	1.76E − 08	1.87E − 08	1.74E − 08	1.76E − 08	2.21E − 08	1.98E − 08
^{134m}Cs	1.00	6.72E − 12	6.28E − 12	6.42E − 12	6.91E − 12	6.57E − 12	6.22E − 12	2.89E − 11	1.33E − 11
^{135}Cs	1.00	1.91E − 09	1.91E − 09	1.91E − 09	1.91E − 09	1.91E − 09	1.91E − 09	1.93E − 09	1.91E − 09
^{136}Cs	1.00	3.04E − 09	2.65E − 09	2.62E − 09	2.95E − 09	2.71E − 09	2.74E − 09	3.52E − 09	3.04E − 09
^{137}Cs	1.00	1.39E − 08	1.24E − 08	1.27E − 08	1.32E − 08	1.26E − 08	1.26E − 08	1.45E − 08	1.35E − 08
^{138}Cs	1.00	8.00E − 12	8.00E − 12	8.53E − 12	7.37E − 12	6.47E − 12	5.73E − 12	1.57E − 10	5.25E − 11
^{139}Ba	1.00E − 01	1.56E − 12	5.17E − 13	3.89E − 13	8.59E − 13	4.38E − 13	2.66E − 13	3.57E − 10	1.08E − 10
^{140}Ba	1.00E − 01	9.96E − 10	1.59E − 10	6.63E − 11	4.39E − 10	5.53E − 10	5.25E − 11	7.37E − 09	2.56E − 09
^{141}Ba	1.00E − 01	2.86E − 12	1.22E − 12	1.10E − 12	1.47E − 12	1.27E − 12	2.25E − 13	1.84E − 10	5.65E − 11
^{142}Ba	1.00E − 01	9.88E − 12	2.52E − 12	1.67E − 12	3.00E − 12	1.24E − 12	2.71E − 13	8.89E − 11	3.01E − 11
^{140}La	1.00E − 03	1.34E − 09	1.80E − 10	4.01E − 11	2.81E − 10	9.77E − 11	6.40E − 12	6.26E − 09	2.28E − 09
^{141}La	1.00E − 03	3.77E − 12	7.07E − 13	2.72E − 13	1.07E − 12	6.06E − 13	5.29E − 14	1.24E − 09	3.74E − 10
^{142}La	1.00E − 03	6.99E − 11	1.54E − 11	8.40E − 12	1.93E − 11	7.40E − 12	1.16E − 12	5.20E − 10	1.79E − 10
^{141}Ce	3.00E − 04	1.08E − 10	1.11E − 11	1.43E − 12	3.39E − 11	2.30E − 11	1.80E − 13	2.50E − 09	7.83E − 10
^{143}Ce	3.00E − 04	2.12E − 10	2.32E − 11	3.82E − 12	5.07E − 11	1.61E − 11	4.35E − 13	3.89E − 09	1.23E − 09
^{144}Ce	3.00E − 04	6.98E − 11	1.22E − 11	6.52E − 12	8.92E − 11	1.28E − 10	5.15E − 12	1.88E − 08	5.68E − 09
^{143}Pr	3.00E − 04	8.99E − 18	1.09E − 18	1.91E − 19	1.03E − 12	1.03E − 12	2.66E − 20	4.22E − 09	1.27E − 09
^{147}Nd	3.00E − 04	1.79E − 10	1.87E − 11	2.44E − 12	5.05E − 11	2.22E − 11	2.64E − 13	3.76E − 09	1.18E − 09
^{147}Pm	3.00E − 04	6.86E − 15	7.45E − 16	1.96E − 16	2.09E − 11	2.61E − 10	3.12E − 17	9.08E − 10	2.83E − 10
^{148}Pm	3.00E − 04	4.72E − 10	6.11E − 11	1.19E − 11	9.85E − 11	3.49E − 11	1.85E − 12	9.32E − 09	2.94E − 09
^{148}Pm	3.00E − 04	2.18E − 09	2.59E − 10	4.44E − 11	4.41E − 10	1.74E − 10	6.47E − 12	4.75E − 09	2.07E − 09
^{149}Pm	3.00E − 04	9.19E − 12	1.02E − 12	1.62E − 13	2.27E − 12	9.59E − 13	1.78E − 14	3.56E − 09	1.07E − 09
^{151}Pm	3.00E − 04	2.11E − 10	2.42E − 11	4.23E − 12	4.94E − 11	1.62E − 11	4.55E − 13	2.49E − 09	8.09E − 10
^{151}Sm	3.00E − 04	2.12E − 14	1.03E − 15	6.52E − 16	2.76E − 11	3.45E − 10	3.27E − 17	3.04E − 10	1.05E − 10
^{153}Sm	3.00E − 04	7.17E − 11	6.91E − 12	7.13E − 13	2.72E − 11	8.38E − 12	2.36E − 14	2.62E − 09	8.07E − 10
^{152}Eu	1.00E − 03	1.33E − 09	2.85E − 10	2.40E − 10	9.19E − 10	2.09E − 09	6.66E − 11	3.92E − 09	1.75E − 09
^{154}Eu	1.00E − 03	1.37E − 09	2.97E − 10	2.16E − 10	1.15E − 09	4.46E − 09	5.71E − 11	6.32E − 09	2.58E − 09
^{155}Eu	1.00E − 03	9.83E − 11	1.44E − 11	9.64E − 12	1.56E − 10	1.29E − 09	1.78E − 12	1.09E − 09	4.13E − 10
^{156}Eu	1.00E − 03	1.22E − 09	1.52E − 10	3.24E − 11	2.56E − 10	1.16E − 10	5.23E − 12	7.04E − 09	2.48E − 09
^{160}Tb	3.00E − 04	1.17E − 09	1.43E − 10	2.72E − 11	2.54E − 10	1.57E − 10	4.29E − 12	4.90E − 09	1.82E − 09
^{166m}Ho	3.00E − 04	2.05E − 09	3.48E − 10	2.16E − 10	8.12E − 10	2.35E − 09	5.53E − 11	4.74E − 09	2.18E − 09
^{181}W	1.00E − 02	7.33E − 11	7.01E − 12	6.23E − 13	3.26E − 11	1.03E − 11	5.41E − 14	2.31E − 10	9.31E − 11
	3.00E − 01	5.36E − 11	7.46E − 12	3.52E − 12	4.86E − 11	4.58E − 11	1.39E − 12	1.84E − 10	7.74E − 11
^{185}W	1.00E − 02	8.74E − 14	8.98E − 15	9.45E − 16	1.64E − 12	4.90E − 12	7.64E − 17	1.79E − 09	5.38E − 10
	3.00E − 01	6.35E − 14	8.78E − 15	3.54E − 15	4.83E − 11	1.47E − 10	1.36E − 15	1.39E − 09	4.28E − 10
^{187}W	1.00E − 02	2.59E − 10	3.22E − 11	6.39E − 12	5.89E − 11	2.12E − 11	7.70E − 13	2.22E − 09	7.46E − 10
	3.00E − 01	1.90E − 10	2.44E − 11	5.80E − 12	5.09E − 11	7.38E − 11	9.00E − 13	1.64E − 09	5.53E − 10
^{210}Pb	2.00E − 01	1.25E − 07	1.25E − 07	1.25E − 07	1.48E − 06	2.16E − 05	1.25E − 07	1.85E − 06	1.45E − 06
^{210}Bi	5.00E − 02	1.97E − 11	1.97E − 11	1.97E − 11	1.97E − 11	1.97E − 11	1.97E − 11	5.72E − 09	1.73E − 09
^{210}Po	1.00E − 01	8.23E − 08	8.23E − 08	8.23E − 08	8.23E − 08	8.23E − 08	8.23E − 08	1.52E − 06	5.14E − 07
^{223}Ra	2.00E − 01	4.26E − 08	4.23E − 08	4.23E − 08	2.80E − 07	2.93E − 06	4.23E − 08	1.10E − 07	1.78E − 07
^{224}Ra	2.00E − 01	2.12E − 08	2.06E − 08	2.05E − 08	1.52E − 07	1.59E − 06	2.05E − 08	7.15E − 08	9.89E − 08
^{225}Ra	2.00E − 01	3.37E − 08	3.37E − 08	3.37E − 08	1.68E − 07	1.78E − 06	3.37E − 08	4.09E − 08	1.04E − 07
^{226}Ra	2.00E − 01	9.16E − 08	9.17E − 08	9.16E − 08	5.98E − 07	6.83E − 06	9.15E − 08	1.03E − 07	3.58E − 07
^{228}Ra	2.00E − 01	1.58E − 07	1.57E − 07	1.57E − 07	6.53E − 07	5.82E − 06	1.57E − 07	1.63E − 07	3.88E − 07
^{225}Ac	1.00E − 03	1.36E − 09	2.73E − 11	3.98E − 12	7.99E − 09	9.94E − 08	5.49E − 13	8.57E − 08	3.00E − 08
^{227}Ac	1.00E − 03	8.31E − 07	1.41E − 10	2.20E − 10	5.40E − 06	6.73E − 05	7.55E − 11	3.08E − 06	3.80E − 06
^{227}Th	2.00E − 04	2.95E − 10	1.40E − 10	1.25E − 10	5.69E − 09	6.84E − 08	1.23E − 10	2.47E − 08	1.03E − 08

(continued)

Table 13.29.1 Committed Dose Equivalent per Unit Intake via Ingestion (Sv/Bq)[a] (Continued)

Nuclide	f1	Gonad	Breast	Lung	R Marrow	Endosteal	Thyroid	Hrem	Heff
^{228}Th	2.00E − 04	2.53E − 09	2.33E − 09	2.31E − 09	1.93E − 07	2.37E − 06	2.30E − 09	3.86E − 08	1.07E − 07
^{229}Th	2.00E − 04	4.69E − 09	4.57E − 09	4.56E − 09	1.91E − 06	2.38E − 05	4.55E − 09	2.80E − 08	9.54E − 07
^{230}Th	2.00E − 04	6.82E − 10	6.80E − 10	6.80E − 10	2.89E − 07	3.60E − 06	6.80E − 10	1.54E − 08	1.48E − 07
^{232}Th	2.00E − 04	1.25E − 09	1.26E − 09	1.25E − 09	1.48E − 06	1.85E − 05	1.21E − 09	1.47E − 08	7.38E − 07
^{234}Th	2.00E − 04	3.12E − 11	3.57E − 12	7.05E − 13	1.84E − 11	2.08E − 11	2.88E − 13	1.23E − 08	3.69E − 09
^{231}Pa	1.00E − 03	1.21E − 10	7.81E − 11	6.80E − 11	5.78E − 06	7.22E − 05	6.33E − 11	1.71E − 08	2.86E − 06
^{233}Pa	1.00E − 03	2.58E − 10	2.71E − 11	3.70E − 12	6.89E − 11	1.02E − 10	4.81E − 13	3.00E − 09	9.81E − 10
^{232}U	5.00E − 02	8.27E − 09	8.33E − 09	8.29E − 09	4.19E − 07	6.63E − 06	8.11E − 09	3.35E − 07	3.54E − 07
	2.00E − 03	3.34E − 10	3.33E − 10	3.32E − 10	1.68E − 08	2.65E − 07	3.25E − 10	2.83E − 08	1.87E − 08
^{233}U	5.00E − 02	2.62E − 09	2.62E − 09	2.62E − 09	7.36E − 08	1.16E − 06	2.62E − 09	1.10E − 07	7.81E − 08
	2.00E − 03	1.07E − 10	1.05E − 10	1.05E − 10	2.95E − 09	4.62E − 08	1.05E − 10	1.78E − 08	7.15E − 09
^{234}U	5.00E − 02	2.59E − 09	2.58E − 09	2.58E − 09	7.21E − 08	1.13E − 06	2.58E − 09	1.09E − 07	7.66E − 08
	2.00E − 03	1.06E − 10	1.03E − 10	1.03E − 10	2.88E − 09	4.52E − 08	1.03E − 10	1.77E − 08	7.06E − 09
^{235}U	5.00E − 02	2.67E − 09	2.49E − 09	2.46E − 09	6.81E − 08	1.05E − 06	2.45E − 09	1.03E − 07	7.19E − 08
	2.00E − 03	3.34E − 10	1.21E − 10	1.01E − 10	2.78E − 09	4.20E − 08	9.82E − 11	1.84E − 08	7.22E − 09
^{236}U	5.00E − 02	2.45E − 09	2.45E − 09	2.45E − 09	6.83E − 08	1.07E − 06	2.45E − 09	1.03E − 07	7.26E − 08
	2.00E − 03	1.00E − 10	9.79E − 11	9.79E − 11	2.73E − 09	4.28E − 08	9.79E − 11	1.67E − 08	6.68E − 09
^{237}U	5.00E − 02	1.75E − 10	2.02E − 11	4.98E − 12	9.50E − 11	4.41E − 10	2.77E − 12	2.59E − 09	8.48E − 10
	2.00E − 03	1.81E − 10	1.81E − 11	2.17E − 12	5.69E − 11	3.39E − 11	2.31E − 13	2.67E − 09	8.57E − 10
^{238}U	5.00E − 02	2.31E − 09	2.31E − 09	2.30E − 09	6.80E − 08	1.01E − 06	2.30E − 09	9.69E − 08	6.88E − 08
	2.00E − 03	1.02E − 10	9.33E − 11	9.22E − 11	2.72E − 09	4.04E − 08	9.20E − 11	1.61E − 08	6.42E − 09
^{237}Np	1.00E − 03	2.46E − 07	1.45E − 10	1.53E − 10	2.18E − 06	2.72E − 05	1.10E − 10	2.10E − 07	1.20E − 06
^{238}Np	1.00E − 03	3.89E − 10	4.81E − 11	1.02E − 11	2.17E − 10	1.77E − 09	1.50E − 12	2.97E − 09	1.08E − 09
^{239}Np	1.00E − 03	1.62E − 10	1.72E − 11	2.40E − 12	4.66E − 11	3.59E − 11	2.07E − 13	2.77E − 09	8.82E − 10
^{238}Pu	1.00E − 03	2.33E − 07	8.41E − 12	8.49E − 12	1.27E − 06	1.58E − 05	7.99E − 12	6.00E − 07	8.65E − 07
	1.00E − 04	2.33E − 08	9.28E − 13	8.50E − 13	1.27E − 07	1.58E − 06	7.99E − 13	7.44E − 08	9.08E − 08
	1.00E − 05	2.33E − 09	1.80E − 13	8.64E − 14	1.27E − 08	1.58E − 07	7.99E − 14	2.18E − 08	1.34E − 08
^{239}Pu	1.00E − 03	2.64E − 07	7.69E − 12	7.74E − 12	1.41E − 06	1.76E − 05	7.49E − 12	6.43E − 07	9.56E − 07
	1.00E − 04	2.64E − 08	8.09E − 13	7.75E − 13	1.41E − 07	1.76E − 06	7.49E − 13	7.77E − 08	9.96E − 08
	1.00E − 05	2.64E − 09	1.21E − 13	7.89E − 14	1.41E − 08	1.76E − 07	7.50E − 14	2.12E − 08	1.40E − 08
^{240}Pu	1.00E − 03	2.64E − 07	7.97E − 12	8.07E − 12	1.41E − 06	1.76E − 05	7.51E − 12	6.43E − 07	9.56E − 07
	1.00E − 04	2.64E − 08	8.82E − 13	8.08E − 13	1.41E − 07	1.76E − 06	7.51E − 13	7.78E − 08	9.97E − 08
	1.00E − 05	2.64E − 09	1.73E − 13	8.22E − 14	1.41E − 08	1.76E − 07	7.51E − 14	2.13E − 08	1.40E − 08
^{241}Pu	1.00E − 03	5.66E − 09	2.52E − 13	4.45E − 13	2.78E − 08	3.48E − 07	1.01E − 13	1.10E − 08	1.85E − 08
	1.00E − 04	5.66E − 10	2.54E − 14	4.45E − 14	2.78E − 09	3.48E − 08	1.01E − 14	1.16E − 09	1.87E − 09
	1.00E − 05	5.66E − 11	2.79E − 15	4.48E − 15	2.78E − 10	3.48E − 09	1.01E − 15	1.85E − 10	2.07E − 10
^{242}Pu	1.00E − 03	2.51E − 07	8.00E − 12	7.88E − 12	1.34E − 06	1.67E − 05	7.29E − 12	6.10E − 07	9.08E − 07
	1.00E − 04	2.51E −08	9.58E − 13	8.00E − 13	1.34E − 07	1.67E − 06	7.30E − 13	7.38E − 08	9.46E − 08
	1.00E − 05	2.51E − 09	2.54E − 13	9.18E − 14	1.34E − 08	1.67E − 07	7.38E − 14	2.02E − 08	1.33E − 08
^{244}Pu	1.00E − 03	2.49E − 07	3.24E − 10	3.23E − 10	1.32E − 06	1.64E − 05	1.50E − 10	6.13E − 07	8,97E − 07
	1.00E − 04	2.53E − 08	7.82E − 11	3.78E − 11	1.33E − 07	1.64E − 06	1.56E − 11	8.15E − 08	9.59E − 08
	1.00E − 05	2.94E − 09	5.36E − 11	9.29E − 12	1.33E − 08	1.65E − 07	2.22E − 12	2.84E − 08	1.58E − 08
^{241}Am	1.00E − 03	2.70E − 07	2.62E − 11	3.36E − 11	1.45E − 06	1.81E − 05	1.32E − 11	6.66E − 07	9.84E − 07
^{242}Am	1.00E − 03	2.66E − 07	1.22E − 11	1.65E − 11	1.41E − 06	1.76E − 05	3.77E − 12	6.20E − 07	9.50E − 07
^{242}Am	1.00E − 03	2.74E − 11	9.38E − 13	1.58E − 13	1.24E − 10	1.52E − 09	2.61E − 14	1.05E − 09	3.81E − 10
^{243}Am	1.00E − 03	2.71E − 07	1.41E − 10	1.95E − 10	1.44E − 06	1.80E − 05	6.80E − 11	6.61E − 07	9.79E − 07
^{242}Cm	1.00E − 03	5.20E − 09	8.95E − 12	8.84E − 12	3.57E − 08	4.46E − 07	8.82E − 12	4.02E − 08	3.10E − 08
^{243}Cm	1.00E − 03	1.73E − 07	6.96E − 11	7.73E − 11	9.81E − 07	1.23E − 05	3.15E − 11	4.97E − 07	6.79E − 07
^{244}Cm	1.00E − 03	1.33E − 07	8.82E − 12	8.81E − 12	7.82E − 07	9.77E − 06	8.44E − 12	4.15E − 07	5.45E − 07
^{245}Cm	1.00E − 03	2.80E − 07	6.80E − 11	8.34E − 11	1.49E − 06	1.86E − 05	3.02E − 11	6.79E − 07	1.01E − 06
^{246}Cm	1.00E − 03	2.77E − 07	3.91E − 11	2.67E − 11	1.48E − 06	1.85E − 05	1.87E − 11	6.76E − 07	1.00E − 06
^{247}Cm	1.00E − 03	2.56E − 07	2.29E − 10	2.66E − 10	1.36E − 06	1.70E − 05	1.20E − 10	6.23E − 07	9.24E − 07
^{248}Cm	1.00E − 03	1.02E − 06	1.10E − 08	6.52E − 09	5.42E − 06	6.75E − 05	3.87E − 09	2.49E − 06	3.68E − 06
^{252}Cf	1.00E − 03	5.39E − 08	1.49E − 09	4.67E − 10	4.69E − 07	5.84E − 06	2.68E − 10	1.58E − 07	2.93E − 07

[a] The coefficients are tabulated in SI units. To convert to the conventional units (mrem/μCi) multiply the table entry by 3.7×10^9.

Table 13.29.2 Committed Dose Equivalent per Unit Intake via Inhalation (Sv/Bq)[a]

Nuclide	Class/f1		Gonad	Breast	Lung	R Marrow	Endosteal	Thyroid	Hrem	Heff
^{3}H	V	1.00E + 00	1.73E − 11	1.73E − 11	1.7E − 11	1.73E − 11	1.73E − 11	1.73E − 11	1.73E − 11	1.73E − 11
^{10}Be	W	5.00E − 03	5.94E − 10	5.94E − 10	4.2E − 08	1.77E − 08	5.26E − 08	5.94E − 10	2.44E − 09	9.75E − 09
	Y	5.00E − 03	2.56E − 10	2.56E − 10	7.8E − 07	7.65E − 09	2.27E − 08	2.56E − 10	2.35E − 09	9.58E − 08
^{11}C	c	1.00E + 00	3.41E − 12	2.98E − 12	3.1E − 12	3.18E − 12	3.03E − 12	2.97E − 12	3.54E − 12	3.29E − 12
	m	1.00E + 00	1.24E − 12	1.08E − 12	1.1E − 12	1.16E − 12	1.10E − 12	1.08E − 12	1.29E − 12	1.20E − 12
	d	1.00E + 00	2.22E − 12	1.94E − 12	2.0E − 12	2.07E − 12	1.97E − 12	1.93E − 12	2.30E − 12	2.14E − 12
^{14}C	c	1.00E + 00	5.64E − 10	5.64E − 10	5.6E − 10	5.64E − 10	5.64E − 10	5.64E − 10	5.64E − 10	5.64E − 10
	m	1.00E + 00	7.83E − 13	7.83E − 13	7.8E − 13	7.83E − 13	7.83E − 13	7.83E − 13	7.83E − 13	7.83E − 13
	d	1.00E + 00	6.36E − 12	6.36E − 12	6.4E − 12	6.36E − 12	6.36E − 12	6.36E − 12	6.36E − 12	6.36E − 12
^{22}Na	D	1.00E + 00	1.77E − 09	1.65E − 09	2.5E − 09	2.73E − 09	3.51E − 09	1.60E − 09	2.00E − 09	2.07E − 09
^{24}Na	D	1.00E + 00	1.78E − 10	1.61E − 10	1.3E − 09	2.13E − 10	2.58E − 10	1.53E − 10	2.35E − 10	3.27E − 10
^{32}P	D	8.00E − 01	4.83E − 10	4.83E − 10	2.5E − 09	5.97E − 09	5.81E − 09	4.83E − 10	7.94E − 10	1.64E − 09
	W	8.00E − 01	3.37E − 10	3.37E − 10	2.6E − 08	4.17E − 09	4.05E − 09	3.37E − 10	1.18E − 09	4.19E − 09
^{41}Ca	W	3.00E − 01	2.43E − 12	2.98E − 12	4.5E − 10	1.62E − 09	3.65E − 09	2.57E − 12	1.53E − 11	3.64E − 10
^{46}Sc	Y	1.00E − 04	1.30E − 09	2.15E − 09	4.6E − 08	2.21E − 09	1.68E − 09	2.02E − 09	4.79E − 09	8.01E − 09
^{51}Cr	D	1.00E − 01	2.71E − 11	1.94E − 11	3.8E − 11	2.68E − 11	2.74E − 11	1.82E − 11	3.55E − 11	2.95E − 11
	W	1.00E − 01	2.21E − 11	1.50E − 11	3.8E − 10	1.87E − 11	1.50E − 11	1.10E − 11	4.93E − 11	7.08E − 11
^{54}Mn	D	1.00E − 01	2.03E − 11	1.58E − 11	5.3E − 10	1.87E − 11	1.39E − 11	1.08E − 11	5.26E − 11	9.03E − 11
		1.00E − 01	8.85E − 10	9.13E − 10	1.2E − 09	1.66E − 09	2.56E − 09	6.52E − 10	2.09E − 09	1.42E − 09
	W	1.00E − 01	7.09E − 10	8.59E − 10	6.7E − 09	1.10E − 09	1.25E − 09	7.40E − 10	1.72E − 09	1.81E − 09
^{56}Mn	D	1.00E − 01	2.19E − 11	1.47E − 11	4.4E − 10	2.36E − 11	2.05E − 11	1.20E − 11	1.25E − 10	1.02E − 10
	W	1.00E − 01	9.46E − 12	7.79E − 12	5.4E − 10	1.02E − 11	8.23E − 12	6.18E − 12	6.50E − 11	8.91E − 11
^{55}Fe	D	1.00E − 01	5.23E − 10	5.09E − 10	5.2E − 10	5.17E − 10	5.14E − 10	5.42E − 10	1.21E − 09	7.26E 10
	W	1.00E − 01	1.79E − 10	1.74E − 10	1.1E − 09	1.76E − 10	1.75E − 10	1.85E − 10	4.37E − 10	3.61E − 10
^{59}Fe	D	1.00E − 01	3.32E − 09	3.01E − 09	3.5E − 09	3.18E − 09	2.91E − 09	2.95E − 09	5.81E − 09	4.00E − 09
	W	1.00E − 01	1.39E − 09	1.26E − 09	1.4E − 08	1.31E − 09	1.11E − 09	1.17E − 09	2.96E − 09	3.30E − 09
^{57}Co	W	5.00E − 02	1.63E − 10	1.56E − 10	4.1E − 09	2.54E − 10	1.97E − 10	1.13E − 10	4.05E − 10	7.12E − 10
	Y	5.00E − 02	1.24E − 10	3.75E − 10	1.7E − 08	5.88E − 10	4.52E − 10	2.71E − 10	8.22E − 10	2.45E − 09
^{60}Co	W	5.00E − 02	4.05E − 09	4.16E − 09	3.6E − 08	4.25E − 09	3.54E − 09	3.72E − 09	7.65E − 09	8.94E − 09
	Y	5.00E − 02	4.76E − 09	1.84E − 08	3.5E − 07	1.72E − 07	1.35E − 08	1.62E − 08	3.60E − 07	5.91E − 08
^{59}Ni	D	5.00E − 02	3.59E − 10	3.46E − 10	3.6E − 10	3.54E − 10	3.51E − 10	3.77E − 10	3.63E − 10	3.58E − 10
	W	5.00E − 02	1.09E − 10	1.05E − 10	1.2E − 09	1.06E − 10	1.05E − 10	1.14E − 10	1.40E − 10	2.48E − 10
	V	1.00E + 01	7.43E − 10	7.15E − 10	7.1E − 10	7.31E 10	7.25E 10	7.80E − 10	7.33E − 10	7.31E − 10
^{63}Ni	D	5.00E − 02	8.22E − 10	8.22E − 10	8.7E − 10	8.22E − 10	8.22E − 10	8.22E − 10	8.59E − 10	8.39E − 10
	W	5.00E − 02	2.47E − 10	2.47E − 10	3.1E − 09	2.47E − 10	2.47E − 10	2.47E − 10	3.67E − 10	6.22E − 10
	V	1.00E + 01	1.70E − 09	1.70E − 09	1.7E − 09	1.70E − 09	1.70E − 09	1.70E − 09	1.70E − 09	1.70E − 09
^{65}Ni	D	5.00E − 02	8.46E − 12	6.48E − 12	3.1E − 10	6.70E − 12	5.79E − 12	5.54E − 12	7.98E − 11	6.55E − 11
	W	5.00E − 02	3.27E − 12	2.95E − 12	3.8E − 10	2.99E − 12	2.38E − 12	2.30E − 12	4.15E − 11	5.99E − 11
	V	1.00E + 01	1.08E − 11	1.21E − 11	6.8E − 10	1.21E − 11	1.14E − 11	1.16E − 11	1.66E − 11	9.32E − 11
^{64}Cu	D	5.00E − 01	1.64E − 11	1.23E − 11	2.0E − 10	1.34E − 11	1.20E − 11	1.16E − 11	6.74E − 11	5.29E − 11
	W	5.00E − 01	1.21E − 11	7.26E − 12	3.4E − 10	7.99E − 12	6.34E − 12	6.10E − 12	7.89E − 11	6.93E − 11
	Y	5.00E − 01	1.24E − 11	6.38E − 12	3.5E − 10	7.12E − 12	5.29E − 12	4.98E − 12	9.20E − 11	7.48E − 11
^{65}Zn	Y	5.00E − 01	2.03E − 09	3.08E − 09	2.1E − 08	3.62E − 09	3.36E − 09	3.02E − 09	4.66E − 09	5.51E − 09
^{69}Zn	Y	5.00E − 01	2.77E − 14	2.77E − 14	8.0E − 11	3.56E − 14	3.43E − 14	2.77E − 14	3.21E − 12	1.06E − 11
^{79}Se	D	8.00E − 01	6.79E − 10	6.79E − 10	8.5E − 10	6.79E − 10	6.79E − 10	6.79E − 10	4.24E − 09	1.77E − 09
	W	8.00E − 01	5.98E − 10	5.98E − 10	9.8E − 09	5.98E − 10	5.98E − 10	5.98E − 10	3.77E − 09	2.66E − 09
^{82}Br	D	1.00E + 00	2.52E − 10	2.37E − 10	7.8E − 10	2.54E − 10	2.31E − 10	2.38E − 10	3.15E − 10	3.31E − 10
	W	1.00E + 00	1.69E − 10	2.10E − 10	1.7E − 09	2.18E − 10	1.92E − 10	2.06E − 10	3.31e − 10	4.13E − 10
^{83}Br	D	1.00E + 00	3.28E − 12	3.29E − 12	1.5E − 10	3.30E − 12	3.29E − 12	3.29E − 12	1.13E − 11	2.33E − 11
	W	1.00E + 00	1.13E − 12	1.14E − 12	1.8E − 10	1.14E − 12	1.14E − 12	1.14E − 12	5.31E − 12	2.41E − 11

[a] The coefficients are tabulated in SI units. To convert to the conventional units (mrem/μCi) multipley the table entry by 3.7×10^{9}.

Note: V Denotes vapor form. c, m, and d denote labelled organic compounds, carbon monoxide, and carbon dioxide, respectively. Committed Dose Equivalant calculated for an AMAD of 1 micron.

Table 13.29.2 Committed Dose Equivalent per Unit Intake via Inhalation (Sv/Bq)[a] (Continued)

Nuclide	Class/f1	Gonad	Breast	Lung	R Marrow	Endosteal	Thyroid	Hrem	Heff
^{86}Rb	D 1.00E + 00	1.34E − 09	1.33E − 09	3.3E − 09	2.32E − 09	4.27E − 09	1.33E − 09	1.38E − 09	1.79E − 09
^{87}Rb	D 1.00E + 00	7.16E − 10	7.16E − 10	1.1E −09	1.27E − 09	2.40E − 09	7.16E − 10	7.20E − 10	8.74E −10
^{88}Rb	D 1.00E + 00	1.31E − 12	1.43E − 12	1.5E − 10	1.45E − 12	1.47E − 12	1.37E − 12	1.38E − 11	2.26E − 11
^{89}Rb	D 1.00E + 10	1.34E − 12	1.73E − 12	6.8E − 11	2.02E − 12	2.54E − 12	1.61E − 12	8.14E − 12	1.16E − 11
^{89}Sr	D 3.00E − 01	4.16E − 10	4.16E − 10	2.2E − 09	5.63E − 09	8.37E − 09	4.16E − 10	1.32E − 09	1.76E − 09
	Y 1.00E − 02	7.95E − 12	7.96E − 12	8.4E − 08	1.07E − 10	1.59E − 10	7.96E − 12	3.97E − 09	1.12E − 08
^{90}Sr	D 3.00E − 01	2.64E − 09	2.64E − 09	3.7E − 09	3.36E − 07	7.27E − 07	2.64E − 09	3.36E − 09	6.47E − 08
	Y 1.00E − 02	2.69E − 10	2.69E − 10	2.9E − 06	3.28E − 08	7.09E − 08	2.69E − 10	5.73E − 09	3.51E − 07
^{91}Sr	D 3.00E − 01	6.41E − 11	4.45E − 11	9.2E − 10	1.23E − 10	1.14E − 10	4.08E − 11	3.33E − 10	2.52E − 10
	Y 1.00E − 02	5.65E − 11	1.74E − 11	2.1E − 09	2.23E − 11	1.27E − 11	9.64E − 12	5.78E − 10	4.49E − 10
^{92}Sr	D 3.00E − 01	3.03E − 11	2.44E − 11	7.1E − 10	3.68E − 11	2.56E − 11	2.19E − 11	2.25E − 10	1.70E − 10
	Y 1.00E − 02	1.02E − 11	6.49E − 12	1.1E − 09	6.98E − 12	4.36E − 12	3.92E − 12	2.90E − 10	2.18E − 10
^{90}Y	W 1.00E − 04	9.52E − 12	9.52E − 12	8.9E − 09	2.79E − 10	2.78E − 10	9.52E − 12	3.40E − 09	2.13E − 09
	Y 1.00E − 04	5.17E − 13	5.17E − 13	9.3E − 09	1.52E − 11	1.51E − 11	5.17E − 13	3.87E − 09	2.28E − 09
^{91}Y	W 1.00E − 04	1.11E − 10	1.11E − 10	5.3E − 08	5.55E − 09	5.54E − 09	1.10E − 10	5.12E − 09	8.72E − 09
	Y 1.00E − 04	8.20E − 12	8.92E − 12	9.9E − 08	3.19E − 10	3.18E − 10	8.50E − 12	4.20E − 09	1.32E − 08
^{91m}Y	W 1.00E − 04	4.33E − 13	7.13E − 13	4.2E − 11	3.94E − 12	3.79E − 12	6.23E − 13	4.15E − 12	7.09E − 12
	Y 1.00E − 04	3.21E − 13	6.08E − 13	7.0E − 11	7.74E − 13	6.21E − 13	5.02E − 13	3.74E − 12	9.82E − 12
^{92}Y	W 1.00E − 04	4.86E − 12	4.07E − 12	1.2E − 09	1.28E − 11	1.23E − 11	3.69E − 12	1.67E − 10	1.93E − 10
	Y 1.00E − 04	2.61E − 12	1.50E − 12	1.2E − 09	2.07E − 12	1.51E − 12	1.05E − 12	2.03E − 10	2.11E − 10
^{93}Y	W 1.00E − 04	8.65E − 12	5.79E − 12	2.4E − 09	4.14E − 11	4.04E − 11	5.06E − 12	7.74E − 10	5.29E − 10
	Y 1.00E − 04	5.31E − 12	1.74E − 12	2.5E − 09	4.04E − 12	3.14E − 12	9.26E − 13	9.25E − 10	5.82E − 10
^{93}Zr	D 2.00E − 03	2.18E − 11	4.68E − 11	8.7E − 11	1.77E − 07	2.18E − 06	1.74E − 11	8.48E − 11	8.67E − 08
	W 2.00E − 03	5.58E − 12	1.20E − 11	3.3E − 09	4.49E − 08	5.54E − 07	4.45E − 12	1.54E − 10	2.25E − 08
	Y 2.00E − 03	2.82E − 12	1.90E − 11	8.7E − 08	1.93E − 08	2.38E − 07	2.28E − 12	1.73E − 10	2.00E − 08
^{95}Zr	D 2.00E − 03	1.88E − 09	1.91E − 09	2.2E − 09	1.30E − 08	1.03E − 07	1.44E − 09	2.28E − 09	6.39E − 09
	W 2.00E − 03	8.40E − 10	9.32E − 10	1.9E − 08	3.24E − 09	2.17E − 08	7.82E − 10	2.13E − 09	4.29E − 09
	Y 2.00E − 03	5.73E − 10	1.23E − 09	4.1E − 08	1.35E − 09	2.33E − 09	1.16E − 09	2.77E − 09	6.31E − 09
^{97}Zr	D 2.00E − 03	1.83E − 10	1.09E − 10	2.1E − 09	4.99E − 10	5.09E − 10	9.56E − 11	1.15E − 09	7.37E − 10
	W 2.00E − 03	1.70E − 10	5.79E − 11	4.0E − 09	1.43E − 10	1.23E − 10	3.75E − 11	1.72E − 09	1.06E − 09
	Y 2.00E − 03	1.84E − 10	4.70E − 11	4.1E − 09	6.37E − 11	3.50E − 11	2.31E − 11	2.04E − 09	1.17E − 09
^{93m}Nb	W 1.00E − 02	4.16E − 10	3.32E − 11	4.9E − 09	2.85E − 10	7.43E − 10	3.04E − 11	3.95E − 10	8.68E − 10
	Y 1.00E − 02	1.55E − 10	4.36E − 11	6.5E − 08	1.14E − 10	2.84E − 10	1.14E − 11	3.04E − 10	7.90E − 09
^{95}Nb	W 1.00E − 02	4.84E − 10	3.77E − 10	5.5E − 09	6.72E − 10	2.42E − 09	3.14E − 10	9.86E − 10	1.29E − 09
	Y 1.00E − 02	4.32E − 10	4.07E − 10	8.3E − 09	4.42E − 10	5.13E − 10	3.58E − 10	1.07E − 09	1.57E − 09
^{97}Nb	W 1.00E − 02	1.21E − 12	1.50E − 12	1.4E − 10	2.07E − 12	1.79E − 12	1.34E − 12	8.89E − 12	2.08E − 11
	Y 1.00E − 02	8.65E − 13	1.12E − 12	1.6E − 10	1.14E − 12	8.26E − 13	9.20E − 13	1.05E − 11	2.24E − 11
^{93}Mo	D 8.00E − 01	9.27E − 11	7.48E − 11	1.2E − 10	2.11E − 10	8.59E − 10	7.06E − 11	5.70E − 10	2.72E − 10
	Y 5.00E − 02	2.45E − 11	2.82E − 10	6.3E − 08	1.06E − 10	2.35E − 10	1.17E − 11	2.10E − 10	7.68E − 09
^{99}Mo	D 8.00E − 01	1.32E − 10	1.29E − 10	1.2E − 09	3.71E − 10	5.40E − 10	1.17E − 10	9.49E − 10	5.42E − 10
	Y 5.00E − 02	9.51E − 11	2.75E − 11	4.3E − 09	5.24E − 11	4.13E − 11	1.52E − 11	1.74E − 09	1.07E − 09
^{99}Tc	D 8.00E − 01	4.52E − 11	4.52E − 11	3.5E − 10	4.52E − 11	4.52E − 11	1.21E − 09	5.78E − 10	2.77E − 10
	W 8.00E − 01	3.99E − 11	3.99E − 11	1.7E − 08	3.99E − 11	3.99E − 11	1.07E − 09	6.26E − 10	2.25E − 09
^{99m}Tc	D 8.00E − 01	2.77E − 12	2.15E − 12	2.3E − 11	3.36E − 12	2.62E − 12	5.01E − 11	1.02E − 11	8.80E − 12
	W 8.00E − 01	1.70E − 12	1.52E − 12	3.1E − 11	2.39E − 12	1.78E − 12	2.09E − 11	6.34E − 12	7.21E − 12
^{101}Tc	D 8.00E − 01	2.50E − 13	3.03E − 13	2.8E − 11	3.19E − 13	2.80E − 13	7.72E − 12	3.52E − 12	4.84E − 12
	w 8.00E − 01	7.31E − 14	1.52E − 13	3.0E − 11	1.60E − 13	1.36E − 13	2.31E − 12	6.60E − 13	3.94E − 12
^{103}Ru	D 5.00E − 02	7.31E − 10	6.07E − 10	1.0E − 09	6.66E − 10	6.18E − 10	5.97E − 10	1.04E − 09	8.24E − 10
	W 5.00E − 02	3.94E − 10	3.18E − 10	9.9E − 09	3.39E − 10	2.71E − 10	2.75E − 10	1.20E − 09	1.75E − 09
	Y 5.00E − 02	3.07E − 10	3.11E − 10	1.6E − 08	3.19E − 10	2.37E − 10	2.57E − 10	1.25E − 09	2.42E − 09

[a] The coefficients are tabulated in SI units. To convert to the conventional units (mrem/μCi) multipley the table entry by 3.7×10^9.

Note: V Denotes vapor form. c, m, and d denote labelled organic compounds, carbon monoxide, and carbon dioxide, respectively. Committed Dose Equivalant calculated for an AMAD of 1 micron.

Table 13.29.2 Committed Dose Equivalent per Unit Intake via Inhalation (Sv/Bq)[a] (Continued)

Nuclide	Class/f1		Gonad	Breast	Lung	R Marrow	Endosteal	Thyroid	Hrem	Heff
^{105}Ru	D	5.00E − 02	2.70E − 11	1.72E − 11	3.7E − 10	1.88E − 11	1.57E − 11	1.50E − 11	1.40E − 10	9.84E − 11
	W	5.00E − 02	1.57E − 11	8.48E − 12	5.4E − 10	9.50E − 12	6.79E − 12	6.46E − 12	1.36E − 10	1.13E − 10
	Y	5.00E − 02	1.59E − 11	6.61E − 12	5.7E − 10	7.70E − 12	4.62E − 12	4.15E − 12	1.61E − 10	1.23E − 10
^{106}Ru	D	5.00E − 02	1.38E − 08	1.37E − 08	1.8E − 08	1.37E − 08	1.37E − 08	1.37E − 08	1.69E − 08	1.52E − 08
	W	5.00E − 02	4.03E − 09	4.03E − 09	2.1E − 07	4.06E − 09	4.00E − 09	4.01E − 09	1.39E − 08	3.18E − 08
	Y	5.00E − 02	1.30E − 09	1.78E − 09	1.0E − 06	1.76E − 09	1.61E − 09	1.72E − 09	1.20E − 08	1.29E − 07
^{105}Rh	D	5.00E − 02	3.49E − 11	2.70E − 11	3.7E − 10	2.90E − 11	2.71E − 11	2.57E − 11	2.20E − 10	1.28E − 10
	W	5.00E − 02	2.23E − 11	9.19E − 12	9.3E − 10	1.12E − 11	8.25E − 12	6.77E − 12	3.89E − 10	2.37E − 10
	Y	5.00E − 02	2.11E − 11	5.61E − 12	9.6E − 10	7.77E − 12	4.46E − 12	2.88E − 12	4.53E − 10	2.58E − 10
^{107}Pd	D	5.00E − 03	9.45E − 13	9.45E − 13	2.9E − 11	5.11E − 12	1.36E − 11	9.45E − 13	2.15E − 10	6.94E − 11
	W	5.00E − 03	2.43E − 13	2.43E − 13	1.5E − 09	1.31E − 12	3.50E − 12	2.43E − 13	1.17E − 10	2.19E − 10
	Y	5.00E − 03	1.05E − 13	1.05E − 13	2.9E − 08	5.68E − 13	1.51E − 12	1.05E − 13	9.71E − 11	3.45E − 09
^{109}Pd	D	5.00E − 03	9.26E − 12	8.36E − 12	6.6E − 10	2.16E − 11	4.64E − 11	8.09E − 12	4.51E − 10	2.23E − 10
	W	5.00E − 03	3.33E − 12	2.03E − 12	1.2E − 09	4.94E − 12	9.75E − 12	1.69E − 12	4.41E − 10	2.72E − 10
	Y	5.00E − 03	2.13E − 12	5.11E − 13	1.2E − 09	9.82E − 13	9.58E − 13	1.55E − 13	5.04E − 10	2.96E − 10
^{110m}Ag	D	5.00E − 02	3.26E − 09	4.14E − 09	8.1E − 09	4.03E − 09	3.05E − 09	1.70E − 09	2.55E − 08	1.07E − 08
	W	5.00E − 02	2.33E − 09	2.93E − 09	3.2E − 08	2.88E − 09	2.13E − 09	2.01E − 09	1.02E − 08	8.34E − 09
	Y	5.00E − 02	2.43E − 09	7.10E − 09	1.2E − 07	6.74E − 09	5.19E − 09	6.39E − 09	1.51E − 08	2.17E − 08
^{111}Ag	D	5.00E − 02	7.60E − 11	7.48E − 11	1.1E − 09	7.62E − 11	7.37E − 11	7.06E − 11	2.46E − 09	9.12E − 10
	W	5.00E − 02	2.59E − 11	1.89E − 11	7.8E − 09	2.03E − 11	1.78E − 11	1.63E − 11	2.07E − 09	1.57E − 09
	Y	5.00E − 02	1.69E − 11	8.47E − 12	8.7E − 12	9.92E − 12	7.41E − 12	6.19E − 12	2.03E − 09	1.66E − 09
^{113m}Cd	D	5.00E − 02	3.32E − 08	3.32E − 08	3.4E − 08	3.32E − 08	3.32E − 08	3.32E − 08	1.30E − 06	4.13E − 07
	W	5.00E − 02	9.95E − 09	9.95E − 09	4.0E − 08	9.95E − 09	9.95E − 09	9.95E − 09	3.89E − 07	1.27E − 07
	Y	5.00E − 02	4.72E − 09	4.72E − 09	4.1E − 07	4.72E − 09	4.72E − 09	4.72E − 09	1.86E − 07	1.08E − 07
^{115m}Cd	D	5.00E − 02	1.57E − 09	1.57E − 09	3.4E − 09	1.58E − 09	1.57E − 09	1.55E − 09	6.06E − 08	1.95E − 08
	W	5.00E − 02	3.80E − 10	3.78E − 10	4.7E − 08	3.81E − 10	3.74E − 10	3.73E − 10	1.76E − 08	1.11E − 08
	Y	5.00E − 02	1.06E − 10	1.08E − 10	7.8E − 08	1.08E − 10	1.03E − 10	1.05E − 10	7.41E − 09	1.16E − 08
^{123}Sn	D	2.00E − 02	7.52E − 10	7.52E − 10	2.3E − 09	5.73E − 09	1.58E − 08	7.49E − 10	1.88E − 09	2.33E − 09
	W	2.00E − 02	1.81E − 10	1.82E − 10	6.1E − 08	1.36E − 09	3.75E − 09	1.81E − 10	3.70E − 09	8.79E − 09
^{125}Sn	D	2.00E − 02	2.60E − 10	2.28E − 10	2.6E − 09	3.62E − 09	5.19E − 09	2.10E − 10	1.87E − 09	1.56E − 09
	W	2.00E − 02	1.59E − 10	9.37E − 11	2.2E − 08	7.26E − 10	1.07E − 09	7.62E − 11	4.38E − 09	4.18E − 09
^{126}Sn	D	2.00E − 02	1.43E − 08	1.41E − 08	1.6E − 08	5.62E − 08	1.18E − 07	1.31E − 08	1.76E − 08	2.36E − 08
	W	2.00E − 02	4.95E − 09	5.39E − 09	1.5E − 08	1.69E − 08	3.33E − 08	4.90E − 09	1.20E − 08	2.69E − 08
^{124}Sb	D	1.00E − 01	9.15E − 10	6.51E − 10	2.0E − 09	1.53E − 09	3.41E − 09	5.68E − 10	2.10E − 09	1.50E − 09
	W	1.00E − 02	1.04E − 09	8.94E − 10	4.1E − 08	1.09E − 09	1.24E − 09	6.74E − 10	4.18E − 09	6.80E − 09
^{125}Sb	D	1.00E − 01	3.19E − 10	2.51E − 10	6.4E − 10	6.49E − 10	2.73E − 09	2.28E − 10	7.16E − 10	5.75E − 10
	W	1.00E − 02	3.60E − 10	4.16E − 10	2.2E − 08	5.35E − 10	9.78E − 10	3.24E − 10	1.45E − 09	3.30E − 09
^{126}Sb	D	1.00E − 01	9.11E − 10	5.89E − 10	1.8E − 09	1.09E − 09	1.71E − 09	5.08E − 10	1.81E − 09	1.27E − 09
	W	1.00E − 02	1.32E − 09	6.44E − 10	1.4E − 08	7.97E − 10	6.75E − 10	4.80E − 10	3.19E − 09	3.17E − 09
^{127}Sb	D	1.00E − 01	2.34E − 10	1.65E − 10	1.4E − 09	4.94E − 10	5.45E − 10	1.50E − 10	1.09E − 09	6.55E − 10
	W	1.00E − 02	2.52E − 10	9.12E − 11	6.9E − 09	1.61E − 10	1.34E − 10	6.15E − 11	2.33E − 09	1.63E − 09
^{125m}Te	D	2.00E − 01	1.24E − 10	1.07E − 10	4.7E − 10	3.01E − 09	3.21E − 08	9.93E − 11	3.14E − 10	1.52E − 09
	W	2.00E − 01	7.93E − 11	7.08E − 11	1.0E − 08	1.15E − 09	1.18E − 08	3.87E − 11	6.75E − 10	1.97E − 09
^{127}Te	D	2.00E − 01	6.63E − 12	6.49E − 12	2.8E − 10	1.43E − 11	1.44E − 11	6.46E − 12	9.74E − 11	6.74E − 11
	W	2.00E − 01	2.02E − 12	1.88E − 12	4.3E − 10	4.09E − 12	4.09E − 12	1.84E − 12	1.11E − 10	8.60E − 11
^{127m}Te	D	2.00E − 01	2.49E − 10	2.43E − 10	8.9E − 10	1.37E − 08	5.24E − 08	2.39E − 10	6.90E − 10	3.64E − 09
	W	2.00E − 01	1.10E − 10	1.10E − 10	3.3E − 08	5.36E − 09	2.04E − 08	9.66E − 11	1.66E − 09	5.81E − 09
^{129}Te	D	2.00E − 01	1.75E − 12	1.68E − 12	1.3E − 10	1.97E − 12	2.03E − 12	1.63E − 12	2.40E − 11	2.42E − 11
	W	2.00E − 01	5.05E − 13	5.39E − 13	1.5E − 10	6.19E − 13	6.22E − 13	5.09E − 13	7.28E − 12	2.09E − 11
^{129m}Te	D	2.00E − 01	4.12E − 10	4.00E − 10	2.2E − 09	8.77E − 09	2.01E − 08	3.95E − 10	1.47E − 09	2.53E − 09
	W	2.00E − 01	1.78E − 10	1.69E − 10	4.0E − 08	3.10E − 09	7.05E − 09	1.56E − 10	3.27E − 09	6.47E − 09

[a] The coefficients are tabulated in SI units. To convert to the conventional units (mrem/μCi) multipley the table entry by 3.7×10^9.

Note: V Denotes vapor form. c, m, and d denote labelled organic compounds, carbon monoxide, and carbon dioxide, respectively. Committed Dose Equivalant calculated for an AMAD of 1 micron.

Table 13.29.2 Committed Dose Equivalent per Unit Intake via Inhalation (Sv/Bq)[a] (Continued)

Nuclide	Class/f1	Gonad	Breast	Lung	R Marrow	Endosteal	Thyroid	Hrem	Heff
^{131}Te	D 2.00E − 01	6.14E − 12	5.53E − 12	2.5E − 10	6.64E − 12	6.21E − 12	2.63E − 09	5.42E − 11	1.29E − 10
	W 2.00E − 01	2.17E − 12	2.67E − 12	3.0E − 10	2.94E − 12	2.61E − 12	2.66E − 09	2.21E − 11	1.24E − 10
^{131m}Te	D 2.00E − 01	1.93E − 10	1.15E − 10	9.4E − 10	2.39E − 10	6.37E − 10	3.28E − 08	5.63E − 10	1.38E − 09
	W 2.00E − 01	2.34E − 10	9.25E − 11	2.2E − 09	1.41E − 10	2.27E − 10	3.61E − 10	9.46E − 10	1.73E − 09
^{132}Te	D 2.00E − 01	3.77E − 10	3.52E − 10	6.5E − 10	4.95E − 10	1.53E − 09	5.87E − 08	5.65E − 10	2.26E − 09
	W 2.00E − 01	4.15E − 10	3.63E − 10	1.7E − 09	4.27E − 10	7.12E − 10	6.28E − 08	7.89E − 10	2.55E − 09
^{133m}Te	D 2.00E − 01	8.97E − 12	7.82E − 12	1.8E − 10	8.32E − 12	6.94E − 12	2.61E − 09	4.14E − 11	1.17E − 10
	W 2.00E − 01	3.39E − 12	4.91E − 12	2.1E − 10	4.89E − 12	4.13E − 12	2.63E − 09	1.43E − 11	1.10E − 10
^{134}Te	D 2.00E − 01	9.00E − 12	8.72E − 12	6.0E − 11	9.30E − 12	8.58E − 12	5.54E − 10	1.88E − 11	3.44E − 11
	W 2.00E − 01	7.90E − 12	7.96E − 12	6.6E − 11	8.38E − 12	7.78E − 12	5.56E − 10	1.09E − 11	3.23E − 11
^{129}I	D 1.00E + 00	8.69E − 11	2.09E − 10	3.1E − 10	1.40E − 10	1.38E − 10	1.56E − 06	1.18E − 10	4.69E − 08
^{130}I	D 1.00E + 00	2.81E − 11	4.87E − 11	6.0E − 10	4.55E − 11	4.03E − 11	1.99E − 08	8.02E − 11	7.14E − 10
^{131}I	D 1.00E + 00	2.53E − 11	7.88E − 11	6.6E − 10	6.26E − 11	5.73E − 11	2.92E − 07	8.03E − 11	8.89E − 09
^{132}I	D 1.00E + 00	9.95E − 12	1.41E − 11	2.7E − 10	1.40E − 11	1.24E − 11	1.74E − 09	3.78E − 11	1.03E − 10
^{133}I	D 1.00E + 00	1.95E − 11	2.94E − 11	8.2E − 10	2.72E − 11	2.52E − 11	4.86E − 08	5.00E − 11	1.58E − 09
^{134}I	D 1.00E + 00	4.25E − 12	6.17E − 12	1.4E − 10	6.08E − 12	5.31E − 12	2.88E − 10	2.27E − 11	3.55E − 11
^{135}I	D 1.00E + 00	1.70E − 11	2.34E − 11	4.4E − 10	2.24E − 11	2.01E − 11	8.46E − 09	4.70E − 11	3.32E − 10
^{134}Cs	D 1.00E + 00	1.30E − 08	1.08E − 08	1.2E − 08	1.18E − 08	1.10E − 08	1.11E − 08	1.39E − 08	1.25E − 08
^{134m}Cs	D 1.00E + 00	3.61E − 12	3.39E − 12	6.4E − 11	3.76E − 12	3.55E − 12	3.34E − 12	6.90E − 12	1.18E − 11
^{135}Cs	D 1.00E + 00	1.20E − 09	1.20E − 09	1.4E − 09	1.20E − 09	1.20E − 09	1.20E − 09	1.20E − 09	1.23E − 09
^{136}Cs	D 1.00E + 00	1.88E − 09	1.67E − 09	2.3E − 09	1.86E − 09	1.70E − 09	1.73E − 09	2.19E − 09	1.98E − 09
^{137}Cs	D 1.00E + 00	8.76E − 09	7.84E − 09	8.8E − 09	8.30E − 09	7.94E − 09	7.93E − 09	9.12E − 09	8.63E − 09
^{138}Cs	D 1.00E + 00	3.28E − 12	4.02E − 12	1.6E − 10	3.95E − 12	3.55E − 12	3.57E − 12	2.06E − 11	2.74E − 11
^{139}Ba	D 1.00E − 01	2.56E − 12	2.46E − 12	2.5E − 10	3.41E − 12	2.49E − 12	2.40E − 12	4.82E − 11	4.64E − 11
^{140}Ba	D 1.00E − 01	4.30E − 10	2.87E − 10	1.7E − 09	1.29E − 09	2.41E − 09	2.56E − 10	1.42E − 09	1.01E − 09
^{141}Ba	D 1.00E − 01	1.41E − 12	1.47E − 12	1.2E − 10	2.49E − 12	4.73E − 12	1.33E − 12	2.27E − 11	2.18E − 11
^{142}Ba	D 1.00E − 01	2.16E − 12	1.60E − 12	5.5E − 11	1.93E − 12	1.42E − 12	1.27E − 12	1.14E − 11	1.11E − 11
^{140}La	D 1.00E − 03	3.62E − 10	2.05E − 10	1.7E − 09	4.56E − 10	4.03E − 10	1.22E − 10	1.81E − 09	9.33E − 10
	W 1.00E − 03	4.54E − 10	1.45E − 10	4.2E − 09	2.14E − 10	1.41E − 10	6.87E − 11	2.12E − 09	1.31E − 09
^{141}La	D 1.00E − 03	1.01E − 11	9.84E − 12	6.5E − 10	2.93E − 11	1.20E − 10	9.40E − 12	2.28E − 10	1.57E − 10
	W 1.00E − 03	2.89E − 12	2.68E − 12	8.9E − 10	7.06E − 12	2.36E − 11	2.45E − 12	1.43E − 10	1.52E − 10
^{142}La	D 1.00E − 03	1.66E − 11	1.13E − 11	3.0E − 10	1.36E − 10	1.11E − 11	8.74E − 12	8.07E − 11	6.84E − 11
	W 1.00E − 03	5.91E − 12	6.28E − 12	3.5E − 10	6.83E − 12	5.39E − 12	4.91E − 12	3.14E − 11	5.50E − 11
^{141}Ce	W 3.00E − 04	8.44E − 11	7.12E − 11	1.1E − 08	4.19E − 10	3.79E − 09	4.61E − 11	2.36E − 09	2.25E − 09
	Y 3.00E − 04	5.54E − 10	4.46E − 10	1.7E − 08	8.96E − 10	2.54E − 10	2.55E − 10	1.26E − 10	2.42E − 09
^{143}Ce	W 3.00E − 04	7.06E − 11	2.22E − 11	3.5E − 09	7.77E − 11	7.90E − 11	1.21E − 11	1.36E − 09	8.66E − 10
	Y 3.00E − 04	7.53E − 11	1.66E − 11	3.9E − 09	2.96E − 11	1.64E − 11	6.23E − 12	1.42E − 09	9.16E − 10
^{144}Ce	W 3.00E − 04	1.93E − 09	1.97E − 09	1.8E − 07	2.67E − 08	4.54E − 08	1.88E − 09	1.03E − 07	5.84E − 08
	Y 3.00E − 04	2.39E − 10	3.48E − 10	7.9E − 07	2.88E − 09	4.72E − 09	2.92E − 10	1.91E − 08	1.01E − 07
^{143}Pr	W 3.00E − 04	4.25E − 18	2.45E − 18	1.1E − 08	2.73E − 10	2.74E − 10	1.58E − 18	2.25E − 09	2.04E − 09
	Y 3.00E − 04	4.37E − 18	2.22E − 18	1.3E − 08	1.48E − 11	1.49E − 11	1.68E − 18	1.97E − 09	2.19E − 09
^{147}Nd	W 3.00E − 04	7.94E − 11	3.76E − 11	8.4E − 09	4.98E − 10	2.33E − 09	1.94E − 11	1.86E − 09	1.72E − 09
	Y 3.00E − 04	8.41E − 11	3.45E − 11	1.1E − 08	9.19E − 11	3.26E − 10	1.82E − 11	1.76E − 09	1.85E − 09
^{147}Pm	W 3.00E − 04	1.88E − 14	3.15E − 14	9.7E − 09	8.16E − 09	1.02E − 07	1.32E − 14	5.89E − 09	6.97E − 09
	Y 3.00E − 04	8.25E − 15	3.60E − 14	7.7E − 08	1.61E − 09	2.01E − 08	1.98E − 14	1.56E − 09	1.06E − 08
^{148}Pm	W 3.00E − 04	1.96E − 10	7.85E − 11	1.3E − 08	5.11E − 10	4.80E − 10	4.27E − 11	3.88E − 09	2.81E − 09
	Y 3.00E − 04	2.12E − 10	7.19E − 11	1.4E − 08	1.07E − 10	7.08E − 11	3.82E − 11	4.10E − 09	2.95E − 09
^{148}Pm	W 3.00E − 04	1.38E − 09	1.28E − 09	2.3E − 08	2.88E − 09	9.05E − 09	8.79E − 10	5.27E − 09	5.46E − 09
	Y 3.00E − 04	1.19E − 09	1.24E − 09	3.6E − 08	1.36E − 09	1.36E − 09	1.05E − 09	3.58E − 09	6.10E − 09

[a] The coefficients are tabulated in SI units. To convert to the conventional units (mrem/μCi) multipley the table entry by 3.7×10^9.

Note: V Denotes vapor form. c, m, and d denote labelled organic compounds, carbon monoxide, and carbon dioxide, respectively. Committed Dose Equivalant calculated for an AMAD of 1 micron.

Table 13.29.2 Committed Dose Equivalent per Unit Intake via Inhalation (Sv/Bq)[a] (Continued)

Nuclide	Class/f1	Gonad	Breast	Lung	R Marrow	Endosteal	Thyroid	Hrem	Heff
^{149}Pm	W 3.00E − 04	3.16E − 12	8.44E − 13	3.0E − 09	7.94E − 11	8.04E − 11	3.69E − 13	1.24E − 09	7.44E − 10
	Y 3.00E − 04	3.61E − 12	8.20E − 13	3.1E − 09	5.53E − 12	5.01E − 12	3.31E − 13	1.39E − 09	7.93E − 10
^{151}Pm	W 3.00E − 04	6.16E − 11	1.59E − 11	1.6E − 09	5.79E − 11	9.73E − 11	6.69E − 12	7.36E − 10	4.38E − 10
	Y 3.00E − 04	7.17E − 11	1.59E − 11	1.6E − 09	2.72E − 11	1.86E − 11	6.18E − 12	8.39E − 10	4.73E − 10
^{151}Sm	W 3.00E − 04	4.03E − 14	1.49E − 13	3.3E − 09	1.10E − 09	1.38E − 07	1.32E − 14	7.51E − 09	8.10E − 09
^{153}Sm	W 3.00E − 04	2.36E − 11	5.67E − 12	2.1E − 09	6.66E − 11	1.57E − 10	1.51E − 12	8.84E − 10	5.31E − 10
^{152}Eu	W 1.00E − 03	1.31E − 08	1.74E − 08	5.8E − 08	7.91E − 08	2.40E − 07	8.25E − 09	9.99E − 08	5.97E − 08
^{154}Eu	W 1.00E − 03	1.17E − 08	1.55E − 08	7.9E − 08	1.06E − 07	5.23E − 07	7.14E − 09	1.13E − 07	7.73E − 08
^{155}Eu	W 1.00E − 03	3.56E − 10	6.14E − 10	1.2E − 08	1.43E − 08	1.52E − 07	2.40E − 10	1.11E − 08	1.12E − 08
^{156}Eu	W 1.00E − 03	6.12E − 10	3.64E − 10	1.8E − 08	1.14E − 09	2.76E − 09	2.16E − 10	3.91E − 09	3.82E − 09
^{160}Tb	W 3.00E − 04	9.36E − 10	9.63E − 10	3.0E − 08	4.43E − 09	2.47E − 08	6.54E − 10	4.84E − 09	6.75E − 09
^{166m}Ho	W 3.00E − 04	3.05E − 08	4.84E − 08	1.1E − 07	1.61E − 07	8.87E − 07	2.14E − 08	4.50E − 07	2.09E − 07
^{181}W	D 3.00E − 01	1.11E − 11	5.93E − 12	5.3E − 11	5.04E − 11	7.08E − 11	2.71E − 12	7.56E − 11	4.09E − 11
^{185}W	D 3.00E − 01	1.24E − 14	6.15E − 15	3.8E − 10	8.39E − 11	2.55E − 10	2.85E − 15	4.65E − 10	2.03E − 10
^{187}W	D 3.00E − 01	2.99E − 11	8.79E − 12	6.1E − 10	2.32E − 11	9.85E − 11	4.37E − 12	2.66E − 10	1.67E − 10
^{210}Pb	D 2.00E − 01	3.18E − 07	3.18E − 07	3.2E − 07	3.75E − 06	5.47E − 05	3.18E − 07	4.69E − 06	3.67E − 06
^{210}Bi	D 5.00E − 02	1.96E − 10	1.96E − 10	2.5E − 09	1.96E − 10	1.96E − 10	1.96E − 10	1.26E − 08	4.18E − 09
	W 5.00E − 02	6.47E − 11	6.47E − 11	4.3E − 07	6.47E − 11	6.47E − 11	6.47E − 11	5.66E − 09	5.29E − 08
^{210}Po	D 1.00E − 01	4.04E − 07	4.04E − 07	7.3E − 07	4.04E − 07	4.04E − 07	4.04E − 07	7.40E − 06	2.54E − 06
	W 1.00E − 01	1.26E − 07	1.26E − 07	1.3E − 05	1.26E − 07	1.26E − 07	1.26E − 07	2.30E − 06	2.32E − 06
^{223}Ra	W 2.00E − 01	3.38E − 08	3.38E − 08	1.7E − 05	2.24E − 07	2.34E − 06	3.38E − 08	6.14E − 08	2.12E − 06
^{244}Ra	W 2.00E − 01	1.56E − 08	1.54E − 08	6.6E − 06	1.13E − 07	1.17E − 06	1.53E − 08	3.55E − 08	8.53E − 07
^{225}Ra	W 2.00E − 01	3.07E − 08	3.07E − 08	1.7E − 05	1.58E − 07	1.68E − 06	3.07E − 08	3.63E − 08	2.10E − 06
^{226}Ra	W 200E − 01	1.02E − 07	1.02E − 07	1.6E − 05	6.64E − 07	7.59E − 06	1.02E − 07	1.07E − 07	2.32E − 06
^{228}Ra	W 2.00E − 01	1.83E − 07	1.84E − 07	7.2E − 06	7.38E − 07	6.51E − 06	1.83E − 07	1.87E − 07	1.29E − 06
^{225}Ac	D 1.00E − 03	5.22E − 07	7.63E − 11	1.6E − 06	3.72E − 06	4.65E − 05	4.03E − 11	2.53E − 06	2.92E − 06
	W 1.00E − 03	8.70E − 08	5.16E − 11	1.6E − 05	6.19E − 07	7.75E − 06	2.89E − 11	4.53E − 07	2.32E − 06
	Y 1.00E − 03	5.20E − 09	4.66E − 11	1.8E − 05	3.63E − 08	4.53E − 07	2.64E − 11	6.14E − 08	2.19E − 06
^{227}Ac	D 1.00E − 03	3.96E − 04	6.66E − 08	1.2E − 07	2.57E − 03	3.12E − 02	3.59E − 08	1.47E − 03	1.81E − 03
	W 1.00E − 03	9.98E − 05	1.70E − 08	6.8E − 05	6.49E − 04	8.10E − 03	9.22E − 09	3.70E − 04	4.65E − 04
	Y 1.00E − 03	3.56E − 05	1.06E − 08	1.5E − 03	2.33E − 04	2.91E − 03	6.47E − 09	1.34E − 04	3.49E − 04
^{227}Th	W 2.00E − 04	5.36E − 08	5.36E − 08	2.4E − 05	2.43E − 06	2.94E − 05	5.35E − 08	1.47E − 07	4.12E − 06
	Y 2.00E − 04	2.96E − 09	2.98E − 09	3.6E − 05	1.30E − 07	1.58E − 06	2.94E − 09	2.06E − 08	4.37E − 06
^{228}Th	W 2.00E − 04	1.35E − 06	1.35E − 06	9.5E − 05	1.12E − 04	1.37E − 03	1.34E − 06	3.44E − 06	6.75E − 05
	Y 2.00E − 04	2.26E − 07	2.32E − 07	6.9E − 04	1.87E − 05	2.29E − 04	2.30E − 07	6.05E − 07	9.23E − 05
^{229}Th	W 2.00E − 04	2.76E − 06	2.76E − 06	8.0E − 05	1.15E − 03	1.43E − 02	2.76E − 06	7.05E − 06	5.80E − 04
	Y 2.00E − 04	1.18E − 06	1.18E − 06	2.0E − 03	4.60E − 04	5.75E − 03	1.18E − 06	3.02E − 06	4.67E − 04
^{230}Th	W 2.00E − 04	4.08E − 07	4.08E − 07	1.6E − 05	1.73E − 04	2.16E − 03	4.08E − 07	1.05E − 06	8.80E − 05
	Y 2.00E − 04	1.72E − 07	1.72E − 07	3.0E − 04	6.99E − 05	8.71E − 04	1.72E − 07	4.48E − 07	7.07E − 05
^{232}Th	W 2.00E − 04	7.62E − 07	7.72E − 07	1.4E − 05	8.93E − 04	1.11E − 02	7.44E − 07	1.87E − 06	4.43E − 04
	Y 2.00E − 04	5.98E − 07	6.14E − 07	9.4E − 04	4.01E − 04	4.99E − 03	5.99E − 07	5.99E − 07	3.11E − 04
^{234}Th	W 2.00E − 04	1.13E − 10	1.08E − 10	4.7E − 08	4.18E − 09	7.83E − 09	1.03E − 10	5.54E − 09	8.04E − 09
	Y 2.00E − 04	2.11E − 11	1.66E − 11	6.4E − 08	2.56E − 10	6.29E − 10	1.27E − 11	5.80E − 09	9.47E − 09
^{231}Pa	W 1.00E − 03	6.90E − 09	8.79E − 09	1.7E − 05	6.97E − 04	8.70E − 03	7.64E − 09	2.87E − 07	3.47E − 04
	Y 1.00E − 03	3.06E − 09	5.65E − 09	7.5E − 04	2.88E − 04	3.60E − 03	4.45E − 09	2.12E − 07	2.32E − 04
^{233}Pa	W 1.00E − 03	1.29E − 10	8.32E − 11	1.2E − 08	8.21E − 10	7.37E − 09	5.17E − 11	1.47E − 09	2.24E − 09
	Y 1.00E − 03	1.29E − 10	9.20E − 11	1.7E − 08	1.86E − 10	8.28E − 10	5.62E − 11	1.48E − 09	2.58E − 09
^{232}U	D 5.00E − 02	8.00E − 08	8.06E − 08	4.1E − 07	4.06E − 06	6.42E − 05	7.85E − 08	3.11E − 06	3.43E − 06
	W 5.00E − 02	2.51E − 08	2.53E − 08	2.5E − 05	1.23E − 06	1.94E − 05	2.47E − 08	9.76E − 07	4.02E − 06
	Y 2.00E − 03	1.69E − 08	2.66E − 08	1.5E − 03	4.68E − 07	7.14E − 06	2.43E − 08	5.86E − 07	1.78E − 04

[a] The coefficients are tabulated in SI units. To convert to the conventional units (mrem/μCi) multipley the table entry by 3.7×10^9.

Note: V Denotes vapor form. c, m, and d denote labelled organic compounds, carbon monoxide, and carbon dioxide, respectively. Committed Dose Equivalant calculated for an AMAD of 1 micron.

Table 13.29.2 Committed Dose Equivalent per Unit Intake via Inhalation (Sv/Bq)[a] (Continued)

Nuclide	Class/f1		Gonad	Breast	Lung	R Marrow	Endosteal	Thyroid	Hrem	Heff
^{133}U	D	5.00E − 02	2.54E − 08	2.54E − 08	3.2E − 07	7.12E − 07	1.12E − 05	2.54E − 08	9.40E − 07	7.53E − 07
	W	5.00E − 02	7.63E − 09	7.63E − 09	1.6E − 05	2.14E − 07	3.36E − 06	7.63E − 09	2.89E − 07	2.16E − 06
	Y	2.00E − 03	2.69E − 09	2.73E − 09	3.0E − 04	7.39E − 08	1.16E − 06	2.70E − 09	1.08E − 07	3.66E − 05
^{234}U	D	5.00E − 02	2.50E − 08	2.50E − 08	3.2E − 07	6.98E − 07	1.09E − 05	2.50E − 08	9.26E − 07	7.37E − 07
	W	5.00E − 02	7.52E − 09	7.52E − 09	1.6E − 05	2.10E − 07	3.29E − 06	7.52E − 09	2.85E − 07	2.13E − 06
	Y	2.00E − 03	2.65E − 09	2.68E − 09	3.0E − 04	7.22E − 08	1.13E − 06	2.65E − 09	1.06E − 07	3.58E − 05
^{235}U	D	5.00E − 02	2.37E − 08	2.38E − 08	3.0E − 07	6.58E − 07	1.01E − 05	2.37E − 08	8.59E − 07	6.85E − 07
	W	5.00E − 02	7.24E − 09	7.33E − 09	1.5E − 05	1.98E − 07	3.05E − 06	7.22E − 09	2.65E − 07	1.97E − 06
	Y	2.00E − 03	2.84E − 09	5.37E − 09	2.8E − 04	7.15E − 08	1.05E − 06	4.11E − 09	1.02E − 07	3.32E − 05
^{236}U	D	5.00E − 02	2.37E − 08	2.37E − 08	3.0E − 07	6.60E − 07	1.04E − 05	2.37E − 08	8.77E − 07	7.01E − 07
	W	5.00E − 02	7.12E − 09	7.12E − 09	1.5E − 05	1.99E − 07	3.12E − 06	7.12E − 09	2.70E − 07	2.01E − 06
	Y	2.00E − 03	2.51E − 09	2.54E − 09	2.8E − 04	6.83E − 08	1.07E − 06	2.51E − 09	1.00E − 07	3.39E − 05
^{237}U	D	5.00E − 02	5.55E − 11	3.39E − 11	6.1E − 10	4.12E − 10	4.02E − 09	2.62E − 11	8.94E − 10	5.32E − 10
	W	5.00E − 02	7.39E − 11	2.78E − 11	4.3E − 09	1.23E − 10	8.35E − 10	1.39E − 11	1.10E − 09	9.03E − 10
	Y	2.00E − 03	8.15E − 11	2.51E − 11	4.7E − 09	5.23E − 11	6.82E − 11	1.00E − 11	1.19E − 09	9.54E − 10
^{238}U	D	5.00E − 02	2.23E − 08	2.23E − 08	2.8E − 07	6.58E − 07	9.78E − 06	2.22E − 08	8.22E − 07	6.62E − 07
	W	5.00E − 02	6.71E − 09	6.74E − 09	1.4E − 05	1.98E − 07	2.94E − 06	6.71E − 09	2.54E − 07	1.90E − 06
	Y	2.00E − 03	2.42E − 09	2.91E − 09	2.7E − 04	6.88E − 08	1.01E − 06	2.73E − 09	9.61E − 08	3.20E − 05
^{237}Np	W	1.00E − 03	2.96E − 05	1.69E − 08	1.6E − 05	2.62E − 04	3.27E − 03	1.34E − 08	2.34E − 05	1.46E − 04
^{238}Np	W	1.00E − 03	1.99E − 09	4.18E − 11	3.5E − 09	1.69E − 08	2.10E − 07	2.45E − 11	2.55E − 09	1.00E − 08
^{239}Np	W	1.00E − 03	7.45E − 11	1.63E − 11	2.4E − 09	2.08E − 10	2.03E − 09	7.62E − 12	9.59E − 10	6.78E − 10
^{238}Pu	W	1.00E − 03	2.80E − 05	1.00E − 09	1.8E − 05	1.52E − 05	1.90E − 03	9.62E − 10	7.02E − 05	1.06E − 04
	Y	1.00E − 05	1.04E − 05	4.40E − 10	3.2E − 04	5.80E − 05	7.25E − 04	3.86E − 10	2.74E − 05	7.79E − 05
^{239}Pu	W	1.00E − 03	3.18E − 05	9.22E − 10	1.7E − 04	1.69E − 04	2.11E − 03	9.03E − 10	7.56E − 05	1.16E − 04
	Y	1.00E − 05	1.20E − 05	3.99E − 10	3.2E − 04	6.57E − 05	8.21E − 04	3.75E − 10	3.02E − 05	8.33E − 05
^{240}Pu	W	1.00E − 03	3.18E − 05	9.51E − 10	1.7E − 05	1.69E − 04	2.11E − 03	9.05E − 10	7.56E − 05	1.16E − 04
	Y	1.00E − 05	1.20E − 05	4.33E − 10	3.2E − 04	6.57E − 05	8.21E − 04	3.76E − 10	3.02E − 05	8.33E − 05
^{241}Pu	W	1.00E − 03	6.82E − 07	3.06E − 11	7.4E − 09	3.36E − 06	4.20E − 05	1.24E − 11	1.31E − 06	2.23E − 06
	Y	1.00E − 05	2.76E − 07	2.14E − 11	3.2E − 06	1.43E − 06	1.78E − 05	9.15E − 12	6.02E − 07	1.34E − 06
^{242}Pu	W	1.00E − 03	3.02E − 05	9.45E − 10	1.6E − 05	1.61E − 04	2.01E − 03	8.79E − 10	7.18E − 05	1.11E − 04
	Y	1.00E − 05	1.14E − 05	4.35E − 10	3.1E − 04	6.25E − 05	7.81E − 04	3.71E − 10	2.86E − 05	7.92E − 05
^{244}Pu	W	1.00E − 03	2.99E − 05	3.33E − 08	1.6E − 05	1.59E − 04	1.98E − 03	1.82E − 08	7.13E − 05	1.09E − 04
	Y	1.00E − 05	1.13E − 05	2.07E − 08	3.0E − 04	6.19E − 05	7.69E − 04	1.27E − 08	2.84E − 05	7.82E − 05
^{241}Am	W	1.00E − 03	3.25E − 05	2.67E − 09	1.8E − 05	1.74E − 04	2.17E − 03	1.60E − 09	7.82E − 05	1.20E − 04
^{242}Am	W	1.00E − 03	3.21E − 05	1.38E − 09	4.2E − 06	1.69E − 04	2.12E − 03	5.64E − 10	7.48E − 05	1.15E − 04
^{242}Am	W	1.00E − 03	1.94E − 09	2.94E − 12	5.2E − 08	1.32E − 08	1.65E − 07	2.52E − 12	8.54E − 09	1.58E − 08
^{243}Am	W	1.00E − 03	3.26E − 05	1.52E − 08	1.8E − 05	1.73E − 04	2.17E − 03	8.29E − 09	7.74E − 05	1.19E − 04
^{242}Cm	W	1.00E − 03	5.70E − 07	9.44E − 10	1.6E − 05	3.90E − 06	4.87E − 05	9.41E − 10	2.45E − 06	4.67E − 06
^{243}Cm	W	1.00E − 03	2.07E − 05	6.29E − 09	1.9E − 05	1.18E − 04	1.47E − 03	3.83E − 09	5.76E − 05	8.30E − 05
^{244}Cm	W	1.00E − 03	1.59E − 05	1.04E − 09	1.9E − 05	9.38E − 05	1.17E − 03	1.01E − 09	4.78E − 05	6.70E − 05
^{245}Cm	W	1.00E − 03	3.37E − 05	6.69E − 09	1.8E − 05	1.79E − 04	2.24E − 03	3.68E − 09	7.96E − 05	1.23E − 04
^{246}Cm	W	1.00E − 03	3.34E − 05	4.00E − 09	1.8E − 05	1.78E − 04	2.22E − 03	2.26E − 09	7.94E − 05	1.22E − 04
^{247}Cm	W	1.00E − 03	3.07E − 05	2.23E − 08	1.7E − 05	1.63E − 04	2.04E − 03	1.45E − 08	7.30E − 05	1.12E − 04
^{248}Cm	W	1.00E − 03	1.21E − 04	1.07E − 06	6.7E − 05	6.52E − 04	8.12E − 03	4.71E − 07	2.89E − 04	4.47E − 04
^{248}Cf	W	1.00E − 03	5.43E − 06	6.56E − 08	3.7E − 05	5.50E − 05	6.86E − 04	3.38E − 08	1.33E − 05	3.70E − 05
	Y	1.00E − 03	1.09E − 06	6.12E − 08	3.0E − 04	1.10E − 05	1.37E − 04	3.20E − 08	2.73E − 06	4.24E − 05

[a] The coefficients are tabulated in SI units. To convert to the conventional units (mrem/μCi) multipley the table entry by 3.7×10^9.

Note: V Denotes vapor form. c, m, and d denote labelled organic compounds, carbon monoxide, and carbon dioxide, respectively. Committed Dose Equivalant calculated for an AMAD of 1 micron.

Table 13.30 Dose Equivalent for Exposure to Selected Radionuclides Distributed in Environmental Media

The dose coefficients of Tables 13.30.1 through 13.30.4 relate the equivalent dose in organs or tissues of the body to the time integral of the radionuclide's concentration in environment media. (Alternatively the coefficients can be interpreted as the instantaneous dose equivalent rate in the tissue per unit activity concentration.) The tabulations include coefficients for the gonads, breast, lung, red marrow, bone surface, thyroid and skin. The effective dose equivalent is given, computed according to ICRP Publication 26. The coefficients assume the radionuclides were distributed uniformly in air, water, on the ground surface, and within the soil. The coefficients are based on the radiations emitted by the indicated radionuclide and do not include radiations emitted by their radioactive decay product(s). Table 8.3 summarizes information on the nuclear decay of each radionuclide and should be consulted for proper usage of the coefficients.

The time integrated activity, $\tilde{A}_i(T)$, of member i, $i = 1, 2, \ldots$ for the time T is

$$\tilde{A}_i(T) = \prod_{j=1}^{i-1} f_{j,j+1}\lambda_j \sum_{j=1}^{i} \frac{A_j^0[1 - e^{-\lambda_j T}]}{\lambda_j \prod\limits_{\substack{k=1 \\ k \neq j}}^{i} (\lambda_k - \lambda_j)}, \tag{1}$$

where A_i^0 is the activity of member i at time zero, λ_j is the decay constant for member j, $f_{j,j+1}$ denotes the fraction of the nuclear transformations of member j forming member $j + 1$ and

$$\prod_{t=1}^{n} a_i = \begin{cases} a_1 * a_2 * \ldots a_n, & \text{if } n \geq 1 \\ 1, & \text{if } n < 1 \end{cases}$$

Dose coefficients are presented for the following exposure conditions:

- Table 13.30.1 submersion in a contaminated atmospheric cloud
- Table 13.30.2 immersion in contaminated water
- Table 13.30.3 exposure to contaminated ground surfaces
- Table 13.30.4 exposure to contaminated soil.

Table 13.30.1 Dose Coefficient for Submersion in Contaminated Air (Sv s^{-1} Bq^{-1} m^3)[a] (After Federal Guidance Report No. 12)

Nuclide	Gonads	Breast	Lung	R Marrow	Endosteal	Thyroid	Heff	Skin
^{3}H	0.00E + 00	0.00E + 00	0.00E + 00	0.00E + 00	0.00E + 00	0.00E + 00	0.00E + 00	0.00E + 00
^{10}Be	1.16E − 17	1.40E − 17	9.69E − 18	8.24E − 18	3.37E − 17	1.10E − 17	1.12E − 17	1.29E − 14
^{11}C	4.78E − 14	5.47E − 14	4.75E − 14	4.57E − 14	8.43E − 14	4.87E − 14	4.89E − 14	7.91E − 14
^{14}C	2.59E − 19	3.52E − 19	1.53E − 19	1.21E − 19	7.06E − 19	2.19E − 19	2.24E − 19	2.43E − 16
^{22}Na	1.06E − 13	1.20E − 13	1.06E − 13	1.04E − 13	1.66E − 13	1.08E − 13	1.08E − 13	1.33E − 13
^{24}Na	2.12E − 13	2.36E − 13	2.16E − 13	2.16E − 13	2.87E − 13	2.20E − 13	2.18E − 13	2.75E − 13
^{32}P	9.89E − 17	1.16E − 16	9.08E − 17	8.19E − 17	2.48E − 16	9.73E − 17	9.90E − 17	4.49E − 14
^{37}Ar	0.00E + 00	0.00E + 00	0.00E + 00	0.00E + 00	0.00E + 00	0.00E + 00	0.00E + 00	0.00E + 00
^{39}Ar	9.38E − 18	1.14E − 17	7.82E − 18	6.63E − 18	2.74E − 17	8.87E − 18	9.10E − 18	1.07E − 14
^{41}Ar	6.33E − 14	7.16E − 14	6.38E − 14	6.32E − 14	9.08E − 14	6.52E − 14	6.50E − 14	1.01E − 13
^{41}Ca	0.00E + 00	0.00E + 00	0.00E + 00	0.00E + 00	0.00E + 00	0.00E + 00	0.00E + 00	0.00E + 00
^{45}Ca	9.44E − 19	1.22E − 18	6.64E − 19	5.34E − 19	2.77E − 18	8.40E − 19	8.63E − 19	1.46E − 15
^{46}Sc	9.77E − 14	1.11E − 13	9.76E − 14	9.62E − 14	1.46E − 13	1.00E − 13	9.98E − 14	1.17E − 13
^{51}Cr	1.47E − 15	1.69E − 15	1.45E − 15	1.37E − 15	3.04E − 15	1.49E − 15	1.51E − 15	1.75E − 15
^{54}Mn	4.01E − 14	4.55E − 14	4.00E − 14	3.91E − 14	6.23E − 14	4.11E − 14	4.09E − 14	4.67E − 14
^{56}Mn	8.37E − 14	9.46E − 14	8.45E − 14	8.37E − 14	1.22E − 13	8.64E − 14	8.61E − 14	1.51E − 13
^{55}Fe	0.00E + 00	0.00E + 00	0.00E + 00	0.00E + 00	0.00E + 00	0.00E + 00	0.00E + 00	0.00E + 00
^{59}Fe	5.83E − 14	6.59E − 14	5.85E − 14	5.79E − 14	8.51E − 14	6.00E − 14	5.97E − 14	7.13E − 14
^{57}Co	5.47E − 15	6.36E − 15	5.21E − 15	4.59E − 15	1.63E − 14	5.46E − 15	5.61E − 15	6.63E − 15
^{60}Co	1.23E − 13	1.39E − 13	1.24E − 13	1.23E − 13	1.78E − 13	1.27E − 13	1.26E − 13	1.45E − 13
^{59}Ni	0.00E + 00	0.00E + 00	0.00E + 00	0.00E + 00	0.00E + 00	0.00E + 00	0.00E + 00	0.00E + 00
^{63}Ni	0.00E + 00	0.00E + 00	0.00E + 00	0.00E + 00	0.00E + 00	0.00E + 00	0.00E + 00	0.00E + 00
^{65}Ni	2.72E − 14	3.07E − 14	2.74E − 14	2.72E − 14	3.93E − 14	2.80E − 14	2.79E − 14	7.18E − 14
^{64}Cu	8.89E − 15	1.02E − 14	8.84E − 15	8.52E − 15	1.56E − 14	9.06E − 15	9.10E − 15	1.64E − 14
^{65}Zn	2.84E − 14	3.21E − 14	2.84E − 14	2.80E − 14	4.18E − 14	2.92E − 14	2.90E − 14	3.29E − 14
^{69}Zn	2.19E − 17	2.62E − 17	1.91E − 17	1.66E − 17	6.09E − 17	2.11E − 17	2.16E − 17	1.81E − 14
^{79}Se	3.47E − 19	4.67E − 19	2.11E − 19	1.67E − 19	9.60E − 19	2.96E − 19	3.03E − 19	3.71E − 16
^{82}Br	1.27E − 13	1.44E − 13	1.27E − 13	1.24E − 13	1.99E − 13	1.30E − 13	1.30E − 13	1.54E − 13
^{83}Br	3.74E − 16	4.29E − 16	3.69E − 16	3.54E − 16	6.75E − 16	3.80E − 16	3.82E − 16	1.85E − 14
^{84}Br	9.16E − 14	1.02E − 13	9.27E − 14	9.26E − 14	1.28E − 13	9.50E − 14	9.41E − 14	1.88E − 13
^{83m}Kr	1.71E − 18	5.05E − 18	1.64E − 19	3.83E − 19	2.25E − 18	6.43E − 19	1.50E − 18	3.56E − 17
^{85m}Kr	7.31E − 15	8.41E − 15	7.04E − 15	6.43E − 15	1.88E − 14	7.33E − 15	7.48E − 15	2.24E − 14
^{85}Kr	1.17E − 16	1.34E − 16	1.14E − 16	1.09E − 16	2.20E − 16	1.18E − 16	1.19E − 16	1.32E − 14
^{87}Kr	4.00E − 14	4.50E − 14	4.04E − 14	4.00E − 14	6.02E − 14	4.13E − 14	4.12E − 14	1.37E − 13
^{88}Kr	9.90E − 14	1.11E − 13	1.01E − 13	1.00E − 13	1.39E − 13	1.03E − 13	1.02E − 13	1.35E − 13
^{86}Rb	4.71E − 15	5.34E − 15	4.71E − 15	4.64E − 15	7.05E − 15	4.84E − 15	4.81E − 15	4.85E − 14
^{88}Rb	3.26E − 14	3.67E − 14	3.31E − 14	3.30E − 14	4.62E − 14	3.37E − 14	3.36E − 14	1.83E − 13
^{89}Rb	1.03E − 13	1.17E − 13	1.04E − 13	1.04E − 13	1.48E − 13	1.07E − 13	1.06E − 13	1.87E − 13
^{89}Sr	7.73E − 17	9.08E − 17	7.08E − 17	6.39E − 17	1.94E − 16	7.60E − 17	7.73E − 17	3.69E − 14
^{90}Sr	7.78E − 18	9.49E − 18	6.44E − 18	5.44E − 18	2.28E − 17	7.33E − 18	7.53E − 18	9.20E − 15
^{91}Sr	3.38E − 14	3.83E − 14	3.37E − 14	3.31E − 14	5.20E − 14	3.47E − 14	3.45E − 14	8.14E − 14
^{92}Sr	6.61E − 14	7.48E − 14	6.67E − 14	6.62E − 14	9.49E − 14	6.82E − 14	6.79E − 14	8.56E − 14
^{90}Y	1.89E − 16	2.20E − 16	1.77E − 16	1.62E − 16	4.44E − 16	1.87E − 16	1.90E − 16	6.24E − 14
^{91m}Y	2.49E − 14	2.85E − 14	2.48E − 14	2.39E − 14	4.28E − 14	2.54E − 14	2.55E − 14	3.11E − 14
^{91}Y	2.56E − 16	2.93E − 16	2.50E − 16	2.41E − 16	4.56E − 16	2.60E − 16	2.60E − 16	3.85E − 14
^{92}Y	1.27E − 14	1.44E − 14	1.27E − 14	1.25E − 14	1.95E − 14	1.30E − 14	1.30E − 14	1.14E − 13

Table 13.30.1 Dose Coefficient for Submersion in Contaminated Air (Sv s^{-1} Bq^{-1} m^3)[a] (Continued)

Nuclide	Gonads	Breast	Lung	R Marrow	Endosteal	Thyroid	Heff	Skin
^{93}Y	4.67E − 15	5.30E − 15	4.68E − 15	4.58E − 15	7.58E − 15	4.79E − 15	4.80E − 15	8.50E − 14
^{93}Zr	0.00E + 00	0.00E + 00	0.00E + 00	0.00E + 00	0.00E + 00	0.00E + 00	0.00E + 00	0.00E + 00
^{95}Zr	3.53E − 14	4.01E − 14	3.51E − 14	3.43E − 14	5.62E − 14	3.61E − 14	3.60E − 14	4.50E − 14
^{97}Zr	8.80E − 15	9.99E − 15	8.81E − 15	8.64E − 15	1.38E − 14	9.03E − 15	9.02E − 15	5.55E − 14
^{93m}Nb	6.33E − 18	1.31E − 17	2.55E − 19	1.18E − 18	6.92E − 18	3.43E − 18	4.44E − 18	4.28E − 17
^{95m}Nb	2.88E − 15	3.31E − 15	2.77E − 15	2.59E − 15	6.60E − 15	2.89E − 15	2.93E − 15	1.12E − 14
^{95}Nb	3.66E − 14	4.16E − 14	3.65E − 14	3.56E − 14	5.79E − 14	3.75E − 14	3.74E − 14	4.30E − 14
^{97m}Nb	3.47E − 14	3.95E − 14	3.46E − 14	3.38E − 14	5.54E − 14	3.56E − 14	3.55E − 14	4.16E − 14
^{97}Nb	3.11E − 14	3.55E − 14	3.10E − 14	3.01E − 14	5.11E − 14	3.18E − 14	3.18E − 14	6.51E − 14
^{93}Mo	3.59E − 17	7.46E − 17	1.44E − 18	6.69E − 18	3.93E − 17	1.95E − 17	2.52E − 17	2.43E − 16
^{99}Mo	7.13E − 15	8.13E − 15	7.06E − 15	6.82E − 15	1.24E − 14	7.27E − 15	7.28E − 15	3.14E − 14
^{99m}Tc	5.75E − 15	6.65E − 15	5.49E − 15	4.91E − 15	1.63E − 14	5.75E − 15	5.89E − 15	7.14E − 15
^{99}Tc	1.74E − 18	2.20E − 18	1.29E − 18	1.05E − 18	5.17E − 18	1.57E − 18	1.62E − 18	2.74E − 15
^{101}Tc	1.57E − 14	1.80E − 14	1.54E − 14	1.46E − 14	3.21E − 14	1.59E − 14	1.61E − 14	4.77E − 14
^{103}Ru	2.19E − 14	2.51E − 14	2.18E − 14	2.10E − 14	3.89E − 14	2.24E − 14	2.25E − 14	2.77E − 14
^{105}Ru	3.72E − 14	4.24E − 14	3.70E − 14	3.59E − 14	6.28E − 14	3.80E − 14	3.81E − 14	6.73E − 14
^{106}Ru	0.00E + 00	0.00E + 00	0.00E + 00	0.00E + 00	0.00E + 00	0.00E + 00	0.00E + 00	0.00E + 00
^{103m}Rh	1.25E − 17	2.15E − 17	1.87E − 18	2.82E − 18	1.76E − 17	8.55E − 18	8.80E − 18	4.49E − 17
^{105}Rh	3.64E − 15	4.16E − 15	3.57E − 15	3.38E − 15	7.53E − 15	3.68E − 15	3.72E − 15	1.07E − 14
^{106}Rh	1.01E − 14	1.16E − 14	1.01E − 14	9.75E − 15	1.72E − 14	1.03E − 14	1.04E − 14	1.09E − 13
^{107}Pd	0.00E + 00	0.00E + 00	0.00E + 00	0.00E + 00	0.00E + 00	0.00E + 00	0.00E + 00	0.00E + 00
^{109}Pd	2.71E − 16	3.52E − 16	1.94E − 16	1.74E − 16	7.02E − 16	2.46E − 16	2.51E − 16	2.15E − 14
^{110m}Ag	1.33E − 13	1.51E − 13	1.33E − 13	1.30E − 13	2.05E − 13	1.36E − 13	1.36E − 13	1.57E − 13
^{110}Ag	1.75E − 15	2.00E − 15	1.73E − 15	1.67E − 15	3.05E − 15	1.78E − 15	1.78E − 15	8.22E − 14
^{111}Ag	1.26E − 15	1.44E − 15	1.23E − 15	1.17E − 15	2.59E − 15	1.27E − 15	1.29E − 15	2.19E − 14
^{113m}Cd	7.17E − 18	8.76E − 18	5.93E − 18	5.01E − 18	2.10E − 17	6.76E − 18	6.94E − 18	8.48E − 15
^{115m}Cd	1.15E − 15	1.30E − 15	1.14E − 15	1.12E − 15	1.80E − 15	1.18E − 15	1.17E − 15	3.99E − 14
^{123}Sn	3.96E − 16	4.51E − 16	3.91E − 16	3.80E − 16	6.50E − 16	4.04E − 16	4.03E − 16	3.28E − 14
^{125}Sn	1.55E − 14	1.75E − 14	1.55E − 14	1.53E − 14	2.31E − 14	1.59E − 14	1.58E − 14	7.13E − 14
^{126}Sn	2.13E − 15	2.55E − 15	1.85E − 15	1.53E − 15	6.94E − 15	2.03E − 15	2.11E − 15	6.65E − 15
^{124}Sb	8.89E − 14	1.01E − 13	8.97E − 14	8.85E − 14	1.34E − 13	9.15E − 14	9.15E − 14	1.26E − 13
^{125}Sb	1.98E − 14	2.27E − 14	1.95E − 14	1.87E − 14	3.53E − 14	2.01E − 14	2.02E − 14	2.65E − 14
^{126m}Sb	7.33E − 14	8.36E − 14	7.29E − 14	7.07E − 14	1.24E − 13	7.49E − 14	7.50E − 14	1.24E − 13
^{126}Sb	1.35E − 13	1.53E − 13	1.34E − 13	1.30E − 13	2.22E − 13	1.37E − 13	1.37E − 13	1.73E − 13
^{127}Sb	3.26E − 14	3.72E − 14	3.24E − 14	3.14E − 14	5.52E − 14	3.33E − 14	3.33E − 14	5.58E − 14
^{125m}Te	5.96E − 16	8.48E − 16	2.23E − 16	1.86E − 16	1.22E − 15	4.64E − 16	4.53E − 16	1.94E − 15
^{127m}Te	1.90E − 16	2.69E − 16	7.62E − 17	6.43E − 17	3.94E − 16	1.50E − 16	1.47E − 16	8.49E − 16
^{127}Te	2.37E − 16	2.73E − 16	2.32E − 16	2.21E − 16	4.65E − 16	2.40E − 16	2.42E − 16	1.14E − 14
^{129m}Te	1.56E − 15	1.81E − 15	1.46E − 15	1.42E − 15	2.60E − 15	1.56E − 15	1.55E − 15	1.49E − 14
^{129}Te	2.71E − 15	3.12E − 15	2.64E − 15	2.54E − 15	4.88E − 15	2.74E − 15	2.75E − 15	3.57E − 14
^{131m}Te	6.85E − 14	7.78E − 14	6.83E − 14	6.68E − 14	1.09E − 13	7.02E − 14	7.01E − 14	8.85E − 14
^{131}Te	1.99E − 14	2.28E − 14	1.96E − 14	1.88E − 14	3.80E − 14	2.03E − 14	2.04E − 14	6.89E − 14
^{132}Te	1.02E − 14	1.18E − 14	9.65E − 15	8.95E − 15	2.42E − 14	1.02E − 14	1.03E − 14	1.39E − 14
^{133m}Te	1.12E − 13	1.27E − 13	1.12E − 13	1.09E − 13	1.75E − 13	1.15E − 13	1.14E − 13	1.74E − 13
^{133}Te	4.49E − 14	5.10E − 14	4.47E − 14	4.36E − 14	7.50E − 14	4.59E − 14	4.60E − 14	1.06E − 13
^{134}Te	4.16E − 14	4.75E − 14	4.10E − 14	3.94E − 14	7.56E − 14	4.23E − 14	4.24E − 14	6.35E − 14

(continued)

Table 13.30.1 Dose Coefficient for Submersion in Contaminated Air (Sv s^{-1} Bq^{-1} m^3)[a] (Continued)

Nuclide	Gonads	Breast	Lung	R Marrow	Endosteal	Thyroid	Heff	Skin
^{129}I	4.83E − 16	6.66E − 16	2.14E − 16	1.64E − 16	1.10E − 15	3.86E − 16	3.80E − 16	1.10E − 15
^{130}I	1.01E − 13	1.16E − 13	1.01E − 13	9.82E − 14	1.68E − 13	1.04E − 13	1.04E − 13	1.36E − 13
^{131}I	1.78E − 14	2.04E − 14	1.76E − 14	1.68E − 14	3.45E − 14	1.81E − 14	1.82E − 14	2.98E − 14
^{132}I	1.09E − 13	1.24E − 13	1.09E − 13	1.07E − 13	1.73E − 13	1.12E − 13	1.12E − 13	1.58E − 13
^{133}I	2.87E − 14	3.28E − 14	2.86E − 14	2.77E − 14	4.87E − 14	2.93E − 14	2.94E − 14	5.83E − 14
^{134}I	1.27E − 13	1.44E − 13	1.27E − 13	1.25E − 13	1.96E − 13	1.30E − 13	1.30E − 13	1.87E − 13
^{135}I	7.77E − 14	8.79E − 14	7.84E − 14	7.76E − 14	1.13E − 13	8.01E − 14	7.98E − 14	1.11E − 13
^{131m}Xe	4.57E − 16	6.02E − 16	2.67E − 16	2.27E − 16	1.06E − 15	3.91E − 16	3.89E − 16	4.82E − 15
^{133m}Xe	1.42E − 15	1.70E − 15	1.19E − 15	1.10E − 15	3.23E − 15	1.36E − 15	1.37E − 15	1.04E − 14
^{133}Xe	1.61E − 15	1.96E − 15	1.32E − 15	1.07E − 15	5.13E − 15	1.51E − 15	1.56E − 15	4.97E − 15
^{135m}Xe	2.00E − 14	2.29E − 14	1.98E − 14	1.91E − 14	3.50E − 14	2.04E − 14	2.04E − 14	2.97E − 14
^{135}Xe	1.17E − 14	1.33E − 14	1.13E − 14	1.07E − 14	2.57E − 14	1.18E − 14	1.19E − 14	3.12E − 14
^{134m}Cs	9.30E − 16	1.12E − 15	7.84E − 16	6.81E − 16	2.61E − 15	8.88E − 16	9.05E − 16	2.88E − 15
^{134}Cs	7.40E − 14	8.43E − 14	7.37E − 14	7.19E − 14	1.20E − 13	7.57E − 14	7.57E − 14	9.45E − 14
^{135}Cs	6.28E − 19	8.23E − 19	4.19E − 19	3.34E − 19	1.81E − 18	5.50E − 19	5.65E − 19	9.06E − 16
^{136}Cs	1.04E − 13	1.18E − 13	1.04E − 13	1.01E − 13	1.66E − 13	1.07E − 13	1.06E − 13	1.25E − 13
^{137}Cs	7.96E − 18	9.67E − 18	6.68E − 18	5.70E − 18	2.29E − 17	7.55E − 18	7.74E − 18	8.63E − 15
^{138}Cs	1.17E − 13	1.33E − 13	1.19E − 13	1.18E − 13	1.70E − 13	1.21E − 13	1.21E − 13	2.17E − 13
^{137m}Ba	2.82E − 14	3.22E − 14	2.80E − 14	2.73E − 14	4.63E − 14	2.88E − 14	2.88E − 14	3.73E − 14
^{139}Ba	2.13E − 15	2.45E − 15	2.03E − 15	1.87E − 15	5.29E − 15	2.13E − 15	2.17E − 15	6.16E − 14
^{140}Ba	8.41E − 15	9.64E − 15	8.27E − 15	7.93E − 15	1.55E − 14	8.53E − 15	8.58E − 15	2.52E − 14
^{141}Ba	4.06E − 14	4.63E − 14	4.03E − 14	3.91E − 14	7.17E − 14	4.15E − 14	4.16E − 14	1.07E − 13
^{142}Ba	5.04E − 14	5.73E − 14	5.02E − 14	4.91E − 14	8.09E − 14	5.17E − 14	5.15E − 14	8.37E − 14
^{140}La	1.14E − 13	1.29E − 13	1.15E − 13	1.14E − 13	1.69E − 13	1.18E − 13	1.17E − 13	1.66E − 13
^{141}La	2.33E − 15	2.64E − 15	2.34E − 15	2.31E − 15	3.49E − 15	2.39E − 15	2.39E − 15	6.58E − 14
^{142}La	1.40E − 13	1.57E − 13	1.42E − 13	1.42E − 13	1.95E − 13	1.45E − 13	1.44E − 13	2.16E − 13
^{141}Ce	3.38E − 15	3.93E − 15	3.17E − 15	2.83E − 15	9.41E − 15	3.35E − 15	3.43E − 15	1.02E − 14
^{143}Ce	1.28E − 14	1.47E − 14	1.23E − 14	1.17E − 14	2.52E − 14	1.28E − 14	1.29E − 14	3.96E − 14
^{144}Ce	8.53E − 16	1.01E − 15	7.69E − 16	6.68E − 16	2.49E − 15	8.33E − 16	8.53E − 16	2.93E − 15
^{143}Pr	2.13E − 17	2.55E − 17	1.86E − 17	1.62E − 17	5.93E − 17	2.05E − 17	2.10E − 17	1.76E − 14
^{144m}Pr	3.25E − 16	4.20E − 16	2.00E − 16	1.56E − 16	8.16E − 16	2.81E − 16	2.79E − 16	5.08E − 16
^{144}Pr	1.90E − 15	2.15E − 15	1.90E − 15	1.87E − 15	2.99E − 15	1.95E − 15	1.95E − 15	8.43E − 14
^{147}Nd	6.13E − 15	7.12E − 15	5.82E − 15	5.40E − 15	1.32E − 14	6.12E − 15	6.19E − 15	1.95E − 14
^{147}Pm	7.48E − 19	9.56E − 19	5.45E − 19	4.46E − 19	2.18E − 18	6.75E − 19	6.93E − 19	8.11E − 16
^{148m}Pm	9.47E − 14	1.08E − 13	9.42E − 14	9.14E − 14	1.58E − 13	9.68E − 14	9.68E − 14	1.18E − 13
^{148}Pm	2.81E − 14	3.19E − 14	2.83E − 14	2.79E − 14	4.24E − 14	2.89E − 14	2.89E − 14	7.97E − 14
^{149}Pm	5.30E − 16	6.07E − 16	5.17E − 16	4.89E − 16	1.10E − 15	5.36E − 16	5.41E − 16	2.19E − 14
^{151}Pm	1.48E − 14	1.70E − 14	1.44E − 14	1.37E − 14	2.99E − 14	1.50E − 14	1.51E − 14	3.32E − 14
^{151}Sm	5.20E − 20	8.80E − 20	7.08E − 21	1.13E − 20	7.09E − 20	3.58E − 20	3.61E − 20	1.90E − 19
^{153}Sm	2.33E − 15	2.82E − 15	1.97E − 15	1.62E − 15	7.29E − 15	2.22E − 15	2.28E − 15	1.45E − 14
^{152}Eu	5.53E − 14	6.29E − 14	5.50E − 14	5.37E − 14	8.89E − 14	5.66E − 14	5.65E − 14	6.90E − 14
^{154}Eu	6.00E − 14	6.81E − 14	5.99E − 14	5.87E − 14	9.43E − 14	6.15E − 14	6.14E − 14	8.29E − 14
^{155}Eu	2.49E − 15	2.95E − 15	2.22E − 15	1.85E − 15	8.09E − 15	2.41E − 15	2.49E − 15	3.39E − 15
^{156}Eu	6.57E − 14	7.42E − 14	6.63E − 14	6.56E − 14	9.58E − 14	6.78E − 14	6.75E − 14	9.98E − 14
^{160}Tb	5.42E − 14	6.16E − 14	5.40E − 14	5.28E − 14	8.59E − 14	5.56E − 14	5.54E − 14	7.34E − 14
^{166m}Ho	8.28E − 14	9.43E − 14	8.19E − 14	7.92E − 14	1.44E − 13	8.44E − 14	8.45E − 14	9.90E − 14
^{181}W	1.45E − 15	1.76E − 15	1.19E − 15	9.10E − 16	5.00E − 15	1.35E − 15	1.40E − 15	1.84E − 15

Table 13.30.1 Dose Coefficient for Submersion in Contaminated Air (Sv s^{-1} Bq^{-1} m^3)[a] (Continued)

Nuclide	Gonads	Breast	Lung	R Marrow	Endosteal	Thyroid	Heff	Skin
^{185}W	5.53E − 18	6.72E − 18	4.61E − 18	3.83E − 18	1.70E − 17	5.21E − 18	5.37E − 18	4.52E − 15
^{187}W	2.24E − 14	2.56E − 14	2.21E − 14	2.12E − 14	4.00E − 14	2.27E − 14	2.28E − 14	4.09E − 14
^{207}Tl	1.60E − 16	1.84E − 16	1.55E − 16	1.47E − 16	3.03E − 16	1.62E − 16	1.62E − 16	3.06E − 14
^{208}Tl	1.72E − 13	1.92E − 13	1.75E − 13	1.74E − 13	2.42E − 13	1.78E − 13	1.77E − 13	2.34E − 13
^{209}Tl	9.95E − 14	1.13E − 13	1.00E − 13	9.86E − 14	1.55E − 13	1.02E − 13	1.02E − 13	1.59E − 13
^{209}Pb	8.37E − 18	1.02E − 17	6.98E − 18	5.93E − 18	2.43E − 17	7.91E − 18	8.12E − 18	9.35E − 15
^{210}Pb	6.19E − 17	8.18E − 17	4.25E − 17	3.14E − 17	1.95E − 16	5.42E − 17	5.64E − 17	1.28E − 16
^{211}Pb	2.44E − 15	2.79E − 15	2.42E − 15	2.34E − 15	4.19E − 15	2.49E − 15	2.49E − 15	3.06E − 14
^{212}Pb	6.75E − 15	7.76E − 15	6.46E − 15	5.92E − 15	1.68E − 14	6.75E − 15	6.87E − 15	1.35E − 14
^{214}Pb	1.16E − 14	1.33E − 14	1.13E − 14	1.06E − 14	2.44E − 14	1.17E − 14	1.18E − 14	2.77E − 14
^{210}Bi	3.32E − 17	3.95E − 17	2.95E − 17	2.60E − 17	8.98E − 17	3.22E − 17	3.29E − 17	2.30E − 14
^{211}Bi	2.17E − 15	2.49E − 15	2.13E − 15	2.01E − 15	4.44E − 15	2.19E − 15	2.22E − 15	3.07E − 15
^{212}Bi	9.02E − 15	1.02E − 14	9.03E − 15	8.87E − 15	1.39E − 14	9.26E − 15	9.24E − 15	4.05E − 14
^{213}Bi	6.25E − 15	7.16E − 15	6.17E − 15	5.91E − 15	1.17E − 14	6.35E − 15	6.39E − 15	3.39E − 14
^{214}Bi	7.44E − 14	8.42E − 14	7.51E − 14	7.43E − 14	1.09E − 13	7.67E − 14	7.65E − 14	1.28E − 13
^{210}Po	4.08E − 19	4.63E − 19	4.06E − 19	3.97E − 19	6.39E − 19	4.18E − 19	4.16E − 19	4.81E − 19
^{211}Po	3.73E − 16	4.24E − 16	3.71E − 16	3.62E − 16	5.97E − 16	3.82E − 16	3.81E − 16	4.47E − 16
^{212}Po	0.00E + 00	0.00E + 00	0.00E + 00	0.00E + 00	0.00E + 00	0.00E + 00	0.00E + 00	0.00E + 00
^{213}Po	0.00E + 00	0.00E + 00	0.00E + 00	0.00E + 00	0.00E + 00	0.00E + 00	0.00E + 00	0.00E + 00
^{214}Po	4.00E − 18	4.54E − 18	3.98E − 18	3.89E − 18	6.27E − 18	4.09E − 18	4.08E − 18	4.71E − 18
^{216}Po	8.12E − 19	9.23E − 19	8.09E − 19	7.91E − 19	1.27E − 18	8.32E − 19	8.29E − 19	9.57E − 19
^{218}Po	4.39E − 19	4.98E − 19	4.37E − 19	4.28E − 19	6.81E − 19	4.50E − 19	4.48E − 19	7.56E − 19
^{217}At	1.45E − 17	1.65E − 17	1.43E − 17	1.37E − 17	2.67E − 17	1.47E − 17	1.48E − 17	1.86E − 17
^{218}At	1.26E − 16	1.60E − 16	9.67E − 17	7.25E − 17	4.23E − 16	1.14E − 16	1.19E − 16	2.12E − 16
^{219}Rn	2.62E − 15	3.00E − 15	2.56E − 15	2.43E − 15	5.44E − 15	2.65E − 15	2.68E − 15	3.38E − 15
^{220}Rn	1.81E − 17	2.07E − 17	1.80E − 17	1.74E − 17	3.13E − 17	1.85E − 17	1.85E − 17	2.20E − 17
^{222}Rn	1.87E − 17	2.14E − 17	1.86E − 17	1.79E − 17	3.31E − 17	1.90E − 17	1.91E − 17	2.28E − 17
^{221}Fr	1.43E − 15	1.64E − 15	1.38E − 15	1.27E − 15	3.48E − 15	1.44E − 15	1.46E − 15	2.02E − 15
^{223}Fr	2.30E − 15	2.72E − 15	2.07E − 15	1.80E − 15	6.29E − 15	2.24E − 15	2.29E − 15	2.30E − 14
^{223}Ra	5.97E − 15	6.91E − 15	5.70E − 15	5.16E − 15	1.54E − 14	5.96E − 15	6.09E − 15	8.87E − 15
^{224}Ra	4.61E − 16	5.28E − 16	4.47E − 16	4.17E − 16	1.07E − 15	4.64E − 16	4.71E − 16	6.35E − 16
^{225}Ra	3.24E − 16	4.24E − 16	1.96E − 16	1.42E − 16	9.20E − 16	2.77E − 16	2.79E − 16	3.01E − 15
^{226}Ra	3.08E − 16	3.54E − 16	2.95E − 16	2.70E − 16	7.95E − 16	3.09E − 16	3.15E − 16	4.79E − 16
^{228}Ra	0.00E + 00	0.00E + 00	0.00E + 00	0.00E + 00	0.00E + 00	0.00E + 00	0.00E + 00	0.00E + 00
^{225}Ac	7.08E − 16	8.28E − 16	6.64E − 16	5.83E − 16	2.07E − 15	6.99E − 16	7.21E − 16	9.40E − 16
^{227}Ac	5.78E − 18	6.98E − 18	5.22E − 18	4.59E − 18	1.68E − 17	5.60E − 18	5.82E − 18	1.10E − 17
^{228}Ac	4.67E − 14	5.30E − 14	4.66E − 14	4.56E − 14	7.39E − 14	4.79E − 14	4.78E − 14	7.88E − 14
^{227}Th	4.80E − 15	5.53E − 15	4.61E − 15	4.27E − 15	1.12E − 14	4.81E − 15	4.88E − 15	6.50E − 15
^{228}Th	9.12E − 17	1.09E − 16	8.33E − 17	7.32E − 17	2.64E − 16	8.88E − 17	9.20E − 17	1.50E − 16
^{229}Th	3.77E − 15	4.42E − 15	3.50E − 15	3.03E − 15	1.15E − 14	3.70E − 15	3.83E − 15	5.41E − 15
^{230}Th	1.80E − 17	2.38E − 17	1.43E − 17	1.22E − 17	5.29E − 17	1.63E − 17	1.74E − 17	4.51E − 17
^{231}Th	5.39E − 16	6.79E − 16	4.35E − 16	3.70E − 16	1.63E − 15	5.00E − 16	5.22E − 16	2.52E − 15
^{232}Th	9.34E − 18	1.36E − 17	6.37E − 18	5.52E − 18	2.60E − 17	7.90E − 18	8.72E − 18	3.44E − 17
^{234}Th	3.38E − 16	4.03E − 16	3.01E − 16	2.49E − 16	1.12E − 15	3.25E − 16	3.38E − 16	7.50E − 16
^{231}Pa	1.71E − 15	1.99E − 15	1.62E − 15	1.52E − 15	3.64E − 15	1.70E − 15	1.72E − 15	2.44E − 15
^{233}Pa	9.16E − 15	1.05E − 14	8.88E − 15	8.27E − 15	2.08E − 14	9.21E − 15	9.35E − 15	1.66E − 14

(continued)

Table 13.30.1 Dose Coefficient for Submersion in Contaminated Air (Sv s^{-1} Bq^{-1} m^3)[a] (Continued)

Nuclide	Gonads	Breast	Lung	R Marrow	Endosteal	Thyroid	Heff	Skin
^{234m}Pa	7.05E − 16	8.05E − 16	6.94E − 16	6.70E − 16	1.24E − 15	7.18E − 16	7.19E − 16	5.48E − 14
^{234}Pa	9.14E − 14	1.04E − 13	9.09E − 14	8.86E − 14	1.50E − 13	9.35E − 14	9.34E − 14	1.24E − 13
^{232}U	1.55E − 17	2.32E − 17	9.84E − 18	8.99E − 18	3.86E − 17	1.29E − 17	1.42E − 17	5.92E − 17
^{233}U	1.69E − 17	2.22E − 17	1.35E − 17	1.24E − 17	4.12E − 17	1.55E − 17	1.63E − 17	4.57E − 17
^{234}U	8.79E − 18	1.44E − 17	4.38E − 18	4.20E − 18	1.99E − 17	6.69E − 18	7.63E − 18	4.25E − 17
^{235}U	7.05E − 15	8.11E − 15	6.75E − 15	6.15E − 15	1.84E − 14	7.05E − 15	7.20E − 15	8.64E − 15
^{236}U	6.10E − 18	1.10E − 17	2.18E − 18	2.33E − 18	1.19E − 17	4.19E − 18	5.01E − 18	3.57E − 17
^{238}U	4.39E − 18	8.54E − 18	9.96E − 19	1.24E − 18	7.40E − 18	2.72E − 18	3.41E − 18	2.91E − 17
^{240}U	4.92E − 17	8.04E − 17	1.84E − 17	1.71E − 17	1.05E − 16	3.61E − 17	3.93E − 17	3.12E − 15
^{237}Np	1.04E − 15	1.26E − 15	9.02E − 16	7.69E − 16	3.20E − 15	9.94E − 16	1.03E − 15	1.54E − 15
^{239}Np	7.53E − 15	8.73E − 15	7.18E − 15	6.50E − 15	2.00E − 14	7.52E − 15	7.69E − 15	1.60E − 14
^{240m}Np	1.58E − 14	1.80E − 14	1.57E − 14	1.53E − 14	2.61E − 14	1.62E − 14	1.62E − 14	5.93E − 14
^{238}Pu	6.56E − 18	1.27E − 17	1.06E − 18	1.68E − 18	9.30E − 18	4.01E − 18	4.88E − 18	4.09E − 17
^{239}Pu	4.84E − 18	7.55E − 18	2.65E − 18	2.67E − 18	9.47E − 18	3.88E − 18	4.24E − 18	1.86E − 17
^{240}Pu	6.36E − 18	1.23E − 17	1.09E − 18	1.65E − 18	9.26E − 18	3.92E − 18	4.75E − 18	3.92E − 17
^{241}Pu	7.19E − 20	8.67E − 20	6.48E − 20	5.63E − 20	2.19E − 19	6.98E − 20	7.25E − 20	1.17E − 19
^{242}Pu	5.34E − 18	1.03E − 17	9.69E − 19	1.43E − 18	7.90E − 18	3.32E − 18	4.01E − 18	3.27E − 17
^{243}Pu	1.02E − 15	1.21E − 15	9.28E − 16	7.84E − 16	3.23E − 15	9.91E − 16	1.03E − 15	8.15E − 15
^{244}Pu	4.10E − 18	8.23E − 18	4.23E − 19	8.80E − 19	5.29E − 18	2.39E − 18	2.97E − 18	2.69E − 17
^{241}Am	8.58E − 16	1.07E − 15	6.74E − 16	5.21E − 16	2.87E − 15	7.83E − 16	8.18E − 16	1.28E − 15
^{242}Am	6.09E − 16	7.30E − 16	5.51E − 16	4.77E − 16	1.88E − 15	5.94E − 16	6.15E − 16	8.20E − 15
^{243}Am	2.19E − 15	2.61E − 15	1.92E − 15	1.55E − 15	7.47E − 15	2.09E − 15	2.18E − 15	2.75E − 15
^{242}Cm	7.83E − 18	1.48E − 17	1.13E − 18	1.89E − 18	1.06E − 17	4.91E − 18	5.69E − 18	4.29E − 17
^{243}Cm	5.77E − 15	6.68E − 15	5.50E − 15	5.00E − 15	1.50E − 14	5.76E − 15	5.88E − 15	9.79E − 15
^{244}Cm	6.90E − 18	1.33E − 17	7.08E − 19	1.46E − 18	8.82E − 18	4.19E − 18	4.91E − 18	3.91E − 17
^{245}Cm	3.88E − 15	4.55E − 15	3.63E − 15	3.17E − 15	1.18E − 14	3.84E − 15	3.96E − 15	5.36E − 15
^{247}Cm	1.47E − 14	1.68E − 14	1.44E − 14	1.38E − 14	2.83E − 14	1.49E − 14	1.50E − 14	1.79E − 14
^{248}Cm	4.75E − 18	9.12E − 18	5.17E − 19	1.02E − 18	6.17E − 18	2.90E − 18	3.39E − 18	2.67E − 17
^{252}Cf	6.85E − 18	1.21E − 17	1.42E − 18	1.91E − 18	1.04E − 17	4.64E − 18	5.06E − 18	3.08E − 17

[a] The coefficients are tabulated in SI units. To convert to conventional units (mrad/y per $\mu Ci/m^3$), multiply table entry by 3.7×10^9. Note that this is for a hemispherical infinite cloud.

Table 13.30.2 Dose Coefficient for Immersion in Contaminated Water (Sv s^{-1} Bq^{-1}) (After Federal Guidance Report No. 12)

Nuclide	Gonads	Breast	Lung	R Marrow	Endosteal	Thyroid	Heff	Skin
^{3}H	0.00E + 00	0.00E + 00	0.00E + 00	0.00E + 00	0.00E + 00	0.00E + 00	0.00E + 00	0.00E + 00
^{10}Be	2.24E − 20	2.73E − 20	1.86E − 20	1.57E − 20	6.52E − 20	2.11E − 20	2.17E − 20	1.37E − 17
^{11}C	1.04E − 16	1.19E − 16	1.03E − 16	9.93E − 17	1.85E − 16	1.06E − 16	1.06E − 16	1.47E − 16
^{14}C	5.10E − 22	6.96E − 22	2.96E − 22	2.35E − 22	1.37E − 21	4.29E − 22	4.39E − 22	2.55E − 19
^{22}Na	2.30E − 16	2.61E − 16	2.30E − 16	2.25E − 16	3.62E − 16	2.35E − 16	2.35E − 16	2.78E − 16
^{24}Na	4.59E − 16	5.12E − 16	4.67E − 16	4.68E − 16	6.23E − 16	4.77E − 16	4.73E − 16	5.59E − 16
^{32}P	1.90E − 19	2.24E − 19	1.73E − 19	1.56E − 19	4.79E − 19	1.86E − 19	1.90E − 19	4.79E − 17
^{37}Ar	0.00E + 00	0.00E + 00	0.00E + 00	0.00E + 00	0.00E + 00	0.00E + 00	0.00E + 00	0.00E + 00
^{39}Ar	1.82E − 20	2.23E − 20	1.50E − 20	1.27E − 20	5.30E − 20	1.71E − 20	1.76E − 20	1.13E − 17
^{41}Ar	1.37E − 16	1.55E − 16	1.38E − 16	1.37E − 16	1.97E − 16	1.41E − 16	1.41E − 16	1.88E − 16
^{41}Ca	0.00E + 00	0.00E + 00	0.00E + 00	0.00E + 00	0.00E + 00	0.00E + 00	0.00E + 00	0.00E + 00
^{45}Ca	1.85E − 21	2.39E − 21	1.28E − 21	1.03E − 21	5.38E − 21	1.64E − 21	1.68E − 21	1.53E − 18
^{46}Sc	2.12E − 16	2.40E − 16	2.11E − 16	2.08E − 16	3.18E − 16	2.18E − 16	2.16E − 16	2.49E − 16
^{51}Cr	3.23E − 18	3.69E − 18	3.15E − 18	2.99E − 18	6.69E − 18	3.26E − 18	3.30E − 18	3.82E − 18
^{54}Mn	8.71E − 17	9.89E − 17	8.66E − 17	8.48E − 17	1.36E − 16	8.92E − 17	8.88E − 17	1.01E − 16
^{56}Mn	1.81E − 16	2.05E − 16	1.83E − 16	1.81E − 16	2.65E − 16	1.87E − 16	1.86E − 16	2.68E − 16
^{55}Fe	0.00E + 00	0.00E + 00	0.00E + 00	0.00E + 00	0.00E + 00	0.00E + 00	0.00E + 00	0.00E + 00
^{59}Fe	1.26E − 16	1.43E − 16	1.27E − 16	1.25E − 16	1.85E − 16	1.30E − 16	1.29E − 16	1.50E − 16
^{57}Co	1.22E − 17	1.42E − 17	1.16E − 17	1.01E − 17	3.64E − 17	1.21E − 17	1.25E − 17	1.47E − 17
^{60}Co	2.67E − 16	3.02E − 16	2.68E − 16	2.66E − 16	3.86E − 16	2.75E − 16	2.74E − 16	3.11E − 16
^{59}Ni	0.00E + 00	0.00E + 00	0.00E + 00	0.00E + 00	0.00E + 00	0.00E + 00	0.00E + 00	0.00E + 00
^{63}Ni	0.00E + 00	0.00E + 00	0.00E + 00	0.00E + 00	0.00E + 00	0.00E + 00	0.00E + 00	0.00E + 00
^{65}Ni	5.88E − 17	6.66E − 17	5.93E − 17	5.87E − 17	8.55E − 17	6.06E − 17	6.04E − 17	1.11E − 16
^{64}Cu	1.94E − 17	2.21E − 17	1.92E − 17	1.85E − 17	3.41E − 17	1.97E − 17	1.98E − 17	2.92E − 17
^{65}Zn	6.15E − 17	6.97E − 17	6.15E − 17	6.07E − 17	9.10E − 17	6.32E − 17	6.29E − 17	7.12E − 17
^{69}Zn	4.24E − 20	5.10E − 20	3.66E − 20	3.18E − 20	1.18E − 19	4.07E − 20	4.16E − 20	1.91E − 17
^{79}Se	6.82E − 22	9.22E − 22	4.08E − 22	3.24E − 22	1.87E − 21	5.79E − 22	5.93E − 22	3.90E − 19
^{82}Br	2.76E − 16	3.14E − 16	2.75E − 16	2.70E − 16	4.34E − 16	2.83E − 16	2.82E − 16	3.28E − 16
^{83}Br	8.09E − 19	9.27E − 19	7.96E − 19	7.64E − 19	1.46E − 18	8.21E − 19	8.25E − 19	2.01E − 17
^{84}Br	1.98E − 16	2.22E − 16	2.01E − 16	2.00E − 16	2.78E − 16	2.06E − 16	2.04E − 16	3.16E − 16
^{83m}Kr	3.99E − 21	1.18E − 20	3.83E − 22	8.93E − 22	5.24E − 21	1.50E − 21	3.49E − 21	8.31E − 20
^{85m}Kr	1.62E − 17	1.86E − 17	1.55E − 17	1.41E − 17	4.17E − 17	1.62E − 17	1.65E − 17	3.38E − 17
^{85}Kr	2.51E − 19	2.89E − 19	2.45E − 19	2.34E − 19	4.72E − 19	2.54E − 19	2.55E − 19	1.41E − 17
^{87}Kr	8.67E − 17	9.77E − 17	8.75E − 17	8.66E − 17	1.31E − 16	8.95E − 17	8.93E − 17	1.97E − 16
^{88}Kr	2.14E − 16	2.41E − 16	2.18E − 16	2.18E − 16	3.03E − 16	2.22E − 16	2.21E − 16	2.68E − 16
^{86}Rb	1.02E − 17	1.15E − 17	1.02E − 17	1.00E − 17	1.53E − 17	1.05E − 17	1.04E − 17	5.76E − 17
^{88}Rb	7.04E − 17	7.93E − 17	7.14E − 17	7.11E − 17	9.99E − 17	7.28E − 17	7.26E − 17	2.38E − 16
^{89}Rb	2.24E − 16	2.53E − 16	2.26E − 16	2.24E − 16	3.21E − 16	2.31E − 16	2.30E − 16	3.31E − 16
^{89}Sr	1.50E − 19	1.76E − 19	1.36E − 19	1.23E − 19	3.76E − 19	1.47E − 19	1.49E − 19	3.94E − 17
^{90}Sr	1.51E − 20	1.85E − 20	1.23E − 20	1.04E − 20	4.41E − 20	1.42E − 20	1.46E − 20	9.71E − 18
^{91}Sr	7.33E − 17	8.32E − 17	7.30E − 17	7.16E − 17	1.13E − 16	7.51E − 17	7.48E − 17	1.30E − 16
^{92}Sr	1.43E − 16	1.62E − 16	1.44E − 16	1.43E − 16	2.06E − 16	1.48E − 16	1.47E − 16	1.75E − 16
^{90}Y	3.61E − 19	4.22E − 19	3.36E − 19	3.07E − 19	8.56E − 19	3.58E − 19	3.63E − 19	6.67E − 17
^{91m}Y	5.42E − 17	6.19E − 17	5.38E − 17	5.19E − 17	9.37E − 17	5.52E − 17	5.54E − 17	6.59E − 17
^{91}Y	5.35E − 19	6.13E − 19	5.22E − 19	5.04E − 19	9.44E − 19	5.43E − 19	5.44E − 19	4.12E − 17
^{92}Y	2.74E − 17	3.11E − 17	2.74E − 17	2.69E − 17	4.22E − 17	2.81E − 17	2.81E − 17	1.38E − 16

(continued)

Table 13.30.2 Dose Coefficient for Immersion in Contaminated Water (Sv s^{-1} Bq^{-1}) (Continued)

Nuclide	Gonads	Breast	Lung	R Marrow	Endosteal	Thyroid	Heff	Skin
^{93}Y	1.01E − 17	1.14E − 17	1.01E − 17	9.86E − 18	1.64E − 17	1.03E − 17	1.03E − 17	9.66E − 17
^{93}Zr	0.00E + 00	0.00E + 00	0.00E + 00	0.00E + 00	0.00E + 00	0.00E + 00	0.00E + 00	0.00E + 00
^{95}Zr	7.66E − 17	8.72E − 17	7.61E − 17	7.42E − 17	1.23E − 16	7.83E − 17	7.82E − 17	9.36E − 17
^{97}Zr	1.91E − 17	2.17E − 17	1.91E − 17	1.87E − 17	3.01E − 17	1.96E − 17	1.96E − 17	7.04E − 17
^{93m}Nb	1.48E − 20	3.08E − 20	5.97E − 22	2.76E − 21	1.62E − 20	8.05E − 21	1.04E − 20	1.01E − 19
^{95m}Nb	6.32E − 18	7.30E − 18	6.06E − 18	5.66E − 18	1.46E − 17	6.33E − 18	6.43E − 18	1.58E − 17
^{95}Nb	7.95E − 17	9.04E − 17	7.90E − 17	7.72E − 17	1.26E − 16	8.13E − 17	8.11E − 17	9.32E − 17
^{97m}Nb	7.55E − 17	8.59E − 17	7.50E − 17	7.31E − 17	1.21E − 16	7.72E − 17	7.70E − 17	8.93E − 17
^{97}Nb	6.76E − 17	7.71E − 17	6.72E − 17	6.53E − 17	1.12E − 16	6.90E − 17	6.91E − 17	1.10E − 16
^{93}Mo	8.43E − 20	1.75E − 19	3.38E − 21	1.57E − 20	9.21E − 20	4.57E − 20	5.92E − 20	5.71E − 19
^{99}Mo	1.55E − 17	1.77E − 17	1.53E − 17	1.48E − 17	2.71E − 17	1.58E − 17	1.58E − 17	4.26E − 17
^{99m}Tc	1.28E − 17	1.48E − 17	1.21E − 17	1.08E − 17	3.63E − 17	1.28E − 17	1.31E − 17	1.56E − 17
^{99}Tc	3.39E − 21	4.32E − 21	2.48E − 21	2.01E − 21	1.00E − 20	3.06E − 21	3.14E − 21	2.88E − 18
^{101}Tc	3.43E − 17	3.93E − 17	3.36E − 17	3.18E − 17	7.07E − 17	3.47E − 17	3.51E − 17	7.16E − 17
^{103}Ru	4.78E − 17	5.47E − 17	4.73E − 17	4.56E − 17	8.52E − 17	4.86E − 17	4.89E − 17	5.85E − 17
^{105}Ru	8.10E − 17	9.23E − 17	8.03E − 17	7.78E − 17	1.37E − 16	8.26E − 17	8.27E − 17	1.20E − 16
^{106}Ru	0.00E + 00	0.00E + 00	0.00E + 00	0.00E + 00	0.00E + 00	0.00E + 00	0.00E + 00	0.00E + 00
^{103m}Rh	2.95E − 20	5.06E − 20	4.37E − 21	6.63E − 21	4.13E − 20	2.01E − 20	2.07E − 20	1.06E − 19
^{105}Rh	7.97E − 18	9.12E − 18	7.78E − 18	7.37E − 18	1.66E − 17	8.05E − 18	8.14E − 18	1.62E − 17
^{106}Rh	2.19E − 17	2.50E − 17	2.17E − 17	2.11E − 17	3.75E − 17	2.23E − 17	2.24E − 17	1.30E − 16
^{107}Pd	0.00E + 00	0.00E + 00	0.00E + 00	0.00E + 00	0.00E + 00	0.00E + 00	0.00E + 00	0.00E + 00
^{109}Pd	6.09E − 19	7.96E − 19	4.27E − 19	3.81E − 19	1.56E − 18	5.47E − 19	5.59E − 19	2.34E − 17
^{110m}Ag	2.88E − 16	3.27E − 16	2.87E − 16	2.82E − 16	4.46E − 16	2.95E − 16	2.94E − 16	3.38E − 16
^{110}Ag	3.72E − 18	4.26E − 18	3.67E − 18	3.54E − 18	6.48E − 18	3.79E − 18	3.79E − 18	8.99E − 17
^{111}Ag	2.75E − 18	3.15E − 18	2.68E − 18	2.54E − 18	5.69E − 18	2.78E − 18	2.81E − 18	2.49E − 17
^{113m}Cd	1.39E − 20	1.71E − 20	1.14E − 20	9.57E − 21	4.06E − 20	1.31E − 20	1.34E − 20	8.95E − 18
^{115m}Cd	2.47E − 18	2.81E − 18	2.46E − 18	2.41E − 18	3.88E − 18	2.53E − 18	2.52E − 18	4.38E − 17
^{123}Sn	8.44E − 19	9.61E − 19	8.32E − 19	8.11E − 19	1.38E − 18	8.61E − 19	8.59E − 19	3.53E − 17
^{125}Sn	3.35E − 17	3.79E − 17	3.35E − 17	3.30E − 17	5.02E − 17	3.44E − 17	3.43E − 17	9.57E − 17
^{126}Sn	4.83E − 18	5.81E − 18	4.15E − 18	3.43E − 18	1.57E − 17	4.60E − 18	4.76E − 18	1.04E − 17
^{124}Sb	1.93E − 16	2.19E − 16	1.94E − 16	1.92E − 16	2.91E − 16	1.98E − 16	1.98E − 16	2.49E − 16
^{125}Sb	4.32E − 17	4.95E − 17	4.23E − 17	4.07E − 17	7.75E − 17	4.38E − 17	4.39E − 17	5.46E − 17
^{126m}Sb	1.60E − 16	1.82E − 16	1.58E − 16	1.53E − 16	2.70E − 16	1.63E − 16	1.63E − 16	2.28E − 16
^{126}Sb	2.92E − 16	3.33E − 16	2.90E − 16	2.82E − 16	4.86E − 16	2.99E − 16	2.99E − 16	3.60E − 16
^{127}Sb	7.09E − 17	8.09E − 17	7.02E − 17	6.80E − 17	1.21E − 16	7.23E − 17	7.24E − 17	1.02E − 16
^{125m}Te	1.40E − 18	2.00E − 18	5.20E − 19	4.35E − 19	2.85E − 18	1.09E − 18	1.06E − 18	3.59E − 18
^{127m}Te	4.47E − 19	6.33E − 19	1.76E − 19	1.49E − 19	9.20E − 19	3.51E − 19	3.44E − 19	1.38E − 18
^{127}Te	5.16E − 19	5.93E − 19	5.04E − 19	4.79E − 19	1.01E − 18	5.21E − 19	5.26E − 19	1.24E − 17
^{129m}Te	3.40E − 18	3.97E − 18	3.18E − 18	3.08E − 18	5.70E − 18	3.40E − 18	3.39E − 18	1.81E − 17
^{129}Te	5.91E − 18	6.81E − 18	5.73E − 18	5.50E − 18	1.07E − 17	5.96E − 18	5.99E − 18	4.16E − 17
^{131m}Te	1.49E − 16	1.69E − 16	1.48E − 16	1.45E − 16	2.38E − 16	1.52E − 16	1.52E − 16	1.83E − 16
^{131}Te	4.35E − 17	4.98E − 17	4.27E − 17	4.08E − 17	8.35E − 17	4.42E − 17	4.44E − 17	9.96E − 17
^{132}Te	2.26E − 17	2.62E − 17	2.12E − 17	1.96E − 17	5.37E − 17	2.25E − 17	2.28E − 17	2.90E − 17
^{133m}Te	2.43E − 16	2.76E − 16	2.42E − 16	2.37E − 16	3.81E − 16	2.49E − 16	2.48E − 16	3.30E − 16
^{133}Te	9.75E − 17	1.11E − 16	9.71E − 17	9.45E − 17	1.64E − 16	9.97E − 17	9.99E − 17	1.71E − 16
^{134}Te	9.06E − 17	1.04E − 16	8.91E − 17	8.56E − 17	1.66E − 16	9.21E − 17	9.24E − 17	1.22E − 16
^{129}I	1.14E − 18	1.57E − 18	4.99E − 19	3.84E − 19	2.56E − 18	9.06E − 19	8.91E − 19	2.29E − 18

Table 13.30.2 Dose Coefficient for Immersion in Contaminated Water (Sv s^{-1} Bq^{-1}) (Continued)

Nuclide	Gonads	Breast	Lung	R Marrow	Endosteal	Thyroid	Heff	Skin
^{130}I	2.21E − 16	2.52E − 16	2.19E − 16	2.13E − 16	3.67E − 16	2.25E − 16	2.25E − 16	2.77E − 16
^{131}I	3.90E − 17	4.46E − 17	3.83E − 17	3.65E − 17	7.58E − 17	3.95E − 17	3.98E − 17	5.53E − 17
^{132}I	2.38E − 16	2.70E − 16	2.37E − 16	2.31E − 16	3.78E − 16	2.43E − 16	2.43E − 16	3.10E − 16
^{133}I	6.25E − 17	7.13E − 17	6.20E − 17	6.01E − 17	1.06E − 16	6.37E − 17	6.39E − 17	9.96E − 17
^{134}I	2.76E − 16	3.13E − 16	2.75E − 16	2.70E − 16	4.26E − 16	2.83E − 16	2.82E − 16	3.63E − 16
^{135}I	1.68E − 16	1.91E − 16	1.70E − 16	1.68E − 16	2.46E − 16	1.74E − 16	1.73E − 16	2.17E − 16
^{131m}Xe	1.06E − 18	1.40E − 18	6.06E − 19	5.12E − 19	2.43E − 18	8.99E − 19	8.93E − 19	6.02E − 18
^{133m}Xe	3.17E − 18	3.82E − 18	2.63E − 18	2.41E − 18	7.23E − 18	3.02E − 18	3.04E − 18	1.32E − 17
^{133}Xe	3.69E − 18	4.50E − 18	2.97E − 18	2.41E − 18	1.16E − 17	3.43E − 18	3.54E − 18	7.89E − 18
^{135m}Xe	4.36E − 17	4.99E − 17	4.31E − 17	4.15E − 17	7.67E − 17	4.43E − 17	4.45E − 17	5.80E − 17
^{135}Xe	2.56E − 17	2.93E − 17	2.48E − 17	2.33E − 17	5.68E − 17	2.57E − 17	2.61E − 17	4.86E − 17
^{134m}Cs	2.10E − 18	2.54E − 18	1.75E − 18	1.51E − 18	5.87E − 18	2.00E − 18	2.03E − 18	4.52E − 18
^{134}Cs	1.61E − 16	1.83E − 16	1.60E − 16	1.56E − 16	2.62E − 16	1.64E − 16	1.64E − 16	1.97E − 16
^{135}Cs	1.23E − 21	1.62E − 21	8.08E − 22	6.44E − 22	3.52E − 21	1.07E − 21	1.10E − 21	9.52E − 19
^{135}Cs	2.27E − 16	2.57E − 16	2.25E − 16	2.20E − 16	3.62E − 16	2.32E − 16	2.31E − 16	2.68E − 16
^{137}Cs	1.54E − 20	1.88E − 20	1.28E − 20	1.09E − 20	4.43E − 20	1.46E − 20	1.49E − 20	9.12E − 18
^{138}Cs	2.55E − 16	2.87E − 16	2.57E − 16	2.55E − 16	3.70E − 16	2.63E − 16	2.62E − 16	3.81E − 16
^{137m}Ba	6.13E − 17	6.99E − 17	6.09E − 17	5.91E − 17	1.01E − 16	6.26E − 17	6.26E − 17	7.65E − 17
^{139}Ba	4.66E − 18	5.38E − 18	4.43E − 18	4.05E − 18	1.16E − 17	4.65E − 18	4.73E − 18	6.85E − 17
^{140}Ba	1.83E − 17	2.10E − 17	1.80E − 17	1.72E − 17	3.40E − 17	1.86E − 17	1.87E − 17	3.79E − 17
^{141}Ba	8.85E − 17	1.01E − 16	8.76E − 17	8.48E − 17	1.57E − 16	9.02E − 17	9.05E − 17	1.66E − 16
^{142}Ba	1.10E − 16	1.25E − 16	1.09E − 16	1.06E − 16	1.77E − 16	1.12E − 16	1.12E − 16	1.54E − 16
^{140}La	2.47E − 16	2.80E − 16	2.50E − 16	2.47E − 16	3.67E − 16	2.55E − 16	2.54E − 16	3.22E − 16
^{141}La	4.99E − 18	5.66E − 18	5.01E − 18	4.95E − 18	7.46E − 18	5.13E − 18	5.12E − 18	7.31E − 17
^{142}La	3.03E − 16	3.40E − 16	3.08E − 16	3.07E − 16	4.25E − 16	3.14E − 16	3.12E − 16	4.06E − 16
^{141}Ce	7.52E − 18	8.77E − 18	7.01E − 18	6.23E − 18	2.10E − 17	7.45E − 18	7.62E − 18	1.55E − 17
^{143}Ce	2.80E − 17	3.22E − 17	2.68E − 17	2.54E − 17	5.56E − 17	2.81E − 17	2.83E − 17	5.93E − 17
^{144}Ce	1.92E − 18	2.27E − 18	1.71E − 18	1.48E − 18	5.59E − 18	1.86E − 18	1.91E − 18	4.35E − 18
^{143}Pr	4.12E − 20	4.95E − 20	3.55E − 20	3.08E − 20	1.15E − 19	3.95E − 20	4.04E − 20	1.87E − 17
^{144m}Pr	7.53E − 19	9.78E − 19	4.58E − 19	3.56E − 19	1.89E − 18	6.49E − 19	6.45E − 19	1.16E − 18
^{145}Pr	4.04E − 18	4.58E − 18	4.05E − 18	3.98E − 18	6.34E − 18	4.15E − 18	4.15E − 18	9.23E − 17
^{147}Nd	1.35E − 17	1.57E − 17	1.28E − 17	1.18E − 17	2.93E − 17	1.35E − 17	1.36E − 17	2.92E − 17
^{147}Pm	1.52E − 21	1.94E − 21	1.10E − 21	9.01E − 22	4.41E − 21	1.37E − 21	1.40E − 21	8.52E − 19
^{148m}Pm	2.06E − 16	2.35E − 16	2.04E − 16	1.98E − 16	3.46E − 16	2.10E − 16	2.10E − 16	2.50E − 16
^{148}Pm	6.10E − 17	6.92E − 17	6.12E − 17	6.03E − 17	9.23E − 17	6.26E − 17	6.26E − 17	1.21E − 16
^{149}Pm	1.15E − 18	1.32E − 18	1.12E − 18	1.06E − 18	2.39E − 18	1.16E − 18	1.17E − 18	2.39E − 17
^{151}Pm	3.25E − 17	3.73E − 17	3.15E − 17	2.98E − 17	6.59E − 17	3.27E − 17	3.30E − 17	5.51E − 17
^{151}Sm	1.22E − 22	2.07E − 22	1.66E − 23	2.67E − 23	1.67E − 22	8.42E − 23	8.50E − 23	4.29E − 22
^{153}Sm	5.31E − 18	6.43E − 18	4.42E − 18	3.62E − 18	1.65E − 17	5.02E − 18	5.15E − 18	1.90E − 17
^{152}Eu	1.20E − 16	1.37E − 16	1.19E − 16	1.16E − 16	1.94E − 16	1.23E − 16	1.23E − 16	1.45E − 16
^{154}Eu	1.30E − 16	1.48E − 16	1.30E − 16	1.27E − 16	2.06E − 16	1.34E − 16	1.33E − 16	1.66E − 16
^{155}Eu	5.63E − 18	6.70E − 18	4.98E − 18	4.13E − 18	1.83E − 17	5.43E − 18	5.61E − 18	7.32E − 18
^{156}Eu	1.42E − 16	1.61E − 16	1.44E − 16	1.42E − 16	2.08E − 16	1.47E − 16	1.46E − 16	1.90E − 16
^{160}Tb	1.18E − 16	1.34E − 16	1.17E − 16	1.15E − 16	1.88E − 16	1.21E − 16	1.20E − 16	1.48E − 16
^{166m}Ho	1.80E − 16	2.06E − 16	1.78E − 16	1.72E − 16	3.15E − 16	1.84E − 16	1.84E − 16	2.14E − 16
^{181}W	3.34E − 18	4.07E − 18	2.71E − 18	2.07E − 18	1.14E − 17	3.10E − 18	3.22E − 18	4.27E − 18

(continued)

Table 13.30.2 Dose Coefficient for Immersion in Contaminated Water (Sv s^{-1} Bq^{-1}) (Continued)

Nuclide	Gonads	Breast	Lung	R Marrow	Endosteal	Thyroid	Heff	Skin
^{185}W	1.15E − 20	1.40E − 20	9.52E − 21	7.88E − 21	3.53E − 20	1.08E − 20	1.11E − 20	4.76E − 18
^{187}W	4.88E − 17	5.58E − 17	4.80E − 17	4.60E − 17	8.79E − 17	4.95E − 17	4.97E − 17	7.31E − 17
^{207}Tl	3.34E − 19	3.85E − 19	3.22E − 19	3.08E − 19	6.27E − 19	3.37E − 19	3.38E − 19	3.27E − 17
^{208}Tl	3.73E − 16	4.17E − 16	3.79E − 16	3.78E − 16	5.27E − 16	3.87E − 16	3.84E − 16	4.66E − 16
^{209}Tl	2.16E − 16	2.45E − 16	2.17E − 16	2.14E − 16	3.39E − 16	2.22E − 16	2.22E − 16	2.97E − 16
^{209}Pb	1.62E − 20	1.98E − 20	1.34E − 20	1.13E − 20	4.71E − 20	1.53E − 20	1.57E − 20	9.88E − 18
^{210}Pb	1.44E − 19	1.91E − 19	9.78E − 20	7.22E − 20	4.50E − 19	1.26E − 19	1.31E − 19	3.00E − 19
^{211}Pb	5.30E − 18	6.05E − 18	5.24E − 18	5.07E − 18	9.14E − 18	5.40E − 18	5.41E − 18	3.56E − 17
^{212}Pb	1.49E − 17	1.72E − 17	1.42E − 17	1.30E − 17	3.73E − 17	1.49E − 17	1.52E − 17	2.35E − 17
^{214}Pb	2.54E − 17	2.91E − 17	2.47E − 17	2.32E − 17	5.38E − 17	2.56E − 17	2.59E − 17	4.49E − 17
^{210}Bi	6.41E − 20	7.65E − 20	5.64E − 20	4.95E − 20	1.74E − 19	6.19E − 20	6.33E − 20	2.44E − 17
^{211}Bi	4.75E − 18	5.45E − 18	4.64E − 18	4.39E − 18	9.79E − 18	4.80E − 18	4.85E − 18	6.17E − 18
^{212}Bi	1.95E − 17	2.22E − 17	1.96E − 17	1.92E − 17	3.02E − 17	2.00E − 17	2.00E − 17	5.47E − 17
^{213}Bi	1.36E − 17	1.56E − 17	1.34E − 17	1.28E − 17	2.57E − 17	1.38E − 17	1.39E − 17	4.43E − 17
^{214}Bi	1.61E − 16	1.83E − 16	1.63E − 16	1.61E − 16	2.38E − 16	1.66E − 16	1.66E − 16	2.32E − 16
^{210}Po	8.86E − 22	1.01E − 21	8.80E − 22	8.61E − 22	1.39E − 21	9.06E − 22	9.03E − 22	1.04E − 21
^{211}Po	8.10E − 19	9.22E − 19	8.05E − 19	7.85E − 19	1.30E − 18	8.28E − 19	8.27E − 19	9.59E − 19
^{212}Po	0.00E + 00	0.00E + 00	0.00E + 00	0.00E + 00	0.00E + 00	0.00E + 00	0.00E + 00	0.00E + 00
^{213}Po	0.00E + 00	0.00E + 00	0.00E + 00	0.00E + 00	0.00E + 00	0.00E + 00	0.00E + 00	0.00E + 00
^{214}Po	8.68E − 21	9.86E − 21	8.63E − 21	8.43E − 21	1.37E − 20	8.88E − 21	8.85E − 21	1.02E − 20
^{216}Po	1.76E − 21	2.00E − 21	1.75E − 21	1.71E − 21	2.77E − 21	1.81E − 21	1.80E − 21	2.07E − 21
^{218}Po	9.52E − 22	1.08E − 21	9.47E − 22	9.27E − 22	1.49E − 21	9.75E − 22	9.71E − 22	1.37E − 21
^{217}At	3.15E − 20	3.61E − 20	3.11E − 20	2.98E − 20	5.87E − 20	3.20E − 20	3.22E − 20	3.89E − 20
^{218}At	2.92E − 19	3.71E − 19	2.21E − 19	1.66E − 19	9.71E − 19	2.64E − 19	2.75E − 19	4.94E − 19
^{219}Rn	5.73E − 18	6.57E − 18	5.60E − 18	5.29E − 18	1.20E − 17	5.79E − 18	5.85E − 18	7.10E − 18
^{220}Rn	3.94E − 20	4.51E − 20	3.91E − 20	3.78E − 20	6.86E − 20	4.02E − 20	4.03E − 20	4.73E − 20
^{222}Rn	4.07E − 20	4.66E − 20	4.03E − 20	3.88E − 20	7.25E − 20	4.14E − 20	4.16E − 20	4.90E − 20
^{221}Fr	3.16E − 18	3.62E − 18	3.03E − 18	2.79E − 18	7.73E − 18	3.16E − 18	3.22E − 18	4.09E − 18
^{223}Fr	5.16E − 18	6.12E − 18	4.59E − 18	3.98E − 18	1.41E − 17	4.99E − 18	5.11E − 18	2.78E − 17
^{223}Ra	1.32E − 17	1.53E − 17	1.26E − 17	1.13E − 17	3.43E − 17	1.32E − 17	1.35E − 17	1.77E − 17
^{224}Ra	1.01E − 18	1.16E − 18	9.79E − 19	9.11E − 19	2.36E − 18	1.02E − 18	1.03E − 18	1.30E − 18
^{225}Ra	7.57E − 19	9.94E − 19	4.54E − 19	3.28E − 19	2.13E − 18	6.46E − 19	6.49E − 19	3.83E − 18
^{226}Ra	6.82E − 19	7.86E − 19	6.50E − 19	5.92E − 19	1.77E − 18	6.81E − 19	6.95E − 19	9.31E − 19
^{228}Ra	0.00E + 00	0.00E + 00	0.00E + 00	0.00E + 00	0.00E + 00	0.00E + 00	0.00E + 00	0.00E + 00
^{225}Ac	1.58E − 18	1.86E − 18	1.47E − 18	1.29E − 18	4.63E − 18	1.56E − 18	1.61E − 18	2.05E − 18
^{227}Ac	1.30E − 20	1.57E − 20	1.16E − 20	1.02E − 20	3.77E − 20	1.25E − 20	1.30E − 20	2.23E − 20
^{228}Ac	1.01E − 16	1.15E − 16	1.01E − 16	9.89E − 17	1.61E − 16	1.04E − 16	1.04E − 16	1.44E − 16
^{227}Th	1.06E − 17	1.22E − 17	1.01E − 17	9.34E − 18	2.49E − 17	1.06E − 17	1.07E − 17	1.36E − 17
^{228}Th	2.04E − 19	2.45E − 19	1.85E − 19	1.62E − 19	5.92E − 19	1.98E − 19	2.05E − 19	3.18E − 19
^{229}Th	8.46E − 18	9.95E − 18	7.78E − 18	6.71E − 18	2.58E − 17	8.28E − 18	8.56E − 18	1.14E − 17
^{230}Th	4.09E − 20	5.43E − 20	3.20E − 20	2.73E − 20	1.20E − 19	3.68E − 20	3.94E − 20	1.01E − 19
^{231}Th	1.22E − 18	1.55E − 18	9.75E − 19	8.28E − 19	3.69E − 18	1.13E − 18	1.18E − 18	3.79E − 18
^{232}Th	2.14E − 20	3.13E − 20	1.44E − 20	1.24E − 20	5.90E − 20	1.80E − 20	1.99E − 20	7.65E − 20
^{234}Th	7.65E − 19	9.16E − 19	6.76E − 19	5.58E − 19	2.53E − 18	7.34E − 19	7.64E − 19	1.33E − 18
^{231}Pa	3.75E − 18	4.39E − 18	3.54E − 18	3.33E − 18	8.06E − 18	3.73E − 18	3.78E − 18	5.18E − 18
^{233}Pa	2.01E − 17	2.32E − 17	1.95E − 17	1.81E − 17	4.61E − 17	2.02E − 17	2.05E − 17	3.01E − 17

Table 13.30.2 Dose Coefficient for Immersion in Contaminated Water (Sv s^{-1} Bq^{-1}) (Continued)

Nuclide	Gonads	Breast	Lung	R Marrow	Endosteal	Thyroid	Heff	Skin
^{234m}Pa	1.49E − 18	1.71E − 18	1.47E − 18	1.42E − 18	2.61E − 18	1.52E − 18	1.52E − 18	5.92E − 17
^{234}Pa	1.99E − 16	2.26E − 16	1.97E − 16	1.92E − 16	3.29E − 16	2.03E − 16	2.03E − 16	2.51E − 16
^{232}U	3.55E − 20	5.33E − 20	2.20E − 20	2.02E − 20	8.77E − 20	2.93E − 20	3.22E − 20	1.31E − 19
^{233}U	3.79E − 20	5.02E − 20	2.98E − 20	2.73E − 20	9.26E − 20	3.46E − 20	3.64E − 20	9.56E − 20
^{234}U	2.03E − 20	3.35E − 20	9.87E − 21	9.50E − 21	4.54E − 20	1.53E − 20	1.75E − 20	9.55E − 20
^{235}U	1.56E − 17	1.80E − 17	1.49E − 17	1.35E − 17	4.08E − 17	1.56E − 17	1.59E − 17	1.89E − 17
^{236}U	1.42E − 20	2.56E − 20	4.94E − 21	5.30E − 21	2.72E − 20	9.67E − 21	1.16E − 20	8.19E − 20
^{238}U	1.03E − 20	2.00E − 20	2.29E − 21	2.88E − 21	1.72E − 20	6.34E − 21	7.95E − 21	6.83E − 20
^{240}U	1.14E − 19	1.88E − 19	4.20E − 20	3.91E − 20	2.41E − 19	8.35E − 20	9.11E − 20	3.52E − 18
^{237}Np	2.35E − 18	2.86E − 18	2.02E − 18	1.71E − 18	7.20E − 18	2.24E − 18	2.32E − 18	3.43E − 18
^{239}Np	1.67E − 17	1.94E − 17	1.58E − 17	1.43E − 17	4.45E − 17	1.66E − 17	1.70E − 17	2.75E − 17
^{240m}Np	3.44E − 17	3.92E − 17	3.41E − 17	3.32E − 17	5.71E − 17	3.51E − 17	3.51E − 17	8.38E − 17
^{238}Pu	1.53E − 20	2.99E − 20	2.43E − 21	3.89E − 21	2.16E − 20	9.36E − 21	1.14E − 20	9.55E − 20
^{239}Pu	1.10E − 20	1.74E − 20	5.88E − 21	5.94E − 21	2.15E − 20	8.75E − 21	9.60E − 21	4.26E − 20
^{240}Pu	1.49E − 20	2.88E − 20	2.49E − 21	3.82E − 21	2.15E − 20	9.15E − 21	1.11E − 20	9.13E − 20
^{241}Pu	1.62E − 22	1.96E − 22	1.44E − 22	1.25E − 22	4.92E − 22	1.56E − 22	1.62E − 22	2.50E − 22
^{242}Pu	1.25E − 20	2.41E − 20	2.21E − 21	3.30E − 21	1.83E − 20	7.74E − 21	9.35E − 21	7.60E − 20
^{243}Pu	2.30E − 18	2.73E − 18	2.07E − 18	1.75E − 18	7.27E − 18	2.23E − 18	2.31E − 18	1.01E − 17
^{244}Pu	9.63E − 21	1.93E − 20	9.83E − 22	2.06E − 21	1.24E − 20	5.61E − 21	6.96E − 21	6.32E − 20
^{241}Am	1.98E − 18	2.48E − 18	1.53E − 18	1.18E − 18	6.55E − 18	1.80E − 18	1.88E − 18	2.98E − 18
^{242}Am	1.37E − 18	1.64E − 18	1.23E − 18	1.06E − 18	4.21E − 18	1.33E − 18	1.38E − 18	9.65E − 18
^{243}Am	5.00E − 18	5.97E − 18	4.33E − 18	3.48E − 18	1.69E − 17	4.74E − 18	4.94E − 18	6.31E − 18
^{242}Cm	1.83E − 20	3.47E − 20	2.59E − 21	4.38E − 21	2.48E − 20	1.15E − 20	1.33E − 20	1.00E − 19
^{243}Cm	1.28E − 17	1.48E − 17	1.21E − 17	1.10E − 17	3.35E − 17	1.27E − 17	1.30E − 17	1.85E − 17
^{244}Cm	1.62E − 20	3.12E − 20	1.65E − 21	3.41E − 21	2.07E − 20	9.83E − 21	1.15E − 20	9.19E − 20
^{245}Cm	8.69E − 18	1.02E − 17	8.08E − 18	7.02E − 18	2.64E − 17	8.57E − 18	8.84E − 18	1.14E − 17
^{247}Cm	3.20E − 17	3.67E − 17	3.15E − 17	3.00E − 17	6.23E − 17	3.24E − 17	3.27E − 17	3.86E − 17
^{248}Cm	1.11E − 20	2.14E − 20	1.21E − 21	2.38E − 21	1.44E − 20	6.80E − 21	7.96E − 21	6.28E − 20
^{252}Cf	1.60E − 20	2.83E − 20	3.24E − 21	4.40E − 21	2.41E − 20	1.08E − 20	1.18E − 20	7.11E − 20

Table 13.30.3 Dose Coefficient for Exposure to Contaminated Ground Surface ($Sv\ s^{-1}\ Bq^{-1}\ m^{3}$) (After Federal Guidance Report No. 12)

Nuclide	Gonads	Breast	Lung	R Marrow	Endosteal	Thyroid	Heff	Skin
^{3}H	0.00E + 00	0.00E + 00	0.00E + 00	0.00E + 00	0.00E + 00	0.00E + 00	0.00E + 00	0.00E + 00
^{10}Be	4.78E − 19	4.99E − 19	3.22E − 19	2.86E − 19	1.19E − 18	3.63E − 19	4.12E − 19	3.06E − 16
^{11}C	1.06E − 15	1.02E − 15	9.66E − 16	9.75E − 16	1.47E − 15	1.01E − 15	1.01E − 15	4.15E − 15
^{14}C	2.22E − 20	2.52E − 20	8.65E − 21	7.25E − 21	4.63E − 20	1.25E − 20	1.61E − 20	7.46E − 20
^{22}Na	2.20E − 15	2.10E − 15	2.02E − 15	2.06E − 15	2.90E − 15	2.05E − 15	2.10E − 15	2.60E − 15
^{24}Na	3.73E − 15	3.55E − 15	3.49E − 15	3.60E − 15	4.61E − 15	3.29E − 15	3.61E − 15	1.03E − 14
^{32}P	3.18E − 18	3.19E − 18	2.54E − 18	2.40E − 18	6.90E − 18	2.71E − 18	2.91E − 18	8.26E − 15
^{37}Ar	0.00E + 00	0.00E + 00	0.00E + 00	0.00E + 00	0.00E + 00	0.00E + 00	0.00E + 00	0.00E + 00
^{39}Ar	3.94E − 19	4.12E − 19	2.63E − 19	2.32E − 19	9.82E − 19	2.97E − 19	3.38E − 19	2.24E − 16
^{41}Ar	1.25E − 15	1.19E − 15	1.16E − 15	1.20E − 15	1.59E − 15	1.15E − 15	1.20E − 15	6.04E − 15
^{41}Ca	0.00E + 00	0.00E + 00	0.00E + 00	0.00E + 00	0.00E + 00	0.00E + 00	0.00E + 00	0.00E + 00
^{45}Ca	5.93E − 20	6.50E − 20	2.96E − 20	2.48E − 20	1.40E − 19	3.78E − 20	4.61E − 20	1.61E − 19
^{46}Sc	2.01E − 15	1.92E − 15	1.85E − 15	1.90E − 15	2.59E − 15	1.89E − 15	1.93E − 15	2.28E − 15
^{51}Cr	3.23E − 17	3.13E − 17	2.94E − 17	2.96E − 17	5.02E − 17	3.01E − 17	3.08E − 17	3.68E − 17
^{54}Mn	8.50E − 16	8.12E − 16	7.77E − 16	7.96E − 16	1.11E − 15	8.07E − 16	8.12E − 16	9.65E − 16
^{56}Mn	1.64E − 15	1.57E − 15	1.52E − 15	1.56E − 15	2.10E − 15	1.50E − 15	1.58E − 15	1.02E − 14
^{55}Fe	0.00E + 00	0.00E + 00	0.00E + 00	0.00E + 00	0.00E + 00	0.00E + 00	0.00E + 00	0.00E + 00
^{59}Fe	1.17E − 15	1.12E − 15	1.08E − 15	1.11E − 15	1.50E − 15	1.08E − 15	1.12E − 15	1.34E − 15
^{57}Co	1.17E − 16	1.14E − 16	1.08E − 16	1.04E − 16	2.95E − 16	1.10E − 16	1.15E − 16	1.38E − 16
^{60}Co	2.45E − 15	2.34E − 15	2.27E − 15	2.33E − 15	3.11E − 15	2.25E − 15	2.35E − 15	2.76E − 15
^{59}Ni	0.00E + 00	0.00E + 00	0.00E + 00	0.00E + 00	0.00E + 00	0.00E + 00	0.00E + 00	0.00E + 00
^{63}Ni	0.00E + 00	0.00E + 00	0.00E + 00	0.00E + 00	0.00E + 00	0.00E + 00	0.00E + 00	0.00E + 00
^{65}Ni	5.35E − 16	5.11E − 16	4.97E − 16	5.11E − 16	6.83E − 16	4.87E − 16	5.15E − 16	7.23E − 15
^{64}Cu	1.97E − 16	1.89E − 16	1.79E − 16	1.81E − 16	2.72E − 16	1.87E − 16	1.87E − 16	3.93E − 16
^{65}Zn	5.78E − 16	5.51E − 16	5.31E − 16	5.47E − 16	7.39E − 16	5.38E − 16	5.53E − 16	6.52E − 16
^{69}Zn	8.12E − 19	8.36E − 19	5.88E − 19	5.35E − 19	1.95E − 18	6.46E − 19	7.18E − 19	2.02E − 15
^{79}Se	2.83E − 20	3.18E − 20	1.15E − 20	9.59E − 21	6.04E − 20	1.62E − 20	2.07E − 20	9.10E − 20
^{82}Br	2.67E − 15	2.55E − 15	2.45E − 15	2.50E − 15	3.15E − 15	2.51E − 15	2.55E − 15	3.05E − 15
^{83}Br	8.61E − 18	8.31E − 18	7.69E − 18	7.71E − 18	1.27E − 17	8.07E − 18	8.13E − 18	2.09E − 15
^{84}Br	1.66E − 15	1.58E − 15	1.54E − 15	1.59E − 15	2.08E − 15	1.49E − 15	1.60E − 15	1.28E − 14
^{83m}Kr	6.16E − 19	1.05E − 18	1.40E − 20	6.21E − 20	3.80E − 19	8.51E − 20	3.80E − 19	1.29E − 17
^{85m}Kr	1.57E − 16	1.53E − 16	1.44E − 16	1.42E − 16	3.20E − 16	1.45E − 16	1.52E − 16	1.36E − 15
^{85}Kr	2.82E − 18	2.74E − 18	2.45E − 18	2.43E − 18	4.47E − 18	2.59E − 18	2.64E − 18	8.00E − 16
^{87}Kr	7.61E − 16	7.27E − 16	7.06E − 16	7.22E − 16	9.99E − 16	6.86E − 16	7.32E − 16	1.35E − 14
^{88}Kr	1.80E − 15	1.72E − 15	1.69E − 15	1.73E − 15	2.28E − 15	1.59E − 15	1.74E − 15	4.43E − 15
^{86}Rb	9.74E − 17	9.30E − 17	8.92E − 17	9.15E − 17	1.27E − 16	9.08E − 17	9.31E − 17	7.72E − 15
^{88}Rb	6.16E − 16	5.89E − 16	5.75E − 16	5.91E − 16	7.85E − 16	5.50E − 16	5.95E − 16	1.67E − 14
^{89}Rb	1.99E − 15	1.90E − 15	1.85E − 15	1.90E − 15	2.52E − 15	1.81E − 15	1.91E − 15	1.21E − 14
^{89}Sr	2.49E − 18	2.51E − 18	1.98E − 18	1.86E − 18	5.43E − 18	2.11E − 18	2.27E − 18	6.66E − 15
^{90}Sr	3.33E − 19	3.50E − 19	2.19E − 19	1.93E − 19	8.31E − 19	2.49E − 19	2.84E − 19	1.40E − 16
^{91}Sr	7.08E − 16	6.76E − 16	6.48E − 16	6.64E − 16	9.25E − 16	6.67E − 16	6.77E − 16	7.53E − 15
^{92}Sr	1.30E − 15	1.24E − 15	1.21E − 15	1.24E − 15	1.64E − 15	1.18E − 15	1.25E − 15	1.86E − 15
^{90}Y	5.75E − 18	5.72E − 18	4.76E − 18	4.57E − 18	1.17E − 17	5.02E − 18	5.32E − 18	1.05E − 14
^{91m}Y	5.50E − 16	5.27E − 16	5.01E − 16	5.07E − 16	7.52E − 16	5.23E − 16	5.23E − 16	9.52E − 16
^{91}Y	6.11E − 18	5.96E − 18	5.31E − 18	5.29E − 18	1.01E − 17	5.44E − 18	5.74E − 18	6.92E − 15
^{92}Y	2.65E − 16	2.53E − 16	2.43E − 16	2.48E − 16	3.50E − 16	2.46E − 16	2.53E − 16	1.39E − 14

Table 13.30.3 Dose Coefficient for Exposure to Contaminated Ground Surface ($Sv\ s^{-1}\ Bq^{-1}\ m^3$) (Continued)

Nuclide	Gonads	Breast	Lung	R Marrow	Endosteal	Thyroid	Heff	Skin
^{93}Y	9.51E − 17	9.14E − 17	8.74E − 17	8.90E − 17	1.33E − 16	8.61E − 17	9.12E − 17	1.23E − 14
^{93}Zr	0.00E + 00	0.00E + 00	0.00E + 00	0.00E + 00	0.00E + 00	0.00E + 00	0.00E + 00	0.00E + 00
^{95}Zr	7.59E − 16	7.25E − 16	6.92E − 16	7.06E − 16	1.00E − 15	7.22E − 16	7.23E − 16	8.91E − 16
^{97}Zr	1.82E − 16	1.74E − 16	1.67E − 16	1.71E − 16	2.43E − 16	1.68E − 16	1.74E − 16	8.27E − 15
^{93m}Nb	1.72E − 18	2.21E − 18	4.95E − 20	2.02E − 19	1.28E − 18	3.36E − 19	9.39E − 19	9.70E − 18
^{95m}Nb	6.81E − 17	6.85E − 17	5.61E − 17	5.67E − 17	1.11E − 16	5.75E − 17	6.26E − 17	1.09E − 16
^{95}Nb	7.85E − 16	7.49E − 16	7.16E − 16	7.32E − 16	1.03E − 15	7.47E − 16	7.48E − 16	9.05E − 16
^{97m}Nb	7.47E − 16	7.14E − 16	6.82E − 16	6.96E − 16	9.85E − 16	7.11E − 16	7.12E − 16	1.08E − 15
^{97}Nb	6.78E − 16	6.49E − 16	6.18E − 16	6.28E − 16	9.06E − 16	6.45E − 16	6.45E − 16	5.56E − 15
^{93}Mo	9.79E − 18	1.26E − 17	2.81E − 19	1.15E − 18	7.29E − 18	1.91E − 18	5.34E − 18	5.51E − 17
^{99}Mo	1.55E − 16	1.49E − 16	1.40E − 16	1.42E − 16	2.21E − 16	1.46E − 16	1.47E − 16	3.76E − 15
^{99m}Tc	1.24E − 16	1.20E − 16	1.13E − 16	1.10E − 16	2.86E − 16	1.14E − 16	1.21E − 16	1.44E − 16
^{99}Tc	9.74E − 20	1.06E − 19	5.29E − 20	4.48E − 20	2.38E − 19	6.52E − 20	7.80E − 20	2.43E − 19
^{101}Tc	3.44E − 16	3.33E − 16	3.13E − 16	3.15E − 16	5.35E − 16	3.21E − 16	3.28E − 16	5.26E − 15
^{103}Ru	4.87E − 16	4.68E − 16	4.43E − 16	4.48E − 16	6.80E − 16	4.63E − 16	4.63E − 16	6.16E − 16
^{105}Ru	8.07E − 16	7.73E − 16	7.36E − 16	7.48E − 16	1.10E − 15	7.66E − 16	7.69E − 16	4.48E − 15
^{106}Ru	0.00E + 00	0.00E + 00	0.00E + 00	0.00E + 00	0.00E + 00	0.00E + 00	0.00E + 00	0.00E + 00
^{103m}Rh	2.18E − 18	2.54E − 18	2.32E − 19	3.38E − 19	2.31E − 18	7.86E − 19	1.25E − 18	6.88E − 18
^{105}Rh	7.98E − 17	7.74E − 17	7.26E − 17	7.30E − 17	1.25E − 16	7.44E − 17	7.62E − 17	1.76E − 16
^{106}Rh	2.23E − 16	2.14E − 16	2.03E − 16	2.05E − 16	3.09E − 16	2.11E − 16	2.12E − 16	1.42E − 14
^{107}Pd	0.00E + 00	0.00E + 00	0.00E + 00	0.00E + 00	0.00E + 00	0.00E + 00	0.00E + 00	0.00E + 00
^{109}Pd	1.58E − 17	1.74E − 17	5.86E − 18	5.82E − 18	2.69E − 17	9.00E − 18	1.12E − 17	2.87E − 15
^{110m}Ag	2.77E − 15	2.65E − 15	2.54E − 15	2.60E − 15	3.62E − 15	2.61E − 15	2.65E − 15	3.22E − 15
^{110}Ag	4.04E − 17	3.89E − 17	3.62E − 17	3.64E − 17	5.92E − 17	3.78E − 17	3.82E − 17	1.27E − 14
^{111}Ag	2.81E − 17	2.72E − 17	2.54E − 17	2.54E − 17	4.43E − 17	2.61E − 17	2.67E − 17	2.75E − 15
^{113m}Cd	3.09E − 19	3.24E − 19	2.02E − 19	1.78E − 19	7.69E − 19	2.30E − 19	2.63E − 19	1.55E − 16
^{115m}Cd	2.45E − 17	2.35E − 17	2.22E − 17	2.26E − 17	3.04E − 17	2.27E − 17	2.34E − 17	7.00E − 15
^{123}Sn	8.85E − 18	8.55E − 18	7.86E − 18	7.94E − 18	1.32E − 17	8.07E − 18	8.37E − 18	5.71E − 15
^{125}Sn	3.14E − 16	3.00E − 16	2.89E − 16	2.96E − 16	4.08E − 16	2.91E − 16	3.01E − 16	9.21E − 15
^{126}Sn	5.99E − 17	6.08E − 17	4.57E − 17	4.06E − 17	1.73E − 16	4.96E − 17	5.47E − 17	8.07E − 17
^{124}Sb	1.78E − 15	1.70E − 15	1.65E − 15	1.69E − 15	2.30E − 15	1.63E − 15	1.71E − 15	5.20E − 15
^{125}Sb	4.53E − 16	4.38E − 16	4.00E − 16	4.02E − 16	6.50E − 16	4.22E − 16	4.25E − 16	5.97E − 16
^{126m}Sb	1.60E − 15	1.53E − 15	1.46E − 15	1.48E − 15	2.18E − 15	1.52E − 15	1.52E − 15	8.61E − 15
^{126}Sb	2.92E − 15	2.79E − 15	2.66E − 15	2.71E − 15	3.92E − 15	2.77E − 15	2.78E − 15	5.33E − 15
^{127}Sb	7.10E − 16	6.81E − 16	6.47E − 16	6.56E − 16	9.73E − 16	6.74E − 16	6.76E − 16	2.85E − 15
^{125m}Te	5.24E − 17	5.76E − 17	1.78E − 17	1.36E − 17	1.01E − 16	3.10E − 17	3.61E − 17	9.45E − 17
^{127m}Te	1.63E − 17	1.79E − 17	5.57E − 18	4.34E − 18	3.13E − 17	9.66E − 18	1.13E − 17	5.20E − 17
^{127}Te	5.48E − 18	5.33E − 18	4.88E − 18	4.87E − 18	8.57E − 18	5.09E − 18	5.18E − 18	5.40E − 16
^{129m}Te	4.33E − 17	4.32E − 17	3.22E − 17	3.18E − 17	6.49E − 17	3.66E − 17	3.78E − 17	2.27E − 15
^{129}Te	6.51E − 17	6.36E − 17	5.52E − 17	5.52E − 17	9.63E − 17	5.90E − 17	6.01E − 17	5.74E − 15
^{131m}Te	1.44E − 15	1.38E − 15	1.31E − 15	1.34E − 15	1.94E − 15	1.34E − 15	1.37E − 15	2.20E − 15
^{131}Te	4.29E − 16	4.13E − 16	3.90E − 16	3.92E − 16	6.74E − 16	4.01E − 16	4.10E − 16	8.36E − 15
^{132}Te	2.45E − 16	2.43E − 16	2.06E − 16	2.01E − 16	4.58E − 16	2.15E − 16	2.28E − 16	2.99E − 16
^{133m}Te	2.32E − 15	2.22E − 15	2.13E − 15	2.18E − 15	3.09E − 15	2.17E − 15	2.22E − 15	1.01E − 14
^{133}Te	9.34E − 16	8.96E − 16	8.57E − 16	8.73E − 16	1.29E − 15	8.66E − 16	8.94E − 16	1.01E − 14
^{134}Te	9.12E − 16	8.78E − 16	8.24E − 16	8.32E − 16	1.35E − 15	8.57E − 16	8.67E − 16	2.16E − 15
^{129}I	3.55E − 17	3.84E − 17	1.48E − 17	1.07E − 17	7.91E − 17	2.28E − 17	2.58E − 17	5.80E − 17

(continued)

Table 13.30.3 Dose Coefficient for Exposure to Contaminated Ground Surface ($Sv\ s^{-1}\ Bq^{-1}\ m^3$) (Continued)

Nuclide	Gonads	Breast	Lung	R Marrow	Endosteal	Thyroid	Heff	Skin
^{130}I	2.20E − 15	2.11E − 15	2.01E − 15	2.04E − 15	2.96E − 15	2.09E − 15	2.10E − 15	4.29E − 15
^{131}I	3.94E − 16	3.81E − 16	3.58E − 16	3.60E − 16	5.90E − 16	3.71E − 16	3.76E − 16	6.43E − 16
^{132}I	2.32E − 15	2.22E − 15	2.12E − 15	2.17E − 15	3.06E − 15	2.19E − 15	2.21E − 15	7.54E − 15
^{133}I	6.27E − 16	6.01E − 16	5.72E − 16	5.80E − 16	8.55E − 16	5.94E − 16	5.97E − 16	4.55E − 15
^{134}I	2.64E − 15	2.52E − 15	2.42E − 15	2.48E − 15	3.45E − 15	2.48E − 15	2.53E − 15	9.85E − 15
^{135}I	1.53E − 15	1.46E − 15	1.42E − 15	1.46E − 15	1.95E − 15	1.40E − 15	1.47E − 15	4.83E − 15
^{131m}Xe	2.76E − 17	2.97E − 17	1.25E − 17	9.79E − 18	5.88E − 17	1.83E − 17	2.06E − 17	4.44E − 17
^{133m}Xe	4.89E − 17	5.06E − 17	3.15E − 17	2.87E − 17	9.51E − 17	3.76E − 17	4.07E − 17	6.93E − 17
^{133}Xe	5.20E − 17	5.34E − 17	3.71E − 17	3.12E − 17	1.51E − 16	4.19E − 17	4.61E − 17	6.93E − 17
^{135m}Xe	4.48E − 16	4.30E − 16	4.04E − 16	4.08E − 16	6.23E − 16	4.24E − 16	4.24E − 16	1.41E − 15
^{135}Xe	2.53E − 16	2.47E − 16	2.30E − 16	2.30E − 16	4.23E − 16	2.33E − 16	2.42E − 16	2.09E − 15
^{134m}Cs	3.01E − 17	3.08E − 17	2.06E − 17	1.83E − 17	7.16E − 17	2.40E − 17	2.59E − 17	4.14E − 17
^{134}Cs	1.60E − 15	1.53E − 15	1.46E − 15	1.48E − 15	2.12E − 15	1.52E − 15	1.52E − 15	2.17E − 15
^{135}Cs	4.38E − 20	4.85E − 20	2.02E − 20	1.69E − 20	1.00E − 19	2.68E − 20	3.33E − 20	1.27E − 19
^{136}Cs	2.18E − 15	2.09E − 15	2.00E − 15	2.04E − 15	2.95E − 15	2.05E − 15	2.09E − 15	2.54E − 15
^{137}Cs	3.31E − 19	3.47E − 19	2.22E − 19	1.97E − 19	8.15E − 19	2.51E − 19	2.85E − 19	2.75E − 16
^{138}Cs	2.27E − 15	2.17E − 15	2.11E − 15	2.17E − 15	2.90E − 15	2.06E − 15	2.19E − 15	1.52E − 14
^{137m}Ba	6.17E − 16	5.90E − 16	5.61E − 16	5.70E − 16	8.27E − 16	5.87E − 16	5.86E − 16	1.65E − 15
^{139}Ba	4.79E − 17	4.69E − 17	4.27E − 17	4.17E − 17	9.73E − 17	4.33E − 17	4.59E − 17	1.03E − 14
^{140}Ba	1.91E − 16	1.85E − 16	1.70E − 16	1.71E − 16	2.81E − 16	1.79E − 16	1.80E − 16	1.95E − 15
^{141}Ba	8.52E − 16	8.20E − 16	7.80E − 16	7.91E − 16	1.23E − 15	7.88E − 16	8.15E − 16	1.06E − 14
^{142}Ba	1.05E − 15	1.01E − 15	9.61E − 16	9.80E − 16	1.44E − 15	9.79E − 16	1.01E − 15	4.80E − 15
^{140}La	2.24E − 15	2.14E − 15	2.08E − 15	2.13E − 15	2.89E − 15	2.03E − 15	2.16E − 15	8.24E − 15
^{141}La	4.74E − 17	4.54E − 17	4.35E − 17	4.44E − 17	6.43E − 17	4.27E − 17	4.54E − 17	1.08E − 14
^{142}La	2.54E − 15	2.42E − 15	2.37E − 15	2.44E − 15	3.19E − 15	2.27E − 15	2.46E − 15	1.17E − 14
^{141}Ce	7.71E − 17	7.56E − 17	6.80E − 17	6.48E − 17	1.80E − 16	6.98E − 17	7.38E − 17	1.32E − 16
^{143}Ce	2.98E − 16	2.90E − 16	2.60E − 16	2.56E − 16	4.99E − 16	2.72E − 16	2.79E − 16	3.99E − 15
^{144}Ce	2.17E − 17	2.15E − 17	1.80E − 17	1.64E − 17	5.64E − 17	1.90E − 17	2.03E − 17	2.61E − 17
^{143}Pr	7.93E − 19	8.16E − 19	5.75E − 19	5.23E − 19	1.91E − 18	6.31E − 19	7.01E − 19	2.00E − 15
^{144m}Pr	1.62E − 17	1.69E − 17	9.29E − 18	6.79E − 18	4.36E − 17	1.18E − 17	1.30E − 17	2.67E − 17
^{144}Pr	3.96E − 17	3.81E − 17	3.61E − 17	3.66E − 17	5.65E − 17	3.56E − 17	3.78E − 17	1.27E − 14
^{147}Nd	1.48E − 16	1.45E − 16	1.28E − 16	1.23E − 16	2.90E − 16	1.36E − 16	1.39E − 16	1.10E − 15
^{147}Pm	4.37E − 20	4.79E − 20	2.20E − 20	1.86E − 20	1.02E − 19	2.80E − 20	3.41E − 20	1.20E − 19
^{148m}Pm	2.06E − 15	1.97E − 15	1.88E − 15	1.91E − 15	2.80E − 15	1.95E − 15	1.96E − 15	2.62E − 15
^{148}Pm	5.71E − 16	5.46E − 16	5.27E − 16	5.40E − 16	7.42E − 16	5.26E − 16	5.48E − 16	8.36E − 15
^{149}Pm	1.19E − 17	1.16E − 17	1.07E − 17	1.07E − 17	1.95E − 17	1.10E − 17	1.13E − 17	2.97E − 15
^{151}Pm	3.31E − 16	3.20E − 16	2.97E − 16	2.96E − 16	5.46E − 16	3.08E − 16	3.15E − 16	2.07E − 15
^{151}Sm	8.66E − 21	1.00E − 20	1.01E − 21	1.39E − 21	9.63E − 21	3.33E − 21	5.03E − 21	2.53E − 20
^{153}Sm	6.71E − 17	6.72E − 17	5.37E − 17	4.51E − 17	2.06E − 16	5.73E − 17	6.22E − 17	7.12E − 16
^{152}Eu	1.16E − 15	1.11E − 15	1.05E − 15	1.07E − 15	1.63E − 15	1.07E − 15	1.10E − 15	1.75E − 15
^{154}Eu	1.24E − 15	1.18E − 15	1.14E − 15	1.16E − 15	1.69E − 15	1.15E − 15	1.19E − 15	2.91E − 15
^{155}Eu	6.09E − 17	6.01E − 17	5.34E − 17	4.71E − 17	1.90E − 16	5.48E − 17	5.90E − 17	7.04E − 17
^{156}Eu	1.28E − 15	1.23E − 15	1.19E − 15	1.22E − 15	1.66E − 15	1.17E − 15	1.23E − 15	5.05E − 15
^{160}Tb	1.13E − 15	1.08E − 15	1.03E − 15	1.06E − 15	1.54E − 15	1.05E − 15	1.08E − 15	1.88E − 15
^{166m}Ho	1.78E − 15	1.71E − 15	1.63E − 15	1.65E − 15	2.56E − 15	1.68E − 15	1.70E − 15	2.11E − 15
^{181}W	4.06E − 17	4.06E − 17	3.49E − 17	2.77E − 17	1.51E − 16	3.51E − 17	3.93E − 17	4.79E − 17

Table 13.30.3 Dose Coefficient for Exposure to Contaminated Ground Surface ($Sv\ s^{-1}\ Bq^{-1}\ m^3$) (Continued)

Nuclide	Gonads	Breast	Lung	R Marrow	Endosteal	Thyroid	Heff	Skin
^{185}W	2.12E − 19	2.22E − 19	1.43E − 19	1.25E − 19	5.64E − 19	1.61E − 19	1.84E − 19	1.57E − 18
^{187}W	4.92E − 16	4.73E − 16	4.48E − 16	4.50E − 16	7.40E − 16	4.67E − 16	4.69E − 16	2.03E − 15
^{207}Tl	4.04E − 18	3.96E − 18	3.44E − 18	3.40E − 18	6.99E − 18	3.62E − 18	3.76E − 18	5.21E − 15
^{208}Tl	3.09E − 15	2.94E − 15	2.88E − 15	2.96E − 15	3.90E − 15	2.75E − 15	2.98E − 15	9.77E − 15
^{209}Tl	1.97E − 15	1.88E − 15	1.83E − 15	1.87E − 15	2.69E − 15	1.78E − 15	1.90E − 15	9.87E − 15
^{209}Pb	3.50E − 19	3.67E − 19	2.34E − 19	2.07E − 19	8.69E − 19	2.64E − 19	3.01E − 19	2.94E − 16
^{210}Pb	3.02E − 18	3.59E − 18	1.64E − 18	1.27E − 18	8.31E − 18	1.87E − 18	2.48E − 18	1.98E − 17
^{211}Pb	5.33E − 17	5.12E − 17	4.84E − 17	4.91E − 17	7.54E − 17	5.03E − 17	5.08E − 17	4.64E − 15
^{212}Pb	1.47E − 16	1.44E − 16	1.34E − 16	1.32E − 16	3.01E − 16	1.35E − 16	1.43E − 16	1.88E − 16
^{214}Pb	2.54E − 16	2.47E − 16	2.32E − 16	2.31E − 16	4.24E − 16	2.37E − 16	2.44E − 16	9.10E − 16
^{210}Bi	1.17E − 18	1.20E − 18	8.80E − 19	8.11E − 19	2.74E − 18	9.54E − 19	1.05E − 18	3.42E − 15
^{211}Bi	4.79E − 17	4.64E − 17	4.37E − 17	4.37E − 17	7.64E − 17	4.49E − 17	4.58E − 17	5.55E − 17
^{212}Bi	1.87E − 16	1.79E − 16	1.71E − 16	1.75E − 16	2.46E − 16	1.74E − 16	1.79E − 16	5.35E − 15
^{213}Bi	1.39E − 16	1.34E − 16	1.26E − 16	1.27E − 16	2.06E − 16	1.31E − 16	1.32E − 16	4.23E − 15
^{214}Bi	1.46E − 15	1.40E − 15	1.36E − 15	1.39E − 15	1.88E − 15	1.33E − 15	1.41E − 15	8.48E − 15
^{210}Po	8.69E − 21	8.30E − 21	7.94E − 21	8.12E − 21	1.14E − 20	8.26E − 21	8.29E − 21	1.11E − 20
^{211}Po	7.98E − 18	7.63E − 18	7.29E − 18	7.44E − 18	1.06E − 17	7.57E − 18	7.61E − 18	1.12E − 17
^{212}Po	0.00E + 00	0.00E + 00	0.00E + 00	0.00E + 00	0.00E + 00	0.00E + 00	0.00E + 00	0.00E + 00
^{213}Po	0.00E + 00	0.00E + 00	0.00E + 00	0.00E + 00	0.00E + 00	0.00E + 00	0.00E + 00	0.00E + 00
^{214}Po	8.52E − 20	8.13E − 20	7.78E − 20	7.96E − 20	1.12E − 19	8.10E − 20	8.13E − 20	1.09E − 19
^{216}Po	1.73E − 20	1.65E − 20	1.58E − 20	1.62E − 20	2.27E − 20	1.64E − 20	1.65E − 20	2.20E − 20
^{218}Po	9.31E − 21	8.88E − 21	8.50E − 21	8.70E − 21	1.22E − 20	8.83E − 21	8.88E − 21	1.17E − 20
^{217}At	3.17E − 19	3.05E − 19	2.89E − 19	2.91E − 19	4.70E − 19	3.00E − 19	3.03E − 19	4.11E − 19
^{218}At	4.74E − 18	5.34E − 18	3.17E − 18	2.49E − 18	1.49E − 17	3.36E − 18	4.18E − 18	2.32E − 17
^{219}Rn	5.74E − 17	5.56E − 17	5.23E − 17	5.25E − 17	9.18E − 17	5.37E − 17	5.49E − 17	6.64E − 17
^{220}Rn	4.00E − 19	3.84E − 19	3.65E − 19	3.69E − 19	5.51E − 19	3.81E − 19	3.81E − 19	5.21E − 19
^{222}Rn	4.15E − 19	3.98E − 19	3.78E − 19	3.81E − 19	5.79E − 19	3.95E − 19	3.95E − 19	5.20E − 19
^{221}Fr	3.08E − 17	3.02E − 17	2.81E − 17	2.79E − 17	5.86E − 17	2.82E − 17	2.98E − 17	3.67E − 17
^{223}Fr	6.03E − 17	6.08E − 17	5.00E − 17	4.50E − 17	1.58E − 16	5.16E − 17	5.65E − 17	2.72E − 15
^{223}Ra	1.32E − 16	1.29E − 16	1.20E − 16	1.16E − 16	2.90E − 16	1.22E − 16	1.28E − 16	1.67E − 16
^{224}Ra	9.94E − 18	9.70E − 18	9.07E − 18	9.05E − 18	1.76E − 17	9.13E − 18	9.57E − 18	1.16E − 17
^{225}Ra	1.63E − 17	1.74E − 17	9.40E − 18	6.74E − 18	4.72E − 17	1.15E − 17	1.33E − 17	3.25E − 17
^{226}Ra	6.64E − 18	6.52E − 18	6.06E − 18	5.95E − 18	1.36E − 17	6.06E − 18	6.44E − 18	8.12E − 18
^{228}Ra	0.00E + 00	0.00E + 00	0.00E + 00	0.00E + 00	0.00E + 00	0.00E + 00	0.00E + 00	0.00E + 00
^{225}Ac	1.66E − 17	1.67E − 17	1.42E − 17	1.36E − 17	4.08E − 17	1.45E − 17	1.58E − 17	3.08E − 17
^{227}Ac	1.89E − 19	2.12E − 19	1.14E − 19	1.13E − 19	3.71E − 19	1.25E − 19	1.57E − 19	7.43E − 19
^{228}Ac	9.71E − 16	9.30E − 16	8.88E − 16	9.08E − 16	1.30E − 15	9.03E − 16	9.28E − 16	4.75E − 15
^{227}Th	1.09E − 16	1.08E − 16	9.60E − 17	9.46E − 17	2.03E − 16	9.78E − 17	1.04E − 16	1.56E − 16
^{228}Th	2.71E − 18	2.99E − 18	1.81E − 18	1.77E − 18	5.67E − 18	1.92E − 18	2.35E − 18	9.74E − 18
^{229}Th	8.95E − 17	9.03E − 17	7.64E − 17	7.18E − 17	2.34E − 16	7.79E − 17	8.54E − 17	1.57E − 16
^{230}Th	1.05E − 18	1.33E − 18	3.52E − 19	3.74E − 19	1.65E − 18	4.46E − 19	7.50E − 19	7.17E − 18
^{231}Th	2.42E − 17	2.75E − 17	1.12E − 17	1.08E − 17	4.78E − 17	1.41E − 17	1.85E − 17	8.58E − 17
^{232}Th	8.47E − 19	1.12E − 18	1.74E − 19	2.09E − 19	1.06E − 18	2.68E − 19	5.51E − 19	6.86E − 18
^{234}Th	8.90E − 18	9.15E − 18	7.11E − 18	6.40E − 18	2.63E − 17	7.34E − 18	8.32E − 18	1.72E − 17
^{231}Pa	4.65E − 17	4.83E − 17	3.41E − 17	3.44E − 17	7.16E − 17	3.69E − 17	4.07E − 17	1.07E − 16
^{233}Pa	2.05E − 16	2.01E − 16	1.83E − 16	1.82E − 16	3.66E − 16	1.88E − 16	1.95E − 16	2.70E − 16

(continued)

Table 13.30.3 Dose Coefficient for Exposure to Contaminated Ground Surface ($Sv\ s^{-1}\ Bq^{-1}\ m^3$) (Continued)

Nuclide	Gonads	Breast	Lung	R Marrow	Endosteal	Thyroid	Heff	Skin
^{234m}Pa	1.61E − 17	1.56E − 17	1.43E − 17	1.44E − 17	2.52E − 17	1.47E − 17	1.53E − 17	9.39E − 15
^{234}Pa	1.93E − 15	1.85E − 15	1.76E − 15	1.79E − 15	2.68E − 15	1.80E − 15	1.84E − 15	3.89E − 15
^{232}U	1.62E − 18	2.09E − 18	2.71E − 19	3.61E − 19	1.78E − 18	4.89E − 19	1.01E − 18	1.10E − 17
^{233}U	1.04E − 18	1.28E − 18	3.20E − 19	3.61E − 19	1.33E − 18	4.42E − 19	7.16E − 19	5.94E − 18
^{234}U	1.25E − 18	1.64E − 18	1.40E − 19	2.21E − 19	1.22E − 18	3.21E − 19	7.48E − 19	9.09E − 18
^{235}U	1.53E − 16	1.51E − 16	1.38E − 16	1.36E − 16	3.14E − 16	1.39E − 16	1.48E − 16	1.94E − 16
^{236}U	1.12E − 18	1.49E − 18	8.56E − 20	1.67E − 19	9.84E − 19	2.54E − 19	6.50E − 19	8.45E − 18
^{238}U	9.65E − 19	1.29E − 18	5.59E − 20	1.28E − 19	8.09E − 19	2.04E − 19	5.51E − 19	7.42E − 18
^{240}U	7.02E − 18	8.73E − 18	9.78E − 19	1.26E − 18	8.22E − 18	2.21E − 18	4.23E − 18	3.74E − 17
^{237}Np	3.38E − 17	3.61E − 17	2.18E − 17	2.02E − 17	7.96E − 17	2.45E − 17	2.87E − 17	8.36E − 17
^{239}Np	1.71E − 16	1.69E − 16	1.50E − 16	1.46E − 16	3.65E − 16	1.53E − 16	1.63E − 16	2.63E − 16
^{240m}Np	3.46E − 16	3.34E − 16	3.10E − 16	3.16E − 16	4.66E − 16	3.21E − 16	3.27E − 16	7.44E − 15
^{238}Pu	1.49E − 18	1.93E − 18	7.87E − 20	1.94E − 19	1.22E − 18	3.40E − 19	8.38E − 19	9.64E − 18
^{239}Pu	6.14E − 19	7.77E − 19	7.87E − 20	1.20E − 19	5.81E − 19	1.78E − 19	3.67E − 19	3.67E − 18
^{240}Pu	1.43E − 18	1.85E − 18	7.81E − 20	1.87E − 19	1.18E − 18	3.28E − 19	8.03E − 19	9.18E − 18
^{241}Pu	2.31E − 21	2.51E − 21	1.42E − 21	1.39E − 21	4.81E − 21	1.57E − 21	1.93E − 21	7.06E − 21
^{242}Pu	1.18E − 18	1.53E − 18	6.60E − 20	1.57E − 19	9.84E − 19	2.73E − 19	6.67E − 19	7.61E − 18
^{243}Pu	2.53E − 17	2.55E − 17	2.13E − 17	1.95E − 17	7.24E − 17	2.19E − 17	2.41E − 17	1.18E − 16
^{244}Pu	9.98E − 19	1.30E − 18	4.65E − 20	1.25E − 19	8.05E − 19	2.23E − 19	5.58E − 19	6.49E − 18
^{241}Am	3.25E − 17	3.52E − 17	2.01E − 17	1.68E − 17	9.30E − 17	2.21E − 17	2.75E − 17	8.32E − 17
^{242}Am	1.82E − 17	1.91E − 17	1.22E − 17	1.18E − 17	4.08E − 17	1.35E − 17	1.57E − 17	2.55E − 16
^{243}Am	5.49E − 17	5.54E − 17	4.76E − 17	4.13E − 17	1.86E − 16	4.78E − 17	5.35E − 17	7.60E − 17
^{242}Cm	1.70E − 18	2.14E − 18	1.05E − 19	2.28E − 19	1.47E − 18	4.38E − 19	9.56E − 19	9.38E − 18
^{243}Cm	1.32E − 16	1.31E − 16	1.14E − 16	1.12E − 16	2.73E − 16	1.17E − 16	1.25E − 16	1.90E − 16
^{244}Cm	1.57E − 18	1.98E − 18	9.00E − 20	2.04E − 19	1.34E − 18	3.98E − 19	8.78E − 19	8.70E − 18
^{245}Cm	9.21E − 17	9.22E − 17	7.73E − 17	7.38E − 17	2.29E − 16	7.99E − 17	8,70E − 17	1.46E − 16
^{247}Cm	3.26E − 16	3.15E − 16	2.96E − 16	2.97E − 16	4.86E − 16	3.07E − 16	3.10E − 16	3.79E − 16
^{248}Cm	1.07E − 18	1.35E − 18	6.26E − 20	1.40E − 19	9.18E − 19	2.73E − 19	6.00E − 19	5.92E − 18
^{252}Cf	1.26E − 18	1.54E − 18	1.12E − 19	1.88E − 19	1.21E − 18	3.86E − 19	7.22E − 19	5.75E − 18

Table 13.30.4 Dose Coefficient for Exposure to Contaminated Soil (Sv Bq^{-1} s^{-1} m^3)[a] (After Federal Guidance Report No. 12)

Nuclide	Gonads	Breast	Lung	R Marrow	Endosteal	Thyroid	Heff	Skin
^{3}H	0.00E + 00	0.00E + 00	0.00E + 00	0.00E + 00	0.00E + 00	0.00E + 00	0.00E + 00	0.00E + 00
^{10}Be	6.12E − 21	6.45E − 21	5.17E − 21	4.63E − 21	1.60E − 20	4.90E − 21	5.76E − 21	3.17E − 20
^{11}C	3.40E − 17	3.48E − 17	3.04E − 17	3.00E − 17	5.15E − 17	2.83E − 17	3.21E − 17	3.80E − 17
^{14}C	8.60E − 23	9.61E − 23	5.41E − 23	4.28E − 23	2.34E − 22	5.64E − 23	7.20E − 23	1.27E − 22
^{22}Na	7.69E − 17	7.84E − 17	7.00E − 17	6.98E − 17	1.07E − 16	6.54E − 17	7.32E − 17	8.41E − 17
^{24}Na	1.59E − 16	1.59E − 16	1.47E − 16	1.49E − 16	1.97E − 16	1.40E − 16	1.52E − 16	1.73E − 16
^{32}P	6.64E − 20	6.90E − 20	5.85E − 20	5.53E − 20	1.40E − 19	5.48E − 20	6.31E − 20	5.20E − 18
^{37}Ar	0.00E + 00	0.00E + 00	0.00E + 00	0.00E + 00	0.00E + 00	0.00E + 00	0.00E + 00	0.00E + 00
^{39}Ar	4.92E − 21	5.19E − 21	4.14E − 21	3.70E − 21	1.29E − 20	3.93E − 21	4.62E − 21	2.41E − 20
^{41}Ar	4.68E − 17	4.74E − 17	4.30E − 17	4.32E − 17	6.08E − 17	4.03E − 17	4.47E − 17	5.29E − 17
^{41}Ca	0.00E + 00	0.00E + 00	0.00E + 00	0.00E + 00	0.00E + 00	0.00E + 00	0.00E + 00	0.00E + 00
^{45}Ca	3.74E − 22	4.06E − 22	2.79E − 22	2.31E − 22	1.07E − 21	2.75E − 22	3.35E − 22	4.79E − 22
^{46}Sc	7.09E − 17	7.25E − 17	6.52E − 17	6.52E − 17	9.57E − 17	6.06E − 17	6.79E − 17	7.83E − 17
^{51}Cr	9.82E − 19	1.01E − 18	8.77E − 19	8.57E − 19	1.72E − 18	8.18E − 19	9.34E − 19	1.08E − 18
^{54}Mn	2.89E − 17	2.96E − 17	2.64E − 17	2.63E − 17	4.01E − 17	2.45E − 17	2.76E − 17	3.20E − 17
^{56}Mn	6.20E − 17	6.27E − 17	5.69E − 17	5.71E − 17	8.11E − 17	5.35E − 17	5.92E − 17	7.60E − 17
^{55}Fe	0.00E + 00	0.00E + 00	0.00E + 00	0.00E + 00	0.00E + 00	0.00E + 00	0.00E + 00	0.00E + 00
^{59}Fe	4.27E − 17	4.35E − 17	3.93E − 17	3.94E − 17	5.64E − 17	3.67E − 17	4.09E − 17	4.69E − 17
^{57}Co	2.77E − 18	2.87E − 18	2.49E − 18	2.28E − 18	7.32E − 18	2.32E − 18	2.68E − 18	3.01E − 18
^{60}Co	9.08E − 17	9.22E − 17	8.36E − 17	8.39E − 17	1.18E − 16	7.82E − 17	8.68E − 17	9.94E − 17
^{59}Ni	0.00E + 00	0.00E + 00	0.00E + 00	0.00E + 00	0.00E + 00	0.00E + 00	0.00E + 00	0.00E + 00
^{63}Ni	0.00E + 00	0.00E + 00	0.00E + 00	0.00E + 00	0.00E + 00	0.00E + 00	0.00E + 00	0.00E + 00
^{65}Ni	2.01E − 17	2.04E − 17	1.85E − 17	1.86E − 17	2.62E − 17	1.73E − 17	1.92E − 17	2.71E − 17
^{64}Cu	6.34E − 18	6.49E − 18	5.67E − 18	5.59E − 18	9.54E − 18	5.29E − 18	5.99E − 18	6.95E − 18
^{65}Zn	2.07E − 17	2.11E − 17	1.90E − 17	1.91E − 17	2.76E − 17	1.77E − 17	1.98E − 17	2.28E − 17
^{69}Zn	1.28E − 20	1.34E − 20	1.10E − 20	1.01E − 20	3.08E − 20	1.04E − 20	1.21E − 20	4.94E − 19
^{79}Se	1.18E − 22	1.31E − 22	7.62E − 23	6.05E − 23	3.25E − 22	7.87E − 23	9.96E − 23	1.69E − 22
^{82}Br	9.22E − 17	9.42E − 17	8.40E − 17	8.37E − 17	1.28E − 16	7.83E − 17	8.78E − 17	1.01E − 16
^{83}Br	2.64E − 19	2.71E − 19	2.36E − 19	2.32E − 19	4.08E − 19	2.20E − 19	2.50E − 19	7.98E − 19
^{84}Br	6.79E − 17	6.82E − 17	6.27E − 17	6.34E − 17	8.62E − 17	5.95E − 17	6.50E − 17	8.91E − 17
^{83m}Kr	2.57E − 22	4.21E − 22	2.74E − 23	3.51E − 23	2.24E − 22	4.79E − 23	1.62E − 22	3.47E − 21
^{85m}Kr	4.22E − 18	4.37E − 18	3.79E − 18	3.59E − 18	9.34E − 18	3.53E − 18	4.06E − 18	4.86E − 18
^{85}Kr	8.10E − 20	8.31E − 20	7.20E − 20	7.05E − 20	1.30E − 19	6.73E − 20	7.65E − 20	2.03E − 19
^{87}Kr	2.95E − 17	2.97E − 17	2.70E − 17	2.71E − 17	3.94E − 17	2.56E − 17	2.81E − 17	4.94E − 17
^{88}Kr	7.42E − 17	7.43E − 17	6.82E − 17	6.89E − 17	9.39E − 17	6.49E − 17	7.08E − 17	8.20E − 17
^{86}Rb	3.42E − 18	3.50E − 18	3.15E − 18	3.15E − 18	4.62E − 18	2.93E − 18	3.28E − 18	9.00E − 18
^{88}Rb	2.45E − 17	2.46E − 17	2.25E − 17	2.27E − 27	3.13E − 17	2.13E − 17	2.34E − 17	5.78E − 17
^{89}Rb	7.66E − 17	7.74E − 17	7.05E − 17	7.09E − 17	9.90E − 17	6.63E − 17	7.32E − 17	9.48E − 17
^{89}Sr	5.12E − 20	5.32E − 20	4.50E − 20	4.25E − 20	1.08E − 19	4.22E − 20	4.86E − 20	3.70E − 18
^{90}Sr	4.02E − 21	4.25E − 21	3.37E − 21	3.00E − 21	1.06E − 20	3.21E − 21	3.77E − 21	1.50E − 20
^{91}Sr	2.44E − 17	2.50E − 17	2.24E − 17	2.23E − 17	3.37E − 17	2.08E − 17	2.33E − 17	3.24E − 17
^{92}Sr	4.90E − 17	4.96E − 17	4.51E − 17	4.53E − 17	6.35E − 17	4.23E − 17	4.68E − 17	5.37E − 17
^{90}Y	1.34E − 19	1.39E − 19	1.19E − 19	1.14E − 19	2.63E − 19	1.12E − 19	1.28E − 19	9.91E − 18
^{91m}Y	1.78E − 17	1.83E − 17	1.60E − 17	1.58E − 17	2.65E − 17	1.49E − 17	1.69E − 17	1.96E − 17
^{91}Y	1.82E − 19	1.86E − 19	1.66E − 19	1.63E − 19	2.82E − 19	1.55E − 19	1.74E − 19	4.16E − 18
^{92}Y	9.27E − 18	9.46E − 18	8.48E − 18	8.47E − 18	1.27E − 17	7.91E − 18	8.85E − 18	3.01E − 17

(continued)

Table 13.30.4 Dose Coefficient for Exposure to Contaminated Soil (Sv Bq^{-1} s^{-1} m^3)[a] (Continued)

Nuclide	Gonads	Breast	Lung	R Marrow	Endosteal	Thyroid	Heff	Skin
^{93}Y	3.39E − 18	3.44E − 18	3.09E − 18	3.09E − 18	4.82E − 18	2.91E − 18	3.24E − 18	1.81E − 17
^{93}Zr	0.00E + 00	0.00E + 00	0.00E + 00	0.00E + 00	0.00E + 00	0.00E + 00	0.00E + 00	0.00E + 00
^{95}Zr	2.54E − 17	2.60E − 17	2.31E − 17	2.29E − 17	3.59E − 17	2.14E − 17	2.42E − 17	2.80E − 17
^{97}Zr	6.40E − 18	6.51E − 18	5.83E − 18	5.82E − 18	8.88E − 18	5.46E − 18	6.09E − 18	1.26E − 17
^{93m}Nb	1.03E − 21	1.41E − 21	2.51E − 23	1.12E − 22	6.70E − 22	1.37E − 22	5.57E − 22	5.26E − 21
^{95m}Nb	1.78E − 18	1.85E − 18	1.59E − 18	1.54E − 18	3.52E − 18	1.49E − 18	1.71E − 18	1.97E − 18
^{95}Nb	2.64E − 17	2.70E − 17	2.40E − 17	2.39E − 17	3.71E − 17	2.23E − 17	2.51E − 27	2.91E − 17
^{97m}Nb	2.50E − 17	2.57E − 17	2.27E − 17	2.26E − 17	3.53E − 17	2.11E − 17	2.38E − 17	2.77E − 17
^{97}Nb	2.24E − 17	2.29E − 17	2.02E − 17	2.01E − 17	3.22E − 17	1.88E − 17	2.13E − 17	2.66E − 17
^{93}Mo	5.84E − 21	8.00E − 21	1.42E − 22	6.37E − 22	3.80E − 21	7.78E − 22	3.16E − 21	2.99E − 20
^{99}Mo	4.99E − 18	5.12E − 18	4.52E − 18	4.47E − 18	7.51E − 18	4.20E − 18	4.75E − 18	6.85E − 18
^{99m}Tc	3.05E − 18	3.17E − 18	2.75E − 18	2.55E − 18	7.62E − 18	2.55E − 18	2.95E − 18	3.33E − 18
^{99}Tc	7.37E − 22	7.93E − 22	5.74E − 22	4.85E − 22	2.11E − 21	5.58E − 22	6.72E − 22	9.09E − 22
^{101}Tc	1.05E − 17	1.08E − 17	9.37E − 18	9.16E − 18	1.83E − 17	8.74E − 18	9.97E − 18	1.35E − 17
^{103}Ru	1.56E − 17	1.60E − 17	1.39E − 17	1.37E − 17	2.37E − 17	1.30E − 17	1.47E − 17	1.70E − 17
^{105}Ru	2.65E − 17	2.72E − 17	2.40E − 17	2.37E − 17	3.90E − 17	2.23E − 17	2.52E − 17	3.04E − 17
^{106}Ru	0.00E + 00	0.00E + 00	0.00E + 00	0.00E + 00	0.00E + 00	0.00E + 00	0.00E + 00	0.00E + 00
^{103m}Rh	2.27E − 21	2.77E − 21	2.69E − 22	3.61E − 22	2.31E − 22	6.23E − 22	1.30E − 21	6.22E − 21
^{105}Rh	2.42E − 18	2.50E − 18	2.16E − 18	2.11E − 18	4.27E − 18	2.02E − 18	2.30E − 18	2.66E − 18
^{106}Rh	7.29E − 18	7.46E − 18	6.56E − 18	6.49E − 18	1.08E − 17	6.12E − 18	6.91E − 18	2.71E − 17
^{107}Pd	0.00E + 00	0.00E + 00	0.00E + 00	0.00E + 00	0.00E + 00	0.00E + 00	0.00E + 00	0.00E + 00
^{109}Pd	1.09E − 19	1.16E − 19	8.62E − 20	7.85E − 20	2.65E − 19	8.30E − 20	9.94E − 20	9.65E − 19
^{110m}Ag	9.64E − 17	9.84E − 17	8.80E − 17	8.78E − 17	1.32E − 16	8.20E − 17	9.19E − 17	1.06E − 16
^{110}Ag	1.26E − 18	1.30E − 18	1.14E − 18	1.12E − 18	1.91E − 18	1.06E − 18	1.20E − 18	1.58E − 17
^{111}Ag	8.40E − 19	8.67E − 19	7.49E − 19	7.32E − 19	1.47E − 18	7.00E − 19	7.99E − 19	1.72E − 18
^{113m}Cd	3.70E − 21	3.91E − 21	3.10E − 21	2.76E − 21	9.76E − 21	2.95E − 21	3.47E − 21	1.81E − 20
^{115m}Cd	8.31E − 19	8.49E − 19	7.60E − 19	7.58E − 19	1.16E − 18	7.09E − 19	7.94E − 19	4.87E − 18
^{123}Sn	2.83E − 19	2.90E − 19	2.59E − 19	2.57E − 19	4.11E − 19	2.41E − 19	2.71E − 19	3.14E − 18
^{125}Sn	1.13E − 17	1.15E − 17	1.04E − 17	1.04E − 17	1.52E − 17	9.68E − 18	1.08E − 17	2.07E − 17
^{126}Sn	8.24E − 19	8.66E − 19	7.10E − 19	6.09E − 19	2.56E − 18	6.69E − 19	7.89E − 19	9.21E − 19
^{124}Sb	6.58E − 17	6.66E − 17	6.00E − 17	6.01E − 17	8.77E − 17	5.65E − 17	6.26E − 17	7.38E − 17
^{125}Sb	1.38E − 17	1.42E − 17	1.24E − 17	1.22E − 17	2.12E − 17	1.15E − 17	1.31E − 17	1.52E − 17
^{126m}Sb	5.24E − 17	5.37E − 17	4.73E − 17	4.68E − 17	769E − 17	4.40E − 17	4.98E − 17	6.20E − 17
^{126}Sb	9.64E − 17	9.88E − 17	8,72E − 17	8.65E − 17	1.40E − 16	8.11E − 17	9.16E − 17	1.07E − 16
^{127}Sb	2.32E − 17	2.38E − 17	2.09E − 17	2.07E − 17	3.42E − 17	1.95E − 17	2.20E − 17	2.61E − 17
^{125m}Te	1.19E − 19	1.39E − 19	3.97E − 20	3.26E − 20	2.07E − 19	5.47E − 20	8.11E − 20	1.95E − 19
^{127m}Te	4.09E − 20	4.71E − 20	1.64E − 20	1.39E − 20	7.35E − 20	2.06E − 20	2.92E − 20	6.86E − 20
^{127}Te	1.62E − 19	1.66E − 19	1.44E − 19	1.41E − 19	2.69E − 19	1.34E − 19	1.53E − 19	2.51E − 19
^{129m}Te	1.05E − 18	1.08E − 18	9.36E − 19	9.27E − 19	1.52E − 18	8.74E − 19	9.91E − 19	2.46E − 18
^{129}Te	1.87E − 18	1.92E − 18	1.67E − 18	1.65E − 18	2.89E − 18	1.56E − 18	1.77E − 18	4.81E − 18
^{131m}Te	4.91E − 17	5.02E − 17	4.49E − 17	4.47E − 17	6.92E − 17	4.18E − 17	4.69E − 17	5.45E − 17
^{131}Te	1.34E − 17	1.38E − 17	1.22E − 17	1.19E − 17	2.19E − 17	1.13E − 17	1.28E − 17	2.04E − 17
^{132}Te	6.07E − 18	6.32E − 18	5.39E − 18	5.19E − 18	1.23E − 17	5.04E − 18	5.80E − 18	6.72E − 18
^{133m}Te	8.07E − 17	8.24E − 17	7.37E − 17	7.35E − 17	1.12E − 16	6.88E − 17	7.70E − 17	9.42E − 17
^{133}Te	3.20E − 17	3.27E − 17	2.91E − 17	2.89E − 17	4.67E − 17	2.72E − 17	3.05E − 17	4.26E − 17
^{134}Te	2.87E − 17	2.94E − 17	2.58E − 17	2.55E − 17	4.48E − 17	2.40E − 17	2.73E − 17	3.17E − 17

Table 13.30.4 Dose Coefficient for Exposure to Contaminated Soil (Sv Bq^{-1} s^{-1} m^3)[a] (Continued)

Nuclide	Gonads	Breast	Lung	R Marrow	Endosteal	Thyroid	Heff	Skin
^{129}I	9.74E − 20	1.13E − 19	3.81E − 20	2.84E − 20	1.94E − 19	4.88E − 20	6.93E − 20	1.48E − 19
^{130}I	7.29E − 17	7.46E − 17	6.58E − 17	6.53E − 17	1.05E − 16	6.13E − 17	6.92E − 17	8.06E − 17
^{131}I	1.22E − 17	1.26E − 17	1.09E − 17	1.07E − 17	2.01E − 17	1.02E − 17	1.16E − 17	1.34E − 17
^{132}I	7.92E − 17	8.09E − 17	7.20E − 17	7.16E − 17	1.11E − 16	6.70E − 17	7.54E − 17	8.98E − 17
^{133}I	2.06E − 17	2.11E − 17	1.85E − 17	1.83E − 17	3.02E − 17	1.73E − 17	1.95E − 17	2.40E − 17
^{134}I	9.21E − 17	9.41E − 17	8.42E − 17	8.40E − 17	1.26E − 16	7.85E − 17	8.79E − 17	1.06E − 16
^{135}I	5.75E − 17	5.82E − 17	5.28E − 17	5.30E − 17	7.51E − 17	4.95E − 17	5.48E − 17	6.39E − 17
^{131m}Xe	1.43E − 19	1.57E − 19	9.47E − 20	8.54E − 20	3.02E − 19	9.72E − 20	1.21E − 19	1.85E − 19
^{133m}Xe	7.44E − 19	7.81E − 19	6.33E − 19	6.07E − 19	1.47E − 18	5.99E − 19	6.96E − 19	8.48E − 19
^{133}Xe	5.71E − 19	6.05E − 19	4.71E − 19	3.98E − 19	1.76E − 18	4.50E − 19	5.36E − 19	6.50E − 19
^{135m}Xe	1.42E − 17	1.46E − 17	1.27E − 17	1.25E − 17	2.14E − 17	1.19E − 17	1.34E − 17	1.57E − 17
^{135}Xe	7.44E − 18	7.71E − 18	6.66E − 18	6.47E − 18	1.41E − 17	6.21E − 18	7.11E − 18	8.60E − 18
^{134m}Cs	4.12E − 19	4.32E − 19	3.50E − 19	3.19E − 19	1.05E − 18	3.31E − 19	3.89E − 19	4.65E − 19
^{134}Cs	5.33E − 17	5.46E − 17	4.83E − 17	4.80E − 17	7.59E − 17	4.50E − 17	5.07E − 17	5.87E − 17
^{135}Cs	2.33E − 22	2.55E − 22	1.66E − 22	1.35E − 22	6.65E − 22	1.66E − 22	2.05E − 22	3.11E − 22
^{136}Cs	7.45E − 17	7.63E − 17	6.81E − 17	6.78E − 17	1.05E − 16	6.34E − 17	7.12E − 17	8.22E − 17
^{137}Cs	4.27E − 21	4.50E − 21	3.61E − 21	3.25E − 21	1.09E − 20	3.43E − 21	4.02E − 21	9.34E − 20
^{138}Cs	8.72E − 17	8.80E − 17	7.99E − 17	8.04E − 17	1.13E − 16	7.54E − 17	8.31E − 17	1.09E − 16
^{137m}Ba	2.03E − 17	2.08E − 17	1.83E − 17	1.82E − 17	2.91E − 17	1.70E − 17	1.93E − 17	2.26E − 17
^{139}Ba	1.25E − 18	1.30E − 18	1.13E − 18	1.07E − 18	2.67E − 18	1.05E − 18	1.21E − 18	1.02E − 17
^{140}Ba	5.85E − 18	5.98E − 18	5.20E − 18	5.12E − 18	9.15E − 18	4.86E − 18	5.52E − 18	6.87E − 18
^{141}Ba	2.84E − 17	2.91E − 17	2.58E − 17	2.55E − 17	4.33E − 17	2.41E − 17	2.71E − 17	4.00E − 17
^{142}Ba	3.59E − 17	3.67E − 17	3.29E − 17	3.27E − 17	5.09E − 17	3.06E − 17	3.43E − 17	4.13E − 17
^{140}La	8.46E − 17	8.54E − 17	7.73E − 17	7.77E − 17	1.11E − 16	7.29E − 17	8.06E − 17	9.45E − 17
^{141}La	1.73E − 18	1.75E − 18	1.58E − 18	1.59E − 18	2.31E − 18	1.49E − 18	1.65E − 18	1.18E − 17
^{142}La	1.05E − 16	1.05E − 16	9.63E − 17	9.73E − 17	1.32E − 16	9.15E − 17	9.99E − 17	1.21E − 16
^{141}Ce	1.77E − 18	1.84E − 18	1.58E − 18	1.47E − 18	4.34E − 18	1.47E − 18	1.70E − 18	1.94E − 18
^{143}Ce	8.36E − 18	8.62E − 18	7.46E − 18	7.30E − 18	1.39E − 17	6.96E − 18	7.93E − 18	1.06E − 17
^{144}Ce	4.01E − 19	4.19E − 19	3.52E − 19	3.20E − 19	1.05E − 18	3.30E − 19	3.84E − 19	4.43E − 19
^{143}Pr	1.24E − 20	1.30E − 20	1.07E − 20	9.83E − 21	3.01E − 20	1.01E − 20	1.18E − 20	5.10E − 19
^{144m}Pr	9.24E − 20	1.02E − 19	5.99E − 20	5.06E − 20	1.94E − 19	6.23E − 20	7.69E − 20	1.19E − 19
^{144}Pr	1.42E − 18	1.43E − 18	1.29E − 18	1.29E − 18	1.96E − 18	1.22E − 18	1.35E − 18	1.65E − 17
^{147}Nd	3.78E − 18	3.90E − 18	3.35E − 18	3.23E − 18	6.67E − 18	3.13E − 18	3.58E − 18	4.34E − 18
^{147}Pm	2.96E − 22	3.20E − 22	2.25E − 22	1.91E − 22	8.31E − 22	2.21E − 22	2.68E − 22	3.75E − 22
^{148m}Pm	6.77E − 17	6.94E − 17	6.12E − 17	6.06E − 17	9.87E − 17	5.69E − 17	6.43E − 17	7.45E − 17
^{148}Pm	2.07E − 17	2.10E − 17	1.89E − 17	1.89E − 17	2.78E − 17	1.77E − 17	1.97E − 17	2.90E − 17
^{149}Pm	3.51E − 19	3.62E − 19	3.14E − 19	3.07E − 19	6.19E − 29	2.93E − 19	3.34E − 19	1.30E − 18
^{151}Pm	9.75E − 18	1.01E − 17	8.73E − 18	8.53E − 18	1.66E − 17	8.15E − 18	9.28E − 18	1.12E − 17
^{151}Sm	9.38E − 24	1.14E − 23	8.79E − 25	1.37E − 24	8.76E − 24	2.48E − 24	5.27E − 24	2.46E − 23
^{153}Sm	9.00E − 19	9.49E − 19	7.55E − 19	6.53E − 19	2.58E − 18	7.18E − 19	8.47E − 19	1.11E − 18
^{152}Eu	3.93E − 17	4.01E − 17	3.59E − 17	3.58E − 17	5.54E − 17	3.35E − 17	3.75E − 17	4.33E − 17
^{154}Eu	4.30E − 17	4.39E − 17	3.94E − 17	3.93E − 17	5.98E − 17	3.68E − 17	4.11E − 17	4.81E − 17
^{155}Eu	1.02E − 18	1.06E − 18	8.85E − 19	7.68E − 19	3.06E − 18	8.31E − 19	9.75E − 19	1.12E − 18
^{156}Eu	4.85E − 17	4.91E − 17	4.45E − 17	4.48E − 17	6.34E − 17	4.19E − 17	4.63E − 17	5.58E − 17
^{160}Tb	3.87E − 17	3.96E − 17	3.55E − 17	3.53E − 17	5.43E − 17	3.30E − 17	3.70E − 17	4.28E − 17
^{166m}Ho	5.78E − 17	5.94E − 17	5.24E − 17	5.18E − 17	8.70E − 17	4.88E − 17	5.51E − 17	6.38E − 17

(continued)

Table 13.30.4 Dose Coefficient for Exposure to Contaminated Soil (Sv Bq^{-1} s^{-1} m^3)[a] (Continued)

Nuclide	Gonads	Breast	Lung	R Marrow	Endosteal	Thyroid	Heff	Skin
^{181}W	4.37E − 19	4.72E − 19	3.56E − 19	2.77E − 19	1.48E − 18	3.43E − 19	4.09E − 19	4.98E − 19
^{185}W	2.47E − 21	2.61E − 21	2.06E − 21	1.80E − 21	6.97E − 21	1.96E − 21	2.32E − 21	2.85E − 21
^{187}W	1.55E − 17	1.59E − 17	1.40E − 17	1.37E − 17	2.36E − 17	1.30E − 17	1.47E − 17	1.76E − 17
^{207}Tl	1.11E − 19	1.14E − 19	1.00E − 19	9.83E − 20	1.82E − 19	9.35E − 20	1.06E − 19	2.53E − 18
^{208}Tl	1.28E − 16	1.29E − 16	1.18E − 16	1.19E − 16	1.63E − 16	1.13E − 16	1.23E − 16	1.41E − 16
^{209}Tl	7.27E − 17	7.34E − 17	6.63E − 17	6.64E − 17	9.91E − 17	6.25E − 17	6.92E − 17	8.35E − 17
^{209}Pb	4.41E − 21	4.65E − 21	3.72E − 21	3.33E − 21	1.15E − 20	3.53E − 21	4.14E − 21	3.91E − 20
^{210}Pb	1.51E − 20	1.70E − 20	1.03E − 20	7.48E − 21	4.68E − 20	1.06E − 20	1.31E − 20	2.26E − 20
^{211}Pb	1.73E − 18	1.77E − 18	1.56E − 18	1.54E − 18	2.57E − 18	1.45E − 18	1.64E − 18	3.91E − 18
^{212}Pb	3.93E − 18	4.09E − 18	3.52E − 18	3.35E − 18	8.30E − 18	3.28E − 18	3.77E − 18	4.32E − 18
^{214}Pb	7.54E − 18	7.78E − 18	6.74E − 18	6.56E − 18	1.34E − 17	6.29E − 18	7.18E − 18	8.38E − 18
^{210}Bi	2.03E − 20	2.12E − 20	1.77E − 20	1.64E − 20	4.71E − 20	1.66E − 20	1.93E − 20	1.20E − 18
^{211}Bi	1.45E − 18	1.49E − 18	1.29E − 18	1.26E − 18	2.50E − 18	1.20E − 18	1.37E − 18	1.58E − 18
^{212}Bi	6.58E − 18	6.70E − 18	6.00E − 18	5.99E − 18	8.99E − 18	5.61E − 18	6.27E − 18	1.13E − 17
^{213}Bi	4.33E − 18	4.45E − 18	3.87E − 18	3.80E − 18	6.90E − 18	3.61E − 18	4.10E − 18	6.47E − 18
^{214}Bi	5.52E − 17	5.57E − 17	5.05E − 17	5.07E − 17	7.24E − 17	4.75E − 17	5.25E − 17	6.51E − 17
^{210}Po	2.94E − 22	3.01E − 22	2.68E − 22	2.67E − 22	4.10E − 22	2.49E − 22	2.80E − 22	3.25E − 22
^{211}Po	2.68E − 19	2.75E − 19	2.44E − 19	2.42E − 19	3.80E − 19	2.27E − 19	2.55E − 19	2.96E − 19
^{212}Po	0.00E + 00	0.00E + 00	0.00E + 00	0.00E + 00	0.00E + 00	0.00E + 00	0.00E + 00	0.00E + 00
^{213}Po	0.00E + 00	0.00E + 00	0.00E + 00	0.00E + 00	0.00E + 00	0.00E + 00	0.00E + 00	0.00E + 00
^{214}Po	2.88E − 21	2.95E − 21	2.63E − 21	2.61E − 21	4.02E − 21	2.44E − 21	2.75E − 21	3.18E − 21
^{216}Po	5.85E − 22	6.00E − 22	5.34E − 22	5.32E − 22	8.16E − 22	4.96E − 22	5.58E − 22	6.48E − 22
^{218}Po	3.16E − 22	3.24E − 22	2.89E − 22	2.88E − 22	4.39E − 22	2.68E − 22	3.02E − 22	3.50E − 22
^{217}At	1.00E − 20	1.03E − 20	8.98E − 21	8.83E − 21	1.57E − 20	8.37E − 21	9.49E − 21	1.10E − 20
^{218}At	3.43E − 20	3.77E − 20	2.63E − 20	1.97E − 20	1.14E − 19	2.59E − 20	3.13E − 20	4.45E − 20
^{219}Rn	1.73E − 18	1.79E − 18	1.55E − 18	1.51E − 18	3.05E − 18	1.44E − 18	1.65E − 18	1.90E − 18
^{220}Rn	1.30E − 20	1.33E − 20	1.16E − 20	1.15E − 20	1.93E − 20	1.08E − 20	1.23E − 20	1.42E − 20
^{222}Rn	1.33E − 20	1.36E − 20	1.19E − 20	1.17E − 20	2.02E − 20	1.11E − 20	1.26E − 20	1.45E − 20
^{221}Fr	8.55E − 19	8.89E − 19	7.67E − 19	7.36E − 19	1.79E − 18	7.15E − 19	8.22E − 19	9.41E − 19
^{223}Fr	1.12E − 19	1.17E − 18	9.76E − 19	9.00E − 19	2.56E − 18	9.18E − 19	1.06E − 18	2.05E − 18
^{223}Ra	3.37E − 18	3.49E − 18	3.01E − 18	2.84E − 18	7.33E − 18	2.81E − 18	3.23E − 18	3.70E − 18
^{224}Ra	2.86E − 19	2.97E − 19	2.56E − 19	2.48E − 19	5.67E − 19	2.39E − 19	2.74E − 19	3.14E − 19
^{225}Ra	7.32E − 20	8.30E − 20	4.20E − 20	2.98E − 20	1.96E − 19	4.59E − 20	5.90E − 20	9.88E − 20
^{226}Ra	1.76E − 19	1.83E − 19	1.58E − 19	1.50E − 19	3.93E − 19	1.47E − 19	1.70E − 19	1.94E − 19
^{228}Ra	0.00E + 00	0.00E + 00	0.00E + 00	0.00E + 00	0.00E + 00	0.00E + 00	0.00E + 00	0.00E + 00
^{225}Ac	3.54E − 19	3.67E − 19	3.15E − 19	2.89E − 19	9.05E − 19	2.94E − 19	3.41E − 19	3.90E − 19
^{227}Ac	2.76E − 21	2.88E − 21	2.43E − 21	2.22E − 21	7.20E − 21	2.27E − 21	2.65E − 21	3.22E − 21
^{228}Ac	3.36E − 17	3.43E − 17	3.07E − 17	3.06E − 17	4.70E − 17	2.86E − 17	3.20E − 17	3.87E − 17
^{227}Th	2.92E − 18	3.03E − 18	2.60E − 18	2.50E − 18	5.77E − 18	2.43E − 18	2.79E − 18	3.22E − 18
^{228}Th	4.42E − 20	4.26E − 20	3.91E − 20	3.58E − 20	1.13E − 19	3.65E − 20	4.25E − 20	5.08E − 20
^{230}Th	6.88E − 21	7.38E − 21	5.72E − 21	5.03E − 21	1.91E − 20	5.41E − 21	6.47E − 21	9.79E − 21
^{231}Th	2.07E − 19	2.19E − 19	1.72E − 19	1.51E − 19	6.02E − 19	1.63E − 19	1.95E − 19	2.56E − 19
^{232}Th	3.07E − 21	3.38E − 31	2.36E − 21	2.04E − 21	8.51E − 21	2.26E − 21	2.79E − 21	5.55E − 21
^{234}Th	1.34E − 19	1.41E − 19	1.17E − 19	1.01E − 19	4.17E − 19	1.10E − 19	1.29E − 19	1.50E − 19
^{231}Pa	1.08E − 18	1.11E − 18	9.52E − 19	9.26E − 19	1.96E − 18	8.90E − 19	1.02E − 18	1.20E − 18
^{233}Pa	5.73E − 18	5.91E − 18	5.11E − 18	4.93E − 18	1.10E − 17	4.77E − 18	5.46E − 18	6.28E − 18

Table 13.30.4 Dose Coefficient for Exposure to Contaminated Soil (Sv Bq^{-1} s^{-1} m^3)[a] (Continued)

Nuclide	Gonads	Breast	Lung	R Marrow	Endosteal	Thyroid	Heff	Skin
^{234m}Pa	5.02E − 19	5.15E − 19	4.57E − 19	4.52E − 19	7.64E − 19	4.26E − 19	4.80E − 19	8.27E − 18
^{234}Pa	6.48E − 17	6.63E − 17	5.91E − 17	5.87E − 17	9.34E − 17	5.50E − 17	6.18E − 17	7.18E − 17
^{232}U	5.38E − 21	5.92E − 21	4.05E − 21	3.64E − 21	1.32E − 20	3.89E − 21	4.83E − 21	9.78E − 21
^{233}U	8.00E − 21	8.47E − 21	6.73E − 21	6.32E − 21	1.75E − 20	6.34E − 21	7.48E − 21	1.08E − 20
^{234}U	2.53E − 21	2.89E − 21	1.64E − 21	1.47E − 21	5.96E − 21	1.62E − 21	2.15E − 21	5.99E − 21
^{235}U	4.00E − 18	4.16E − 18	3.59E − 18	3.40E − 18	9.04E − 18	3.35E − 18	3.86E − 18	4.40E − 18
^{236}U	1.46E − 21	1.76E − 21	7.46E − 22	6.81E − 22	2.99E − 21	7.77E − 22	1.15E − 21	4.61E − 21
^{238}U	8.19E − 22	1.06E − 21	2.34E − 22	2.18E − 22	1.32E − 21	2.91E − 22	5.52E − 22	3.55E − 21
^{240}U	1.04E − 20	1.24E − 20	4.38E − 21	3.59E − 21	2.16E − 20	5.07E − 21	7.62E − 21	2.67E − 20
^{237}Np	4.37E − 19	4.59E − 19	3.78E − 19	3.34E − 19	1.25E − 18	3.55E − 19	4.17E − 19	5.03E − 19
^{239}Np	4.19E − 18	4.35E − 18	3.75E − 18	3.53E − 18	9.52E − 18	3.50E − 18	4.03E − 18	4.61E − 18
^{240m}Np	1.14E − 17	1.16E − 17	1.03E − 17	1.02E − 17	1.64E − 17	9.58E − 18	1.08E − 17	1.72E − 17
^{238}Pu	1.26E − 21	1.60E − 21	2.99E − 22	3.32E − 22	1.57E − 21	4.04E − 22	8.10E − 22	5.09E − 21
^{239}Pu	1.82E − 21	1.99E − 21	1.31E − 21	1.25E − 21	3.40E − 21	1.27E − 21	1.58E − 21	3.38E − 21
^{240}Pu	1.21E − 21	1.55E − 21	2.93E − 22	3.18E − 22	1.58E − 21	3.95E − 22	7.85E − 22	4.87E − 21
^{241}Pu	3.28E − 23	3.42E − 23	2.89E − 23	2.60E − 23	9.16E − 23	2.70E − 23	3.16E − 23	3.78E − 23
^{242}Pu	1.04E − 21	1.32E − 21	2.75E − 22	2.93E − 33	1.41E − 21	3.57E − 22	6.85E − 22	4.08E − 21
^{243}Pu	4.43E − 19	4.62E − 19	3.90E − 19	3.44E − 19	1.27E − 18	3.65E − 19	4.26E − 19	4.96E − 19
^{244}Pu	7.00E − 22	9.29E − 22	7.05E − 23	1.06E − 22	6.55E − 22	1.50E − 22	4.04E − 22	3.27E − 21
^{241}Am	2.53E − 19	2.74E − 19	2.01E − 19	1.57E − 19	8.43E − 19	1.94E − 19	2.34E − 19	3.10E − 19
^{242}Am	2.77E − 19	2.89E − 19	2.45E − 29	2.19E − 19	7.86E − 19	2.29E − 19	2.67E − 19	3.37E − 19
^{243}Am	7.91E − 19	8.36E − 19	6.82E − 19	5.68E − 19	2.60E − 18	6.43E − 19	7.60E − 19	8.80E − 19
^{242}Cm	1.48E − 21	1.87E − 21	2.87E − 22	3.45E − 22	1.61E − 21	4.42E − 22	9.15E − 22	5.49E − 21
^{243}Cm	3.25E − 18	3.37E − 18	2.91E − 18	2.75E − 18	7.26E − 18	2.71E − 18	3.12E − 18	3.58E − 18
^{244}Cm	1.19E − 21	1.54E − 21	1.05E − 22	1.71E − 22	1.06E − 21	2.59E − 22	6.74E − 22	4.89E − 21
^{245}Cm	1.88E − 18	1.95E − 18	1.68E − 18	1.52E − 18	5.12E − 18	1.56E − 18	1.82E − 18	2.06E − 18
^{247}Cm	1.01E − 17	1.03E − 17	8.96E − 18	8.78E − 18	1.65E − 17	8.36E − 18	9.53E − 18	1.10E − 17
^{248}Cm	8.22E − 22	1.06E − 21	8.01E − 23	1.23E − 22	7.65E − 22	1.85E − 22	4.70E − 22	3.35E − 21
^{252}Cf	1.42E − 21	1.71E − 21	4.09E − 22	4.34E − 22	1.96E − 21	5.45E − 22	9.41E − 22	4.12E − 21

[a] A uniform infinite distribution.

Table 13.31 Maximum Committed Dose Equivalent to Any Organ for Adults per Becquerel of Intake from a Puncture (From NCRP 111, 1991)

Radionuclide	(Sv/Bq)	Radionuclide	(Sv/Bq)
^{3}H (as $^{3}H_2O$)	1.7×10^{-11}	^{90}Sr	1.4×10^{-6}
^{3}H (elemental)	—	^{99m}Tc	1.1×10^{-10}
^{14}C	5.6×10^{-10}	^{111}In	2.1×10^{-8}
^{22}Na	5.5×10^{-9}	^{123}I	4.4×10^{-9}
^{24}Na	—	^{125}I	3.4×10^{-7}
^{32}P	1.0×10^{-8}	^{131}I	4.8×10^{-7}
^{35}S	9.5×10^{-11}	^{133}Xe	—
^{36}Cl	8.0×10^{-10}	^{137}Cs	1.4×10^{-8}
^{45}Ca	1.7×10^{-8}	^{147}Pm	3.3×10^{-4}
^{57}Co	1.5×10^{-9}	^{192}Ir	1.0×10^{-7}
^{59}Fe	1.8×10^{-8}	^{201}Tl	2.7×10^{-10}
^{60}Co	4.3×10^{-8}	^{204}Tl	4.6×10^{-9}
^{67}Ga	1.6×10^{-7}		

[a] Computed from oral and f_1 values of ICRP Publication 30, 1979a—does not include skin as an organ.

Table 13.32 Dose Reduction Factors for Inhalation (From NRPB, 1988)

Details of Study	Reduction Factor	Location
Windscale fire, iodine-131 aerosol, 1961	0.2 or better	
SO_2 experiments, Netherlands, 1965	0.1	
Particulate studies, USA, 1971	0.4	private houses
	0.3–0.5	offices
	0.2–0.3	public building
Industrial dusts/aerosols, USA, 1976 and 1980	0.1–0.5	various building types
Beryllium-7 aerosol experiments, Denmark, 1986	0.3	
	0.2	with building airing
	0.5	non-depositing gas with building airing
Beryllium-7 aerosol experiments, Finland, 1987	0.2–0.5	flats
	0.4–0.9	wooden villa
Chernobyl measurements, Denmark, 1987	0.4	particulate iodine-131
	0.3	cesium-137

Table 13.33 Dose Reduction Factors for Cloud Gamma Exposure (From NRPB, 1988)

Details of Study	Reduction Factor		Location
Reactor accident energy spectrum, 9 cm concrete, 1978	0.5		
Reactor accident energy spectrum, USA, 1987	0.9		wooden house, no basement
	0.6		masonry house, no basement
	0.2 or less		large office (away from doors and windows)
	0.4		basement of masonry house
Large multi-story buildings, concrete walls, tile or flat roof, France, 1986	0.1	story 1 (0.5 MeV)	
	0.1–0.2	story 4 (0.5 MeV)	
	0.1–0.2	story 5 (0.5 MeV)	
	0.1–0.2	story 1 (4 MeV)	
	0.2–0.3	story 4 (4 MeV)	
	0.4–0.7	story 5 (4 MeV)	
Typical dwelling, brick, concrete and stone, France, 1987	0.08–0.1	mean (0.5 MeV)	
	0.03–0.17	extreme (0.5 MeV)	
	0.24–0.32	mean (5 MeV)	
	0.05–0.51	extreme (5 MeV)	
Nordic work, 1985	0.3–0.5		wooden houses
	0.03–0.05		cellars
	0.01–0.5		ground floor flats
Calculation of shielding factors for a reactor accident energy spectrum, Israel, 1987	0.33		buildings
	0.05		underground shelter

Table 13.34 Dose Reduction Factors for Deposited Gamma Exposure (From NRPB, 1988)

Details of Study		Reduction Factor	Location
Review of early experimental data, all away from doors and windows, 1977		0.57	1 and 2 story wood frame house
		0.29	1 and 2 story block or brick house
		0.07	3 or 4 story, 1st/2nd floors
		0.01	upper floor, multistory structure
		0.0005–0.03	basements
Calculated shielding factors based on building from France, UK and Denmark, 1984	France	0.025–0.09	houses
		0.006–0.04	multistory
	UK	0.06	semi-detached
		0.008–0.03	multistory
		0.3–0.4	lightweight houses
		0.05–0.2	modern houses
		0.04–0.1	traditional houses
	Denmark	0.1–0.3	houses
		0.01–0.1	multistory
Calculated shielding factors for ^{137}Cs in FRG, 1987	dry deposit	2E − 4 – 7E − 4	basement
		0.5–1.0	prefab
		0.1–0.2	semi-detached
		0.02–0.05	multistory
	wet deposit	5E − 5 – 1E − 3	basement
		0.3–0.5	prefab
		0.07–0.15	semi-detached
		7E − 4 – 5E − 3	multistory
Calculated shielding factors for a reactor accident energy spectrum, Israel, 1987		0.07	buildings
		0.01	underground shelter

Table 13.35 Effective Dose Equivalent (Corrected to Account for *Radioactive Decay* and *Weathering*) Due to an Initial Uniform Concentration of 1 pCi/m^2 on Ground Surface (After EPA 520/1-75-001A, 1990)

	Integrated Dose (Weathering Factor Included)[a]		
Radionuclide	**Year 1 (mrem per pCi/m^2)[c]**	**Year 2 (mrem per pCi/m^2)[c]**	**0–50 Year (mrem per pCi/m^2)[c]**
Zr-95	3.3E − 05	4.0E − 07	3.4E − 05
Nb-95	b	b	b
Ru-103	7.1E − 06	0	7.1E − 06
Ru-106	1.2E − 05	3.7E − 06	1.8E − 05
Te-132	3.2E − 06	0	3.2E − 06
I-131	1.3E − 06	0	1.3E − 06
I-132	b	b	b
I-133	2.1E − 07	0	2.1E − 07
I-135	1.6E − 07	0	1.6E − 07
Cs-134	1.0E − 04	4.7E − 05	2.4E − 04
Cs-137	4.5E − 05	2.9E − 05	6.1E − 04
Ba-140	1.1E − 05	0	1.1E − 05
La-140	b	b	b

[a] Estimated at 1 meter above contaminated ground surface.

[b] Radionuclides that have short-lived daughters (Zr/Nb-95, Te/I-132, Ru/Rh-106, Cs-137/Ba-137m, Ba/La-140) are assumed to quickly reach equilibrium. The *integrated* dose factors listed are the effective gamma dose due to the parent and the daughter. Based on data from reference (U.S. Dept. Energy 1988)

[c] $1 \frac{mrem}{pCi/m^2} = 0.27 \frac{mSv}{Bq/m^2}$

Table 13.36 Gender-Specific and Average Risk Coefficients and Organ Weighting Factors (After Xu and Reece, 1996)

Organ	Risk Coefficient		Weighting Factor by This Study		Weighting Factor by Williams et al.[a] (1985)		ICRP 26 Average	
	Female (10^{-4} Sv^{-1})	Male (10^{-4} Sv^{-1})	Female	Male	Female	Male	Risk (10^{-4} Sv^{-1})	Weighting Factor
Gonads	40	40	0.25	0.25	0.210	0.286	40	0.25
Breast	50	0	0.30	0.00	0.263	0.000	25	0.15
Lung	20	20	0.12	0.12	0.106	0.143	20	0.12
Red bone marrow	20	20	0.12	0.12	0.106	0.143	20	0.12
Thyroid	7	3	0.04	0.02	0.026	0.036	5	0.03
Bone surface	5	5	0.03	0.03	0.030	0.030	5	0.03
Remainder	50	50	0.30	0.30	0.263	0.356	50	0.30
Totals	192	138	1.16	0.84	1.000	1.000	165	1.00

[a] Rounded to three decimal places, therefore totals are 1.000.

Table 13.37 Geometry Factors, g(m) with the Gamma Source in the Thyroid (After Tsoulfanidis and Shrestha, 1995)

Organ E(MeV)	Thyroid		Breasts		Lungs		Brain		Fetus		Kidneys	
	g(m)	Rel. Err (%)	g(m)	Rel. Err (%)	g(m)	Rel. Err (%)	g(m)	Rel. Err (%)	g(m)	Rel. Err (%)	g(m)	Rel. Err (%)
0.05	2.01E − 01	0.2	4.05E − 05	3	2.70E − 04	2	2.24E − 04	1	5.85E − 07	13	2.62E − 06	16
0.1	1.50E − 01	0.6	8.10E − 05	6	3.96E − 04	3	3.27E − 04	2	1.91E − 06	16	1.25E − 05	16
0.2	1.35E − 01	0.6	7.69E − 05	5	3.10E − 04	3	2.86E − 04	2	2.91E − 06	11	1.48E − 05	16
0.5	1.28E − 01	0.6	8.47E − 05	4	2.79E − 04	3	2.87E − 04	2	5.54E − 06	6	2.03E − 05	11
1	1.27E − 01	0.6	1.02E − 04	4	2.94E − 04	3	3.15E − 04	2	7.65E − 06	5	3.24E − 05	8
1.5	1.27E − 01	0.6	1.15E − 04	5	3.04E − 04	3	3.44E − 04	2	1.05E − 05	5	3.55E − 05	8
2	1.28E − 01	0.6	1.22E − 04	5	3.10E − 04	3	3.79E − 04	2	1.28E − 05	5	3.25E − 05	8
2.5	1.27E − 01	0.6	1.33E − 04	5	3.15E − 04	3	3.94E − 04	2	1.47E − 05	5	4.15E − 05	8
3	1.29E − 01	0.6	1.39E − 04	5	3.29E − 04	3	4.03E − 04	2	1.66E − 05	5	4.71E − 05	8
3.5	1.29E − 01	0.6	1.45E − 04	5	3.37E − 04	4	4.17E − 04	2	1.80E − 05	5	4.44E − 05	9
4	1.30E − 01	0.6	1.55E − 04	5	3.44E − 04	4	4.25E − 04	2	1.93E − 05	5	5.02E − 05	9
4.5	1.30E − 01	0.6	1.53E − 04	5	3.46E − 04	4	4.31E − 04	2	1.97E − 05	5	4.48E − 05	9
5	1.31E − 01	0.6	1.60E − 04	4	3.53E − 04	4	4.32E − 04	2	2.22E − 05	5	4.23E − 05	9
Organ Volume (m^3)	1.97E − 05		1.85E − 03		2.94E − 03		1.47E − 03		2.63E − 03		2.84E − 04	

The dose rate in the target organ in Sv per s is found by multiplying the geometry factor g(m) by the following four quantities:
(a) the constant 1.602E − 13 Joules per MeV
(b) the activity concentration in the source organ in Bq per cubic meter
(c) the photon energy (E) in MeV
(d) the mass-energy absorption coefficient in the tissue of the target organ in square meters per kg for photons of energy E.

Table 13.38 Geometry Factors, g(m) with the Gamma Source in the Brain (After Tsoulfanidis and Shrestha, 1995)

Organ E(MeV)	Thyroid		Breasts		Lungs		Brain		Fetus		Kidneys	
	g(m)	Rel. Err (%)	g(m)	Rel. Err (%)	g(m)	Rel. Err (%)	g(m)	Rel. Err (%)	g(m)	Rel. Err (%)	g(m)	Rel. Err (%)
0.05	1.58E − 02	2	1.75E − 03	2	1.04E − 03	3	1.14E + 00	0.03	2.70E − 05	7	2.95E − 05	16
0.1	2.38E − 02	3	2.61E − 03	3	2.42E − 03	4	8.42E − 01	0.07	5.52E − 05	8	1.29E − 04	16
0.2	2.11E − 02	3	2.53E − 03	2	2.18E − 03	3	6.83E − 01	0.06	7.48E − 05	6	1.51E − 04	16
0.5	2.19E − 02	4	2.98E − 03	2	2.37E − 03	2	9.21E − 01	0.06	9.56E − 05	4	2.52E − 04	11
1	2.45E − 02	5	3.69E − 03	2	3.08E − 03	2	6.11E − 01	0.06	1.76E − 04	3	4.22E − 04	8
1.5	2.65E − 02	6	4.01E − 03	3	3.55E − 03	2	6.13E − 01	0.06	2.48E − 04	2	5.84E − 04	8
2	2.77E − 02	6	4.41E − 03	3	3.99E − 03	2	6.16E − 01	0.06	3.54E − 04	2	7.32E − 04	8
2.5	2.83E − 02	6	4.58E − 03	3	4.28E − 03	2	6.14E − 01	0.06	4.13E − 04	2	9.32E − 04	8
3	2.94E − 02	6	4.77E − 03	3	4.54E − 03	2	6.25E − 01	0.06	4.68E − 04	2	8.60E − 04	8
3.5	2.93E − 02	7	4.89E − 03	3	4.77E − 03	2	6.26E − 01	0.06	5.25E − 04	2	1.06E − 03	9
4	2.95E − 02	7	5.11E − 03	3	4.97E − 03	2	6.34E − 01	0.06	6.05E − 04	2	1.08E − 03	9
4.5	3.14E − 02	7	5.18E − 03	3	5.12E − 03	2	6.34E − 01	0.06	6.29E − 04	2	1.18E − 03	9
5	3.21E − 02	7	5.27E − 03	3	5.30E − 03	2	6.38E − 01	0.06	6.48E − 04	2	1.26E − 03	9
Organ Volume (m^3)	1.97E − 05		1.85E − 03		2.94E − 03		1.47E − 03		2.63E − 03		2.84E − 04	

The dose rate in the target organ in Sv per s is found by multiplying the geometry factor g(m) by the following four quantities:
(a) the constant 1.602E − 13 Joules per MeV
(b) the activity concentration in the source organ in Bq per cubic meter
(c) the photon energy (E) in MeV
(d) the mass-energy absorption coefficient in the tissue of the target organ in square meters per kg for photons of energy E

Table 13.39 Mass Attenuation Coefficients (μ/ρ), Mass Energy Absorption Coefficients (μ_{en}/ρ), and Electron Mass Stopping Powers (S/ρ) for Av. Soft Tissue (After ICRU 46, 1992)

	Adult Male ICRU-44			Adult Female ICRU-44		
Energy (MeV)	μ/ρ ($m^2\ kg^{-1}$)	μ_{en}/ρ ($m^2\ kg^{-1}$)	S/ρ ($MeV\ m^2\ kg^{-1}$)	μ/ρ ($m^2\ kg^{-1}$)	μ_{en}/ρ ($m^2\ kg^{-1}$)	S/ρ ($MeV\ m^2\ kg^{-1}$)
0.010	4.86E − 01	4.38E − 01	2.26E + 00	4.55E − 01	4.09E − 01	2.27E + 00
0.015	1.55E − 01	1.23E − 01	1.65E + 00	1.46E − 01	1.14E − 01	1.66E + 00
0.020	7.60E − 02	4.94E − 02	1.32E + 00	7.22E − 02	4.59E − 02	1.32E + 00
0.030	3.61E − 02	1.42E − 02	9.66E − 01	3.50E − 02	1.32E − 02	9.69E − 01
0.040	2.62E − 02	6.43E − 03	7.78E − 01	2.57E − 02	6.04E − 03	7.81E − 01
0.050	2.23E − 02	3.98E − 03	6.60E − 01	2.21E − 02	3.79E − 03	6.63E − 01
0.060	2.03E − 02	3.06E − 03	5.80E − 01	2.02E − 02	2.95E − 03	5.82E − 01
0.080	1.82E − 02	2.54E − 03	4.76E − 01	1.81E − 02	2.50E − 03	4.77E − 01
0.100	1.69E − 02	2.51E − 03	4.12E − 01	1.69E − 02	2.49E − 03	4.13E − 01
0.150	1.49E − 02	2.74E − 03	3.24E − 01	1.49E − 02	2.74E − 03	3.25E − 01
0.200	1.36E − 02	2.95E − 03	2.79E − 01	1.36E − 02	2.95E − 03	2.80E − 01
0.300	1.18E − 02	3.17E − 03	2.36E − 01	1.18E − 02	3.17E − 03	2.36E − 01
0.400	1.05E − 02	3.26E − 03	2.15E − 01	1.06E − 02	3.26E − 03	2.16E − 01
0.500	9.62E − 03	3.28E − 03	2.04E − 01	9.63E − 03	3.28E − 03	2.04E − 01
0.600	8.90E − 03	3.26E − 03	1.96E − 01	8.90E − 03	3.27E − 03	1.97E − 01
0.800	7.81E − 03	3.18E − 03	1.89E − 01	7.82E − 03	3.19E − 03	1.89E − 01
1.000	7.02E − 03	3.08E − 03	1.85E − 01	7.03E − 03	3.08E − 03	1.85E − 01
1.500	5.72E − 03	2.81E − 03	1.83E − 01	5.72E − 03	2.82E − 03	1.83E − 01
2.000	4.91E − 03	2.59E − 03	1.84E − 01	4.91E − 03	2.59E − 03	1.84E − 01
3.000	3.94E − 03	2.26E − 03	1.87E − 01	3.94E − 03	2.26E − 03	1.88E − 01
4.000	3.37E − 03	2.04E − 03	1.92E − 01	3.37E − 03	2.04E − 03	1.92E − 01
5.000	3.00E − 03	1.89E − 03	1.96E − 01	3.00E − 03	1.89E − 03	1.96E − 01
6.000	2.74E − 03	1.78E − 03	1.99E − 01	2.73E − 03	1.78E − 03	2.00E − 01
8.000	2.39E − 03	1.63E − 03	2.06E − 01	2.39E − 03	1.63E − 03	2.06E − 01
10.000	2.18E − 03	1.54E − 03	2.13E − 01	2.17E − 03	1.53E − 03	2.13E − 01
15.000	1.90E − 03	1.41E − 03	2.28E − 01	1.89E − 03	1.40E − 03	2.28E − 01
20.000	1.77E − 03	1.35E − 03	2.42E − 01	1.75E − 03	1.34E − 03	2.42E − 01
30.000	1.66E − 03	1.28E − 03	2.69E − 01	1.64E − 03	1.27E − 03	2.69E − 01
40.000	1.62E − 03	1.26E − 03	2.95E − 01	1.60E − 03	1.25E − 03	2.94E − 01
50.000	1.61E − 03	1.24E − 03	3.21E − 01	1.59E − 03	1.23E − 03	3.20E − 01
60.000	1.61E − 03	1.21E − 03	3.47E − 01	1.59E − 03	1.20E − 03	3.46E − 01
80.000	1.63E − 03	1.19E − 03	3.99E − 01	1.61E − 03	1.18E − 03	3.96E − 01
100.000	1.65E − 03	1.17E − 03	4.51E − 01	1.63E − 03	1.16E − 03	4.48E − 01

Table 13.40 Proton Stopping Powers (MeV m^2 kg^{-1}) for Body Tissues (After ICRU 46, 1992)

Energy (MeV)	Av. Soft Tissue Adult Male (ICRU-44)	Av. Soft Tissue Adult Female (ICRU-44)
1.00	2.62E + 01	2.63E + 01
1.50	1.96E + 01	1.98E + 01
2.00	1.59E + 01	1.60E + 01
3.00	1.17E + 01	1.18E + 01
4.00	9.42E + 00	9.47E + 00
5.00	7.92E + 00	7.96E + 00
6.00	6.87E + 00	6.90E + 00
8.00	5.46E + 00	5.49E + 00
10.00	4.57E + 00	4.59E + 00
15.00	3.29E + 00	3.30E + 00
20.00	2.60E + 00	2.61E + 00
30.00	1.87E + 00	1.88E + 00
40.00	1.49E + 00	1.49E + 00
50.00	1.24E + 00	1.25E + 00
60.00	1.08E + 00	1.08E + 00
80.00	8.61E − 01	8.64E − 01
100.00	7.28E − 01	7.30E − 01
150.00	5.43E − 01	5.45E − 01
200.00	4.48E − 01	4.50E − 01
300.00	3.51E − 01	3.52E − 01
400.00	3.02E − 01	3.03E − 01
500.00	2.74E − 01	2.74E − 01

Table 13.41 Neutron Kerma Factors (Gy m²) for Body Tissues (After ICRU 46, 1992)

Energy (MeV)	Av. Soft Tissue Adult Male (ICRU-44)	Av. Soft Tissue Adult Female (ICRU-44)
2.53E − 08	2.18E − 17	1.94E − 17
3.60E − 07	5.83E − 18	5.19E − 18
6.30E − 06	1.46E − 18	1.31E − 18
1.10E − 04	1.50E − 18	1.47E − 18
2.00E − 03	2.10E − 17	2.12E − 17
3.60E − 02	3.12E − 16	3.16E − 16
9.40E − 02	6.44E − 16	6.51E − 16
1.35E − 01	8.15E − 16	8.24E − 16
1.85E − 01	9.85E − 16	9.96E − 16
2.70E − 01	1.22E − 15	1.24E − 15
3.70E − 01	1.46E − 15	1.47E − 15
5.40E − 01	1.71E − 15	1.74E − 15
7.40E − 01	2.00E − 15	2.03E − 15
9.40E − 01	2.32E − 15	2.34E − 15
1.35E + 00	2.72E − 15	2.75E − 15
1.85E + 00	3.12E − 15	3.15E − 15
2.70E + 00	3.60E − 15	3.65E − 15
3.70E + 00	4.40E − 15	4.46E − 15
5.40E + 00	4.58E − 15	4.63E − 15
7.40E + 00	5.45E − 15	5.48E − 15
9.40E + 00	5.75E − 15	5.83E − 15
1.35E + 01	6.61E − 15	6.66E − 15
1.85E + 01	7.42E − 15	7.53E − 15
2.70E + 01	7.74E − 15	7.89E − 15

References

Berger, M.J. ''Distribution of absorbed dose around point sources of electrons and beta particles in water and other media,'' MIRD Pamphlet No. 7, *J Nucl Med,* Suppl. **53**:3; 1971.

Cross, W.G., Freedman, N.O., Wong, P.Y. ''Beta-ray dose distributions from point sources in an infinite water medium,'' *Health Physics,* **63**(2):160–171; 1992a.

Cross, W.G., Ing, H., Freedman, N.O., Mainville, J. *Tables of Beta Ray Dose Distributions in Water, Air and Other Media.* Atomic Energy of Canada Limited. AECL-7617; Chalk River Nuclear Laboratories; Chalk River, Ontario; 1982.

Cross, W.G., Freedman, N.O., and Wong, P.Y. ''Beta-ray dose distributions from skin contamination,'' *Radiation Protection Dosimetry,* **40**(3):149–168; 1992b.

Department of Energy. *External Dose Rate Conversion Factors for Calculation of Dose to the Public.* DOE/EH-0070; U.S. Department of Energy; Washington, DC; July 1988.

Eckerman, K.F. *A Code to Review the External Dose Rate Coefficients of DOE/EH-00700.* DFext Code Ver.; Kiawah; Oak Ridge National Laboratory: Oak Ridge, TN; 1991.

Eckerman, K.F., Wolbarst, A.B., Richardson, A.C.B. *Limiting Values of Radionuclide Intake and Air Concentration and Dose Conversion Factors for Inhalation, Submersion and Ingestion.* Federal Guidance Report 11, EPA-520/1-88-020; Environmental Protection Agency; Washington, DC; 1988.

Ehrlich, M. ''Choice of conversion factors to the shallow and deep dose equivalent for use in a U.S. personnel dosimetry performance testing program,'' *Radiation Protection Dosimetry,* **1**:271–275; 1981.

Environmental Protection Agency. *Manual of Protective Actions for Nuclear Incidents.* EPA 520/1-75-0001-A; Washington, DC; 1990.

Faw, R.E. ''Absorbed doses to skin from radionuclide sources on the body surface,'' *Health Physics,* **63**(4):443–448; 1992.

Holaday, D.A., Rushing, D.E., Coleman, R.D., Woolrich, P.F., Kusnets, H.L., Bale, W.F. *Control of Radon and Daughters in Uranium Mines and Calculations of Biological Effects.* U.S. Public Health Service Publication No. 494. U.S. Government Printing Office; Washington, DC; 1957.

International Commission on Radiation Units and Measurements (ICRU). *Measurement of Dose Equivalents from External Photon and Electron Radiations.* Report 47; Bethesda, MD; 1992.

International Commission on Radiation Units and Measurements (ICRU). *Photon, Electron, Proton and Neutron Interaction Data for Body Tissues.* Report 46; Bethesda, MD; 1992.

International Commission on Radiological Protection. *1990 Recommendations of the International Commission on Radiological Protection.* ICRP Publication 60; Pergamon Press; Oxford; 1990.

International Commission on Radiological Protection. *Data for Use in Protection Against External Radiation.* ICRP Publication 51; Pergamon Press; Oxford; 1987.

International Commission on Radiological Protection. *Statement from the 1985 Paris Meeting of the International Commission on Radiological Protection.* Publication 45; Pergamon Press; Oxford; 1985b.

International Commission on Radiological Protection. *Recommendations of the International Commission on Radiological Protection.* Publication 26; Pergamon Press; Oxford; 1977.

International Commission on Radiological Units. *Determination of Dose Equivalents Resulting from External Radiation Sources.* ICRU Report 39; Bethesda, MD; 1985a.

Kearfott, K.J., Zhu, M. ''A comparison of values of annual limits on intake presented in ICRP 61 and 10 CFR part 20,'' *Health Physics,* **70**(4):552–555; 1996.

Kocher, D.C., Eckerman, K.F. ''Electron dose-rate conversion factors for external exposure of the skin for uniformly deposited activity on the body surface,'' *Health Physics,* **53**:135–141; 1987.

Kocher, D.C., Eckerman, K.F. ''Electron dose-rate conversion factors for external exposure of the skin,'' *Health Physics,* **40:** 467; 1981.

National Academy of Science, National Research Council. *Health Risks of Radon and Other Internally Deposited Alpha Emitters.* Committee on the Biological Effects of Ionizing Radiation BEIR IV. National Academy Press; Washington, DC; 1988.

National Council on Radiation Protection and Measurements. *Developing Radiation Emergency Plans for Academic, Medical or Industrial Facilities.* NCRP Report 111; Bethesda, MD; 1991.

National Council on Radiation Protection and Measurements. *Conceptual Basis for Calculations of Absorbed Dose Distributions.* NCRP Report No. 108; Bethesda, MD; 1991.

National Council on Radiation Protection and Measurements. *Relative Biological Effectiveness of Radiation of Different Quality.* NCRP Report No. 104; Bethesda, MD; 1990.

National Council on Radiation Protection and Measurements. *Limit for Exposure to ''Hot Particles'' on the Skin.* NCRP Report 106; Bethesda, MD; 1989.

National Radiological Protection Board. *Radiation Protection Bulletin No. 97.* Oxon, U.K.; Nov. 1988.

Nuclear Regulatory Commission. *Generic Environmental Impact Statement for License Renewal of Nuclear Plants.* Draft Report for Comment. NUREG-1437; Washington, DC; August 1991.

Nuclear Regulatory Commission. ''10CFR part 20 et al. standards for protection against radiation: final rule,'' *Federal Register,* **56:**98:23360–23474; Washington, DC; May 21, 1991.

Tsoulfanidis, N., Shrestha, B. ''Geometry factors used for the calculation of gamma dose received by various organs of a human phantom,'' *Radiation Protection Management,* **12**(4):56–66; 1995.

Whitton, J.T. ''New values for epidermal thickness and their importance,'' *Health Physics,* **24:**1; 1973.

Xu, X.G., Reece, W.D. ''Sex-specific tissue weighting factors for effective dose equivalent calculations,'' *Health Physics,* **70**(1):106. 81–86, 1996.

Yoder, C., Bartlett, W.T., Courtney, J.W., Hoolser, C.D., Holland, J.A., Hogan, B.T., ''Confirmation of Conversion Factors Relating to Exposure and Dose-Equivalent Index,'' NUREG/CR-1057; PNL-3219; Richland, WA; 1979.

CHAPTER 14

NUCLEAR TRANSPORTATION INCLUDING SHIPMENT OF LOW-LEVEL WASTE

This chapter outlines the basic requirements of the Federal regulations which are applicable to shippers of radioactive materials and low-level wastes for land disposal. It is not intended to be a *complete* outline of *all* of the applicable regulations. Persons engaged in or contemplating the shipment of radioactive materials should obtain complete copies of the pertinent regulations. Relevant paragraph numbers in the Federal regulations are cited in the outline. The outline for transportation of radioactive materials was provided by Alfred W. Grella; material on waste disposal by Timothy W. Osborne.

TABLE OF CONTENTS

Table 14.1 Statutory Basis of DOT and NRC Regulations[a]

DOT—Dept. of Transportation Act of 1967, P.L. 89-670
DOT—Transportation Safety Act of 1974, P.L. 93-633
DOT—Hazardous Materials Transportation Uniform Safety Act of 1990
NRC—Atomic Energy Act of 1954, P.L. 83-703
NRC—Energy Reorganization Act 42 U.S.C. 5841

Table 14.2 International Standards and Regulations

U.S. regulations are based upon the international standards as issued by the International Atomic Energy Agency (IAEA) in its 1985 edition of Safety Series No. 6, ''Regulations for the Safe Transport of Radioactive Materials.''

[NOTE: Most countries and international transport organizations base their regulations on the IAEA rules. There are significant differences in the USDOT implementation of these rules. Generally these differences are of the nature of added flexibility for domestic shipments. Hence care must be taken to consult the appropriate national authorities for international shipments.]

Table 14.3 International Transport Organizations

The following international transport organizations issue regulations on hazardous and radioactive materials transportation, based on the 1985 IAEA standards:

Water—International Maritime Organization (IMO)
Air International Civil Aviation Organization (ICAO)
—International Air Transport Association (IATA)
Various Conventions, e.g., in Europe for rail, road, and inland water modes.

Table 14.4 U.S. Regulators—Applicable Codes of Federal Regulations

U.S. Department of Transportation (DOT)—49 CFR Parts 170–178
U.S. Nuclear Regulatory Commission (NRC)—10 CFR Part 71
U.S. Postal Service—U.S. Postal Service Publication #6
Various State Regulatory Agencies—Usually adopt DOT regulations by reference, which apply in cases where the transportation is not subject to Federal jurisdiction, e.g., intrastate shipments.

[a] Outline of Nuclear Transportation Regulations, Tables 14.1 through 14.14 and Figures 14.1 through 14.5 adapted from personal communication by A.W. Grella, 1991.

Table 14.5 Main Headings of DOT's 49 CFR "Hazardous Materials Regulations"

49 CFR 106	Rulemaking Procedures
49 CFR 107	Hazardous Material Program Procedures
49 CFR 171	General Information, Regulations and Definitions
49 CFR 172	Hazardous Materials Tables, Hazardous Materials Communications Requirements and Emergency Response Information Requirements
49 CFR 173	Shippers-General Requirements for Shipments and Packaging
49 CFR 174	Carriage by Rail*
49 CFR 175	Carriage by Aircraft*
49 CFR 176	Carriage by Vessel*
49 CFR 177	Carriage by Public highway*
49 CFR 178	Shipping Container Specifications

* NOTE: Modal carrier requirements are not included in this outline.

Table 14.6 Main Headings of NRC's 10 CFR Part 71 Regulations

Subpart A	General Provisions [NOTE: Section 71.5 effectively subjects all *NRC Licensees* to the DOT's 49 CFR regulations applicable to shippers and carriage of radioactive materials as a private carrier. (Common and Contract carriers are not subject to NRC regulation-10 CFR 30.13, 40.12 and 70.12)]
Subpart B	Exemptions [NOTE: extremely important exemptions include the exemption, with certain exceptions, from Part 71 requirements of any packages having less than a Type A (an A_1 or A_2) quantity, LSA* or SCO* materials, or less than 15 grams of a fissile radioactive material]
Subpart C	General Licenses [NOTE: The general license in 71.12 is the authorization for any NRC licensee to use any package which has been certified by NRC as meeting 10CFR71 technical standards]
Subpart D	Application for Package Approval
Subpart E	Package Approval Standards
Subpart F	Package, Specification, and LSA-III Tests
Subpart G	Operating Controls and Procedures
Subpart H	Quality Assurance
Appendix A	Determination of A_1 and A_2 (See also 49CFR 173.435)

* See Table 14.9A.

Table 14.7 Method of Limiting Package Activity

Safety in transport of radioactive materials is accomplished mainly by requiring the proper type of packaging, depending upon the type, quantity and form of the material. The system is based upon the setting of limits for activity in *Type A packaging*, i.e., that which must be designed and tested to resist normal transport conditions without leakage. *Type B packaging*, therefore, is that which must be designed and tested to retain its contents during both normal and accident conditions.

A_1 means the maximum amount of *special form* (encapsulated or massive solid metal) material allowed in a *Type A package*, such that its escape from the packaging would cause only a direct radiation hazard.

A_2 means the maximum amount of *normal form* or *non-special* form material allowed in a *Type A package*, such that its escape from the packaging would present both a radiation and a contamination hazard.

Table 14.7.1 Examples of A_1 and A_2 Values

(From 49 CFR 173.435)

Symbol of Radionuclide		A_1 (Special Form)		A_2 (Normal Form)	
		TBq	Ci	TBq	Ci
^{14}C	Carbon (6)	40	1080	2	54.1
^{137}Cs	Cesium (55)	2	54.1	0.5	13.5
^{99}Mo	Molybdenum (42)	0.6	16.2	0.5	13.5
^{235}U	Uranium (92)	unlimited	unlimited	unlimited	unlimited
^{226}Ra	Radium (88)	0.3	8.11	0.02	0.541
^{239}Pu	Plutonium (94)	2	54.1	0.0002	0.00541
^{35}S	Sulfur (16)	40	1080	2	54.1
^{60}Co	Cobalt (27)	0.4	10.8	0.4	10.8
^{90}Sr	Strontium (38)	0.2	5.41	0.1	2.7
^{241}Am	Americium (95)	2	54.1	0.0002	0.00541
^{192}Ir	Iridium (77)	1	27	0.5	13.5

Note: Quantities exceeding A_1 or A_2 require *Type B packaging*.

Table 14.8 Types of Packaging

A. *Excepted Packaging*—must be only "strong, tight"
- Limited quantities (173.421)
- Instruments and articles (173.424)
- Articles containing natural uranium or thorium (173.426)
- *Empty* packaging containing residual radioactive material (173.428)
- Mailable packages—USPS publication #6—same requirements as limited quantity and instruments/articles, except that 1/10th of activity is permitted in package

Table 14.8.1 Activity Limits for Limited Quantities, Instruments and Articles (173.423)

Nature of Contents	Instruments and Articles		
	Instrument and Article Limits	Package Limits	Materials Package Limits[a]
Solids			
Special form	10^{-2} A_1	A_1	10^{-3} A_1
Other forms	10^{-2} A_2	A_2	10^{-3} A_2
Liquids			
Tritiated water			
<0.0037 TBq/L (<0.1 Ci/liter)	—	—	37 TBq (1,000 curies)
0.0037 to 0.037 TBq/L (0.1 Ci to 1.0 Ci/L)	—	—	3.7 TBq (100 curies)
>0.037 TBq/L (>1.0 Ci/liter)	—	—	0.037 TBq (1 curie)
Other liquids	10^{-3} A_2	10^{-1} A_2	10^{-4} A_2
Gases			
Tritium	2 10^{-2} A_2	2 10^{-1} A_2	2 10^{-2} A_2
Special form	10^{-3} A_1	10^{-2} A_1	10^{-3} A_1
Other forms	10^{-3} A_2	10^{-2} A_2	10^{-3} A_2

[a] For mixture of radionuclides see Section 173.433 (b).

Table 14.8.2 Common Aspects of the ''Exceptions''

- Packages are still regulated, but are excepted from specification packaging, marking and labeling requirements
- No shipping papers are required, but certification statement with appropriate words referencing applicable exception paragraph of regulations must be ''in'' or ''on'' the package
- Activity in package or instrument is limited to table in 173.423
- Dose rate at outside of package must not exceed 0.5 mrem/hr
- Outside of inner package marked ''RADIOACTIVE'', unless there is no inner, then outer must be so marked

B. *Type A Packages*—Design and Test Requirements (173.24, 173.24a, 173.410, 173.412, 173.461, 173.463, 173.465, 173.466, 178.608)

- Authorized packages (173.415)
  [As a practical matter, the only DOT specification *Type A package* listed is the DOT-7A, which is a total performance-oriented specification (178.350). It is self-approved by the user. A record of the testing or evaluation of the package against the specification must, however, be maintained on file by the shipper]
- The DOT-7A specification requires a package to meet some general design objectives (173.24, 173.410, 173.412) and some specific performance tests (173.465, 173.466). The primary tests are a water spray test, a free drop test, a stacking test, and a penetration test.

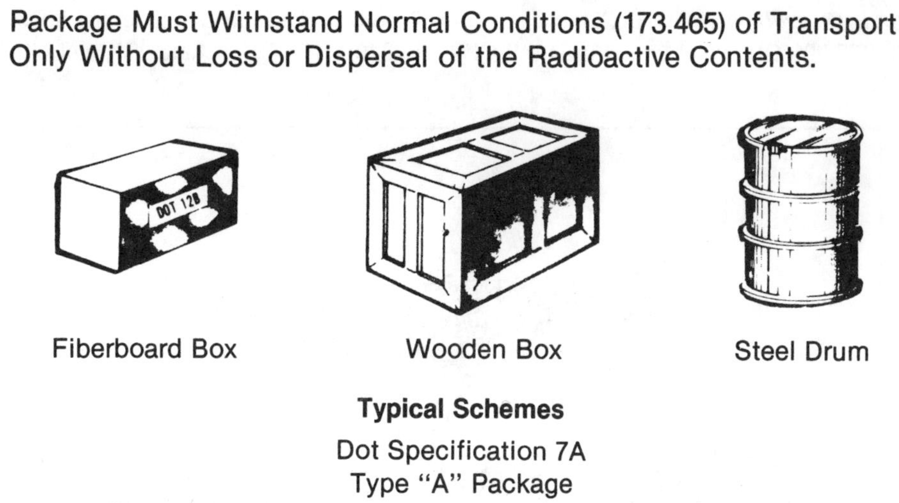

Figure 14.1 Typical Type A (DOT Specification 7A) Packaging

C. *Type B Packages*—Design, test, approval, and certification requirements are in 10 CFR 71 of NRC regulations.

- Authorized packages (173.416)
  [Except for several DOT specifications, e.g., DOT-6M, 20WC, 21WC, 20PF, used under the NRC general license of 10 CFR 71.14, most Type B packages are those which are certified by NRC pursuant to 10 CFR 71]
- Quality Assurance Program approval (10 CFR 71, Subpart H)
- DOT requirements for use of NRC-certified packages (49 CFR 173.471)

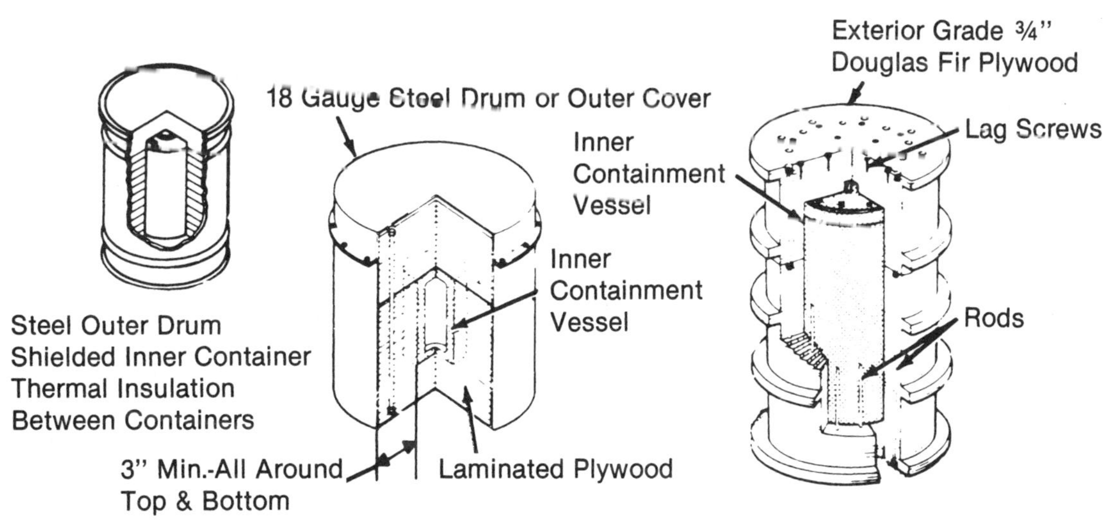

Figure 14.2 Typical (Small) Type B Packaging Schemes

D. *Highway Route Control Quantity* (HRCQ) package—A Type B package containing either 3000 A_1 or 3000 A_2 or 1000 TBq (27,000 Ci), whichever is least (49 CFR 173.22(c), 173.403(1), and 371, and 10 CFR 71.97).

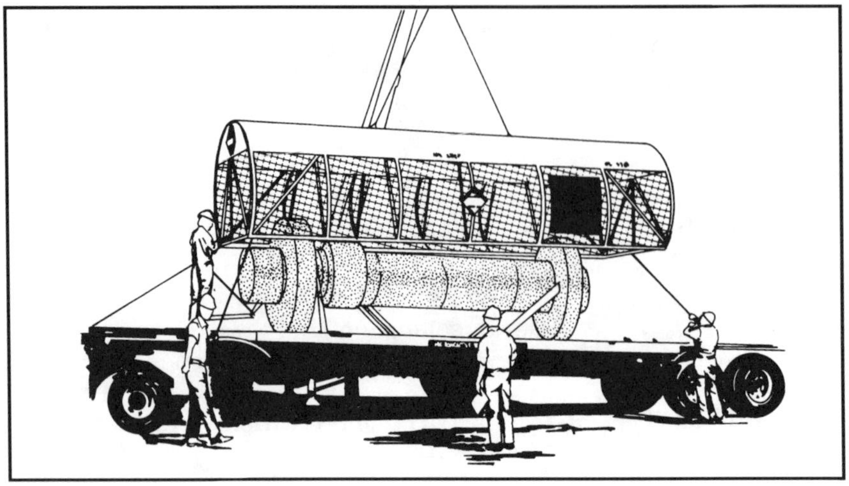

Figure 14.3 HRCQ Spent Fuel Shipment

Table 14.9 Low Specific Activity and Surface Contaminated Object Shipments

A. Definition—*Low Specific Activity* (LSA) materials are limited to those in which the activity must be either 'distributed throughout' or 'essentially uniformly distributed', depending on the material category. *Surface Contaminated Objects* (SCO) are non-radioactive solids with surface contamination. LSA materials and SCOs are categorized into classes, depending on the kind and activity level of the material. Examples, without all the restrictions specified, are:

LSA-I:
- Mill tailings, contaminated earth, concrete, solid activated material less than 10^{-6} A_2/g
- Ores containing uranium or thorium, or concentrates of such ores.

LSA-II:
- Solids or gases less than 10^{-4} A_2/g, or liquids less than 10^{-5} A_2/g.
- Water with a tritium concentration less than 0.8 TBq/liter (20 Ci/L).

LSA-III:
- Material that meets certain specific tests (173.468).

SCO-I:
- Non-fixed contamination does not exceed 4 Bq/cm^2 (beta, gamma, low toxicity alphas), 0.4 Bq/cm^2 (alpha).
- Fixed contamination does not exceed 4×10^4 Bq/cm^2 (beta, gamma, low toxicity alphas), 4×10^3 Bq/cm^2 (alpha).

SCO-II:
- Non-fixed contamination does not exceed 400 Bq/cm^2 (beta, gamma, low toxicity alphas), 40 Bq/cm^2 (alpha).
- Fixed contamination does not exceed 8×10^5 Bq/cm^2 (beta, gamma, low toxicity alphas), 8×10^4 Bq/cm^2 (alpha).

B. *Shipment of LSA materials*
- Specification 7A or IP-1, IP-2, or IP-3 (Industrial Package) may be used depending on the LSA/SCO class, total activity, form (solid, liquid, gas), and shipment control (exclusive versus non-exclusive use). Tables 8 and 9 (173.427) specify the type of industrial package and the conveyance activity limits.
- "Strong tight" packaging which must retain its contents without leakage during normal transport conditions can be used for exclusive use shipments, subject to certain retrictions depending on the LSA or SCO class.

C. *LSA or SCO Exceeding A_2 in the package*— 10CFR71 exempts such shipments from the NRC Type B requirements if it is an exclusive use shipment, subject to certain added requirements (10CFR71.52). This provision expires on April 1, 1999.

Table 14.10 Fissile Radioactive Materials

- *Definition*—173.403(j)—any materials containing one or more fissile radionuclides, e.g., Pu-238, Pu-239, Pu-241, U-233, or U-235. Natural or depleted uranium are not fissile materials.
- *Packaging*—fissile materials are controlled by assigning an appropriate TI and controlling the mode of transport (exclusive or non-exclusive use) to provide nuclear criticality safety during transportation. Packages must be designed and evaluated to provide both radiological safety and nuclear safety. Those used are typically NRC-certified as *Type A Fissile* or *Type B Fissile* (173.417, 173.420, 173.453, 173.457, 173.459 and 10CFR71, many parts).

Table 14.11 Radiation Limits

A. On packages shipped as *non-exclusive use* (173.441(a))
- At any point on surface—200 mrem/hr
- At one meter from package surface—10 mrem/hr

  [NOTE: the radiation level at one meter from the surface of a package is referred to as the *transport index* (173.403(b)]

B. On packages and vehicles shipped as *exclusive use* (173.441(b) and 10CFR71.47)
- At any point on package surface—200 mrem/hr, except for a closed transport vehicle *only*—1000 mrem/hr
- At two meters (6.6 ft) from lateral surfaces of vehicle—10 mrem/hr
- At all external surfaces of vehicle—200 mrem/hr
- In occupied area of vehicle—2 mrem/hr (with certain exceptions)

Table 14.12 Limits for Allowable Removable (Non-Fixed) Contamination on Packages and Areas After Cleanup of a Spill (Removable External Radioactive Contamination—Wipe Limits[a])

	Maximum Permissible Limits		
Contaminant	**Bq/cm² [b]**	**μCi/cm² [c]**	**dpm/cm² [d]**
Beta/gamma-emitting radionuclides and low toxicity alpha emitters	0.41	10^{-5}	22
All other alpha-emitting radionuclides	0.04	10^{-6}	2.2

[a] As averaged over 300 cm^2.
[b] Bq/cm^2 = becquerels per square centimeter.
[c] $\mu Ci/cm^2$ = microcuries per square centimeter.
[d] dpm/cm^2 = disintegrations per minute per square centimeter.
The limits stated in the table apply to the *wipe sample*. (A useful reference on contamination limits and surveys is NRC Information Notice No. 85-46.)

Table 14.13 Hazardous Materials Communications and Emergency Response Information Requirements—49 CFR Part 172

Subpart A—General
Subpart B—Tables of hazardous material, their description, proper shipping name, class, label, packaging and other requirements (172.101)
Subpart C—Shipping Papers
Subpart D—Marking
Subpart E—Labeling
Subpart F—Placarding
Subpart G—Emergency Response Information
Subpart H—Training
Subpart I—Radiation Protection Program

Table 14.13.1 Most Commonly Used Shipping Names for Radioactive Materials[a] (From Hazardous Materials Table, Section 172.101)

Radioactive Material, Excepted Package—Limited Quantity of Material	UN 2910
Radioactive Material, Excepted Package—Instruments, *or* articles[c]	UN 2910
Radioactive Material, Excepted Package—Empty Packaging	UN 2910
Radioactive Material, Fissile, n.o.s.	UN 2918
Radioactive Material, Low Specific Activity *or* LSA, n.o.s.[c]	UN 2912
Radioactive Material, Surface Contaminated Object *or* SCO, n.o.s.[c]	UN 2913
Radioactive Material, Special Form, n.o.s.	UN 2974
Radioactive Material, n.o.s.	UN 2982
Uranium Hexafluoride, Fissile (*Containing more than 1% U-235*)[c]	UN 2977
Uranium Hexafluoride, Low Specific Activity	UN 2978

[a] Refer to Section 172.101 for other proper shipping names.
[b] n.o.s. means "not otherwise specified."
[c] Italicized words are not part of the proper shipping name.

Table 14.13.2 Shipping Papers (49 CFR Part 172)

Subpart C—Shipping Papers—172.200–172.205

- General requirements—include the following:
  (1) Proper shipping name from Section 172.101;
  (2) Hazard class (172.202 (a)(2)), hazard class from Column 3, Section 172.101, except when the hazard class is contained in the shipping name;
  (3) Identification number (172.202 (a)(3)) from Column 3A, Section 172.101;
  (4) Net quantity of material by weight or volume as stated in Sections 172.202(a)(4) and (c). For *most* radioactive materials packages, it is not required to list the weight or volume. The requirements of Section 172.203(d) provide better indications of potential hazards and controls required. These requirements include the package contents as measured in curies and the transport index. A listing of weight or volume measurements for radioactive materials is *usually* needed only for establishing transportation charges;
- Specific requirements for radioactive materials shipping paper descriptions (172.203(d)) include the following:
  (1) Radionuclide(s) contained in package (abbreviations are allowed). For a mixture of radionuclides, only those radionuclides which comprise 1% or more of the total activity in the package must be listed;
  (2) Physical and chemical form of material, or statement that the material is "special form" (if it is special form). A generic description of material, such as protein, carbohydrate, enzyme, or organic salt, is authorized if exact chemical form is difficult to specify;
  (3) Activity in appropriate SI units, e.g., Bq., which may be followed by customary units, e.g., curies (Ci), millicuries (mCi), or microcuries (μCi). If the package contains a *Highway Route Controlled Quantity*, those words must also be shown on the shipping papers;
  (4) Category of RADIOACTIVE labels applied to package;
  (5) Transport index of the package if labeled RADIOACTIVE Yellow-II or RADIOACTIVE Yellow-III;
  (6) The information required in Section 172.203(d)(7) must be included if the shipment is *fissile* radioactive material;
  (7) The identification markings shown on the package must appear on the shipping paper if the package is approved and certified by the Nuclear Regulatory Commission or the Department of Energy, or is certified by DOT or other National Competent Authority for international shipment.
  (8) Other information as required by the mode of transportation or subsidiary hazard of the material (172.203).
  (9) Exclusive use requirements, if applicable

Table 14.13.3 Marking Requirements

Subpart D—Marking Requirements—172.300–172.338, primarily 172.310

Required package markings for Radioactive materials, unless excepted, include:

- Proper Shipping Name—from 172.101
- UN Hazard Identification Number
- Name/Address of consignor or consignee
- ''Type A'' or ''Type B,'' as appropriate
- ''This Side Up'' or ''This End Up'' with arrows, if a liquid
- DOT Package Specification Number or NRC Certificate Identification Number
- ''USA,'' if intended for export
- ''RQ,'' if a ''Reportable Quantity'' (172.101, App. Table 2)

Table 14.13.4 Labeling Requirements (49 CFR Part 172)

Subpart E—Labeling requirements (172.400–172.450, particularly 172.403)

Radioactive-White I
(See §172.436)

Radioactive-Yellow II
(See §172.438)

Radioactive-Yellow III
(See §172.440)

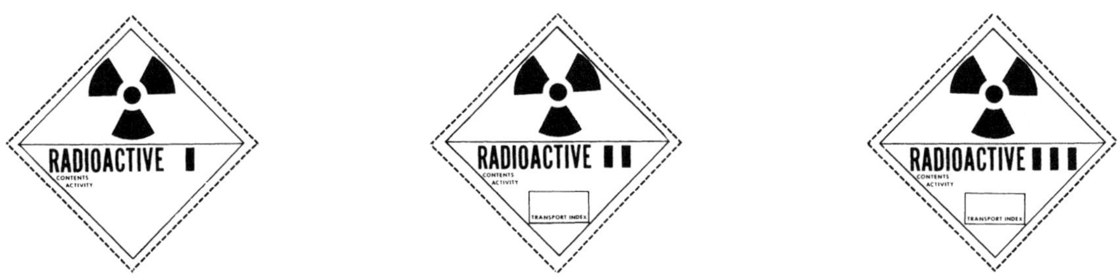

Figure 14.4 Radioactive Materials Package Labels

Table 14.13.4.1 Radioactive Materials Packages Labeling Criteria (172.403)

Transport Index (T.I)	Radiation Level at Package Surface (RL)	Label Category[a]
0[b]	RL ≤ 0.005 mSv/h (RL ≤ 0.5 mrem/h)	White-I
0 < T.I. ≤ 1.0	0.005 mSv/h < RL ≤ 0.5 mSv/h (0.5 mrem/h < RL ≤ 50 mrem/h)	Yellow-II
1.0 < T.I. ≤ 10	0.5 mSv/h < RL ≤ 2 mSv/h (50 mrem/h < RL ≤ 200 mrem/h)	Yellow-III
T.I. > 10	2 mSv/h < RL ≤ 10 mSv/h (200 mrem/h < RL ≤ 1000 mrem/h)	Yellow-III (Must be shipped under exclusive use provisions; see 173.441(b)

[a] Any package containing a ''Highway Route Controlled Quantity'' (173.403) (Table 14.8 (D) of this chapter) must be labeled as Radioactive Yellow-III.

[b] If the measured TI is not greater than 0.05, the value may be considered zero.

Table 14.13.5 Placarding (49 CFR Part 172)

Subpart F—Placarding (172.500–172.558)
Vehicle must be placarded on all four sides of vehicle or the cargo-carrying body, as follows:
• If any quantity of packages bearing the RADIOACTIVE-YELLOW III labels is present on the vehicle (172.504, Table 1)
• By the shipper, when loading and preparing an exclusive-use shipment of LSA or SCO materials (172.504, Table 1, footnote 1)

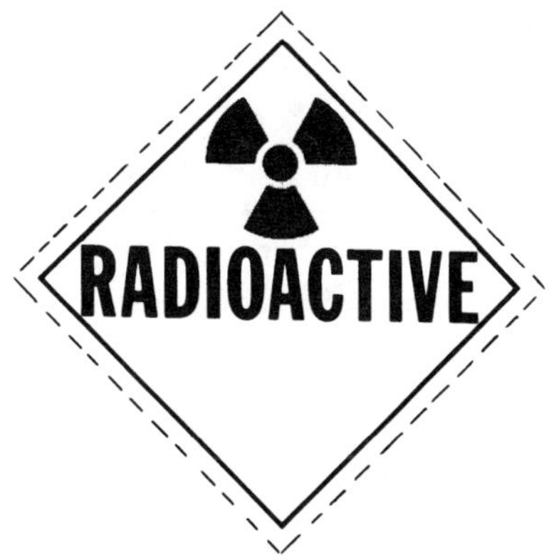

Figure 14.5 Placard Format (172.556)

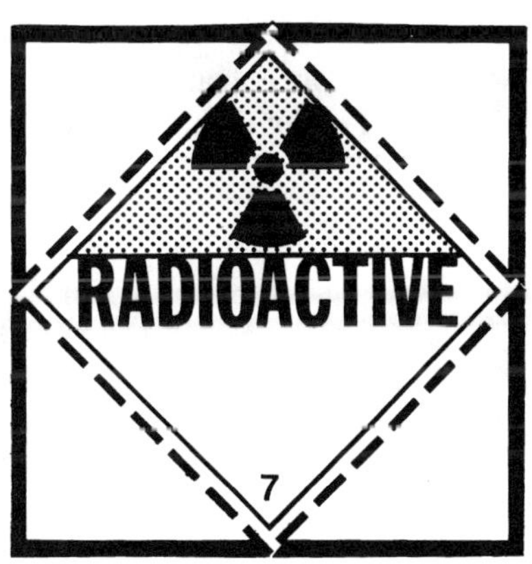

Figure 14.6 Placard for a ''Highway Route Control Quantity'' Shipment

For a ''Highway route control quantity'' shipment, the Radioactive placard must be displayed on a white background 14″ square, surrounded by a rectangular 1″ black border (172.507 and 172.527).

Table 14.13.6 Emergency Response Information (49 CFR 172)

Subpart G—Emergency response information (172.600–172.604)

- Shipper must provide technical name of material and emergency response mitigation information on shipping papers. Information must be on vehicles and maintained at all locations where shipment is handled during transportation. (172.604)
- Shipper must provide emergency response telephone number on shipping papers. Number must be monitored at all times the shipment is in transit. Number must be for a person or agency which is either knowledgeable of or has access to a person having the applicable emergency response information. (172.604)
- Telephone number may be that of an agent which is capable of and agrees to furnish the emergency response information.

Table 14.13.7 Training and Radiation Protection Program

Subpart H—Training: Initial and recurrent training must be provided.

Subpart T—Radiation Protection Program: Required (with certain exceptions) if a worker transports packages totaling in excess of 200 TI in a year.[a]

[a] Editorial Note: Subpart T withdrawn September, 1997.

Table 14.14.1 Classification of Wastes for Near Surface Disposal Long-Lived Radionuclides (From NRC 10 CFR 61.55, 1991)

Classification determined by long-lived radionuclides. If waste contains only radionuclides listed in this table, classification shall be determined as follows:

Radionuclide	Concentration (Curies per Cubic Meter)	Concentration (Millicuries per 55 Gallon Drum)[a]
^{14}C	8	1,699
^{14}C in activated metal	80	16,990
^{59}Ni in activated metal	220	46,720
^{94}Nb in activated metal	0.2	42
^{99}Tc	3	637
^{129}I	0.08	17
Alpha emitting transuranic nuclides with half life greater than 5 years	100[b]	34[c]
^{241}Pu	3,500[b]	1190[c]
^{242}Cm	20,000[b]	6804[c]

[a] A 55 gallon drum contains 7.5 cubic feet (0.21 cubic meters).
[b] Units are nanocuries per gram.
[c] Assuming a solidified drum containing 750 lbs of cement (340,500 grams).

Table 14.14.1 Rules

If Concentration $<0.1 \times$ Table $\rightarrow$ **Class A**
If Concentration $>0.1 \times$ Table and Concentration $<$ Table $\rightarrow$ **Class C**
If Concentration $>$ Table $\rightarrow$ **Not acceptable for near surface disposal**

Table 14.14.2 Classification of Wastes for Near Surface Disposal of Short-Lived Radionuclides

(From NRC 10 CFR 61.55, 1991)

Classification determined by short-lived radionuclides. If waste does not contain any of the radionuclides listed in Table 14.14.1, classification shall be determined based on the concentrations shown in this table.

	Part 61 Concentration (Curies per Cubic Meter)			Calculated Concentration (Millicuries per 55 Gallon Drum)[b]		
Radionuclide	**Col 1**	**Col 2**	**Col 3**	**Col 1**	**Col 2**	**Col 3**
Total of all nuclides with less than 5 year half life	700	[a]	[a]	148,663	[a]	[a]
^{3}H	40	[a]	[a]	8,495	[a]	[a]
^{60}Co	700	[a]	[a]	148,663	[a]	[a]
^{63}Ni	3.5	70	700	743	14,866	148,663
^{63}Ni in activated metal	35	700	7000	7,433	148,663	1,486,630
^{90}Sr	0.04	150	7000	8.5	31,856	1,486,630
^{137}Cs	1	44	4600	212	9,345	976,931

[a] There are no limits established for these radionuclides in Class B or C wastes. These wastes shall be Class B unless the concentrations of other nuclides in this table determine the waste to be Class C independent of these nuclides.
[b] A 55 gallon drum contains 7.5 cubic feet (0.21 cubic meters).

Table 14.14.2 Rules

If Concentration < Col 1 → **Class A**
If Concentration > Col 1 and Concentration < Col 2 → **Class B**
If Concentration > Col 2 and Concentration < Col 3 → **Class C**
If Concentration > Col 3 → **Not acceptable for near surface disposal**

Additional Rules for Tables 14.14.1 and 14.14.2

1. For wastes containing mixtures of radionuclides in Table 1:	Use Sum of Fractions Rule
2. If wastes contain *no* Table 1 radionuclides:	Use Table 2 to classify
3. If wastes contain *no* Table 1 or Table 2 radionuclides:	It is Class **A**
4. For wastes containing mixtures of radionuclides in Table 2:	Use Sum of Fractions Rule
5. For wastes containing mixtures of Table 1 and Table 2 radionuclides:	If concentration $< 0.1 \times$ Table 1, use Table 2 to classify If concentration $\geq 0.1 \times$ Table 1 & $<$ Table 1 & $\leq$ Col 3 of Table 2 then it is CLASS **C**

Table 14.15 A Brief Summary of Requirements for Low Level Waste Transfer for Disposal at Land Disposal Facilities and Manifests[a] (From Timothy O. Osborne, Personal Communication, 1996)

Appendix F to 10 CFR 20 (''Requirements for Low-Level-Waste Transfer for Disposal at Land Disposal Facilities and Manifests'') indicates requirements for the manifest, certification, and control and tracking of low level waste transfer to land disposal sites.

Effective March 1, 1998, transfer for disposal and manifests is governed by APPENDIX G to 10 CFR 20 (''REQUIREMENTS FOR LOW-LEVEL-WASTE TRANSFER FOR DISPOSAL AT LAND DISPOSAL FACILITIES AND MANIFESTS'') This section requires the use of the following forms:

NRC Form 540 ''Uniform Low-Level Radioactive Waste Manifest (Shipping Paper)'' [and NRC Form 540A (Continuation Page)]

NRC Form 541 ''Uniform Low-Level Radioactive Waste Manifest (Container and Waste Description)'' [and NRC Form 541A (Continuation Page)] and if necessary:

NRC Form 542 ''Uniform Low-Level Radioactive Waste Manifest (Manifest Index and Regional Compact Tabulation)

NRC Forms 540 (and 540A) must be completed and must physically accompany the pertinent waste shipment. Upon agreement between shipper and consignee, NRC Forms 541 and 542 may be completed, transmitted and stored in electronic media with the capability for producing legible, accurate, and complete records on the respective forms.

Licensees are not required to comply with the manifesting requirements of Appendix F (or G) when they ship:

LLW for processing and expect its return prior to disposal. LLW sent to a waste processor that becomes the processor's ''residual waste''.

The licensee or the licensed waste collector or processor must classify the waste according to Section 61.55 (''Waste Classification'') of 10CFR Part 61 (''Licensing Requirements for Land Disposal of Radioactive Waste''). Section 61.55 defines radioactive waste suitable for land disposal as falling into one of three categories—i.e., *Class A* waste, *Class B* waste, and *Class C* waste. Wastes are determined to fall into one of the three classes by comparison to limiting concentrations of particular radionuclides as set forth in Table 1 (see Table 14.1.15.1) and Table 2 (see Table 14.15.2) of Section 61.55.

Wastes determined to fall into one of the classes mustbe labeled as such in accordance with Section 61.57 (''Labeling''). Waste generators and waste processors must record on shipment manifests a description of the transferred waste, and must also carry out a quality control program to assure that classification of waste is carried out in a proper manner.

All three classes of waste are required to meet certain minimum requirements as set forth in paragraph 61.56(a) of Section 61.56 (''Waste Characteristics'') which are intended to facilitate handling of waste at the disposal site and provide protection of public health and safety. Class B and Class C wastes, however, are required to meet more rigorous requirements on waste stability. These stability requirements are set forth in paragraph 61.56(b) of Section 61.56. Class C waste must be also identified to allow for additional disposal procedures to be carried out at the disposal site to provide protection to a potential inadvertent intruder. Finally, wastes having concentrations of particular radionuclides exceeding those allowed for Class C waste are generally considered unacceptable for near surface disposal.

The reader is directed toward pertinent parts of the Nuclear Regulatory Commission's 10 CFR 20 and 10 CFR 61 for details, only a brief summary is presented here.

Manifest: The shipment manifest shall contain the name, address, and telephone number of the person generating the waste. The manifest shall also include the name, address, and telephone number or the name and EPA hazardous waste identification number of the person transporting the waste to the land disposal facility. The manifest must also indicate as completely as practicable: a physical description of the waste, the volume, radionuclide identity and quantity, the total radioactivity, and the principal chemical form. The solidification agent must be specified. Waste containing more than 0.1% chelating agents by weight must be identified and the weight percentage of the chelating agent estimated. Wastes classified as Class A, Class B, or Class C in § 61.55 must be clearly identified as such in the manifest.

The total quantity of the radionuclides ^{3}H, ^{14}C, ^{99}Tc, and ^{129}I must be listed. These radionuclides, as well as the other radionuclides listed in Section 61.55, are used to determine the classification status of radioactive waste. Controlled disposal of wastes containing these radionuclides is considered important in assuring that the performance objectives of Subpart C of the Part 61 regulation are met. Additional information may be required for shipment to a particular disposal facility depending upon facility specific license conditions.

[a] This summary is based on a personal communication from T. Osbourne.

Table 14.15 A Brief Summary of Requirements for Low Level Waste Transfer for Disposal at Land Disposal Facilities and Manifests[a] (Continued)

Certification: The waste generator must certify the waste is properly classified, described, packaged, marked, and labeled, and are in a proper condition for transportation according to applicable Department of Transportation regulations.

Control and Tracking: The generator shall maintain a quality control program and a tracking program as detailed in 10CFR20, Appendix F.

Waste classification: To classify waste for disposal and fill out shipment manifests, a licensee must make two basic determinations: (1) whether the waste is acceptable for near surface disposal, and (2) if acceptable for near surface disposal, whether the waste is classified as Class A, Class B, or Class C waste. Another determination is whether the waste complies with any additional waste form, package, or content requirement which may be in place at the particular disposal facility to which the waste is to be shipped.

Waste is determined to be generally unacceptable for near surface disposal if it contains any radionuclides in concentrations exceeding the limits established in Tables 1 and 2 of Section 61.55. If determined to be acceptable for near surface disposal, waste is determined to be Class A, Class B, or Class C based upon the radionuclide concentration limits and procedure set forth in Table 1 (see Table 14.15.1) and Table 2 (see Table 14.15.2) of 10CFR 61.55.

All generators must carry out a compliance program to assure proper classification of waste. The NRC regulatory staff is prepared to be flexible in the adaptation of a particular program to a particular waste generating facility. A principal consideration for the acceptability of a particular program will be whether a reasonable effort has been made to ensure a realistic representation of the distribution of radionuclides within waste, given physical limitations, and to classify waste in a consistent manner. The staff considers a reasonable target for determining measured or inferred radionuclide concentrations is that the concentrations are accurate to within a factor of 10.

There are at least four basic methods which may be potentially used either individually or in combination by licensees:

- Materials accountability
- Classification by source
- Gross radioactivity measurements
- Direct measurement of individual radionuclides

Materials accountability. A given quantity (and resulting concentration) of radioactive material may be known to be contained within a given waste or may be inferred through determining the difference between the quantity of radioactive material entering and exiting a given process.

Classification by source. This method is similar to the above method and involves determining the radionuclide content and classification of waste through knowledge and control of the source of the waste.

Gross radioactivity measurements. Measurement of gross radioactivity is an acceptable method for all classes of waste provided that:

- The gross radioactivity measurements are correlated on a consistent basis with the distribution of radionuclides within the particular waste stream analyzed, and
- The radionuclide distributions are initially determined and periodically verified by direct measurement techniques.

Licensees carrying out gross radioactivity measurements to assure compliance with the waste classification requirement must establish a program to correlate and calibrate measured radioactivity levels with radionuclide concentrations in wastes prepared for shipment. This program must at a minimum take into account waste package and detector geometry, shielding and attenuation effects, the effective gamma energies of the emitted photons, and the number of photons per decay.

Measurement of specific radionuclides. In using this method, licensees may directly measure individual radionuclides or may establish an inferential measurement program whereby concentrations of radioisotopes which cannot be readily measured are projected through ratioing to concentrations of radioisotopes which can be readily measured.

Radionuclide concentrations should be determined based upon the volume or weight of the final waste form. The lower limit of detection of a measurement technique for direct measurement of a particular radionuclide should be no more than 0.01 times the concentration for that radionuclide listed in Table 1, and 0.01 times the smallest concentration for that radionuclide listed in Table 2.

For most facilities and for most Class B and C waste types a confirmatory analysis should be performed on at least an annual basis. Confirmatory analyses for Class A wastes should be performed on at least a biannual basis.

[a] This summary is based on a personal communication from T. Osbourne.

(continued)

Table 14.15 A Brief Summary of Requirements for Low Level Waste Transfer for Disposal at Land Disposal Facilities and Manifests[a] (Continued)

Concentration Averaging: Paragraph 61.55(a)(8) states that the concentration of a radionuclide may be averaged over the volume of the waste, or the weight of the waste if the concentration units are expressed as nanocuries per gram. An NRC Technical Position (NRC, 1995) addressed this issue in more detail.

Most waste streams may be considered to be homogeneous for the purpose of waste classification. Contaminated trash waste streams, which are composed of a variety of miscellaneous materials, may be considered homogeneous for the purpose of waste classification when placed and compacted within shipping containers. The activity of small concentrated sources within the trash, such as small check sources or gauges, may be averaged over the trash volume with certain restrictions. In determining the classification it is always permissible to base the classification on the highest classification of any component of the mixture.

In many cases the volume used for waste classification purposes may be considered to correspond to the volume of the waste container. Care needs to be taken, however, to differentiate between the volume of the waste form and the volume of the waste container if the latter is significantly larger (e.g., greater than 10%).

Classification of absorbed liquids should be based on the volume and mass of the liquids prior to absorption. Classification of solidified liquids would be based on the volume and mass of the solidified waste mass.

The regulatory position of the Nuclear Regulatory Commission needs to be consulted in these and all other matters concerning the shipment, transfer or disposal of low level waste material for land disposal.

[a] This summary is based on a personal communication from T. Osbourne.

Table 14.15.1 Barnwell Waste Management Facility Changes in Acceptance Criteria (From Personal Communication, Timothy W. Osborne, 1996)

1. Condition 39.A

Waste containing radioisotopes with halflives greater than 5 years and having a specific activity greater than 1 microcurie/cubic centimeter must be stabilized. (This includes biological and DAW waste streams)

Following are package limits to meet this standard:

Package Type	Package Volume (cu.ft.)	Activity Limit (mCi)
55 gal drum	7.5	212
30 gal drum	4.01	113
85 gal drum	11.6	328

2. Sealed Sources:

The following sealed sources can be accepted by CNSI without specific approval from SC DHEC:

Radionuclide	Total Activity
^{14}C	100 μCi
^{59}Ni	100 μCi
^{94}Nb	0.1 μCi
^{99}Tc	10 μCi
^{129}I	0.1 μCi
Table II radionuclides	10 Ci

The sources must be processed by encapsulating with a minimum of 4 inches of cement on all sides of the sources. The cement must have a minimum compressive strength of 2,500 psi.

Small quantity sources with radionuclides other than Radium and Transuranics with activities which do not exceed Class A limits (determined using a source volume of 1 cubic centimeter) may be disposed as Class A waste packaged as DAW.

Table 14.16 Interstate Compact Groupings (From Personal Communication, Timothy W. Osborne, 1996)

1. Regional Compacts

APPALACHIAN COMPACT[a]:
- *Pennsylvania (Host)*
- Delaware
- Maryland
- West Virginia

CENTRAL INTERSTATE COMPACT[a]:
- *Nebraska (Host)*
- Arkansas
- Louisiana
- Oklahoma
- Kansas

CENTRAL MIDWEST COMPACT[a]:
- *Illinois (Host)*
- Kentucky

MIDWEST COMPACT[a]:
- *Ohio (Host)*
- Iowa
- Indiana
- Minnesota
- Missouri
- Wisconsin

NORTHEAST COMPACT[a]:
- *Connecticut (Host)*
- *New Jersey (Host)*

NORTHWEST COMPACT[b]:
- *Washington (Host)*
- Alaska
- Hawaii
- Idaho
- Montana
- Oregon
- Utah
- Wyoming

ROCKY MOUNTAIN COMPACT[a,d]:
- *Nevada (Host)*
- Colorado
- New Mexico

SOUTHEAST COMPACT[a]:
- *North Carolina (Host)*
- Alabama
- Florida
- Georgia
- Mississippi
- Tennessee
- Virginia

SOUTHWESTERN COMPACT[a]:
- *California (Host)*
- Arizona
- North Dakota
- South Dakota

TEXAS COMPACT[a]:
- *Texas (Host)*
- Maine
- Vermont

2. Unaffiliated States/Regions[c]

- Massachusetts
- Michigan
- New Hampshire
- New York
- South Carolina[c]
- Puerto Rico
- Rhode Island
- District of Columbia

[a] Non-Sited Regional Compacts are those Compacts of States approved by Congress that do not currently have an operational LLW disposal Facility.

[b] Sited Regional Compacts are those Compacts of States approved by Congress that do have an operational LLW disposal facility.

[c] Unaffiliated States/Regions are those States/Regions that are not a member of a Regional Compact and that are pursuing LLW disposal capacity or other LLW disposal arrangements independently. South Carolina continues to operate its LLW site as a national facility (with some restrictions), subject to certain monetary goals and waste origin restrictions.

[d] Has a contract with the Northwest Compact for waste disposal.

References

Department of Transportation. *A Review of the Department of Transportation Regulations for Transportation of Radioactive Materials*. Pamphlet; Washington; DC.

Department of Transportation. *Hazardous Materials Regulations*. 49 CFR; Government Printing Office, Washington, DC.

- Subpart I, Radioactive Materials, Section 173.400 through 173.478,
- Subparts B-F, Part 172 (All sections dealing with radioactive materials communications requirements),
- Parts 174.700, 175.700, 176.700 and 177.700, sections dealing with carrier requirements for radioactive materials shipments.

Grella, A.W., ''Regulation of nuclear waste transportation,'' In *Radioactive Waste Technology*. Moghissi, A.A., et al., eds.; Society of Mechanical Engineers; 407–421, 1986.

Nuclear Regulatory Commission. *Packaging and Transportation of Radioactive Materials*. 10 CFR Part 71; Government Printing Office; Washington, DC.

Nuclear Regulatory Commission Appendix F. *Requirements for Low Level Waste Transfer for Disposal at Land Disposal Facilities and Manifests*. Code of Federal Regulations 10 CFR Part 20 et al. *FR*23468–23470; U.S. Government Printing Office; Washington, DC; Tuesday, May 21, 1991.

Nuclear Regulatory Commission. *Clarification of Several Aspects of Removable Radioactive Surface Contamination Limits for Transportation Packages*. Information Notice 85–46; USNRC; Washington, DC, 20555; June 10, 1985.

Nuclear Regulatory Commission. *Licensing Requirements for Land Disposal of Radioactive Waste*. Code of Federal Regulations 10 CFR Part 61; U.S. Government Printing Office; Washington, DC; 1991.

Nuclear Regulatory Commission. ''Transportation Regulators: Compatibility with the International Atomic Energy Agency (IAEA),'' *Federal Register*. Proposal to revise 10 CFR 71; Government Printing Office; Washington, DC; 21550; June 8, 1988.

Nuclear Regulatory Commission. ''Transportation Regulations: Compatibility with the Regulations of the International Atomic Energy Agency, Notice of Proposed Rule,'' *Federal Register*. 49 CFR Part 171, et al., Part II; Government Printing Office; Washington, DC; Nov. 14, 1989.

Nuclear Regulatory Commission. *Technical Position on Concentration Averaging and Encapsulation*. Letter to Licensees; Division of Waste Management; January 17, 1995.

Osborne, T.O., Personal Communication; 1996.

CHAPTER 15

IONIZING RADIATION BIOEFFECTS AND RISKS

Radiation protection requires an understanding of the prompt and late biological effects of radiation and numerical estimates of radiation risks. This chapter presents the characteristics of the ''acute radiation syndrome'' which can occur if an individual is exposed to high doses of radiation, and the effects of high levels of radiation on the skin. It also describes the late bioeffects of low levels of low LET radiation on individuals and the whole population. These risks are quantified and are put in perspective by comparison to other societal hazards.

Several national and international groups, including the National Academy of Sciences, National Research Council Committee on the Biological Effects of Ionizing Radiation (BEIR), and the United Nations Scientific Committee on the Effects of Atomic Radiation (UNSCEAR) have reviewed the available data on the effects of radiation on humans, primarily effects associated with low energy transfer (LET) radiation, and reported their conclusions in several reports, the conclusions of which are summarized in this text. In some cases their conclusions have been interpreted by other bodies, i.e., the International Commission on Radiation Protection (ICRP) in order to set limits for protection of radiation workers and the public. These data have been presented elsewhere in this text (Chapter 4). Comparisons are given between the various reports of UNSCEAR, the ICRP and the BEIR committees.

The BEIR IV report (NAS/NRC, 1988) on health risks of internally deposited alpha emitters addresses radon (Rn), polonium (Po), radium (Ra), thorium (Th), uranium (U), and the transuranic elements, principally plutonium (Pu), with a major proportion devoted to the analysis for estimating the lung cancer risk from radon.

In deriving risk estimates for exposure to low levels of ionizing radiation the BEIR V Committee (NAS/NRC, 1988) performed its own evaluations of available data rather than relying solely on information in the scientific literature. For the most part, estimates on radiation risk of cancer induction are based on human data from studies of the following exposed populations: survivors of the atomic bombings in Japan; x-rayed tuberculosis patients, and persons exposed during treatment for ankylosing spondylitis, cervical cancer, and tinea capitas. The Committee based its nominal estimates of cancer risk primarily on data from the Life Span Study of the Japanese atomic bomb survivors, using data from other studies for estimation of incidence or mortality risks for specific sites.

Heritable effects of ionizing radiation exposure have not been ''clearly'' demonstrated in humans, but genetic effects of radiation on the reproductive cells of the mouse have been quantitated. The Committee's estimates of genetic risk in humans is based on extrapolation of mice data to humans and is thus ''highly uncertain''. An additional uncertainty arises from the lack of knowledge of the contribution from disorders of complex genetic origins.

Data on the frequency of severe mental retardation in the Japanese atomic bomb survivors is not sufficiently precise to define a dose response relationship for the exposed fetus. However, findings of an excess frequency of mental retardation in children exposed at 8–15 weeks of gestational age suggests that there may be no threshold for the effect during the period when the fetal brain is in its most sensitive stage of development.

BEIR IV and BEIR V risk estimates for excess cancer mortality, hereditary effects and severe mental retardation are provided in tables in this chapter.

The 1990 recommendations of the ICRP are based on the UNSCEAR 1988. The analysis of radiation risk employed by the ICRP in its recent recommendations is abstracted and also presented in this chapter.[a]

TABLE OF CONTENTS

[a] This chapter was composed and updated by William A. Mills.

Table 15.1 Acute Radiation Syndrome (After IAEA 88, 1988)

Grouping	Range of Doses (Gy)
1. Hematopoietic	1–10
a. From 0 to 0.25 Gy: No clinical symptoms but a slightly increased frequency of chromosome aberrations may be detected in lymphocytes.	
b. From 0.25 to 1 Gy: Either no symptoms or transient nausea. Biological tests may reveal a lymphopenia accompanied in some cases by slight thrombopenia. Cytogenetic changes in lymphocytes are readily detected. Some studies have shown slight changes in the patient's electroencephalogram.	
2. Gastrointestinal	10–20
3. Cardiovascular or Toxemic	20–50
4. Nervous System	Above 50

Table 15.1.1 Acute and Delayed Noncancer Effects of Low LET Radiation and Approximate Single Doses for 50% Incidence in People (Lushbaugh 1981, USNRC, 1975)

Irradiation	Health Effect		Rad Dose for 50% Incidence[a,b]
Whole Body (External)	Anorexia		150
	Nausea		210
	Fatigue		220
	Vomiting		280
	Epilation		300
	Diarrhea		350
	Hemorrhage		400
	Mortality		345
Thorax (External)	Pneumonitis		1050
	Mortality		1700[c]
Lung (Internal)	Mortality		>10,000[c]
Abdomen (External)	Mortality		>1500
Gastrointestinal Tract (Internal)	Mortality		>3000[c]
Reproductive Organs (External)	Sterility	Males (temporary)	80
		Females (permanent)	200

[a] Doses at which 10% incidence would be expected are approximately one fourth of those listed. Protraction of the radiation exposure increases the dose required for each level of effect. For example, one mathematical model for predicting mortality estimates the 50% lethal dose in rad by using the expression:

$$LD_{50} - 345\ t^{0.26}$$

where t is the time in weeks over which the radiation is delivered and 345 rad is the 50% lethal dose for low LET radiation delivered in less than one week. The equivalent 10% and 90% lethal dose values are 110 rad and 585 rad, respectively. (Lushbaugh 1981)

[b] To obtain Gy dose divide by 100.

[c] Projected from studies in laboratory animals.

Table 15.2 Clinical Course of Acute Radiation Syndrome (Courtesy IAEA from Safety Series No. 88, 1988)

Acute Radiation Syndrome	Approximate Duration (for hematopoietic syndrome)
Time from exposure to symptoms	Minutes to hours
Prodromal phase	1–7 days
Latent phase	7–21 days
Critical phase	From second or third week up to the seventh week
Recovery	8–15 weeks
Symptoms and Signs in Prodromal Stage of Acute Radiation Syndrome (in approximate order of increasing severity)	
Anorexia	Shock
Nausea	Oliguria
Vomiting	Ataxia
Weakness and fatigue	Disorientation
Prostration	Coma
Diarrhea	Death
Conjunctivitis	
Erythema	
Hyperesthesia, paraesthesia	
Symptoms and Signs in Critical Phase of Acute Radiation Syndrome	
Fever	Infection
Abdominal pain	Purpura
Abdominal distention	Hemorrhage
Scalp pain	Weight loss
Epilation	

Salient features of the haematopoietic form of the acute radiation symdrome in man

Haematopoietic form	Characteristic signs and symptoms	Underlying pathology
Prodromal phase	Anorexia Nausea Vomiting	
Bone marrow depression phase	Purpura Haemorrhage Susceptibility to infection	Bone marrow aplasia Leukopenia Thrombocytopenia Anaemia

Severity of reaction

0 2 4 6 8 Weeks post-exposure

Salient features of the gastrointestinal form of the acute radiation syndrome

Gast-ointestinal form	Characteristic signs and symptoms	Underlying pathology
Prodromal phase	Anorexia Nausea Vomiting	
Radiation induced enterocolitis	Fever Diarrhoea Disturbance of electrolyte balance	Mitotic arrest in epithelium Denudation and ulceration of intestinal wall

Severity of reaction

0 2 4 6 8 20 12 Days post-exposure

Central nervous system form of the acute radiation syndrome

Cerebral form	Characteristic signs and symptoms	Underlying pathology
Prodromal phase	Anorexia Nausea Vomiting	
Inflammatory reactions	Apathy Lethargy Somnolence	Vasculitis Meningitis Encephalitis Brain oedema
Convulsive phase	Tremor Convulsions Ataxia	Pyknosis of cerebellar granule cells

Severity of reaction

0 2 4 6 8 20 12

Hours post-exposure

Figure 15.1 Acute Radiation Syndrome Features. Cardiovascular and toxemic syndromes are not included (From Upton, 1969, with permission of author)

Table 15.2.1 Skin Effects after Single-Fraction Irradiation (With Permission From Wagner et al., 1994)

Effect	Single-Dose Threshold (Gy)	Onset	Peak
Temporary epilation	3	~3 wk	
Permanent epilation	7	~3 wk	
Early transient erythema	2	hours	~24 h
Main erythema	6	~10 d	~2 wk
Dry desquamation	10	~4 wk	~5 wk
Moist desquamation	15	~4 wk	~5 wk
Late erythema	15	~6–10 wk	
Secondary ulceration	20	>6 wk	
Dermal necrosis	18	>10 wk	
Dermal atrophy	11	>14 wk	
Telangiectasia	12	>52 wk	
Invasive fibrosis	10		

(With permission from Wagner, L.K., Eifel, P.J., and Geise, R.A.; ''Patented Biological Effects Following High X-Ray Dose Interventional Procedures; Journal of Vascular and Interventional Radiology 5:71–84, 1994.)

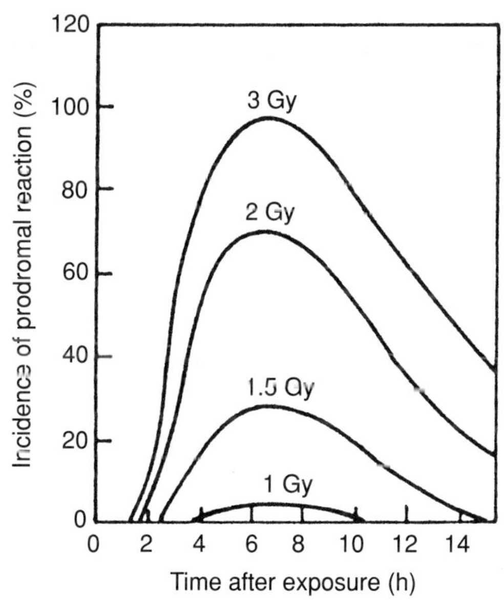

Figure 15.2 Estimated Incidence and Timing of Prodromal Symptoms in Man in Relation to Absorbed Doses Received at a Low Linear Energy Transfer (LET) (Courtesy IAEA from Safety Series 88, 1988)

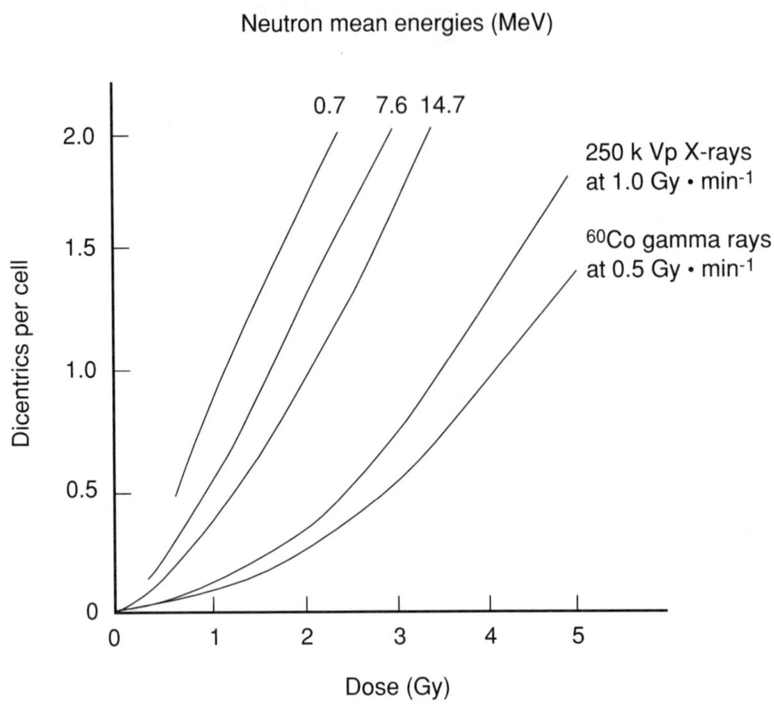

Figure 15.3 Relationship Between Dicentric Yield and Acute Exposure to Several Types of Radiation (From Lloyd, 1981, with permission)

Table 15.3 Radon (After National Academy of Science/National Research Council, BEIR IV, 1988)

Regardless of whether the primary source is radon in air or radon in potable water, the risk of cancer due to exposure to radon is the risk of lung cancer following inhalation of radon progeny. [To assess the associated inhalation lung cancer risk from radon in water, the most accepted transport ratio of radon in air to radon in water is on the order of 10^{-4} (Nazaroff et al., 1988)]. The BEIR IV Committee considered two approaches for deriving inhalation risk estimates for radon in air: a dosimetric approach based on modeling the dose to target cells in the respiratory tract and an epidemiologic approach based directly on the ''substantial'' body of available human data. The Committee chose the epidemiological approach, analyzing four sets of underground miner data.

For radon progeny in air the BEIR IV Committee recommends an age specific relative risk, time since exposure, model of the form:

BEIR IV: RELATIVE RISK MODEL FOR RADON PROGENY

$$r(a) = r_0(a)\{1 + 0.025\gamma(a)[W_1 + 0.5 W_2]\}$$

where,
- a = specific age of individual at risk;
- $r(a)$ = age specific lung cancer mortality rate;
- $r_0(a)$ = age specific baseline lung cancer mortality rate;
- $\gamma(a)$ = 1.2, when ''a'' is <55 y, 1.0, when ''a'' is 55–65 y, and 0.4, when ''a'' is ≥65 y;
- W_1 = working level months, WLM, incurred between 5 and 15 y before age ''a''
- W_2 = working level months, WLM, incurred 15 or more years before age ''a''

In this general relative risk model, $r_0(a)$ is the total lung cancer mortality rate from all causative agents, not just the rate due to radon exposure. Designating the lifetime probability of lung cancer mortality in a nonexposed person to radon as R_0 and that of an exposed person as R_e, the ratio of lifetime risks R_e/R_0 is the proportional increased lifetime risk associated with exposure to radon progeny and the excess risk is R_e-R_0. It is important to note that the excess relative risk due to radon in this model varies with time since exposure (TSE); thus, cumulative exposure occurring 15 or more years prior to age (a) is discounted by 50%. This discounting of prior exposures is, in principle, consistent with the model adopted earlier by the National Council on Radiation Protection and Measurements which included a factor for diminishing of risk from prior exposures with a half time of 20 years (NCRP 1988).

In calculating R_e/R_0, the BEIR IV Committee considered confounding factors of sex and smoking status, assuming cigarette smoking to have a multiplicative interaction with radon exposure. No adjustments were made in baseline rates (R_0) for levels of ''ambient radon progeny,'' concluding that ''this correction would be small'' compared with the overall uncertainty in the estimates. Interestingly, the Committee included estimates for an exposure rate of 0.1 WLM/y, which represents a relatively small increase in the U.S. ''ambient'' average indoor exposure rate of 0.2 WLM/y.

Table 15.3.1 provides BEIR IV modified estimates (See Table 15.3.4) of increased risk of lung cancer mortality due to radon exposure, according to sex and designation as smoker or nonsmoker. Smokers are assumed to be only cigarette smokers who start their habit at the age of 18 and continue at a steady state consumption rate for life. For comparable smoking status, males have about a 2× greater excess risk than females, and for both sexes, smokers have about a 10× greater excess risk than nonsmokers.

Table 15.3.1 Increase in Lifetime Risks of Lung Cancer Death Resulting from Exposure to Radon Daughters[a] (After National Academy of Sciences/National Research Council BEIR IV, 1988)

	Males						Females					
Exposure Rate	Nonsmokers			Smokers			Nonsmokers			Smokers		
(WLM/yr)	R_e/R_0	R_e	R_e-R_0	R_e/R_0	R_e	R_e-R_0	R_e/R_0	R_e	R_e-R_0	R_e/R_0	R_e	R_e-R_0
0	1.0	0.0112	0	1.0	0.123	0	1.0	0.00603	0	1.0	0.0582	0
0.1	1.06	0.0118	0.0006	1.05	0.129	0.006	1.06	0.00637	0.00034	1.06	0.0614	0.0032
0.2	1.11	0.0124	0.0012	1.10	0.135	0.012	1.11	0.00672	0.00069	1.11	0.0646	0.0064
0.3	1.16	0.0131	0.0019	1.15	0.141	0.018	1.17	0.00706	0.00103	1.16	0.0678	0.0096
0.4	1.22	0.0137	0.0025	1.20	0.147	0.024	1.23	0.00741	0.00138	1.22	0.0710	0.0128
0.5	1.27	0.0143	0.0031	1.24	0.153	0.030	1.28	0.00775	0.00172	1.27	0.0742	0.0160
0.6	1.33	0.0149	0.0037	1.29	0.159	0.036	1.34	0.00809	0.00206	1.33	0.0773	0.0191
0.8	1.44	0.0161	0.0049	1.39	0.170	0.047	1.46	0.00878	0.00275	1.44	0.0836	0.0254
1.0	1.54	0.0173	0.0061	1.48	0.182	0.059	1.57	0.00946	0.00343	1.54	0.0898	0.0316
1.5	1.82	0.0204	0.0092	1.70	0.209	0.086	1.85	0.0112	0.00517	1.80	0.105	0.0468
2.0	2.08	0.0234	0.0122	1.91	0.235	0.112	2.14	0.0129	0.00687	2.06	0.120	0.0618
2.5	2.35	0.0264	0.0152	2.12	0.260	0.137	2.42	0.0146	0.00857	2.32	0.135	0.0768
3.0	2.62	0.0294	0.0182	2.31	0.284	0.161	2.70	0.0163	0.0103	2.56	0.149	0.0908
3.5	2.89	0.0324	0.0212	2.49	0.306	0.183	2.98	0.0180	0.0112	2.81	0.163	0.105
4.0	3.15	0.0354	0.0242	2.66	0.328	0.205	3.26	0.0197	0.0137	3.04	0.177	0.119
4.5	3.41	0.0383	0.0271	2.83	0.348	0.225	3.55	0.0214	0.0154	3.28	0.191	0.133
5.0	3.68	0.0413	0.0301	2.99	0.368	0.245	3.83	0.0231	0.0171	3.51	0.204	0.146
10.0	6.24	0.0700	0.0588	4.24	0.521	0.398	6.59	0.0398	0.0338	5.56	0.324	0.266

[a] R_0 = Baseline risk relative to persons of the same sex and smoking status. Value is not corrected for risk associated with average ambient radon daughter exposure rate of 0.2 WLM/y.
R_e = Total risk of lung cancer mortality.
R_e-R_0 = Excess risk of lung cancer mortality associated with annual radon daughter exposure rate.
Note: The Table is modified from that shown in BEIR IV by the added column for R_e-R_0 (i.e., the added risk due to the radon exposure rate).

It is noteworthy that although the ratio of lifetime risks R_e/R_0 was the Committee's preferred measure of increased risk, it considered the number of years lost because of radon exposure also as a measure of risk. The Committee provided similar table entries of estimates for the differences between the expected years of life from birth for a ''nonexposed'' subject (L_0) and that of an exposed subject (L_e), where L_0 is the average lifetime of nonsmokers. For a lifetime exposure range of 0.1 WLM/y to 10. WLM/y values of L_0-L_e range from about 3 days to 10 months in male nonsmokers, 1.6 years to 9 years in male smokers, 2 days to 7 months in female nonsmokers, and 10 months to 6 years in female smokers. According to the Committee, the number of years of life lost by those who actually die of lung cancer is typically about 15 years for males and 18 years for females.

For convenience in transposing from ''traditional'' units for expressing radon concentrations (e.g., pCi/L) to SI International System of units (e.g., Bq/m^3), selected values of exposure rate and corresponding R_e/R_0 ratios are shown in Table 15.3.2.

Table 15.3.2 Lifetime Risk of Lung Cancer Mortality for Lifetime Exposure to Radon Concentrations Expressed in Traditional and SI Units (After National Academy of Sciences/National Research Council BEIR IV, 1988)

Exposure[a]			Males		Females	
			Ratio = $\frac{\text{Total Lung Cancer Risk } (R_e)}{\text{Baseline Lung Cancer Risk } (R_0)}$			
$pCi\ L^{-1}$	$Bq\ m^{-3(b)}$	Exposure Rate ($WLM\ y^{-1}$)	Nonsmoker $R_0 = 0.0112$	Smoker $R_0 = 0.123$	Nonsmoker $R_0 = 0.00603$	Smoker $R_0 = 0.0582$
0	0	0[c]	1.00	1.00	1.00	1.00
0.7	25	0.1	1.06	1.05	1.06	1.06
2	74	0.3	1.16	1.15	1.17	1.16
4	150	0.6	1.33	1.29	1.34	1.33
10	370	1.5	1.82	1.70	1.85	1.80
20	740	3.0	2.62	2.31	2.70	2.56
30	1100	4.5	3.41	2.83	3.55	3.28
67	2500	10.0	6.24	4.24	6.59	5.56

[a] Neglecting ''ambient'' radon background level.
Conversion assumptions for Exposure Rate/Exposure:
$[R_n\ DP]$ to $[R_n]$ equilibrium = 0.4
WL to $[R_n]$ = 0.01 WL/pCi L^{-1}
Year at 1 WL = 51.5 WLM/y
Indoor ''home'' occupancy = 75%

[b] 1 pCi/L = 37 Bq/m^3

[c] Included are indoor $[R_n]$ = 1.5 pCi L^{-1} or 0.2 WLM y^{-1}.

BEIR IV also provided lifetime risk coefficients for various ages at which exposure to radon progeny begins and ends, taking into account a 10 year latency period for lung cancer to be manifested. At the start of exposure ages ranged from 0 to 60 years. At the end of exposure ages ranged from 10 to 110 years. As an example, Table 15.3.3 shows values for males and females continuously exposed during the appropriate time period to a rate of 1 WLM/y.

Table 15.3.3 Lifetime Risks (R_e/R_0) for Various Age Dependent Radon Exposure Periods[a] (After National Academy of Sciences/National Research Council BEIR IV, 1988)

Males
Exposure Rate = 1.00 WLM/yr

	Age (yr) Exposure Ends								
Age (yr) Started	10	20	30	40	50	60	70	80	110
0	1.076	1.151	1.226	1.305	1.391	1.460	1.496	1.509	1.512
10		1.076	1.151	1.231	1.318	1.388	1.424	1.437	1.440
20			1.076	1.157	1.244	1.314	1.351	1.364	1.367
30				1.081	1.169	1.240	1.276	1.290	1.293
40					1.088	1.160	1.197	1.211	1.213
50						1.072	1.109	1.123	1.126
60							1.038	1.052	1.054

Females
Exposure Rate = 1.00 WLM/yr

	Age (yr) Exposure Ends								
Age (yr) Started	10	20	30	40	50	60	70	80	110
0	1.082	1.165	1.248	1.338	1.432	1.504	1.539	1.555	1.560
10		1.083	1.166	1.256	1.351	1.422	1.458	1.473	1.479
20			1.084	1.174	1.269	1.341	1.376	1.392	1.397
30				1.090	1.186	1.258	1.293	1.309	1.314
40					1.096	1.168	1.203	1.219	1.224
50						1.072	1.108	1.124	1.129
60							1.036	1.052	1.057

[a] Smoking status of population unspecified.

Assuming an equal number of males and females in a given population with an unspecified smoking characterization, the BEIR IV nominal lifetime risk of lung cancer mortality due to lifetime exposure to radon progeny is **350 cancer deaths per 10^6 person WLM.**

However, this value is based on the BEIR IV Committee's assumption ''. . .that an exposure of 1 WLM in a home and exposure to 1 WLM in a mine have equivalent potency in causing lung cancer.'' Since the publication of BEIR IV, a NAS/NRC Panel has examined this assumption in regard to dosimetric considerations and concluded that the dose per unit exposure delivered to target cells in the respiratory tract for those exposed in the home environment should be reduced by about 30% for adults of both sexes and by 20% or less for infants and children aged 10 or less (NAS/NRC 1991). Thus, for a life span of 70 years, the reduction is about 30%, and for the home environment the reduced BEIR IV risk coefficient becomes about **250 cancer deaths per 10^6 person WLM.**

Table 15.3.4 shows averaged dosimetric modifying factors given in the NAS/NRC Panel's report.

Table 15.3.4 Dosimetric Modifying Factors for Converting Radon Risk Estimates for Miners to Members in the General Population (After National Academy of Sciences/National Research Council, 1991)

Subject Category	Modifying Factor[a]
Infant, age 1 mo	0.69
Child, age 1 year	0.94
Child, age 5–10 yr	0.78
Female (adult)	0.67
Male (adult)	0.71
Average lifetime	0.71

[a] Averaged for secretory and basal target cells.

It is clear that smoking status plays a key role in attempting to estimate an individual's risk from radon exposure. The principal cause of lung cancer in the U.S. is cigarette smoking. Annual lung cancer mortality rates in the U.S. track very well with U.S. cigarette consumption. Of the estimated 143,000 lung cancer deaths expected in 1991, 83%, or about 120,000, can be attributed to cigarette smoking (85% among men and 75% among women). (American Cancer Society, 1991)

If one assumes a per capita radon progeny exposure rate of 0.2 WLM/y for a U.S. population of 250 million and the reduced BEIR IV risk coefficient, an estimated 12,000 lung cancer deaths in 1991 can be attributed to radon exposure. However, 10,000 of these cases would occur in smokers and only about 2,000 in nonsmokers, including those at risk from "environmental tobacco smoke" in the home. The vast majority of these radon-attributable lung cancers are associated with radon progeny exposures below the U.S. Environmental Protection Agency's indoor radon guide of 4 pCi/L.

The UNSCEAR review generally supports risk estimates and the relative risk model reported in BEIR V. The report suggests that a less than multiplicative risk model may underestimate risk to nonsmokers and overestimate risk to smokers; also, that confounding carcinogens found in underground mine environments, such as asbestos, require further evaluation. Two notable conclusions reported are (i) ". . . little direct evidence on the risks of lung cancer resulting from residential exposure to radon," (geographical studies being difficult to interpret, rendering) ". . . them unsuitable for use in risk estimation;" and (ii) ". . . no consistent evidence that radon causes cancer in tissues other than lung."

Table 15.4 Radium

Radium toxicity has been studied for more than a half century and continues to be of great interest, not only for its radioepidemiological significance but also because of its ubiquity in our environment. The history of radiation protection is intimately associated with epidemiologic studies of radium toxicity.

Until the introduction of the concept of effective dose equivalent (now effective dose) by the ICRP in 1977, occupational limits in radiation protection for internal emitters were based on a level of safety associated with a ^{226}Ra body burden equal to 0.1 μCi. The selection of this body burden value was done because at or below this level no increase in bone cancer was observed in the extensive studies of radium-dial painters. Maximum permissible body burdens (MPBB) and maximum permissible concentrations (MPC) in air or water for other internally deposited radionuclides were determined by dosimetric comparisons to this radium level of 0.1 μCi. Limits for the public were assumed to be 1/10 of the occupational limit.

ICRP Publication 26 recommended a different approach to controlling exposures resulting from internally deposited radionuclides. Under the ICRP's approach, the limits for internally deposited radionuclides are based on comparisons to total body risk associated with an acute (in time) exposure to low-LET radiation. Since effective dose is dependent on two quantitatively uncertain weighting factors, organ radiosensitivity and an alpha quality factor, this approach seems, at least for risk assessment, less sound scientifically than the earlier approach using body burden, concentrations, absorbed dose, and critical organs. For protection against radium risks, the earlier approach appears to be especially appropriate.

The biological endpoints associated with the ingestion of radium (the primary pathway for human intake) are bone sarcomas and facial carcinomas; specifically carcinomas of the paranasal sinuses and mastoids. Facial carcinomas are considered to be due, at least partially, to exposure to radon and its progeny resulting from the decay of ^{226}Ra deposited in bone. It is noteworthy that except perhaps for the irradiation of bone sarcomas by the shorter half-life injected ^{224}Ra, leukemia has not been shown to be a discernable risk following radium ingestion.

Although the BEIR IV Committee offered a lifetime ^{224}Ra risk estimate for bone sarcoma of 2×10^{-4} rad, the Committee, unfortunately, chose not to suggest risk coefficients for the radium nuclides of general interest in the practice of radiation protection, i.e., radium-226 and radium-228. Studies of injected ^{224}Ra has limited application to radiation protection because of its short half life that limits exposure to bone surfaces and does not become a source of long-term exposure to bone.

In addition to a risk coefficient for ^{224}Ra, Table 15.4.1 shows risk coefficients for ^{226}Ra and ^{228}Ra derived from BEIR IV and Mays et al. but not presented in these documents as recommended values *per se*.

Only bone sarcomas and sinus carcinomas have been found as a result of radium deposition in skeleton and ''any practical threshold, if it exists at all, cannot be greater than 1 Gy. Skeletal deposition does not result in a risk of leukemia. Studies of geographical association between the level of ^{226}Ra in ground or drinking waters ''. . . are not convincing and, in fact, are typical of geographical correlation studies.'' Studies of radium injected patients and workers show a lifetime excess absolute bone cancer risk of 0.05% per Sv and a minimum latency no more than 3 years, independent of sex and age at exposure.

Table 15.4.1 Radium—Risk Coefficients and Latency for Radium Ingestion

Radium-226		
Bone Cancer[a]	37×10^{-6}/rad (skeletal)	5 y latency
Facial Carcinoma	52×10^{-6}/rad (skeletal)[b]	10 y latency
Radium-228		
Bone Cancer[a]	88×10^{-6}/rad (skeletal)	11 y latency
Radium-224		
Bone Cancer	200×10^{-6}/rad (skeletal)	5 y latency

[a] Values taken from BEIR IV, Table 7A-2.

[b] Based on facial carcinomas to bone sarcomas ratio of 1.4 (Mays 1985).

Table 15.5 Polonium

There are over 25 isotopes of polonium, all of which are radioactive and most of which are alpha emitters. The important radioisotopes of interest to radiation protection are ^{210}Po, ^{214}Po, and ^{218}Po, with the latter two being important as progeny from the decay of ^{222}Rn. ^{210}Po is a major contributor to the internal dose received from natural radionuclides in the body, the other isotope being ^{40}K. Radiation protection interests in ^{210}Po result from its use in experimental work, as a source of neutrons from the (α, n) reaction, and in consumer applications, such as static eliminator devices. Polonium in tobacco has been implicated as a contributing factor in the induction of lung cancer in smokers.

No direct evidence of health effects from exposure to polonium exists. Therefore, estimates applicable to risk assessments for radiation protection must be obtained indirectly from results with other alpha emitters. The BEIR IV report concluded, that the toxicity of polonium is comparable to plutonium-239 and about 5 times that of ^{226}Ra. Risk is presented in Table 15.4.1 for ^{226}Ra. Over very long exposure times and very low doses, its toxicity approaches that of ^{226}Ra. This implies ^{210}Po tumor risk estimates of the order of 10^{-5}/rad.

Among a cohort of US workers monitored for ^{210}Po, mortality was less than expected and no significant dose-response trend was observed for all cancer or specific cancers.

Table 15.6 Thorium—Lifetime Excess Cancer Risks from Thorotrast (Courtesy National Academy of Sciences/National Research Council from BEIR IV, 1988)

Tissue	Risk Coefficient Per 10^6 Person Rad (tissue)	Latency (yr)
Liver	260–300	20
Bone Marrow (Leukemia)	50–60	5
Bone	55–120	10

Considerable uncertainty exists in these estimates because of nonuniform tissue distribution, the chemistry of thorium, and incomplete follow up in the epidemiologic studies. As concluded by BEIR IV, "The extent to which these risk numbers apply to thorium radionuclides in other forms is unknown."

There is strong evidence of liver cancer resulting from injected Thorotrast that is retained in the body more or less indefinitely. The minimum latency period is about 10 years and the risk appears independent of sex but higher among those injected at younger ages. The absolute excess risk of malignant liver cancer is estimated to be about 300×10^{-4} per Gy or 15×10^{-4} per Sv.

Table 15.7 Uranium

The major pathway for uranium transport to humans is through ingestion, principally of food, although water is an important source in some geographical areas. The uptake by the GI tract is low, about 1% even for soluble materials. Although the skeleton is the major site of deposition, the biological half life in bone is short, attaining equilibrium between intake and excretion. Other organ sites of depositions of natural uranium are the lung, liver, and kidney.

Health concerns are not limited to its radiation toxicity due to alpha particle decay, but also included its chemical toxicity in inducing kidney damage, i.e., a nephrotoxic effect. The BEIR IV Committee concluded that it is premature to provide a risk estimate for the probability of developing renal damage from uranium, but noted that estimates for a threshold concentration range from 3 to ≤ 0.1 μg/g depending upon the choice of animal species and metabolic model.

Both animal and epidemiologic studies support the conclusion that the induction of bone sarcoma is the most probable health effect following human exposure to uranium, especially to high specific activity uranium such as reactor produced ^{233}U. There is a suggestion of risk of lung cancer in humans from chronic inhalation of uranium dust in the workplace; however, the Committee concluded that quantification of this risk ''. . . cannot be determined from published epidemiological studies because of confounding factors and the limited power of the surveys. . .''

The likelihood of bone sarcomas being induced in the general population from exposure to environmental natural uranium concentrations is ''virtually zero'' when the estimate is based on a quadratic dose response relationship. Even assuming a linear dose-response relationship and a constant nonoccupational intake of 1 pCi/day (estimated average U.S. daily intake from food and water consumption), the risk is relatively low. Mays et al. reported a **Lifetime risk of bone sarcoma = 1.5 × 10^{-6}/pCi day^{-1}** or about 1 × 10^{-5}/rad (Mays 1985).

However, perhaps more importantly, the BEIR IV Committee concluded that, ''. . . exposure to natural uranium is unlikely to be a significant health risk in the population and may well have no measurable effect.''

No health hazards specific to uranium workers in the nuclear industry (not including miners exposed to radon) have been identified. The number of deaths observed from lung cancer in uranium millers is found to be less than expected and no excess of bone cancer has been observed. However, there is evidence of non-leukemia cancer in hematopoietic tissues.

Table 15.8 Transuranic Elements

Transuranic (TRU) elements are actinides with atomic numbers from 93 (neptunium) through 103 (lawrencium). Most have isotopes with half lives of the order of minutes or less and, thus, are not of substantive health concern. The nuclides of greater interest in radiation protection are ^{237}Np, ^{238}Pu and ^{239}Pu, ^{241}Am, and ^{244}Cm. The most studied of these elements in regard to biological effects is plutonium, especially plutonium in the form of plutonium oxide ($^{239}PuO_2$) which is highly insoluble.

Studies of nuclear workers exposed to plutonium provide ''no clear evidence'' of cancer.

Transuranic Elements Risk Estimates (After National Academy of Sciences/National Research Council from BEIR IV, 1988)

Organ	Cancer Deaths Per 10^6 Person Rad	Human Data Base
Lung	500[a]	Radon progeny
Bone	80–1100	Radium
Liver	300	Thorotrast

[a] Panel modified BEIR IV: 250 cases per 10^6 person WLM.

Table 15.9 Iodine

Risk estimation for radiation-induced thyroid cancer is based primarily on studies of children exposed to x-rays for the treatment of a variety of benign diseases such as thymic enlargement and *tinea capitas*. Data from experimental animal studies and limited human data (e.g., Marshall Islanders exposed to weapon testing fallout) suggest however, that ^{131}I is less of a carcinogen than x-rays; probably due to differences in dose rate and distribution of dose within the thyroid (NCRP 80). The NCRP recommends that the organ dose received from ^{131}I be considered no more that ⅓ as effective as the organ dose received from external radiation. Its model for thyroid cancer risk estimation allows also for sex and age differences.

''No studies have yet provided evidence that an increase in thyroid cancer can be attributed to ^{131}I.'' Most of the evidence relates to adult patients treated with ^{131}I and to thyroid cancer following external radiation. The possibility of substantial risk to children remains of major concern and requires further study, especially children exposed following the Chernobyl nuclear power station accident. Risk estimates cited by UNSCEAR 1994 for thyroid cancer in the a-bomb survivors are:

Mortality—0.094 per Sv, 90%CI (<0.1–0.4), excess relative risk;
—1.2 × 10^4 person-years per Sv, 90%CI (<0.03–0.02), excess absolute risk;
Incidence—1.2 per Sv, 90%CI (0.05–2.1), excess relative risk;
—1.6 per Sv, 90%CI (0.8–2.5), excess absolute.
Effective doses are neutron weighted doses based on an RBE = 10.

The relative risk effectiveness of ^{131}I compared to external radiation is between zero and 0.5 based on human experience, attributable to protraction of the iodine dose and its distribution in thyroid tissue.

Radioiodine Thyroid Cancer (Excess Lifetime Risk Per 10^6 Persons Rad[a]) (Courtesy NCRP from Report 80, 1985)

Exposure Age of Population[b]	Source of Irradiation	Total Cases[c]		Deaths[c]	
		Male	Female	Male	Female
≤18 y	^{125}I, ^{131}I	5	10	0.5	1
	External x- or γ-rays, ^{132}I, ^{133}I, ^{135}I	15	30	1.5	3
>18 y	^{125}I, ^{131}I	3	7	0.3	0.7
	External x- or γ-rays, ^{132}I, ^{133}I, ^{135}I	8	20	0.8	2

[a] Thyroid doses from 6 to 1500 rad; 5 y minimum latency.
[b] Median ages: ≤18 y 9.2 M, 9.3 F
>18 y 38.6 M, 41.4 F
[c] Rounded values.

Table 15.10 Strontium

NCRP has published a comprehensive review of strontium radiobiology (NCRP 1991). Animal studies suggest that the organs at risk from internally deposited strontium, primarily ^{90}Sr, seek bone and blood forming tissues, resulting in the risk of bone sarcomas and leukemia. However, these effects have been observed only at doses of thousands of rad, and the nonlinear dose response curve is similar to that observed for the radium dial painters. The NCRP concluded that, ''The dose response relationships for ^{90}Sr induced bone sarcomas in animal studies are in concordance with but do not prove the existence of a threshold.'' Based on comparisons to ^{226}Ra human data on bone sarcomas and the Japanese A bomb survivor's leukemia data, the NCRP suggested the following risk estimates, and value ranges, as applicable to populations exposed to radiostrontium at low doses and dose rates.

An excess risk of leukemia is reported in a cohort of 28,000 using water contaminated with fission products discharged into the Techa River from the fuel reprocessing facility in the former Soviet Union. Bone marrow doses up to 3 Gy and exposures up to 1 mGy per hour on river banks are reported.

Cancer Risk from Internally Deposited Strontium (Courtesy NCRP from Report 110, 1991)

	Risk Estimate	Range
Bone sarcoma	1 case per 10^6 person rad	0–500
Leukemia	3–6 cases per 10^6 person rad	0–1600

Table 15.11 Summary: Risk Coefficients for Internally Deposited Radionuclides (Tissue/Organ Dose)

Radon	
Lung	350 cancer deaths per 10^6 person WLM (underground miners) 250 cancer deaths per 10^6 person WLM (modified for general population)
Polonium	
^{210}Po	order of 1 cancer death per 10^5 tissue rad
Radium	
^{224}Ra Bone	200 cancer deaths per 10^6 tissue rad (skeletal)
^{226}Ra Bone & Facial	90 cancer deaths per 10^6 tissue rad (skeletal)
^{228}Ra Bone	90 cancer deaths per 10^6 tissue rad (skeletal)
Thorium	
$^{232}ThO_2$	
Liver	300 cancer deaths per 10^6 tissue rad
Bone Marrow	50 leukemia deaths per 10^6 tissue rad
Bone	90 cancer deaths per 10^6 tissue rad
Uranium	
Bone	1 cancer death per 10^6 persons at 1pCi/d (Nephrotoxicity Threshold 3 to ≤ 1 μg/g) of renal tissue
Transuranic Elements	
Lung	700 cancer deaths per 10^6 person rad
Bone	80–1100 cancer deaths per 10^6 person rad
Liver	300 cancer deaths per 10^6 person rad
Iodine	
Thyroid	1 cancer death per 10^6 person rad
Strontium	
Bone	1 cancer death per 10^6 person rad
Bone Marrow	3 cancer deaths per 10^6 person rad

Table 15.12 Carcinogenic Effects—Estimates of Health Risk from Exposure to Low Levels of Ionizing Radiation: BEIR V (Reprinted with permission from *Health Effects of Exposure to Low Levels of Ionizing Radiation: BEIR V*, c. 1990 by the National Academy of Sciences. Published by National Academy Press, Washington, DC)

Table 15.12.1 Cancer Excess Mortality by Age at Exposure and Site for 100,000 Persons of Each Age Exposed to 10 rem (0.1 Sv)[a]

Males

Age at Exposure	Total	Leukemia	Nonleukemia	Respiratory	Digestive	Other
5	1,276	111	1,165	17	361	787
15	1,144	109	1,035	54	369	612
25	921	36	885	124	389	372
35	566	62	504	243	28	233
45	600	108	492	353	22	117
55	616	166	450	393	15	42
65	481	191	290	272	11	7
75	258	165	93	90	5	—
85	110	96	14	17	—	—
Average[b]	770	110	660	190	170	300

Females

Age at Exposure	Total	Leukemia	Nonleukemia	Breast	Respiratory	Digestive	Other
5	1,532	75	1,457	129	48	655	625
15	1,566	72	1,494	295	70	653	476
25	1,178	29	1,149	52	125	679	293
35	557	46	511	43	208	73	187
45	541	73	468	20	277	71	100
55	505	117	388	6	273	64	45
65	386	146	240	—	172	52	16
75	227	127	100	—	72	26	3
85	90	73	17	—	15	4	—
Average[b]	810	80	730	70	150	290	220

[a] Instantaneous exposure

[b] Averages are weighted for the age distribution in a stationary population having 1980 U.S. mortality rates and have been rounded to the nearest 10.

Table 15.12.2 Total Cancer Excess Mortality for All Sites for 100,000 Persons Exposed to 10 rem (0.1 Sv)[a] Averaged for All Ages[b]

Leukemia	100
Nonleukemia	700
Total	800

[a] Instantaneous Exposure

[b] Averages are weighted for the age distribution in a stationary population having 1980 U.S. mortality rates and have been rounded to the nearest 10. Assumes equal populations of males and females.

Table 15.12.3 Total Cancer Excess Mortality for 100,000 Persons Each Continuously Exposed for a Lifetime at a Dose-Equivalent Rate of 0.1 rem per year (0.001 Sv y^{-1}) (Two significant numbers)

	Male	Female	Sex Average[a]
Leukemia	70	60	60
Nonleukemia	450	540	500
Total	520	600	560

[a] Half male and half female population.

Table 15.12.4 Total Cancer Excess Mortality for 100,000 Persons Each Continuously Exposed From Age 18 Until Age 65 at a Dose-Equivalent Rate of 1 rem per year (0.01 Sv y^{-1}) (Two significant numbers)

	Male	Female	Sex Averaged
Leukemia	400	310	360
Nonleukemia	2500	2800	2600
Total	2900	3100	3000

Table 15.12.5 Risks for Low Dose Rate, Low LET Radiation

The Committee recognized that its models for risk estimation were derived from acute exposures either as a single instantaneous exposure or fractionated with high dose rates and that application of its models to continuous low dose rates requires consideration of a dose rate effectiveness factor (DREF). The Committee's ''single best estimate'' of DREF for leukemia is 2.1 (based on human data) and for life shortening and tumorigenesis is 4 (based on laboratory animal studies). The risk estimates for leukemia given above include a DREF of 2 for leukemia, but not the DREF value of 4 for tumorigenesis. If this DREF value of 4 is applied to the nonleukemia risk estimates shown in the above BEIR V Table 15.12.1, the following excess cancer mortality risk estimates for the weighted 1980 U.S. age distribution are derived for low dose rate exposures.

Total Excess Cancer Mortality Risks Estimates for the Weighted 1980 U.S. Age Distribution for Low Dose Rate, Low LET Radiation—100,000 Persons Each Exposed to 10 rem (0.1 Sv)
(Two significant numbers)

	Male	Female	Sex Averaged[a]
Leukemia	110	80	100
Nonleukemia[b]	160	180	170
Total	270	260	270

[a] Half male and half female
[b] DREF of 4 applied to Table 15.12.1 risks. See Table 15.19 for summary DREF factors.

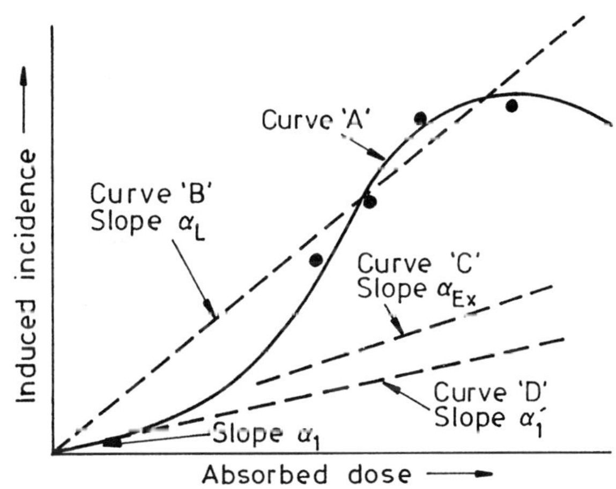

Figure 15.4 Schematic Curves of Incidence Versus Absorbed Dose (Courtesy NCRP from Report 64, 1980)

Table 15.12.6 Characteristics of Life Span Study Population

In considering the findings of the BEIR V Committee it is important to note the number of cancer deaths that can be attributed to radiation exposure in the A bomb survivors study population. Shimizu, et al. report that over the time period from 1950 to 1985, there were a total of 3,435 cancer deaths in a study population of 41,719 survivors who were exposed to a DS86 shielded kerma dose ≥ 0.01 Gy (average dose 0.30 Gy). Of the 3,435 total cancer deaths the estimated excess attributable to exposure is 340, of which 80 are leukemia cases. The total number of leukemia deaths in this population is 144. The table below provides further details on the tissue distribution of these cancer deaths.

Cancer Deaths and Estimated Cancer Deaths Attributable to Radiation in A Bomb Survivors

(With permission Journal of the American Medical Association from Shimizu, et al. *J. Am. Med. Assn.* **264**:601 1990 copyright 1990, American Medical Association)

	Total	Control Population (Exposure: 0 Gy)	Exposed Population (≥ 0.01 Gy)		
			Total	Attributable Risk (%)	Number of Attributable Cancers
Population Size	75,991	34,272	41,719		
Cancer Deaths	5,936	2,501	3,435		340
Leukemia	202	58	144	55	80
Nonleukemia	5,734	2,443	3,291	8	260
Stomach	2,007	854	1,153	6	73
Colon	232	103	129	15	19
Lung	638	253	385	11	44
Breast	156	57	96	22	22
Urinary Tract	133	49	84	23	19
Multiple Myeloma	36	13	23	33	7
(Other Solid Cancers)					(76)

Table 15.13 Heritable Effects—Estimates of Health Risk from Exposure to Low Levels of Ionizing Radiation: BEIR V

By extrapolation from mouse to man, the BEIR V Committee estimates that at least 100 rad (1 Gy) of the low dose rate, low LET radiation is required to double the spontaneous mutation ratio in man. A doubling dose of 100 rem approximates the lower 95% confidence limit for the data from atomic bomb survivors in Japan and the Committee regards the estimates of risk given in the following table ''. . . as being too high rather than too low.'' The table below gives the estimated genetic effects of an average population exposure of 1 rem/30 year generation.

Estimated Genetic Effects of 1 Rem Per Generation (After NAS/NRC BEIR V, 1990)

Type of Disorder	Current Incidence Per 10^6 Liveborn Offspring	Additional Cases Per 10^6 Liveborn Offspring Per Rem Per Generation	
		1st Generation	Equilibrium
Autosomal dominant			
Clinically severe	2500	5–20	25
Clinically mild	7500	1–15	75
X-linked recessive	400	<1	<5
Autosomal recessive	2500	<1	very slow increase
Chromosomal			
Unbalanced translocations	600	<5	very little increase
Trisomies	3800	<1	<1
Congenital abnormalities	20,000–30,000	10	10–100
Others of complex etiology	Hundreds of 1000s	Not Estimated	

Based on the above a conservative estimate of risk of heritable effects, excluding any disorders of complex etiology, the risk of heritable effects is less than 50 additional cases per 10^6 liveborn offspring per average population exposure of 1 rem/30 year generation (first generation) and less than 200 additional cases at generational equilibrium.

Table 15.14 Mental Retardation—Estimates of Health Risks from Exposure to Low Levels of Ionizing Radiation: BEIR V

In humans mental retardation is the best documented consequence of irradiation of the mammalian embryo and fetus during the period of major organogenesis relating to brain development. Among the Japanese atomic bomb survivors irradiated in utero, the prevalence of radiation related mental retardation was highest in those irradiated between 8 and 15 weeks after conception. In this group, the increase appeared to be consistent with a linear, non-threshold response but the data do not exclude a threshold value in the range of 20–40 rad. The diminution in intelligence score under the linear model is about 20–30 points per 100 rad. Figure 15.5 shows the percentage of severe mental retardation observed in the atomic bomb survivors at various fetal doses.

Table 15.15 Summary: BEIR V

Total cancer excess deaths per 10^5 persons receiving instantaneous exposure of 10 rem	800
Total cancer excess deaths per 10^5 persons per lifetime exposure rate of 0.1 rem per year	560
Additional heritable effects per 10^6 liveborn per 1 rem exposure over 30 y generation period	50 (1st generation) 200 (equilibrium)
Diminution in intelligence score per 100 rad in utero exposure	20–30 IQ points

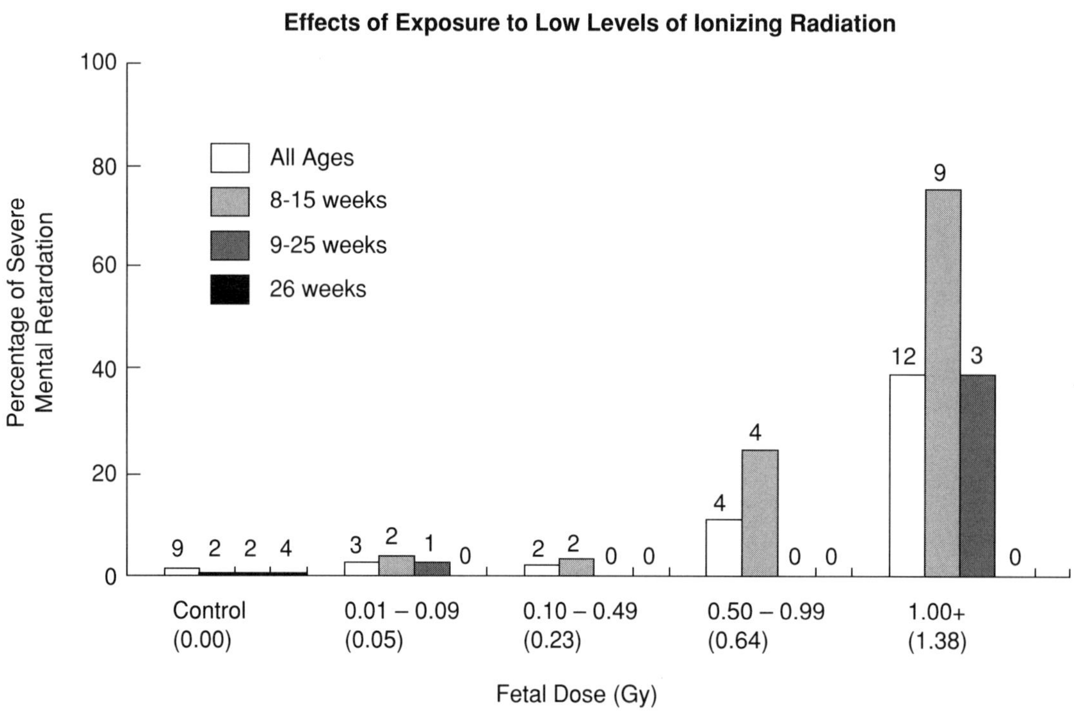

Figure 15.5 Percentages of Severe Mental Retardation at Various Fetal Doses in the Combined Hiroshima and Nagasaki Data. The number of cases is given at the top of the histogram. (With permission RERF from Otake et al., 1987)

Table 15.16 Radiation Risk Models Employed by ICRP Publication No. 60 (1990) (After Vennart, 1991)

Cancer
The ICRP 1990 recommendations employ risk models based on UNSCEAR 1988 Japanese Atomic Bomb survivor observations which, because 60% are still living, require models to predict lifetime risks of radiation from the data presently available. Two models are employed: the so-called ''multiplicative'' which assumes that radiation increases the normal risk of dying of cancer by a constant factor; and a second model which assumes that the risk of dying of cancer following irradiation increases by a constant amount at any age (''additive'' model). These models are illustrated in Figure 15.6.
The projected lifetime risk of fatal cancer estimated by UNSCEAR for the whole Japanese population is 4–11% per Gy of low LET radiation, and 4–8% per Gy for Japanese of working age. The difference reflects the greater sensitivity of young people to radiation-induced cancer. The lower values of the range are for the *additive* model and the higher for the *multiplicative* one. The ICRP employs the higher value of the range.
The ICRP recommends use of a Dose and Dose Rate Effectiveness Factor (DDREF) of 2 for low doses and low dose rates, the bottom end of the values suggested by UNSCEAR, a range for the DDREF of namely 2 to 10.
The lifetime risks of fatal cancer from radiation now recommended by the ICRP are 5×10^{-2} per Sv for a population and 4×10^{-2} per Sv for workers. (The 1977 ICRP value was 1.25×10^{-2} per Sv).

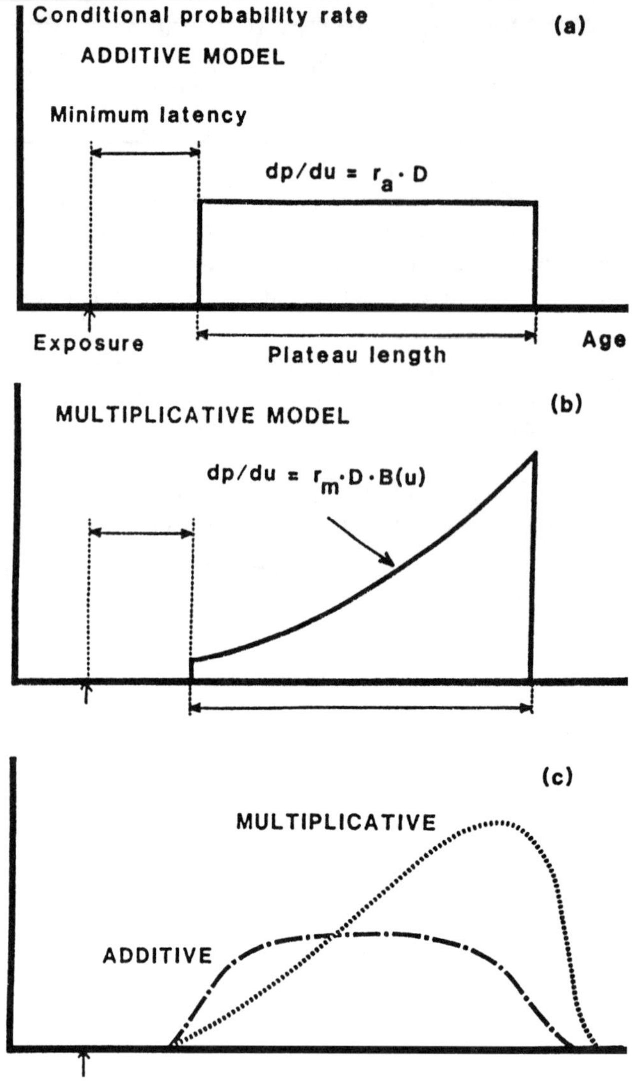

Figure 15.6 Illustration of the Two Simple Projection Models. (Courtesy ICRP 1991)

Figures (a) and (b) show the stylized models. Figure (c) indicates possible curve shapes under more realistic assumptions.

(a) The simple *additive* model: The excess conditional probability rate (of death from cancer) after a single radiation dose, *D*, is assumed to be proportional to the dose, but first after a minimum latency period and over a ''plateau'' period of time. (b) The simple *multiplicative* model: The excess probability rate is also assumed to be proportional to the background rate of cancer death, *B(u)*.

Hereditary Diseases

Risks are derived from animal experiments since human epidemiological studies provide no quantitative information beyond perhaps an upper bound of the risk.

The UNSCEAR 1988 risk for severe hereditary effects to children and grandchildren of exposed individuals is 0.3 $\times 10^{-2}$ per Sv. For all descendants of the irradiated parents it will be 1.2 $\times 10^{-2}$ per Sv. These do not include allowance for disorders of multifactorial origin.

Making allowances for disorders of multifactorial origin, and assuming 40% of an individual's life is genetically significant, the ICRP estimates that the probability of radiation risks of severe hereditary effects in all descendants of a whole population to be 1 $\times 10^{-2}$ per Sv. For workers it is 0.6 $\times 10^{-2}$ per Sv because a smaller fraction of the working life is genetically significant.

For radiation-induced genetic disease the detriment is increased by a factor of 0.8 for the adult worker and 1.3 for the whole population to account for non-fatal hereditary effects.

Detriment

In the earlier ICRP recommendations no allowance was made for the effect of non-fatal cancers on the total detriment. The present recommendations make allowances for the relative loss of life expected for cancers in different organs of the body.

Nominal probability coefficients for the somatic and severe hereditary detriments are presented in the table below.

Table 15.16.1 Nominal Probability Coefficients for Stochastic Effects

	Detriment (10^{-2} Sv^{-1})			
Exposed Population	**Fatal Cancers**	**Non-Fatal Cancers**	**Severe Hereditary Effects**	**Total**
Adult Workers	4.0	0.8	0.8	5.6
Whole Population	5.0	1.0	1.3	7.3

The total detriment (somatic and hereditary effect) allowing for an effect of non-fatal diseases is 7.3 $\times 10^{-2}$/Sv for a whole population and 5.6 $\times 10^{-2}$/Sv for adult workers.

This is 3 to 4 times greater than the 1977 ICRP recommendations.

Ante-natal Exposure Effects

Information now available yields the following conclusions

- Exposure of the embryo in first 3 weeks is likely to result in undetectable death of the conceptus.
- After 3 weeks, effects are deterministic with a threshold estimated to be about 0.1 Gy.
- Irradiation in the period 8–15 weeks (during development of the brain) may reduce the child's IQ by 30 points per Sv.

Table 15.17 Carcinogenic Effects—Risk Coefficients Adopted by the ICRP 1990[a] (After Clark, R.H., 1991)

	ICRP 1990		
Organ or Tissue	**Fatal Cancer (% Sv^{-1})**	**Lethality (%)**	**Loss of Life (y)**
Bladder	0.30	50	9.8
Bone surface	0.05	70	15.0
Breast	0.20	50	18.2
Colon	0.85	55	12.5
Liver	0.15	95	15.0
Lung	0.85	95	13.5
Oesophagus	0.30	95	11.5
Ovary	0.10	70	16.8
Skin	0.02	0.2	15.0
Stomach	1.10	90	12.4
Thyroid	0.08	10	15.0
Red bone marrow	0.50	99	30.9
Remainder	0.50	71	13.7
Subtotal	5.0	—	—
Hereditary defects	1.0[a]	—	20.0
Total		←7.2 (weighted)→	

[a] All generations

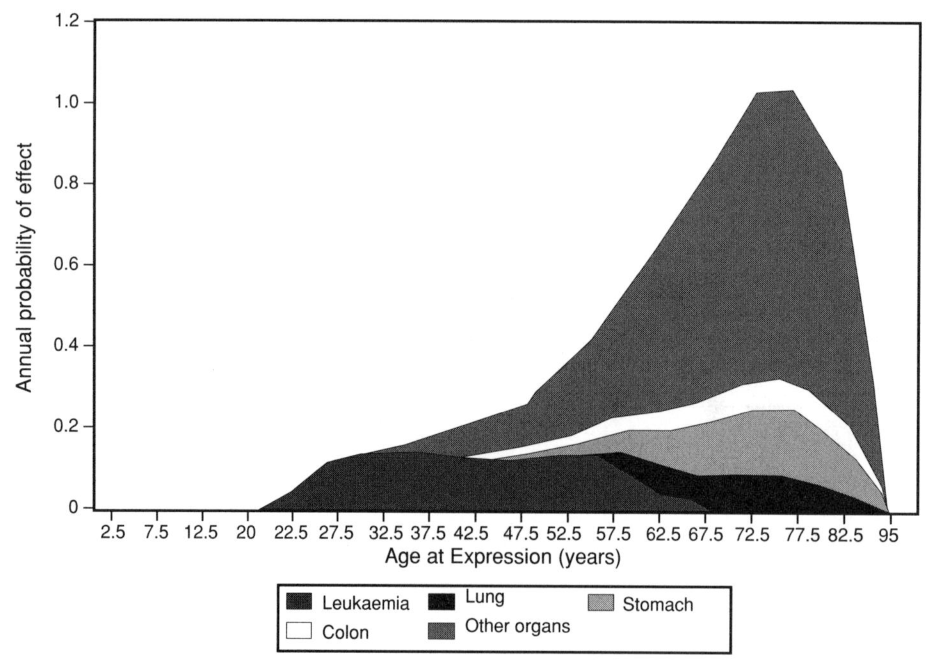

Figure 15.7 Attributable Fatal Cancer Probability (ICRP 1990 Model) to a Male Following a Single Low Dose Exposure of 1 mSv at Age 20 Broken Down According to Cancer Type (With permission publisher from Webb, 1991)

Table 15.18 Comparison of Radiation Risk Estimates from Various Sources—Projected Excess Cumulative Lifetime Mortality from Cancer, All Types Combined, Attributable to 1 Gy Acute Whole-Body Low-LET Irradiation of the General Population. (Courtesy ICRP from Annals, 1991)

Source of Estimate	Additive Risk Projection Model (deaths per 10,000 persons)[a]	Multiplicative Risk Projection Model (deaths per 10,000 persons)[a]
BEIR I, 1972	120[b]	620[b]
UNSCEAR, 1977	250[b]	—
BEIR III, 1980	80[c]–250[b]	230[c]–500[b]
NUREG, 1985	290[c]	520[c]
UNSCEAR, 1988	400[b,d]–500[b,e]	700[b,e]–100[b,d]
BEIR V, 1989	—	885[b,f]

[a] Values rounded; estimates based largely on follow-up of Japanese A bomb survivors, analyzed with T65D dosimetry prior to 1988 and with DS-86 dosimetry thereafter.
[b] Linear dose-incidence model.
[c] Estimate based on linear-quadratic dose-incidence model.
[d] Estimate for Japanese population, based on age specific risk coefficients.
[e] Estimate for Japanese population, based on age-averaged risk coefficient.
[f] Estimate for U.S. population, based on modified multiplicative model employing the following assumptions:

Based on a single exposure to radiation, and on a lifetable weighted average over each of the ages listed, in a stationary population having U.S. mortality rates.

Based on the sum of cancers of respiratory tract, digestive tract, breast, and other organs.

Values rounded to nearest 10.

The age specific cancer risk y(d) was expressed as:

$$y(d) = y_0[1 + f(d)g(\beta)]$$

where y_0 denotes the age specific background risk of death due to a specific cancer for an individual at an age, which also depends upon the individual's sex and year of birth, f(d) represents a function of the dose (d).

The expression of cancer mortality risk employed in ICRP Publication 60 is based on primary risk coefficients given in the 1988 United Nations Scientific Committee on the Effects of Atomic Radiation Report.

UNSCEAR 1994 reports lifetime cancer mortality risks, based on a constant relative risk model that allows for age at exposure and sex, of 11% per Sv for solid tumors and 1% per Sv for leukemia (weighted neutron dose, [10]RBE. Comparable UNSCEAR 1988 estimates are 10% and 1%, respectively. The 1994 Committee states that the use of nominal values of 5% per Sv for radiation risk of cancer mortality in a population of all ages, and a value of 4% for and adult working population, remains valid.

Table 15.19 Summary of Dose-Rate Effectiveness Factors for Low-LET Radiation (From National Academy of Sciences BEIR V, 1990)

Source of Data	Observed Full Range of Values	Limited for Narrow Range of Values	Single Best Estimate
Human leukemia (present report)	—	—	2.1
BEIR III	—	—	2.0 to 2.5
Laboratory animal studies			
Specific locus mutation	3–10	3–7	5
Reciprocal transloc.	5–10	5–7	5
Life shortening	3–10	3–5	4
Tumorigenesis	2–10	2–5	4

Table 15.20 Radiological Risks Compared (From EPA *Federal Register*, 1989)

	Annual Effective Dose Equivalent (mrem)	Lifetime Risk
Regulatory Risk		
Federal guidance[c] (1960) (Individual, long term)	500	1.5×10^{-2}
ICRP Advisory[a,c] (1987) (all sources)	100	3×10^{-3}
NCRP Advisory[b,c] (1985) (all sources)	100	3×10^{-3}
British Advisory[c] (1987) (all sources)	50	1.5×10^{-3}
NCRP Advisory[b,c] (1984) (air sources)	25	7×10^{-4}
NRC goal for nuclear power plants[c] (current)	5	1.5×10^{-4}
EPA drinking water standards (1976)	4	1.2×10^{-4}
Background Risk		
Natural background (total)	300	1×10^{-2}
Natural background (total non-radon)	100	3×10^{-3}
Yearly round trip flight N.Y. to L.A. (70 years)	7	2×10^{-4}
Remaining fallout from atomic tests	4	1.2×10^{-4}

[a] International Commission on Radiological Protection
[b] National Council on Radiation Protection and Measurement
[c] Risks stated are the maximum allowed. These regulatory decisions presume that all exposures will be kept ''as low as reasonably achievable.''

Table 15.20.1 Comparison of NCRP Report No. 91 (NCRP, 1987), ICRP Publication 60 (ICRP, 1991a) and NCRP Report No. 116 (NCRP, 1993)

Recommendations, Risk Values and Other Factors	NCRP Report No. 91 (NCRP, 1987)	ICRP Publication 60 (ICRP, 1991a)	NCRP Report No. 116 (NCRP, 1993)
Assumed Radiation Risks			
Workers	1.25×10^{-2} Sv^{-1} for fatal cancer[a]	4.0×10^{-2} Sv^{-1} for fatal cancer 0.8×10^{-2} Sv^{-1} nonfatal cancer detriment	4.0×10^{-2} Sv^{-1} for fatal cancer 0.8×10^{-2} Sv^{-1} nonfatal cancer detriment
	0.4×10^{-2} Sv^{-1} for severe genetic effects[a]	0.8×10^{-2} Sv^{-1} for severe genetic effects	0.8×10^{-2} Sv^{-1} for severe genetic effects
Members of the Public	(not specifically addressed)	5.0×10^{-2} Sv^{-1} for fatal cancer 1.0×10^{-2} Sv^{-1} for nonfatal cancer 1.3×10^{-2} Sv^{-1} for severe genetic effects	5.0×10^{-2} Sv^{-1} for fatal cancer 1.0×10^{-2} Sv^{-1} for nonfatal cancer 1.3×10^{-2} Sv^{-1} for severe genetic effects
Embryo-fetus	20×10^{-2} Sv^{-1} total detriment (UNSCEAR, 1986)	(not specifically stated)	$\sim 10 \times 10^{-2}$ Sv^{-1}

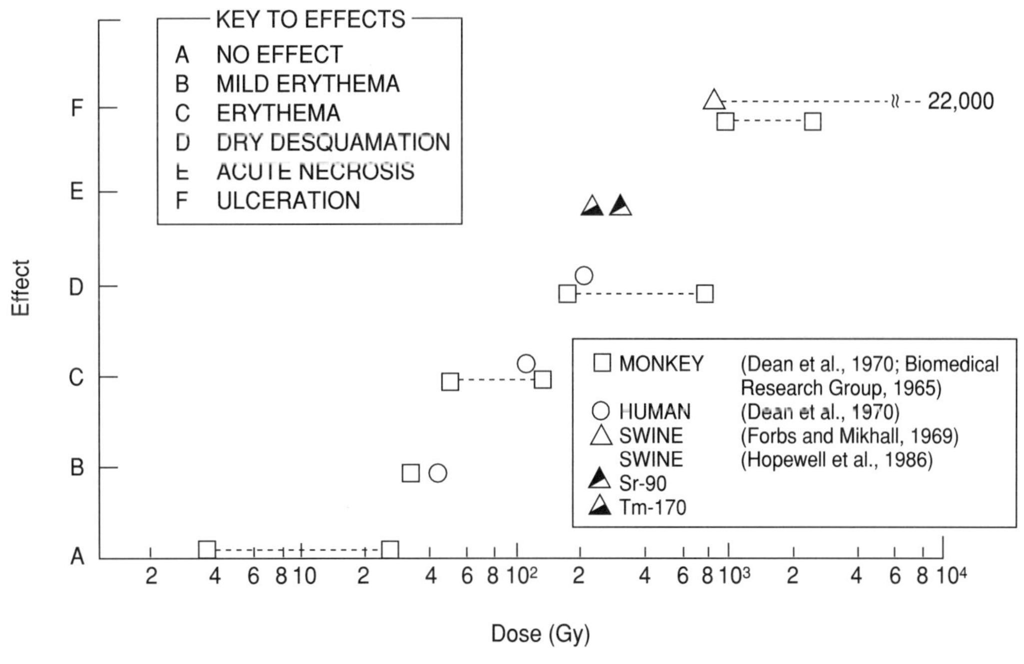

Figure 15.8 Biological Effects of Small Radioactive Particles on the Skin. Doses have been adjusted to a common basis. (Courtesy NCRP from Report 106, 1989)

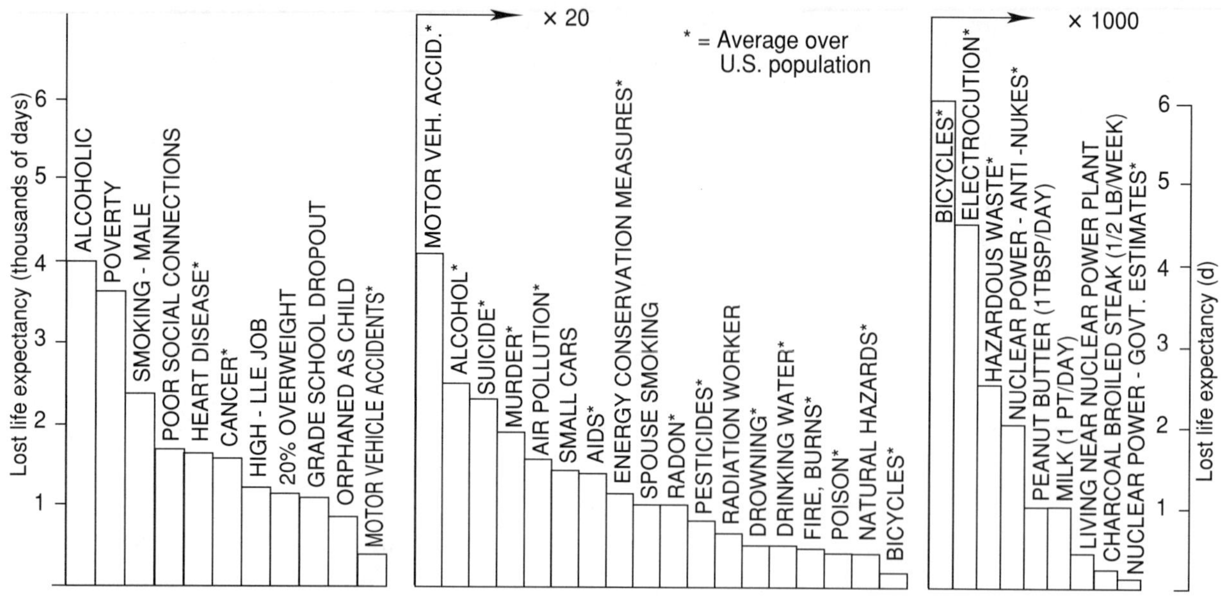

Figure 15.9 Comparison of Risks. Asterisk designates average risk spread over the total U.S. population; others refer to risks of those exposed or participating. The ordinate scale is shown at the left. The heights of the bars are multiplied by 20 in the center section and by 1,000 in the right section. The first bar in each of these reproduces the last bar in the previous section, showing the effect of scale change. (Reproduced from the journal *Health Physics* with permission from the Health Physics Society from Cohen, 1991)

Table 15.21 Loss of Life Expectancy (LLE) From Various Causes of Death in the U.S. Calculated from the U.S. Bureau of the Census (1990) (Reproduced from the journal *Health Physics* with permission from the Health Physics Society from Cohen, 1991)

Disease	LLE (days)	M:F	B:W
Tuberculosis	4.7	2.0	4.2
Viral hepatitis	3.3	1.6	1.0
Cancer—all types	1.247 (3.4 y)	1.21	0.85
Lip, oral, pharynx	22	2.14	1.29
Digestive organs	269	1.16	0.96
Respiratory	343	2.25	0.85
Breast	109	0.006	0.78
Genital organs	113	1.26	1.17
Urinary organs	114	1.86	0.61
Leukemia	46	1.29	0.65
Diabetes	82 (2.7 mo)	0.74	1.45
Nutrition deficiency	3.50	0.64	1.08
Cardiovascular	2,043 (5.6 y)	1.02	0.82
Heart disease	1,607 (4.4 y)	1.10	0.80
Cerebrovascular	250 (8 mo)	0.69	0.96
Atherosclerosis	24	0.64	0.58
Pneumonia	103 (3.3 mo)	1.03	0.76
Influenza	2.3	0.67	0.22
Chronic pulmonary	164 (5.4 mo)	1.68	0.48
Bronchitis	7.3	1.29	0.35
Emphysema	32	1.95	0.36
Asthma	11.3	0.68	1.87
Ulcer	11.8	0.96	0.71
Appendicitis	1.2	1.00	2.00
Liver diseases	81 (2.7 mo)	1.88	1.20
Gallbladder	4.7	0.85	0.62
Nephritis	41 (1.3 mo)	1.06	1.61
Accidents	365	2.33	1.09
Motor vehicle	205	2.61	0.89
All other	158	2.08	1.30
Suicide	115	3.80	0.47
Homicide	93	3.40	5.70

M:F = male:female; B:W = black:white

Table 15.22 Deaths per Year and Loss of Life Expectancy (LLE) Due to Various Types of Accidents for Average Citizens of U.S. For work-related accidents, LLE are for those exposed 2000 h y^{-1} from ages 18–65 (Reproduced from the journal *Health Physics* with permission from the Health Physics Society from Cohen, 1991)[a]

Accident Type	1988 Deaths	LLE (days)
All accidents	96,000	366
Motor vehicle	49,000	207
Home	22,500	74
Work	10,600	60
Public	18,000	60
Falls	12,000	28
Poison (solid, liquid)	5,300	20
Drowning	5,000	24
Fire, burns	5,000	20
Suffocation	3600	28
Firearms	1400	6.5
Poison (gas)	1000	4.0
Electric current	850	4.5
Explosives	250	1.6
Knives, razors	120	0.7
Machinery	1250	6.5
Falling objects	900	6.0
Venom (plant and animal)	60	0.4
Injury by animals	95	0.6
Motor vehicle	49000	207
Collisions	21200	87
Non-Collision	13900	61
Pedestrians	8800	36
Fixed objects	3300	14
Pedalcycle	1100	5.7
Railroad	600	2.5
Home	22500	74
Falls	6500	13
Poison (solid, liquid)	4300	16
Poison (gas)	600	2.6
Fire, burns	4100	17
Suffocation	2900	9.1
Drowning	800	4.2
Firearms	800	3.8
All other	2500	7.9

Table 15.22 Deaths per Year and Loss of Life Expectancy (LLE) Due to Various Types of Accidents for Average Citizens of U.S. For work-related accidents, LLE are for those exposed 2000 h y^{-1} from ages 18–65 **(Continued)**[a]

Accident Type	1988 Deaths	LLE (days)
Public	18000	60
Falls	4100	9.3
Drowning	2900	14.0
Fire, burns	600	2.1
Firearms	500	2.2
Air transport	900	3.7
Water transport	800	3.3
Railroad	300	1.3
Other transport	200	0.9
All other	7700	22.8
Work (occupation)	10600	60[b]
All (114×10^6)	10600	60
Agriculture	1500	320
Mine, quarry	200	167
Construction	2200	227
Manufacturing	1100	40
Transportation, utility	1400	160
Trade	1100	27
Services	1500	27
Government	1600	60

[a] Calculated from NSC 1989.
[b] This column represents risk to workers in that occupation.

Table 15.23 Fatal Accident Rates in Various Industries, 1976 and 1991 (From NCRP Report 116, 1993)

	Mean rate 1976[a] (10^{-4} y^{-1})	Mean rate 1991[b] (10^{-4} y^{-1})
All groups	1.42	0.90
Trade	0.64	0.40
Manufacture	0.89	0.40
Service	0.86	0.40
Government	1.11	0.90
Transport and public utilities	3.13	2.20
Construction	5.68	3.10
Mines and quarries	6.25	4.30
Agriculture (1973–80)	5.41	4.40

[a] Reference NSC (1976).
[b] Reference NSC (1992).

References

American Cancer Society (ACS) *Cancer facts and figures—1991.* American Cancer Society, Atlanta, Georgia; 1991.

Casarett, A.P. *Radiation Biology.* Prentice Hall, Inc.; Englewood Cliffs, N.J.; 220; 1968.

Clark, R.H. "1990 Recommendations of ICRP," Supplement to the *Radiological Protection Bulletin,* No. 199; National Radiological Protection Board; 1991.

Cohen, B.L. "Catalog of Risks Extended and Updated," *Health Physics,* **61:**317–335; 1991.

Dean, P.N., Langham, J., Holland, L.M. "Skin response to a point source of fissioned uranium-235 carbide," *Health Phys.* **19:**3; 1970.

Environmental Protection Agency. *National Emission Standards for Hazardous Air Pollutants: Regulation of Radionuclides.* Proposed Rule Making 40CFR Part 61; Federal Register; Tuesday, March 7, 1989.

International Atomic Energy Agency (IAEA). *Medical Handling of Accidentally Exposed Individuals.* Safety Series No. 88; Vienna, Austria; 1988.

International Commission on Radiological Protection (ICRP). *1990 Recommendations of the International Commission on Radiological Protection.* ICRP Publication 60; Pergamon Press; 1991.

International Commission on Radiological Protection (ICRP). *Risks Associated with Ionizing Radiations.* Annals of the ICRP, Volume 22, No. 1; Pergamon Press; 1991.

Lloyd, D.C., Purrott, R.J. "Chromosome aberration analysis in radiological protection dosimetry," *Radiat Prot Dosim* **1:** 19–28; 1981.

Lushbaugh, C.C. *The Impact of Estimates of Human Radiation Tolerance Upon Radiation Emergency Management.* Proceedings of the NCRP Symposium, The Control of Exposure of the Public to Ionizing Radiation in the Event of Accident or Attack. Reston, VA; April 27–29, 1981.

Mays, C.W., Rowland, R.E., Stehney, A.F. "Cancer risk from the lifetime intake of radium and uranium isotopes." *Health Physics* **48:**635; 1985.

Nazaroff, W.N., Doyle, S.M., Nero, A.V., Jr., Sexton, R.G. "Radon entry via potable water." In *Radon and Its Decay Products in Indoor Air.* Nazaroff, W.N., Nero, A.V., Jr., eds. John Wiley and Sons, New York: 131–155; 1988.

National Academy of Sciences/National Research Council (NAS/NRC). *Health risks of radon and other internally deposited alpha-emitters: BEIR IV.* National Academy Press; Washington, D.C.; 1988.

National Academy of Sciences/National Research Council (NAS/NRC). *Health effects of exposure to low levels of ionizing radiation: BEIR V.* National Academy Press; Washington, D.C.; 1990.

National Academy of Sciences/National Research Council (NAS/NRC). *Comparative Dosimetry of Radon in Mines and Homes.* National Academy Press; Washington, D.C.; 1991.

National Council on Radiation Protection and Measurements (NCRP). *Influence of Dose and its Distribution in Time on Dose-Response Relationships of Low LET Radiations.* NCRP Report No. 64; Bethesda, Maryland; 1980.

National Council on Radiation Protection and Measurements (NCRP). *Induction of thyroid cancer by ionizing radiation.* NCRP Report No. 80; Bethesda, Maryland; 1985.

National Council on Radiation Protection and Measurements (NCRP). *Limit for Exposure to "Hot Particles" on the skin.* NCRP Report No. 106; Bethesda, MD; 1989.

National Council on Radiation Protection and Measurements (NCRP). *Limitation of Exposure to Ionizing Radiation.* NCRP Report No. 116; Bethesda, MD; March 31, 1993.

National Council on Radiation Protection and Measurements (NCRP). *Selected aspects of strontium radiobiology.* NCRP Report No. 110; Bethesda, Maryland; 1991.

National Safety Council (NSC). *Accident Facts*. Chicago, IL; 1976, 1989, 1992.

Nuclear Regulatory Commission. *Reactor Safety Study*. WASH-1400; National Technical Information Service; Springfield, VA; 1975.

Nuclear Regulatory Commission. *Generic Environmental Impact Statement for License Renewal of Nuclear Plants*. Draft Report for Comment; Washington, DC; 1991.

Otake, M., Yoshimaru, H., Schull, W.J. *Severe mental retardation among the prenatally exposed survivors of the atomic bombing of Hiroshima and Nagasaki: A comparison of the old and new dosimetry system*. Radiation Effects Research Foundation, RERF Technical Report 16–87; Hiroshima, Japan; 1987.

Shimizu, Y., Schull, W.J., Kato, H. "Cancer risk among atomic bomb survivors," *J Am Med Assn* **264:**601; 1990.

United Nations Scientific Committee on the Effects of Atomic Radiation (UNSCEAR). *1994 Report to the General Assembly, with Scientific Annexes*. United Nations, New York; 1994.

United Nations Scientific Committee on the Effects of Atomic Radiation (UNSCEAR).*1988 Report to the General Assembly, with Annexes*. United Nations, New York; 1988.

Upton, A.C. *Radiation Injury*; Chicago; 1969.

Vennart, J. "The 1990 recommendations of the International Commission on Radiological Protection," *J Radiol Prot* **11**(3): 199–203; 1991.

Wagner, L.K., Eifel, P.J., Geiss, R.A. "Potential biological effects following high x-ray dose international procedures," *J Vasc Interv Radiol* **5:**71–84; 1994.

Webb, G.A.M. "Quantification of radiation detriment," *J Radiol Prot* **11**(3):163–171; 1991.

CHAPTER 16

NON-IONIZING RADIATION

This chapter contains tables and figures relating to: (1) radiofrequency and microwave radiation and Extremely Low Frequency (ELF)/Very Low Frequency (VLF) fields; (2) visible, ultraviolet and infrared radiation (so-called ''optical radiations'') as well as laser (coherent) light; (3) ultrasound; and (4) heat and noise exposures. The units, terminology, hazards and standards for these classes of non-ionizing radiation and physical agents are discussed. Greatest emphasis is placed on the potential hazards and safety aspects of devices using/emitting these energies. The American Conference of Governmental Industrial Hygienist's (ACGIH) Threshold Limit Values (TLVs) recommends occupational threshold levels for each of the radiation types discussed above. The reader is directed to the ACGIH document for the TLVs.

The reader is directed to Chapter 4 Section 3 for standards and regulations for laser products, ultrasound and ultraviolet lamps. The recently published revision of Herman Cember's *Introduction to Health Physics—Third Edition* includes an excellent discussion of lasers, radiofrequency radiation and microwaves (Chapter 14). Explanations of biological effects and calculational methods are provided there. Another important source for those involved in laser safety is the Laser Institute of America located in Orlando, FL. The Institute frequently updates relevant materials and provides training sessions.

SECTION 1 RF/MICROWAVE

TABLE OF CONTENTS

Table 16.1 Sources (and Examples) of Non-Ionizing Electromagnetic Radiation (Energy) and Ultrasonic Energy (Personal communication Z. Glazer, 1991)

Optical Energy

Visible "light" (projector; spotlights and floodlights)

Infrared (objects heated to high temperature, heating sources, lamp filaments, molten metal, thermotherapy)

Ultraviolet (electric arcs in metal welding and cutting; fabrication, control and occupational use of fluorescent and mercury vapor lamps; tanning booths; UV sterilization; natural exposure to sunlight; phototherapy)

Lasers [coherent energy], (microwelding and microfinishing; drilling; building; precision measurements; telemetry, holography; telecommunications; guidance systems; light shows; research in nuclear fusion; isotope separation and spectroscopy; medical photocoagulation; microsurgery; transillumination; and cauterization)

Microwave and Radiofrequency Energy

Radiofrequency (broadcasting and telecommunications; radar; air traffic control; meteorology; metallurgy, food processing; sterilization; scientific research and medicine)

Microwave (radar installations; broadcasting stations; television transmitters; microwave ovens; diathermy units)

Extremely Low Frequency (ELF)/Very Low Frequency (VLF) (high voltage transmission and power lines, many electrical appliances containing motors, video display terminals (VDTs).

Ultrasonic (US) Energy

Industrial (cleaning; machining; welding plastics; emulsifying; flow detection, electronic signal processing and sonar detection)

Medical (physical therapy; fetal cephalometry, placental localization; detection of intra-uterine life, diagnosis of multiple pregnancy; and dental hygiene)

Consumer/Airborne US (bug, bird, and rodent control; burglar alarms; traffic control, and dog whistles)

Table 16.1.1 General Radiation Phenomena (From Repacholi, 1988, with permission)

Non-ionizing radiation is often emitted in a pulse mode characterized by the *duty factor d.* Instantaneous *radiant power,* P_{inst}, during pulses will then exceed temporal average radiant power, P_{av}, by the factor 1/d. Frequency spectra are characterized by *bandwidth* Δf and *center frequency* f_c. Attenuation phenomena can be quantified using the concepts of *amplitude* and *power level difference* in decibels (dB), whose advantage is their additivity when different attenuation phenomena are combined. Attenuation coefficients may be stated equivalently in reciprocal meters or in dB/m; if the *power attenuation coefficient* is given as $\alpha = 1\ m^{-1}$, the corresponding value is 4.343 dB/m.

Table 16.1.2 Electromagnetic Radiation and Fields (ELF) (From Repacholi, 1988, with permission)

Extremely low frequency electromagnetic phenomena adverse to the human body (frequencies of the order of 100 Hz) require indications of *electric field strength E* and *magnetic field strength H* in free space, and currents induced in the body may be characterized by *current density J*. Exposure limits are formulated in terms of free space E and H values.

At higher frequencies the radiative properties of electromagnetic fields become more pronounced, manifested by the phenomena of reflection, transmission, scattering and absorption in biological structures. A distinction must be made between the radiation field existing in space in the absence of the exposed body (''free field'') and the radiation field in the presence of the exposed body. In the second case it is necessary to distinguish further between the radiation field within and in the vicinity of the exposed body.

For radiofrequencies below 10 MHz, exposure limits are expressed in terms of the ''effective electric field strength'', E_{eff}, and the ''effective magnetic field strength'', H_{eff}. Effective field strengths are determined in the ''free field'', i.e., in the absence of an absorbing or scattering body. Since, in the near field, the phase relationship between the directional components of a field strength is usually unknown, the ''effective field strength'' is obtained by adding the squares of the amplitudes of the vertical and the horizontal components and taking the square root of this sum.

At frequencies higher than 10 MHz, basic exposure limits have been formulated with partial reference to the thermal mechanism of radiation action. This is made possible by applying the quantity *specific absorption rate (SAR)* in W/kg. The advantage of this choice of the quantity is that exposure limits can be stated by one number for a large region of frequencies. SAR is a quantity which is defined locally (for a small amount of tissue), and the concept is extended to include spatial peak SAR as well as temporal peak SAR, and SAR averaged over part of an organ or the whole body.

Although there are good reasons to state ''basic exposure limits'' in terms of SAR, practical measurement is often performed with instruments calibrated to measure *surface power density* (abbr.: power density) in W/cm^2. It is therefore practical to state ''derived exposure limits'' in terms of power density. The definition given in the list uses the concept of a small receptor sphere which offers the same cross sectional area to all directions of incidence. Since in the far field $E/H = 377\ \Omega$, we have $E{\cdot}H = E^2/(377\ \Omega)$, so that is is possible to use instruments which are sensitive to E.

Table 16.1.3 Electromagnetic Quantities (Courtesy IRPA from *Non-Ionizing Radiations*, 1988)

Quantity	Symbol	Definition	Remarks	Name of Unit	Symbol
Quantities Describing General Radiation Phenomena					
duty factor	d	ratio between the pulse duration and the pulse period of a pulse train	dimensionless quantity	1	
bandwidth	Δf	difference $f_1 - f_2$ of the frequencies f_1 and f_2 at which the amplitude spectrum is 50% (−6 dB) of its maximum value		hertz	Hz
center frequency	f_c	arithmetic mean $(f_1 + f_2)/2$ of the frequencies defining bandwidth		hertz	Hz
amplitude level difference	L_F	$L_F = 20 \lg(F_1/F_2)$ where F_1 and F_2 represent two amplitudes of the same kind	example: field strength level difference L_E	decibel	dB
power level difference	L_P	$L_P = 10 \lg(P_1/P_2)$ where P_1 and P_2 represent two powers of the same kind	if $P_1/P_2 = (F_1/F_2)^2$, then $L_P = L_F$	decibel	dB
Quantities Describing Electromagnetic Radiation and Fields					
electric field strength	E	force, exerted by an electric field on an electric point charge, divided by the charge		volt per meter	V/m
electric flux density	D	the factor whose divergence is equal to the volume density of electric charge		coulomb per square meter	C/m^2
permittivity	ϵ	electric flux density divided by electric field strength	relative permittivity: $\epsilon_r = \epsilon/\epsilon_0$	farad per meter	F/m
current density	J	the vector whose integral over a given surface is the current through the surface		ampere per square meter	A/m^2

(continued)

Table 16.1.3 Electromagnetic Quantities (Continued)

Quantity	Symbol	Definition	Remarks	Name of Unit	Symbol
Quantities Describing Electromagnetic Radiation and Fields (continued)					
magnetic field strength	H	the vector whose curl is equal to the current density	1 Oe ≙ 79.577 A/m	ampere per meter	A/m
magnetic flux density	B	the vector whose vector product with an element of current gives the force on this element	1 T = 1 V s/m^2 1 G ≙ 0.0001 T	tesla	T
permeability	μ	magnetic flux density divided by magnetic field strength	relative permeability: $\mu_r = \mu/\mu_0$	henry per meter	H/m
radiant energy	Q	energy emitted, transferred or received in the form of electromagnetic radiation		joule	J
radiant power	P	power emitted, transferred or received in the form of electromagnetic radiation		watt	W
surface power density	ψ	radiant power incident on a small sphere divided by cross section area of sphere	distinction: momentary and average power density	watt per square meter	W/m^2
power per solid angle	I	radiant power leaving a source in an element of solid angle at a given direction, divided by that solid angle	the optical analogue is "radiant intensity"	watt per steradian	W/sr
specific absorption	SA	quotient dW/dm of incremental energy dW, absorbed in matter of mass dm	the ionizing radiation analog is "absorbed dose"	joule per kilogram	J/kg
specific absorption rate	SAR	time derivative of the specific absorption: SAR = d(SA)/dt	ionizing radiation analog is "absorbed dose rate"	watt per kilogram	W/kg
power attenuation coefficient	α	factor of distance x in exponential attenuation law $\psi = \psi_0 \exp(-\alpha x)$	$\alpha_a + \alpha_s$ from absorption and scattering	reciprocal meter	m^{-1}

Table 16.1.4 Use of Radiofrequency and Microwave Radiation

Use	Frequency	Exposure Groups
Metallurgy, welding, melting and tempering	Below 3 MHz	Factory workers in furniture veneering and auto industry
Heating, drying, gluing polymerization, and sterilization of dielectrics	3–30 MHz	Workers in auto, wood, chemical and food industries
Food and drug processing	3–30 MHz	Microwave oven operators and maintenance workers
Broadcasting, radio communication, radionavigation, radar	Below 3 MHz to 300 MHz	Electronic engineers and technicians; air and seaport personnel, radar mechanics and operators
Medicine	30–3000 MHz	Microwave diathermy operators
TV, air traffic control, radar, telecommunication, telemetry	30–3000 MHz	Broadcasting transmitter and TV personnel. Radar mechanics and operators. Inhabitants in vicinity of radar installations and TV transmitters
Microwave ovens, food industry and at home	300–3000 MHz	Microwave oven operators, members of households
Microwave point-to-point	300 MHz–30 GHz	Operators and technicians
Altimeters, air- and ship-borne radar, satellite communication	3–30 GHz	Air, marine, coast guard and shipboard personnel
Radioastronomy, radiometeorology, space research, nuclear physics and radiospectroscopy	30–300 GHz	Astronomers, scientists

Table 16.1.5 Radiofrequency and Microwave Band Designations (After Cember, 1996; NCRP Report No. 119, 1993)

Band	Frequency	Description
SELF	0 to 3E − 05	Sub-extremely-low frequency
ELF	3E − 05 to 3E − 04	Extremely low frequency
VF	3E − 04 to 3E − 03	Voice frequency
VLF	3E − 03 to 3E − 02	Very low frequency
LF	3E − 02 to 3E − 01	Low frequency
MF	3E − 01 to 3	Medium frequency
HF	3 to 3E + 01	High frequency
VHF	3E + 01 to 3E + 02	Very high frequency
UHF	3E + 02 to 3E + 03	Ultrahigh frequency
SHF	3E + 03 to 3E + 04	Superhigh frequency
EHF	3E + 04 to 3E + 05	Extremely high frequency
SEHF	3E + 05 to 3E + 06	Supra-extremely-high frequency

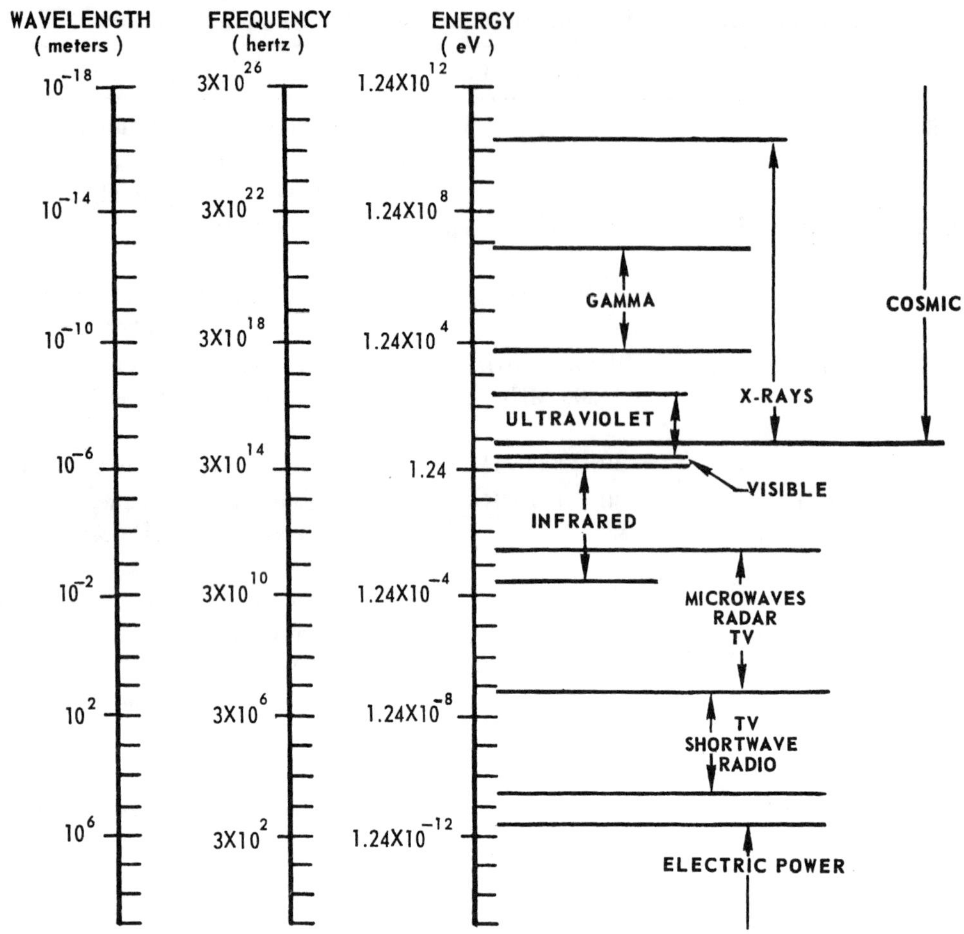

Figure 16.1 The Electromagnetic Spectrum. See Figure 16.2.3 for an expanded view of the ultraviolet region.

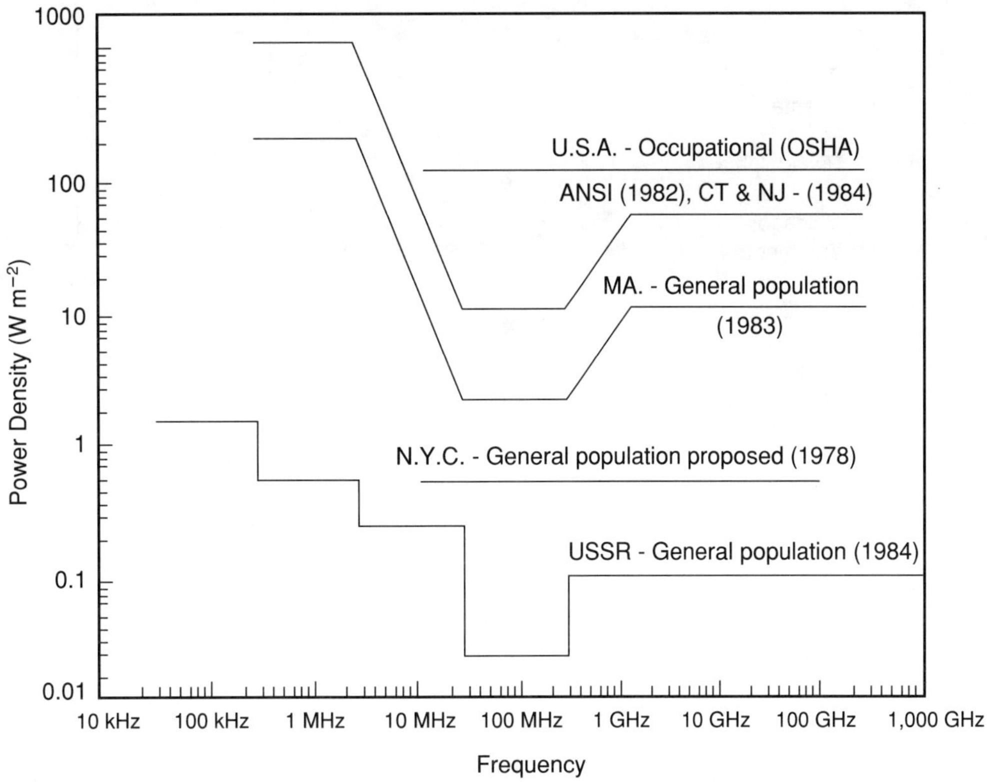

Figure 16.1.1 Various Radiofrequency/Microwave Standards and Recommendations for Continuous Exposure. (Reproduced from the journal *Health Physics* with permission from the Health Physics Society from Petersen, 1991)

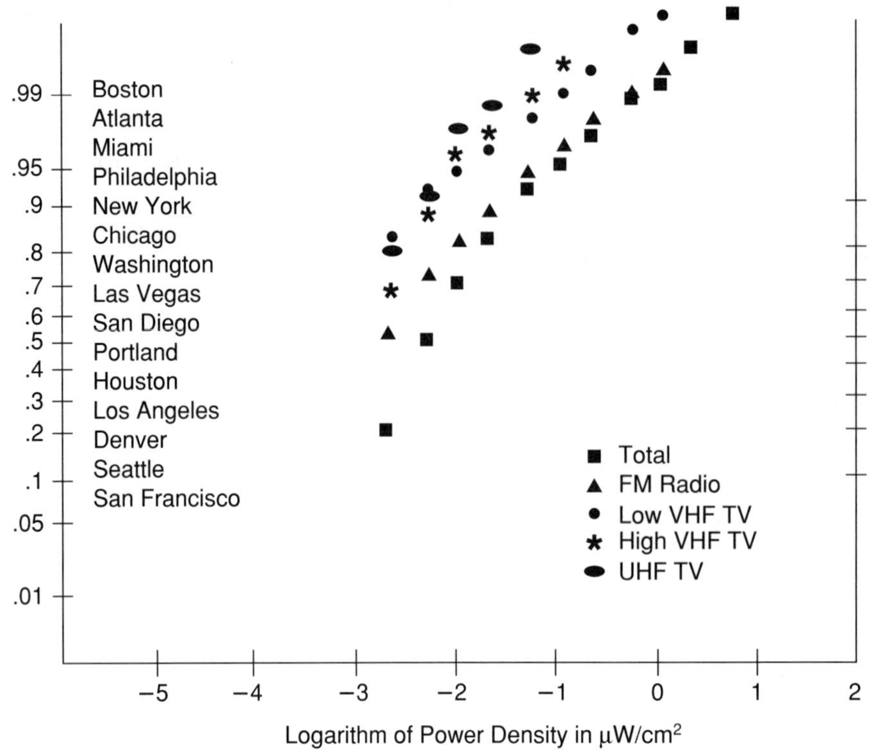

Figure 16.1.2 Cumulative Population Exposure for 15 Cities. (From Hankin, 1986)

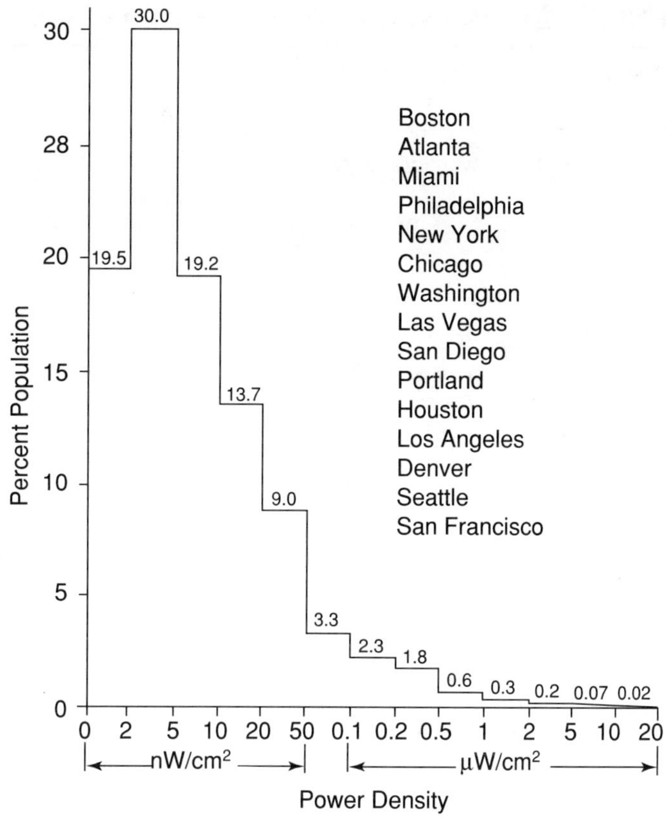

Figure 16.1.3 Differential Fraction of Population Exposed Within Given Power Density Intervals (15 Cities) (From Hankin, 1986)

Table 16.1.6 Limits of Exposure to 50/60 Hz Electric and Magnetic Fields (Reproduced from the journal *Health Physics* with permission from the Health Physics Society from IRPA/INIRC, 1990)

Exposure Characteristics	Electric Field Strength $kV\ m^{-1}$ (rms)	Magnetic Flux Density mT (rms)
Occupational		
Whole working day	10	0.5
Short term	30[a]	5[b]
For limbs	—	25
General Public		
Up to 24 h d^{-1}[c]	5	0.1
Few hours per day[d]	10	1

[a] The duration of exposure to fields between 10 and 30 $kV\ m^{-1}$ may be calculated from the formula $t \leq 80/E$, where t is the duration in hours per work day and E is the electric field strength in $kV\ m^{-1}$.

[b] Maximum exposure duration is 2 h per work day.

[c] This restriction applies to open spaces in which members of the general public might reasonably be expected to spend a substantial part of the day, such as recreational areas, meeting grounds, and the like.

[d] These values can be exceeded for a few minutes per day provided precautions are taken to prevent indirect coupling effects.

Table 16.1.7 ICNIRP Limits of Exposure to Static Magnetic Fields (After ICNIRP, 1994)

Exposure Characteristics	Magnetic Flux Density
Occupational	
Whole working day (time-weighted average)	200 mT
Ceiling value	2 T
Limbs	5 T
General Public	
Continuous exposure	40 mT

Caution: People with cardiac pacemakers and other implanted electrically activated devices, or with ferromagnetic implants, may not be adequately protected by the limits given here. The majority of cardiac pacemakers are unlikely to be affected from exposure to fields below 0.5 mT. People with some ferromagnetic implants or electrically activated devices (other than cardiac pacemakers) may be affected by fields above a few mT. When magnetic flux densities exceed 3 mT, precautions should be taken to prevent hazards from flying metallic objects.

Analog watches, credit cards, magnetic tapes, computer disks, etc. may be adversely affected by exposures to 1 mT, but this is not a safety concern for humans.

General Public: occasional access of members of the public to special facilities where magnetic flux densities exceed 40 mT can be allowed under appropriately controlled conditions provided that the appropriate occupational exposure limit is not exceeded.

Table 16.1.8 Exposure Limits to Radiofrequency Electromagnetic Fields (After Cember, 1996)

Frequency, f(MHz)	Unperturbed RMS Field Strength: Electric $E(V\ m^{-1})$	Unperturbed RMS Field Strength: Magnetic $H(A\ m^{-1})$	Equivalent Plane Wave Power Density: $P_{eq}(W\ m^{-2})$	Equivalent Plane Wave Power Density: $P_{eq}(mW\ m^{-2})$
Occupational				
0.1–1	614	1.6/f	—	—
>1–10	614/f	1.6/f	—	—
>10–400	61	0.16	10	1
>400–2,000	$3f^{0.5}$	$0.008f^{0.5}$	f/40	f/400
>2,000–300,000	137	0.36	50	5
General Public				
0.1–1	87	$0.23/f^{0.5}$	—	—
>1–10	$87/f^{0.5}$	$0.23/f^{0.5}$	—	—
>10–400	27.5	0.073	2	0.2
>400–2,000	$1.375f^{0.5}$	$0.0037f^{0.5}$	f/200	f/2000
>2,000–300,000	61	0.16	10	1

RMS = Root Mean Square

Hazards of RF burns should be eliminated by limiting currents from contact with metal objects. In most situations, this may be achieved by reducing the E values from 614 to 194 $V\ m^{-1}$ in the range from 0.1 to 1 MHz and from 614/f to $194/f^{0.5}$ in the range from >1 to 10 Mhz.

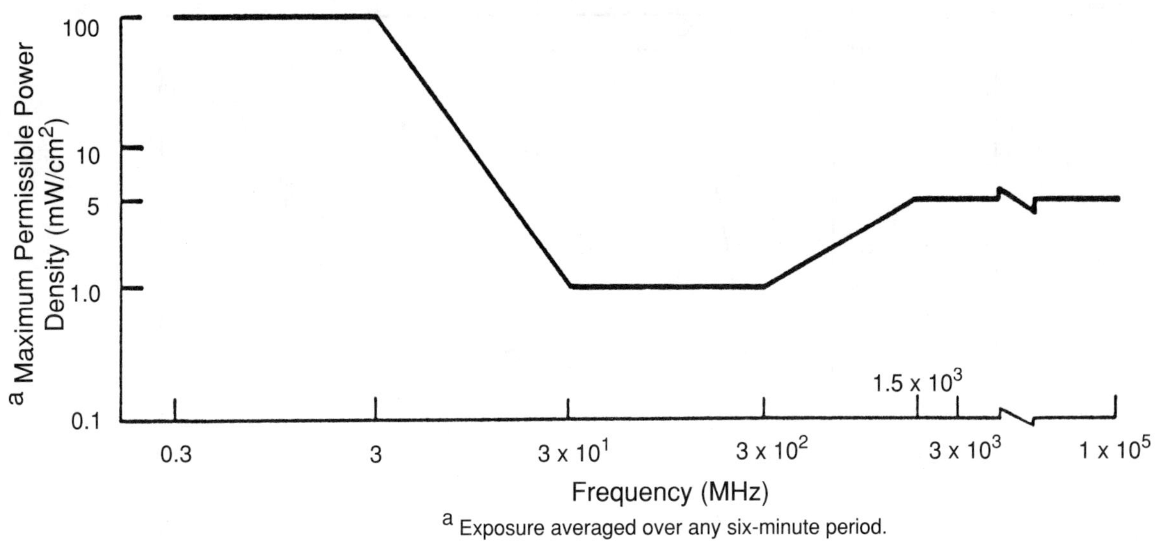

Figure 16.1.4 Radiofrequency Protection Guide. (From *Instrumentation for Non-Ionizing Radiation Measurement,* Conference of Radiation Control Directors, Inc., HHS Publication FDA 84-8222, U.S. Dept. of Health and Human Services, 1984 after ANSI C95.1-1982.

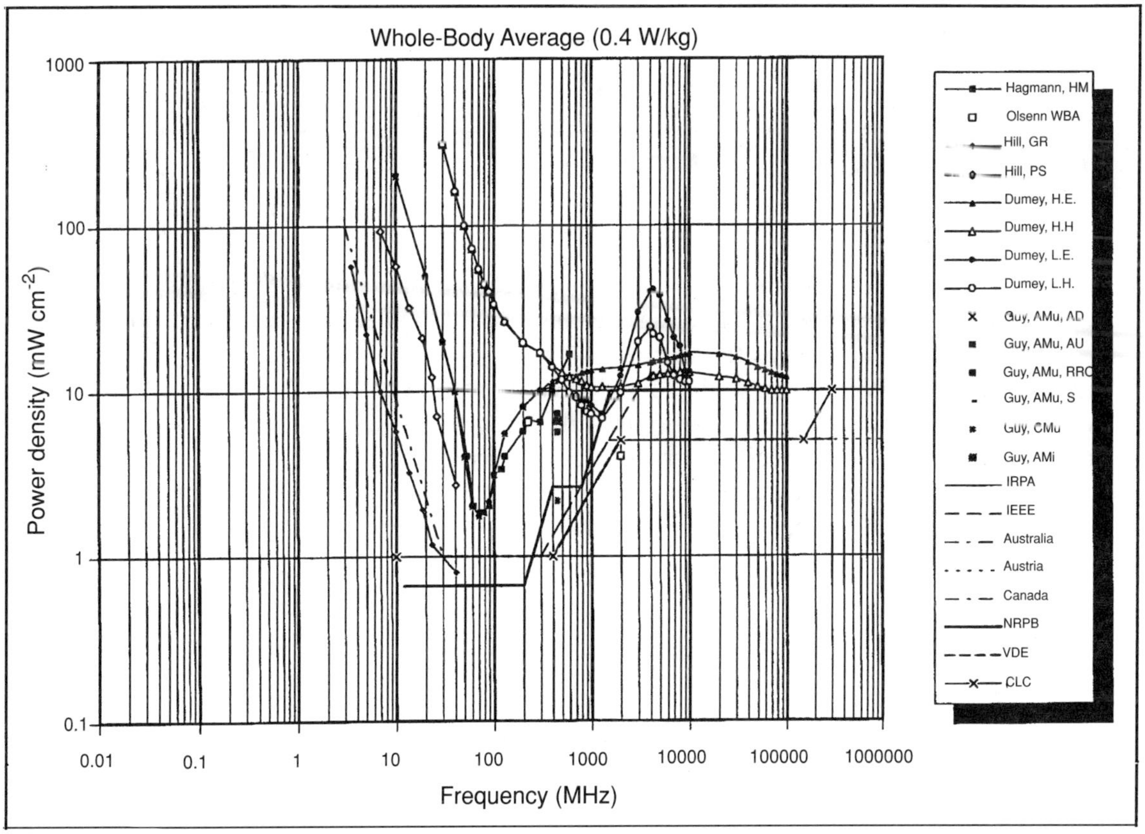

Figure 16.1.5 Power Density that is Reported to Cause a Whole-Body Average SAR of 0.4 W kg^{-1} and Exposure Limits Given in Some Current Standards. (From Garn and Gabriel, 1995, with permission)

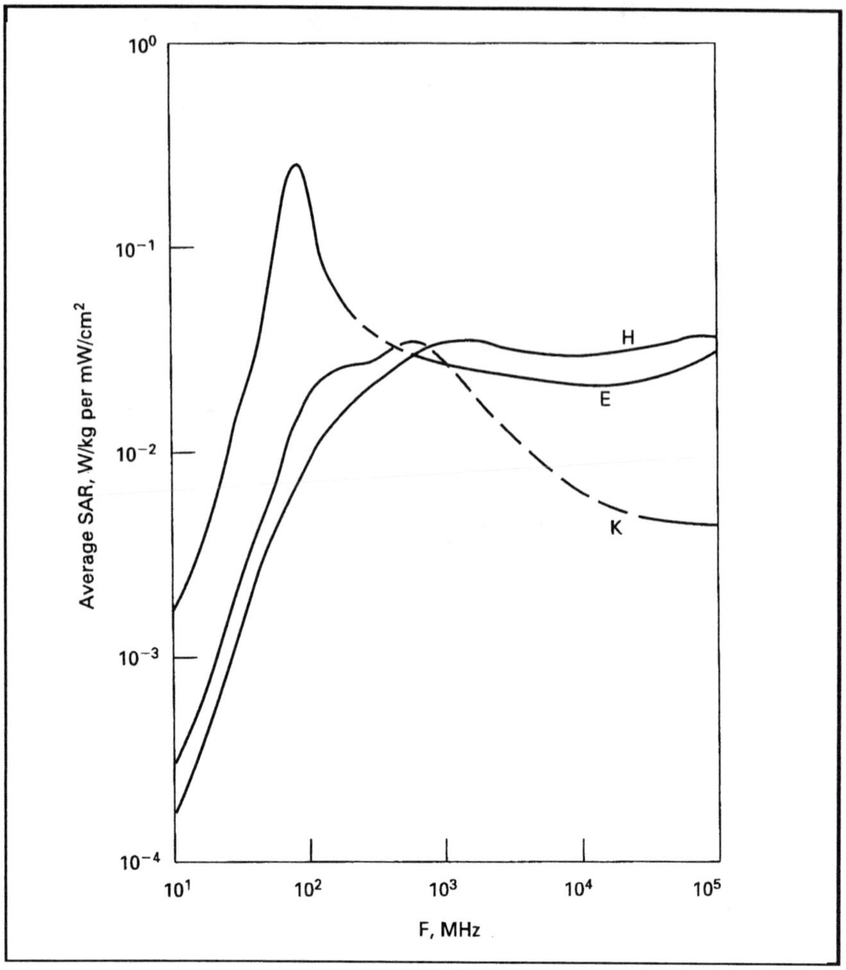

Figure 16.1.6 Whole-Body Average SAR as a Function of Frequency.
The graph displays model results for an average person exposed to three different orientations of a 1 mW cm^{-2} non-ionizing radiation field as follows:

curve E electric field parallel to the long dimension of the person
curve H electric field perpendicular to the long dimension of the person
curve K electric field between the first two orientations.

An absorption resonance (dependent upon wavelength and absorber dimensions) occurs at about 70 Mhz for humans. (From Cember, 1996; NCRP 119, 1994)

SECTION 2 LIGHT AND LASERS

TABLE OF CONTENTS

Table 16.2.1 Optical Radiation (From Repacholi, 1988, with permission)

Due to the small penetration depths of visible and UV light in most materials, the real inclination angles of source and receptor surfaces with respect to radiation directions have to be considered in defining characteristic quantities (see figure 16.2.2). Thus, quantities *radiant exitance M* (for emission) and *irradiance E* (for reception) relate the emitted or received power with the true area of the surface, whatever its inclination. But there are also quantities relating radiant power with solid angle *(radiant intensity I)* and with solid angle and cross sectional area perpendicular to the radiation *(radiance L)*. The latter represents power density in 5-dimensional phase space. Furthermore, radiance is a quantity of practical importance in laser light protection, because coherent light may have high radiance values in small cross section areas and solid angles. Focused by the eye lens, near-parallel laser light may hit very small areas of the retina.

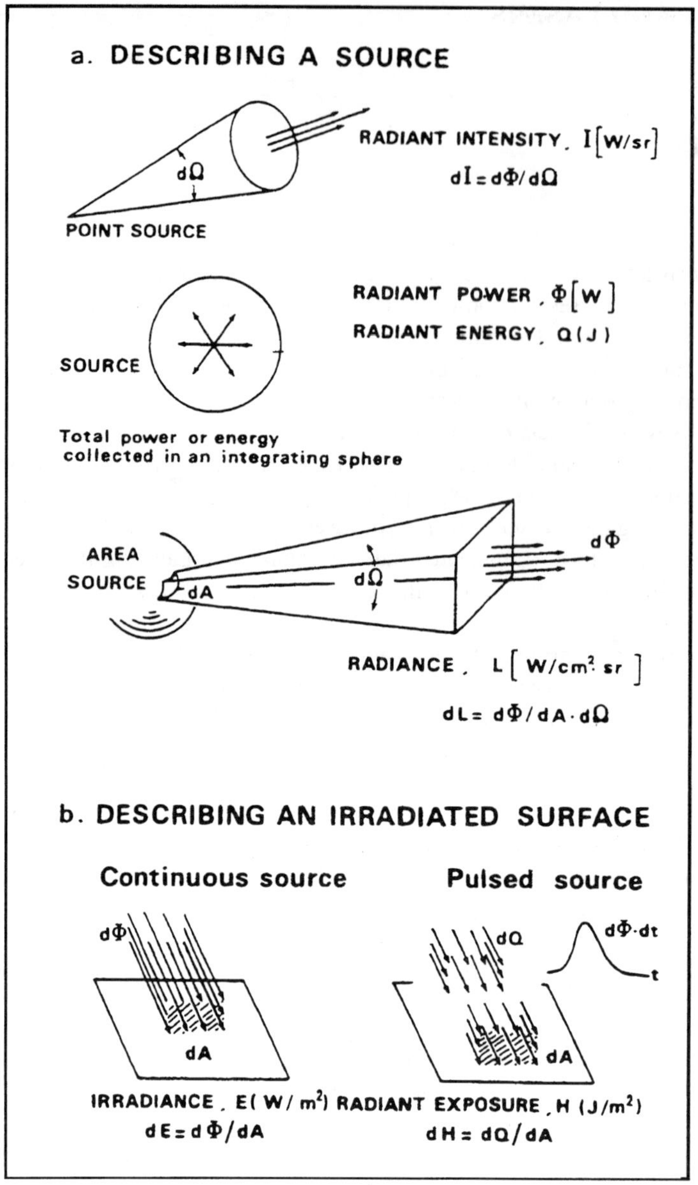

Figure 16.2.1 Schematic Representation of Important Radiometric Terms. (From LIA, 1996)

Table 16.2.2 Optical Radiation Quantities[a,b]

Quantity	Symbol	Definition	Remarks	Name of Unit	Symbol
Radiometric Quantities					
Radiant energy	Q	energy emitted, transferred or received as optical radiation		joule	J
Radiant power	P, ϕ	power emitted, transferred or received as optical radiation		watt	W
Radiant intensity	I	for a source in a given direction, the radiant power leaving the source in an element of solid angle, divided by that element of solid angle	characteristic of a radiation source	watt per steradian	W/sr
Radiant exitance	M	at a point of a surface, the radiant power leaving an element of the surface divided by the area of that element	characteristic of a radiation source	watt per square meter	W/m^2
Radiance	L	at a point of a surface and in a given direction, the radiant intensity dI at an element dA of the surface, divided by the orthogonal projection area da of this element on a plane perpendicular to the given direction: $L = dI/da$	characteristic of a radiation field	watt per square meter steradian	$W/(m^2sr)$
Irradiance	E	at a point of a surface the radiant power incident on an element of the surface, divided by the area of that element	characteristic of a radiation receptor	watt per square meter	W/m^2
Radiant exposure	H	time integral of the irradiance	characteristic of a radiation receptor	joule per square meter	J/m^2
Photometric Quantities					
Quantity of light	Q	time integral of luminous flux		lumen second	lm s
Luminous flux	ϕ	integral of lumous intensity over solid angle		lumen	lm
Luminous intensity	I	basic quantity	characteristic of a radiation source	candela	cd
Luminous exitance	M	at a point of the surface, the luminous flux leaving an element of the surface, divided by the area of that element	characteristic of a radiation source	lumen per square meter	lm/m^2
Luminance	L	at a point of a surface and in a given direction, the luminous intensity of an element of the surface, divided by the orthogonal projection area of this element on a plane perpendicular to the given direction	characteristic of a radiation field	candela per square meter	cd/m^2
Illuminance	E	at a point of a surface, the luminous flux incident on an element of the surface, divided by the area of that element	characteristic of a radiation receptor	lux	lx
Light exposure	H	time integral of illuminance	characteristic of a radiation receptor	lux second	lx s

[a] The lists of the radiometric and photometric quantities are arranged in sequential order, so that correspondences can be easily seen: *Radiant energy* is analog with *quantity of light, radiant power* with *luminous intensity* and so on. Each of these quantities has a spectral distribution function which may be characterized by index λ, for instance ϕ_λ. Another index may be used for radiometric (e) and photometric quantities (υ). The photometric quantities are formally obtained by weighting the radiometric quantities with the spectral response function $V(\lambda)$ of the light adapted eye. This is shown here for the example of spectral luminous flux, $\phi_{\upsilon\lambda}$, and spectral radiant power $\phi_{\upsilon\lambda}$:

$$\phi_{\upsilon\lambda} = K_m V(\lambda)\phi_{\upsilon\lambda}$$

where K_m = 680 lm/W is the maximum spectral luminous efficacy and $V(\lambda)$ the spectral luminous efficiency (relative values). Similarly, limits of exposure for the skin and eye to UV radiation can be expressed in terms of the ''effective irradiance'' whereby the irradiance of a broadband source is weighted by a spectral effectiveness function S_λ.

[b] Interaction with Matter. In the case of ionizing radiation there is the possibility to neatly separate quantities describing the radiation field (''radiometric quantities'') from the ''dosimetric'' quantities involving interaction of radiation with matter, especially with the human body. These two are connected by ''interaction coefficients''. In the case of non-ionizing radiation there exists a similar set of interaction coefficients such as the *attenuation coefficient* α, *absorption coefficient* α_α and *scattering coefficient* α_s. This list could be further supplemented by reflection factor, transmission factor, refractive index etc. (see INIRC 1985). However, as we have seen, the ''dosimetric quantities'' useful in non-ionizing radiation work are not so uniform in concept as in the case of ionizing radiation. This is due to the large multiplicity of physical effects and measuring techniques present. Thus, attempts of unification of quantities and units for non-ionizing radiation will find their natural limit here.

Table 16.2.3 Conversion Between Irradiance Units

		W/M^2	mW/cm^2	$\mu W/cm^2$
1 W/m^2	=	1	0.1	100
1 mW/cm^2	=	10	1	10^3
1 $\mu W/cm^2$	=	0.01	10^{-3}	1
1 erg/(cm^2 s)	=	10^{-3}	10^{-4}	0.1
1 erg/(m^2 s)	=	10^{-7}	10^{-8}	10^{-5}

Similar conversions hold for radian exposure units, if watts (W) are replaced by joules (J) in the table.

Table 16.2.4 Ultraviolet Radiation Spectrum

The UVR[a] spectrum may be divided into three major components which induce significantly different biological effects:

UV-A wavelengths from 400 nm to 320nm (synonyms: long wave UVR, near UVR, black light);

UV-B 320 to 280 nm (synonyms: middle UVR, ''sunburn'' radiation);

UV-C 280nm to 20 nm (synonyms: short wave UVR, far UVR, germicidal radiation).

Wavelengths below 200 nm are of little biological significance, since radiation in this region (''vacuum UVR'') is absorbed in very short pathlengths in air.

NOTE: The components of the UV spectrum are shown in Figure 16.2.2.

[a] UVR = UV radiation

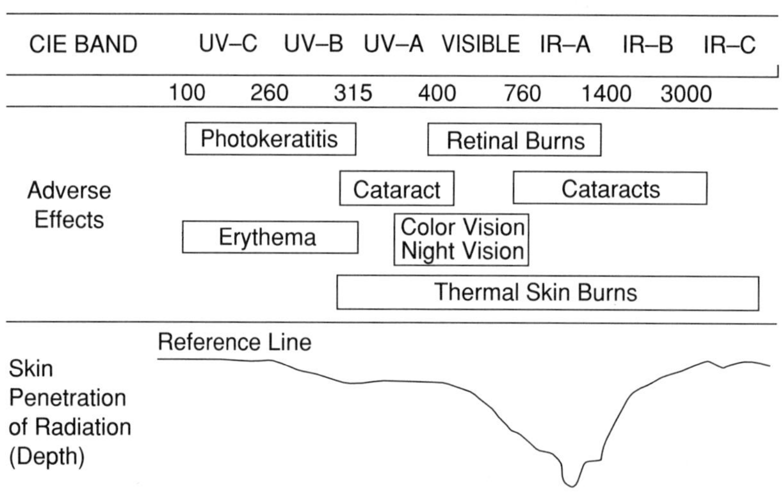

Figure 16.2.2 The Adverse Effects of Optical Radiation. The precise positions of the boxes outlining the effects will vary slightly depending upon the criteria for stating that an effect can occur. For example, photokeritit is can be the result of excessive exposure to UV-A, although the levels required to elicit the effect would be more than a thousand times the threshold level at 270 nm. (From LIA, 1996)

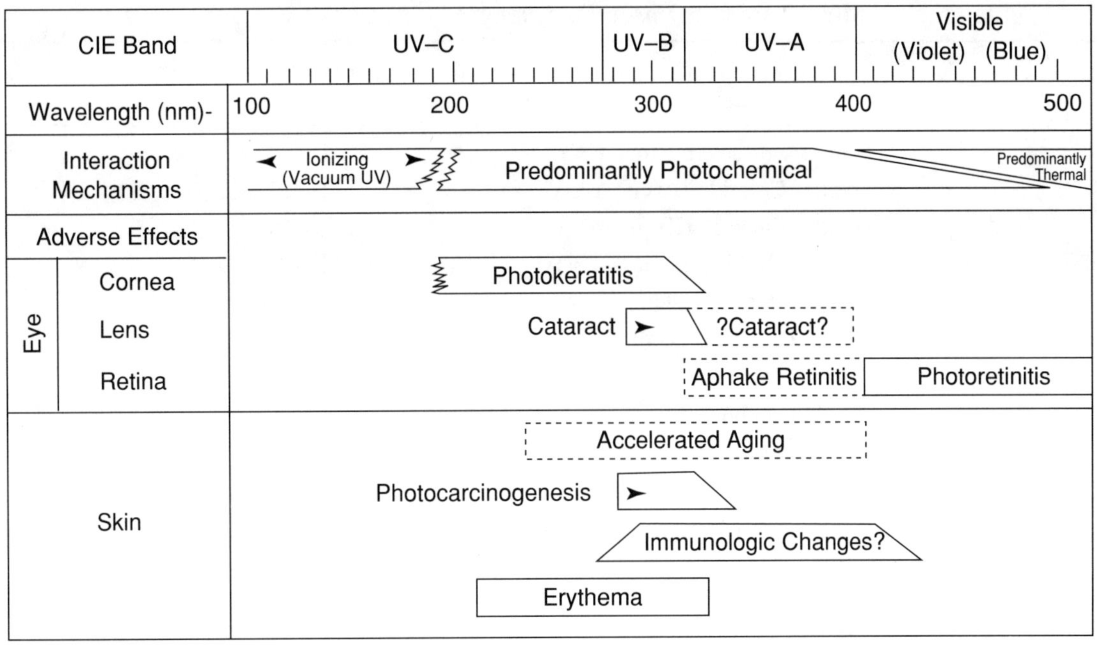

Figure 16.2.3 CIE Spectral Band Designations and Bioeffects in the Ultraviolet Region. (From LIA, 1996, with permission)

Table 16.2.5 Most Common Laser Wavelengths (After OSHA Instruction PUB 8-1.7, 1991)

Laser Type	Wavelength (μmeters)
Argon Fluoride (Excimer-UV)	0.193
Krypton Chloride (Excimer-UV)	0.222
Krypton Fluoride (Excimer-UV)	0.248
Xenon Chloride (Excimer-UV)	0.308
Xenon Fluoride (Excimer-UV)	0.351
Helium Cadmium (UV)	0.325
Nitrogen (UV)	0.337
Helium Cadmium (violet)	0.441
Krypton (blue)	0.476
Argon (blue)	0.488
Copper Vapor (green)	0.510
Argon (green)	0.514
Krypton (green)	0.528
Frequency Doubled	
Helium Neon (green)	0.543
Krypton (yellow)	0.568
Copper Vapor (yellow)	0.570
Helium Neon (yellow)	0.594
Helium Neon (orange)	0.610
Gold Vapor (red)	0.627
Helium Neon (red)	0.633
Krypton (red)	0.647
Rhodamine 6G Dye (tunable)	0.570–0.650
Ruby (Cr:AI03)(red)	0.694
Gallium Arsenide (diode-NIR)	0.840
ND:YAG (NIR)	1.064
Helium Neon (NIR)	1.15
ND:YAG (NIR)	1.33
Erbium (NIR)	1.504
Helium Neon (NIR)	3.39
Hydrogen Fluoride (NIR)	2.70
Carbon Dioxide (FIR)	9.6
Carbon Dioxide (FIR)	10.6

UV: Ultraviolet (0.200–0.400 μm)
VIS: Visible (0.400–0.700 μm)
NIR: Near infrared (0.700–1.400 μm)
FIR: Far Infrared (1.400–30.0 μm)

Table 16.2.6 Laser Types For Current Applications (After OSHA Instruction PUB 8-1.7, 1991)

Laser Media	Wavelength (nanometers)	Major Laser Applications
Ruby laser	6943	Satellite ranging, medical, drilling holes
Neodymium-YAG	1064	Various laser metal processing, welding, medical (surgery, eye), military (ranging)
Carbon dioxide	10,600	Materials processing, surgery, laser fusion
Argon ion gas	488–514, 351 & 363	Laser eye treatments, photoetching, laser entertainment Medical: cell counters, medical diagnosis
Helium neon	6328	UPC checkout systems, lab alignment, construction alignment, videodisc
Gallium arsenide	840	Communications, infrared beacons, compact disk players, printers
Krypton ion gas	4762, 5280, 5682, & 8471	Entertainment, holography, diagnostics
Dye lasers such as: Rhodamine 6-G	Tunable: 400–600	Spectroscopy, IC circuit etching, special photography, ophthalomology

Table 16.2.7 Summary of Laser-Engineered Safety Features and Labeling Requirements (From *Federal Register* **39:** 172, September 4, 1974)

	Class I	Class II	Class III	Class IV
Safety Feature				
Protective housing	X	X	X	X
Safety interlock	X	X	X	X
Remote connector			X	X
Key control			X	X
Emisssion indicator		X	X	X
Beam attenuator		X	X	X
Label				
Certification and manufacturer	X	X	X	X
Class designation and warning logotype		X	X	X
Aperture label		X	X	X
Radiation output		X	X	X
Non-interlocked protective housing		X	X	X

Table 16.2.8 Occupational Safety and Health Administration Exposure Level Limits for Light Intensities (From 29CFR 1926.54)

No employee shall be exposed to light intensities above	
Viewing Orientation	**Light Intensity**
Direct Staring	1 microwatt per cm^2
Incidental observation	1 milliwatt per cm^2
Diffuse reflected light	2.5 watts per cm^2

Table 16.2.9 Fluorescent Lighting and Malignant Melanoma (Reproduced from the journal *Health Physics* with permission of the Health Physics Society)

During the last 20 years, epidemiological studies of the incidence of malignant melanoma of the skin have suggested an etiologic role of ultraviolet radiation (UVR) (Anaise et al. 1978; Beral and Robinson 1981; Dubin et al. 1986; Fears et al. 1976; Gallagher et al. 1987; Green et al. 1986; Holman et al. 1986; Klepp and Magnus 1979; Kripke 1979; Lee 1985; MacKie 1987; Sober 1987).

More recently, some concern has arisen regarding the potential role that UVR emitted from fluorescent lighting could play in the etiology of malignant melanoma. This concern developed from published reports of epidemiological studies of the incidence of malignant melanoma in various occupations. An initial study, conducted in Australia by Beral et al. (1982), indicated that indoor office workers who reported working for many years under fluorescent lights had a higher incidence of malignant melanoma than those who reported they did not and those who worked outdoors. Further epidemiological studies specifically designed to test the hypothesis that exposure to UVR from artificial sources correlated with malignant melanoma incidence have shown either a positive correlation (Elwood 1986; English et al. 1985; Pasternack et al. 1983) or no significant correlation (Pasternack et al. 1983; Rigel et al. 1983; Sorahan and Grimley 1985; Swerdlow et al. 1988). The results of these studies and problems in their methodologies have been reviewed (Muel et al. 1988).

Despite the fact that Beral's original reported correlation was greatest for malignant melanoma occurrences on the trunk which is normally covered by clothes, it has been speculated that the weak UVR emissions of fluorescent lamps could explain the correlation. This hypothesis would require an indirect mechanism, such as a general UVR effect upon the immune system (Kripke 1979).

An obvious difficulty in all of the above studies has been the estimation of indoor vs. outdoor exposure to UVR and reliance on the recollections of both patients and matched controls of the characteristics of indoor lighting. In an ongoing study in Queensland, Australia,[a] very poor correlation was found between the recollections of patients and controls about the types of artificial lighting to which they had been exposed and the descriptions provided by a lighting engineer familiar with the buildings where the patients and controls had worked. It is therefore likely that one cannot completely rely upon the results found in such studies. From a theoretical point of view, it is far more likely that alternative theories are more valid to explain the clear increase in incidence of malignant melanoma of the skin among these indoor workers.

Recreational and social habits of indoor workers may increase the likelihood that they would sustain severe, acute overexposure to sunlight on untanned, normally covered regions of the skin (Carlton-Foss 1982; Holman et al. 1986; MacKie and Aitchison 1982). The very low incidence of melanoma lesions on lease-exposed areas of the skin (e.g., buttocks and women's breasts) and the high incidence of appearance on normally covered areas of the body (e.g., the trunk) argues for the hypothesis of an etiology related to acute overexposure to sunlight and against the hypothesis of an etiology related to direct fluorescent light exposure. The role of UVB in an indirect photochemical mechanism remains unresolved (Wiskemann et al. 1986).

The very low contribution of UVB (280–315 nm) and UVC (100–280 nm) radiation (CIE 1983; Cole et al. 1985; Diethelm 1970; Muel et al. 1988; Sliney and Wolbarsht 1980; Whillock et al. 1988) to the emissions from fluorescent lighting also argues against this exposure as a major or very significant etiology. Plastic diffusers serve as shields and will further attenuate UVB and UVC emissions (Cole et al. 1985; Whillock et al. 1988). Even if individuals were exposed to the UVR from unshielded fluorescent lamps, the exposure from these would be only a small fraction of exposure to solar UVR (Muel et al. 1988).

At least one health authority has suggested that where people are concerned about the UVR emitted by fluorescent lamps, absorbing plastic diffusers may be fitted to effectively remove it (FDA 1988). However, the reported health benefits of low-level exposure to UVB (e.g., vitamin D production, adaptation to further exposure) have been used to argue in favor of people regularly receiving a small amount of UVB (Health Council of the Netherlands 1986).

Considering all of the above arguments, INIRC concludes that UVR exposure from indoor fluorescent lighting should not be considered a malignant melanoma risk. Lamp manufacturers should be aware of this issue and not allow the current low levels of emission of UVB from fluorescent lighting to increase.

[a] Private communication (1988), R. MacLennan, Queensland, Australia.

Table 16.2.10 Alleged Radiation Risks from Visual Display Units

A Statement by the International Non-Ionizing Radiation Committee[a] of the International Radiation Protection Association (Reproduced from the journal *Health Physics* with the permission of the Health Physics Society)

Visual display units (VDUs) have become a major element in the modern work environment as an interface between man and computer. The discussion as to whether work at VDUs can affect human health has been centered on different types of effects, such as eye damage or discomforts, neck and shoulder discomfort, different stress reactions, skin disorders and adverse reproductive outcomes. In this context, much concern has been expressed in the media in relation to the possibility of radiation hazards due to VDUs based on cathode ray tubes (CRTs). This aspect will be covered in the present document, while the reader is referred to other texts for a discussion on the influence of various ergonomic factors on health (see e.g. World Health Organization 1987).

A number of careful scientific studies have been focused on the measurement of electromagnetic radiation or fields due to the VDUs, while some limited attention has also been given to acoustic radiation; several publications also address the topic of health risk assessment (see reference list).

(1) Soft x-ray radiation is produced within the CRT. The glass material of the tube, however, effectively prevents any leakage of x-ray radiation outside of the tube during operation. Thus, x-ray radiation from VDUs is not detectable with normal measuring instruments.

(2) Ultraviolet radiation in the near region (UV-A) can be detected from certain VDUs. The levels are, however, insignificant compared to present occupational standards (10 W/m^2) (International Radiation Protection Association 1985) and also insignificant compared to emission from other sources (e.g., sunlight through windows). In one investigation, VDU operators were found to be exposed to lower levels of UVA than those not working with VDUs, attributable to the fact that the former often draw the window curtains.

(3) Visible radiation can be measured and is necessary in order to perform the intended function of the CRT—to provide a visual display. Luminance levels recorded are far below current exposure limits, thus precluding (according to present knowledge) the possibility of pathological injury due to excessive exposure. There are ergonomic considerations of light emission from the display, such as flicker, contrast glare or readability. These are, however, not considered in this context.

(4) Infrared (IR) radiation is emitted from all warm bodies, and since all surfaces of the VDU are at room temperature or slightly above, IR radiation can be detected, although at levels far below any levels of concern for potential hazards.

(5) In the extremely low frequency and the radiofrequency regions, electric and magnetic fields have been detected. The dominant sources are the power supply and the vertical and horizontal sweep arrangements (at frequencies of some 50–80 Hz and 15–35 kHz, respectively). Compared to fields in many industrial or household situations, the fields around VDUs do not correspond to high exposure situations. These fields do not appear to represent any risk factor when evaluated by comparison with current standards, guidelines and recommendations for occupational exposure.

(6) In some countries, a number of VDU operators have experienced skin disorders. The relationship of these to VDU work is not known. Electrostatic fields at VDU workplaces have been suggested as a possible cause of skin disorders. Research conducted hitherto has indicated that the electrostatic charge of the operator might be a relevant factor. A relationship between electrostatic fields and skin disorders must, however, still be regarded as hypothetical.

(7) Airborne ultrasonic (acoustical) radiation is produced in VDUs as a result of mechanical vibrations generated in the core of the flyback transformer (responsible for the horizontal sweep of some 15–35 kHz). The sound pressure levels found are considerably below existing exposure limits (75 dB) (International Radiation Protection Association 1984). Some sensitive individuals may detect this sound or subharmonic as an annoying factor.

Effects which have been suggested as caused by exposure to electromagnetic radiation or fields include adverse pregnancy outcome or cataracts. Comparison of the occurrence of cataracts or of adverse pregnancy outcome among VDU operators to those of controls have failed to show an excess occurrence due to VDU work.

In conclusion, and based on current biomedical knowledge, there are no health hazards associated with radiation or fields from VDUs. Thus, there is no scientific basis to justify shielding or radiation monitoring of VDUs. However, since a large number of people are involved in VDU work, it is important that further knowledge is attained on certain areas where our knowledge must be regarded as incomplete. These areas include: (a) further investigations into the possibility that skin disorders may be related to VDU work, and if so, the factor(s) involved; and (b) the possibility of interactions between low frequency magnetic fields and biological systems. Considerations should be given to magnetic fields in various situations and should not be restricted to VDU work situations.

Measures should be taken to ensure that VDU work places are ergonomically well designed. This includes aspects of the VDU, the work station and work environment, as well as work organization. Visual screening examination is also valuable, in ensuring that the operator has adequate visual acuity, and that any corrective glasses are suitable for use at the VDU working distance.

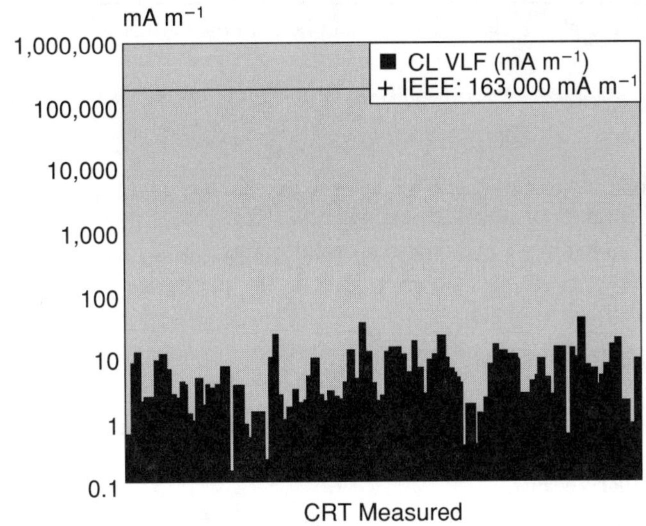

VDT VLF magnetic field intensities measured at operator positions as compared to ANSI/IEEE C95.1-1991 (ANSI, 1991) exposure guidelines.

The bold line indicates the ANSI/IEEE exposure guideline of 163,000 mA m^{-1}

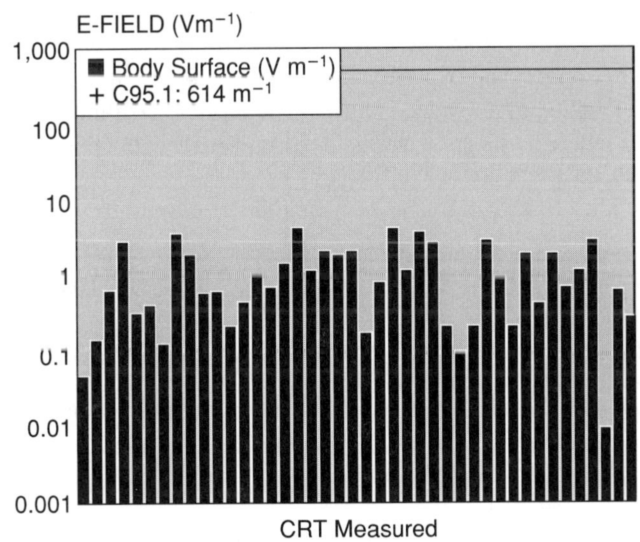

VDT VLF electric field intensities measured at operators' body surface as compared to ANSI/IEEE C95.1-1991 (ANSI, 1991) exposure guidelines.

The bold line indicates the ANSI/IEEE exposure guideline of 614 V m^{-1}

Figure 16.2.4 Illustrations of VDT VLF Magnetic and Electric Field Intensities at Operator's Positions Compared to ANSI/IEEE Exposure Guidelines. (From Haes and Fitzgerald, 1995, with permission, *Health Physics*)

Table 16.2.11 Laser Safety Precautions (From Sliney and Wolbarsht, 1980 with permission of author)

The safety rules accompanying the above classifications can be summarized as follows:

Class I Controls

No user safety rules are necessary.

Class II Controls

a. Never permit a person to continuously stare into the laser source if exposure levels exceed the applicable permissible exposure level for the duration of intended staring.
b. Never point the laser at an individual's eye unless a useful purpose exists and the exposure level and duration will not exceed the permissible limit.

Class III Controls

a. Do not aim the laser at an individual's eye.
b. Permit only experienced personnel to operate the laser.
c. Enclose as much of the beam path as possible. Even a transparent enclosure will prevent individuals from placing their head or reflecting objects within the beam path. Terminations should be used at the end of the useful paths of the direct and any secondary beams.
d. Shutters, polarizers, and optical filters should be placed at the laser exit port to reduce the beam power to the minimal useful level.
e. Control spectators.
f. A warning light or buzzer should indicate laser operation. This is especially needed if the beam is not visible, i.e., for infrared lasers.
g. Do not permit laser tracking of nontarget vehicles or aircraft.
h. Operate the laser only in a restricted area—for example, in a closed room without windows, and place a warning sign on the door.
i. Place the laser path well above or well below the eye level of any sitting or standing observers whenever possible. The laser should be mounted firmly to assure that the beam travels only along its intended path.
j. Always use proper laser eye protection if a potential eye hazard exists for the direct beam or a specular reflection.
k. A key switch should be installed to minimize tampering by unauthorized individuals.
l. The beam or its specular reflection should never be directly viewed with optical instruments such as binoculars or telescopes, unless with sufficient protective filters.
m. Remove all unnecessary mirror-like surfaces from within the vicinity of the laser beam path.

Class IV Controls

a. Fortunately, these high power lasers are seldom used outside of research laboratories and restricted industrial environments where personnel access is carefully controlled.
b. These lasers should only be operated within a localized enclosure, or in a controlled workplace, or where the beam is directed into outer space. If a complete local enclosure is not possible, laser operation indoors should be in a light tight room with interlocked entrances to assure that the laser cannot emit while a door is open.
c. Eye protection is needed for all individuals working within the controlled area. If the laser beam irradiance is sufficient to be a serious skin or fire hazard, a suitable shielding should be used between the laser beam and any personnel.
d. Remote firing with video monitoring or other remote (safe) viewing techniques should be chosen when feasible.
e. Outdoor high power laser devices such as satellite laser transmission systems and laser radar (LIDAR) should have positive stops on the azimuth and elevation traverse to assure that the beam cannot intercept occupied areas or non-target aircraft.
f. Beam shutters, beam polarizers, and beam filters should always be limited to use by authorized personnel only. The flashlamps is optical pump systems should be shielded to eliminate any direct viewing.
g. Backstops should be diffusely reflecting, fire resistant target materials where feasible. Safety enclosures should be used around microwelding and microdrilling work place to contain hazardous reflections from the work area. Microscopic viewing systems used to study the work areas should ensure against hazardous levels of reflection of laser irradiation back through the optics.

Table 16.2.12 Intrabeam Protection Standards for Eye and Skin Exposure to Laser Radiation

(After LIA, 1993)

CW Lasers Laser Type	Primary Wavelength (nm)	Protection Standard: Eye	Protection Standard: Skin
Helium-Cadmium	441.6	2.5 mW cm^{-2} for 0.25 s	0.2 W cm^{-2} for t > 10 s
Helium-Neon	632.8	10 C_B mJ cm^{-2} for 10 to 10^4 s	
Argon	488 and 514.5	C_B μW cm^{-2} for t > 10^4 s	
Krypton	647.1		
Frq Doubled Nd:YAG	532		0.2 W cm^{-2} for t > 10 s
Nd:YAG	1064	2.84 mW cm^{-2} for t > 100 s	1.0 W cm^{-2} for t > 10 s
Gallium-Arsenide at room temperature	905	1.46 mW cm^{-2} for t > 100 s	0.5 W cm^{-2} for t > 10 s
Helium-Cadmium	325	1 J cm^{-2} for t > 10 s	1 J cm^{-2} for 10 to 10^3 s
Nitrogen	337.1		1 mW cm^{-2} for t > 10^3 s
Carbon Dioxide	10,600	0.1 W cm^{-2} for t > 10 s	0.1 W cm^{-2} for t > 10 s

Pulsed Lasers Laser Type	Primary Wavelength (nm)	Pulse Duration	Protection Standard: Eye	Protection Standard: Skin
Normal Pulsed Ruby	694.3	~1 ms	10^{-5} J cm^{-2}	0.2 J cm^{-2}
Q-switched Ruby	694.3	5–10 ns	5×10^{-7} J cm^{-2}	0.02 J cm^{-2}
Q-switched, Frq Doubled Nd:YAG	532	5–100 ns	5×10^{-7} J cm^{-2}	0.02 J cm^{-2}
Rhodamine 6G Dye	~500–70	9.5–20 μs	5×10^{-7} J cm^{-2}	0.06–0.07 J cm^{-2}
Normal Pulsed Nd:YAG	1064	~1 ms	5×10^{-5} J cm^{-2}	0.06–0.07 J cm^{-2}
Q-switched Nd:YAG	1064	5–100 ns	5×10^{-6} J cm^{-2}	0.1 J cm^{-2}

Table 16.2.13 Maximum Permissible Exposures for Lasers (After Cember, 1996; ANSI Z136.1, 1993; ACGIH, 1990)

Wavelength (λ) μm	Exposure Time (t) Seconds	MPE (based on a 7-mm Maximum Pupil Diameter for Averaging the Radiant Exposure)
Direct Ocular Exposures—Intrabeam Viewing		
0.40–0.700	1E − 09 to 1.8E − 05	5E − 07 J cm^{-2}
	1.8E − 05 to 10	$1.8t^{0.75}$E − 03 Jcm^{-2}
0.40–0.550	10 to 1E + 04	1E − 02 J cm^{-2}
0.550–0.700	10 to (10 × $10^{[20(\lambda-0.550)]}$)	$1.8t^{0.75}$E − 03 J cm^{-2}
	(10 × $10^{[20(\lambda-0.550)]}$) to 1E + 04	10C_BE − 03 J cm^{-2}
0.400–0.700	1E + 04 to 3E + 04	C_BE − 06 W cm^{-2}
C_B = 1 for λ = 0.400–0.550 μm and C_B = $10^{[15(\lambda-0.550)]}$ for λ = 0.550–0.700 μm		
Viewing a Diffuse Reflection of a Laser Beam or an Extended Source Laser		
0.315–0.400	1E − 09 to 10	$0.56t^{0.25}$ J cm^{-2}
	10 to 1E + 03	1 J cm^{-2}
	1E + 03 to 3E + 04	0.001 W cm^{-2}
0.400–0.700	1E − 09 to 10	10 $t^{0.33}$ J cm^{-2} sr^{-1}
0.400–0.550	10 to 1E + 04	21 J cm^{-2} sr^{-1}
0.550–0.700	10 to (10 × $10^{[20(\lambda-0.550)]}$)	3.83 $t^{0.75}$ J cm^{-2} sr^{-1}
	(10 × $10^{[20(\lambda-0.550)]}$) to 1E + 04	21 C_B J cm^{-2} sr^{-1}
0.400–0.700	1E + 04 to 3E + 04	2.1 C_B tE-03 W cm^{-2} sr^{-1}
Skin Exposure to a Laser Beam		
0.315–0.400	1E − 09 to 10	$0.56t^{0.25}$ J cm^{-2}
	10 to 1 E + 03	1 J cm^{-2}
	1E + 03 to 3E + 04	0.001 W cm^{-2}
0.4–1.4	1E − 09 to 1 E − 07	0.02 C_A J cm^{-2}
	1E − 07 to 10	1.1 $C_A t^{0.25}$ J cm^{-2}
	10 to 3E + 04	0.2 C_A W cm^{-2}
1.4–1000	1E − 09 to 1E − 07	0.01 J cm^{-2}
	1E − 07 to 10	$0.56t^{0.25}$ J cm^{-2}
	>10	0.1 W cm^{-2}

C_A = 1 for $\lambda < 0.700$ μm and C_A = $10^{[2(\lambda-0.700)]}$ for λ = 0.700–1.049 μm and C_A = 5 for λ = 1.050–1.400 μm.

Photobiological Spectral Domain		Eye Effects	Skin Effects
Ultraviolet C	(0.200-0.280 μm)		Erythma (sunburn) Skin Cancer
Ultraviolet B	(0.280-0.315μm)	Photokeratitis	Accelerated Skin Aging Increased Pigmentation
Ultraviolet A	(0.315-0.400 μm)	Photochemical UV Cataract	Pigment Darkening
Visible	(0.400-0.780 μm)	Photochemical & Thermal Retinal Injury	Photosensitive Reactions
Infrared A	(0.780-1.400 μm)	Cataract, Retinal Burns	Skin Burns
Infrared B	(1.400-3.000 μm)	Corneal Burn Aqueous Flare IR Cataract	
Infrared C	(3.000-1000 μm)	Corneal Burn Only	

Figure 16.2.5 Summary of Basic Biological Effects of Light. (From OSHA Instruction PUB 8-1.7, 1991)

SECTION 3 ULTRASOUND

TABLE OF CONTENTS

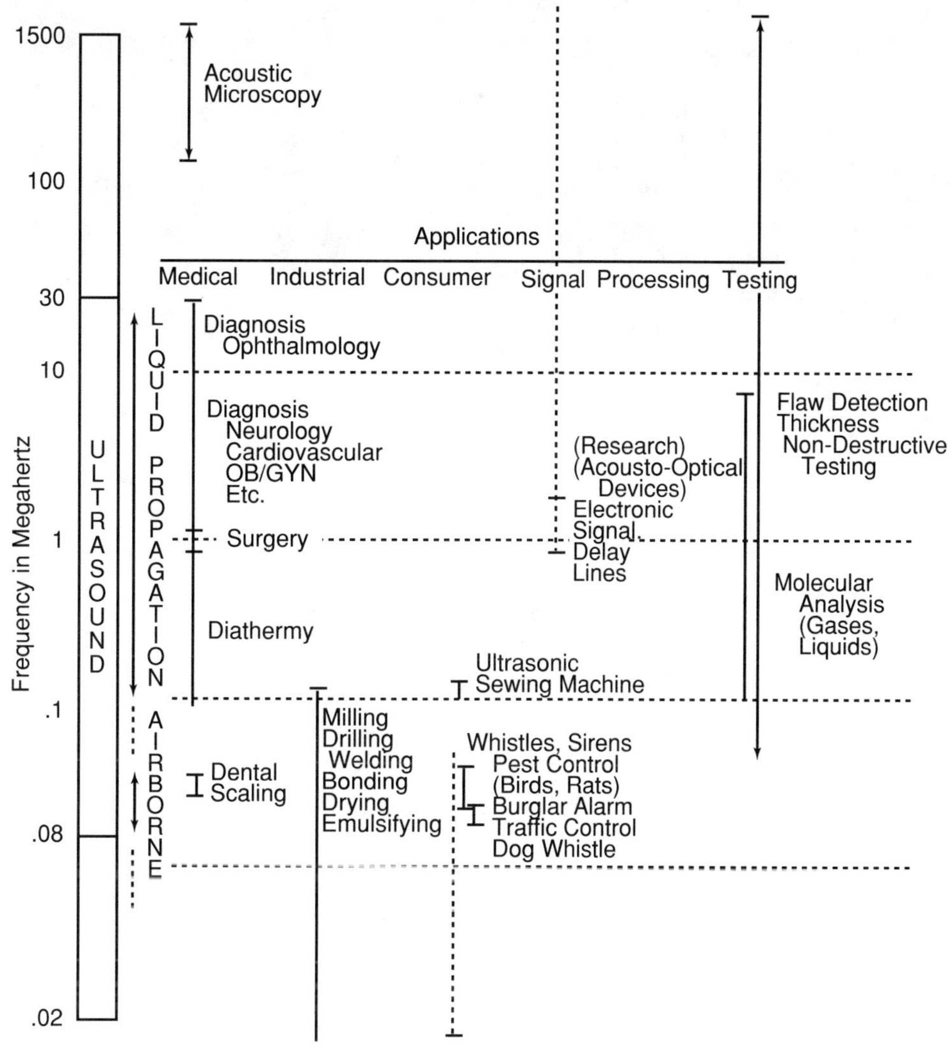

Figure 16.3.1 The Ultrasound Spectrum with Applications. (From FDA 84-8222, 1984)

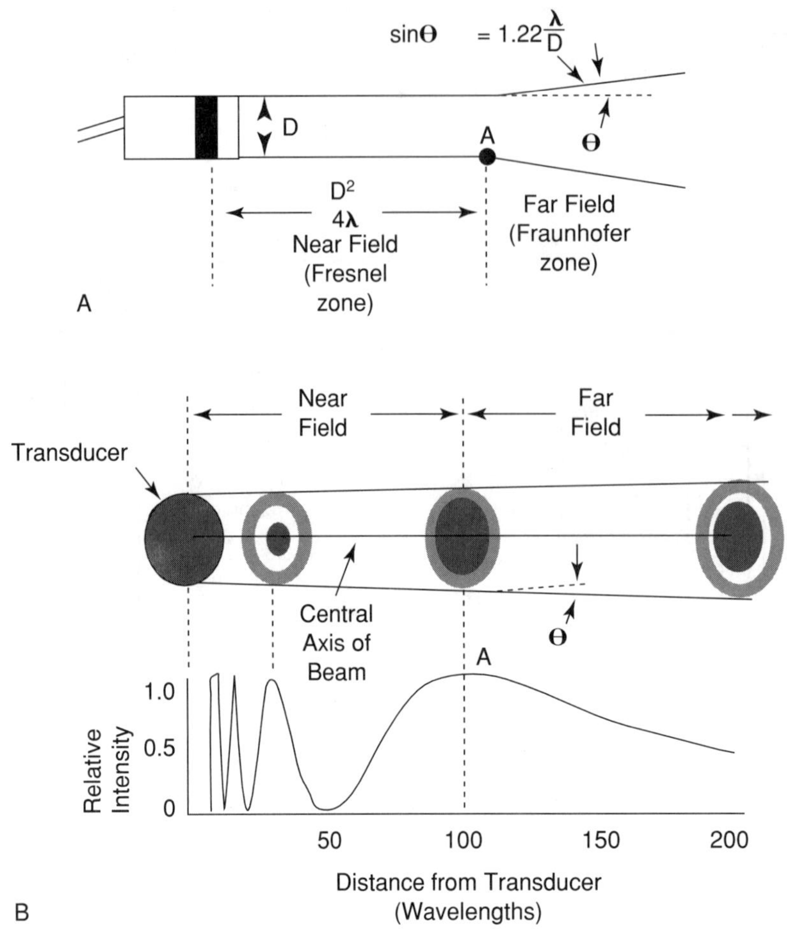

Figure 16.3.2 Structure of Ultrasound Fields. (a) Near and far fields relative to the transducer. (b) Field distirbution of an ideal piston source generating a continuous wave-this transducer has diameter of 10 wavelengths. The ring diagrams represent the cross-sectional intensity distribution at selected positions along the central axis of the beam. (From Health and Welfare Canada Safety Code 23, 1980)

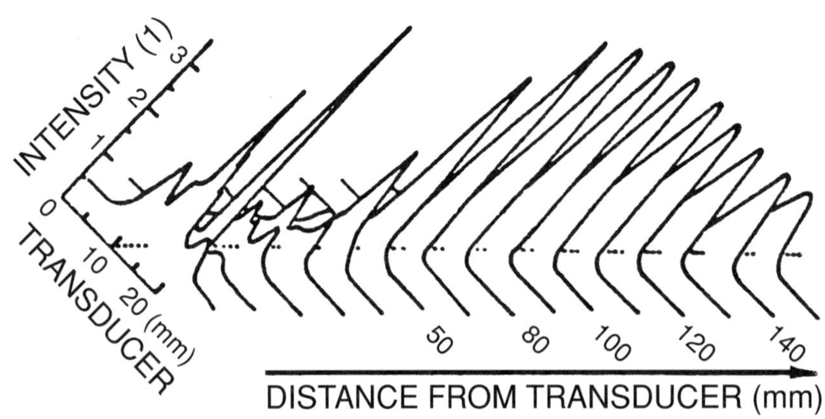

Figure 16.3.3 A Three Dimensional Representation of the Ultrasound Intensity Distribution Across the Transducer at Various Distances from the Crystal. (From Health and Welfare Canada Safety Code 23, 1980)

Table 16.3.1 Ultrasound Acoustic Parameters

Acoustic Output	Time/Frequency Characteristics of Ultrasound Field	Spatial Distribution of Ultrasonic Field
Intensities (maximum and average in space in time)	Type of waveform (cw or pulsed)	Transducer type (focusing or non-focussing)
Total Power (maximum and average in time)	Pulse duration and repetition rate	Radiating area/ beam width
	Pulse shape	Beam profile (axial and transverse)
	Frequency (center)	Focussing characteristics (if focussed)
	Pulse spectrum (bandwidth)	Focal area/ beam width
		Depth of focus
		Focal Length

Table 16.3.2 Medical Ultrasound Fields—Exposure Parameters

The parameters listed are for a fixed transducer, especially a circular one generating a well defined beam. For pulsed operation the temporal average symbolized by I_{SPTA}, I_{SATA}, or I_T is the overall value, i.e., the averaging interval is a complete repetition period.

Symbol	Name and/or Description
W	Total emitted acoustil power (time averaged).
$I_{SPTA} = I(SPTA)$	Spatial peak temporal average intensity. Temporal average at the spatial peak.
$I_{SATA} - I(SATA)$	Time average intensity spatially averaged over ''effective cross section'' of beam.
$I_{SATA,T} = I(SATA, T) = I_T$	Time average intensity at radiating face of transducer spatially averaged over effective area.
$I_{SPPA} = I(SPPA)$	Spatial peak pulse average intensity. Intensity at spatial peak, time averaged over pulse duration.
I_p	For a pulse, highest of the maxima of the instantaneous intensity at the spatial peak.
I_m	Spatial peak intensity averaged over largest half cycle of a pulse; equal to $I_p/2$ for nearly sinusoidal oscillations. For simplicity called ''maximum intensity.''

Table 16.3.3 Decibel Notation

The need often arises for comparing intensity or pressure levels; for example, when considering the amount of reflection or absorption which an ultrasonic field has undergone. In this case, it may be an advantage to express the ratio of intensities or pressures as a logarithm because this affords a simple method of expressing numbers that extends over many orders of magnitude and because the arithmetic product of two or more quantities are obtained by the addition of the logarithms. The decibel (dB) is the logarithmic unit most commonly used for expressing the ratio of two quantities.

It is important to realize that since the decibel unit is only a relative measurement, a reference level must also be stated to obtain an absolute value. For example, an intensity of 16 dB above 1 W/cm^2 is equal to 39.81 W/cm^2. A reference level usually used for audible sound is 20 micro-pascals which corresponds to the weakest sound a human being can hear.

The formulae for the decibel and reference levels sometimes used are as follows:

Decibel Formulae and Reference Levels Sometimes Used

Quantity	Formula	Reference Level[a]
Sound pressure	20 log (p/p_0) dB	20 μPa (in air) 1 μPa (in other media)
Acceleration	20 log (a/a_0) dB	1 μm/s^2
Velocity	20 log (v/v_0) dB	1 nm/s
Force	10 log (F/F_0) dB	1 μN
Power	10 log (P/P_0) dB	1 pW
Intensity	10 log (I/I_0) dB	1 pW/m^2
Energy density	10 log (W/W_0) dB	1 pJ/m^3
Energy	10 log (E/E_0) dB	1 pJ
Voltage	20 log (V/V_0) dB	

[a] Note that a change of 3 dB changes power, intensity, force, and energy by a factor of 2, and sound pressure, acceleration, velocity, and voltage by a factor of the square root of 2 or 1.41. A change of an additional 3 dB to make 6 dB represents a power ratio of 2^2 or 4 and sound pressure a ratio of 2.

In biological effects literature, reference is often made to the neper. The neper is a logarithmic unit corresponding to a reduction in amplitude (e.g., pressure amplitude) to 1/e of the initial value, i.e.,

$$\text{nepers} = \log_e (P/P_0)$$

Since this corresponds to a change of -8.686 dB, we can say that 1 neper = 8.686 dB.

Table 16.3.4 Ultrasound—Units, Relationships, and Conversion Factors

Term	Units	Symbol	Equivalent Units or Comment
Angular frequency	hertz (Hz)	ω	$\omega = 2\pi f$
Power	watt (W)	P	J/s
Propagation constant	cm^{-1}	k	$2\pi/\lambda$
Intensity[a]	watts/sq. meter (W/m^2)	I	
Speed of sound in the medium	meters/second (m/s)	c	
Force	newton (N)	F	kg/s^2
Pressure	pascal (Pa)	p	N/m^2
Particle displacement	meter (m)	s	
Particle velocity	meters/second (m/s)	v	
Particle acceleration	meter/sq. second (m/s^2)	a	
Characteristic acoustic impedance	rayls (r)	Z	$kg/(s^1m^2)$
Amplitude attenuation coefficient	nepers/cm	α	8.686 dB/cm
Amplitude absorption coefficient	nepers/cm	α_a	8.686 dB/cm
Intensity attenuation coefficient	nepers/cm	μ	2α
Wavelength	meter (m)	λ	
Frequency	hertz (Hz)	f	1/s
Energy	joule (J)	E	N m (= W s)
Density	kg/m^3	ρ	
Area	sq. meters (m^2)	A	

[a] In practice, it is more convenient to express intensity in units of watts per square centimeter (W/cm^2) or milliwatts per square centimeter (mW/cm^2).

Table 16.3.5 Ultrasound—Relationship of Terms

Particle Displacement

$$s = s_0 \sin(\omega t - kx)$$

where s_0 = maximum displacement amplitude
$\omega = 2\pi f$ = angular frequency
$k = 2\pi/\lambda$ = wave number
s = displacement amplitude

Particle Velocity

$$v = \partial s/\partial t = v_0 \cos(\omega - kx)$$

where $v_o = \omega s_0$ = velocity amplitude
$k = 2\pi/\lambda$ = propagation constant

Particle Acceleration

$$a = \partial v/\partial t = -a_o \sin(\omega t - kx)$$

where $a_o = \omega^2 s_0$ = acceleration amplitude

Acoustic Pressure

$$\partial p/\partial x = -\rho a, \quad \text{hence}$$
$$p = p_0 \cos(\omega t - kx)$$

where $p_0 = \dfrac{c\omega^2 s_0}{k} = \rho c \omega s_0$ = pressure amplitude
c = propagation velocity

Specific Acoustic Impedance

$$Z = P_0 v_0, \quad \text{hence}$$
$$Z = \rho c$$

Energy Density

The total kinetic energy of a single oscillating particle (at maximum velocity) is

$$e = m v_0^2/2$$
m = mass if the particle
v_0 = particle velocity amplitude

hence the energy density (E) of the sound field is

$$E = \rho v_0^2/2 \text{ or, using } Z = P_0/v_0 = \rho c$$
$$E = \rho p_0^2/2Z^2 = P_0^2/2\rho c^2$$
ρ = mean density of the medium

Intensity[a]

Intensity is equal to the speed of sound in the medium (c), times the total energy

$$I = cE$$

hence, using

$$E = p_0^2/2\rho c^2$$
$$I = p_0^2/2\rho c$$

For a given intensity, the quantities s_0, v_o, a_o and p_o can be calculated from

$$s_0 = 1/\omega(2I/\rho c)^{1/2}$$
$$v_0 = (2I/\rho c)^{1/2}$$
$$a_0 = \omega(2I/\rho c)^{1/2}$$
$$p_0 = (2\rho c I)^{1/2}$$

[a] the above relationships are based on the assumption of a plane continuous (sinusoidal) wave, and I represents the intensity of the wave averaged over one cycle. In such a wave, the instantaneous peak intensity (I_p) is twice the average value, i.e., $I = I_A$ and $I_p = 2I_A$. If the wave consists of short asymmetric pulses, such as those emitted by pulse-echo diagnositic ultrasonic instruments, it is usually not possible to define an average over one cycle. It is therefore necessary to specify the output of such instruments in terms of the instantaneous peak intensity.

$$I_p = p_0^2/\rho c$$

and the particle parameters are now given by

$$s_0 = 1/\omega(I/\rho c)^{1/2}$$
$$v_0 = (I/\rho c)^{1/2}$$
$$a_0 = \omega(I/\rho c)^{1/2}$$
$$p_0 = (\rho c I)^{1/2}$$

Table 16.3.6 Range of Ultrasonic Output Intensities Found in Beams Produced by Medical Ultrasonic Equipment (From FDA 82-8190, 1982)

Type of Equipment	Acoustic Power	Spatial Average, Temporal Average Intensity on the Radiating Surface	Spatial Peak, Temporal Average Intensity	Spatial Peak Pulse Average Intensity	Spatial Peak Temporal Peak Intensity
Static pulse echo scanners and mode equipment	0.1–20 mW	0.01–10 mW/cm^2	0.6–125 mW/cm^2	0.01–160 W/cm^2	0.4–700 W/cm^2
Automatic sector scanners (phased arrays and wobblers)	9–20 mW	0.5–15 mW/cm^2	2–200 mW/cm^2	0.3–75 W/cm^2	0.4–300 W/cm^2
Sequenced linear arrays	0.1–33 mW	0.06–10 mW/cm^2	0.5–12 mW/cm^2	0.3–69 W/cm^2	.4–120 W/cm^2
Pulsed doppler, primarily for cardiac work	8–24 mW	5–32 mW/cm^2	20–290 mW/cm^2	1–14 W/cm^2	2–600 W/cm^2
Doppler instruments, primarily for obstetric applications	1–18 mW	0.26–25 mW/cm^2	0.6–75 mW/cm^2		
Continuous wave doppler primarily for peripheral vascular	6–105 mW	10–400 mW/cm^2			
Therapy continuous	1–25 W	0–4 W/cm^2	0–16 W/cm^2		
Therapy pulsed	.250–4 W	0–1 W/cm^2	0–4 W/cm^2		

Table 16.3.7 Guidelines on Human Exposure to Airborne Ultrasound Basic Concepts (Summary) (After IRPA/INIRC, 1984 with permission)

Airborne ultrasound is usually quantified in terms of sound pressure level (SPL) in decibels (dB), such that:

$$SPL(dB) = 20 \log_{10}(p/p_r),$$

where p is the root mean square acoustic pressure and p_r is the reference pressure. p_r is equivalent to approximately the lowest level of audible sound perceived by humans at the most sensitive frequency (approximately 1 kHz), and is normally taken as equal to 20 micropascals (μPa). 20 μPa is equivalent to an acoustic intensity $I_r = 10^{-12} W/m^2$ in the air.

Since the acoustic intensity (I) is proportional to the square of the acoustic pressure, the sound pressure level can be equivalently expressed by

$$SPL(dB) = 10 \log_{10}(I/I_r).$$

Therefore, doubling the intensity (I) increases the SPL by 3 dB, whereas doubling the pressure (p) increases the SPL by 6 dB.

It should be noted that commonly used sound level meters have an effective complete cut-off above about 20 kHz. Thus special sound level meters are needed for measurements above this frequency.

An octave band contains a range of frequencies, the upper frequency limit being twice the lower frequency limit. The center or mid frequency used to designate each octave is twice the center frequency of the preceding octave band. In this document, one third octave bands are used to geometrically split an octave band into three parts and the mid frequency is used to designate each band.

Table 16.3.8 Interim Guidelines on Limits of Human Exposure to Airborne Ultrasound Levels

(From IRPA/INIRC, 1984 with permission)

A. Limits for Continuous Occupational Exposure to Airborne Ultrasound[a,b]

Mid Frequency of One-Third Octave Band (kHz)	Sound Pressure Level (dB re: 20 μPa)
20	75
25	110
31.5	110
40	110
50	110
63	110
80	110
100	110

[a] The limits apply to continuous exposure to workers for an 8 hour working day. The limits in this table may be increased in accordance with corrections given in Table 16.3.8 B provided the duration of exposure per day does not exceed 4 hours.
[b] The limits recommended in these guidelines may be exceeded for occupational exposure, if workers are provided with ear protectors that reduce ultrasound levels at their ears to the sound pressure given in Table 16.3.8 A.

B. Modification to Occupational Exposure Limits Given for Exposure Durations Not Exceeding 4 Hours Per Day

Total Exposure Duration (h)	Correction to SPL (dB)
2–4	+3
1–2	+6
0–1	+9

C. Limits for Continuous Exposure of the General Public to Airborne Ultrasound[a,b]

Mid Frequency of One-Third Octave Band (kHz)	Sound Pressure Level (dB re: 20 μPa)
20	70
25	100
31.5	100
40	100
50	100
63	100
80	100
100	100

[a] The limits apply to continuous exposure of the general public for up to 24 hours per day.
[b] No exclusions to these limits are recommended for exposure of the general public.

Table 16.3.9 Protective Measures for Ultrasound Equipment (Adapted, by permission, from: *Ultrasound* Geneva, WHO 1982 Environmental Health Criteria, No. 22 pp. 140-144)

For Diagnostic Devices

a. Criteria for imaging effectiveness should be developed and disseminated. Such criteria would help the user in evaluating benefit versus risk and in keeping the output of ultrasonic equipment as low as practicable, consistent with obtaining the necessary diagnostic information.

b. Output levels approaching the lower limits of those used in therapy, i.e., 100 mW/cm^2, should not be employed for diagnostic purposes, unless they can be justified on the basis of providing necessary information that cannot be obtained by other means.

c. Equipment should be designed with adjustable controls so that the operator can use the minimum ultrasound exposure required to obtain an image or other information concerning the organ of interest in each patient.

d. Diagnostic ultrasound should be used in human beings only when there is a valid medical reason. Individuals, and especially pregnant woman, should not be exposed for commercial demonstrations or for routine imaging to produce test images when equipment is being serviced.

For Therapeautic Ultrasound Equipment

a. Accuracy specifications for the output power and the timer are needed, because both directly affect the dose delivered to the patient.

b. No pregnant patient should receive ultrasound therapy in such a way as to expose the fetus directly or indirectly. At present, ultrasound therapy is given to pregnant patients for low back pain. This practice should be discouraged.

c. It is not advisable to use ultrasound over the vertebral column, especially following laminectomies, or when anesthetized areas are involved.

d. Care should be taken when epiphyseal lines in children are exposed to ultrasound, especially when these regions are still at the growing stage.

e. Care should be exercised when treating peripheral vascular disease in the extremities because, with diminished sensation and reduced circulation, the patient may not be aware of overexposure to ultrasound.

f. Ultrasound exposure close to a strong reflecting surface, such as bone, may lead to the formation of standing waves, which may produce blood flow stasis and related effects. In therapy, the ultrasound transducer should be moved over the region of injury to minimized harmful effects from standing waves and possible cavitation.

g. Patient exposure can and should be minimized by:
   (i) testing the patient's skin sensation prior to the application of ultrasound, since patients unable to differentiate between hot and cold will not be able to detect overexposure.
   (ii) using the minimum effective exposure;
   (iii) keeping the energized transducer moving slowly over the treatment region to minimize the risk of undue local temperature elevations;
   (iv) ensuring that the operator is present to terminate the treatment if the patient shows the least sign of distress;
   (v) calibrating equipment regularly.

h. Operator exposure can be minimized by:
   (i) not touching the face of the transducer or applicator when it is emitting ultrasound; and
   (ii) not immersing any part of the operator's body in the water bath while ultrasound is being generated.

For Ultrasound Exposure in Industry

a. Persons exposed to high levels of noise associated with ultrasonic equipment should be protected either by means of devices such as earmuffs, or by constructing acoustic barriers around the equipment to reduce the noise levels.

b. Direct contact exposure to high intensities of liquid borne ultrasound should be avoided. For example, operators should not place their hands in ultrasonic cleaning tanks during operation. Warning signs should be placed at suitable locations.

c. In burglar alarms, the ultrasonic source should be switched off, instead of only the alarm, when the system is not in use.

Table 16.3.10 Ultrasound Properties of Various Media[a] (Reproduced, by permission, from Suess, M.J. and Benwell-Morrison, D.A. ed *Nonionizing Radiation Protection*, 2nd ed. Copenhagen, WHO Regional Office for Europe, 1989 WHO Regional Publications, European Series, No. 29)

Medium	Sound Speed, *c* (compression wave) (m/s)	Characteristic Acoustic Impedance, *z* (kg/(s m^2))	Attenuation Coefficient α at 1MHz (neper/m)[b]	Frequency Dependence of Attenuation Coefficient, *n*
Air	330	4.50×10^{-2}	15	2
Water	1500	1.50×10^6	0.02	2
Liver	1540	1.54×10^6	8	1.2
Fat	1440	1.40×10^6	5–25	1.4
Lens of eye	—	1.84×10^6	—	—
Blood	1520	1.61×10^6	2.3	1.3
Skeletal muscle	1520	1.70×10^6	10–35	1.1
Skull bone	3360	6.99×10^6	115	1.7
Perspex (Lucite)	2680	3.16×10^6	23	2

[a] Approximate room temperature values for illustrative purposes only. Accurate measurement of ultrasound attenuation in human tissues is difficult, and published data are not always reliable. Furthermore, actual values may show quite marked variability with such factors as temperature.
[b] To convert to ''engineering'' units of dB/cm, the values in this column should be multiplied by 0.087.

Table 16.3.11 Ultrasound Bioeffects (From FDA 78-8048, 1977)

Average[a] Intensity (mW/cm^2)	Total Exposure Time (min)	Test System	Effect Observed
Developmental			
10 (cw)[b]	5	Rat	Delayed neuromuscular development
20 (cw)	300	Rat	Delayed neuromotor reflex development
20 (cw)	300	Rat	Altered emotional behavior
40 (cw)	300	Mouse	Fetal abnormalities
125 (cw)	3	Mouse	Postpartum mortality
500–5,000 (cw)	0.17–3	Mouse	Reduced fetal weight
Hematological and Vascular			
50 (cw)	1.5	Rabbit eye	Vascular changes
65 (cw)	5	Human blood	Decreased in vitro clotting time
500 (cw)	2	Canine bone	Hemorrhage
500 (cw)	>0.1	Chick embryo	Blood stasis
Neurological and Behavioral			
1.5 (P)[c]	360	Canine CNS	Increased GOT levels in cerebrospinal fluid
3 (P)		Primate CNS	Altered EEG response
10 (cw)[d]	5	Rat	Delayed neuromotor reflex development
20 (cw)	300	Rat	Delayed neuromotor reflex development
20 (cw)	300	Rat	Altered emotional behavior
Genetic			
4 (P)[c]	10	HeLa cells	Decreased incorporation of nucleic acid precursors
200 (cw)	1	Vicia root	Chromosomal aberrations
200 (cw)	15	Calf thymus	DNA strand degradation
400 (cw)	3	Calf thymus & salmon sperm DNA	DNA strand degradation

[a] Spatial and temporal average
[b] Continuous wave ultrasound
[c] Pulsed ultrasound
[d] Continuous wave ultrasound-evoked EEG response appeared immediately upon start of sonication but disappeared after 3 min. exposure.

References

American Conference of Governmental Industrial Hygienists. *1990–1991 Threshold Limit Values for Chemical Substances and Physical Agents and the Biological Exposure Indexes.* pp 7–121; Cincinnati, OH; 1990.

American National Standards Institute (ANSI). *ANSI Z136.1-1993 American National Standard for Safe Use of Lasers.* LIA; Orlando, FL; 1993.

Cember, H. *Introduction to Health Physics - Third Edition.* McGraw-Hill; New York, NY; 1996.

Food and Drug Administration. *Symposium on Biological Effects and Characterization of Ultrasound Sources.* U.S. Dept. HEW Publication; FDA 78-8048; 1977.

Food and Drug Administration. *Instrumentation for Non-Ionizing Radiation Measurement.* Conference of Radiation Control Program Directors. FDA 84-8222; Public Health Service, Department of Health and Human Services; Rockville, MD; 1984.

Food and Drug Administration. *Federal Performance Standards for Laser Products.* 21 CFR Section 1040; Center for Devices and Radiological Health; Rockville, MD.

Garn, H., Gabriel, C. ''Present Knowledge About Specific Absorption Rates Inside a Human Body Exposed to Radiofrequency Electromagnetic Fields,'' *Health Physics,* **68**(2):147–156; 1995.

Glazer, Z. ''Non-ionizing radiation control,'' *Handbook of Management of Radiation Protection Programs,* Miller, K.L. (Ed.) CRC Press (1991 in press).

Glazer, Z. Personal Communication, 1991.

Glazer, Z.G., Dodge, C.H. in *Risk/Benefit Analysis,* Steneck, N.H., Ed.; San Francisco Press, Inc.; San Francisco, CA; 1982.

Haes, D.L., Fitzgerald, M.R. ''Video display terminal very low frequency measurments: The need for protocols in assessing VDT user 'dose','' *Health Physics,* **68**(4):572–578; 1995.

Hankin, N.N. *The Radiofrequency Radiation Environment: Environmental Exposure Levels and RF Radiation Emitting Sources.* EPA 520/1-85-014; July 1986.

Health and Welfare Canada. *Guidelines for the Safe Use of Ultrasound Part 1 (Medical and Paramedical Applications).* Safety Guide 23; 80-EHD-59; 1980.

International Commission on Non-Ionizing Radiation Protection (ICNIRP). ''Guidelines on Limits of Exposure to Static Magnetic Fields,'' *Health Physics,* **66**(1):100–106; 1994.

International Radiation Protection Association (IRPA) and International Non-Ionizing Radiation Committee (INRC). ''Interim Guidelines on Limits of Human Exposure to Airborne Ultrasound,'' *Health Physics,* **46**(4):969–974; 1984.

International Radiation Protection Association (IRPA). ''Guidelines on limits of exposure to radiofrequency electromagnetic fields in the frequency range from 100 kHz to 300 GHz,'' *Health Physics,* **54**(1):115–123; 1988.

International Radiation Protection Association (IRPA) and International Non-Ionizing Radiation Committee (INRC). ''Interim guidelines on limits of exposure to 50/60 Hz electric and magnetic fields,'' *Health Physics,* **58**(1):113–122; 1990.

Laser Institute of America (LIA). *Laser Safety Guide - Ninth Edition.* Edited by David H. Sliney. LIA; Orlando, FL; 1993.

Laser Institute of America (LIA). *Industrial Laser Safety Reference Guide.* LIA; Orlando, FL; 1996.

Occupational Safety and Health Administration (OSHA). *OSHA Instruction PUB 8-1.7 Guidelines for Laser Safety and Hazard Assessment.* LIA; Orlando, FL; 1991.

National Council on Radiation Protection and Measurements (NCRP). *A Practical Guide to the Determination of Human Exposure to Radiofrequency Fields.* Report No. 119; Bethesda, MD; 1993.

Pearson, A.J., Grainger, K.J.L., Whillock, M.J., Driscoll, C.M.H. *Hazard Assessment of Optical Radiation Sources used in Some Consumer Products.* NRPB Bullentin 126; National Radiation Protection Board; Oxon, UK; October 1991.

Peterson, R.C. ''Radiofrequency/microwave protection guides,'' *Health Physics,* **61**(1):59–67; 1991.

Repacholi, M.H.(Ed), ''Non-ionizing Radiations: Physical Characteristics, Biological Effects and Health Hazard Assessment,'' International Radiation Protection Association/International Non-Ionizing Radiation Committee Publication. Proceeding of the International Non-Ionizing Radiation Workshop; Melbourne, Australia; April 5–9, 1988. Available from: Australian Radiation Laboratory, Lower Plenty Road, Yallambie, Victoria, Australia, 3085.

Sliney, D., Wolborsht, M. *Safety with Lasers and Other Optical Sources.* Plenum Press; New York, NY; 1980.

Stewart H., Stratmeyer, M.E. An Overview of Ultrasound: Theory, Measurement, Medical Applications and Biological Effects. Food and Drug Administration; Public Health Services; U.S. Dept. of HEW; Rockville, MD; 1982.

World Health Organization. *Ultrasound (Executive Summary).* WHO Environmental Health Criteria 22; UN Environmental Program and the International Radiation Protection Association; Geneva; 1982.

World Health Organization. *Non-Ionizing Radiation Protection.* 2nd ed., Suess, M.J., Benwell-Morison, ed; WHO Regional Publication European Series 29; Geneva; 1989.

GLOSSARIES

GLOSSARY—IONIZING RADIATION

Ablation—The functional destruction of an organ through surgery or exposure to large doses of radiation.

Absorbed Dose—The amount of *ionizing radiation* energy absorbed in matter, including human tissue. The units of *absorbed dose* are the *rad* and the *gray (Gy).*

Absorber—Any material that absorbs or lessens the intensity of *ionizing radiation. Neutron* absorbers (like boron, hafnium, and cadmium) are used in *control rods* for *reactors*. Concrete and steel absorb *gamma rays* and neutrons in reactor *shields*. A thin sheet of paper or metal will absorb or weaken *alpha particles* and all except the most energetic *beta particles*. (See *control rod; shielding*.)

Absorption—The process by which the number of particles or *photons* entering a body of matter is reduced or *attenuated* by interaction with the matter. (See *neutron capture*.)

Absorption factor—Ratio of entry to exit dose.

Access Hatch (air lock)—An airtight door system that preserves the pressure integrity of a reactor *containment* building while allowing access to personnel and equipment.

Activation—The process of making a material *radioactive* by bombardment with *neutrons, protons*, or other *nuclear radiation*. (See *induced radioactivity*.)

Activation Product—*Radioactivity* that is created when stable substances are bombarded by *neutrons*. For example, *stable isotope* cobalt-59 (^{59}Co or Co-59) becomes the *radioactive isotope* cobalt-60 (^{60}Co or Co-60) under *neutron* bombardment. See *induced radioactivity*.

Activity—The rate of transformation (or "disintegration" or "decay") of radioactive material. The units of activity are the *curie (Ci)* and the *becquerel (Bq)*.

Activity Median Aerodynamic Diameter (AMAD)—The diameter of a unit density sphere with the same terminal settling velocity in air as that of the aerosol particle whose activity is the median for the entire aerosol.

Acute Exposure—The absorption of a relatively large amount of radiation (or intake of radioactive material) over a short period of time.

Acute Health Effects—Prompt radiation effects (those that would be observable within a short period of time) for which the severity of the effect varies with the dose, and for which a practical threshold exists.

Acute Radiation Sickness (Syndrome)—See *radiation sickness (syndrome).*

Added Filtration—Any filtration which is in addition to the inherent filtration.

Adult—An individual 18 or more years of age.

Agreement State—Any State with which the U.S. Nuclear Regulatory Commission or the U.S. Atomic Energy Commission has entered into an effective agreement under subsection 274b. of the Atomic Energy Act of 1954, as amended (73 Stat. 689).

Airborne Radioactive Material—Radioactive material dispersed in the air in the form of dusts, fumes, particulates, mists, vapors, or gases.

Airborne Radioactivity Area—A room, enclosure, or area in which airborne radioactive materials exist in concentrations—

(1) In excess of the specified *derived air concentrations* (DACs)

(2) To such a degree that an individual present in the area without respiratory protective equipment could exceed, during the hours an individual is present in a week, an intake of 0.6 percent of the *annual limit on intake* (ALI) or 12 DAC-hours.

Air Lock—See *access hatch.*

Air Sampler—Apparatus used for air sampling.

Air Sampling—The collection and analysis of samples of air to detect the presence of, identify the composition of, or measure the concentration of *radioactive* substances, particulate matter or chemical pollutants.

ALARA (acronym for "as low as is reasonably achievable")—Making every reasonable effort to maintain exposures to *radiation* as far below the dose limits as is practical consistent with the purpose for which the activity is undertaken, taking into account the state of technology, the economics of improvements in relation to state of technology, the economics of improvements in relation to benefits to the public health and safety, and other societal and socioeconomic considerations, and in relation to utilization of nuclear energy and radioactive materials in the public interest.

Alpha Particle—A positively charged particle ejected spontaneously from the *nuclei* of some *radioactive* elements. It is identical to a helium *nucleus* that has a *mass number* of 4 and an electrostatic charge of +2.

Aluminum Equivalent—The thickness of type 1100 aluminum alloy[a] affording the same attenuation, under specified conditions, as the material in question.

Analytical X-Ray Equipment—Equipment used for *x-ray* diffraction or fluorescence analysis.

Analytical X-Ray System—A group of components utilizing x- or gamma rays to determine the elemental composition or to examine the microstructure of materials.

Anion—Negatively charged *ion*. (See *ionization*.)

Annual Limit on Intake (ALI)—The derived limit for the amount of radioactive material taken into the body of an adult worker by inhalation or ingestion in a year. ALI is the smaller value of intake of a given radionuclide in a year by the reference man that would result in a *committed effective dose equivalent* of 5 rem (0.05 Sv) or a *committed dose equivalent* of 50 rem (0.5 Sv) to any individual organ or tissue. The ALI given by ICRP 1991 are based on limiting the committed effective dose from an intake in a single year to 20 mSv.

Annual Reference Levels of Intake (ARLI)[b]—The activity of a radionuclide that, taken into the body during a year, would provide a committed effective dose to a person, represented by *Reference Man*, equal to 20 mSv. The ARLI is expressed in *becquerels (Bq)*.

Anti-Contamination Clothes (Anti-Cs) ***or Protective Clothes***—Protective clothing worn by radiation workers used to intercept radioactive materials which would otherwise contaminate the worker's skin or clothing that he wears outside the radioactivity area. The Anti-Cs may include laboratory coats, coveralls, caps, gloves, and shoes or shoe covers and are removed when the worker leaves the radioactivity area.

Atom—The smallest particle of an *element* that cannot be divided or broken up by chemical means. It consists of a central core called the *nucleus*, which contains *protons* and *neutrons*. *Electrons* revolve in orbits in the region surrounding the nucleus.

Atomic Energy—Energy released in *nuclear reactions*. Of particular interest is the energy released when a *neutron* initiates the breaking up or *fissioning* or an *atom*'s *nucleus* into smaller pieces (*fission*), or when two nuclei are joined together under millions of degrees of heat (*fusion*). It is more correctly called "*nuclear energy*."

Atomic Number—The number of *protons* (or number of positive charges) in the nucleus of an atom. The number of protons determines what an atom is chemically, and, hence, identifies it as belonging to a certain chemical element.

Atomic Weight—See *mass number*.

Attenuation—The process by which a beam of radiation is reduced in intensity when passing through some material. It is the combination of absorption and scattering processes and leads to a decrease in flux density of the beam when projected through matter.

Attenuation Coefficient—Of a substance, for a parallel beam of specified radiation: the quantity μ, in the expression μdx for the fraction removed by attenuation in passing through a thin layer of thickness dx of that substance. It is a function of the energy of the radiation. As dx is expressed in terms of length, mass per unit area, moles or atoms per unit area, μ is called the linear, mass, molar, or atomic attenuation coefficient respectively.

Auxiliary Building—Building at a *nuclear power plant*, frequently located adjacent to the *reactor containment* building, that houses most of the reactor auxiliary and safety systems, such as *radioactive waste* systems, chemical and volume control systems, and emergency cooling water systems.

Auxiliary Feedwater—Backup *feedwater* supply used during nuclear plant *startup* and *shutdown*; also known as *emergency feedwater*. (See *feedwater*.)

Background Radiation—Radiation that occurs naturally in the environment. Background radiation consists of cosmic radiation from outer space, radiation from the radioactive elements in rocks and soil, and radiation from radon and its decay products in the air we breathe.

Backscatter factor—Ratio of number of backscattered electrons to the number of incident electrons.

Beam Limiting Device—A device which provides a means to restrict the dimensions of the *x-ray* field.

Beta Particle—A negatively charged particle that is emitted by certain radioactive atoms. A beta particle is identical to the electron.

Becquerel—A unit, in the International System of Units (SI), of measurement of radioactivity equal to one transformation per second.

Binding Energy—The minimum energy required to separate a *nucleus* into its component *neutrons* and *photons*.

Bioassay (radiobioassay)—The determination of kinds, quantities or concentrations, and, in some cases, the locations of radioactive material in the human body, whether by direct measurement (in vivo counting) or by analysis and evaluation of materials excreted or removed from the human body.

---

[a] The nominal chemical composition of type 1100 aluminum alloy is 99.00% minimum aluminum, 0.12% copper.

[b] Introduced by NCRP (1993) to be secondary and derived units corresponding to a 20 mSv committed effective dose.

Biological Half-life—The time required for a biological system, such as that of a human, to eliminate by natural processes half the amount of a substance (such as a *radioactive* material) that has entered it.

Biological Shield—A mass of *absorbing* material placed around a *reactor* or *radioactive* source to reduce the *radiation* to a level safe for humans.

Body Burden—The amount of *radioactive* material which if deposited in the total body will produce the maximum permissible dose rate to the body organ considered the critical organ.

Boiling Water Reactor (BWR)—A *nuclear reactor* in which water is allowed to boil in the reactor core. The resulting steam is used directly to drive a turbine and electrical generator. About one-third of the operating nuclear power reactors in the U.S. are BWR's.

Bone Seeker—A radionuclide that tends to accumulate in the bones when it is introduced into the body. An example is *strontium*-90 which behaves chemically like calcium.

Brachytherapy—A method of radiation therapy in which sealed sources are utilized to deliver a radiation dose at a distance of up to a few centimeters, by surface, intracavitary, or interstitial application.

Breeder—A *reactor* that produces more nuclear fuel than it consumes. A *fertile material*, such as *uranium*-238, when bombarded by *neutrons*, is transformed into a *fissile material*, such as *plutonium*-239, which can be used as fuel. (See *fissile, fissionable* and *fertile material*.)

Bremsstrahlung—Secondary *electromagnetic radiation* (*x-rays*) produced by deceleration of charged particles through matter.

Btu—A British thermal unit. The amount of heat required to change the temperature of one pound of water one degree Fahrenheit at sea level.

Buffer Zone—An expanded portion of the restricted zone selected for temporary radiation protection controls until the stability of radioactivity levels in the area is confirmed.

Buildup Factor—In the passage of radiation through a medium, the ratio of the total value of a specified radiation quantity at any point to the contribution to that value from radiation reaching the point through the medium without having undergone a collision.

Buildup Factor, Energy Absorption, B_A—A photon buildup factor in which the quantity of interest is the absorbed or deposited energy in the shield medium. The energy response function is that of absorption in the material.

Buildup Factor, Exposure, B_D—A photon buildup factor in which the quantity of interest is exposure. The energy response function is that of absorption in air.

BWR—A *boiling water reactor*.

Byproduct Material—

(1) Any radioactive material (except *special nuclear material*) yielded in, or made *radioactive* by, exposure to the radiation incident to the process of producing or utilizing special nuclear material; and

(2) The tailings or wastes produced by the extraction or concentration of uranium or thorium from ore processed primarily for its source material content, including discrete surface wastes resulting from uranium solution extraction processes. Underground ore bodies depleted by these solution extraction operations do not constitute *byproduct material* within this definition.

Cabinet Radiography—Industrial radiography conducted in an enclosure or cabinet shielded so that radiation levels at every location on the exterior meet the limitations specified in the regulations.

Cabinet X-Ray System—An *x-ray* system with the *x-ray* tube installed in an enclosure independent of existing architectural structures except the floor on which it may be placed. The cabinet *x-ray* system is intended to contain at least that portion of a material being irradiated, provide radiation attenuation, and exclude personnel from its interior during generation of radiation. Included are all *x-ray* systems designed primarily for the inspection of carry-on baggage at airline, railroad, and bus terminals, and in similar facilities. An *x-ray* tube used within a shielded part of a building, or *x-ray* equipment which may temporarily or occasionally incorporate portable shielding, is not considered a cabinet *x-ray* system.

Calibration—The check or correction of the accuracy of a measuring instrument to assure proper operational characteristics. (See *counter*.)

CANDU—Canadian Deuterium Uranium-heavy water moderated natural uranium fuel reactor manufactured by Canada.

Carrier—A person engaged in the transportation of passengers or property by land or water as a common, contract, or private carrier, or by civil aircraft.

Cask—A heavily *shielded* container used to store and/or ship *radioactive materials*. Lead and steel are common materials used in the manufacture of casks.

Cation—A positively charged *ion*. (See *ionization*.)

Cephalometric Device—A device intended for the radiographic visualization and measurement of the dimensions of the human head.

Certified Health Physicist—A health physicist who has completed certain requirements of study and professional experience, which the American Board of Health Physics considers to constitute an adequate foundation in health physics, and has passed an examination designed to test competence in this field. (A small number of *Certifid Health Physicists* were ''grandfathered.'')

Chain Reaction—A reaction that stimulates its own repetition. In a *nuclear fission* chain reaction, a fissionable *nucleus* absorbs a *neutron* and fissions, releasing additional neutrons. These in turn can be absorbed by other fissionable nuclei, releasing still more neutrons. A fission chain reaction is self-sustaining when the number of neutrons released in a given time equals or exceeds the number of neutrons lost by absorption in nonfissionable material or by escape from the system.

Charged Particle—An *ion.* An elementary particle carrying a positive or negative electric charge.

Chemical Compound—See *compound.*

Chemical Recombination—Following an *ionization* event, the positive and negatively charged *ion* pairs may or may not realign themselves to form the same chemical substance they formed before ionization. Thus, chemical recombination could change the chemical composition of the material bombarded by *radiation.*

China Syndrome—The hypothetical result of a *power reactor* core melt accident in which molten fuel melts through the reactor *pressure vessel* and the bottom of the *containment* building and into the earth ''all the way to China.''

Chronic Exposure—The absorption of radiation (or intake of radioactive materials over a long period of time, i.e., over a lifetime).

Cladding—The thin-walled metal tube that forms the outer jacket of a nuclear *fuel rod.* It prevents corrosion of the fuel by the *coolant* and the release of *fission products* into the coolant. Aluminum, stainless steel and zirconium alloys are common cladding materials.

Class (or Lung Class or Inhalation Class)—A classification scheme for inhaled material according to its rate of clearance from the pulmonary region of the lung. Materials are classified as D, W, or Y, which applies to a range of clearance halftimes; for Class D (Days) of less than 10 days, for Class W (Weeks) from 10 to 100 days, and for Class Y (Years) of greater than 100 days.

Cleanup System—A system used for continuously filtering and demineralizing the *reactor coolant system* to reduce *contamination* levels and minimize corrosion.

Cloudshine—Gamma radiation from radioactive materials in an airborne plume.

Coastdown—An action that permits the *reactor* power level to decrease gradually as the fuel in the *core* is depleted.

Cold Neutrons—Neutrons in thermal equilibrium with an environment cooled well below 20°C, typically at 20–50 Kelvin.

Cold Shutdown—The term used to define a *reactor coolant system* at atmospheric pressure and at a temperature below 212°F following a reactor *cooldown.* (See *control rod.*)

Collective Dose—The sum of the individual *doses* received in a given period of time by a specified population from *exposure* to a specified radiation practice or source of radiation. The usual units of collective dose are the person-*rem* or the person-*sievert.*

Collimator—A device used to limit the size, shape, and direction of the primary radiation beam.

Committed Dose Equivalent ($H_{T,50}$)—The *dose equivalent* to organs or tissues of reference (T) that will be received from an intake of radioactive material by an individual during the 50-year period following the intake. The ICRP defines this as the *committed equivalent dose.* The units of the *committed dose equivalent* are the *rem* or the *sievert.*

Committed Effective Dose ($H_{E,50}$)[c]—The sum of the products of the *weighting factors* applicable to each of the body organs or tissues that are irradiated and the *committed equivalent dose* to these organs or tissues ($H_{E,50} = \Sigma W_T H_{T,50}$). The unit of committed effective dose is the *sievert.*

Committed Equivalent Dose ($H_{T,50}$)[c]—The *equivalent dose* to organs or tissues of reference (T) that will be received from an intake of radioactive material by an individual during the 50-year period following the intake. The unit of committed equivalent dose is the *sievert.*

Compound—A chemical combination of two or more *elements* combined in a fixed and definite proportion by weight.

Compton effect—Absorption or attenuation effect observed for X- or gamma-radiation in which the incident photon interacts with an orbital electron on the absorber atom to produce a recoil electron and a photon of energy less than the incident photon.

Computed Tomography—The production of a tomogram by the acquisition and computer processing of *x-ray* transmission data.

Condensate—Water that has been produced by the cooling of steam in a condenser.

Condenser—A large *heat exchanger* designed to cool exhaust steam from a *turbine* below the boiling point so that it can be returned to the heat source as water. In a *pressurized water reactor,* the water is returned to the *steam generator.* In a *boiling water reactor,* it returns to the *reactor core.* The heat removed from the steam by the condenser is transferred to a circulating water system and is exhausted to the environment, either through a *cooling tower* or directly into a body of water. (See *cooling tower.*)

---

[c] Quantities recommended by ICRP (1991). Tissue weighting factors recommended by ICRP (1977) and ICRP (1991) differ in the tissues included and the numerical values of the respective factors.

Contamination—The deposition of unwanted *radioactive* material on the surfaces of structures, areas, objects, or personnel.

Containment—A gas-tight shell or other enclosure around a *nuclear reactor* to confine *radioactive materials* that otherwise might be released to the atmosphere in the event of an accident.

Continuous Air Monitor (CAM)—A system which continuously samples air and continuously provides analysis and readout to determine airborne radioactivity concentrations with time.

Control Rod—A rod, plate or tube containing a material such as hafnium, boron, etc., used to control the power of a *nuclear reactor*. By absorbing *neutrons*, a control rod prevents the neutrons from causing further *fission*. (See *poison*.)

Controlled Area—An area outside of a *restricted area* but inside the site boundary, access to which can be limited for any reason.

Control Room (Building)—The area in a nuclear power plant from which most of the plant power production and emergency safety equipment can be operated by remote control.

Coolant—A substance circulated through a *nuclear reactor* to remove or transfer heat. The most commonly used coolant in the United States is water. Other coolants include *heavy water*, air, carbon dioxide, helium, liquid sodium and sodium-potassium alloy.

Cooldown—The gradual decrease in reactor fuel rod temperature caused by the removal of heat from the *reactor coolant system*.

Cooling Tower—A *heat exchanger* designed to aid in the cooling of water that was used to cool exhaust steam exiting the *turbines* of a power plant. Cooling towers transfer exhaust heat into the air instead of into a body of water.

Core—The central portion of a *nuclear reactor* containing the *fuel elements, moderator*, neutron *poisons* and support structures.

Core Melt Accident—See *China syndrome*.

Correction Factor, Shield Tissue Interface—A correction factor to be applied to the basic infinite-medium exposure buildup factor to correct for the scattering in a tissue phantom after emerging from a shield.

Cosmic Radiation—Penetrating *ionizing radiation*, both particulate and electromagnetic, originating in space. Secondary cosmic rays, formed by interactions in the earth's atmosphere, account for about 45 to 50 *millirem* annually.

Counter—A general designation applied to *radiation detection instruments* or *survey meters* that detect and measure radiation. The signal that announces an *ionization* event is called a count. (See *Geiger-Mueller counter*.)

Critical Mass—The smallest mass of *fissionable material* that will support a self-sustaining *chain reaction*.

Critical Organ—The body organ receiving a *radionuclide* or radiation *dose* that results in the greatest overall damage to the body.

Criticality—A term used in *reactor* physics to describe the state when the number of neutrons released by fission is exactly balanced by the neutrons being absorbed (by the fuel and poisons) and escaping the reactor core. A reactor is said to be "critical" when it achieves a self-sustaining nuclear *chain reaction*.

Crud—A colloquial term for corrosion and wear products (rust particles, etc.) that become *radioactive* under a *radiation* flux. (See *induced radioactivity*.)

Cumulative Dose—The total *dose* resulting from repeated exposures of *radiation* to the same region, or to the whole body, over a period of time.

Curie (Ci)—The basic unit of *activity*. A quantity of any radionuclide that undergoes an average transformation rate of 37 billion transformations per second. One curie is the approximate *activity* of 1 gram of *radium*. Named for Marie and Pierre Curie, who discovered radium in 1898.

Decay Chain—A sequential radioactive transformation process characteristic of some radionuclides. A *radionuclide* produces a radioactive *decay product* which in turn forms another radioactive product, etc., until eventually a stable nuclide is formed.

Decay Product or "Daughter" Product—The nuclide produced by the transformation of a radioactive nuclide.

Decay Heat—The heat produced by the *decay* of *radioactive fission products* after the *reactor* has been shut down. (See *residual heat*.)

Decay, Radioactive—The decrease in the amount of any *radioactive* material with the passage of time, due to the spontaneous emission from the atomic nuclei of either *alpha* or *beta particles*, often accompanied by *gamma radiation*. (See *half-life; radioactive*.)

Declared Pregnant Woman—A woman who has voluntarily informed her employer, in writing, of her pregnancy and the estimated date of conception.

Decontamination—The reduction or removal of contaminating radioactive material from a structure, area, object, or person. Decontamination may be accomplished by (1) treating the surface to remove or decrease the *contamination;* or (2) letting the material stand so that the *radioactivity* is decreased as a result of radioactive decay.

Decontamination factor—The ratio of the initial activity to the final activity.

Deep-dose equivalent (H_d)—As defined by the *NRC*, the *dose equivalent* estimated for a tissue depth of 1 cm. The deep-dose equivalent applies to external whole-body exposure and is intended to represent the upper limit to the dose received by the major organs and tissues of the body other than skin and lens of the eye.

Delayed Health Effects—Radiation effects which are manifested long after the relevant exposure. The vast majority are stochastic, that is, the severity is independent of dose and the probability is assumed to be proportional to the dose, without threshold.

Depleted Uranium—*Uranium* having a percentage of *uranium*-235 smaller than the 0.7% found in *natural uranium.* It is obtained from *spent* (used) *fuel elements* or as by-product *tails*, or residues, from uranium *isotope separation.* (See *mill tailings.*)

Deposition Probability (in lung region)—The fraction of the activity or mass of an inhaled aerosol which is deposited in a particular region of the lung.

Derived Air Concentration (DAC)[b]—The concentration of a given radionuclide in air which, if breathed by the *reference man* for a working year of 2,000 hours under conditions of light work (inhalation rate 1.2 cubic meters of air per hour), results in an intake of one ALI.

Derived Air Concentration-Hour (DAC-hour)[b]—The product of the concentration of radioactive material in air (expressed as a fraction or multiple of the *derived air concentration* for each radionuclide) and the time of exposure to that radionuclide, in hours. A licensee may take 2,000 DAC-hours to represent one ALI equivalent to a *committed effective dose equivalent* of 5 rems (0.05 Sv).

Derived Reference Air Concentrations (DRAC)[b]—The *ARLI* of a radionuclide divided by the volume of air inhaled by Reference Man in a working year (i.e., 2.4×10^3 m^3). The unit of DRAC is Bq m^{-3}.

Derived Response Level (DRL)—A level of *radioactivity* in an environmental medium that would be expected to produce a dose equal to its corresponding *Protective Action Guide.*

Design-Basis Accident—A postulated accident that a nuclear facility must be designed and built to withstand without loss to the systems, structures and components necessary to assure public health and safety.

Design-Basis Phenomena—Earthquakes, tornadoes, hurricanes, floods, etc., that a nuclear facility must be designed and built to withstand without loss to the systems, structures, and components necessary to assure public health and safety. (See *seismic Category I.*)

Detector—A material or device that is sensitive to *radiation* and can produce a response signal suitable for measurement or analysis. A *radiation detection instrument.* (See *counter.*)

Deterministic Effect—Health effects, the severity of which varies with the dose and for which a threshold is believed to exist. Radiation induced cataract formation is an example of a *deterministic effect.*

Deuterium—An *isotope* of hydrogen with one *proton* and one *neutron* in the *nucleus.* (See *heavy water.*)

Deuteron—The *nucleus* of *deuterium.* It contains one *proton* and one *neutron.*

Diagnostic X-Ray System—An *x-ray* system designed for irradiation of any part of the human body for the purpose of diagnosis or visualization.

Differential Pressure (DP)—The difference in pressure between two points of a system, such as between the inlet and outlet of a pump.

Disintegration—See *decay, radioactive.*

Doppler Coefficient—See *fuel temperature coefficient of reactivity.*

Dose or Radiation Dose—A generic term that means *absorbed dose, equivalent dose, effective dose, committed equivalent dose, committed effective dose*, or *total effective dose*, as defined elsewhere in this section.

Dose Conversion Factor—Any factor that is used to change an environmental measurement to *dose* in the units of concern. Frequently used as the factor that expresses the *committed effective dose equivalent* to a person from the intake (inhalation or ingestion) of a unit activity of a given radionuclide.

Dose Equivalent (H_T)—The product of the absorbed dose in tissue, *quality factor*, and all other necessary modifying factors at the location of interest. The units of *dose equivalent* are the rem and sievert (Sv). The ICRP defines this as the *equivalent dose.*

Dose Rate—The *radiation dose* delivered per unit of time. Measured, for example, in *rem* or Sv per hour.

Dosimeter—A portable instrument for measuring and registering the total accumulated exposure to *ionizing radiation.* (See *dosimetry.*)

Dosimetry—The theory and application of the principles and techniques involved in the measurement and recording of *radiation doses.* Its practical aspect is concerned with the use of various types of radiation instruments with which measurements are made. See *film badge; survey meter.*)

Dosimetry Processor—An individual or an organization that processes and evaluates individual monitoring equipment in order to determine the *radiation dose* delivered to the equipment.

Drywell—The *containment* structure enclosing a *boiling water reactor* vessel and its recirculation system. The drywell provides both a pressure suppression system and a *fission product* barrier under accident conditions.

Effective Dose (E)[c]—The sum over specified tissues of the products of the equivalent dose in a tissue (T) and the weighting factor for that tissue (W_T), i.e., $E = \Sigma W_T H_T$.

---

[b] Introduced by NCRP (1993) to be secondary and derived units corresponding to a 20 mSv committed effective dose.

[c] Quantities recommended by ICRP (1991). Tissue weighting factors recommended by ICRP (1977) and ICRP (1991) differ in the tissues included and the numerical values of the respective factors.

Effective Dose Equivalent (H_E)—The sum of the products of the *dose equivalent* to the organ or tissue (H_T) and the *weighting factors* (W_T) applicable to each of the body organs or tissues that are irradiated ($H_E = \Sigma W_T H_T$). The ICRP defines this as the *effective dose.*

Effective Half-life—The time required for the amount of a *radioactive* element deposited in a living organism to be diminished 50 percent as a result of the combined action of radioactive *decay* and biological elimination. (See *biological half-life.*)

Efficiency, Plant—The percentage of the total energy content of a power plant's fuel that is converted into electricity. The remaining energy is lost to the environment as heat.

Electrical Generator—An electromagnetic device that converts mechanical (rotational) energy into electrical energy. Most large electrical generators are driven by steam or water *turbine* systems.

Electromagnetic Radiation—Energy being propagated by a traveling wave motion resulting from changing electric or magnetic fields. Familiar electromagnetic radiations range from *x-rays* and *gamma rays* of short wavelength, through the ultraviolet, visible and infrared regions, to radar, radio waves of relatively long wavelength. The *ionizing* electromagnetic radiations are *gamma rays* and *x-rays.*

Electron—A subatomic particle with a negative charge. The electron circles the nucleus of an atom.

Electron Volt (eV)—Customary unit for expressing the energy of ionizing radiation. One eV is equal to the energy of one electron moving through a potential difference of one volt.

Element—One of the 111 known chemical substances that cannot be broken down further without changing its chemical properties. Some examples include hydrogen, nitrogen, gold, lead and *uranium.*

Elimination—Removal of material from the body via urine, feces, sweat or exhalation. Excretion usually refers to elimination via urine or feces.

Embryo/Fetus—The developing human organism from conception until the time of birth. More accurately; embryo: 2 wk (when implantation occurs)-8 wk; fetus: end of wk 8-term.

Emergency Core Cooling System (ECCS)—Reactor system components (pumps, valves, heat exchangers, tanks and piping) that are specifically designed to remove residual heat from the reactor *fuel rods* should the normal core cooling system (*reactor coolant system*) fail.

Emergency Feedwater—See *auxiliary feedwater.*

Energy Absorption Coefficient—Of a substance, for a parallel beam of specified radiation: the quantity μ_{en} in the expression $\mu_{en}dx$ for the fraction removed by attenuation in passing through a thin layer of thickness *dx* of that substance. It is a function of energy of the radiation. As *dx* is expressed in terms of length, mass per unit area, moles per unit area, or atoms per unit area, μ_{en} is called the linear, mass, molar, or atomic energy absorption coefficient. NOTE: It is that part of the attenuation coefficient resulting from energy absorption only, and is equal to the product of the energy transfer coefficient and 1-g, where *g* is the fraction of the energy of secondary charged particles that is lost to bremsstrahlung in the material.

Engineered Barrier—A man-made structure or device that is intended to improve the land disposal facility's ability to meet performance objectives.

Enrichment—See *isotopic enrichment.*

Entrance or Access Point—Any location through which an individual could gain access to radiation areas or to radioactive materials. This includes entry or exit portals of sufficient size to permit human entry, irrespective of their intended use.

Entrance Exposure Rate—The *exposure* per unit time at the point where the center of the useful beam enters the patient.

Equivalent Dose (H_T)[c]—A quantity used for radiation-protection purposes that takes into account the different probability of effects which occur with the same absorbed dose delivered by radiations with different W_R values. It is defined as the product of the averaged absorbed dose in a specified organ or tissue (D_T) and the radiation weighting factor (W_R). The unit of equivalent dose is joules per kilogram (J kg^{-1}) and its name is the sievert (Sv).

Evacuation—The urgent removal of people from an area to avoid or reduce high-level, short-term exposure, usually from the plume or from deposited activity. Evacuation may be a preemptive action taken in response to a facility condition rather than an actual release.

Excretion Function—A function describing the time dependence of the quantity of material eliminated in urine or feces per day.

Excursion—A sudden, very rapid rise in the power level of a *reactor* caused by *supercriticality.* Excursions are usually quickly suppressed by the *negative temperature coefficient,* the *fuel temperature coefficient* or the *void coefficient* (depending on reactor design), and by rapid insertion of *control rods.*

Exposure—A measure of the ionization produced in air by x- or gamma radiation; the sum of electric charges on all ions of one sign produced in air when all electrons liberated by photons in a volume of air are completely stopped in air, divided by the mass of the air in the volume; units of exposure in air is the roentgen or coulomb per kilogram (SI units).

---

[c] Quantities recommended by ICRP (1991). Tissue weighting factors recommended by ICRP (1977) and ICRP (1991) differ in the tissues included and the numerical values of the respective factors.

Exposure—The quotient of dQ by dm where *dQ* is the absolute value of the total charge of the ions of one sign produced in air when all the electrons (negatrons and positrons) liberated by photons in a volume element of air having mass *dm* are completely stopped in air. The unit of *exposure* is the coulomb per kilogram (C/kg). One roentgen is equal to 2.58×10^{-4} coulomb per kilogram.

Exposure—Being exposed to *ionizing radiation* or to radioactive material.

Extendable Deadtime—Deadtime initiated by every incoming event.

External Contamination—Radioactive materials deposited on the outside of the body.

External Dose—That portion of the *dose equivalent* received from radiation sources outside the body.

Extremity Dose—Dose to a limb of the body, especially a hand or a foot.

Eye Dose Equivalent—Applies to the external exposure of the lens of the eye and is taken as the *dose equivalent* at a tissue depth of 0.3 centimeter (300 mg cm^{-3}).

Fast Fission—*Fission* of a heavy *atom* (such as *uranium*-238) when it absorbs a high-energy (*fast*) *neutron*. Most *fissionable materials* need *thermal* (slow) neutrons in order to fission.

Fast Neutron—A *neutron* released during fission with *kinetic energy* greater than its surroundings.

Fast Reactor—A *reactor* in which the *fission chain reaction* is sustained primarily by *fast neutrons* rather than by slow-moving neutrons. Fast reactors contain little or no *moderator* to slow down the neutrons from the speeds at which they are ejected from fissioning *nuclei*.

Feedwater—Water supplied to the *reactor pressure vessel* (in a *BWR*) or the *steam generator* (in a *PWR*) that removes heat from the reactor fuel rods by boiling and becoming steam. The steam becomes the driving force for the plant *turbine* generator.

Fertile Material—A material, which is not itself *fissile* (fissionable by *thermal neutrons*), that can be converted into a fissile material by irradiation in a *reactor*. There are two basic fertile materials, *uranium*-238 and *thorium*-232. When these fertile materials capture neutrons, they are converted into fissile *plutonium*-239 and *uranium*-233, respectively.

Film Badge—A pack of photographic film used for approximate measurement of *radiation* exposure for *personnel monitoring* purposes. The badge may contain two or three films of differing sensitivity, and it may contain a filter that shields part of the film from certain types of radiation.

Fissile Material—Although sometimes used as a synonym for *fissionable material*, this term has acquired a more restricted meaning; namely, any material fissionable by *thermal* (slow) *neutrons*. The three primarily fissile materials are *uranium*-233, *uranium*-235 and *plutonium*-239.

Fission—The splitting of a *nucleus* into at least two other nuclei and the release of a relatively large amount of energy. Two or three *neutrons* are usually released during this type of transformation.

Fission Gases—Those *fission products* that exist in the gaseous state. Primarily the *noble gases* (krypton, xenon, etc.).

Fission Products—The nuclei (fission fragments) formed by the fission of heavy elements, plus the *nuclides* formed by the fission fragments' radioactive *decay*.

Fissionable Material—Commonly used as a synonym for *fissile material*, the meaning of this term has been extended to include material that can be fissioned by fast *neutrons*, such as *uranium*-238.

"Flea"—See *hot particle*.

Fluence—The number of radioactive particles, neutrons, or photons per unit cross-sectional area.

Fluoroscopic Imaging Assembly—A subsystem in which *x-ray* photons produce a fluoroscopic image. It includes the image receptors(s) such as the image intensifier and spot film device, electrical interlocks, if any, and structural material providing linkage between the image receptor and diagnostic source assembly.

Flux—A term applied to the amount of some type of *radiation* crossing a certain area per unit time. The unit of flux is the number of particles, energy, etc., per square centimeter per second.

Flux Density—The flux density at a point is the number of radioactive particles, neutrons, or photons passing per unit time, per unit area of the beam.

Frisker—A detector used to search a person for radioactive contamination on the body or clothing.

"Frisking"—Searching a person's clothing or body with a radiation detector.

Fuel Cycle—The series of steps involved in supplying fuel for nuclear *power reactors*. It can include mining, milling, *isotopic enrichment*, fabrication of fuel elements, use in a *reactor*, chemical reprocessing to recover the *fissionable material* remaining in the *spent fuel*, reenrichment of the fuel material, refabrication into new *fuel elements*, and waste disposal.

Fuel "Flea"—A small, high specific activity, radioactive fragment arising from nuclear fuel fragments.

Fuel Pellet—Cylinders into which nuclear fuel (*fissionable material*) is formed for use in a *nuclear reactor*. A fuel pellet is about the size of your fingertip.

Fuel Reprocessing—The processing of reactor fuel to separate the unused *fissionable material* from waste material.

Fuel Rod—A long slender tube that holds a number of fuel pellets.

Fuel Rod Bundle or Fuel Element—An assembly of fuel rods. Fuel rod bundles are loaded individually into the reactor core.

Fuel Temperature Coefficient of Reactivity—The physical property of fuel *pellet* material (*uranium*-238) that causes the uranium to absorb more *neutrons* without fissioning as fuel *pellet* temperature increases. This acts to stabilize *power reactor* operations. Also known as the *Doppler coefficient*.

Fusion (Thermonuclear Reaction)—A *nuclear reaction* characterized by joining together of light *nuclei* to form heavier nuclei, the energy for the reactions being provided by violent thermal agitation of particles at very high temperatures. If the colliding particles are properly chosen, there will be a release of energy from the reaction. The energy of the stars is derived from such reactions.

Gap—The space inside a reactor *fuel rod* that exists between the fuel *pellet* and the fuel rod *cladding*.

Gamma Radiation or Gamma Ray—Gamma radiation is high-energy, short-wavelength *electromagnetic radiation* emitted from the *nucleus*. A gamma ray is a discrete packet of electromagnetic energy. Gamma radiation frequently accompanies *alpha* and *beta* emissions and always accompanies *nuclear fission*. Gamma rays are very penetrating and are best stopped or *shielded* against by dense materials, such as lead or uranium. Gamma rays are identical to *x-rays*, but have a nuclear origin, rather than an atomic origin.

Gas-Cooled Reactor—A *nuclear reactor* in which a gas is the *coolant*.

Gases—Normally formless fluids that completely fill the space and take the shape of their container.

Gaseous Diffusion (plant)—A method of *isotopic separation* based on the fact that *gas atoms* or *molecules* with different masses will diffuse through a porous barrier (or membrane) at different rates. This method is used to separate *uranium*-235 from *uranium*-238; it requires large gaseous diffusion plants and enormous amounts of electric power.

Geiger-Mueller Counter—A *radiation* detection and measuring instrument. It consists of a gas-filled tube containing electrodes, between which there is an electrical voltage but no current flowing. When *ionizing radiation* passes through the tube, a short, intense pulse of current passes from the negative electrode to the positive electrode and is measured or counted. The number of pulses per second measures the intensity of radiation. It was named for Hans Geiger and W. Mueller who invented it in the 1920s. It is sometimes called simply a Geiger counter, or a G-M counter.

General Purpose Radiographic X-Ray System—Any radiographic *x-ray* system which, by design, is not limited to radiographic examination of specific anatomical regions.

Genetic Effect—An effect in a descendant resulting from the modification of genetic material in a parent.

Geometry Factor—The solid angle subtended by a detector plane frontal area with respect to a point source, or vice versa.

Gonad Shield—A protective barrier for the testes or ovaries.

Graphite—A form of carbon, similar to the lead used in pencils, used as a *moderator* in some *nuclear reactors*.

Groundshine—Gamma radiation from radioactive materials deposited on the ground.

Gray (Gy)—The SI unit of *absorbed dose*. One gray is equal to an *absorbed dose* of 1 J kg^{-1} (100 rad).

Half-life—The time in which half the *atoms* of a particular *radioactive* substance disintegrate to another nuclear form. Measured half-lives vary from millionths of a second to billions of years. Also called physical half-life.

Half-life, Biological—The time required for the body to eliminate half of the material taken in by natural biological means.

Half-life, Effective—The time required for a *radionuclide* contained in a biological system, such as a human or an animal, to reduce its activity by half as a combined result of radioactive *decay* and biological elimination.

Half-Thickness—The thickness of any given *absorber* that will reduce the intensity of a beam of *radiation* to one-half its initial value. (See *attenuation; shielding.*)

Half-time, biological (T_b)—The time in which half the quantity of a material in a compartment, in an organ or in the whole body is eliminated by biological processes.

Half-time, effective (T_e)—The time taken for the activity of a radioactive material in a compartment, in an organ or in the whole body to be reduced to half its value by a combination of biological elimination and radioactive decay.

$$\frac{1}{T_e} = \frac{1}{T_b} + \frac{1}{T_R}$$

Half-time, physical (T_R)—The time taken for the activity of a radionuclide to lose half its value by radioactive decay.

Head, Reactor Vessel—The removable top section of a reactor *pressure vessel*. It is bolted in place during power operation and removed during refueling to permit access of fuel-handling equipment to the *core*.

Healing Arts Screening—The testing of human beings using *x-ray* machines for the detection or evaluation of health indications when such tests are not specifically and individually ordered by a licensed practitioner of the healing arts legally authorized to prescribe such *x-ray* tests for the purpose of diagnosis or treatment.

Health Physicist—A scientist whose goal is to protect people and the environment from unnecessary exposure to radiation.

Health Physics—The science concerned with recognition, evaluation and control of health hazards from *ionizing* and *non-ionizing radiation*.

Health Physics Technician—An individual skilled in the application of radiation monitoring and radiation survey techniques to the extent that he/she is capable of assuming responsibility for routine monitoring and survey operations once the radiation protection aspects of the operation have been programmed under the guidance of a qualified expert. Usually has a high school degree and may have several years of technical college credit.

Heat Exchanger—Any device that transfers heat from one fluid (liquid or gas) to another fluid or to the environment.

Heat Sink—Anything that absorbs heat; usually part of the environment, such as the air, a river or outer space.

Heatup—The rise in temperature of the reactor *fuel rods* resulting from an increase in the rate of fission in the *core*.

Heavy Water (D_2O)—Water containing significantly more than the natural proportions (1 in 6500) of heavy hydrogen (*deuterium*) atoms to ordinary hydrogen atoms. Heavy water is used as a *moderator* in some *reactors* because it slows down neutrons effectively and also has a low probability for *absorption* of *neutrons*.

Heavy-Water-Moderated Reactor—A *reactor* that uses *heavy water* as its *moderator*. Heavy water is an excellent moderator and thus permits the use of inexpensive (unenriched) *uranium* as a fuel.

HEPA Filters—High Efficiency Particulate Air filters used to filter radioactive dusts from the air.

High Radiation Area—An area, accessible to individuals, in which radiation levels could result in an individual receiving a *dose equivalent* in excess of 0.1 rem (1 mSv) in 1 hour at 30 centimeters from the radiation source or from any surface that the radiation penetrates.

Hot—A colloquial term meaning highly *radioactive*.

Hot Particle—Also called a ''*flea*''. A small, discrete, high specific activity radioactive particle. Hot particles may originate from activation of corrosion or wear products circulating in the primary coolant (activation ''*flea*'') or may arise from nuclear fuel fragments (*fuel ''fleas''*).

Hot Spot—The region in a *radiation/contamination* area in which the level of radiation/contamination is noticeably greater than in neighboring regions in the area.

Image Intensifier—A device, installed in its housing, which instantaneously converts an *x-ray* pattern into a corresponding light image of higher energy density.

Image Receptor—Any device, such as a fluorescent screen or radiographic film, which transforms incident *x-ray* photons either into a visible image or into another form which can be made into a visible image by further transformations.

Incident Phase—This guidance distinguishes three phases of an incident (or accident):

(1) *Early Phase*: The period at the beginning of a nuclear incident when immediate decisions for effective use of protective actions are required, and must be based primarily on predictions of radiological conditions in the environment. This phase may last from hours to days. For the purpose of dose projection, it is assumed to last for four days.

(2) *Intermediate Phase*: The period beginning after the incident source and releases have been brought under control and reliable environmental measurements are available for use as a basis for decisions on additional protective actions and extending until these protective actions are terminated. This phase may overlap the early and late phases and may last from weeks to many months. For the purpose of dose projection, it is assumed to last for one year.

(3) *Late Phase*: The period beginning when recovery action designed to reduce radiation levels in the environment to permanently acceptable levels are commenced, and ending when all recovery actions have been completed. This period may extend from months to years (also referred to as the recovery phase).

Individual—Any human being.

Individual Monitoring—

(1) The assessment of *dose equivalent* by the use of devices designed to be worn by an individual;

(2) The assessment of *committed effective dose equivalent* by *bioassay* (see *Bioassay*) or by determination of the time-weighted air concentrations to which an individual has been exposed, i.e., DAC-hours; or

(3) The assessment of *dose equivalent* by the use of survey data.

Individual Monitoring Devices (individual monitoring equipment)—Devices designed to be worn by a single individual for the assessment of *dose equivalent* such as film badges, thermoluminescent dosimeters (TLDs), pocket ionization chambers, and personal (''lapel'') air sampling devices.

Induced Radioactivity—*Radioactivity* that is created when stable substances are bombarded by *neutrons* or other particles. For example, the *stable isotope cobalt*-59 becomes the radioactive isotope *cobalt*-60 under *neutron* bombardment.

Industrial Radiography—The examination of the macroscopic structure of materials by nondestructive methods using sources of ionizing radiation to produce radiographic images.

Inherent Filtration—The filtration of the useful beam provided by the permanently installed components of the tube housing assembly.

Intake—Quantity of material entering the body, the principal routes being inhalation, by ingestion or through intact or wounded skin.

Internal Bremsstralung—That originating within a decaying atom.

Internal Dose—That portion of the *dose equivalent* received from radioactive material taken into the body.

Internal Dosimetry—Calculation of the dose to a person from radioactive materials deposited in, or in transit through, the body.

Internal Radioactivity—Radioactive materials inside the body. The body always contains naturally occurring radioactivity; it may or may not also have internal contamination.

Investigation Level (for intake of radionuclides)—Level of *committed dose equivalent* or *intake* above which the result is regarded as sufficiently important to justify further investigation. Investigation levels are defined for routine monitoring, IL_R, and for special or operational monitoring, IL_S. Derived investigation levels, DIL_R and DIL_S, are values of body or organ content or elimination rate that correspond to investigation levels, IL_R and IL_S. These values are calculated by means of defined models of *intake*, deposition, *uptake*, retention and *elimination*.

Ion—An *atom* that has too many or too few *electrons*, causing it to be chemically active; an electron that is not associated (in orbit) with a *nucleus*. (See *ionization*.)

Ion Pair—A pair of atoms or molecules, one with a negative charge and one with a positive charge.

Ionization—The process of adding one or more *electrons* to, or removing one or more electrons from, *atoms* or *molecules*, thereby creating *ions*. High temperatures, electrical discharges, or nuclear radiations can cause ionization.

Ionization Chamber—An instrument that detects and measures *ionizing radiation* by measuring the electrical current that flows when radiation ionizes gas in a chamber, making the gas a conductor of electricity. (See *counter*.)

Ionizing Radiation—Any *radiation* capable of displacing electrons from atoms or molecules, thereby producing *ions*. Examples: *alpha, beta, gamma, x-rays* and *neutrons*.

Irradiation—Exposure to *radiation*.

Isotone—One of several different *nuclides* having the same number of neutrons in their nuclei.

Isotope—One of two or more *atoms* with the same number of *protons*, but different numbers of *neutrons*, in their *nuclei*. Thus, *carbon*-12, *carbon*-13 and *carbon*-14 are isotopes of the *element* carbon, the numbers denoting the approximate *atomic weights*. Isotopes have very nearly the same chemical properties, but often different physical properties (for example, *carbon*-12 and -13 are *stable*, carbon-14 is *radioactive*.

Isotope Separation—The process of separating isotopes from one another, or changing their relative abundances, as by *gaseous diffusion* or electromagnetic separation. Isotope separation is a step in the *isotopic enrichment* process.

Isotopic Enrichment—A process by which the relative abundances of the *isotopes* of a given *element* are altered, thus producing a form of the element that has been enriched in one particular isotope and depleted in its other isotopic forms.

Kerma (k)—The quotient of dE_{tr} by dm (dE_{tr}/dm), where dE_{tr} is the sum of the initial kinetic energies of all the charged ionizing particles liberated by uncharged ionizing particles in a material of mass dm. The SI unit is J kg^{-1}. The special name of this unit is the gray, Gy.

Kilo-—A prefix that multiplies a basic unit by 1000. Example: 1 kilometer = 1000 meters.

Kiloelectron Volt (keV)—A unit of energy equal to the energy of one electron moving through a potential difference of 1000 volts. One keV = 1000 eV.

Kilovolt (kV)—The unit of electrical potential equal to 1000 volts.

Kinetic Energy—The energy that a body possesses by virtue of its mass and velocity; the energy of motion.

kVp—(See *Peak tube potential*)

Land Disposal Facility—The land, buildings, and equipment which is intended to be used for the disposal of wastes into the subsurface of the land.

LD 50/60—The *dose* of *radiation* expected to cause death within 60 days to 50 percent of those exposed. Generally accepted as 500 *rad* (5 Gy) received over a short period of time.

Leakage Radiation—Radiation emanating from the diagnostic or therapeutic source assembly except for:

(1) the useful beam, and

(2) radiation produced when the exposure switch or timer is not activated.

Licensed Material—*Source material, special nuclear material*, or *byproduct material* received, possessed, used, transferred or disposed of under a general or specific license issued by the Nuclear Regulatory Commission (or an *Agreement State*).

Licensee—The holder of a license.

Licensing State—Any State with regulations equivalent to the Suggested State Regulations for Control of Radiation relating to, and an effective program for, the regulatory control of NARM and which has been granted final designation by the Conference of Radiation Control Program Directors, Inc.

Light Water—Ordinary water (H_2O) as distinguished from *heavy water* (D_2O).

Light-Water Reactor—A term used to designate *reactors* using ordinary water as *coolant*, including *boiling water reactors* (BWRs) and *pressurized water reactors* (PWRs), the most common types used in the United States.

Limits (dose limits)—The permissible upper bounds of *radiation doses*.

Linear Energy Transfer (LET)—An expression of the energy lost by a charged particle per unit distance traveled in a material (in keV μm^{-1} or other units of energy and length). The value of LET is determined by the material and the type and energy of the charged particle. Effectiveness in producing a biological effect per unit *absorbed dose* (i.e., *quality factor or Q*) increases with the LET in tissue (or water). Electrons (and beta particles) and x and gamma rays (which produce electrons as their initial interactions in tissue) are referred to as ''low'' LET radiations and have been assigned Q's of 1.

Heavy charged particles (such as alpha particles) and neutrons (which produce heavy charged particles in their initial interactions in tissue) are known as ''high'' LET radiations and have been assigned values of Q ranging from 2 to 20.

Lixiscope—A portable light intensified imaging device using a sealed source.

Loop—In a *pressurized water reactor*, the *coolant* flow path through piping from the reactor *pressure vessel* to the *steam generator*, to the reactor coolant pump, and back to the reactor pressure vessel. Large PWRs may have as many as four separate loops.

Lost or Missing Licensed Material—*Licensed material* whose location is unknown. It includes material that has been shipped but has not reached its destination and whose location cannot be readily traced in the transportation system.

Low Population Zone (LPZ)—An area of low population density often required around a nuclear installation. The number and density of residents is of concern in emergency planning so that certain protective measures (such as notification and instructions to residents) can be accomplished in a timely manner.

Lung Class (D, W or Y)—A classification scheme for inhaled material according to its rate of clearance from the pulmonary region of the lung.

Mass-Energy Equation—The equation developed by Albert Einstein which is usually given as $E = mc^2$, showing that, when the energy of a body changes by an amount E (no matter what form the energy takes), the mass, m, of the body will change by an amount equal to E/c^2. The factor c^2, the square of the speed of light in a vacuum, may be regarded as the conversion factor relating units of mass and energy. The equation predicted the possibility of releasing enormous amounts of energy by the conversion of mass to energy. It is also called the Einstein equation.

Mass Number—The number of *nucleons* (*neutrons* and *protons*) in the *nucleus* of an *atom*. Also known as the *atomic weight* of an atom.

Mega-—A prefix that multiplies a basic unit by 1,000,000.

Megacurie—One million curies. (See *curie*.)

Mean Free Path—The average distance that photons of a given energy travel before an interaction in a given medium occurs. It is equal to the reciprocal of the attenuation coefficient. Thus, the distance x in ordinary units can be converted into the dimensionless distance $\mu\chi$, the number of *mean free path lengths (mfp)*.

Mean Lifetime—An average lifetime related to the biologic or the effective *half-time*, or the physical *half-life*. Effective *mean lifetime* = 1.443 × effective half-time.

Member of the Public—An individual in a *controlled* or *unrestricted area*. However, an *individual* is not a member of the public during any period in which the *individual* receives an occupational dose.

Micro-—A prefix that divides a basic unit into one million parts.

Microcurie—A one-millionth part of a curie. (See *curie*.)

Microsecond—A one-millionth part of a second.

Mill Tailings—Naturally *radioactive* residue from the processing of *uranium* ore into *yellowcake* in a mill. Although the milling process recovers about 93 percent of the uranium, the residues, or tailings, contain several radioactive elements, including *uranium*, *thorium*, *radium*, *polonium* and *radon*.

Milli-—A prefix that divides a basic unit by 1000.

Million Electron Volts (MeV)—A unit of energy equal to the energy of one electron moving through a potential difference of one-million volts. One MeV = 1,000 keV = 1,000,000 eV.

Millirem—A one-thousandth part of a rem. (See *rem*.)

Milliroentgen—A one-thousandth part of a roentgen. (See *roentgen*.)

Millisievert—A one-thousandth part of a *sievert*. (See *sievert*.)

Minor—An *individual* less than 18 years of age.

Moderator—A material, such as ordinary water, *heavy water*, or graphite, used in a *reactor* to slow down high-velocity *neutrons*, thus increasing the likelihood of *fission*.

Moderator Temperature Coefficient of Reactivity—The property of a reactor *moderator* to slow down fewer *neutrons* as its temperature increases. This acts to stabilize *power reactor* operations.

Molecule—A group of *atoms* held together by chemical forces. A molecule is the smallest unit of a compound that can exist by itself and retain all its chemical properties.

Monitoring (radiation monitoring, radiation protection monitoring)—The measurement of radiation levels, concentrations, surface area concentrations or quantities of radioactive material and the use of the results of these measurements to evaluate potential *exposures* and *doses*.

Nano-—A prefix that divides a basic unit by one billion.

Nanocurie—One billionth part of a *curie*.

NARM—Any Naturally occurring or Accelerator produced Radioactive Material. It does not include byproduct, source, or special nuclear material.[d]

---

[d] For the purpose of meeting the definition of a Licensing State by the Conference of Radiation Control Program Directors, Inc. (CRCPD). NARM only refers to discrete sources of NARM. Diffuse sources of NARM are excluded from consideration by the CRCPD for Licensing State designation purposes.

Natural Radiation—See *background radiation.*

Natural Uranium—*Uranium* as found in nature. It contains 0.7 percent *uranium*-235, 99.3 percent *uranium*-238 and a trace of *uranium*-234.

Near Surface Disposal Facility—A land disposal facility in which waste is disposed of within approximately the upper 30 meters of the earth's surface.

Negative Temperature Coefficient—See *moderator temperature coefficient.*

Neutron—An uncharged particle with a mass comparable to (only slightly greater than) that of the *proton*, and found in the *nucleus* of every *atom* heavier than hydrogen.

Neutron Capture—The process in which an atomic *nucleus* absorbs or captures a *neutron*. The product of neutron capture is often *radioactive* (see *activation product*).

Neutron Chain Reaction—A process in which some of the neutrons released in one *fission* event cause other fissions to occur. There are three types of chain reactions:

(1) Nonsustaining chain reaction—An average of less than one *fission* is produced by the neutrons released by each previous fission (reactor *subcriticality*.)

(2) Sustaining chain reaction—An average of exactly one *fission* is produced by the neutrons released by each previous fission (reactor *criticality*.)

(3) Multiplying chain reaction—An average of more than one *fission* is produced by the neutrons released by previous fission (reactor *supercriticality*.)

Neutron Generation—The release, *thermalization* and *absorption* of fission neutrons by a *fissile material* and the *fission* of that material producing a second generation of neutrons. In a typical reactor system, there are about 40,000 generations of neutrons every second.

Neutron Leakage—Neutrons that escape from the vicinity of the *fissionable material* in a reactor core. Neutrons that leak out of the fuel region are no longer available to cause fission and must be *absorbed* by *shielding* placed around the reactor *pressure vessel* for that purpose.

Neutron, Slow—See *neutron, thermal.*

Neutron Source—A *radioactive material* (*decays* by neutron emission) that can be inserted into a *reactor* to ensure that a sufficient quantity of neutrons is available to start a *chain reaction* and register on neutron detection equipment.

Neutron, Thermal—A *neutron* that has (by collision with other particles) reached an energy state equal to that of its surroundings. (See *thermalization.*)

Noble Gas—A gaseous chemical *element* that does not readily enter into chemical combination with other elements. An inert gas. These are He, Ne, Ar, Kr, Xe, and Rn.

Non-extendable Deadtime—deadtime initiated by every registered event.

Non-Vital Plant Systems—Systems at a nuclear facility that may or may not be necessary for the operation of the facility (i.e., power production), but that would have little or no effect on public health and safety should they fail. These systems are not *safety related.*

NORM—Naturally Occurring Radioactive Materials.

Normal Form Radioactive Material—Radioactive material which has not been demonstrated to qualify as *special form radioactive material.*

Nozzle—As used in *PWR*s and *BWR*s, the interface for fluid (inlet or outlet) between reactor plant components (*pressure vessel, coolant* pumps, *steam generators*, etc.) and their associated piping systems.

Nuclear Disintegration—See *decay, radioactive*

Nuclear Energy—The energy liberated by a *nuclear reaction* (*fission* or *fusion*) or by radioactive *decay.*

Nuclear Fission—See *fission.*

Nuclear Force—A powerful short-ranged attractive force that holds together the particles inside an atomic *nucleus.*

Nuclear Fusion—See *fusion.*

Nuclear Incident—An event or series of events, either deliberate or accidental, leading to the release, or potential release, into the environment of radioactive materials in sufficient quantity to warrant consideration of *protective actions.*

Nuclear Power Plant—An electrical generating facility using a *nuclear reactor* as its power (heat) source.

Nuclear Radiation—See *radiation, nuclear.*

Nuclear Reaction—See *reaction, nuclear.*

Nuclear Reactor—See *reactor, nuclear.*

Nucleon—Common name for a constituent particle of the atomic *nucleus.* At present, applied to *protons* and *neutrons* but may include any other particles found to exist in the nucleus.

Nucleus (or Atomic Nucleus); *Nuclei* (plural)—The small, central, positively charged region of an *atom* that carries essentially all the mass. Except for the *nucleus* of ordinary (light) hydrogen, which has a single *proton*, all atomic nuclei contain both protons and *neutrons*. The number of protons determines the total positive charge, or *atomic number*; this is the same for all the atomic nuclei of a given chemical *element*. The total number of *neutrons* and *protons* is called the mass number. (See *isotope.*)

Nuclide—A general term referring to any known *isotope*, either *stable* (about 290) or unstable (about 2200), of any chemical *element.*

NVLAP—National Voluntary Laboratory Accreditation Program. A program of the National Institute of Standards and Technology to accredit various types of laboratories, including those providing personnel dosimetry services. NVLAP accreditation for personnel dosimetry assures the facility has met accepted standards for quality.

Occupational Radiation Exposure—The radiation exposure or *dose* to an individual in the course of employment in which the individual's assigned duties involve *exposure* to radiation and to radioactive materials. *Occupational dose* does not include *dose* received from: *background radiation*, as a patient from medical practices; from voluntary participation in medical research programs; or as a member of the general public.

Operating Basis Earthquake—An earthquake that could be expected to affect the plant site, but for which the plant power production equipment is designed to remain functional without undue risk to public health and safety. (See *design-basis phenomenon*.)

Open Beam Configuration—An analytical *x-ray* system in which an individual could accidentally place some part of his body in the primary beam path during normal operation.

Oralloy—*Uranium* enriched in the *isotope uranium*-235. This material is an excellent *fission* fuel and is capable of sustaining a *chain reaction*.

Organ or Tissue Weighting Factor (W_T)—A factor that indicates the ratio of the risk of stochastic effects attributable to irradiation of a given organ or tissue (T) to the total risk when the whole body is uniformly irradiated.

Packaging—The assembly of components necessary to ensure compliance with the packaging requirements. It may consist of one or more receptacles, absorbent materials, spacing structures, thermal insulation, radiation shielding, and devices for cooling or absorbing mechanical shocks. The vehicle, tie-down system, and auxiliary equipment may be designated as part of the packaging.

Pair production—An absorption process for X- or gamma-radiation in which the incident photon is annihilated in the vicinity of the nucleus of the absorbing atom with subsequent production of an electron and positron pair. The reaction only occurs for incident photon energies exceeding 1.02 MeV. This is an example of direct conversion of energy into matter according to Einstein's equation: $E = mc^2$. It only occurs when a gamma-ray passes close to a nucleus which appears to act as a catalyst for the process.

Parent—A *radionuclide* that upon radioactive *decay* or disintegration yields a specific nuclide (the *daughter*).

Particle Accelerator—Any machine capable of accelerating electrons, protons, deuterons, or other charged particles in a vacuum and of discharging the resultant particulate or other radiation into a medium at energies usually in excess of 1 MeV.

Parts Per Million (ppm)—Parts (*molecules*) of a substance contained in a million parts of air (or water) by volume.

Peak Tube Potential—The maximum value of the potential difference across the *x-ray* tube during an exposure.

Pellet, Fuel—As used in *PWRs* and *BWRs*, a pellet is a small cylinder approximately ⅜-inch in diameter and ⅝-inch in length consisting of *uranium* fuel in a ceramic form—uranium dioxide, UO_2. Typical fuel pellet *enrichments* range from 2 to 3.5 percent *uranium*-235.

Periodic Table—An arrangement of chemical *elements* in order of increasing *atomic number*. Elements of similar properties are placed one under the other, yielding groups or families of elements. Within each group, there is a variation of chemical and physical properties, but in general there is a similarity of chemical behavior within each group. (See Figure 2.1)

Person—

(1) Any *individual*, corporation, partnership, firm, association, trust, estate, public or private institution, group, Government agency other than the Nuclear Regulatory Commission or the Department of Energy (except that the Department shall be considered a person within the meaning of the regulations in 10 CFR chapter I to the extent that its facilities and activities are subject to the licensing and related regulatory authority of the Nuclear Regulatory Commission.

(2) Any legal successor, representative, agent, or agency of the foregoing.

Personnel Monitoring or Personal Monitoring—The continuous measurement of an individual's exposure to external radiation by means of suitable devices, such as *film badges*, *TLD* badges, *pocket dosimeters* or electronic dosimeters worn on the individual's person.

Phantom—A volume of material behaving in a manner similar to tissue with respect to the attenuation and scattering of radiation.

Photodosimetry—The determination of the cumulative *dose* of *ionizing radiation* by use of photographic film.

Photoelectric effect—A process by which a photon ejects an electron form an atom. All the energy of the photon is absorbed in ejecting the electron and in imparting kinetic energy to it; a characteristic X-ray (or Auger electron) is subsequently produced when the vacated shell is filled by another orbital electron.

Photon—A quantum (or packet) of energy emitted in the form of *electromagnetic radiation*. *Gamma rays* and *x-rays* are examples of photons.

Phototimer—A method for controlling radiation *exposures* to image receptors by the amount of radiation which reaches a radiation monitoring device(s). The radiation monitoring device(s) is part of an electronic circuit which controls the duration of time the *x-ray* tube is activated.

Pico—A prefix that divides a basic unit by one trillion.

Picocurie—One trillionth (10^{-12}) part of a *curie*.

Pig—A container (usually lead) used to ship or store *radioactive* materials. The thick walls protect the person handling the container from *radiation*. Large containers are commonly called *casks*.

Pile—A *nuclear reactor*; called a pile because the earliest reactor were "piles" of graphite and uranium blocks.

Planned Special Exposure—An infrequent *exposure* to *radiation*, separate from and in addition to the annual *dose limits*.

Plutonium (Pu)—A heavy, radioactive, manmade metallic *element* with *atomic number* 94. Its most important *isotope* is *fissile plutonium*-239, which is produced by *neutron* irradiation of *uranium*-238.

Pocket Dosimeter—A small *ionization* detection instrument that indicates radiation exposure directly. An auxiliary charging device is usually necessary.

Poison—In *reactor* physics, a material other than *fissionable material* in the vicinity of the reactor *core* that will absorb neutrons. The addition of poisons, such as *control rods* or boron, into the reactor is said to be an addition of negative *reactivity*.

Pool Reactor—A *reactor* in which the *fuel elements* are suspended in a pool of water that serves as the *reflector, moderator* and *coolant*. Popularly called a "swimming pool reactor," it is used for research and training, not for electrical generation.

Position Indicating Device—A device on dental *x-ray* equipment used to indicate the beam position and to establish a definite source-surface (skin) distance. It may or may not incorporate or serve as a beam limiting device.

Positron—Particle equal in mass, but opposite in charge, to the *electron*; a positive electron.

Power Reactor—A *reactor* designed to produce heat for electric generation, as distinguished from reactors used for research, for producing *radiation* or *fissionable materials*, or for reactor component testing.

Pressure Vessel—A strong-walled container housing the *core* of most types of *power reactors*; it usually also contains the *moderator*, neutron *reflector*, *thermal shield* and *control rods*.

Pressurized Water Reactor (PWR)—A *nuclear reactor* in which heat is transferred from the core to a heat exchanger (the steam generator) by high-temperature water kept under high pressure in what is known as the primary system. Steam generated from water in a secondary circuit is used to drive a turbine and electrical generator. About two-thirds of the operating nuclear power reactors in the U.S. are PWR's.

Pressurizer—A tank or vessel that acts as a head tank (or surge volume) to control the pressure in a *pressurized water reactor*.

Primary System—See *reactor coolant system*.

Prodromal Effects—The forewarning symptoms of more serious health effects.

Projected Dose—Future dose calculated for a specified time period on the basis of estimated or measured initial concentrations of radionuclides or exposure rates and in the absence of *protective actions*.

Proportional Counter—An instrument in which an electronic detection system receives pulses that are proportional to the number of *ions* formed in a gas-filled tube by *ionizing radiation*.

Protective Action—An activity conducted in response to an incident or potential incident to avoid or reduce radiation dose to members of the public (sometimes called a protective measure).

Protective Action Guide (PAG)—The *projected dose* to *reference man* (or standard man), or other defined individual, from an accidental release of radioactive material at which a specific *protective action* to reduce or avoid that dose is warranted.

Protective Barrier—A barrier of radiation absorbing material(s) used to reduce radiation exposure. The types of protective barriers are as follows:

(1) *Primary Protective Barrier* means the material, excluding filters, placed in the useful beam, for protection purposes, to reduce the radiation exposure.

(2) *Secondary protective barrier* means a barrier sufficient to attenuate the stray radiation to the required degree.

Proton—An elementary nuclear particle with a positive electric charge located in the *nucleus* of an *atom*. (See *atomic number*.)

Public Dose—The *dose* received by a member of the public from *exposure* to *radiation* and to radioactive material released by a licensee, or to another source of radiation either within a licensee's *controlled area* or in *unrestricted areas*. It does not include *occupational dose* or *doses* received from *background radiation*, as a patient from medical practices, or from voluntary participation in medical research programs.

PWR—A *pressurized water reactor*.

Quality Factor (Q)—A numerical factor assigned to describe the average effectiveness of a particular kind (and sometimes energy) of radiation in producing biological effects in the human. The factor used to derive *equivalent dose* from *absorbed dose*. X- and gamma rays, electrons, and beta particles have been assigned Q's of 1. Protons, alpha particles, other heavy (mass number $\geqslant$1) charged particles and neutrons have been assigned values of Q ranging from 2 to 20.

Quantum Theory—The concept that energy is radiated intermittently in units of definite magnitude called quanta, and absorbed in a like manner. (See *photon*.)

Quarter—A period of time equal to one-fourth of the year observed by the licensee (approximately 13 consecutive weeks), providing that the beginning of the first quarter in a year coincides with the starting date of the year and that no day is omitted or duplicated in consecutive quarters.

Rad—The special unit of *absorbed dose*. One *rad* is equal to an *absorbed dose* of 0.01 J kg^{-1} (0.01 gray).

Radiac—An acronym derived from "radioactivity detection indication and computation," a generic term applying to radiological instruments or equipment.

Radiation (ionizing radiation)—*Alpha particles, beta particles, gamma rays, x-rays, neutrons*, high-speed electrons, high-speed protons, and other particles capable of producing ions. Radiation, as used in this part, does not include non-ionizing radiation, such as radio- or microwaves, or visible, infrared, or ultraviolet light.

Radiation Area—An area, accessible to *individuals*, in which radiation levels could result in an *individual* receiving a *dose equivalent* in excess of 0.005 rem (0.05 mSv) in 1 hour at 30 centimeters from the radiation source or from any surface that the radiation penetrates.

Radiation Controlled Area—An area inside a facility for which access is controlled, and for which special conditions may be prescribed, because of the potential for radiation, airborne radioactivity or radioactive contamination.

Radiation Detection Instrument—A device that detects the presence of *ionizing radiation*. Some radiation detectors also identify characteristics of the radiation.

Radiation Exposure Permit (REP) or ***Radiation Work Permit*** (RWP)—Document generated prior to an activity potentially involving exposure of workers to radiation. It describes the work location and work to be performed and presents the results of preliminary radiation, contamination and/or airborne radioactivity measurements. It prescribes conditions for entry to and work in the area such as requirements for protective clothing, shielding, ventilation, and radiation/radioactivity survey and monitoring. It may specify individual and/or collective dose limits for the job and may specify occupancy times (''stay times''). It provides for appropriate authorizing signatures.

Radiation Machine—Any device capable of producing radiation except those which produce radiation only from radioactive material.

Radiation Monitoring—See *monitoring*.

Radiation Shielding—Reduction of *radiation* by interposing a shield of absorbing material between any radioactive source and a person, work area or radiation-sensitive device.

Radiation Sickness (Syndrome)—The complex of symptoms characterizing the disease known as radiation injury, resulting from excessive exposure of the whole body (or large part) to *ionizing radiation*. The earliest of these symptoms are nausea, fatigue, vomiting, and diarrhea, which may be followed by loss of hair (epilation), hemorrhage, inflammation of the mouth and throat, and general loss of energy. In severe cases, where the radiation exposure has been relatively large, death may occur within two to four weeks. Those who survive six weeks after the receipt of a single large *dose* of *radiation* may generally be expected to recover.

Radiation Source—Usually a manmade sealed source of *radiation* used in teletherapy, *radiography*, as a power source for batteries, or in various types of industrial gauges. Machines such as accelerators and radioisotope generators and natural *radionuclides* may be considered sources.

Radiation Standards—Exposure standards, permissible concentrations, rules for safe handling, regulations for transportation, regulations for industrial control of radiation and control of *radioactive* material by legislative means.

Radiation Syndrome—See *radiation sickness (syndrome)*.

Radiation Therapy Simulation System—A radiographic or fluoroscopic *x-ray* system intended for localizing the volume to be exposed during radiation therapy and confirming the position and size of the therapeutic irradiation field.

Radiation Warning Symbol—An officially prescribed symbol (a magenta trefoil) on a yellow background that must be displayed where certain quantities of *radioactive* materials are present or where certain *doses* of *radiation* could be received.

Radiation Weighting Factor (W_R)—A factor used for radiation-protection purposes that accounts for differences in biological effectiveness between different radiations. The *radiation weighting factor* (W_R) is independent of the *tissue weighting factor* (W_T).

Radioactive—Exhibits *radioactivity*; undergoes *radioactive decay*.

Radioactive Contamination—Deposition of *radioactive* material in any place where it may harm persons or equipment.

Radioactive Isotope—A *radioisotope*.

Radioactive Series—A succession of *nuclides*, each of which transforms by radioactive *disintegration* into the next until a *stable* nuclide results. The first member is called the *parent*, the intermediate members are called *daughters*, and the final *stable* member is called the end product.

Radioactive Waste—See *waste, radioactive*.

Radioactivity—The process of undergoing spontaneous transformation of the nucleus, generally with the emission of *alpha* or *beta particles*, often accompanied by gamma rays. The term is also used to designate *radioactive* materials.

Radiographer—Any individual who performs or personally supervises industrial radiographic operations and who is responsible to the licensee or registrant for assuring compliance with the requirements of these regulations and all license and/or certificate of registration conditions.

Radiographic Exposure Device—Any instrument containing a sealed source fastened or contained therein, in which the sealed source or shielding thereof may be moved, or other wise changed, from a shielded to unshielded position for purposes of making a radiographic exposure.

Radiograph—An image receptor on which the image is created directly or indirectly by an *x-ray* pattern and results in a permanent record.

Radiographic Imaging System—Any system whereby a permanent or semi-permanent image is recorded on an image receptor by the action of ionizing radiation.

Radiography—The making of shadow images on photographic film by the action of *ionizing radiation*.

Radioisotope—A *radioactive isotope*; i.e. an unstable *isotope* that undergoes spontaneous transformation, emitting *radiation*. Approximately 2500 natural and artificial radioisotopes have been identified.

Radiological Survey—The evaluation of the *radiation* hazards accompanying the production, use, or existence of *radioactive materials* under a specific set of conditions. Such evaluation customarily includes a physical survey of the disposition of materials and equipment, measurements or estimates of the levels of *radiation* that may be involved, and a sufficient knowledge of processes affecting these materials to predict hazards resulting from unexpected or possible changes in materials or equipment.

Radiology—That branch of medicine dealing with the diagnostic and therapeutic applications of radiant energy, including *x-rays* and *radioisotopes*.

Radionuclide—A *radioactive nuclide*.

Radiosensitivity—The relative susceptibility of cells, tissues, organs, organisms, or other substances to the injurious action of *radiation*.

Radium (Ra)—A *radioactive* metallic *element* with *atomic number* 88. As found in nature, the most common *isotope* has a mass number of 226. It occurs in minute quantities associated with *uranium* in pitchblende, carnotite and other minerals.

Radon (Rn)—A *radioactive element* that is one of the heaviest gases known. Its *atomic number* is 86. Radon with a *mass number* of 222, is a *daughter* of *radium*-226.

Reaction—Any process involving a chemical or nuclear change.

Reactivity—A term expressing the departure of a *reactor* system from *criticality*. A positive reactivity addition indicates a move toward *supercriticality* (power increase). A negative reactivity addition indicates a move toward *subcriticality* (power decrease).

Reactor Coolant System—The cooling system used to remove energy from the reactor *core* and transfer that energy either directly or indirectly to the steam *turbine*.

Reactor, Nuclear—A device in which nuclear *fission* may be sustained and controlled in a self-supporting nuclear *reaction*. The varieties are many, but all incorporate certain features, including *fissionable material* or fuel, a *moderating* material (unless the reactor is operated on *fast neutrons*), a *reflector* to conserve escaping neutrons, provisions for removal of heat, measuring and controlling instruments, and protective devices.

Recording Level (for intake of radionuclides)—Level of *committed dose equivalent* or *intake* above which the result is of sufficient interest to be worth keeping and interpreting. Recording levels are defined for routine monitoring, RL_R, and for special or operational monitoring, RL_S. Derived recording levels, DRL_R and DRL_S, are values of body or organ content or elimination rate that correspond to recording levels, RL_R and RL_S. The values are calculated by means of defined models of *intake*, *deposition*, *uptake*, *retention* and *elimination*.

Recovery—The process of reducing radiation exposure rates and concentrations of radioactive material in the environment to levels acceptable for unconditional occupancy or use.

Recycling—The reuse of slightly contaminated materials, chiefly metals, with or without decontamination or processing.

Reentry—Temporary entry into a restricted zone under controlled conditions.

Reference Man—A hypothetical aggregation of human physical and physiological characteristics arrived at by international consensus. These characteristics may be used by researchers and public health workers to standardize results of experiments and to relate biological insult to a common base.

Reflector—A layer of material immediately surrounding a reactor *core* that scatters back (or reflects) into the core many *neutrons* that would otherwise escape. The returned neutrons can then cause more *fissions* and improve the neutron economy of the reactor. Common reflector materials are graphite, beryllium, water and *natural uranium*.

Relocation—The removal or continued exclusion of people (households) from contaminated areas to avoid chronic radiation exposure.

Rem—The special unit of any of the quantities expressed as *dose equivalent*. The *dose equivalent* in *rem* in equal to the absorbed *dose* in *rad* multiplied by the *quality factor* (1 *rem* = 0.01 *sievert*).

Reprocessing—The reuse of *fissionable material* after it has been recovered by chemical processing from *spent or depleted* reactor fuel, reenriched and then refabricated into new fuel elements.

Respirator—A device covering the mouth and nose to prevent the inhalation of radioactive materials.

Respiratory Protective Device—An apparatus, such as a respirator, used to reduce the individual's *intake* of *airborne radioactive materials*.

Restricted Area—An area, access to which is limited by the licensee for the purpose of protecting individuals against undue risks from *exposure* to *radiation* and *radioactive materials*. *Restricted area* does not include areas used as residential quarters, but separate rooms in a residential building may be set apart as a restricted area.

Restricted Zone—An area with controlled access from which the population has been relocated.

Retained Quantity—In a specific organ or tissue, the quantity of deposited material in that organ or tissue at a given time after intake, deposition or uptake. Material taken up by body fluids is known as systemic material. The quantity in the whole body is the sum of systemic material and material retained within the respiratory and the gastrointestinal tracts.

Retention Function—A function describing the time dependence of the retained quantity.

Return—The reoccupation of areas cleared for unrestricted residence or use.

Roentgen (r)—A unit of exposure to *ionizing radiation.* It is that amount of *gamma* or *x-rays* required to produce *ions* carrying 1 electrostatic unit of electrical charge in 1 cubic centimeter of dry air under standard conditions. Named after Wilhelm Roentgen, German scientist who discovered *x-rays* in 1895.

Roentgen Equivalent Man (or mammal)—See *rem.*

Routine Workplace Radiation Survey—A regularly scheduled (routine) evaluation of radiological conditions and potential hazards incident to the production, use, transfer, release, disposal, or presence of radioactive material or other sources of *radiation.* When appropriate, such an evaluation includes a physical survey of the location of radioactive material and measurements or calculations of levels of radiation, or concentrations or quantities of radioactive material present.

Safeguards—The protection of *special nuclear material* (SNM) to prevent theft, loss or sabotage. (See *special nuclear material.*)

Safe Shutdown Earthquake—A design-basis earthquake. (See *design-basis phenomenon.*)

Safety Injection—The rapid insertion of a chemically soluble neutron *poison* (such as boric acid) into the *reactor coolant system* to ensure *reactor shutdown.* (See *shutdown.*)

Safety Related—The managerial controls, administrative documents, operating procedures, systems, structures and components that have been designed to mitigate the consequences of postulated accidents that could cause undue risk to public health and safety.

Safety Rod—See *control rod*; *scram.*

Sanitary sewerage—A system of public sewers for carrying off waste water and refuse, but excluding sewage treatment facilities, septic tanks, and leach fields owned or operated by the licensee.

Scattered Radiation—*Radiation* that, during its passage through a substance, has been changed in direction. It may also have been modified by a decrease in energy. It is one form of *secondary radiation.*

Scattered Radiation—Radiation that, during passage through matter, has been deviated in direction.

Scintillation Detector or Counter—The combination of phosphor, photomultiplier tube, and associated electronic circuits for counting light emissions produced in the phosphor by *ionizing radiation.* (See *counter.*)

Scram—Sudden shutting down of a *nuclear reactor,* usually by rapid insertion of *control rods,* either automatically or manually by the reactor operator.

Sealed Source—Radioactive material that is permanently bonded or fixed in a capsule or matrix designed to prevent release and dispersal of the radioactive material under the most severe conditions which are likely to be encountered in normal use and handling.

Secondary Radiation—*Radiation* originating as the result of absorption of other radiation in matter. It may be either electromagnetic or particulate in nature.

Secondary System—The *steam generator* tubes, *steam turbine, condenser* and associated pipes, pumps and heaters used to convert the heat energy of the *reactor coolant system* into mechanical energy for electrical generation. Most commonly used in reference to *pressurized water reactors.*

Seismic Category I—A term used to define structures, systems and components that are designed and built to withstand the maximum potential (earthquake) stresses for the particular region that a nuclear plant is sited.

Self-Reading Pocket Dosimeter (SRPD)—A small radiation detection instrument that indicates radiation exposure directly. It is usually worn in a shirt pocket and can be read by the wearer.

Shallow-Dose Equivalent (H_S)—Which applies to the external exposure of the skin or an extremity, is taken as the *dose equivalent* at a tissue depth of 0.007 centimeter (7 mg cm^2) averaged over an area of 1 square centimeter.

Sheltering—The use of a structure for radiation protection from an airborne plume and/or deposited radioactive materials.

Shielded Room Radiography—Industrial radiography conducted in a room shielded so that radiation levels at every location on the exterior meet the limitations specified in the regulations.

Shielding—Any material or obstruction that absorbs *radiation* and thus tends to protect personnel or materials from the effects of *ionizing radiation.*

Short-Lived Daughters—Radioactive progeny of radioactive isotopes that have *half-lives* on the order of a few hours or less.

Shutdown—A decrease in the rate of *fission* (and heat production) in a reactor (usually by the insertion of *control rods* into the *core*). See *subcriticality.*

SID—See *Source image receptor distance.*

Sievert—The SI unit of any of the quantities expressed as *dose equivalent.* The *dose equivalent* in *sieverts* is equal to the *absorbed dose* in *gray* multiplied by the *quality factor* (1 *Sv* = 100 *rem*).

Site Boundary—That line beyond which the land or property is not owned, leased, or otherwise controlled by the licensee.

Site Closure and Stabilization—Those actions that are taken upon completion of operations that prepare the disposal site for custodial care and that assure that the disposal site will remain stable and will not need ongoing active maintenance.

Skyshine—Radiation emitted over an open-topped shielded enclosure and reflected by air so as to radiate people on the outside.

Smear or Smear Test—A method of determining the removable contamination on a surface. The suspected area is wiped with a filter paper and the radioactivity in the paper is measured. Also called a *wipe test.*

Somatic Effects of Radiation—Effects of radiation limited to the exposed individual, as distinguished from genetic effects, which may also affect subsequent unexposed generations.

Source Image Receptor Distance**—**The distance from the source to the center of the input surface of the image receptor.

Source Material**—**

(1) Uranium or thorium or any combination of uranium and thorium in any physical or chemical form; or

(2) Ores that contain, by weight, one-twentieth of 1 percent (0.05 percent), or more, of uranium, thorium, or any combination of uranium and thorium. *Source material* does not include *special nuclear material.*

Special Form Radioactive Material**—**Radioactive material which satisfies the following conditions:

(1) It is either a single solid piece or is contained in a sealed capsule that can be opened only by destroying the capsule;

(2) The piece or capsule has at least one dimension not less than 5 millimeters (0.197 inch); and

(3) It satisfies the test requirements specified by the U.S. Nuclear Regulatory Commission.

Special Nuclear Material**—**

(1) Plutonium, *uranium*-233, uranium enriched in the isotope 233 or in the isotope 235, and any other material that the Nuclear Regulatory Commission determines to be *special nuclear material*, but does not include *source material*; or

(2) Any material artificially enriched by any of the foregoing but does not include *source material.*

Spectroscopic Analysis or Spectrometric Analysis**—**Any one of a number of instrumental methods for determining the constituents in a sample. In the context of radioactivity analysis, alpha, beta, and gamma-ray spectrometers are used to identify and quantitate the radionuclide constituents in a sample.

Spent (Depleted) Fuel**—**Uranium fuel that has been used and then removed from the reactor. Spent fuel from nuclear power plants typically contains most of the original *uranium*-238, about 25 percent of the original *uranium*-235, transuranic elements (formed by neutron capture) and fission products. Spent fuel is highly radioactive.

Spent Fuel Pool**—**An underwater storage and cooling facility for *fuel elements* that have been removed from a *reactor.*

SSD**—**The distance between the source and the skin of the patient.

Stable Atom**—**An atom that will not spontaneously change to another atom (i.e., it will not undergo radioactive transformation).

Startup**—**An increase in the rate of *fission* (and heat production) in a reactor usually by the removal of control rods from the core). (See *supercriticality.*)

Stay Time**—**The period during which personnel may remain in a *restricted area* before accumulating some permissible *dose.*

Steam Generator**—**The *heat exchanger* used in some *reactor* designs to transfer heat from the primary (*reactor coolant*) system to the secondary (steam) system. This design permits heat exchange with little or no contamination of the secondary system equipment.

Stochastic Effects**—**Health effects that occur randomly and for which the probability of the effect occurring, rather than its severity, is assumed to be a linear function of dose without threshold. Hereditary effects and cancer incidence are examples of *stochastic effects.*

Subcriticality**—**The condition of a *nuclear reactor* system when the rate of production of *fission neutrons* is lower than the rate of production in the previous generation due to increased *neutron leakage* and *poisons.*

Subcritical Mass**—**An amount of *fissionable material* insufficient in quantity or of improper geometry to sustain a fission *chain reaction.*

Supercriticality**—**The condition for increasing the level of operation of a *reactor.* The rate of fission *neutron* production exceeds all neutron losses, and the overall neutron population increases. (See *critical mass; criticality.*)

Supercritical Reactor**—**A *reactor* in which the power level is increasing.

Superheating**—**The heating of a vapor, particularly steam, to a temperature much higher than the boiling point at the existing pressure. This is done in some power plants to improve efficiency and to reduce water damage to the *turbine.*

Survey**—**An evaluation of the radiological conditions and potential hazards incident to the production, use, transfer, release, disposal, or presence of radioactive material or other sources of *radiation.* When appropriate, such an evaluation includes a physical survey of the location of radioactive material and measurements or calculations of levels of radiation, or concentrations or quantities of radioactive material present.

Survey Meter**—**Any portable *radiation detection instrument* especially adapted for inspecting an area to establish the existence and amount of *radioactive* material present. (See *counter.*)

Tailings, Tails**—**See *mill tailings.*

Technique Factors**—**The following conditions of operation:

(1) For capacitor energy storage equipment, peak tube potential in kV and quantity of charge in mAs;

(2) For field emission equipment rated for pulsed operation, peak tube potential in kV, and number of *x-ray* pulses;

(3) For CT *x-ray* systems designed for pulsed operation, peak tube potential in kV, scan time in seconds, and either tube current in mA, *x-ray* pulse width in seconds, and the number of *x-ray* pulses per scan, or the product of tube current, *x-ray* pulse width, and the number of *x-ray* pulses in mAs;

(4) For CT *x-ray* systems not designed for pulsed operation, peak tube potential in kV, and either tube current in mA and scan time in seconds, or the product of tube current and exposure time in mAs and the scan time when the scan time and exposure time are equivalent; and

(5) For all other equipment, peak tube potential in kV, and either tube current in mA and exposure time in seconds, or the product of tube current and exposure time in mAs.

Technologically Enhanced**—**Substance which because of processing contains more naturally occurring radioactive material than originally found in nature.

Teletherapy**—**Therapeutic irradiation in which the source of radiation is at a distance from the body.

Tenth Thickness**—**The thickness of a given material that will decrease the amount (or *dose*) of *radiation* to one-tenth of the amount incident upon it. Two-tenth thicknesses will reduce the dose received by a factor of 10 × 10; i.e., 100, and so on. (See *shielding*.)

Terrestrial Radiation**—**The portion of *natural radiation* (background) that is emitted by naturally occurring *radioactive* materials in the earth.

Thermal Breeder Reactor**—**A *breeder reactor* in which the *fission chain reaction* is sustained by thermal neutrons. (See *neutron, thermal*.)

Thermalization**—**The process undergone by high-energy (fast) neutrons as they lose energy by collision. (See *neutron, thermal*.)

Thermal Neutron**—**See *neutron, thermal*.

Thermal Reactor**—**A reactor in which the *fission chain reaction* is sustained primarily by thermal neutrons. Most current reactors are thermal reactors.

Thermal Shield**—**A layer or layers of high-density material located within a reactor *pressure vessel* or between the vessel and the *biological shield* to reduce radiation heating in the vessel and the biological shield.

Thermonuclear**—**An adjective referring to the process in which very high temperatures are used to bring about the *fusion* of light nuclei, such as those of the hydrogen *isotopes*, *deuterium* and *tritium*, with the accompanying liberation of energy. (See *fusion*.)

Tissue Weighting Factor (W_T)—See *Organ or Tissue Weighting Factor*.

Thermoluminescence Dosimeter (TLD)**—**a crystalline material which, when heated after having been exposed to radiation, emits light in proportion to the radiation dose previously received. Numerous materials make effective TLD's; three examples include lithium fluoride (LiF), calcium fluoride with a Mn impurity (CaF_2:Mn) and lithium borate ($Li_2B_4O_7$).

Tomogram**—**The depiction of the *x-ray* attenuation properties of a section through the body.

Total Effective Dose Equivalent (TEDE)—The sum of the *deep-dose equivalent* (for external exposures) and the *committed effective dose equivalent* (for internal exposures).

Transport Index**—**The dimensionless number, rounded up to the first decimal place, placed on the label of a package to designate the degree of control to be exercised by the carrier during transportation. The transport index is the number expressing the maximum radiation level in millirem per hour at 1 meter from the external surface of the package.

Transient**—**A change in the *reactor coolant system* temperature and/or pressure due to a change in power output of the *reactor*. Transients can be caused by adding or removing neutron *poisons*, by increasing or decreasing the electrical load on the *turbine generator*, or by accident conditions.

Transition**—**A nuclear change from one energy state to another, generally accompanied by the emission of particles. Often called a decay, or a disintegration.

Transuranic Elements**—**Elements with atomic numbers higher than that of uranium (92).

Trip, Reactor**—**See *scram*.

Tritium**—**A radioactive *isotope* of hydrogen (one *proton*, two *neutrons*). Because it is chemically identical to natural hydrogen, tritium can easily be taken into the body by any ingestion path. *Decays* by *beta* emission. Its radioactive *half-life* is about 12½ years.

Tube**—**An *x-ray* tube, unless otherwise specified.

Turbine**—**A rotary engine made with a series of curved vanes on a rotating shaft. Usually turned by water or steam. Turbines are considered to be the most economical means to turn large electrical generators.

Turbine Generator (TG)—A steam (or water) *turbine* directly connected to an electrical generator. The two devices are often referred to as one unit.

Type A Quantity**—**A quantity of radioactive material, the aggregate radioactivity of which does not exceed A_1 for special form radioactive material or A_2 for normal form radioactive material.

Type B Quantity**—**A quantity of radioactive material greater than a *Type A quantity*.

Ultraviolet**—***Electromagnetic radiation* of a wavelength between the shortest visible violet and low-energy *x-rays*.

Unstable Atom**—**An atom that will spontaneously transform to another atom (radioactive).

Unrestricted Area**—**An area, access to which is neither limited nor controlled by the *licensee*.

Uptake**—**Quantity of material transferred from the site of intake to body organs or tissues.

Uranium (U)—A radioactive element with the *atomic number* 92, and as found in natural ores, an *atomic weight* of approximately 238. The two principal natural *isotopes* are *uranium*-235 (0.7 percent of natural uranium), which is *fissile*, and *uranium*-238 (99.3 percent of natural uranium), which is *fissionable* by fast neutrons and is *fertile*. *Natural uranium* also includes a minute amount of *uranium*-234.

Uranium Enrichment**—**See *isotopic enrichment*.

***Uranium Fuel Cycle*—**The operations of milling of uranium ore, chemical conversion of uranium, isotopic enrichment of uranium, fabrication of uranium fuel, generation of electricity by a light-water-cooled *nuclear power plant* using uranium fuel, and reprocessing of spent uranium fuel to the extent that these activities directly support the production of electrical power for public use. *Uranium fuel cycle* does not include mining operations, operations at waste disposal sites, transportation of radioactive material in support of these operations, and the reuse of recovered non-uranium *special nuclear* and *by product materials* from the cycle.

Uranium Millings (Tails)—See *mill tailings.*

***Vapor*—**The gaseous form of substances that are normally in liquid or solid form.

***Very High Radiation Area*—**An area, accessible to *individuals*, in which radiation levels could result in an individual receiving an *absorbed dose* in excess of 500 rad (5 Gy) in 1 hour at 1 meter from a radiation source or from any surface that the radiation penetrates. (Note: At very high doses received at high dose rates, units of *absorbed dose* (e.g., *rad* and *gray*) are appropriate, rather than units of *dose equivalent* (e.g., *rem* and *siever*).

***Vessel*—**See *pressure vessel.*

***Vital Plant Systems*—**See *safety related.*

***Void*—**An area of lower density in a moderating system (such as steam bubbles in water) that allows more *neutron leakage* than does the more dense material around it. (See *moderator; void coefficient; neutron leakage.*)

***Void Coefficient of Reactivity*—**Property of a reactor plant moderating system where, as temperature increases in the system, *neutron leakage* increases due to an increase in the number and size of *voids* (steam bubbles) in the *moderator.*

***Waste, Radioactive*—**Solid, liquid and gaseous materials from nuclear operations that are radioactive or become radioactive and for which there is no further use. Wastes are generally classified as high level (having radioactivity concentrations of hundreds of thousands of *curies* per gallon or cubic foot), low level (in the range of 1 *microcurie* per gallon or cubic foot), or intermediate level (between these extremes).

***Weathering Factor*—**The fraction of radioactivity remaining after being affected by average weather conditions for a specified period of time.

***Week*—**Seven consecutive days starting on Sunday.

***Well Bore*—**A drilled hole in which wireline service operations or subsurface tracer studies are performed.

***Well Logging*—**All operations involving the lowering and raising of measuring devices or tools which may contain sources of radiation into well bores or cavities for the purpose of obtaining information about the well or adjacent formations.

***Whole Body*—**For purposes of external exposure, head, trunk (including male gonads), arms above the elbow, or legs above the knee.

***Whole Body Counter*—**A device used to identify and measure the radioactivity in the body (*body burden*). It uses a sensitive radiation detector (or array of detectors) located outside the body to measure the radiation emitted by the radioactive materials inside the body. It is useful for detecting those radionuclides that have radiations that are sufficiently penetrating to be detected outside the body.

***Whole-Body Exposure*—**An exposure of the body to radiation, in which the entire body rather than an isolated part is irradiated. Where a *radioisotope* is uniformly distributed throughout the body tissues, rather than being concentrated in certain parts, the irradiation can be considered as a whole-body exposure.

***Wipe Test*—**See *Smear or Smear Test.*

***Wireline*—**A cable containing one or more electrical conductors which is used to lower and raise logging tools in the well bore.

***Wireline Service Operation*—**Any evaluation or mechanical service which is performed in the well bore using devices on a wireline.

***Working Level (WL)*—**Any combination of *polonium*-218, *lead*-214, *bismuth*-214, and *polonium*-214 (the short-lived progeny of radon) in 1 liter of air, under ambient temperature and pressure that results in the ultimate emission of 1.3×10^5 MeV of alpha particle energy. This is about the total amount of energy released over a long period of time by the short-lived daughters in equilibrium with 100 pCi of radon.

***Working Level Month (WLM)*—**A cumulative exposure, equivalent to exposure to one working level for a working month (170 h), *i.e.*, 2×10^{-5} Jh $m^{-3} \times 170$ h $= 3.5 \times 10^{-3}$ Jh m^{-3}.

***X-Ray Control*—**A device which controls input power to the *x-ray* high voltage generator and/or the *x-ray* tube. It includes equipment such as timers, phototimers, automatic brightness stabilizers, and similar devices, which control the technique factors of an *x-ray* exposure.

***X-Ray Equipment*—**An *x-ray* system, subsystem, or component thereof. Types of *x-ray* equipment are as follows:

(1) *Mobile x-ray* equipment means *x-ray* equipment mounted on a permanent base with wheels and/or casters for moving while completely assembled.

(2) *Portable x-ray* equipment means *x-ray* equipment designed to be hand carried.

(3) *Stationary x-ray* equipment means *x-ray* equipment which is installed in a fixed location.

X-Ray High Voltage Generator—A device which transforms electrical energy from the potential supplied by the *x-ray* control to the tube operating potential. The device may also include means for transforming alternating current to direct current, filament transformers for the *x-ray* tube(s), high voltage switches, electrical protective devices, and other appropriate elements.

X-Ray System—An assemblage of components for the controlled production of *x-rays*. It includes minimally an *x-ray* high voltage generator, an *x-ray* control, a tube housing assembly, a beam limiting device, and the necessary supporting structures. Additional components which function with the system are considered integral parts of the system. *X-ray subsystem* means any combination of two or more components of an *x-ray* system.

X-Rays—Penetrating *electromagnetic radiation* having a wavelength that is much shorter than that of visible light. Rays produced by excitation of the *electron* field around certain nuclei are called characteristic *x-rays*. Electromagnetic rays that are produced as the result of deceleration of charged particles as they pass near the nucleus are called continuous *x-rays* (or *Bremsstrahlung*). *X-rays* are identical to *gamma rays*, but originate outside the nucleus.

Year—The period of time beginning in January used to determine compliance with the provisions of Nuclear Regulatory Commission regulations. The *licensee* may change the starting date of the year used to determine compliance by the *licensee* provided that the change is made at the beginning of the year and that no day is omitted or duplicated in consecutive years.

Yellowcake—A product of the *uranium* milling process, yellowcake is a solid uranium-oxygen compound (U_3O_8) that takes its name from its color and texture. Yellowcake is the feed material used for fuel *enrichment* and fuel *pellet* fabrication.

References

International Commission on Radiological Protection. *Recommendations of the International Commission on Radiological Protection*. ICRP Publication 60; Pergamon Press; Elmsford, NY; 1977, 1991.

U.S. Nuclear Regulatory Commission. *Glossary of Terms Nuclear Power and Reactors*. NUREG-0770; 1981.

U.S. Nuclear Regulatory Commission 10 CFR Part 20 et al. ''Standards for protection against radiation, final rule,'' *Federal Register*. *56*(98):23360; U.S. Government Printing Office; Washington, DC; May 21, 1991.

National Council on Radiation Protection and Measurements. *Limitation of Exposure to Ionizing Radiation NCRP Report No. 116*. National Council on Radiation Protection and Measurements; Bethesda, Maryland; 1993.

GLOSSARY—LIGHT AND LASERS

Accommodation—The ability of the eye to change its power and thus focus for different object distances.

Angstrom (Å)—A unit of measure of *wavelength* equal to 10^{-10} meter, 0.1 nanometer, of 10^{-4} micrometer, no longer widely used.

Area S—Potentially hazardous zone for *specular reflections* around a target.

Area T—Hazardous area for viewing a *diffuse reflection* of an emergent laser beam in front of a laser.

Attenuation—Decrease in the radiant flux of any optical beam as it passes through an absorbing or scattering medium.

Beam Diameter (D_L)—The distance between diametrically opposed points in the cross section of a circular beam where the power per unit area is 1/e times (37 percent) that at the peak.

Beam Divergence (ϕ)—Angle of beam spread measured in radians or milliradians (1 milliradian = 3.4 minutes of arc or approximately 1 mil). For small angles where the chord is approximately equal to the arc, the increase in the diameter of the beam is numerically equal to 1,000th of the range in meters multiplied by the number of milliradians of beam divergence. That is, at 1,000 meters range a beam divergence of 2 milliradians would give a beam diameter 2 meters wider than the emergent beam diameter.

Beam Splitter—An optical device using controlled reflection to produce two beams from a single incident beam.

Biennial Vision Screening Examination—*Vision screening examination* using multiphasic vision screening equipment every 2 years.

Classification Duration (T_{max})—The maximum duration of exposure inherent in the design of the *laser device*.

Closed Installation—any location where lasers are used which will be closed to unprotected personnel during laser operation.

CW Laser—Continuous-wave laser, as distinguished from a *pulsed laser*. A laser emitting for a period in excess of 0.25 second.

Controlled Area—An area where the occupancy and activity of those within are subject to control and supervision for the purpose of protection from optical radiation hazards.

Data Quality Objective (DQO)—The definition of the multiple aspects of the analytical process to achieve the desired analytical results, e.g., precisions, bios, etc.

Diffuse Reflection—Takes place when different parts of a beam incident on a surface are reflected over a wide range of angles.

Distance Z—Downrange distance along the approved lines of sight. Distance Z is always greater than or equal to the NOHD.

Duty Cycle—Ratio of "on time" to total exposure duration for a repetitively pulsed laser.

Electromagnetic Radiation—The propagation of varying electric and magnetic fields through space at the velocity of light.

Emergent Beam Diameter (a)—Diameter of the laser beam at the exit aperture of the system in centimeters (cm); for a Gaussian beam, the diameter at 1/e peak intensity values.

Enclosed Laser System—Any *laser* or *laser system* located within an enclosure which does not permit emission of hazardous optical radiation from the enclosure.

Energy (Q)—The capacity for doing work. *Energy* is commonly used to characterize the output from *pulsed lasers*, and it is generally measured in joules (J).

Extended Source—An *extended source* of radiation can be resolved into a geometrical image in contrast with a point source of radiation, which cannot be resolved into a geometrical image.

Gas Laser—A type of laser in which the laser action takes place in a gas medium, usually operated as a CW laser.

Hertz (Hz)—Unit of frequency, (i.e., "cycles per second").

Infrared Radiation—*Electromagnetic radiation* with *wavelengths* which lie within the range of 0.7 to 1000 μm. This region is often broken into three spectral banks by *wavelength*: IR-A (0.7–0.78 to 1.4 μm), IR-B (1.4 μm to 3 μm), and IR-C (3 μm to 1 mm).

Integrated Radiance (L_p)—Product of the exposure duration times the *radiance*. Also known as pulsed radiance (W s)(cm^{-2} sr^{-1}) = J(cm^{-2} sr^{-1}).

Intensity—*Radiant exposure* or *irradiance*.

Intrabeam Viewing—Viewing the laser source from within the beam. The beam may either be direct or specularly reflected.

Irradiance (E)—Power per unit area on a given surface, in units of watts per square centimeter (W cm^{-2}).

Joule (J)—A unit of energy (1 watt-second) used normally in describing a single pulsed output of a laser; it is equal to one watt-second or 0.239 calories.

Joule cm^{-2} (J cm^{-2})—A unit of *radiant exposure* used in measuring the amount of energy per unit area of absorbing surface or per unit area of a laser beam.

***Lambertian Surface*—**An ideal diffuse surface whose emitted or reflected *radiance* (brightness) is independent of the viewing angle.

***Laser*—**A source of intense, coherent, directional beam of optical radiation. Also, an acronym for *light amplification by stimulated emission of radiation.* A *laser* usually is composed of an energy source, a resonant cavity and active lasing medium.

***Laser Device*—**Either a laser or a laser system.

Laser Safety Danger Zone (LSDZ)—The ground area that requires control during laser operation. Unauthorized personnel are not permitted and laser eye protectors are required for personnel who may engage in intrabeam viewing within this area.

***Laser System*—**An assembly of electrical, mechanical, and optical components that includes a laser.

***Laser Controlled Area*—**Any area which contains one or more lasers and in which the activity of personnel is subject to control and supervision.

***Light*—**Visible radiation (400 nm to 700–780 nm).

Micrometer (μm)—Formerly termed "micron", a measure of length equal to 10^{-6} m.

Nanometer (nm)—Unit of length equal to 10^{-9} m.

***Nominal Ocular Hazard Distance (NOHD)*—**The *NOHD* is the distance from the operating laser at which the *radiant exposure* or *irradiance* within the beam equals the applicable exposure limit.

***Ocular Surveillance Examination*—**A professional eye evaluation performed by an ophthalmologist, optometrist, or physician skilled in funduscopy and biomicroscopy of the eye.

***Open Installation*—**Any location where lasers are used which will be open to operating personnel during laser operation and may or may not specifically restrict entry to casuals.

***Optical Density (OD)*—**A logarithmic expression for the *attenuation* produced by an attenuating medium, such as an eye protection filter.

$$OD = \log_{10} \phi_o/\phi_t$$

Where ϕ_o is the incident power and ϕ_t is the transmitted power at a specific *wavelength* (λ).

***Optically Pumped Lasers*—**A type of laser that derives energy from another optical radiation source such as a xenon flash lamp (coherent light sources have also been used).

***Output Power and Output Energy*—**The laser *output power* is used primarily to rate *CW lasers* since the *energy* delivered per unit time remains relatively constant (output measured in watts). In contrast, pulsed lasers deliver their energy impulses in pulses and their effects may best be categorized by energy output per pulse. [The power output level of *CW lasers* is usually expressed in milliwatts (mW = 1/1000 watts) or watts, *pulsed lasers* in the megawatt (MW = million watts) or gigawatt range (GW = billion watts]. Pulsed energy output is usually expressed in joules or millijoules (mJ = 1/100 J) per pulse.

***Point Source of Optical Radiation*—**Ideally, a source with infinitesimal dimensions. Practically, a source of radiation whose dimensions are small compared with the viewing distance.

Power (W) the time rate at which energy is transferred. Usually expressed in watts (joules per second); also termed *Radiant Flux.*

***PRF*—**Abbreviation for *pulse repetition frequency.*

***Pulse Duration*—**Duration of a *pulsed laser* flash; it may be measured in terms of milliseconds (ms = 10^{-3}s), microseconds (μs = 10^{-6}s), or nanoseconds (ns = 10^{-9}s). The time interval between the half peak power points on the leading and trailing edges of the pulse.

***Pulsed Laser*—**A laser that delivers its energy in short pulses, as distinct from a *CW laser.* For the purpose of this guide, a laser which emits for less than 0.25 second.

***Q-Switched Laser*—**Also known as *Q-spoiled*—is a laser capable of extremely high peak powers for very short durations (pulse length of several nanoseconds.).

***Quantum Mechanics*—**Branch of science dealing with atomic and subatomic particles.

***Q-switched Laser*—**A laser capable of extremely high peak powers for very short durations (pulse duration of several nanoseconds). A laser with a pulse width between 1 ns and 18 μs.

***Radian*—**A unit of angular measure equal to the angle subtended at the center of a circle by an arc whose length is equal to the radius of the circle.

One (1) Radian = 57.3 Degrees
Or 2π Radians = 360 Degrees

Radiance (L)—Radiant flux (*radiant power*) output per unit solid angle per unit area (W sr^{-1} cm^{-2}); radiometric brightness.

Radiant Energy (Q)—*Energy* in the form of electromagnetic waves usually expressed in units of joules (watt-seconds). Commonly used to describe the output of *pulsed lasers.*

Radiant Exposure (H)—The *energy* per unit area incident upon a given surface in a given time interval. It is used to express exposure dose to *pulsed laser* radiation and is commonly expressed in J cm^{-2}.

Radiant Intensity (I)—Radiant power in a given direction. Radiant flux emitted from the source per unit solid angle (steradian), in the direction of propagation, usually expressed in W sr^{-1}.

Radiant Power (ϕ)—The time rate of flow of radiant energy. Units of watts. Commonly used to describe the output of *CW lasers* or the average radiant output power of *repetitively pulsed lasers.*

Reflectance or Reflectivity (ρ)—The ratio of reflected radiant flux to incident radiant flux.

Repetitively Pulsed Laser—A *pulsed laser* with reoccurring pulsed output. The frequency of the pulses is termed *pulse repetition frequency* (*PRF*). *Repetitively pulsed lasers* have properties similar to *CW laser* if the *PRF* or duty cycle is very high.

Scintillation—In laser work, this term is frequently used to describe the effect upon a laser beam by atmospheric turbulence.

Scotoma—Loss of vision in part of the visual field; blind spot.

Semi-Conductor or Injection Diode Laser—A class of lasers that produces relatively low average power outputs.

Shall—Indicates a requirement that is necessary or essential to meet the currently accepted standards of protection or Federal rules and regulations.

Should—Indicates an advisory recommendation that is to be applied when practicable.

Solid Angle (Ω)—The ratio of the area on the surface of a sphere to the square of the radius of that sphere. It is expressed in steradians (sr).

Specular or Regular Reflection—A mirror-like reflection.

Steradian (sr)—The unit of measure for a solid angle. There are 4π steradians in a sphere.

Transmittance or transmissivity (τ)—The ratio of total transmitted *radiant power* to total incident *radiant power.*

Ultraviolet Radiation—*Electromagnetic radiation* with wavelengths between soft *x-rays* and visible, violet light. This region is often broken down into three spectral bands by wavelength: UV-A (315-400 nm), UV-B (280–315 nm), and UV-C (200–280 nm).

Visible Radiation (light)—*Electromagnetic radiation* which can be detected by the human eye. It is commonly used to describe wavelengths which lie in the range between 400 nm and 700–780 nm.

Vision Screening Examination—A battery of visual tests which may be accomplished by a trained technician. The testing is generally done with a stereoscopic type instrument for measuring visual acuity, phorias, stereopsis, and color perception.

Watt (W)—The unit of power, or radiant flux; one Joule per second. Used principally with *CW lasers.*

Watt $\boldsymbol{cm^{-2}}$ (W cm^{-2})—A unit of *irradiance* used in measuring the amount of power per area of absorbing surface, or per cross sectional area of a *CW laser* beam.

Wavelength (λ)—The distance between two points in a periodic wave which have the same phase is termed one wavelength. The velocity of light (3×10^{10} cm s^{-1}) divided by frequency (in Hz) equals *wavelength* (in cm).

References

Army Environmental Hygiene Agency. *Laser and Optical Hazards Course Manual*. Aberdeen Proving Ground, MD; 1985.

GLOSSARY—DEFINITIONS OF QUALITY ASSURANCE TERMS

Analyte is "the specific component measured in a chemical analysis; also called analate."

Audit/Appraisal is a planned and documented activity performed in accordance with procedures to determine, by examination and evaluation of objective evidence, the adequacy of and extent to which applicable elements of the quality assurance program have been developed, documented, and effectively implemented in accordance with specified requirements.[a]

Blank is "the measured value obtained when a specified component of a sample is not present during the measurement. In such a case, the measured value/signal for the component is believed to be due to artifacts, hence should be deducted from a measured value to give a net value due to the component contained in a sample. The blank measurement must be made so that the correction process is valid."[a]

Blind Sample is "a sample submitted for analysis whose composition is known to the submitter but unknown to the analyst. A blind sample thus is one way to test proficiency of a measurement process."[b]

Calibrant is "a substance used to calibrate or to establish the analytical response of a measurement system."

Calibration is the "comparison of a measurement standard or instrument with another standard or instrument to report or eliminate by adjustment any variation (deviation) in the accuracy of the item being compared."

Certified Reference Material (CRM) is "a reference material one or more of whose property values are certified by a technically valid procedure, accompanied by or traceable to a certificate or other documentation which is issued by a certifying body."

Certified Value is "the value that appears in a certificate as the best estimate of the value for a property of a reference material."

Check Standard is "in physical calibration, an artifact measured periodically, the results of which typically are plotted on a control chart to evaluate the measurement process."

Coefficient of Variation is "the standard deviation divided by the average value of the parameter measured."

Composite Sample is "a sample composed of two or more increments selected to represent a population of interest."

Control Chart is "a graphical plot of test results with respect to time or sequence of measurement together with limits within which they are expected to lie."

Control Limits are "the limits shown on a control chart beyond which it is highly improbable that a point could lie."

Control Sample is "a material of known composition that is analyzed concurrently with test samples to evaluate a measurement process (see also *check standard*)."

Double Blind refers to "a sample, known by the submitter but submitted to an analyst in such a way that neither its composition nor its identification as a check sample are known to the latter."[b]

Duplicate Measurement is "a second measurement made on the same (or identical) sample of material to assist in the evaluation of measurement variance."

Duplicate Sample is "a second sample randomly selected from a population of interest (see also split sample) to assist in the evaluation of sample variance."

Error—the difference between the true value and the measured value of a quantity or parameter.

Increment is "an individual portion of material collected by a single operation of a sampling device, from parts of a lot separated in time or space. Increments may be either tested individually or combined (composited) and tested as a unit."

Intercalibration is "the process, procedures, and activities used to ensure that the several laboratories engaged in a monitoring program can produce compatible data. When compatible data outputs are achieved and this situation is maintained, the laboratories can be said to be intercalibrated."

Limiting Mean is "the value approached by the average as the number of measurements, made by a stable measurement process, increases indefinitely."

Method is "an assemblage of measurement techniques and the order in which they are used."

Outlier is "a value which appears to deviate markedly from other members of the sample in which it occurs."

Primary Standard is "a substance or artifact, the value of which can be accepted (within specific limits) without question when used to establish the value of the same or related property of another material."

---

[a] This definition of "blank" is applicable to certain uses in quality assurance, but this term is also commonly used with other, somewhat different meanings.

[b] These definitions of "blind sample" and "double blind" are applicable to certain uses in quality assurance, but these terms are also commonly used with other, somewhat different meanings.

Procedure is "a set of systematic instructions for using a method of measurement or of sampling or of the steps or operations associated with such."

Protocol is "a procedure specified to be used when performing a measurement or related operation, as a condition to obtain results that could be acceptable to the specifier."

Quality Assurance involves all those planned and systematic actions necessary to provide adequate confidence that a facility, structure, system, or component will perform satisfactorily and safely in service.[c]

Quality Control, which is included within Quality Assurance, comprises all those actions necessary to control and verify the features and characteristics of a material, process, product, or service to specified requirements.[c]

Random Errors—errors that vary in a nonreproducible way around the limiting mean. These errors can be treated statistically by use of the laws of probability.

Reference Material (RM) is "a material or substance one or more properties of which are sufficiently well established to be used for the calibration of an apparatus, the assessment of a measurement method, or for the assignment of values to materials."

Reference Method is "a method which has been specified as capable, by virtue of recognized accuracy, of providing primary reference data."

Relative Standard Deviation is "the coefficient of variation, expressed as a percentage."

Repeatability of Measurement "The closeness of the agreement between the results of successive measurements of the same quantity carried out by the same method, by the same observer, with the same measuring instruments, in the same laboratory, at quite short intervals of time."[c]

Replicate is "a counterpart of another, usually referring to an analytical sample or a measurement. It is the general case for which duplicate is the special case consisting of two samples or measurement."

Reproducibility of Measurements "The closeness of the agreement between the results of measurements of the same quality, where the individual measurements are made:

- by different methods, with different measuring instruments,
- by different observers, in different laboratories,
- after intervals of time that are quite long compared with the duration of a single measurement, and
- under different normal conditions of use of the instruments employed."

"The term reproducibility is also used when some of the factors listed above are different in the individual measurements; these factors should be specified in detail in each particular case."[c]

Sample is "a portion of a population or lot. It may consist of an individual or groups of individuals. It may refer to objects, materials, or to measurement, conceivable as part of a larger group that could have been considered."

Split Sample is "a replicate portion or sub-sample of a total sample obtained in such a manner that it is not believed to differ significantly from other portions of the same sample."

Standard is "a substance or material, the properties of which are believed to be known with sufficient accuracy to permit its use to evaluate the same property of another. In chemical measurements, it often describes a solution or substance, commonly prepared by the analyst, to establish a calibration curve or the analytical response function of an instrument."

Standard Method is "a method (or procedure) of test developed by a standards-writing organization, based on consensus opinion or other criteria, and often evaluated for its reliability by a collaborative testing procedure."

Standard Reference Material is "a reference material distributed and certified by the National Institute of Standards and Technology."

Standardization, in analytical chemistry, is "the assignment of a compositional value to one standard on the basis of another standard."

Systematic Errors—Errors that are reproducible and tend to bias a result in one direction. Their causes can be assigned, at least in principle, and they can have both constant and variable components. Generally these errors cannot be treated statistically.

Technique is "a physical or chemical principle utilized separately or in combination with other techniques to determine the composition (analysis) of materials."

Traceability is "the ability to trace the source of uncertainty of a measurement or a measured value."

Uncertainty—the range of values within which the true value is estimated to lie. It is a best estimate of possible inaccuracy due to both random and systematic errors.

Validation is "the process by which a sample, measurement method, or a piece of data is deemed to be useful for a specific purpose."

Warning Limits are "the limits shown on a control chart within which most of the test results are expected to lie (within a 95% probability) while the system is in a state of statistical control."

---

[c] Defined by the International Organization of Legal Metrology (IOLM, 1976).

References

Department of Energy. *Quality Assurance.* DOE Order DOE 5700.6B; Washington, DC; September 1986.

Environmental Monitoring Laboratory (EML). *Procedures Manual.* HASL-300, 27th Edition, Vol. 1; U.S. DOE; New York, NY; 1990.

International Organization of Legal Metrology (IOLM). *Vocabulary of Legal Terms.* Paris; 1976.

Taylor, J.K. *Handbook for SRM Users*, National Bureau of Standards Special Publication 260-100; Gaithersburg, MD; September 1985.

Energy Density, Dissipated—The electromagnetic energy that is converted to other forms of energy, such as heat, in an infinitesimal volume of a medium divided by that volume. This energy is not directly recoverable in the form of electromagnetic energy. *Dissipated energy density* is expressed in units of joule per cubic meter (J/m^3).

Energy Density, Stored—The energy stored in the electromagnetic fields in an infinitesimal volume of a medium divided by that volume. This energy is recoverable in the form of electromagnetic energy. *Stored energy density* is expressed in units of joule per cubic meter (J/m^3).

Energy Flux Density—The rate of energy transport into a small sphere divided by the cross-sectional area of that sphere. *Energy flux density* is expressed in units of watt per square meter (W/m^2). For ionizing radiation, this quantity is now called the energy fluence rate.

Far Field Region—The region of an antenna in which the field per unit solid angle is constant. In this region the field has a predominantly plane-wave character, i.e., locally very uniform distributions of electric field strength and magnetic field strength in planes transverse to the direction of propagation. For large antennas especially, the far field region is also referred to as the *Fraunhofer region.*

Fraunhofer Region—See *far field region.*

Free Space—An ideal, perfectly homogeneous medium having a *relative permittivity* and *permeability* of unity and in which there is nothing to reflect, refract, or absorb energy, i.e., a perfect vacuum.

Fresnel Region—The radiating *near field region* of a large antenna. The *Fresnel region* usually is taken to exclude the *reactive near field region* immediately adjacent to the antenna where much of the stored energy associated with the field of an antenna is located. See also *antenna, field regions of, reactive near field region,* and *radiating near field region.*

Impedance, Characteristic—The ratio of voltage to current at a point along a uniform section of a two or more conductor transmission line that is free of standing wave components, i.e., for a wave traveling in one direction. *Characteristic impedance* is expressed in units of ohm (Ω).

Impedance, Intrinsic—The *wave impedance* for a plane wave in an unbounded medium. Its value depends only on the properties of the medium. *Intrinsic impedance* is expressed in units of ohm (Ω).

Impedance, Wave—The ratio of the *electric field strength* to the corresponding *magnetic field strength* of a propagating wave at a point. For a plane wave, the *wave impedance* is the same as the *intrinsic impedance.* In a waveguide, there is a wave impedance associated with each mode of propagation supported by the structure. *Wave impedance* is expressed in units of ohm (Ω).

Incident Wave—See *wave, incident.*

Ionizing Radiation—Radiation having a sufficiently large photon energy to directly ionize atomic or molecular systems with a single quantum event. It is to be distinguished from non-ionizing radiation that may lead to the ionization of these systems through multiple quantum events.

Intrinsic Impedance—See *impedance, intrinsic.*

Irradiance—The energy flux density of an electromagnetic wave incident upon the surface. *Irradiance* is expressed in units of watt per square meter (W/m^2).

Isotropic—Having the same properties in all directions.

Isotropic Antenna—A hypothetical antenna radiating or receiving equally in all directions, representing a convenient reference for expressing directional properties of actual antennas.

Lobe (Antenna)—A portion of the radiation pattern between adjacent minima.

Loss Tangent—The ratio of the imaginary part of the complex *relative permittivity* of a medium to its real part.

Magnetic Dipole—A current flowing in an infinitesimally small loop. When the current is oscillating, the dipole becomes an elementary radiating *magnetic dipole.*

Magnetic Dipole Moment—A vector, the magnitude of which is equal to the product of the current flowing in a loop and the area of the current loop, and whose direction is perpendicular to the plane of the loop and obeys the righthand rule. *Magnetic dipole moment* is expressed in units of ampere square meter ($A\ m^2$).

Magnetic Field Strength—A field vector, H, that is equal to the product of the *magnetic flux density* and the reciprocal of the *permeability. Magnetic field strength* is expressed in units of ampere per meter (A/m).

Magnetic Flux Density—A vector field quantity, B, that results in a force, F, that acts on a moving charge or charges. When B is vector-multiplied by velocity, v, at which an infinitesimal unit test charge, q, is moving, the result is the force which acts on the test charge divided by q.

$$\frac{F}{q} = (v \times B)$$

Magnetic flux density is expressed in units of tesla (T), formerly weber per square meter (Wb/M^2).

Magnetic Susceptibility—The ratio of the *magnetization* at a point in a medium to the *magnetic field strength* at that point.

Magnetization (Magnetic Polarization)—The difference between the *magnetic flux density* in a medium and the *magnetic flux density* in a vacuum for the same *magnetic field strength*, all divided by the *permeability* of vacuum. *Magnetization* is expressed in units of ampere per meter (A/m).

Mode (Cavity or Transmission Line)—An electromagnetic field pattern within a cavity or transmission line that is determined by the geometrical configuration of the structure and the wavelength of the *electromagnetic wave* within the structure.

Near Field Region—A region in the field of an *antenna*, located near the *antenna*, in which the electric and magnetic fields do not have a substantially plane-wave character, but vary considerably from point to point. The term *near field region* is only vaguely defined and has different meanings for large and small *antennas*. The *near field region* is further subdivided into the *reactive near field region*, which is closest to the *antenna* and contains most or nearly all of the stored energy associated with the field of the *antenna*, and the *radiating near field region*. See also: *antenna, field region of, reactive near field, ''Fresnel region*, and *far field region.*

Non-Thermal Effect—A change in a medium or system that is not directly associated with heat production when electromagnetic energy is absorbed.

Permeability—The ratio of the *magnetic flux density* to the *magnetic field strength* at a point. *Permeability* is expressed in units of henry per meter (H/m).

Permeability, Relative—The ratio of the *permeability* of a medium at a point to that of vacuum.

Permittivity—The ratio of the *electric flux density* to the *electric field strength* at a point. *Permittivity* is expressed in units of farad per meter (F/m).

Permittivity, Relative—The ratio of the permittivity of a medium at a point to that of vacuum.

Phase Coefficient (phase constant) (see *propagation coefficient*)—The imaginary part (β) of the *propagation coefficient* that describes the change of phase of a field component with distance in the direction of propagation. The *phase coefficient* is expressed in units of radian per meter (rad/m) or degree per meter.

Phasor—A spatially dependent complex scalar or vector field parameter. A *phasor* is commonly used to represent *electromagnetic fields* under single frequency, steady state conditions. Phasor notation greatly facilitates mathematical manipulation in field problems and in the graphical representation of field quantities.

Plane Wave—See *wave, plane.*

Polarization, Electric—See *electric polarization.*

Polarization (Electromagnetic Wave)—The directional and time characteristics of the electric field vector associated with a propagating wave.

Polarization, Magnetic—See *magnetization.*

Polarization, Plane of—The plane containing the electric field of a propagating wave.

Power—The rate of change of energy with time. Typically used to describe the rate of energy flow across a surface or the rate of change of energy from one form to another. Power is expressed in units of watt (W).

Power Density—See *energy flux density* and *Poynting vector.*

Power Density, Plane Wave Equivalent—A quantity that is associated with any *electromagnetic wave* that is equal in magnitude to the *power density* of a *plane wave* that has the same *electric* (E) or *magnetic* (H) *field strength.*

$$S = E^2/120\pi = 120\pi H^2 \ (W/m^2)$$

Power Gain (antenna)—The ratio of the power per unit solid angle radiated in a given direction and at a given frequency to the power per unit solid angle radiated by a hypothetical isotropic, lossless radiator for the same input power to both *antennas. Power gain* is a function of direction, frequency, distance, and polarization. When ''gain'' is used without qualifications, the maximum value of *power gain* is usually implied, i.e., the asymptotic value approached with increasing distance in the direction of maximum power per unit solid angle.

Poynting Vector—A field vector quantity, $\mathbf{S}$, equal to the vector product of the electric field strength, $\mathbf{E}$, and the *magnetic field strength*, $\mathbf{H}$, that represents the magnitude and the direction of the electromagnetic energy flux density.

$$S = E \times H$$

When applied to a propagating wave, the integral of S over any surface represents the instantaneous power transmitted through the surface. S is in the direction of propagation. The *Poynting vector* is expressed in units of watt per square meter (W/m^2).

Propagation Coefficient (propagation constant) (See *attenuation coefficient, phase coefficient*)—A complex quantity, the real part of which (*attenuation coefficient*) describes the change in magnitude and the imaginary part of which (*phase coefficient*) describes the change in phase with distance of a field component in the direction of propagation of an electromagnetic wave.

Radiating Near-Field Region—The region in the field of an *antenna* where the *radiation field* (see definition) predominates over the reactive field but lacks substantial plane-wave character and is complicated in structure. The term *radiating near-field region* generally is associated with large antennas where the largest dimension of the antenna is very much greater than the free space wavelength. The *radiating near field region* lies between the *reactive near field region* and the *far-field region*. Also see *antenna, field regions of, near-field region*, and *radiation field.*

Radiation Field—Collectively, the components of the total electromagnetic field produced by an *antenna* that include, only and all, the energy propagated away from the *antenna*. The *radiation field* is not in the category of a "field region" of an *antenna* in that it is understood to exclude the fields that contain reactive energy (energy that enters the space but returns to the *antenna*), although such reactive fields coexist with *radiation fields* at the same locations. In most of the *radiation field* both E and H vary inversely with distance from the *antenna*. Also see *antenna, field regions of* and *radiation near field region.*

Radiation Pattern—The angular distribution of the radiating portion of the electromagnetic fields in the vicinity of an *antenna.* The *radiation pattern* may refer to such quantities as power per unit solid angle, *electric* or *magnetic field strengths*, polarization or phase.

Reactive Near-Field Region—The region in the field of an *antenna* in which reactive fields are significant, i.e., in which most of the stored electromagnetic energy associated with the *antenna* is located. In the reactive near-field region, E and H may vary rapidly from point to point. This region starts immediately at the *antenna* and extends from it for only a short distance, less than or equal to the free space wavelength. The fields can be inductive or capacitive in nature and relate to the inductance or capacitance of the *antenna* itself. Inductive and capacitive fields can coexist near one *antenna*; in some instances one of them can predominate strongly over the other. In the course of a cycle, a portion of this energy is not propagated beyond the near field, but is interchanged periodically between the *antenna* and the near field and, hence, is considered to be stored energy. Also see *antennas, field regions of, "near-field region, Fresnel region*, and *radiating near-field region.*

Reflected Wave—See *wave, reflected.*

Reflection Coefficient—The ratio of the electric or magnetic field strength phasors associated with the reflected wave to that associated with the incident wave.

Refracted Wave—See *wave, transmitted.*

Relative Permeability—See *permeability, relative.*

Relative Permittivity—See *permittivity, relative.*

Relaxation Spectrum—The variation of *relative permittivity* with angular frequency, uniquely described by a monotonic decrease of the real component with increasing angular frequency, the maximum slope occurring when the product of angular frequency and the relaxation time is unity, and characterized by a maximum in the imaginary component at the same angular frequency where the slope of the real component is maximum.

Relaxation Time—The time, after a static electric field has been applied to a dielectric, required for the *electric polarization* to reach (e—1)/e of the steady state value. For a dielectric that exhibits a *relaxation spectrum*, the average *relaxation time* is equal to the reciprocal of the angular frequency for which the imaginary part of the *relative permittivity* is a maximum. The *relaxation time* is expressed in units of second(s).

Resonance Spectrum—The variation of *relative permittivity* with angular frequency uniquely described by a dispersion of the real part around a resonant angular frequency characteristic of the system and a maximum in the imaginary component in the same frequency region. The dispersion of the real part exhibits a maximum below the resonant angular frequency and a minimum above it. In the limit of maximal damping, a *resonance spectrum* approaches a *relaxation spectrum* and the frequency dependence of the real part becomes monotonic.

Scattering—The process that causes waves incident on discontinuities or boundaries in media to be changed in direction, frequency, phase or polarization.

Solar Constant—The mean value of the total solar *irradiance* at normal incidence outside the atmosphere of the earth at the mean solar distance (W/m^2).

Specific Absorption (SA)—The quotient of the incremental energy (dW) absorbed by (dissipated in) an incremental mass (dm) contained in a volume element (dV) of a given density (ρ).

$$SA = \frac{dW}{dm} = \frac{dW}{\pi dV}$$

The *specific absorption* is expressed in units of joule per kilogram (J/kg).

Specific Absorption Rate (SAR)—The time derivative of the incremental energy (dW) absorbed by (dissipated in) an incremental mass (dm) contained in a volume element (dV) of a given density (π).

$$SAR = \frac{d}{dt}\left(\frac{dW}{dm}\right) = \frac{d}{dt}\left(\frac{dW}{\rho dV}\right)$$

The *specific absorption* rate is expressed in units of watt per kilogram (W/kg). In view of the proliferation of terms for describing the *electromagnetic radiation* conditions in biological materials and the discipline-oriented interpretation of these terms, it is recommended that the name *specific absorption rate* be used for the quantity defined here, rather than such names as ''absorbed power density per unit mass.''

Spectral Irradiance—*Irradiance* per unit wavelength interval. *Spectral irradiance* is expressed in units of watt per square meter meter (W/m^2m).

Spherical Wave—See *wave, spherical.*

Standing Wave—The field pattern generated by two equal-amplitude propagating waves traveling in opposite directions. A *standing wave* pattern is characterized by spatial points or planes of maximum field amplitude and other spatial points or planes of zero field amplitude displaced along the direction of propagation.

Standing Wave Ratio—The ratio of maximum field strength along the direction of propagation of two waves travelling in opposite directions.

Survey Instrument—A portable device used for measuring a field component.

Thermal Effect—A change in a medium or system that is directly associated with heat production when electromagnetic energy is absorbed.

Thermogram—A spatial representation of the temperature distribution within a medium.

Transmission Coefficient—The ratio of the electric or magnetic field strength phasors associated with a transmitted wave to that associated with an incident wave.

Transmission Line—A physical structure for guiding electromagnetic energy. Common examples are: wire pairs, coaxial lines, strip lines, and waveguides.

Wave, Electromagnetic—A wave characterized by variations of electric and magnetic fields.

Wave, Incident—A wave, traveling through a medium in a specified direction, directed toward a reference point, toward a discontinuity in the medium, or toward a medium of different propagation characteristics.

Wave, Impedance—See *impedance, wave.*

Wave, Plane—A wave with parallel planar surfaces of constant phase.

Wave, Reflected—A wave in a medium produced by a wave in that medium incident on a discontinuity in the medium or on a boundary of a different medium, excluding the incident wave.

Wave, Spherical—A wave with concentric spherical surfaces of constant phase.

Wave, Standing—See *standing wave.*

Wave, Transmitted (refracted wave)—A wave produced by an incident wave that continues beyond a discontinuity in a medium or beyond a boundary between two different media.

Wave, Transverse Electric (TE)—An *electromagnetic wave* in which the *electric field strength* is everywhere perpendicular to the direction of propagation.

Wave, Transverse Electromagnetic (TEM)—An *electromagnetic wave* in which the *electric field strength* is everywhere perpendicular to the *magnetic field strength* and both lie in a plane perpendicular to the direction of propagation.

Wave, Transverse Magnetic (TM)—An *electromagnetic wave* in which the *magnetic field strength* is everywhere perpendicular to the direction of propagation.

Waveguide—An enclosed system capable of guiding *electromagnetic waves* from one place to another. Usually it consists of a hollow metallic tube or a solid dielectric material.

References

National Council on Radiation Protection and Measurements. *Radiofrequency Electromagnetic Fields: Properties, Quantities and Units, Biophysical Interaction, and Measurements*. NCRP Report No. 67; Washington, DC 20014; 1981.

GLOSSARY—ULTRASOUND

A-Mode (Amplitude-Mode)—A method of *echo signal* display in which time is represented along the horizontal axis and *echo amplitude* is displayed along the vertical axis.

AB-Mode (Amplitude Brightness-Mode)—A method of data presentation on the oscilloscope screen in which one coordinate represents time (depth) and the *amplitude* of the echo signal is displayed as both a deflection along the other coordinate and as a brightening of the display spot.

Absolute Maximum—Means the largest possible value of a specified quantity either for an individual instrument or for all instruments of a given generic type. This value shall include effects of inaccuracies and imprecision of the measurement process(es) used to determine it.

Absolute Minimum—Means the smallest possible value of a specified quantity either for an individual instrument or for all instruments of a given generic type. This value shall include effects of inaccuracies and imprecision of the measurement process(es) used to determine it.

Absorbed Dose—The thermal energy imparted to matter by *absorption* of *acoustic* radiation per unit mass (or per unit volume) or irradiated material at the site of interest.

Absorption—The process by which *acoustic* radiation imparts energy locally to the medium through which it propagates, by conversion of *acoustic energy* to heat. *Absorption* contributes to *attenuation.*

Acoustic, Acoustical—The qualifying adjectives ''acoustic'' and ''acoustical'' mean containing, producing, arising from, actuated by, related to, or associated with *sound. Acoustic* is used when the term being qualified designates something that has the properties, dimensions, or physical characteristics associated with sound waves; *acoustical* is used when the term being qualified does not designate explicitly something that has such properties, dimensions, or physical characteristics.

Note 1: The following examples qualify as having the properties or physical characteristics associated with sound waves and hence would take *acoustic: impedance*, output (sound power), energy wave, medium, *signal, transducer.*

Note 2: The following examples do not have the requisite physical characteristics and therefore take *acoustical*: method, engineer, symbol, problem, measurement.

Note 3: As illustrated in the preceding notes, usually the generic term is modified by *acoustical*, whereas the specific technical implication calls for *acoustic.*

Acoustic Attenuation—*Amplitude* reduction of the *acoustic signal* as a function of time or of propagation includes the effects of *absorption, scattering, reflection, refraction* and *diffraction.*

Acoustic Energy—Mechanical energy transported by an *acoustic wave*. The units are those of *acoustic power* times time, the joule (J) (Watt-second) in standard international units.

Acoustic Field—A distribution (in space and time) of *acoustic energy.*

Acoustic Holography—See *Holography.*

Acoustic Impedance—A vector quantity formed by taking the ratio of the instantaneous *acoustic pressure* at a surface to the instantaneous volume velocity at the surface in an *acoustic field.* (See also *specific acoustic impedance, characteristic acoustic impedance.*)

Acoustic Impedance Match (Colloquial)—The condition of equal *characteristic* of *acoustic impedance* of contiguous media, avoiding *reflection* of *acoustic energy* at the *interface*. (See *Impedance Ratio.*)

Acoustic Impedance Mismatch—A condition of unequal *characteristic acoustic impedances* of contiguous media, causing *reflection* of acoustic energy at the *interface*. (See *Impedance Ratio.*)

Acoustic Intensity—See *Intensity.*

Acoustic Lens—A refractive element employed to redirect *acoustic* wavelets or rays in order to increase or decrease *acoustic energy* density in a prescribed volume or to modify phase coherence at a receiving *transducer.*

Acoustic Power—*Acoustic energy* transported per unit time (usually a temporal average is quoted) (1 joule per second). (See *Average Acoustic Power.*)

Acoustic Pressure—The instantaneous value of the total pressure minus the ambient pressure.

Acoustics—The science of sound, including its production, transmission and effects.

Acoustic Shadow—A manifestation of reduced *acoustic signal amplitude* in or returning from regions lying beyond an attenuating object. It is important to distinguish between acoustic shadows and regions of low reflectivity.

Acoustic Streaming—An acoustically generated time-independent transport of fluid within the body of the sonified fluid or tissue.

Acoustic Wave—A mechanical disturbance which propagates through a continuous medium.

Acoustic Waveform—See *Waveform.*

Acoustic Wavefront—The surface of equal phase in a propagating *wave.*

Acoustic Wavelength—The distance between any two adjacent points at which the phase, at the same instant, differs by 2π; it corresponds to the distance travelled by the *wave* during one cycle; $\lambda = c/f$, where λ is the wavelength, c is the speed of sound, and f is the *frequency*. For water or tissue at 1 MHz, the wavelength is approximately 1.5 mm.

Amplitude—The magnitude of the envelope of a first order electrical or *acoustic waveform* (e.g., voltage or *acoustic pressure* in linear acoustics).

Amplitude Modulated Waveform—A *waveform* in which the carrier *wave* is modified in *amplitude* by a *signal* wave as a means of transmitting information. For measurement purposes the AIUM-NEMA standard defines it as a waveform in which the *amplitude modulation factor* is greater than 5%.

Amplitude Modulation Factor—The value of the expression $100 \times (|A|—|B|)/|A|$, expressed as a percentage, where $|A|$ and $|B|$ are the absolute maximum and minimum amplitudes of the envelope of a modulated *acoustical* or electrical carrier (first order quantity), respectively.

Angle of Incidence—The angle between the axis of an acoustic beam encountering an interface, and the vector normal (perpendicular) to the interface.

Attenuation—See *Acoustic Attenuation.*

Attenuation Coefficient—The relative change in the *acoustic wave amplitude* per unit path length in a medium. Commonly employed units are dB/cm, and Neper/cm.

Attenuator—A device which reduces the *signal* by a specified amount, e.g., 10 dB steps.

Average Acoustic Power—The power output from an *acoustic transducer* averaged over a period of time which is either long compared to, or exactly equal to, the period of pulses or variations in power.

Average Intensity—See *Intensity.*

Axial Resolution—The minimum separation of reflectors, required along the direction of sound *travel*, such that each can be separately distinguished on the display. (Same as *Depth Resolution, Longitudinal Resolution*, and *Range Resolution.*)

Azimuthal Resolution—The minimum angular separation between adjacent reflectors at the same *range* such that each can be separately distinguished in the display. The resolution is limited by the *beamwidth* of the *transducer* at that range of the targets. (See *Lateral Resolution.*)

B-Mode (Brightness-Mode)—A method of display on an oscilloscope screen in which the *intensity* of the *echo* is represented by modulation of the brightness of the spot and in which the position of the echo, displayed in the x-y plane, is determined from the position of the *transducer* and the transit time of the acoustic pulse.

B-Scan—A misnomer for a *B-mode scan* or image; scanning with *B-mode* display.

Backscattered Energy—The portion of the incident *acoustic energy* reflected from a small (compared to the *wavelength*) target back toward the reflector source; to be distinguished from *specular reflection* where the reflector dimension may be large compared to a wavelength.

Bandwidth—The transmitted *bandwidth* is the difference in the frequencies, F_1 and F_2, at which the magnitude in the acoustic pressure spectrum is 71% (−3 dB) of its maximum value. The pulse–echo bandwidth is the difference in frequencies, F_1 and F_2, at which the magnitude of the pulse–echo response from a planar reflector at a specified range is 50% (−6 db) of its maximum value. (AIUM Standard for Testing Single Element Pulse-Echo Ultrasonic Transducers. American Institute of Ultrasound in Medicine, 6161 N. May Ave., Suite 45W, Oklahoma City, OK 73112.)

Beam—The directed *acoustic field* produced by a *transducer.*

Beam Axis—A straight line joining the points of maximum *sound pressure amplitude*, at increasing distances from the source in the *far field*, and extending back to the *transducer assembly* surface. In pulse-echo situations, the above points of maximum spatial pressure amplitude are replaced by the points of maximum pulse–echo response from a specified reflector.

Beam Cross-Sectional Area—The area of that portion of a surface, in a plane perpendicular to the *beam axis*, that is bounded by that contour of the pulse–echo *amplitude* from a specified point or line reflector which is 25% (−12 dB) of the maximum *transducer signal* in that plane. Transmitted beam cross-sectional area is the area on the surface of a plane perpendicular to the *beam axis* consisting of all points where the *acoustic pressure* is greater than 50% of the maximum acoustic pressure in that plane.

Beam Cross-Sectional Profile—The *sound pressure amplitude* distribution along a line perpendicular to the beam axis. (See also *Pulse–Echo Response Profile.*)

Beam Divergence—The full angle of *beam* spread in a particular plane through the *beam axis*. The orientation of the plane must be specified.

Beam Pattern—The directional response pattern of a *transducer* used for *sound* emission and/or reception is a description, often presented graphically, of the response of the transducer as a function of the direction of the transmitted or incident sound waves in a specified plane and at a specified *frequency.* A complete description of the *beam pattern* of a transducer would require three-dimensional presentation. The beam pattern is often shown as the response relative to the maximum response. (USA Standard S1.1-1971 (R-196) ''Acoustical Terminology'' published by American National Standards Institute, 1430 Broadway, New York, NY 10018.)

Beam Uniformity Ratio—The ratio of the *Spatial Peak–Temporal Average Intensity* (SPTA) to the *Spatial Average–Temporal Average Intensity* (SATA) where both quantities are measured in a plane perpendicular to the beam axis. (See *Spatial Average.*)

Beam Width (Transmission)—The transverse distance between points on a specified *beam cross-sectional profile* where the *acoustic pressure* is a specified fraction of the maximum acoustic pressure on the profile. This may also be expressed as the angle formed between lines from the location of these two points to the point of intersection of the *beam axis* and the surface of the *transducer assembly.*

C-Mode (Constant Range-Mode)—A method of display of cross-sectional echo data in which the plane imaged is at a constant range from the *transducer* and is perpendicular to the interrogating beam.

Cathode Ray Tube (CRT)—An electron beam tube designed for two-dimensional display of signals as a function of their coordinates in space, time, or both. It consists of an electron source (gun), a means for deflecting the electronic beam in the x and y directions, and a phosphorous screen upon which the position of the electron beam is visible. The brightness of the display can be modulated by varying the current to the electron source, or the voltage on the grid of the CRT.

Cavitation (Acoustically-Induced)—A phenomenon produced by *sound* in liquid or liquid-like media involving bubbles or cavities containing gas or vapor.

Center Frequency—The frequency by $(F_1 + F_2)/2$, where F_1 and F_2 are the frequencies used in defining *bandwidth.* Generally, the frequency at which the *amplitude* spectrum is a maximum.

Centroid of a Surface—The point whose coordinates are the mean value of the coordinates of the surface.

Characteristic Acoustic Impedance—The *specific acoustic impedance* for plane waves in a lossless medium equal to the produce (pc) of the undisturbed density (p) and the speed of sound (c) of the medium.

Compressional Wave—A *wave* motion which is characterized by changes of density in the medium. (See *Longitudinal Wave* as an example.

Contact Coupling—*Acoustical* coupling of a *transducer* by direct contact with the skin, using liquid or gel to exclude air from the space between the *transducer* and skin.

Continuous Wave (c.w.) Ultrasound—A *wave* of (almost) constant *amplitude* which persists for a large number of cycles. (AIUM-NEMA Safety Standard for Diagnostic Ultrasound Equipment National Electronic Manufacturers Association, 2101 L Street NW, Washington, DC 20037.)

Coupling Methods—The method by which *ultrasound* is transmitted from a transducer to the subject and vice versa. These methods include: (1) *Contact Coupling*, (2) *Immersion Coupling*, and (3) *Liquid Coupling.*

Crystal—A colloquial term for the piezoelectric element of the *transducer.* Most piezoelectric elements are made of polycrystalline materials.

D-Mode—A display method in which only moving targets are displayed through their *Doppler frequency shifts.* If a scan is made it is referred to as scanned D-mode imaging.

Damping—Any mechanism which removes mechanical or electrical energy from the *transducer.* This can include internal absorption in the transducer as well as electrical or mechanical loading of a transducer to produce a more rapid decrease in the trailing edge of the *transmitted acoustic pulse* and the received echoes. Damping is used to improve *axial resolution.*

Dead Time—The time interval between the start of the *transmitter complex* and the arrival of the first identifiable *echo.* The dead time is determined primarily by a characteristic of the receiving amplifier and may be controlled by minimizing the *amplitude* of the *transmitter pulse* reaching the amplifier and adjusting the recovery time of the amplifier.

Decibel—A unit used for expressing the ratio of two like quantities, such as electrical *signal* amplitudes or *sound* energies. The decibel unit is only a relative measurement of the intensity of signals or sound energy levels and does not specify any definite voltage, *power* or *intensity*, unless one of several conventional reference levels is used and stated. The equations for expressing the decibel are as follows: $n(dB) = 20 \log_{10}(P_1/P_2)$; $n(dB) = 10 \log_{10}(W_1/W_2)$; $n(dB) = 20 \log_{10}(V_1/V_2)$; $n(dB) = 10 \log_{10}(I_1/I_2)$; where n is the number of decibels, P_1 and P_2 designate two ultrasonic pressure levels, W_1 and W_2 designate two power levels, V_1 and V_2 designate two voltage levels, and I_1 and I_2 designate two intensity levels.

Delivered Acoustic Energy—The product of *acoustic power* and *exposure time* at the prescribed site.

Delivered Acoustic Pulse Energy—See *Energy Per Pulse.*

Depth—The distance along the *sound* path from the point of entry into the patient or other object being examined to the point of interest. Distance along the time axis of the display is assumed to correspond proportionally to depth in the tissue.

Depth of Focus—The distance along the *beam axis*, for a focusing *transducer assembly*, from the point where the *beam cross-sectional area* first becomes equal to four times the *focal area* to the point beyond the *focal surface* where the beam cross-sectional area again becomes equal to four times the focal area. Specify whether the depth of focus is measured in one way or round trip (pulse-echo) conditions. (See also *Focal Zone.*)

Diffraction—A redistribution in space of the *intensity* of waves that results from the presence of inhomogeneities causing variations of the *amplitude* and/or phase of the waves. Thus, the ultrasonic field which appears in and near the geometric shadow of an obstacle typically has a complex spatial distribution which is explained by diffraction.

Directivity Pattern—A *beam pattern* expressed in polar coordinates.

Dispersion—The dependence of propagation speed upon *frequency*. Dispersion is responsible, to a small extent, for the changes in shape of a *pulse waveform* as it propagates.

Display Format—The manner in which information is presented to the diagnostician, e.g., *A-mode, B-mode, C-mode*, etc.

Displayed Beam Width—The length of the displayed image of a point target, measured normal to the direction of the axis of propagation. See also *Beam Cross-Sectional Area* and *Pulse Echo Response Profile*.

Doppler Effect—A shift in observed *frequency* (and *wave-length*), caused by relative motions among sources, receivers, and the propagation medium when there is a component of relative motion parallel to the *beam axis*.

Doppler Frequency Shift—The difference between the frequencies of transmitted and received waves, being proportional to the speed of relative motion between the *transducer*(s) and the target (reflector(s)).

Doppler Ultrasound—Application of the *Doppler Effect* in *ultrasound* to detect movement of a reflecting boundary relative to the source from a change of the *frequency* of the reflected *wave*.

Doppler Velocity Signal—A *signal* whose instantaneous voltage corrected for the angle between the beams, is proportional to the instantaneous *Doppler frequency shift*, derived by a frequency-to-voltage conversion of the Doppler signal.

Dosimetry—The quantitative determination of spatial and temporal field distributions in media of interest (usually tissues).

Duty Factor—The product of the *pulse duration* and the *pulse repetition rate*.

Dynamic Imaging—Imaging of an object in motion, a technique which is frequently referred to as imaging at a *real time rate*.

Echo—Acoustic signal received from *scattering* elements or a specular reflector.

Echo Ranging—A technique for measuring distances in materials of known *acoustic* velocity by measuring the transit time for the sound to propagate from the *transducer* to the target and return. Echo ranging techniques, in particular pulse-echo ultrasound, form the basis for most of the ultrasonic visualization systems.

Echo (Signal) Shaping—Image modification in which the *echo waveform* is changed using techniques such as *limiting* and *differentiation*.

Echo Strength—See *Magnitude of Echoes*.

Energizing Pulse (Transmitter Pulse)—An electrical pulse used to excite (or ''shock'') an ultrasonic *transducer*. Frequently, the pulse is a ''spike'' whose *rise time* is short compared to the natural period for the fundamental resonant oscillations of the transducer.

Energy Per Pulse—The ratio of the *average acoustic power* to the pulse repetition rate, measured in joules.

Entrance Beam Dimensions—The dimensions of the *beam cross-sectional* area where the beam enters the patient. For contact transducers these dimensions can be taken as the dimensions of the radiating element, if so stated.

Envelope—A continuous curve connecting the peaks of the successive cycles of the *waveform*.

Exposure Time—The total amount of time the *transducer assembly* is delivering ultrasonic energy to the subject. In a *pulse waveform* this includes time between pulses.

Far Field (Fraunhofer Zone)—That region of the field in which the *acoustic energy* flow along the beam axis proceeds essentially as though coming from a point source located in the vicinity of the *transducer assembly*. (Note: For an unfocused transducer assembly, the far field commonly is ascribed to ranges greater than $S/\pi\lambda$, where S is the *radiating cross-sectional* and λ is the *acoustic wavelength* in the medium.)

Focal Area—The area of the *focal surface*.

Focal Length—The axial distance from the centroid of the radiating surface of a *focusing transducer assembly* to the *focal surface*.

Focal Surface—The surface containing the smallest of all *beam cross-sectional areas* of a *focusing transducer assembly*.

Focal Zone—The volume lying within the *depth of focus* and the perimeters of the *beam cross-sectional areas*.

Focusing Transducer Assembly—A *transducer assembly* for which the ratio of the smallest *beam cross-sectional area* to *radiating cross-sectional area* is less than 0.5 or 0.25 transducer *beam* diameter. Also see *Transducer*.

Fractional Bandwidth—The *bandwidth* divided by the *center frequency*.

Fraunhofer Zone (Far Field)—See *Far Field*.

Frequency—Number of cycles of a periodic process per unit of time, usually expressed in Hertz (Hz), or multiples such as Megahertz (1 MHz = 10^6 Hz).

Fresnel Zone (Near Field)—See *Near Field*.

Gain—The ratio of the output to input of an amplifying system, generally expressed in decibels (dB).

Geometrical Focal Length—The distance along the beam axis from the center of the face of the transducer or lens to the geometrical focal point.

Geometrical Focal Point—The point of intersection of the greatest number of rays from the active transmitting element(s) of the *transducer*. Each ray is perpendicular to a small element of given surface area and may be refracted by lenses and/or reflected by mirrors.

***Gray Scale*—**A term describing the property of a display in which intensity information is recorded as variations in the brightness. The number of intensity levels differing in luminance by $\sqrt{2}$ or the number of distinguishable gray scale levels with a specified test pattern is a measure of the output *dynamic range* of the display. The dynamic range of the *signal* input to the display amplifier(s) is related to the output gray scale luminance by the gray scale transfer function. Logarithmic and other non-linear amplifiers are used to provide dynamic range compression and modify the gray scale transfer function.

***Half-Power Distance*—**The distance an *ultrasonic beam* must travel in a medium to reduce its power to one-half of its original value. (See *Half-Value Layer.*)

***Half Value Layer*—**A layer of a specified substance whose thickness is the *half-power distance.*

***Hard Copy*—**A permanent visual record on materials such as paper or film, as opposed to an image on an oscilloscope screen or magnetic tape.

***Harmonic*—**A whole number multiple of the fundamental *frequency* of a periodic quantity. For example, the second harmonic of a 1 MHz wave is 2 MHz. (Subharmonics also are possible; e.g., at ½, ⅓, etc., of the fundamental frequency.)

***Hertz*—**The standard unit of *frequency* equal to one cycle per second.

***Holography*—**A two-stage process of imaging. The object to be visualized is uniformly irradiated with *ultrasound* (or light) and the reflected or transmitted waves are sampled over a large area. The resulting image or hologram is generated by recording the sum of the reflected or transmitted waves and a reference *wave* or *signal*. This resulting image is an *interference* pattern where the contours are lines of constant phase. Although holograms contain three-dimensional data, they are usually reconstructed in *acoustics* so that only two dimensions are displayed.

***Immersion Coupling*—**A method of coupling an *ultrasonic transducer* to an object by placing both in a bath of the coupling medium.

***Impedance*—**See *Acoustic Impedance*.

***Impedance Ratio*—**The ratio Z_1/Z_2, where Z_1 and Z_2 are the specific *acoustic* impedances of two contiguous media respectively.

***Instantaneous Acoustic Power*—**The *acoustic power* at an instant in time.

***Intensity*—**A quantity related to *acoustic power* transmitted in a specified direction per unit area normal to this direction at the point considered. The particular intensity intended should be specified as defined below.

Instantaneous Intensity—The instantaneous *acoustic power* transmitted in a specified direction per unit is normal to this direction at the point considered. For measurement purposes, this point is restricted to where it is reasonable to assume that the *acoustic pressure* and *particle velocity* are in phase, viz, in the *far-field* or the area of the focus. Under such conditions, the intensity can be expressed as:

$$I = \frac{P^2}{2\rho c}$$

where P is the instantaneous acoustic pressure, ρ is the density of the medium, and c is the *speed of sound* in the medium.

Pulse Average Intensity—The time-average of *instantaneous intensity* at a point in space, when averaged over the *pulse duration.* (May be calculated approximately as the ratio of the *temporal average intensity* to the *duty factor.*)

Spatial-Average Intensity—The same as *spatial-average, temporal average intensity.* Generally, this parameter is used when specifying the intensity for *continuous wave (cw) ultrasound.*

Spatial Average-Pulse Average Intensity (SAPA)—The *pulse average intensity* averaged over the *beam cross-sectional area.* (May be calculated as the ratio of *acoustic power* to the product of *duty factor* and beam cross-sectional area.)

Spatial Average-Temporal Average Intensity (SATA)—The *temporal average intensity* averaged over the *beam cross-sectional area.* (May be calculated as the ratio of *acoustic power* to the beam cross-sectional area.)

Spatial Peak-Pulse Average Intensity (SPPA)—The value of the *pulse average intensity* at the point in the acoustic field where the pulse average intensity is a maximum, or is a local maximum within a specified region.

Spatial Peak-Temporal Average Intensity (SPTA)—The value of the *temporal average intensity* at the point in the *acoustic field* where the temporal average intensity is a maximum, or is a local maximum within a specified region.

Spatial Peak-Temporal Peak Intensity (SPTP)—The value of *temporal peak intensity* at the point in the acoustical field where the temporal peak intensity is a maximum, or is a local maximum within a specified region.

Temporal Average Intensity—The time-average of *instantaneous intensity* at a point in space; equal to the mean value of the instantaneous intensity at the point considered. For non-auto-scanning systems, the average is taken over one or more *pulse repetition periods*. For auto-scanning systems, the instantaneous intensity is averaged over one or more *scan* repetition periods for a specified operating mode.

Temporal Peak Intensity—The peak value of the *instantaneous* intensity at the point considered.

***Interface*—**The surface forming the boundary between two media having different properties.

***Interference*—**The phenomenon in which two or more waves of the same or harmonically-related *frequency(ies)* add together or cancel each other, according to their amplitude and phases.

***Isotropic*—**Having non-directional properties (i.e., physical properties that are independent of direction). For example, the *speed of sound* is not a function of the direction of propagation through an isotropic material. In contrast, the *velocity of sound* in muscle differs when propagating parallel to the fibers from that propagating at right angles to the fiber orientation; thus, muscle is anisotropic.

***Lateral Resolution*—**The minimum separation of reflectors in a direction normal to the *beam axis* at which the individual reflectors can be distinguished in the display. (See *Azimuthal Resolution.*)

Limiting (Clipping)—A technique which does not permit a voltage level to exceed a specified value.

***Linear Scan*—**The motion of a *transducer* at constant speed along a straight line at right angles to the *beam.*

***Liquid Coupling*—**A technique using a liquid, such as water, to couple the *transducer* to the object. (See *Coupling Method.*) The method is used with focused transducers so that focus can be moved with respect to the tissue.

Longitudinal Wave*—Wave* motion for which the *particle* displacement in the medium is normal to the wavefront.

M-Mode (Motion-Mode)—A method of display in which tissue depth is displayed along one axis and time is displayed along the second axis. The second axis displays time at a rate of physiological interest. M-mode is used frequently to display echocardiographic data when the changes in range of echoes corresponding to heart wall and valve motion are displayed as a function of time. The *intensity* of the echoes may be displayed by modulation of the brightness of the *CRT* image, or the shading of the *hard copy.*

***Megahertz*—**One million cycles per second (10^6 Hz); see *Hertz.*

***Monochromatic*—**Having a single *frequency*; from analogy with light.

Near Field (Fresnel Zone)—A region of an *acoustic field* lying between the *transducer* and an axial point at approximately 0.7 times the range to the last axial pressure maximum. For a plane disc transducer this pressure maximum occurs approximately at a range of $S/\pi\lambda$, where S is the *radiating cross-sectional area* of the transducer and λ is the *wavelength.* In the near field it is necessary to consider both *amplitude* and phase in describing the field parameter distributions.

***Neper*—**A logarithmic unit expressing the *amplitude* ratio of two like quantities equal to the natural logarithm (ln = log e) of the amplitude ratio of the two quantities: In A_1/A_2 = amplitude ratio in Nepers (Np) = 8.686 decibels (dB).

***On-Time*—**The sum of *pulse duration* during the total time that the *transducer* is acoustically coupled to the subject or other object of interest. Contrasted with ''off-time'' which is the sum of intervals between pulses when the transducer is not electrically driven. Total Time = On-Time + Off-Time.

Peak Instantaneous Intensity = See *Intensity.*

***Peak Intensity*—**See *Intensity.*

***Peak Spatial Average Temporal Intensity*—**See *Intensity* and *Spatial Peak–Temporal Average Intensity (SPTA).*

***Peak Spatial-Peak Temporal Intensity*—**See *Intensity* and *Spatial Peak Temporal Peak Intensity (SPTP).*

***Peak Temporal-Average Spatial Intensity*—**See *Intensity* and *Spatial Average Temporal Peak Intensity (SATP).*

***Phantom*—**A passive device which simulates some parameters of the human body, and allows meaningful measurements of *ultrasound* system parameters, or visualization of simulated anatomical features.

***Piezoelectric Effect*—**The property, exhibited by all electrically asymmetrical crystals, of generating electrical potentials when mechanically stressed. Conversely, these crystals generate mechanical strains when electrically stressed. This effect is the basis of electromechanical transduction of energy in *transducers.*

Power—Acoustic or Ultrasonic. The quantity of energy flow per unit time, expressed in watts. One watt is equivalent to a rate of flow of energy of 1 joule per second.

***Pressure*—**See *Acoustic Pressure.*

***Pulse Average Intensity*—**See *Intensity.*

***Pulse Average Ultrasonic Power*—**See *Ultrasonic Power.*

***Pulse Duration*—**The time interval beginning when the absolute value of the *acoustic pressure* exceeds 32% (−10 dB) of the maximum absolute value of the acoustic pressure and ending at the last time the absolute value of acoustic pressure returns to this value. This term is preferable to *pulse length.*

***Pulse Echo Response Profile*—**The spatial response of a pulse echo system to a small defined reflector.

***Pulse-Echo Technique*—**See *Echo Ranging.*

***Pulse Length*—**See *Pulse Duration.*

Pulse Repetition Frequency (PRF)—The repetition rate of the pulses of a pulse-echo system; the inverse of the *pulse repetition period.* Typically, the PRF of a system may be in the range from 1.5 kHz to 5 kHz.

***Pulse Repetition Period*—**The time interval between the same point on the *waveform* of two successive pulses.

***Pulse Repetition Rate*—**See *Pulse Repetition Frequency.*

***Pulse Waveform*—**A *waveform* in which B (defined as the *amplitude modulation factor*) is equal to 100% for a time greater than the *pulse duration.*

***Radial Mode*—**A mode of oscillation of an *acoustic wave* propagating radially in a disc transducer; it does not contribute to the desired acoustic output of the transducer. Therefore, it is regarded as a parasitic oscillation.

***Radiating Cross-Sectional Area*—**The *beam cross-sectional area* at the surface of the *transducer assembly.*

Radiation Force—The constant unidirectional force exerted on an interface by an incident *acoustic wave*. The force results from the transfer to the second medium of momentum carried by the wave to the *interface*. The term radiation pressure is a misnomer for this force.

Real-Time—A characteristic of a system whose output keeps pace with changes in input.

Real-Time Display—A display for which the image is continuously renewed, keeping pace with changes in the object, and in which storage or processing time does not delay appreciably the image presentation.

Real-Time Ultrasonic Visualization System—A system presenting *real-time* ultrasonic images. Real-time displays present the *acoustic* data at the time it is received without a discernible delay for processing, and at a *frame rate* which is sufficient to enable the operator to appreciate relative motion between the tissue and the *transducer*. The high data rate characteristic of real-time displays results in the continuously updated image analogous to television, so that moving structures, such as the heart and heart valves, can be visualized. The high frame rate is also useful when using the scanning system in the search mode.

Reflected Acoustic Pulse—See *Echo*.

Reflection—Reversal of the direction of propagation of a component of a *wave* that is propagating in one medium and encounters an extended interface with another medium of different *acoustic* properties. The amplitude of the reflected wave is related to the characteristic acoustic impedances across the interface. The angle of the reflection from a plane interface which is large compared to the *acoustic wavelength* is equal to the angle (between the wave vector and normal to the interface) of the incident wave in accordance with Snell's law.

Reflection Coefficient (Amplitude)—The ratio of the reflected to the incident *wave pressure amplitudes* at normal incidence $R = (Z_2 - Z_1)/(Z_2 + Z_1)$, where Z_1 and Z_2 are the characteristic acoustic impedances of the first and second media, respectively.

Reflection Mode Imaging—A technique which makes use of the reflected *acoustic energy* to produce the image data. Also called *Echo Ranging*.

Refraction—The phenomenon of changing the direction of propagation as an obliquely incident *acoustic wave* propagates from a medium of one acoustic velocity to a second medium of differing acoustic velocity.

Registration Accuracy—A quality of the display related to the accuracy of representation of the position of *acoustic* targets. It generally refers to display errors produced by *refraction*, position sensing and computation devices for the *B-mode* scanning arm, or inadequacy of the *CRT* spot in representing the location of *echo*-producing interfaces.

Rejection—A technique to improve the apparent *signal*-to-noise ratio by eliminating low amplitude signals from a display. This technique emphasizes strong echoes at the expense of noise and weaker echoes.

Relaxation—A class of processes in which *acoustic energy* is absorbed in a medium.

Resolution—A measure of the ability of a system to display distinguishable images of two closely spaced structures as discrete targets. (Also see *Azimuthal Resolution, Lateral Resolution, Axial (Longitudinal) Resolution.*)

Reverberation—The phenomenon of multiple reflections within a closed system. This phenomenon causes echoes to be misplaced in the display, thereby presenting false information. Multiple reflections may be identified in an image by moving the *transducer* relative to the object. The multiple reflections will move faster than the primary echoes because the primary echoes move a distance on the display which is equivalent to twice the incremental distance, while the first multiple reflection moves a distance equivalent to four times the increment.

Rise Time—The time taken for a pulse or *echo amplitude* to increase from 10% to 90% of its peak value.

Sagittal Plane—Any one of a set of anterior-posterior planes parallel to the long axis of the body.

Scale Factor—Generally, a transfer function between the input and output of a system. In *ultrasound* diagnosis, it commonly refers to the ratio of the displayed size of an object to the real size of the object.

Scan—The moving of an *acoustic beam* to produce an image, for which the *transducer* and the display movements are synchronized in space and time.

Scan Repetition Frequency—See *Scan Repetition Rate*.

Scan Repetition Rate—The repetition rate of a complete frame, sector, or scan. The term applies to automatic scanning systems only. Also see *Frame Rate*.

Scanner—A device to move an *acoustic beam* relative to a target. This is accomplished by using the beam steering and focusing capability of *phased array* system or by mechanically moving a *transducer*.

Scattering—The diffuse *reflection, refraction* or *diffraction of ultrasound* in many directions from irregular surfaces or inhomogeneities within a medium. The discontinuities are dimensionally comparable to or smaller than an *acoustic wavelength*; e.g., small spheres in the path of a *plane wave* give rise to complex reflection, refraction and diffraction behavior called Scattering. In an ultrasonic visualization system, by far the largest number of reflective objects in a specimen are scatterers. Visualization of scattering sources provides a much more complete picture than visualization of specular reflections. For this reason, images based on scattered *acoustic energy* are easier to interpret, but systems with higher sensitivity and greater *dynamic range (gray scale)* are required to display the weak scattered signals.

Sector Scan—A system of scanning in which the *transducer* or transmitted *beam* is rotated through an angle, the center of rotation being near or behind the surface of the transducer.

Sensitivity—The minimum *signal* that can be satisfactorily detected generally limited by the input noise level of the system.

Shear Wave—*Wave* motion with *particle* movements perpendicular to the propagation direction. Shear waves propagate in solids but are highly attenuated in liquid systems. Shear waves are generated when a *longitudinal wave* impinges obliquely on soft tissue-bone interfaces and partially account for the heating of the periosteum and bone at this location.

Short Axis Scan—A *scan* parallel to the short axis of the heart obtained from *cross-sectional echocardiography* with a *transducer* scanning a plane at right angles to the *long axis* of the heart (base to apex).

Side Lobe—A diffractive characteristic of an *acoustic beam* in which secondary, off-axis maxima occur in the near or far *acoustic field*, or in the *focal zone*. The presence of side lobes tends to cause target ambiguity and limit the *resolution*.

Signal (Electrical)—The information content of the electrical variation voltage or current in a circuit. Signal-to-noise ratio is a statement of *sensitivity*.

Single Sweep Scan—A *scan* mode in which only a single pass of the transducer over the tissue to be examined is used. This scan mode may be used where relative motion of tissues could be expected and where this motion would obscure the desired detail.

Sonar—Applied to medical *ultrasound*, the term ''sonar'' is the generic term for echo ranging. Acronym from SOund NAvigation Ranging.

Sonography—Any imaging method using *sound* and yielding a graphical representation of the subject. This is a more inclusive term than *echography* in as much as transmission sonography is also included.

Sound Pressure Amplitude—The deviation from the ambient value of the pressure in a medium due to the presence of an *acoustic wave*. It usually refers to the peak instantaneous wave pressure, but also may be the general instantaneous, or root-mean-square (rms) pressure. The pressure amplitude of an acoustic wave may be measured with a linear device such as a hydrophone. In a plane progressive (*cw*) *wave, intensity* (I) and maximum pressure amplitude (P) are related by $I = P^2/2\rho c$ where ρ and c are the mean density and speed of sound of the medium, respectively.

Spatial Average—See *Intensity*.

Spatial Average-Pulse Average Intensity (SAPA)—See *Intensity*.

Spatial Average-Temporal Average Intensity (SATA)—See *Intensity*.

Spatial Peak-Temporal Average Intensity (SPTA)—See *Intensity*.

Spatial Peak-Temporal Peak Intensity (SPTP)—See *Intensity*.

Specific Acoustic Impedance—The ratio of instantaneous *acoustic pressure* to instantaneous *particle velocity*. For plane progressive *wave* in a lossless medium, the specific acoustic impedance is numerically equal to the *characteristic acoustic impedance*.

Speed of Sound—The speed of sound, c, in a fluid medium is determined by the properties of the propagation medium; $c = \sqrt{K/\rho}$, where ρ is the mean density of the medium and K is the *adiabatic bulk modulus*. The speed of sound is the product of the frequency (f) and the wavelength (λ): $c = f\lambda$. Also, $c = Z/\rho$, where Z is the *characteristic acoustic impedance* (a scalar quantity).

Spiral C-Mode Scanner—Apparatus to perform scanning in a spiral motion so that from a selected site on the body surface, scans are made corresponding to sections parallel to the surface at varying depths.

Superposition Principle—If a linear physical system is acted upon by a number of independent influences, the resultant influence is the sum of the independent influences. Any linear *wave* phenomenon can be analyzed by simple addition to scalar contributions from some distribution of simple sources, properly selected in phase and *amplitude* to represent the physical situation. The vector quantities can then be determined from the basic equations by taking gradients. This principle is applied in *phase array* transducers to generate the appropriate wave amplitude and phase relationships throughout the field.

Tri-Scanning (Time-Motion)—See *M-Mode*.

Temporal Average Intensity—See *Intensity*.

Temporal-Average Ultrasonic Power—See *Average Acoustic Power*.

Temporal-Maximum Ultrasonic Power—U.S. Therapy Standards name for *Pulse-Average Ultrasonic Power* (see *Ultrasonic Power*).

Temporal Peak Intensity—See *Intensity*.

Test Object—A passive device which provides echoes and permits evaluation of one or more parameters of an *ultrasound* system, but does not necessarily duplicate the acoustical properties of the human body. See also *Phantom*.

Theoretical Angular Beam Width—The computed angle subtended by two *far field*, off-axis points in a plane containing the *beam axis*, where the computed quantity (specified pressure, velocity or *intensity*) is at its first zero (or some other specified value) of its axial magnitude; the angular *beam width* is computed on the basis of continuous excitation unless otherwise specified.

Through-Transmission Imaging—The process of imaging by transmitting the *sound* field through the specimen and receiving the transmitted energy on a far surface or a receiving *transducer* or array. See also *Holography* and *Transsonogram*.

T-M Mode—Synonym for *M-Mode*.

***Transceiver*—**A *transducer* used both for transmission and reception of *acoustic energy*. This is the customary configuration for *ultrasound* visualization equipment. (In contrast, typical *CW* Doppler equipment is an example of instruments which use a separate transmitter and receiver.)

***Transceiver Voltage Response*—**The ratio of the *amplitude* of the energizing pulse with the *transceiver* attached to the amplitude of the *echo* from a perfect-planar *reflector*.

***Transducer*—**A device capable of converting *energy* from one form to another. Specifically in ultrasonics, the device used to convert electrical energy to mechanical energy and, reciprocally, to convert mechanical energy to electrical energy. If, in the application, the device performs both functions, the term may be left unqualified. If the device is used only to transmit or to receive, the device should be referred to as the ''transmitting'' or ''receiving'' transducer.

***Transducer Assembly*—**That portion of a fully assembled ultrasonic diagnostic product which is designed to emit and/or receive ultrasonic radiation and which includes one or more ultrasonic transducers and any associated housing.

***Transducer Dynamic Response*—**See *Dynamic Response*.

***Transition Zone*—**That portion of the *acoustic field* between *Fresnel Zone* (*near field*) and the *Fraunhofer Zone* (*far field*) which encompasses the last maximum occurring along the *beam axis*. The transition zone has no distinct boundaries but is sometimes referred to in the literature.

***Transmitted Acoustic Pulse*—**The *acoustic* pulse transmitted into the coupling medium due to the applied energizing pulse.

***Transmitter Pulse*—**See *Energizing Pulse*.

***Transverse Wave*—**See *Shear Wave*.

***Two Dimensional Echocardiography*—**B-Mode imaging of the heart.

***Ultrasonic Power*—**(See also *Acoustic Power* and *Power*.) In the North American Therapy Standards *Ultrasonic Power* is defined as ''the total power emitted in the form of ultrasonic radiation by the applicator averaged over each cycle of the ultrasonic radiation carrier wave''. *Pulse-Average* (or *Temporal-Maximum*), *Ultrasonic Power* is equal to one-half the instantaneous power, and is also numerically equal to the *Temporal Average Ultrasonic Power* of a cw waveform having the same instantaneous power. *Temporal Average Ultrasonic Power* is the time average of the *Instantaneous Power* at a point in space.

***Ultrasonic Shadow*—**See *Acoustic Shadow*.

***Ultrasonogram*—**Any image obtained from ultrasonic examination methods. The term may be qualified by adjectives appropriate to the field of application. The term includes both *echograms* and *transsonograms*.

Ultrasound*—Acoustic* radiation at frequencies above the range of human hearing (conventionally, above 20 kHz).

***Unipolar Pulse or Waveform*—**A *waveform* which has either positive or negative excursions from the base-line but not both. A unipolar waveform can be produced by rectification of radio frequency signals.

***Velocity of Sound*—**(See *Speed of Sound*.) The term ''velocity'' implies both direction and speed; the term ''speed of sound'' should be used where direction is of no concern.

***Video Signal*—**The rectified and often filtered *echo* signals in an ultrasonic visualization system generally are referred to as ''video signals'' by analogy with television nomenclature.

Watt Per Square Centimeter (W/cm^2)—The unit of Intensity (10^4 W/m^2).

***Wave*—**See *Acoustic Wave*.

***Waveform*—**The representation of an *acoustical* or electrical parameter as a function of time.

***Wavelength*—**See *Acoustic Wavelength*.

References

Health and Welfare. *Guidelines for the Safe Use of Ultrasound Part I (Medical and Paramedical Applications).* Safety Code 23, 80-EHD-59; Canada; 1980.

INDEX